PDR®
14
EDITION
1993

PHYSICIANS' DESK REFERENCE FOR NONPRESCRIPTION DRUGS®

Director of Production:
MARJORIE A. DUFFY

Assistant Director of Production:
CARRIE WILLIAMS

Production Manager:
KIMBERLY V. HILLER

Format Editor:
MILDRED M. SCHUMACHER

Production Coordinator:
ELIZABETH A. KARST

Art Associate:
JOAN K. AKERLIND

Product Manager:
CURTIS ALLEN

Sales Manager:
CHARLIE J. MEITNER

Account Managers:
JEFFREY M. KELLER
JAMES R. PANTALEO
MICHAEL S. SARAJIAN
JOANNE C. TERZIDES

Commercial Sales Manager:
ROBIN B. BARTLETT

Direct Marketing Manager:
ROBERT W. CHAPMAN

Manager, Professional Data:
MUKESH MEHTA, R.Ph.

Index Editor:
ADELE L. DOWD

Officers of Medical Economics Data Production, Co.: **President and Chief Executive Officer**, Norman R. Snesil; **Executive Vice President**: Mark L. Weinstein; **Senior Vice President and Chief Financial Officer**, J. Crispin Ashworth; **Senior Vice President of Business Development**, Stephen J. Sorkenn; **Vice President of Product Management**, Curtis B. Allen; **Vice President of Sales and Marketing**, Thomas F. Rice; **Vice President of Operations**, John R. Ware; **Vice President of Information Systems and Services**, Edward J. Zecchini

ISBN 1-56363-16-8

MEDICAL ECONOMICS DATA

Foreword to the Fourteenth Edition

Welcome to the fourteenth edition of the PHYSICIANS' DESK REFERENCE For NONPRESCRIPTION DRUGS®, the over-the-counter drug companion to the Physicians' Desk Reference. The shift of some drug ingredients and dosage forms from prescription to over-the-counter status is continuing. It is the goal of the PHYSICIANS' DESK REFERENCE For NONPRESCRIPTION DRUGS® to provide detailed labeling information to help ensure appropriate use of these products. Manufacturers of these nonprescription drug products have included inactive ingredients as well as active ingredients to alert those who may have sensitivity to certain ingredients.

The PHYSICIANS' DESK REFERENCE For NONPRESCRIPTION DRUGS® is published annually by Medical Economics Data, a division of Medical Economics Company, Inc., with the cooperation of the manufacturers whose products are described in the Product Information and Diagnostics, Devices and Medical Aids Sections. It is organized in a similar manner to the PHYSICIANS' DESK REFERENCE with a Manufacturers' Index, Product Name Index, Product Category Index, and Active Ingredients Index-all color coded for quick reference. Descriptive labeling appears in the Product Information Section and Diagnostics, Devices and Medical Aids Section.

The function of the publisher is the compilation, organization, and distribution of this information. Each product description has been prepared by the manufacturer, and edited and approved by the manufacturer's medical department, medical director, and/or medical consultant. In organizing and presenting the material in PHYSICIANS' DESK REFERENCE For NONPRESCRIPTION DRUGS®, the publisher does not warrant or guarantee any of the products described herein or perform any independent analysis in connection with any of the product information contained herein. PHYSICIANS' DESK REFERENCE For NONPRESCRIPTION DRUGS® does not assume, and expressly disclaims, any obligation to obtain and include information other than that provided to it by the manufacturer. In making this material available it should be understood that the publisher is not advocating the use of any product described herein. Besides the information given here, additional information on any product may be obtained through the manufacturer.

MEDICAL ECONOMICS DATA

Contents

MEDICAL ECONOMICS DATA

SECTION 1

Manufacturers' Index

The manufacturers whose names appear in this index have provided information concerning their products in either the Product Information Section, Product Identification Section, or the Diagnostics, Devices and Medical Aids Section.

Included in this index are the names and addresses of manufacturers, individuals or departments to whom you may address inquiries, a partial list of products as well as emergency telephone numbers wherever available.

The symbol ◆ indicates that the product is shown in the Product Identification Section.

PAGE

ALLERGAN PHARMACEUTICALS **502**
A Division of Allergan, Inc.
2525 Dupont Drive
P.O. Box 19534
Irvine, CA 92713-9534
Address Inquiries to:
Scientific Information/Medical Compliance (800) 433-8871
(714) 752-4500
For Medical Emergencies Contact:
Scientific Information/Medical Compliance (714) 752-4500
OTC Products Available
Cellufresh Lubricant Ophthalmic Solution
Celluvisc Lubricant Ophthalmic Solution
Lacri-Lube NP Lubricant Ophthalmic Ointment
Lacri-Lube S.O.P. Sterile Ophthalmic Ointment
Refresh P.M. Lubricant Ophthalmic Ointment
Tears Plus Lubricant Ophthalmic Solution

ALMAY, INC. **503**
625 Madison Avenue
New York, NY 10022
Address inquiries to:
Center for Professional Services
(800) 334-8332
OTC Products Available
Almay Anti-Itch Lotion
Almay Eyelid Cleansing Pads
Almay Hydrocortisone Antipruritic Cream
Almay Hydrocortisone Antipruritic Lotion
Almay Protective Eye Treatment SPF 12
Almay Protective Face Cream SPF 15
Almay Therapeutic Body Treatment
Almay Therapeutic Face Lotion
Almay Therapeutic Shampoo

APOTHECON **403, 505**
A Bristol-Myers Squibb Company
P.O. Box 4500
Princeton, NJ 08543-4500
(609) 987-6800
Address inquiries to:
Apothecon Customer Service Dept.
P.O. Box 5250
Princeton, NJ 08543-5250
(800) 321-1335
Orders for Apothecon Products may be placed by:
1. Calling toll-free (800) 631-5244
Between 8:30 AM-6:00 PM EST
2. Mailing your purchase orders to:
Apothecon
Attn: Customer Service Dept.
P.O. Box 5250
Princeton, NJ 08543-5250
3. Orders may be telefaxed to:
Customer Service Dept.
FAX (800) 523-2965
OTC Products Available
◆Colace
◆Peri-Colace

B. F. ASCHER & COMPANY, INC. **403, 506**
15501 West 109th Street
Lenexa, KS 66219
Mailing Address: P.O. Box 717
Shawnee Mission, KS 66201-0717
Address inquiries to:
Joan F. Bowen (913) 888-1880
OTC Products Available
◆Ayr Saline Nasal Drops
◆Ayr Saline Nasal Mist
◆Itch-X Gel
◆Mobigesic Analgesic Tablets
◆Mobisyl Analgesic Creme
◆Pen•Kera Creme
Unilax Stool Softener/Laxative Softgel Capsules

ASTRA PHARMACEUTICAL PRODUCTS, INC. **403, 507**
50 Otis Street
Westboro, MA 01581-4500
Address inquiries to:
Roy E. Hayward, Jr. (508) 366-1100
For Medical Emergencies Contact:
Dr. William Gray (508) 366-1100
OTC Products Available
◆Xylocaine Ointment 2.5%

AU PHARMACEUTICALS, INC. **507**
P.O. Box 131835
Tyler, TX 75713-1835
Address inquiries to:
Michael Vick (800) 568-2873
For Medical Emergencies Contact:
Christopher Burda, M.D.
(800) 568-2873
OTC Products Available
Aurum Analgesic Lotion
Feminine Gold Analgesic Lotion
Theragold Analgesic Lotion
Therapeutic Gold Analgesic Lotion

AYERST LABORATORIES **508**
Division of American Home Products Corporation
685 Third Avenue
New York, NY 10017-4071

(◆ Shown in Product Identification Section)

For information for Ayerst's consumer products, see product listings under Whitehall Laboratories.
Please turn to Whitehall Laboratories, page 774.

BAKER CUMMINS DERMATOLOGICALS, INC. 403, 508
1950 Swarthmore Avenue
Lakewood, NJ 08701
Address inquiries to:
(908) 905-5200
FAX (908) 905-5255
For Medical Emergencies Contact:
Medical Department (908) 905-5200
(800) 842-6704
FAX (908) 905-5255
OTC Products Available
Acticort Lotion 100
Aqua-A Cream
◆Aquaderm Cream
◆Aquaderm Lotion
Aquaderm Sunscreen Moisturizer (SPF 15 Formula)
Baker's Biopsy Punch (sizes 2, 3, 3.5, 4, 5 and 6 mm)
Baker's DTM
◆P & S Liquid
P & S Plus Tar Gel
◆P & S Shampoo
Panscol Medicated Lotion
Panscol Medicated Ointment
Phacid Shampoo
Snaplets (D, DM, EX, FR, and Multi)
◆Ultra Mide 25
Ultraderm Bath Oil
◆UltraDerm Lotion
◆X-Seb Shampoo
◆X-Seb Plus Conditioning Shampoo
◆X-Seb T Shampoo
◆X-Seb T Plus Conditioning Shampoo

BEACH PHARMACEUTICALS 510
Division of Beach Products, Inc.
Executive Office
5220 South Manhattan Avenue
Tampa, FL 33611 (813) 839-6565
Manufacturing and Distribution
Main Street at Perimeter Road
Conestee, SC 29605
Toll Free 1-(800) 845-8210
Address inquiries to:
Victor De Oreo, R Ph, V.P., Sales
(803) 277-7282
Richard Stephen Jenkins, Exec. V.P.
(813) 839-6565
OTC Products Available
Beelith Tablets

BEIERSDORF INC. 403, 510
P.O. Box 5529
Norwalk, CT 06856-5529
Address inquiries to:
Medical Division (203) 853-8008
FAX (203) 854-8180
OTC Products Available
◆Aquaphor Antibiotic Ointment
◆Aquaphor Healing Ointment
◆Aquaphor Healing Ointment, Original Formula
Basis Facial Cleanser (Normal to Dry Skin)
Basis Intensive Hydrating Oil
Basis Multi Protective Balm
Basis Over Night Recovery Creme
Basis Soap-Combination Skin
Basis Soap-Extra Dry Skin
Basis Soap-Normal to Dry Skin
Basis Soap-Sensitive Skin
◆Eucerin Cleansing Lotion Dry Skin Care
◆Eucerin Dry Skin Care Cleansing Bar
◆Eucerin Dry Skin Care Creme
◆Eucerin Dry Skin Care Daily Facial Lotion SPF 20
◆Eucerin Dry Skin Care Lotion (Fragrance-free)
◆Eucerin Plus Moisturizing Lotion
Nivea Bath Silk Bath Oil
Nivea Bath Silk Bath & Shower Gel (Extra-Dry Skin)
Nivea Bath Silk Bath & Shower Gel (Normal-to-Dry Skin)
Nivea Moisturizing Creme
Nivea Moisturizing Lotion (Extra Enriched)
Nivea Moisturizing Lotion (Original Formula)
Nivea Moisturizing Oil
Nivea Skin Oil
Nivea Sun After Sun Lotion
Nivea Sun SPF 15
Nivea Visage Facial Nourishing Creme
Nivea Visage Facial Nourishing Lotion

BIOLINK INTERNATIONAL INC. 512
1502 Brittain Road
Akron, OH 44310
Address inquiries to:
Professional Services Department
(216) 633-4300
FAX (216) 633-7054
OTC Products Available
BioBars Diet and Fitness Bar
BioClenz Herbal Bowel Activator
BioEner-G-Thin Fat Reducing Energizer
BioTrim High-Fiber Drink
CalLink Calcium and Magnesium Complex
ChildLink (Pediatric version of VitaLink II)
LifeLink Pain Reliever
VitaLink II Multivitamin and Mineral Supplement

THE BIOPRACTIC GROUP II, INC. 512
99 Broad Street
P.O. Box 5300
Phillipsburg, NJ 08865
Address inquiries to:
Customer Service (908) 859-4060
FAX (908) 859-4417
OTC Products Available
Foot Miracle Foot Cream
Skin Miracle Therapeutic Moisturizer
Surgeon's Choice

BLAINE COMPANY, INC. 512
1465 Jamike Lane
Erlanger, KY 41018
Address inquiries to:
Mr. Alex M. Blaine (606) 283-9437
FAX (606) 283-9460
OTC Products Available
Mag-Ox 400
Uro-Mag

BLAIREX LABORATORIES, INC. 513
4810 Tecumseh Lane
P.O. Box 15190
Evansville, IN 47716-0190
Address inquiries to:
Bruce Faulkenberg, R.Ph.
(800) 252-4739
FAX (812) 474-6764
For Medical Emergency Contact:
Bruce Faulkenberg, R.Ph.
(800) 252-4739
FAX (812) 474-6764
OTC Products Available
Broncho Saline
Nasal Moist

BLOCK DRUG COMPANY, INC. 513
257 Cornelison Avenue
Jersey City, NJ 07302
Address inquiries to:
Steve Gattanella (201) 434-3000
For Medical Emergencies Contact:
James Gingold (201) 434-3000
OTC Products Available
Arthritis Strength BC Powder
BC Powder
BC Cold Powder Multi-Symptom Formula (Cold-Sinus-Allergy)
BC Cold Powder Non-Drowsy Formula (Cold-Sinus)
Nytol Tablets
Promise Toothpaste
Cool Gel Sensodyne
Fresh Mint Sensodyne Toothpaste
Original Formula Sensodyne-SC Toothpaste
Tegrin Dandruff Shampoo
Tegrin for Psoriasis Lotion, Skin Cream & Medicated Soap
Tegrin-HC with Hydrocortisone Anti-Itch Ointment

BOCK PHARMACAL COMPANY 404, 516
P.O. Box 8519
St. Louis, MO 63126-0519
Address inquiries to:
(314) 343-0994
OTC Products Available
◆Emetrol

BOIRON USA 404, 516
Headquarters and East Coast Branch
1208 Amosland Road
Norwood, PA 19074
Address inquiries to:
Gina M. Casey
Communications & P.R. Manager
(800) 258-8823
For Medical Emergencies Contact:
Mark Land
Technical Services Department
(800) 258-8823
West Coast Branch
98C West Cochran Street
Simi Valley, CA 93065
(805) 582-9091
Address inquiries to:
Majid Djoudi, R.Ph.
Sales & Technical Dept., West Coast
OTC Products Available
◆Oscillococcinum

BRISTOL-MYERS PRODUCTS 404, 517
A Bristol-Myers Squibb Company
345 Park Avenue
New York, NY 10154
Address Inquiries to:
Bristol-Myers Products Division
Consumer Affairs Department
US Highway 202/206 North
P.O. Box 1279
Somerville, NJ 08876-1279
In Emergencies Call:
(800) 468-7746
OTC Products Available
◆Alpha Keri Moisture Rich Body Oil
Alpha Keri Moisture Rich Cleansing Bar
Alpha Keri Moisturizing Body Lotion
Alpha Keri Moisturizing Spray Mist
Alpha Keri Shower & Bath Gelee
Ammens Medicated Powder
B.Q. Cold Tablets
BAN Antiperspirant Cream Deodorant
BAN Basic Non-Aerosol Antiperspirant Spray
BAN Roll-On Antiperspirant Deodorant
BAN Solid Antiperspirant Deodorant
◆Arthritis Strength Bufferin Analgesic Caplets
◆Extra Strength Bufferin Analgesic Tablets
◆Bufferin Analgesic Tablets and Caplets
◆Bufferin AF Nite Time Analgesic/Sleeping Aid Caplets
◆Allergy-Sinus Comtrex Multi-Symptom Allergy-Sinus Formula Tablets & Caplets
◆Cough Formula Comtrex
◆Comtrex Multi-Symptom Cold Reliever Tablets/Caplets/Liqui-Gels/Liquid
◆Comtrex Multi-Symptom Day-Night Caplet-Tablet
◆Comtrex Multi-Symptom Non-Drowsy Caplets
◆Congespirin For Children Aspirin Free Chewable Cold Tablets
◆Aspirin Free Excedrin Analgesic Caplets
◆Excedrin Extra-Strength Analgesic Tablets & Caplets
◆Excedrin P.M. Analgesic/Sleeping Aid Tablets, Caplets and Liquid
◆Sinus Excedrin Analgesic, Decongestant Tablets & Caplets
4-Way Cold Tablets
◆4-Way Fast Acting Nasal Spray (regular & mentholated) & Metered Spray Pump (regular)
◆4-Way Long Lasting Nasal Spray

(◆ **Shown in Product Identification Section**)

Fostex 10% Benzoyl Peroxide Bar
Fostex 10% Benzoyl Peroxide (Vanish) Gel
Fostex 10% Benzoyl Peroxide Wash
Fostex Medicated Cleansing Bar
Fostex Medicated Cleansing Cream
Keri Facial Soap
◆Keri Lotion - Original Formula
◆Keri Lotion -Silky Smooth with Vitamin E
◆Keri Lotion - Silky Smooth Fragrance Free with Vitamin E
Minit-Rub Analgesic Ointment
Mum Antiperspirant Cream Deodorant
◆No Doz Fast Acting Alertness Aid Tablets
◆No Doz Maximum Strength Caplets
◆Nuprin Ibuprofen/Analgesic Tablets & Caplets
◆Pazo Hemorrhoid Ointment & Suppositories
PreSun 15 Facial Sunscreen
PreSun 15 Lip Protector Sunscreen
PreSun Active 15 and 30 Clear Gel Sunscreens
◆PreSun for Kids Lotion
◆PreSun 23 and For Kids, Spray Mist Sunscreens
PreSun 8 and 15 Moisturizing Sunscreens with KERI
PreSun 25 Moisturizing Sunscreen with KERI Moisturizer
◆PreSun 15 and 29 Sensitive Skin Sunscreens
PreSun 46 Moisturizing Sunscreen
◆Theragran Liquid
◆Theragran Stress Formula
◆Theragran Tablets
◆Theragran-M Tablets with Beta Carotene
◆Therapeutic Mineral Ice, Pain Relieving Gel
◆Therapeutic Mineral Ice Exercise Formula, Pain Relieving Gel
Tickle Roll-On Antiperspirant/Deodorant

BURROUGHS WELLCOME CO. 406, 535
3030 Cornwallis Road
Research Triangle Park, NC 27709
(800) 722-9292
For Medical or Drug Information:
Contact Drug Information Service
Business hours only
(8:15 AM to 4:15 PM EST)
(800) 443-6763
For 24-hour Medical Emergency Information, call (800) 443-6763
For Sales Information:
Contact Sales Distribution Department
Address Other Inquiries to:
Consumer Products Division
OTC Products Available
◆Actifed Plus Caplets
◆Actifed Plus Tablets
◆Actifed Sinus Daytime/Nighttime Caplets
◆Actifed Sinus Daytime/Nighttime Tablets
◆Actifed Syrup
◆Actifed Tablets
Borofax Ointment
◆Empirin Aspirin
◆Marezine Tablets
◆Neosporin Ointment
◆Neosporin Plus Maximum Strength Cream
◆Neosporin Plus Maximum Strength Ointment
◆Nix Creme Rinse
◆Polysporin Ointment
◆Polysporin Powder
◆Sudafed Children's Liquid
◆Sudafed Cough Syrup
◆Sudafed Plus Liquid
◆Sudafed Plus Tablets
◆Sudafed Severe Cold Formula Caplets
◆Sudafed Severe Cold Formula Tablets
◆Sudafed Sinus Caplets
◆Sudafed Sinus Tablets
◆Sudafed Tablets, 30 mg
◆Sudafed Tablets, Adult Strength, 60 mg
◆Sudafed 12 Hour Caplets

CAMPBELL LABORATORIES INC. 543
Address Inquiries to:
Richard C. Zahn, President
P.O. Box 812, FDR Station
New York, NY 10150-0812
(212) 688-7684
OTC Products Available
Herpecin-L Cold Sore Lip Balm

CARE-TECH LABORATORIES 544
3224 South Kingshighway Boulevard
St. Louis, MO 63139
Address inquiries to:
Sherry L. Brereton (314) 772-4610
FAX (314) 772-4613
For Medical Emergencies Contact:
Customer Service (800) 325-9681
Fax (314) 772-4613
OTC Products Available
Barri-Care Antimicrobial Barrier Ointment
CC-500 Antibacterial Skin Cleanser
Care Creme
Clinical Care Dermal Wound Cleanser
Concept
Formula Magic Antibacterial Powder
Just Lotion - Highly Absorbent Aloe Vera Based Skin Lotion
Loving Lather II Antibacterial Skin Cleanser
Loving Lotion Antibacterial Skin & Body Lotion
Orchid Fresh II Perineal/Ostomy Cleanser
Satin Antimicrobial Skin Cleanser
Skin Magic - Antimicrobial Body Rub & Emollient
Soft Skin Non-greasy Bath Oil with Rich Emollients
Swirlsoft Whirlpool Emollient for Dry Skin Conditions
Techni-Care Surgical Scrub
Velvet Fresh Non-irritating Cornstarch Baby Powder

CHATTEM INC., CONSUMER PRODUCTS DIVISION 545
Division of Chattem, Inc.
1715 West 38th Street
Chattanooga, TN 37409
Address Inquiries to:
David A. Robb, Jr. (615) 821-4571
FAX (615) 821-5022
For Medical Emergencies Contact:
Walter Ludwig (615) 821-4571
FAX (615) 821-5022
OTC Products Available
Black-Draught Granulated
Black-Draught Lax-Senna Tablets
Black-Draught Syrup
Blis-To-Sol Liquid
Blis-To-Sol Powder
Flex-all 454 Pain Relieving Gel
Icy Hot Balm
Icy Hot Cream
Icy Hot Stick
Norwich Aspirin
Norwich Aspirin - Maximum Strength
Norwich Enteric Safety Coated Aspirin
Norwich Enteric Safety Coated Aspirin - Maximum Strength
Nullo Deodorant Tablets
Multi-Symptom Pamprin Tablets and Caplets
Maximum Pain Relief Pamprin Caplets
Prēmsyn PMS Caplets
Soltice Quick-Rub

CHESEBROUGH-POND'S INC. 548
33 Benedict Place
Greenwich, CT 06830
Address inquiries to:
Consumer Affairs (800) 243-5804
For Medical Emergencies Contact:
(800) 243-5804
OTC Products Available
Vaseline Intensive Care Moisturizing Sunblock Lotion
Vaseline Intensive Care U.V. Daily Defense Lotion for Hand and Body
Vaseline Intensive Care Lotion Extra Strength
Vaseline Pure Petroleum Jelly Skin Protectant

CHURCH & DWIGHT CO., INC. 549
469 North Harrison Street
Princeton, NJ 08540
Address inquiries to:
Mr. Stephen Lajoie (609) 683-5900
For Medical Emergencies Contact:
Mr. Stephen Lajoie (609) 683-5900
OTC Products Available
Arm & Hammer Pure Baking Soda

CIBA CONSUMER PHARMACEUTICALS 407, 550
Division of CIBA-GEIGY Corporation
Mack Woodbridge II
Woodbridge, NJ 07095
Address inquiries to:
(908) 602-6600
For Medical Emergencies Contact:
(908) 277-5000
OTC Products Available
◆Acutrim 16 Hour Steady Control Appetite Suppressant
◆Acutrim Late Day Strength Appetite Suppressant
◆Acutrim II Maximum Strength Appetite Suppressant
◆Doan's - Extra-Strength Analgesic
◆Extra Strength Doan's P.M.
◆Doan's - Regular Strength Analgesic
◆Dulcolax Suppositories
◆Dulcolax Tablets
◆Eucalyptamint 100% All Natural Ointment
◆Eucalyptamint Muscle Pain Relief Formula
Fiberall Chewable Tablets, Lemon Creme Flavor
◆Fiberall Fiber Wafers - Fruit & Nut
◆Fiberall Fiber Wafers - Oatmeal Raisin
◆Fiberall Powder Natural Flavor
◆Fiberall Powder Orange Flavor
◆Nōstril 1/4% Mild Nasal Decongestant
◆Nōstril 1/2% Regular Nasal Decongestant
◆Nōstrilla Long Acting Nasal Decongestant
◆Nupercainal Hemorrhoidal and Anesthetic Ointment
◆Nupercainal Pain Relief Cream
◆Nupercainal Suppositories
◆Otrivin Nasal Drops
◆Otrivin Pediatric Nasal Drops
◆Privine Nasal Solution and Drops
◆Privine Nasal Spray
◆Q-vel Muscle Relaxant Pain Reliever
◆Slow Fe Tablets
◆Sunkist Children's Chewable Multivitamins - Complete
◆Sunkist Children's Chewable Multivitamins - Plus Extra C
◆Sunkist Children's Chewable Multivitamins - Plus Iron
◆Sunkist Children's Chewable Multivitamins - Regular
◆Sunkist Vitamin C - Chewable
◆Sunkist Vitamin C - Easy to Swallow

COLUMBIA LABORATORIES, INC. 408, 557
4000 Hollywood Boulevard
Hollywood, FL 33021
Address inquiries to:
Professional Services Department
For Medical Emergencies Contact
(305) 964-6666
OTC Products Available
◆Diasorb Liquid
◆Diasorb Tablets
◆Legatrin Tablets
Vaporizer in a Bottle Nasal Decongestant

COPLEY PHARMACEUTICAL INC. 408, 558
25 John Road
Canton, MA 02021
Address inquiries to:
Copley Pharmaceutical Inc.
(617) 821-6111

For Medical Emergencies Contact:
Dr. Antoon (617) 821-6111
OTC Products Available
Alum-Boro Effervescent Tablets and Powder Packets
Bromatapp Extended Release Tablets
Brompheril Extended Release Tablets
Diphenhydramine Hydrochloride Spray 2%
Doxylamine Succinate 25 mg Tabs
Hydrocortisone 0.5% Aerosol and 1.0% Aerosol
◆Lice•Enz Foam Shampoo Aerosol
Miconazole Cream 2% and Spray Powder
Saliv-Aid Oral Lubricant
Simethicone Drops
Tolnaftate 1% Liquid Aerosol
Tolnaftate 1% Powder Aerosol

DEL PHARMACEUTICALS, INC. 408, 558
A Subsidiary of Del Laboratories, Inc.
163 East Bethpage Road
Plainview, NY 11803
Addess inquiries to:
Peter Liman, V.P. Marketing
(516) 293-7070
FAX (516) 293-9018
For Medical Emergencies Contact:
Dr. John Schmermund
(516) 293-7070, Ext. 3545
OTC Products Available
ArthriCare Pain Relieving Rubs
Auro-Dri Ear Drops
Auro Ear Wax Removal Aid
Boil-Ease Antiseptic Drawing Salve
Dermarest Anti-Itch Gels
◆Dermarest DriCort 1% Hydrocortisone Creme
DeTane Desensitizing Lubricant
Diaper Guard Skin Rash Ointment
Exocaine Analgesic Rubs
Off-Ezy Corn Remover
Off-Ezy Wart Remover
Baby Orajel Nighttime Formula
◆Baby Orajel Teething Pain Medicine
◆Baby Orajel Tooth & Gum Cleanser
Denture Orajel Denture Pain Medicine
◆Orajel Maximum Strength Toothache Medication
◆Orajel Mouth-Aid for Canker and Cold Sores
◆Pronto Lice Killing Shampoo Kit
◆Pronto Lice Killing Spray
Propa pH Acne Medication Cleansing Lotion
Skin Shield Liquid Bandage
Stye Ophthalmic Ointment
Tanac Mouth and Lip Sore Medicines
TripTone for Motion Sickness

EFFCON LABORATORIES, INC. 409, 560
P.O. Box 71206
Marietta, GA 30007-1206
Address inquiries to:
Ed R. Burklow (800) 722-2428
FAX (404) 578-8065
For Medical Emergency Contact:
Ed R. Burklow (800) 722-2428
FAX (404) 578-8065
OTC Products Available
◆Pin-X Pinworm Treatment

EMUTECH INTERNATIONAL, INC. 560
4790 Irvine Boulevard
Suite 105-418
Irvine, CA 92720
Address inquiries to:
(714) 552-1015
FAX (714) 552-2927
OTC Products Available
Aloe Up
Cheater's Delight
Kick Start
Renew
Ultra Meal
Vita Fuel

FISONS CONSUMER HEALTH 409, 561
Fisons Corporation
P.O. Box 1212
Rochester, NY 14603
Address inquiries to:
Product Service Department
P.O. Box 1212
Rochester, NY 14603
(716) 475-9000
FAX (716) 274-5304
For Medical Emergencies Contact
Fisons Corporation
(716) 475-9000
OTC Products Available
Allerest Children's Chewable Tablets
Allerest Eye Drops
Allerest Headache Strength Tablets
Allerest 12 Hour Caplets
Allerest 12 Hour Nasal Spray
◆Allerest Maximum Strength Tablets
◆Allerest No Drowsiness Tablets
Allerest Sinus Pain Formula
◆Americaine Hemorrhoidal Ointment
◆Americaine Topical Anesthetic First Aid Ointment
◆Americaine Topical Anesthetic Spray
Bacid Capsules
◆Caldecort Anti-Itch Hydrocortisone Cream
Caldecort Anti-Itch Hydrocortisone Spray
◆Caldecort Light Cream
◆Caldesene Medicated Ointment
◆Caldesene Medicated Powder
Cholan HMB
◆Cruex Antifungal Cream
Cruex Antifungal Powder
◆Cruex Antifungal Spray Powder
Desenex Antifungal Cream
Desenex Antifungal Foam
◆Desenex Antifungal Ointment
◆Desenex Antifungal Powder
Desenex Antifungal Spray Liquid
◆Desenex Antifungal Spray Powder
Desenex Foot & Sneaker Deodorant Powder Plus
◆Desenex Foot & Sneaker Deodorant Spray Powder
Desenex Soap
Emul-O-Balm
Isoclor Liquid
Isoclor Tablets
◆Isoclor Timesule Capsules
Kondremul
Kondremul with Phenylphthalein
Myoflex Analgesic Creme
Sinarest 12 Hour Nasal Spray
Sinarest No Drowsiness Tablets
Sinarest Tablets
Sinarest Extra Strength Tablets
◆Ting Antifungal Cream
◆Ting Antifungal Powder
◆Ting Antifungal Spray Liquid
◆Ting Antifungal Spray Powder
Vitron-C Tablets
Vitron-C Plus Tablets

FISONS CORPORATION PRESCRIPTION PRODUCTS 566
755 Jefferson Road
Rochester, NY 14623

Mailing Address: P.O. Box 1766
Rochester, NY 14603
Address inquiries to:
Professional Services Department
P.O. Box 1766
Rochester, NY 14603
(716) 475-9000
OTC Products Available
Delsym Cough Formula

FLEMING & COMPANY 566
1600 Fenpark Dr.
Fenton, MO 63026
Address inquiries to:
John J. Roth, M.D. (314) 343-8200
For Medical Emergencies Contact:
John R. Roth, M.D. (314) 343-8200
OTC Products Available
Chlor-3 Condiment
Impregon Concentrate
Magonate Tablets and Liquid
Marblen Suspension Peach/Apricot
Marblen Suspension Unflavored
Marblen Tablets
Nephrox Suspension
Nicotinex Elixir
Ocean Nasal Mist
Purge Concentrate

GEBAUER COMPANY 567
9410 St. Catherine Avenue
Cleveland, OH 44104
Address inquiries to:
(800) 321-9348
FAX (216) 271-5335
For Medical Emergencies Contact:
(800) 321-9348
FAX (216) 271-5335
OTC Products Available
Dr. Caldwell Senna Laxative
Salivart Saliva Substitute

GLENBROOK LABORATORIES
See STERLING HEALTH, page 738.

HERALD PHARMACAL, INC. 568
6503 Warwick Road
Richmond, VA 23225
Address inquiries to:
Henry H. Kamps
(804) 745-3400
For Medical Emergencies Contact:
Henry H. Kamps
(804) 745-3400
OTC Products Available
Aqua Glycolic Lotion
Aqua Glycolic Shampoo
Aqua Glyde Cleanser
Aquaray 20 Sunscreen
Cam Lotion

INTER-CAL CORPORATION 568
427 Miller Valley Road
Prescott, AZ 86301
Address inquiries to:
Gerald W. Elders (602) 445-8063
OTC Products Available
Ester-C Tablets, Caplets and Powder

JOHNSON & JOHNSON CONSUMER PRODUCTS, INC. 409, 568
Grandview Road
Skillman, NJ 08558
Address inquiries to:
Customer Information Services
(800) 526-3967
For Medical Emergency Contact:
Customer Information Services
(800) 526-3967
OTC Products Available
Johnson's Baby Diaper Rash Relief
Johnson's Baby Sunblock, SPF 30+
◆K-Y Brand Jelly Personal Lubricant
Purpose Dual Treatment Moisturizer-Fragrance Free
Purpose Dual Treatment Moisturizer-Lightly Scented

JOHNSON & JOHNSON • MERCK CONSUMER PHARMACEUTICALS CO. 409, 569
Camp Hill Road
Fort Washington, PA 19034
Address inquiries to:
Consumer Affairs Department
(215) 233-7000
For Medical Emergencies Contact:
(215) 233-7000
OTC Products Available
◆ALternaGEL Liquid
◆Dialose Tablets
◆Dialose Plus Tablets
◆Effer-Syllium Natural Fiber Bulking Agent
◆Ferancee Chewable Tablets
◆Ferancee-HP Tablets
◆Mylanta Gas Tablets-40 mg
◆Mylanta Gas Tablets-80 mg
◆Maximum Strength Mylanta Gas Tablets-125 mg
◆Mylanta Gelcaps Antacid
◆Mylanta Liquid
◆Mylanta Tablets

(◆ Shown in Product Identification Section)

◆Mylanta Double Strength Liquid
◆Mylanta Double Strength Tablets
◆Mylicon Drops
◆The Stuart Formula Tablets
◆Stuartinic Tablets

KONSYL PHARMACEUTICALS, INC. 574
4200 South Hulen
Ft. Worth, TX 76109
Address inquiries to:
Bill Steiber (817) 763-8011
FAX (817) 731-9389
OTC Products Available
Konsyl Powder
Konsyl-D Powder
Konsyl-Orange Powder

LACTAID INC. 413, 575
Pleasantville, NJ 08232
Address inquiries to:
Alan E Kligerman (609) 645-5100
OTC Products Available
◆Lactaid Caplets (Now marketed by McNeil Consumer Products Co.)
◆Lactaid Drops (Now marketed by McNeil Consumer Products Co.)

LAVOPTIK COMPANY, INC. 575, 793
661 Western Avenue North
St. Paul, MN 55103
Address inquiries to:
661 Western Avenue North
St. Paul, MN 55103 (612) 489-1351
For Medical Emergencies Contact:
B. C. Brainard (612) 489-1351
OTC Products Available
Lavoptik Eye Cup
Lavoptik Eye Wash

LEDERLE LABORATORIES 410, 576
Division of American Cyanamid Co.
One Cyanamid Plaza
Wayne, NJ 07470
Address inquiries on medical matters to:
Professional Services Dept.
Lederle Laboratories
Pearl River, NY 10965
8 AM to 4:30 PM EST
(914) 735-2815
All other inquiries and after hours emergencies
(914) 732-5000
Distribution Centers
ATLANTA
Contact EASTERN (Philadelphia) Distribution Center
CHICAGO
Bulk Address
1100 East Business Center Drive
Mt. Prospect, IL 60056
Mail Address
P.O. Box 7614
Mt. Prospect, IL 60056-7614
(800) 533-3753
(708) 827-8871
DALLAS
Bulk Address
7611 Carpenter Freeway
Dallas, TX 75247
Mail Address
P.O. Box 655731
Dallas, TX 75265 (800) 533-3753
(214) 631-2130
LOS ANGELES
Bulk Address
2300 S. Eastern Avenue
Los Angeles, CA 90040
Mail Address
T.A. Box 2202
Los Angeles, CA 90051
(800) 533-3753
(213) 726-1016
EASTERN (Philadelphia)
Bulk Address
202 Precision Drive
Horsham, PA 19044
Mail Address
P.O. Box 993
Horsham, PA 19044 (800) 533-3753
(215) 672-5400

OTC Products Available
Acetaminophen Capsules, Tablets
◆Caltrate 600
◆Caltrate 600 + Iron & Vitamin D
◆Caltrate 600 + Vitamin D
◆Centrum
◆Centrum, Jr. (Children's Chewable) + Extra C
◆Centrum, Jr. (Children's Chewable) + Extra Calcium
◆Centrum, Jr. (Children's Chewable) + Iron
◆Centrum Liquid
◆Centrum Silver
◆Ferro-Sequels
◆FiberCon
Filibon Prenatal Vitamin Tablets
Gevrabon Liquid
Gevral T Tablets
Incremin with Iron Syrup
◆Protegra Vitamin and Mineral Supplement
◆Stresstabs
◆Stresstabs + Iron, Advanced Formula
◆Stresstabs + Zinc
◆Zincon Dandruff Shampoo

LEVER BROTHERS 411, 582
390 Park Avenue
New York, NY 10022
Address inquiries to:
(212) 688-6000
OTC Products Available
◆Dove Bar
◆Liquid Dove Beauty Wash
◆Lever 2000

MACSIL, INC. 582
1326 Frankford Avenue
Philadelphia, PA 19125
(215) 739-7300
OTC Products Available
Balmex Baby Powder
Balmex Emollient Lotion
Balmex Ointment

MARION MERRELL DOW INC. 583

See SMITHKLINE BEECHAM CONSUMER BRANDS.

MARLYN HEALTH CARE 583
14851 North Scottsdale Road
Scottsdale, AZ 85254 USA
(800) 462-7596
(602) 991-0200
Address inquiries to:
Kelly Easton (602) 991-0200
FAX (602) 991-0551
OTC Products Available
4-Hair
4-Nails
Hep-Forte Capsules
Marlyn Formula 50
Marlyn Formula 50 Mega Forte
Marlyn PMS
Osteo Fem
Pro-Skin-E (Face Capsule)
Pro-Skin Nutribloxx
Wobenzym N

McNEIL CONSUMER PRODUCTS CO. 411, 583
Division of McNeil-PPC, Inc.
Camp Hill Road
Fort Washington, PA 19034
(215) 233-7000
Address inquiries to:
Consumer Affairs Department
Fort Washington, PA 19034
Manufacturing Divisions
Fort Washington, PA 19034
Southwest Manufacturing Plant
4001 N. I-35
Round Rock, TX 78664
OTC Products Available
◆Imodium A-D Caplets and Liquid
◆PediaCare Cold Allergy Chewable Tablets
◆PediaCare Cough-Cold Chewable Tablets
◆PediaCare Cough-Cold Liquid
◆PediaCare Infants' Decongestant Drops
◆PediaCare Night Rest Cough-Cold Liquid
◆Sine-Aid Maximum Strength Sinus Headache Gelcaps, Caplets and Tablets
◆Tylenol acetaminophen Children's Chewable Tablets, Elixir, Suspension Liquid
◆Tylenol Allergy Sinus Medication Maximum Strength Gelcaps and Caplets
◆Children's Tylenol Cold Multi Symptom Liquid Formula and Chewable Tablets
◆Children's Tylenol Cold Plus Cough Multi Symptom Liquid Formula
◆Tylenol Cold & Flu Hot Medication, Packets
◆Tylenol Cold & Flu No Drowsiness Hot Medication, Packets
◆Tylenol Cold Multi Symptom Medication Caplets and Tablets
◆Tylenol Cold Medication, Effervescent Tablets
◆Tylenol Cold Medication No Drowsiness Formula Gelcaps and Caplets
◆Tylenol Cold Night Time Medication Liquid
◆Tylenol Cough Medication Maximum Strength Liquid
◆Tylenol Cough Medication Maximum Strength Liquid with Decongestant
Tylenol, Extra Strength, acetaminophen Adult Liquid Pain Reliever
◆Tylenol, Extra Strength, acetaminophen Gelcaps, Caplets, Tablets
◆Tylenol Headache Plus Pain Reliever with Antacid Caplets
◆Tylenol, Infants' Drops and Infants' Suspension Drops
◆Tylenol, Junior Strength, acetaminophen Coated Caplets, Grape and Fruit Chewable Tablets
◆Tylenol, Maximum Strength, Sinus Medication Gelcaps, Caplets and Tablets
◆Tylenol, Regular Strength, acetaminophen Caplets and Tablets
◆Tylenol PM Extra Strength Pain Reliever/Sleep Aid Gelcaps, Caplets, Tablets

MEAD JOHNSON NUTRITIONALS 601
A Bristol-Myers Squibb Company
2400 W. Lloyd Expressway
Evansville, IN 47721
(812) 429-5000
Address inquiries to:
Scientific Information Section
Medical Department
OTC Products Available
Enfamil Human Milk Fortifier
Enfamil Infant Formula
Enfamil Infant Formula Nursette
Enfamil With Iron Infant Formula
Enfamil Premature Formula
Enfamil Premature Formula With Iron
Fer-In-Sol
HIST 1
HIST 2
HOM 1
HOM 2
LYS 1
LYS 2
Lofenalac Iron Fortified Low Phenylalanine Diet Powder
Low Methionine Diet Powder (Product 3200K)
Low PHE/TYR Diet Powder (Product 3200AB)
MSUD Diet Powder
MSUD 1
MSUD 2
Mono- and Disaccharide-Free Diet Powder (Product 3232A)
Nutramigen Hypoallergenic Protein Hydrolysate Formula
OS 1
OS 2
PKU 1
PKU 2

(◆ Shown in Product Identification Section)

PKU 3
Phenyl-Free Phenylalanine-Free Diet Powder
Poly-Vi-Sol Vitamins, Chewable Tablets and Drops (without Iron)
Poly-Vi-Sol Vitamins, Peter Rabbit Shaped Chewable Tablets (without Iron)
Poly-Vi-Sol Vitamins with Iron, Peter Rabbit Shaped Chewable Tablets
Poly-Vi-Sol Vitamins with Iron, Drops
Pregestimil Iron Fortified Protein Hydrolysate Formula with Medium Chain Triglycerides
ProSobee Soy Formula
ProSobee Soy Formula Nursette
Protein-Free Diet Powder (Product 80056)
Ricelyte Oral Electrolyte Maintenance Solution Made With Rice Syrup Solids
Special Metabolic Diets
Special Metabolic Modules
TYR 1
TYR 2
Tempra 1 Acetaminophen Infant Drops
Tempra 2 Acetaminophen Toddlers Syrup
Tempra 3 Chewable Tablets, Regular or Double-Strength
Trind
Trind-DM
Tri-Vi-Sol Vitamin Drops
Tri-Vi-Sol Vitamin Drops with Iron
UCD 1
UCD 2

MEAD JOHNSON PHARMACEUTICALS
A Bristol-Myers Squibb Company
See APOTHECON.

MENLEY & JAMES LABORATORIES, INC. **414, 601**
Commonwealth Corporate Center
100 Tournament Drive, Suite 310
Horsham, PA 19044-3697
Address inquiries to:
Consumer Affairs Department
(800) 321-1834
OTC Products Available
◆A.R.M. Allergy Relief Medicine Caplets
◆Acnomel Acne Medication Cream
◆Aqua Care Cream
◆Aqua Care Lotion
AsthmaHaler Inhalation Aerosol Epinephrine Bitartrate Bronchodilator
AsthmaNefrin Solution "A" Bronchodilator
◆Benzedrex Inhaler
◆Benzedrex Nasal Spray Regular
◆Benzedrex Nasal Spray 12 Hour Relief
◆Congestac Caplets
◆FemIron Iron Supplement
◆FemIron Multivitamins and Iron
◆Garfield Chewable Multivitamins - Regular
◆Garfield Chewable Multivitamins Plus Extra C
◆Garfield Chewable Multivitamins Plus Iron
◆Garfield Chewable Multivitamins Complete with Minerals
◆Hold DM Cough Suppressant Lozenge
◆Liquiprin Infants' Drops
◆Ornex Caplets
◆Maximum Strength Ornex Caplets
◆Ornex Severe Cold Formula Caplets
◆Serutan Toasted Granules
Troph-Iron Liquid
Trophite Liquid

MILES INC. CONSUMER HEALTHCARE PRODUCTS **414, 609**
1127 Myrtle Street
Elkhart, IN 46514
Address inquiries to:
Director, Consumer Relations
(800) 800-4793
OTC Products Available
◆Alka-Mints Chewable Antacid
◆Alka-Seltzer Effervescent Antacid
◆Alka-Seltzer Effervescent Antacid and Pain Reliever
◆Alka-Seltzer Extra Strength Effervescent Antacid and Pain Reliever
◆Alka-Seltzer (Flavored) Effervescent Antacid and Pain Reliever
◆Alka-Seltzer Plus Cold Medicine
◆Alka-Seltzer Plus Cold & Cough Medicine
◆Alka-Seltzer Plus Night-Time Cold Medicine
◆Alka Seltzer Plus Sinus Allergy Medicine
◆Bactine Antiseptic/Anesthetic First Aid Liquid
◆Bactine First Aid Antibiotic Plus Anesthetic Ointment
◆Bactine Hydrocortisone Anti-Itch Cream
◆Bugs Bunny Children's Chewable Vitamins (Sugar Free)
◆Bugs Bunny Complete Children's Chewable Vitamins + Minerals with Iron and Calcium (Sugar Free)
◆Bugs Bunny With Extra C Children's Chewable Vitamins (Sugar Free)
◆Bugs Bunny Plus Iron Children's Chewable Vitamins (Sugar Free)
◆Domeboro Astringent Solution Effervescent Tablets
◆Domeboro Astringent Solution Powder Packets
◆Flintstones Children's Chewable Vitamins
◆Flintstones Children's Chewable Vitamins With Extra C
◆Flintstones Children's Chewable Vitamins Plus Iron
◆Flintstones Complete With Calcium, Iron & Minerals Children's Chewable Vitamins
◆Miles Nervine Nighttime Sleep-Aid
◆Mycelex OTC Cream Antifungal
◆Mycelex OTC Solution Antifungal
◆Mycelex-7 Vaginal Cream Antifungal
◆Mycelex-7 Vaginal Inserts Antifungal
◆One-A-Day Essential Vitamins
◆One-A-Day Maximum Formula Vitamins and Minerals
◆One-A-Day Plus Extra C Vitamins
◆One-A-Day Stressgard Formula Vitamins
◆One-A-Day Women's Formula Multivitamins with Calcium, Extra Iron, Zinc and Beta Carotene

MURO PHARMACEUTICAL, INC. **619**
890 East Street
Tewksbury, MA 01876-1496
Address inquiries to:
Professional Service Dept.
(800) 225-0974
(508) 851-5981
OTC Products Available
Bromfed Syrup
Guaifed Syrup
Guaitab Tablets
Salinex Nasal Mist and Drops

NATREN INC. **620**
3105 Willow Lane
Westlake Village, CA 91361
Address inquiries to:
Professional Services Department
(800) 992-3323
FAX (805) 371-4742
For Medical Emergency Contact:
Professional Services Department
(800) 992-3323
FAX (805) 371-4742
OTC Products Available
Bifido Factor
Bulgaricum I.B.
Life Start
M.F.A.
Pro-Bifidonate Powder
Pro-Bionate Powder and Capsules
Superdophilus

NATURE'S BOUNTY, INC. **416, 620**
90 Orville Drive
Bohemia, NY 11716
Address inquiries to:
Professional Service Department
(516) 567-9500
(800) 645-5412
FAX (516) 563-1623
OTC Products Available
ABC to Z
Acidophilus
B-Complex +C (Long Acting) Tablets
B-6 50 mg., 100 mg., 200 mg.
B-12 1000 mcg. Tablets
B-12 and B-12 Sublingual Tablets
B-50 Tablets
B-100 Tablets-Ultra B Complex
Beta-Carotene Capsules
Bounty Bears (Children's Chewables)
C-500 mg., C-1000 mg., C-1500 mg. & Time Release Formulas
Calcium Magnesium-Chelated Tablets
E-Oil 25,000 I.U.
◆Ener-B Vitamin B_{12} Nasal Gel Dietary Supplement
EnerVite (High Performance Nutrition)
Ferrous Sulfate Tablets
Garlic Oil 15 gr. & 77 gr.
KLB6 Capsules
l-Lysine 500 mg. Tablets & 1000 mg. Tablets
Lecithin 1200 mg. Capsules
M-KYA (For Leg Cramps)
Niacin 50 mg., 100 mg., & 250 mg.
Oat Bran 850 mg.
Oystercal-500 & Oystercal 500 + D
Ultra Vita-Time Tablets
Vitamin A 10,000 I.U. & 25,000 I.U.
Vitamin E (Natural d-alpha tocopheryl)
Water Pill (Natural Diuretic)
Zinc 10 mg., 25 mg., 50 mg. Tablets

NEUTROGENA DERMATOLOGICS **416, 620**
Division of Neutrogena Corporation
5760 West 96th Street
Los Angeles, CA 90045
Address inquiries to:
Mitchell S. Wortzman, Ph.D.
(310) 642-1150
FAX (310) 337-5557
For Medical Emergencies Contact:
Mitchell S. Wortzman, Ph.D.
9:00AM to 5PM-PCT (310) 216-5345
FAX (310) 337-5557
After Hours (310) 641-8659
OTC Products Available
Neutrogena Acne Mask
Neutrogena Chemical-Free Sunblocker
Neutrogena Cleansing Bar for Acne-prone Skin
Neutrogena Cleansing Bar for Dry Skin (FF)
Neutrogena Cleansing Bar for Oily Skin
Neutrogena Cleansing Bar Original Formula (FF)
◆Neutrogena Cleansing Wash
Neutrogena Lip Moisturizer (SPF 15)
◆Neutrogena Moisture
◆Neutrogena Moisture SPF 15 Untinted
◆Neutrogena Moisture SPF 15 with Sheer Tint
Neutrogena Non-Drying Cleansing Lotion
◆Neutrogena Norwegian Formula Emulsion
◆Neutrogena Norwegian Formula Hand Cream
Neutrogena Rainbath
Neutrogena Shampoo
◆Neutrogena Sunblock SPF 15
◆Neutrogena Sunblock SPF 30
Neutrogena T/Derm Tar Emollient
Neutrogena T/Gel Therapeutic Conditioner
◆Neutrogena T/Gel Therapeutic Shampoo
◆Neutrogena T/Sal Therapeutic Shampoo
Neutrogena Vehicle/N
Neutrogena Vehicle/N Mild

NICHE PHARMACEUTICALS, INC. **622**
300 Trophy Club Drive, #400
Roanoke, TX 76262

(◆ Shown in Product Identification Section)

Address inquiries to:
Steve F. Brandon (817) 491-2770
FAX (817) 491-3533
For Medical Emergencies Contact:
Gerald L. Beckloff, M.D.
(817) 491-2770
FAX (817) 491-3533
OTC Products Available
MagTab SR Caplets

OHM LABORATORIES, INC. 416, 623
P.O. Box 279
Franklin Park, NJ 08823
Address inquiries to:
Arun Heble (908) 297-3030
For Medical Emergencies Contact:
(908) 297-3030
OTC Products Available
Bisacodyl Tablets 5 mg.
◆Cramp End Tablets
Docusate Potassium Capsules
Docusate Potassium with Casanthranol Capsules and Caplets
◆Ibuprohm Ibuprofen Caplets
◆Ibuprohm Ibuprofen Tablets
◆Loperamide Hydrochloride Caplets
Ohmni-Scon Chewable Tablets, Extra Strength
Pseudoephedrine Hydrochloride Tablets 30mg and 60mg
Senna Tablets
Tribuffered Aspirin
Trisudrine Tablets

ORTHO PHARMACEUTICAL CORPORATION 417, 624, 793
Advanced Care Products
Route #202 South
Raritan, NJ 08869 (908) 524-0400
For Medical Emergencies Contact:
Dr. Carole Sampson-Landers
(908) 524-1305
OTC Products Available
◆Advance Pregnancy Test
◆Conceptrol Contraceptive Gel • Single Use Contraceptive
◆Conceptrol Contraceptive Inserts
◆Delfen Contraceptive Foam
◆Fact Plus Pregnancy Test
◆Gynol II Extra Strength Contraceptive Jelly
◆Gynol II Original Formula Contraceptive Jelly
◆Micatin Antifungal Cream
◆Micatin Antifungal Odor Control Spray Powder
◆Micatin Antifungal Powder
◆Micatin Antifungal Spray Liquid
◆Micatin Antifungal Spray Powder
Micatin Jock Itch Cream
Micatin Jock Itch Spray Powder
◆Monistat 7 Vaginal Cream
◆Monistat 7 Vaginal Suppositories
◆Ortho-Gynol Contraceptive Jelly

P & S LABORATORIES 627
210 West 131st Street
Los Angeles, CA 90061

See STANDARD HOMEOPATHIC COMPANY.

PRN LABORATORIES, INC. 627
285 National Place, Unit 127
Longwood, FL 32750
Address inquiries to:
(407) 260-2225
FAX (407) 644-2717
For Medical Emergency Contact:
(407) 260-2225
FAX (407) 644-2717
OTC Products Available
Dia Scan Gel
Pain Free Aloe Vera Gel with Capsaicin
Pain Free Natural with Capsaicin
Pain Freeze Menthol Gel
Pain Stop Extra Strength Lotion
Thera Scan Gel
Top Skin Multi-Purpose Skin Care Lotion

PARKE-DAVIS 417, 627, 793
Consumer Health Products Group
Division of Warner-Lambert Company
201 Tabor Road
Morris Plains, New Jersey 07950
See also Warner-Lambert Company
(201) 540-2000
For product information call:
1-(800) 223-0432
For medical information call:
(201) 540-3950
OTC Products Available
Agoral, Marshmallow Flavor
Agoral, Raspberry Flavor
Alcohol, Rubbing (Lavacol)
Alophen Pills
◆Anusol Hemorrhoidal Suppositories
◆Anusol Ointment
◆Anusol HC-1
◆Benadryl Allergy Sinus Headache Formula
◆Benadryl Anti-Itch Cream, Regular Strength 1% and Maximum Strength 2%
◆Benadryl Cold Tablets
◆Benadryl Cold Nighttime Formula
◆Benadryl Decongestant Elixir
◆Benadryl Decongestant Kapseals
◆Benadryl Decongestant Tablets
◆Benadryl Elixir
◆Benadryl Spray, Maximum Strength 2%
◆Benadryl Spray, Regular Strength 1%
◆Benadryl 25 Kapseals
◆Benadryl 25 Tablets
◆Benylin Cough Syrup
◆Benylin Decongestant
◆Benylin DM Pediatric Cough Formula
◆Benylin Expectorant
◆Caladryl Clear Lotion
◆Caladryl Cream, Lotion, Spray
◆e.p.t. Early Pregnancy Test
◆Gelusil Liquid & Tablets
Lavacol (Rubbing Alcohol)
◆Medi-Flu Caplet, Liquid
◆Medi-Flu Without Drowsiness Caplets
◆Myadec
Proxacol-Hydrogen Peroxide Solution
◆Replens
Siblin Granules
◆Sinutab Sinus Allergy Medication, Maximum Strength Caplets
◆Sinutab Sinus Allergy Medication, Maximum Strength Tablets
◆Sinutab Sinus Medication, Maximum Strength Without Drowsiness Formula, Tablets & Caplets
◆Sinutab Sinus Medication, Regular Strength Without Drowsiness Formula
Tucks Cream
◆Tucks Premoistened Pads
Tucks Take-Alongs

THE PARTHENON COMPANY, INC. 637
3311 West 2400 South
Salt Lake City, UT 84119
Address inquiries to:
(801) 972-5184
FAX (801) 972-4734
For Medical Emergency Contact:
Nick G. Mihalopoulos (801) 972-5184
OTC Products Available
Devrom Chewable Tablets

PERFECTIVE COSMETICS, INC. 637
688 High Ridge Road
P.O. Box 3488
Stamford, CT 06905
(203) 329-1800
(800) 477-7786
FAX (203) 322-5046
OTC Products Available
Perfective Prevention Cream

PFIZER CONSUMER HEALTH CARE DIVISION 419, 638
Division of Pfizer Inc.
100 Jefferson Road
Parsippany, NJ 07054
Address inquiries to:
Research and Development Dept.
(201) 887-2100

OTC Products Available
Ben-Gay External Analgesic Products
Bonine Tablets
◆Desitin Ointment
Rheaban Maximum Strength Tablets
Rid Lice Control Spray
Rid Lice Killing Shampoo
Unisom Nighttime Sleep Aid
Unisom with Pain Relief Nighttime Sleep Aid/Analgesic
◆Visine A.C. Eye Drops
◆Visine EXTRA Eye Drops
◆Visine Eye Drops
◆Visine L.R. Eye Drops
Wart-Off Wart Remover

PLOUGH, INC.

See SCHERING-PLOUGH HEALTHCARE PRODUCTS

POLYMEDICA PHARMACEUTICALS (USA), INC. 642
Subsidiary of PolyMedica Industries, Inc.
2 Constitution Way
Woburn, MA 01801
Address inquiries to:
Dr. Arthur Siciliano (617) 933-2020
FAX (617) 933-7992
For Medical Emergencies Contact:
(617) 933-2020
FAX (617) 933-7992
OTC Products Available
Alconephrin Nasal Decongestant
Azo-Standard
Neopap Pediatric Suppositories

PREMIER, INC. 643
Greenwich Office Park One
Greenwich, CT 06831
Address inquiries to:
Robert Albus (203) 622-1211
FAX (203) 622-0773
For Medical Emergency Contact:
Sergio Nacht, Ph.D. (415) 366-2626
FAX (415) 368-4470
Branch Office
3696 Haven Avenue
Redwood City, CA (415) 366-2626
FAX (415) 368-4470
OTC Products Available
Every Step Foot Deodorant
Exact Cream

PROCTER & GAMBLE 643
P.O. Box 5516
Cincinnati, OH 45201
Address inquiries to:
Arnold P. Austin (800) 358-8707
For Medical Emergencies Contact:
Call collect (513) 751-2823
OTC Products Available
Children's Chloraseptic Lozenges
Vicks Children's Chloraseptic Spray
Chloraseptic Liquid, Cherry, Menthol or Cool Mint
Chloraseptic Lozenges, Cherry, Cool Mint or Menthol
Head & Shoulders Antidandruff Shampoo
Head & Shoulders Antidandruff Shampoo 2-in-1 plus Conditioner
Head & Shoulders Dry Scalp Shampoo
Head & Shoulders Dry Scalp Shampoo 2-in-1 plus Conditioner
Head & Shoulders Intensive Treatment Dandruff Shampoo
Head & Shoulders Intensive Treatment Dandruff Shampoo 2-in-1 plus Conditioner
Metamucil Effervescent Sugar Free, Lemon-Lime Flavor
Metamucil Effervescent Sugar Free, Orange Flavor
Metamucil Powder, Orange Flavor
Metamucil Powder, Regular Flavor
Metamucil Sunrise Smooth, Citrus Flavor
Metamucil Sunrise Smooth, Sugar Free, Citrus Flavor
Metamucil Sunrise Smooth Powder, Orange Flavor

(◆ Shown in Product Identification Section)

Metamucil Sunrise Smooth Powder, Sugar Free, Orange Flavor
Metamucil Wafers, Apple Crisp
Metamucil Wafers, Cinnamon Spice
Oil of Olay Daily UV Protectant SPF 15 Beauty Fluid-Original and Fragrance Free (Olay Co. Inc.)
Oil of Olay Daily UV Protectant SPF 15 Moisture Replenishing Cream-Original and Fragrance Free (Olay Co. Inc.)
Pepto Diarrhea Control
Pepto-Bismol Liquid & Tablets
Maximum Strength Pepto-Bismol Liquid
Percogesic Analgesic Tablets
Vicks Children's NyQuil Nighttime Cold/Cough Medicine
Vicks Children's NyQuil Nighttime Allergy/Head Cold Medicine
Vicks Cough Drops
Extra Strength Vicks Cough Drops
Vicks DayQuil
Vicks DayQuil LiquiCaps
Vicks Formula 44 Cough Medicine
Vicks Formula 44D Cough & Decongestant Medicine
Vicks Formula 44E Cough & Expectorant Medicine
Vicks Formula 44M Multi-Symptom Cough & Cold Medicine
Vicks Inhaler
Vicks NyQuil LiquiCaps Nighttime Cold/Flu Medicine
Vicks NyQuil Nighttime Cold/Flu Medicine - Regular & Cherry Flavor
Vicks Pediatric Formula 44 Cough Medicine
Vicks Pediatric Formula 44d Cough & Decongestant Medicine
Vicks Pediatric Formula 44e Cough & Expectorant Medicine
Vicks Pediatric Formula 44m Multi-Symptom Cough & Cold Medicine
Vicks Sinex Decongestant Nasal Spray (Regular)
Vicks Sinex Decongestant Nasal Ultra Fine Mist
Vicks Sinex Long-Acting Decongestant Nasal Spray
Vicks Sinex Long-Acting Decongestant Nasal Ultra Fine Mist
Vicks VapoRub
Vicks VapoSteam
Vicks Vatronol Nose Drops

REED & CARNRICK 419, 657
Division of Block Drug Company, Inc.
257 Cornelison Avenue
Jersey City, NJ 07302
Address Inquiries to:
Marketing Services
(201) 434-4000
FAX (201) 434-3032
For Medical Emergencies Contact:
Reed & Carnrick Consumer Services
(800) 568-6133
OTC Products Available
◆Phazyme Drops
◆Phazyme Tablets
◆Phazyme-125 Softgels Maximum Strength
◆Phazyme-95 Tablets
ProctoFoam (non-steroid)
Proxigel
R&C Lice Treatment Kit
R&C Shampoo
R&C Spray
Trichotine Liquid Vaginal Douche
Trichotine Powder Vaginal Douche

THE REESE CHEMICAL COMPANY 419, 658
10617 Frank Avenue
Cleveland, OH 44106
Address inquiries to:
George W. Reese, III
(216) 231-6441
OTC Products Available
Bi-Zet Throat Lozenges
Cold Control+ Intense Cold Medicine
Colicon Drops
Dentapaine Gel
Dermatox Skin Lotion
Licide Lice Control Kit
Licide Lice Control Shampoo
Pediatric Formula Cough & Cold Liquid
Pediatric Plus Cough & Cold Liquid
Podactin Anti-Fungal Cream
Redacon DX Pediatric Drops
Red Hearts Vitamin Tonic Tablets
◆Reese's Pinworm Medicine
Sleep-ettes-D Tablets
Theracof Cough & Cold Liquid
Tri-Biozene Ointment

REQUA, INC. 659
Box 4008
1 Seneca Place
Greenwich, CT 06830
Address inquiries to:
Geoffrey Geils (203) 869-2445
(800) 321-1085
FAX (203) 661-5630
OTC Products Available
Charcoaid
Charcoal Tablets
Charcocaps

RHONE-POULENC RORER PHARMACEUTICALS INC. 419, 659
Consumer Pharmaceutical Products
500 Arcola Road
Collegeville, PA 19426-0107
For Medical Emergencies/ Product Information Contact:
Drug Product Safety and Product Information Call (215) 454-8870
For Regulatory Questions Contact:
Margaret Masters
Assoc. Director, Regulatory Control
(215) 628-6085
OTC Products Available
◆Ascriptin A/D Caplets
◆Extra Strength Ascriptin Caplets
◆Regular Strength Ascriptin Tablets
◆Maalox Antacid Caplets
◆Maalox HRF Heartburn Relief Formula Suspension
◆Maalox HRF Heartburn Relief Formula Antacid Tablets
◆Maalox Suspension
◆Maalox Plus Tablets
◆Extra Strength Maalox Plus Suspension
◆Extra Strength Maalox Plus Tablets
◆Perdiem Fiber Granules
◆Perdiem Granules

RICHARDSON-VICKS, INC. 666
See PROCTER & GAMBLE.

ROBERTS PHARMACEUTICAL CORPORATION 420, 666
6 Industrial Way West
Eatonton, NJ 07724
Address inquiries to:
Customer Service Department
(908) 389-1182
FAX (908) 389-1014
(800) 828-2088
For Medical Emergencies Contact:
Medical Services Department
(908) 935-9170
(800) 992-9306
OTC Products Available
Alkets Tablets
Baciguent Topical Cream
Calcium Lactate Tablets
Cheracol Cough Syrup
◆Cheracol-D Cough Formula
Cheracol Nasal Spray Pump
◆Cheracol Plus Head Cold/Cough Formula
Cheracol Sinus
Cheracol Sore Throat Spray
Cheracol Throat Discs
Citrocarbonate Antacid
Clocort Cream with Aloe
Clocort Maximum Strength Cream
Clocream Skin Protectant Cream
Clomycin Antibiotic Ointment
Diostate D Tablets
◆Haltran Tablets
Kasof Capsules
Lipomul Oral Liquid
Myciguent Topical Cream
Orexin Tablets
Orthoxicol Cough Syrup
◆P-A-C Analgesic Tablets
Probec-T Tablets
◆Pyrroxate Capsules
◆Sigtab Tablets
◆Sigtab-M Tablets
Super D Perles
Zymacap Capsules

A. H. ROBINS CONSUMER PRODUCTS DIVISION 420, 671
Subsidiary of American Home Products Corporation
1405 Cummings Drive
Richmond, VA 23220
Address inquiries to:
Consumer Affairs (800) 762-4672
For Medical Emergencies Contact:
Medical Department (804) 257-2000
(day or night)
If no answer, call answering service
(804) 257-7788
OTC Products Available
Allbee with C Caplets
Allbee C-800 Plus Iron Tablets
Allbee C-800 Tablets
◆Anacin Caplets
◆Anacin Tablets
Maximum Strength Anacin Tablets
◆Aspirin Free Anacin Caplets
◆Aspirin Free Anacin Gel Caplets
◆Aspirin Free Anacin Tablets
◆Aspirin Free Anacin P.M. Caplets
◆Chap Stick Lip Balm
◆Chap Stick Medicated Lip Balm
◆Chap Stick Sunblock 15 Lip Balm
◆Chap Stick Petroleum Jelly Plus
◆Chap Stick Petroleum Jelly Plus with Sunblock 15
Dimacol Caplets
Dimetane Elixir
Dimetane Extentabs 8 mg
Dimetane Extentabs 12 mg
Dimetane Tablets
Dimetane Decongestant Caplets
Dimetane Decongestant Elixir
◆Dimetapp Elixir
◆Dimetapp Extentabs
◆Dimetapp Liqui-Gels
◆Dimetapp Tablets
◆Dimetapp Cold & Allergy Chewable Tablets
◆Dimetapp Cold & Flu Caplets
◆Dimetapp DM Elixir
◆Dimetapp Sinus Caplets
◆Robitussin
Robitussin Cough Calmers
◆Robitussin Cough Drops
◆Robitussin Maximum Strength Cough Suppressant
◆Robitussin Maximum Strength Cough & Cold
◆Robitussin Night Relief
◆Robitussin Pediatric Cough & Cold Formula
◆Robitussin Pediatric Cough Suppressant
◆Robitussin-CF
◆Robitussin-DM
◆Robitussin-PE
Z-BEC Tablets

ROSS LABORATORIES 421, 683
Division of Abbott Laboratories USA
P.O. Box 1317
Columbus, OH 43216-1317
Address Inquiries to:
Medical Director (614) 624-3333
OTC Products Available
◆Clear Eyes ACR Astringent/Lubricating Eye Redness Reliever
◆Clear Eyes Lubricating Eye Redness Reliever
◆Ear Drops by Murine—(See Murine Ear Wax Removal System/Murine Ear Drops)
◆Murine Ear Drops
◆Murine Ear Wax Removal System
◆Murine Lubricating Eye Drops

(◆ **Shown in Product Identification Section**)

◆Murine Plus Lubricating Redness Reliever Eye Drops
Pedialyte Oral Electrolyte Maintenance Solution
Rehydralyte Oral Electrolyte Rehydration Solution
Ross Pediatric Nutritional Products
Alimentum Protein Hydrolysate Formula With Iron
Isomil Soy Formula With Iron
Isomil SF Sucrose-Free Soy Protein Formula With Iron
PediaSure Liquid Nutrition for Children
RCF Ross Carbohydrate Free Low-Iron Soy Protein Formula Base
Similac Low-Iron Infant Formula
Similac PM 60/40 Low-Iron Infant Formula
Similac Special Care With Iron 24 Premature Infant Formula
Similac With Iron Infant Formula
◆Selsun Blue Dandruff Shampoo
◆Selsun Blue Dandruff Shampoo Medicated Treatment Formula
◆Selsun Blue Extra Conditioning Formula Dandruff Shampoo
◆Selsun Gold for Women Dandruff Shampoo
◆Tronolane Anesthetic Cream for Hemorrhoids
◆Tronolane Hemorrhoidal Suppositories

RYDELLE LABORATORIES 422, 687
Division of S.C. Johnson & Son, Inc.
1525 Howe Street
Racine, WI 53403
Address inquiries to:
Thomas Conrardy
Consumer Resource Center Director
(414) 631-2000
For Medical Emergencies Contact:
Marvin G. Parker, M.D., F.A.C.P.
(414) 631-2111
OTC Products Available
◆Aveeno Anti-Itch Concentrated Lotion
◆Aveeno Anti-Itch Cream
◆Aveeno Bath Oilated
◆Aveeno Bath Regular
◆Aveeno Cleansing Bar for Acne-Prone Skin
◆Aveeno Cleansing Bar for Combination Skin
◆Aveeno Cleansing Bar for Dry Skin
◆Aveeno Moisturizing Cream
◆Aveeno Moisturizing Lotion
◆Aveeno Shower and Bath Oil
◆Rhulicream
◆Rhuligel
◆Rhulispray

SANDOZ PHARMACEUTICALS/ CONSUMER DIVISION 422, 688
59 Route 10
East Hanover NJ 07936
Address Medical Inquiries To:
Medical Department
Sandoz Pharmaceuticals Corporation
East Hanover, NJ 07936
(201) 503-7500
Other Inquiries To:
(201) 503-7500
FAX (201) 503-8265
OTC Products Available
Acid Mantle Creme
◆BiCozene Creme
Cama Arthritis Pain Reliever
◆Dorcol Children's Cough Syrup
◆Dorcol Children's Decongestant Liquid
◆Dorcol Children's Liquid Cold Formula
◆Ex-Lax Chocolated Laxative Tablets
◆Extra Gentle Ex-Lax Laxative Pills
◆Maximum Relief Formula Ex-Lax Laxative Pills
◆Regular Strength Ex-Lax Laxative Pills
◆Ex-Lax Gentle Nature Laxative Pills
◆Gas-X Chewable Tablets
◆Extra Strength Gas-X Chewable Tablets
◆Tavist-1 12 Hour Relief Medicine
◆Tavist-D 12 Hour Relief Medicine
◆TheraFlu Flu and Cold Medicine
◆TheraFlu Flu, Cold and Cough Medicine
◆TheraFlu Maximum Strength Nighttime Flu, Cold and Cough Medicine
Triaminic Allergy Medicine
Triaminic Chewable Tablets For Children
◆Triaminic Cold Medicine
◆Triaminic Expectorant
◆Triaminic Nite Light
◆Triaminic Syrup
◆Triaminic-12 Maximum Strength 12 Hour Relief
◆Triaminic-DM Syrup
◆Triaminicin Cold, Allergy, Sinus Medicine
◆Triaminicol Multi-Symptom Cold and Cough Medicine
◆Triaminicol Multi-Symptom Relief
Ursinus Inlay-Tabs

SANOFI WINTHROP PHARMACEUTICALS 696
Main Office
90 Park Avenue
New York, NY 10016
(212) 907-2000
Address Medical Inquiries to:
Product Information Services
(800) 446-6267
All Other Information:
Customer Relations/Orders
(800) 223-5511
OTC Products Available
Anti-Rust Tablets
Breonsin Capsules
Bronkolixir
Bronkotabs Tablets
Drisdol
pHisoDerm (See Sterling Health)
Pontocaine Cream
Pontocaine Ointment
Zephiran Chloride Aqueous Solution
Zephiran Chloride Concentrate Solution
Zephiran Chloride Spray
Zephiran Chloride Tinted Tincture
Zephiran Towelettes

SCHERING CORPORATION

See SCHERING-PLOUGH HEALTHCARE PRODUCTS

SCHERING-PLOUGH HEALTHCARE PRODUCTS 423, 698
110 Allen Road
Liberty Corner, NJ 07938
Address product requests to:
Public Relations (908) 604-1969
For Medical Emergencies Contact:
Clinical Department
(901) 320-2998
OTC Products Available
◆A and D Ointment
◆Afrin Cherry Scented Nasal Spray 0.05%
◆Afrin Children's Strength Nose Drops 0.025%
◆Afrin Menthol Nasal Spray, 0.05%
◆Afrin Nasal Spray 0.05% and Nasal Spray Pump
◆Afrin Nose Drops 0.05%
◆Afrin Saline Mist
◆Afrin Tablets
◆Aftate for Athlete's Foot
◆Aftate for Jock Itch
Aspergum
◆Chlor-Trimeton Allergy Decongestant Tablets
◆Chlor-Trimeton Allergy-Sinus Headache Caplets
◆Chlor-Trimeton Allergy Syrup and Tablets
◆Chlor-Trimeton Long Acting Antihistamine and Decongestant Repetabs Tablets
◆Chlor-Trimeton Non-Drowsy Decongestant Tablets - 4 Hour
◆Chooz Antacid Gum
◆Complex 15 Hand & Body Moisturizing Cream
◆Complex 15 Hand & Body Moisturizing Lotion
◆Complex 15 Moisturizing Face Cream
◆Coricidin 'D' Decongestant Tablets
◆Coricidin Tablets
Correctol Extra Gentle Stool Softener
◆Correctol Laxative Tablets
Cushion Grip Denture Adhesive
◆Di-Gel Antacid/Anti-Gas
Drixoral Antihistamine/Nasal Decongestant Syrup
◆Drixoral Cold and Allergy Sustained-Action Tablets
◆Drixoral Cold and Flu Extended-Release Tablets
◆Drixoral Non-Drowsy Formula
◆Drixoral Sinus
◆DuoFilm Liquid
◆DuoFilm Patch
◆DuoPlant Gel
◆Duration 12 Hour Nasal Spray
◆Duration 12 Hour Nasal Spray Pump
◆Feen-A-Mint Gum
◆Feen-A-Mint Laxative Pills
◆Gyne-Lotrimin Vaginal Cream Antifungal
◆Gyne-Lotrimin Vaginal Cream with 7 Disposable Applicators
◆Gyne-Lotrimin Vaginal Inserts
◆Gyne-Moistrin Vaginal Moisturizing Gel
◆Lotrimin AF Antifungal Cream, Lotion and Solution
Muskol Insect Repellent Aerosol Liquid
Muskol Insect Repellent Lotion
Muskol Insect Repellent Pump Spray
Muskol Insect Repellent Roll-on
◆OcuClear Eye Drops (See PDR For Ophthalmology)
St. Joseph Adult Chewable Aspirin (81 mg.)
St. Joseph Aspirin-Free Fever Reducer for Children Chewable Tablets
St. Joseph Cold Tablets for Children
St. Joseph Cough Suppressant for Children
◆Tinactin Aerosol Liquid 1%
◆Tinactin Aerosol Powder 1%
◆Tinactin Antifungal Cream, Solution & Powder 1%
Tinactin Deodorant Powder Aerosol 1%
◆Tinactin Jock Itch Cream 1%
◆Tinactin Jock Itch Spray Powder 1%

SCOT-TUSSIN PHARMACAL CO., INC. 712
50 Clemence Street
Cranston, RI 02920-0217 (USA)
Mailing Address: P.O. Box 8217
Cranston, RI 02920-0217
Address inquiries to:
(401) 942-8555
(401) 942-8556
(800) 638-SCOT (7268)
FAX (401) 942-5690
For Medical Emergency Contact:
Dr. S. G. Scotti
(800) 638-SCOT (7268)
FAX (401) 942-5690
OTC Products Available
Chlorpheniramine Maleate
Febrol DF and Febrol SF
Hayfebrol Allergy Relief Formula
Scot-Tussin Allergy Relief Formula Sugar-Free
Scot-Tussin DM Cough Chasers Lozenges Sugar-Free
Scot-Tussin DM Sugar-Free
Scot-Tussin DM-2 Syrup USP
Scot-Tussin Expectorant Sugar-Free
Scot-Tussin Original Syrup
Scot-Tussin Sugar-Free Original Syrup
Vitalize Sugar-Free Stress Formula

SMITHKLINE BEECHAM CONSUMER BRANDS 426, 712
Unit of SmithKline Beecham, Inc.
P.O. Box 1467
Pittsburgh, PA 15230
Address inquiries to:
Professional Services Department
(800) BEECHAM
(412) 928-1050
OTC Products Available
◆A-200 Lice Control Spray and Kit
◆A-200 Pediculicide Shampoo

(◆ Shown in Product Identification Section)

◆Cēpacol Anesthetic Lozenges (Troches)
◆Cēpacol/Cēpacol Mint Mouthwash/Gargle
◆Cēpacol Dry Throat Lozenges, Cherry Flavor
◆Cēpacol Dry Throat Lozenges, Honey-Lemon Flavor
◆Cēpacol Dry Throat Lozenges, Menthol-Eucalyptus Flavor
◆Cēpacol Dry Throat Lozenges, Original Flavor
◆CĒPASTAT Cherry Flavor Sore Throat Lozenges
◆CĒPASTAT Extra Strength Sore Throat Lozenges
◆CITRUCEL Orange Flavor
◆CITRUCEL Sugar Free Orange Flavor
◆Clear by Design Medicated Acne Gel
◆Contac Continuous Action Decongestant/Antihistamine Capsules
◆Contac Day & Night Cold & Flu - Day Caplets
◆Contac Day & Night Cold & Flu - Night Caplets
◆Contac Maximum Strength Continuous Action Decongestant/Antihistamine Caplets
◆Contac Severe Cold and Flu Formula Caplets
◆Contac Severe Cold & Flu Nighttime
◆Debrox Drops
◆Ecotrin Enteric Coated Aspirin Maximum Strength Tablets and Caplets
◆Ecotrin Enteric Coated Aspirin Regular Strength Tablets and Caplets
◆Feosol Capsules
◆Feosol Elixir
◆Feosol Tablets
◆Gaviscon Antacid Tablets
◆Gaviscon-2 Antacid Tablets
◆Gaviscon Extra Strength Relief Formula Antacid Tablets
◆Gaviscon Extra Strength Relief Formula Liquid Antacid
◆Gaviscon Liquid Antacid
Geritol Complete Tablets
Geritol Extend Caplets
Geritol Liquid - High Potency Iron & Vitamin Tonic
◆Gly-Oxide Liquid
◆Massengill Disposable Douches
Massengill Liquid Concentrate
◆Massengill Medicated Disposable Douche
Massengill Medicated Liquid Concentrate
Massengill Medicated Soft Cloth Towelette
Massengill Powder
Massengill Unscented Soft Cloth Towelette
◆Nature's Remedy Natural Vegetable Laxative Tablets
N'ICE Medicated Sugarless Sore Throat and Cough Lozenges
◆Novahistine DMX
◆Novahistine Elixir
◆Os-Cal 250+D Tablets
◆Os-Cal 500 Chewable Tablets
◆Os-Cal 500 Tablets
◆Os-Cal 500+D Tablets
◆Os-Cal Fortified Tablets
◆Os-Cal Plus Tablets
Oxy Medicated Cleanser
Oxy Medicated Pads - Regular, Sensitive Skin, and Maximum Strength
Oxy Medicated Soap
Oxy Night Watch Nighttime Acne Medication-Maximum Strength and Sensitive Skin Formulas
◆Oxy 10 Benzoyl Peroxide Wash
◆Oxy-5 and Oxy-10 Tinted and Vanishing Formulas with Sorboxyl
Simron Capsules
Simron Plus Capsules
◆Sine-Off Maximum Strength No Drowsiness Formula Caplets
◆Sine-Off Sinus Medicine Tablets-Aspirin Formula
Singlet Tablets
◆Sominex Caplets and Tablets
◆Sominex Pain Relief Formula
Sucrets Children's Cherry Flavored Sore Throat Lozenges
Sucrets Maximum Strength Wintergreen and Sucrets Wild Cherry (Regular Strength) Sore Throat Lozenges
◆Teldrin Timed-Release Allergy Capsules, 12 mg.
◆Throat Discs Throat Lozenges
◆Tums Antacid Tablets
◆Tums Anti-gas/Antacid Formula Tablets, Assorted Fruit
◆Tums E-X Antacid Tablets
Vivarin Stimulant Tablets

SMITHKLINE CONSUMER PRODUCTS

See SMITHKLINE BEECHAM CONSUMER BRANDS.

E. R. SQUIBB & SONS, INC.
A Bristol-Myers Squibb Company
P.O. Box 4000
Princeton, NJ 08543-4000

Theragran line is now being distributed by BRISTOL-MYERS PRODUCTS.

STANDARD HOMEOPATHIC COMPANY **735**
210 West 131st Street
Box 61067
Los Angeles, CA 90061

OTC Products Available
Hyland's Arnicaid Tablets
Hyland's Bed Wetting Tablets
Hyland's Calms Forté Tablets
Hyland's ClearAc Tablets
Hyland's Colic Tablets
Hyland's Cough Syrup with Honey
Hyland's C-Plus Cold Tablets
Hyland's Diarrex Tablets
Hyland's EnurAid Tablets
Hyland's Teething Tablets
Hyland's Vitamin C for Children

STELLAR PHARMACAL CORPORATION **428, 737**
1990 N.W. 44th Street
Pompano Beach, FL 33064-8712

Address inquiries to:
Scott L. Davidson (305) 972-6060
Customer Service & Order Department (800) 845-7827

OTC Products Available
◆Star-Optic Eye Wash
◆Star-Otic Ear Solution

STERLING HEALTH **428, 738**
Division of Sterling Winthrop Inc.
90 Park Avenue
New York, NY 10016
(212) 907-2000

Address medical inquiries to:
Product Information Services
(800) 446-6267

OTC Products Available
◆Bayer Children's Chewable Aspirin
◆Genuine Bayer Aspirin Tablets & Caplets
◆Maximum Bayer Aspirin Tablets & Caplets
◆Extended Release Bayer 8-Hour Aspirin
◆Bayer Plus Aspirin Tablets
◆Extra Strength Bayer Plus Aspirin Caplets
◆Adult Low Strength Bayer Enteric Aspirin Tablets
◆Regular Strength Bayer Enteric Aspirin Caplets
◆Bayer Select Headache Pain Relief Formula
◆Bayer Select Ibuprofen Pain Relief Formula
◆Bayer Select Menstrual Multi-Symptom Formula
◆Bayer Select Night Time Pain Relief Formula
◆Bayer Select Sinus Pain Relief Formula
◆Bronkaid Mist
Bronkaid Mist Suspension
◆Bronkaid Tablets
◆Campho-Phenique Cold Sore Gel
◆Campho-Phenique Liquid
◆Campho-Phenique Triple Antibiotic Ointment Plus Pain Reliever
◆Dairy Ease Caplets and Tablets
◆Dairy Ease Drops
◆Dairy Ease Real Milk
◆Fergon Iron Supplement Tablets
◆Haley's M-O, Regular & Flavored
◆Cramp Relief Formula Midol IB
◆Maximum Strength Multi-Symptom Menstrual Formula Midol
◆Night Time Formula Midol PM
◆PMS Multi-Symptom Formula Midol
◆Regular Strength Multi-Symptom Midol Formula
◆Teen Multi-Symptom Formula Midol
NTZ Long Acting Nasal Spray & Drops 0.05%
◆NāSal Moisturizer AF Nasal Spray
◆NāSal Moisturizer AF Nasal Drops
Neo-Synephrine Maximum Strength 12 Hour Nasal Spray
◆Neo-Synephrine Maximum Strength 12 Hour Nasal Spray Pump
◆Neo-Synephrine Nasal Drops, Pediatric, Mild, Regular & Extra Strength
◆Neo-Synephrine Nasal Sprays, Pediatric, Mild, Regular & Extra Strength
◆pHisoDerm Cleansing Bar
◆pHisoDerm For Baby
◆pHisoDerm Skin Cleanser and Conditioner - Regular, Lightly Scented and Unscented, and Oily Skin Unscented
◆pHisoPUFF
◆Children's Panadol Chewable Tablets, Liquid, Infant's Drops
◆Junior Strength Panadol
◆Maximum Strength Panadol Tablets and Caplets
◆Phillips' Chewable Tablets
◆Phillips' Gelcaps
◆Concentrated Phillips' Milk of Magnesia
◆Phillips' Milk of Magnesia Liquid
◆Stri-Dex Antibacterial Cleansing Bar
◆Stri-Dex Dual Textured Maximum Strength Pads
◆Stri-Dex Dual Textured Regular Strength Pads
Stri-Dex Dual Textured Sensitive Skin Pads
◆Stri-Dex Single Textured Maximum Strength Pads
◆Stri-Dex Super Scrub Pads-Oil Fighting Formula
◆Vanquish Analgesic Caplets
WinGel Liquid

SYNTEX LABORATORIES, INC. **757**
3401 Hillview Avenue
P.O. Box 10850
Palo Alto, CA 94304

Direct General/Sales/Order inquiries for U.S. Marketed products to:
Marketing Information Department
Specify product (415) 855-5050

Direct Medical inquiries on U.S. marketed products to:
Medical Services Department
General Medical Inquiries (415) 855-5545
Adverse Reactions Inquiries (415) 852-1386

OTC Products Available
Carmol 10 Lotion

THOMPSON MEDICAL COMPANY, INC. **431, 757**
222 Lakeview Avenue
West Palm Beach, FL 33401

Address inquiries to:
Consumer Services (800) 352-8466

OTC Products Available
Appedrine, Maximum Strength Tablets
Aqua-Ban, Maximum Strength Plus Tablets
Aqua-Ban Tablets
Arthritis Hot
Aspercreme Creme, Lotion Analgesic Rub
Breathe Free
Control Capsules
◆Cortizone for Kids

(◆ Shown in Product Identification Section)

◆Cortizone-5 Cream and Ointment
Cortizone-5 Wipes
◆Cortizone-10 Cream, Ointment and Liquid
Dexatrim Capsules, Caplets, Tablets
Dexatrim Maximum Strength Caffeine-Free Caplets
Dexatrim Maximum Strength Caffeine-Free Capsules
Dexatrim Maximum Strength Extended Duration Time Tablets
◆Dexatrim Maximum Strength Plus Vitamin C/Caffeine-free Caplets
◆Dexatrim Maximum Strength Plus Vitamin C/Caffeine-free Capsules
Diar Aid Tablets
Encare Vaginal Contraceptive Suppositories
End Lice
Ibuprin
Lactogest Softgel Capsules
NP-27 Cream, Solution, Spray Powder & Powder Antifungal
Prolamine Maximum Strength Capsules
Sleepinal Medicated Night Tea
◆Sleepinal Night-time Sleep Aid Capsules
Sportscreme External Analgesic Rub Cream and Lotion
◆Sportscreme External Analgesic Rub Ice
◆Tempo Soft Antacid with Antigas Action
Tribiotic Plus

TRITON CONSUMER PRODUCTS, INC. 760
561 West Golf Road
Arlington Heights, IL 60005
Address inquiries to:
Karen Shrader (800) 942-2009
For Medical Emergencies Contact
(800) 942-2009
OTC Products Available
MG 217 Medicated Tar Shampoo
MG 217 Medicated Tar-Free Shampoo
MG 217 Psoriasis Ointment and Lotion
ProTech First-Aid Stik
Retro G Medicated Cold Sore Gel
Skeeter Stik Insect Bite Medication
Skeeter Stop 100 Insect Repellent
Tick Away Insect Repellent

UAS LABORATORIES 760
9201 Penn Avenue South #10
Minneapolis, MN 55431
Address inquiries to:
Dr. S. K. Dash (612) 881-1915
(800) 422-3371
OTC Products Available
DDS-Acidophilus

THE UPJOHN COMPANY 432, 761
7000 Portage Road
Kalamazoo, MI 49001
For Medical and Pharmaceutical Information, Including Emergencies:
(616) 329-8244
(616) 323-6615
Pharmaceutical Sales Areas and Distribution Centers
Atlanta (Chamblee)
GA 30341-2626 (404) 451-4822
Boston (Wellesley)
MA 02181 (617) 431-7970
Buffalo (Amherst)
NY 14221 (716) 632-5942
Chicago (Oak Brook Terrace)
IL 60181 (708) 574-3300
Cincinnati, OH 45202
(513) 723-1010
Dallas (Irving)
TX 75062 (214) 256-0022
Denver, CO 80216 (303) 399-3113
Hartford (Enfield)
CT 06082 (203) 741-3421
Honolulu, HI 96818 (808) 422-2777
Kalamazoo, MI 49001
(616) 323-4000
Kansas City (Overland Park)
KS 66210 (913) 469-8863
Memphis, TN 38119 (901) 685-8192
New York (Uniondale)
NY 11553 (516) 745-6100
Orlando, FL 32809 (407) 859-4591
Philadelphia (Berwyn)
PA 19312 (215) 993-0100
Pittsburgh (Bridgeville)
PA 15017 (412) 257-0200
Portland, OR 97232 (503) 232-2133
St. Louis, MO 63141 (314) 872-8626
San Francisco (Foster City)
CA 94404 (415) 377-0203
Shreveport, LA 71129
(318) 688-3700
Simi Valley, CA 93065
(213) 463-8101
Washington, DC 20011
(202) 726-1517
OTC Products Available
◆Cortaid Cream with Aloe
◆Cortaid Lotion
◆Cortaid Ointment with Aloe
◆Cortaid Spray
◆Maximum Strength Cortaid Cream
◆Maximum Strength Cortaid Ointment
◆Maximum Strength Cortaid Spray
Cortef Feminine Itch Cream
◆Doxidan Liqui-Gels
◆Dramamine Chewable Tablets
◆Children's Dramamine
◆Dramamine Tablets
◆Dramamine II Tablets
◆Kaopectate Concentrated Anti-Diarrheal, Peppermint Flavor
◆Kaopectate Concentrated Anti-Diarrheal, Regular Flavor
◆Kaopectate Children's Chewable Tablets
◆Kaopectate Children's Liquid
◆Kaopectate Maximum Strength Caplets
◆Motrin IB Caplets and Tablets
◆Mycitracin Plus Pain Reliever
◆Maximum Strength Mycitracin Triple Antibiotic First Aid Ointment
Phenolax Wafers
Progaine Shampoo
◆Surfak Liqui-Gels
◆Unicap Softgel Capsules & Tablets
Unicap Jr. Chewable Tablets
◆Unicap M Tablets
Unicap Plus Iron Vitamin Formula Tablets
◆Unicap Sr. Tablets
◆Unicap T Tablets

VISION PHARMACEUTICALS, INC. 766
1022 North Main Street
Mitchell, SD 57301
Address inquiries to:
Jane Schoenfelder
(800) 325-6789
(605) 996-7072
OTC Products Available
Anti-Oxidant Skin Treatment Products
Vit-A-Clenz Liquid Cleanser
Vit-A-Clenz Lotion Cleanser
Vit-A-Silk Lotion Moisturizer
Vit-A-Spritz Skin Enhancer
Viva-Drops

WAKUNAGA OF AMERICA CO., LTD. 432, 766
Subsidiary of Wakunaga Pharmaceutical Co., Ltd.
23501 Madero
Mission Viejo, CA 92691
Address inquires to:
(714) 855-2776
OTC Products Available
◆Kyolic
Kyo-Dophilus, Capsules: Acidophilus, Bifidus, S. Faecium
Kyo-Green, Powder: Barley & Wheat Grass, Chlorella, Brown Rice, Kelp
Kyolic Formula 106 Capsules: Aged Garlic Extract Powder (300 mg) & Vitamin E
Kyolic Super Formula 104 Capsules: Aged Garlic Extract Powder (300 mg)
Kyolic Super Formula 105 Capsules: Aged Garlic Extract Powder (200 mg)
Kyolic Super Formula 100 Capsules & Tablets: Aged Garlic Extract Powder (300 mg)
Kyolic Super Formula 100 Tablets: Aged Garlic Extract Powder (270 mg)
◆ Kyolic-Aged Garlic Extract Flavor & Odor Modified Enriched with Vitamins B_1 and B_{12}
Kyolic-Aged Garlic Extract Flavor & Odor Modified Plain
Kyolic-Aged Garlic Extract Liquid Enriched with Vitamin B & Vitamin B_{12}
Kyolic-Aged Garlic Extract Liquid Plain
◆ Kyolic-Formula 101 Capsules: Aged Garlic Extract (270 mg)
Kyolic-Formula 103 Capsules: Aged Garlic Extract Powder (220 mg)
Kyolic-Formula 101 Tablets: Aged Garlic Extract Powder (270 mg)
Kyolic-Super Formula 104, Aged Garlic Extract Powder (300 mg) with Lecithin
Kyolic-Super Formula 103, Capsules: Aged Garlic Extract Powder (220 mg) with Vitamin C, Astragalus, Calcium
Kyolic-Super Formula 105, Capsules: Aged Garlic Extract Powder (250 mg) with Selenium, Vitamins A & E
Kyolic-Super Formula 106, Capsules: Aged Garlic Extract Powder (300 mg) with Vitamin E, Cayenne Pepper, Hawthorn Berry
◆ Kyolic-Super Formula 101 Garlic Plus Tablets & Capsules: Aged Garlic Extract Powder (270 mg) with Brewer's Yeast, Kelp & Algin
Kyolic-Super Formula 102, Tablets & Capsules: Aged Garlic Extract Powder (350 mg) with Enzyme Complex

WALKER PHARMACAL COMPANY 766
4200 Laclede
St. Louis, MO 63108
Address Inquiries to:
Customer Service (314) 533-9600
OTC Products Available
HIKE Antiseptic Ointment
PRID Salve

WALLACE LABORATORIES 432, 766
Half Acre Road
Cranbury, NJ 08512
Address inquiries to:
Wallace Laboratories
Div. of Carter-Wallace, Inc.
P.O. Box 1001
Cranbury, NJ 08512 (609) 655-6000
For Medical Emergencies:
(800) 526-3840
OTC Products Available
◆Maltsupex Liquid, Powder & Tablets
◆Ryna Liquid
◆Ryna-C Liquid
◆Ryna-CX Liquid
◆Syllact Powder

WARNER-LAMBERT COMPANY 433, 769
Consumer Health Products Group
201 Tabor Road
Morris Plains, NJ 07950
Address Inquiries to:
Robert Kohler (201) 540-6705
For Medical Emergencies Call:
(201) 540-2000
OTC Products Available
Bromo-Seltzer
Corn Husker's Lotion
Professional Strength Efferdent
◆Halls Mentho-Lyptus Cough Suppressant Tablets
◆Halls Plus Cough Suppressant Tablets
◆Halls Vitamin C Drops
Listerex Lotion
◆Listerine Antiseptic
◆Cool Mint Listerine Antiseptic
◆Listermint with Fluoride

(◆ Shown in Product Identification Section)

Lubriderm Bath Oil
Lubriderm Body Bar
◆Lubriderm Lotion
◆Rolaids Antacid Tablets
◆Rolaids (Calcium Rich/Sodium Free) Antacid Tablets
◆Extra Strength Rolaids Antacid Plus Anti-Gas Tablets
◆Soothers Throat Drops
Super Anahist Tablets

WATER-JEL TECHNOLOGIES, INC. 772
243 Veterans Boulevard
Carlstadt, NJ 07072
Address inquiries to:
Bob Daniels (201) 507-8300
FAX (201) 507-8325
For Medical Emergencies Contact:
Bob Daniels (201) 507-8300
FAX (201) 507-8325
OTC Products Available
Water-Jel Burn Jel
Water-Jel Burn Wrap
Water-Jel Face Mask for Facial Burns
Water-Jel Fire Blanket Plus
Water-Jel Heat Shield
Water-Jel Sterile Burn Dressings

WELLNESS INTERNATIONAL, INC. 772
1501 Luna, Suite 102
Carrollton, TX 75006
Address inquiries to:
Dr. Clifton Jolly, PhD
(619) 471-0166
FAX (619) 471-2513
For Medical Emergency Contact:
Steven E. Langer, MD
(619) 471-0166
FAX (619) 471-2513
OTC Products Available
Flora-Plus Capsules
Nutra-Lean Shake
Tri-Lean Additive Drink

WHITEHALL LABORATORIES INC. 433, 774, 794
Division of American Home Products Corporation
685 Third Avenue
New York, NY 10017
Address inquiries to:
Consumer Affairs
Professional Samples
(800) 343-0856
Other information
(800) 322-3129
OTC Products Available
◆Advil Cold and Sinus (formerly CoAdvil)
◆Advil Ibuprofen Caplets and Tablets
Anacin Caplets and Tablets (See A.H. Robins Consumer)
Maximum Strength Anacin (See A.H. Robins Consumer)
Aspirin Free Anacin, Maximum Strength (See A.H. Robins Consumer)
◆Baby Anbesol
◆Grape Baby Anbesol
◆Anbesol Gel - Regular Strength
◆Anbesol Gel - Maximum Strength
◆Anbesol Liquid - Regular Strength
◆Anbesol Liquid - Maximum Strength
Arthritis Pain Formula, Maximum Strength Analgesic Caplets (See 1993 Physicians' Desk Reference)
Bronitin Mist and Tablets
◆Clearblue Easy
◆Clearplan Easy
Compound W Gel (See 1993 Physicians' Desk Reference)
Compound W Liquid (See 1993 Physicians' Desk Reference)
◆Denorex Medicated Shampoo and Conditioner
◆Denorex Medicated Shampoo, Extra Strength
◆Denorex Medicated Shampoo, Extra Strength With Conditioners
◆Denorex Medicated Shampoo, Regular & Mountain Fresh Herbal Scent
Dermoplast Lotion (See 1993 Physicians' Desk Reference)
Dermoplast Spray (See 1993 Physicians' Desk Reference)
◆Dristan Allergy
◆Dristan Cold
Dristan Inhaler
◆Dristan Juice Mix-In
◆Dristan Cold, Maximum Strength Multi-symptom Formula
◆Dristan Cold, Maximum Strength No Drowsiness Formula
Dristan Nasal Spray, Regular
Dristan Nasal Spray, Menthol
◆Dristan Saline Spray
◆Dristan Sinus
Dristan 12-hour Nasal Spray
Freezone Solution
Heet Liniment and Spray
InfraRub Analgesic Cream
Kerodex Cream 51 (for dry or oily work)
Kerodex Cream 71 (for wet work)
Momentum Backache Formula
Outgro Solution
Oxipor VHC Psoriasis Lotion
Posture 600 mg (See 1993 Physicians' Desk Reference)
Posture-D 600 mg (See 1993 Physicians' Desk Reference)
◆Preparation H Cleansing Tissues
◆Preparation H Hemorrhoidal Cream
◆Preparation H Hemorrhoidal Ointment
◆Preparation H Hemorrhoidal Suppositories
◆Preparation H Hydrocortisone 1% Cream
◆Primatene Mist
Primatene Mist Suspension
◆Primatene Tablets
Riopan Suspension
Riopan Plus Suspension
◆Riopan Plus 2 Suspension
Semicid (See 1993 Physicians' Desk Reference for picture)
Sleep-eze 3 Tablets
Today Personal Lubricant
◆Today Sponge
Viro-Med Tablets

WINTHROP CONSUMER PRODUCTS
Division of Sterling Winthrop Inc.
90 Park Avenue
New York, NY 10016
See STERLING HEALTH, page 738.

WINTHROP PHARMACEUTICALS
90 Park Avenue
New York, NY 10016
See SANOFI WINTHROP PHARMACEUTICALS, page 696.

WYETH-AYERST LABORATORIES 435, 784
Division of American Home Products Corporation
P.O. Box 8299
Philadelphia, PA 19101
Address inquiries to:
Professional Service (215) 688-4400
For EMERGENCY Medical Information
Day or night call (215) 688-4400

WYETH-AYERST DISTRIBUTION CENTERS

Atlanta, GA—P.O. Box 1773
Paoli, PA 19301-1773
(800) 666-7248
Freight address:
221 Armour Drive NE
Atlanta, GA 30324
Mail DEA order forms to:
P.O. Box 4365
Atlanta, GA 30302

Boston MA—P.O. Box 1773
Paoli, PA 19301-1773
(800) 666-7248
Freight address:
7 Connector Road
Andover, MA 01810
Mail DEA order forms to:
P.O. Box 1776
Andover, MA 01810

Chamblee, GA—P.O. Box 1773
Paoli, PA 19301-1773
(800) 666-7248
Freight address:
3600 American Drive
Chamblee, GA 30341

Chicago, IL—P.O. Box 1773
Paoli, PA 19301-1773
(800) 666-7248
Freight address:
745 N. Gary Avenue
Carol Stream, IL 60188
Mail DEA order forms to:
P.O. Box 140
Wheaton, IL 60189-0140

Dallas, TX—P.O. Box 1773
Paoli, PA 19301-1773
(800) 666-7248
Freight address:
11240 Petal Street
Dallas, TX 75238
Mail DEA order forms to:
P.O. Box 650231
Dallas, TX 75265-0231

Foster City, CA—P.O. Box 1773
Paoli, PA 19301-1773
(800) 666-7248
Freight address:
1147 Chess Drive
Foster City, CA 94404

Hawaii—P.O. Box 1773
Paoli, PA 19301-1773
(800) 666-7248
Mail DEA order forms to:
96-1185 Waihona, Street, Unit C1
Pearl City, HI 96782

Kansas City, MO—P.O. Box 1773
Paoli, PA 19301-1773
(800) 666-7248
Freight address:
1340 Taney Street
North Kansas City, MO 64116
Mail DEA order forms to:
P.O. Box 7588
North Kansas City, MO 64116

Los Angeles, CA—P.O. Box 1773
Paoli, PA 19301-1773
(800) 666-7248
Freight address:
6530 Altura Blvd.
Buena Park, CA 90622
Mail DEA order forms to:
P.O. Box 5000
Buena Park, CA 90622-5000

Philadelphia, PA—P.O. Box 1773
Paoli, PA 19301-1773
(800) 666-7248
Freight address:
31 Morehall Road
Frazer, PA 19355

(◆ Shown in Product Identification Section)

Mail DEA order forms to:
P.O. Box 61
Paoli, PA 19301

Seattle, WA—P.O. Box 1773
Paoli, PA 19301-1773
(800) 666-7248

Freight address:
19255 80th Ave. South
Kent, WA 98032

Mail DEA order forms to:
P.O. Box 5609
Kent, WA 98064-5609

South Plainfield, NJ—P.O. Box 1773
Paoli, PA 19301-1773
(800) 666-7248

Freight address:
4000 Hadley Road
South Plainfield, NJ 07080

OTC Products Available

◆Aludrox Oral Suspension
◆Amphojel Suspension (Mint Flavor)
◆Amphojel Suspension without Flavor
◆Amphojel Tablets
◆Basaljel Capsules
◆Basaljel Suspension
◆Basaljel Tablets
◆Cerose-DM
◆Collyrium for Fresh Eyes
◆Collyrium Fresh
◆Donnagel Liquid and Donnagel Chewable Tablets
◆Nursoy, Soy Protein Isolate Formula for Infants, Concentrated Liquid, Ready-to-Feed, and Powder
◆SMA Iron Fortified Infant Formula, Concentrated, Ready-to-Feed and Powder
◆SMA lo-iron Infant Formula, Concentrated, Ready-to-Feed, and Powder
◆Stuart Prenatal Tablets
◆Wyanoids Relief Factor Hemorrhoidal Suppositories

ZILA PHARMACEUTICALS, INC. **435, 789**
5227 North 7th Street
Phoenix, AZ 85014-2817

Address inquiries to:
Ed Pomerantz,
Vice President, Marketing
(602) 266-6700

OTC Products Available

◆DermaFlex Topical Anesthetic Gel Coating
PeriGel Oral Care System
◆Zilactin Medicated Gel
◆Zilactin-L Liquid

MEDICAL ECONOMICS DATA

SECTION 2

Product Name Index

In this section only described products are listed in alphabetical sequence by brand name or generic name. They have page numbers to assist you in locating the descriptions. For additional information on other products, you may wish to contact the manufacturer directly. The symbol ◆ indicates the product is shown in the Product Identification Section.

A

B

C

D

(◆ Shown in Product Identification Section)

E

F

G

H

I

K

L

M

(◆ Shown in Product Identification Section)

N

O

(◆ Shown in Product Identification Section)

T

(◆ Shown in Product Identification Section)

U

V

W

X

Z

(◆ Shown in Product Identification Section)

MEDICAL ECONOMICS DATA

SECTION 3

Product Category Index

Products described in the Product Information (White) Section are listed according to their classifications. The headings and sub-headings have been determined by the OTC Review process of the U.S. Food and Drug Administration. Classification of products have been determined by the Publisher with the cooperation of individual manufacturers. In cases where there were differences of opinion or where the manufacturer had no opinion, the Publisher made the final decision.

A

ANTI-INFLAMMATORY AGENTS

NON-STEROIDALS

SALICYLATES

OTHER

ANTIOXIDANTS

ANTIPARASITICS

ARTHROPODS

LICE

HELMINTHS

ENTEROBIUS (PINWORM)

ANTIPERSPIRANTS
(see DEODORANTS & DERMATOLOGICALS, ANTIPERSPIRANTS)

ANTIPYRETICS

ANTISEPTICS

ANTITUSSIVES
(see COLD & COUGH PREPARATIONS)

ANTIVIRALS, SYSTEMIC

APPETITE SUPPRESSANTS

ANTITUSSIVES & COMBINATIONS

TOPICAL

EXPECTORANTS & COMBINATIONS

Desitin Ointment (Pfizer Consumer) p 419, 638
Mycitracin Plus Pain Reliever (Upjohn) p 432, 763
Neosporin Ointment (Burroughs Wellcome) p 406, 538
Neosporin Plus Maximum Strength Cream (Burroughs Wellcome) p 406, 539
Neosporin Plus Maximum Strength Ointment (Burroughs Wellcome) p 407, 539
Nupercainal Pain Relief Cream (CIBA Consumer) p 408, 554
Polysporin Ointment (Burroughs Wellcome) p 407, 539
Polysporin Powder (Burroughs Wellcome) p 407, 540
Water-Jel Burn Jel (Water-Jel Technologies) p 772
Water-Jel Sterile Burn Dressings (Water-Jel Technologies) p 772

CLEANSING AGENTS
Almay Eyelid Cleansing Pads (Almay) p 503
Aqua Glyde Cleanser (Herald Pharmacal) p 568
Aveeno Bath Oilated (Rydelle) p 422, 687
Aveeno Bath Regular (Rydelle) p 422, 687
Aveeno Cleansing Bar for Acne-Prone Skin (Rydelle) p 422, 687
Aveeno Cleansing Bar for Combination Skin (Rydelle) p 422, 687
Aveeno Cleansing Bar for Dry Skin (Rydelle) p 422, 687
Aveeno Shower and Bath Oil (Rydelle) p 422, 687
Cam Lotion (Herald Pharmacal) p 568
Concept (Care-Tech) p 544
Dove Bar (Lever Brothers) p 411, 582
Liquid Dove Beauty Wash (Lever Brothers) p 411, 582
Eucerin Cleansing Lotion Dry Skin Care (Beiersdorf) p 404, 511
Eucerin Dry Skin Care Cleansing Bar (Beiersdorf) p 404, 511
Lubriderm Bath Oil (Warner-Lambert) p 770
Massengill Unscented Soft Cloth Towelette (SmithKline Beecham Consumer) p 725
Neutrogena Cleansing Wash (Neutrogena) p 416, 620
Orchid Fresh II Perineal/Ostomy Cleanser (Care-Tech) p 544
Oxy Medicated Cleanser (SmithKline Beecham Consumer) p 729
Oxy Medicated Pads - Regular, Sensitive Skin, and Maximum Strength (SmithKline Beecham Consumer) p 730
Oxy Medicated Soap (SmithKline Beecham Consumer) p 729
Oxy Night Watch Nighttime Acne Medication-Maximum Strength and Sensitive Skin Formulas (SmithKline Beecham Consumer) p 730
Oxy 10 Benzoyl Peroxide Wash (SmithKline Beecham Consumer) p 428, 730
pHisoDerm Cleansing Bar (Sterling Health) p 431, 755
pHisoDerm For Baby (Sterling Health) p 431, 755
pHisoDerm Skin Cleanser and Conditioner - Regular, Lightly Scented and Unscented, and Oily Skin Unscented (Sterling Health) p 431, 754
Satin Antimicrobial Skin Cleanser (Care-Tech) p 545
Stri-Dex Antibacterial Cleansing Bar (Sterling Health) p 431, 756
Techni-Care Surgical Scrub (Care-Tech) p 545

COAL TAR
Denorex Medicated Shampoo and Conditioner (Whitehall) p 434, 776
Denorex Medicated Shampoo, Extra Strength (Whitehall) p 434, 776
Denorex Medicated Shampoo, Extra Strength With Conditioners (Whitehall) p 434, 776
Denorex Medicated Shampoo, Regular & Mountain Fresh Herbal Scent (Whitehall) p 434, 776
MG 217 Medicated Tar Shampoo (Triton Consumer) p 760
MG 217 Psoriasis Ointment and Lotion (Triton Consumer) p 760
Neutrogena T/Derm Tar Emollient (Neutrogena) p 622
Neutrogena T/Gel Therapeutic Shampoo (Neutrogena) p 416, 622
P & S Plus Tar Gel (Baker Cummins Dermatologicals) p 508
Tegrin Dandruff Shampoo (Block) p 515
Tegrin for Psoriasis Lotion, Skin Cream & Medicated Soap (Block) p 515
X-Seb T Shampoo (Baker Cummins Dermatologicals) p 403, 509
X-Seb T Plus Conditioning Shampoo (Baker Cummins Dermatologicals) p 403, 510

CONDITIONING RINSES
Denorex Medicated Shampoo and Conditioner (Whitehall) p 434, 776
Denorex Medicated Shampoo, Extra Strength With Conditioners (Whitehall) p 434, 776

CONTACT DERMATITIS
Care Creme (Care-Tech) p 544
Maximum Strength Cortaid Cream (Upjohn) p 432, 761
Maximum Strength Cortaid Ointment (Upjohn) p 432, 761
Maximum Strength Cortaid Spray (Upjohn) p 432, 761
Satin Antimicrobial Skin Cleanser (Care-Tech) p 545

DANDRUFF MEDICATIONS
Almay Therapeutic Shampoo (Almay) p 504
Denorex Medicated Shampoo and Conditioner (Whitehall) p 434, 776
Denorex Medicated Shampoo, Extra Strength (Whitehall) p 434, 776
Denorex Medicated Shampoo, Extra Strength With Conditioners (Whitehall) p 434, 776
Denorex Medicated Shampoo, Regular & Mountain Fresh Herbal Scent (Whitehall) p 434, 776
Head & Shoulders Antidandruff Shampoo (Procter & Gamble) p 644
Head & Shoulders Antidandruff Shampoo 2-in-1 plus Conditioner (Procter & Gamble) p 644
Head & Shoulders Dry Scalp Shampoo (Procter & Gamble) p 644
Head & Shoulders Dry Scalp Shampoo 2-in-1 plus Conditioner (Procter & Gamble) p 644
Head & Shoulders Intensive Treatment Dandruff Shampoo (Procter & Gamble) p 645
Head & Shoulders Intensive Treatment Dandruff Shampoo 2-in-1 plus Conditioner (Procter & Gamble) p 645
MG 217 Medicated Tar Shampoo (Triton Consumer) p 760
MG 217 Medicated Tar-Free Shampoo (Triton Consumer) p 760
P & S Plus Tar Gel (Baker Cummins Dermatologicals) p 508
P & S Shampoo (Baker Cummins Dermatologicals) p 403, 509
Selsun Blue Dandruff Shampoo (Ross) p 421, 685
Selsun Blue Dandruff Shampoo Medicated Treatment Formula (Ross) p 421, 685
Selsun Blue Extra Conditioning Formula Dandruff Shampoo (Ross) p 421, 685
Selsun Gold for Women Dandruff Shampoo (Ross) p 422, 686
Tegrin Dandruff Shampoo (Block) p 515
X-Seb Shampoo (Baker Cummins Dermatologicals) p 403, 509
X-Seb Plus Conditioning Shampoo (Baker Cummins Dermatologicals) p 403, 509
X-Seb T Shampoo (Baker Cummins Dermatologicals) p 403, 509
X-Seb T Plus Conditioning Shampoo (Baker Cummins Dermatologicals) p 403, 510
Zincon Dandruff Shampoo (Lederle) p 411, 582

DEODORANTS
Desenex Foot & Sneaker Deodorant Powder Plus (Fisons Consumer Health) p 564
Desenex Foot & Sneaker Deodorant Spray Powder (Fisons Consumer Health) p 409, 564

DERMATITIS RELIEF
A and D Ointment (Schering-Plough HealthCare) p 423, 699
Acid Mantle Creme (Sandoz Consumer) p 688
Alpha Keri Moisture Rich Body Oil (Bristol-Myers Products) p 405, 517
Aqua Care Cream (Menley & James) p 414, 602
Aqua Care Lotion (Menley & James) p 415, 602
Aveeno Bath Oilated (Rydelle) p 422, 687
Aveeno Bath Regular (Rydelle) p 422, 687
Aveeno Moisturizing Cream (Rydelle) p 422, 687
Aveeno Moisturizing Lotion (Rydelle) p 422, 687
Aveeno Shower and Bath Oil (Rydelle) p 422, 687
Bactine Hydrocortisone Anti-Itch Cream (Miles Consumer) p 415, 614
Balmex Baby Powder (Macsil) p 582
Balmex Emollient Lotion (Macsil) p 582
Balmex Ointment (Macsil) p 582
BiCozene Creme (Sandoz Consumer) p 422, 688
Caladryl Clear Lotion (Parke-Davis) p 418, 633
Caladryl Cream, Lotion, Spray (Parke-Davis) p 418, 633
Caldecort Anti-Itch Hydrocortisone Cream (Fisons Consumer Health) p 409, 563
Caldecort Anti-Itch Hydrocortisone Spray (Fisons Consumer Health) p 563
Caldecort Light Cream (Fisons Consumer Health) p 409, 563
Caldesene Medicated Ointment (Fisons Consumer Health) p 409, 563
Caldesene Medicated Powder (Fisons Consumer Health) p 409, 563
Cam Lotion (Herald Pharmacal) p 568
Clocream Skin Protectant Cream (Roberts) p 668
Concept (Care-Tech) p 544
Cortaid Cream with Aloe (Upjohn) p 432, 761
Cortaid Lotion (Upjohn) p 432, 761
Cortaid Ointment with Aloe (Upjohn) p 432, 761
Cortaid Spray (Upjohn) p 432, 761
Maximum Strength Cortaid Cream (Upjohn) p 432, 761
Maximum Strength Cortaid Ointment (Upjohn) p 432, 761
Maximum Strength Cortaid Spray (Upjohn) p 432, 761
Cortizone for Kids (Thompson Medical) p 431, 757
Cortizone-5 Cream and Ointment (Thompson Medical) p 431, 757
Cortizone-5 Wipes (Thompson Medical) p 757
Cortizone-10 Cream, Ointment and Liquid (Thompson Medical) p 431, 758
Desitin Ointment (Pfizer Consumer) p 419, 638

Domeboro Astringent Solution Effervescent Tablets (Miles Consumer) p 415, 616
Domeboro Astringent Solution Powder Packets (Miles Consumer) p 415, 616
Eucerin Dry Skin Care Daily Facial Lotion SPF 20 (Beiersdorf) p 404, 511
Massengill Medicated Soft Cloth Towelette (SmithKline Beecham Consumer) p 725
P & S Liquid (Baker Cummins Dermatologicals) p 403, 508
P & S Plus Tar Gel (Baker Cummins Dermatologicals) p 508
P & S Shampoo (Baker Cummins Dermatologicals) p 403, 509
Satin Antimicrobial Skin Cleanser (Care-Tech) p 545
Tegrin-HC with Hydrocortisone Anti-Itch Ointment (Block) p 516
X-Seb Plus Conditioning Shampoo (Baker Cummins Dermatologicals) p 403, 509
X-Seb T Shampoo (Baker Cummins Dermatologicals) p 403, 509
X-Seb T Plus Conditioning Shampoo (Baker Cummins Dermatologicals) p 403, 510

DETERGENTS

pHisoDerm For Baby (Sterling Health) p 431, 755
pHisoDerm Skin Cleanser and Conditioner - Regular, Lightly Scented and Unscented, and Oily Skin Unscented (Sterling Health) p 431, 754
Selsun Blue Dandruff Shampoo (Ross) p 421, 685
Selsun Blue Dandruff Shampoo Medicated Treatment Formula (Ross) p 421, 685
Selsun Blue Extra Conditioning Formula Dandruff Shampoo (Ross) p 421, 685
Selsun Gold for Women Dandruff Shampoo (Ross) p 422, 686
X-Seb Shampoo (Baker Cummins Dermatologicals) p 403, 509
X-Seb Plus Conditioning Shampoo (Baker Cummins Dermatologicals) p 403, 509
X-Seb T Shampoo (Baker Cummins Dermatologicals) p 403, 509
X-Seb T Plus Conditioning Shampoo (Baker Cummins Dermatologicals) p 403, 510
Zincon Dandruff Shampoo (Lederle) p 411, 582

DIAPER RASH RELIEF

Caldesene Medicated Ointment (Fisons Consumer Health) p 409, 563
Caldesene Medicated Powder (Fisons Consumer Health) p 409, 563
Clocream Skin Protectant Cream (Roberts) p 668
Vaseline Pure Petroleum Jelly Skin Protectant (Chesebrough-Pond's) p 548

EMOLLIENTS

A and D Ointment (Schering-Plough HealthCare) p 423, 699
Almay Therapeutic Body Treatment (Almay) p 504
Almay Therapeutic Face Lotion (Almay) p 504
Alpha Keri Moisture Rich Body Oil (Bristol-Myers Products) p 405, 517
Alpha Keri Moisture Rich Cleansing Bar (Bristol-Myers Products) p 517
Aqua Care Cream (Menley & James) p 414, 602
Aqua Care Lotion (Menley & James) p 415, 602
Aqua-A Cream (Baker Cummins Dermatologicals) p 508
Aquaderm Cream (Baker Cummins Dermatologicals) p 403, 508
Aquaderm Lotion (Baker Cummins Dermatologicals) p 403, 508
Aquaderm Sunscreen Moisturizer (SPF 15 Formula) (Baker Cummins Dermatologicals) p 508
Aquaphor Healing Ointment (Beiersdorf) p 403, 511
Aquaphor Healing Ointment, Original Formula (Beiersdorf) p 403, 510
Aveeno Bath Oilated (Rydelle) p 422, 687
Aveeno Bath Regular (Rydelle) p 422, 687
Aveeno Moisturizing Cream (Rydelle) p 422, 687
Aveeno Moisturizing Lotion (Rydelle) p 422, 687
Aveeno Shower and Bath Oil (Rydelle) p 422, 687
Balmex Baby Powder (Macsil) p 582
Balmex Emollient Lotion (Macsil) p 582
Balmex Ointment (Macsil) p 582
Borofax Ointment (Burroughs Wellcome) p 538
Care Creme (Care-Tech) p 544
Carmol 10 Lotion (Syntex) p 757
Chap Stick Lip Balm (Robins Consumer) p 420, 673
Chap Stick Medicated Lip Balm (Robins Consumer) p 420, 673
Chap Stick Sunblock 15 Lip Balm (Robins Consumer) p 420, 674
Chap Stick Petroleum Jelly Plus (Robins Consumer) p 420, 674
Chap Stick Petroleum Jelly Plus with Sunblock 15 (Robins Consumer) p 420, 674
Clocream Skin Protectant Cream (Roberts) p 668
Complex 15 Hand & Body Moisturizing Cream (Schering-Plough HealthCare) p 424, 702
Complex 15 Hand & Body Moisturizing Lotion (Schering-Plough HealthCare) p 424, 703
Complex 15 Moisturizing Face Cream (Schering-Plough HealthCare) p 424, 703
Concept (Care-Tech) p 544
Desitin Ointment (Pfizer Consumer) p 419, 638
Eucerin Dry Skin Care Creme (Beiersdorf) p 404, 511
Eucerin Dry Skin Care Daily Facial Lotion SPF 20 (Beiersdorf) p 404, 511
Eucerin Dry Skin Care Lotion (Fragrance-free) (Beiersdorf) p 404, 511
Herpecin-L Cold Sore Lip Balm (Campbell) p 543
Keri Lotion - Original Formula (Bristol-Myers Products) p 405, 530
Keri Lotion -Silky Smooth with Vitamin E (Bristol-Myers Products) p 405, 530
Keri Lotion - Silky Smooth Fragrance Free with Vitamin E (Bristol-Myers Products) p 405, 530
Lubriderm Bath Oil (Warner-Lambert) p 770
Lubriderm Lotion (Warner-Lambert) p 433, 770
Neutrogena Norwegian Formula Emulsion (Neutrogena) p 416, 621
Neutrogena Norwegian Formula Hand Cream (Neutrogena) p 416, 621
Oil of Olay Daily UV Protectant SPF 15 Beauty Fluid-Original and Fragrance Free (Olay Co. Inc.) (Procter & Gamble) p 647
Oil of Olay Daily UV Protectant SPF 15 Moisture Replenishing Cream-Original and Fragrance Free (Olay Co. Inc.) (Procter & Gamble) p 647
pHisoDerm Cleansing Bar (Sterling Health) p 431, 755
pHisoDerm For Baby (Sterling Health) p 431, 755
pHisoDerm Skin Cleanser and Conditioner - Regular, Lightly Scented and Unscented, and Oily Skin Unscented (Sterling Health) p 431, 754
Pen•Kera Creme (Ascher) p 403, 506
Satin Antimicrobial Skin Cleanser (Care-Tech) p 545
Ultra Mide 25 (Baker Cummins Dermatologicals) p 403, 509
Vaseline Intensive Care Lotion Extra Strength (Chesebrough-Pond's) p 549
Vaseline Pure Petroleum Jelly Skin Protectant (Chesebrough-Pond's) p 548

FOOT CARE

Desenex Foot & Sneaker Deodorant Powder Plus (Fisons Consumer Health) p 564
Desenex Foot & Sneaker Deodorant Spray Powder (Fisons Consumer Health) p 409, 564
Formula Magic Antibacterial Powder (Care-Tech) p 544
Lotrimin AF Antifungal Cream, Lotion and Solution (Schering-Plough HealthCare) p 425, 708

FUNGICIDES

Cruex Antifungal Cream (Fisons Consumer Health) p 409, 563
Cruex Antifungal Powder (Fisons Consumer Health) p 563
Cruex Antifungal Spray Powder (Fisons Consumer Health) p 409, 563
Desenex Antifungal Cream (Fisons Consumer Health) p 564
Desenex Antifungal Foam (Fisons Consumer Health) p 564
Desenex Antifungal Ointment (Fisons Consumer Health) p 409, 564
Desenex Antifungal Powder (Fisons Consumer Health) p 409, 564
Desenex Antifungal Spray Liquid (Fisons Consumer Health) p 564
Desenex Antifungal Spray Powder (Fisons Consumer Health) p 409, 564
Impregon Concentrate (Fleming) p 566
Lotrimin AF Antifungal Cream, Lotion and Solution (Schering-Plough HealthCare) p 425, 708
Massengill Medicated Disposable Douche (SmithKline Beecham Consumer) p 427, 725
Massengill Medicated Liquid Concentrate (SmithKline Beecham Consumer) p 725
Micatin Antifungal Cream (Ortho Pharmaceutical) p 417, 626
Micatin Antifungal Odor Control Spray Powder (Ortho Pharmaceutical) p 417, 626
Micatin Antifungal Powder (Ortho Pharmaceutical) p 417, 626
Micatin Antifungal Spray Liquid (Ortho Pharmaceutical) p 417, 626
Micatin Antifungal Spray Powder (Ortho Pharmaceutical) p 417, 626
Micatin Jock Itch Cream (Ortho Pharmaceutical) p 626
Micatin Jock Itch Spray Powder (Ortho Pharmaceutical) p 626
Mycelex OTC Cream Antifungal (Miles Consumer) p 416, 617
Mycelex OTC Solution Antifungal (Miles Consumer) p 416, 617
Tinactin Aerosol Liquid 1% (Schering-Plough HealthCare) p 426, 711
Tinactin Aerosol Powder 1% (Schering-Plough HealthCare) p 425, 711
Tinactin Antifungal Cream, Solution & Powder 1% (Schering-Plough HealthCare) p 425, 711
Tinactin Deodorant Powder Aerosol 1% (Schering-Plough HealthCare) p 711
Tinactin Jock Itch Cream 1% (Schering-Plough HealthCare) p 425, 711
Tinactin Jock Itch Spray Powder 1% (Schering-Plough HealthCare) p 425, 711
Ting Antifungal Cream (Fisons Consumer Health) p 409, 565
Ting Antifungal Powder (Fisons Consumer Health) p 409, 565

Ting Antifungal Spray Liquid (Fisons Consumer Health) p 409, 565
Ting Antifungal Spray Powder (Fisons Consumer Health) p 409, 565

GENERAL
A and D Ointment (Schering-Plough HealthCare) p 423, 699
Acid Mantle Creme (Sandoz Consumer) p 688
Aveeno Bath Regular (Rydelle) p 422, 687
Aveeno Moisturizing Cream (Rydelle) p 422, 687
Aveeno Moisturizing Lotion (Rydelle) p 422, 687
Bactine First Aid Antibiotic Plus Anesthetic Ointment (Miles Consumer) p 415, 614
Bactine Hydrocortisone Anti-Itch Cream (Miles Consumer) p 415, 614
Balmex Ointment (Macsil) p 582
Caldesene Medicated Ointment (Fisons Consumer Health) p 409, 563
Cortaid Cream with Aloe (Upjohn) p 432, 761
Cortaid Lotion (Upjohn) p 432, 761
Cortaid Ointment with Aloe (Upjohn) p 432, 761
Cortaid Spray (Upjohn) p 432, 761
Maximum Strength Cortaid Cream (Upjohn) p 432, 761
Maximum Strength Cortaid Ointment (Upjohn) p 432, 761
Maximum Strength Cortaid Spray (Upjohn) p 432, 761
Cortizone for Kids (Thompson Medical) p 431, 757
Cortizone-5 Cream and Ointment (Thompson Medical) p 431, 757
Cortizone-5 Wipes (Thompson Medical) p 757
Cortizone-10 Cream, Ointment and Liquid (Thompson Medical) p 431, 758
Desitin Ointment (Pfizer Consumer) p 419, 638
Lubriderm Lotion (Warner-Lambert) p 433, 770
Massengill Unscented Soft Cloth Towelette (SmithKline Beecham Consumer) p 725

HERPES TREATMENT
Campho-Phenique Cold Sore Gel (Sterling Health) p 429, 747
Campho-Phenique Liquid (Sterling Health) p 429, 747
Herpecin-L Cold Sore Lip Balm (Campbell) p 543
Zilactin Medicated Gel (Zila Pharmaceuticals) p 435, 789
Zilactin-L Liquid (Zila Pharmaceuticals) p 435, 789

INSECT BITES & STINGS
Almay Anti-Itch Lotion (Almay) p 503
Aveeno Bath Regular (Rydelle) p 422, 687
Benadryl Anti-Itch Cream, Regular Strength 1% and Maximum Strength 2% (Parke-Davis) p 417, 629
Benadryl Spray, Maximum Strength 2% (Parke-Davis) p 417, 632
Benadryl Spray, Regular Strength 1% (Parke-Davis) p 417, 632
Campho-Phenique Liquid (Sterling Health) p 429, 747
Maximum Strength Cortaid Cream (Upjohn) p 432, 761
Maximum Strength Cortaid Ointment (Upjohn) p 432, 761
Maximum Strength Cortaid Spray (Upjohn) p 432, 761
Cortizone for Kids (Thompson Medical) p 431, 757
Cortizone-5 Cream and Ointment (Thompson Medical) p 431, 757
DermaFlex Topical Anesthetic Gel Coating (Zila Pharmaceuticals) p 435, 789
Dermarest DriCort 1% Hydrocortisone Creme (Del Pharmaceuticals) p 408, 558
Domeboro Astringent Solution Effervescent Tablets (Miles Consumer) p 415, 616
Domeboro Astringent Solution Powder Packets (Miles Consumer) p 415, 616
Itch-X Gel (Ascher) p 403, 506
Massengill Medicated Soft Cloth Towelette (SmithKline Beecham Consumer) p 725

KERATOLYTICS
Carmol 10 Lotion (Syntex) p 757
MG 217 Medicated Tar-Free Shampoo (Triton Consumer) p 760
Neutrogena T/Sal Therapeutic Shampoo (Neutrogena) p 416, 622
Ultra Mide 25 (Baker Cummins Dermatologicals) p 403, 509

MOISTURIZERS
Almay Protective Eye Treatment SPF 12 (Almay) p 504
Almay Protective Face Cream SPF 15 (Almay) p 504
Almay Therapeutic Body Treatment (Almay) p 504
Almay Therapeutic Face Lotion (Almay) p 504
Alpha Keri Moisture Rich Body Oil (Bristol-Myers Products) p 405, 517
Alpha Keri Moisture Rich Cleansing Bar (Bristol-Myers Products) p 517
Aqua Care Cream (Menley & James) p 414, 602
Aqua Care Lotion (Menley & James) p 415, 602
Aqua Glycolic Lotion (Herald Pharmacal) p 568
Aqua-A Cream (Baker Cummins Dermatologicals) p 508
Aquaderm Cream (Baker Cummins Dermatologicals) p 403, 508
Aquaderm Lotion (Baker Cummins Dermatologicals) p 403, 508
Aquaderm Sunscreen Moisturizer (SPF 15 Formula) (Baker Cummins Dermatologicals) p 508
Aquaphor Healing Ointment (Beiersdorf) p 403, 511
Aquaphor Healing Ointment, Original Formula (Beiersdorf) p 403, 510
Aveeno Bath Oilated (Rydelle) p 422, 687
Aveeno Moisturizing Cream (Rydelle) p 422, 687
Aveeno Moisturizing Lotion (Rydelle) p 422, 687
Aveeno Shower and Bath Oil (Rydelle) p 422, 687
Balmex Emollient Lotion (Macsil) p 582
Carmol 10 Lotion (Syntex) p 757
Chap Stick Lip Balm (Robins Consumer) p 420, 673
Chap Stick Medicated Lip Balm (Robins Consumer) p 420, 673
Chap Stick Sunblock 15 Lip Balm (Robins Consumer) p 420, 674
Chap Stick Petroleum Jelly Plus (Robins Consumer) p 420, 674
Chap Stick Petroleum Jelly Plus with Sunblock 15 (Robins Consumer) p 420, 674
Clocream Skin Protectant Cream (Roberts) p 668
Complex 15 Hand & Body Moisturizing Cream (Schering-Plough HealthCare) p 424, 702
Complex 15 Hand & Body Moisturizing Lotion (Schering-Plough HealthCare) p 424, 703
Complex 15 Moisturizing Face Cream (Schering-Plough HealthCare) p 424, 703
Eucerin Dry Skin Care Cleansing Bar (Beiersdorf) p 404, 511
Eucerin Dry Skin Care Creme (Beiersdorf) p 404, 511
Eucerin Dry Skin Care Daily Facial Lotion SPF 20 (Beiersdorf) p 404, 511
Eucerin Dry Skin Care Lotion (Fragrance-free) (Beiersdorf) p 404, 511
Eucerin Plus Moisturizing Lotion (Beiersdorf) p 404, 512
Keri Lotion - Original Formula (Bristol-Myers Products) p 405, 530
Keri Lotion - Silky Smooth with Vitamin E (Bristol-Myers Products) p 405, 530
Keri Lotion - Silky Smooth Fragrance Free with Vitamin E (Bristol-Myers Products) p 405, 530
Lubriderm Bath Oil (Warner-Lambert) p 770
Lubriderm Lotion (Warner-Lambert) p 433, 770
Neutrogena Moisture (Neutrogena) p 416, 621
Neutrogena Moisture SPF 15 Untinted (Neutrogena) p 416, 621
Neutrogena Moisture SPF 15 with Sheer Tint (Neutrogena) p 416, 621
Neutrogena Norwegian Formula Emulsion (Neutrogena) p 416, 621
Neutrogena Norwegian Formula Hand Cream (Neutrogena) p 416, 621
Oil of Olay Daily UV Protectant SPF 15 Beauty Fluid-Original and Fragrance Free (Olay Co. Inc.) (Procter & Gamble) p 647
Oil of Olay Daily UV Protectant SPF 15 Moisture Replenishing Cream-Original and Fragrance Free (Olay Co. Inc.) (Procter & Gamble) p 647
Pen•Kera Creme (Ascher) p 403, 506
Ultra Mide 25 (Baker Cummins Dermatologicals) p 403, 509
Vaseline Intensive Care Moisturizing Sunblock Lotion (Chesebrough-Pond's) p 549
Vaseline Intensive Care U.V. Daily Defense Lotion for Hand and Body (Chesebrough-Pond's) p 549
Vaseline Intensive Care Lotion Extra Strength (Chesebrough-Pond's) p 549
Vaseline Pure Petroleum Jelly Skin Protectant (Chesebrough-Pond's) p 548

POISON IVY, OAK OR SUMAC
Aveeno Anti-Itch Concentrated Lotion (Rydelle) p 422, 687
Aveeno Anti-Itch Cream (Rydelle) p 422, 687
Aveeno Bath Oilated (Rydelle) p 422, 687
Aveeno Bath Regular (Rydelle) p 422, 687
Benadryl Anti-Itch Cream, Regular Strength 1% and Maximum Strength 2% (Parke-Davis) p 417, 629
Benadryl Spray, Maximum Strength 2% (Parke-Davis) p 417, 632
Benadryl Spray, Regular Strength 1% (Parke-Davis) p 417, 632
Caladryl Clear Lotion (Parke-Davis) p 418, 633
Caladryl Cream, Lotion, Spray (Parke-Davis) p 418, 633
Cortaid Cream with Aloe (Upjohn) p 432, 761
Cortaid Lotion (Upjohn) p 432, 761
Cortaid Ointment with Aloe (Upjohn) p 432, 761
Cortaid Spray (Upjohn) p 432, 761
Maximum Strength Cortaid Cream (Upjohn) p 432, 761
Maximum Strength Cortaid Ointment (Upjohn) p 432, 761
Maximum Strength Cortaid Spray (Upjohn) p 432, 761
Cortizone for Kids (Thompson Medical) p 431, 757
Cortizone-5 Cream and Ointment (Thompson Medical) p 431, 757
Cortizone-5 Wipes (Thompson Medical) p 757
Cortizone-10 Cream, Ointment and Liquid (Thompson Medical) p 431, 758
DermaFlex Topical Anesthetic Gel Coating (Zila Pharmaceuticals) p 435, 789

Care Creme (Care-Tech) p 544
DermaFlex Topical Anesthetic Gel Coating (Zila Pharmaceuticals) p 435, 789

OTHER
Bactine Hydrocortisone Anti-Itch Cream (Miles Consumer) p 415, 614
Borofax Ointment (Burroughs Wellcome) p 538
PRID Salve (Walker Pharmacal) p 766
Perfective Prevention Cream (Perfective Cosmetics) p 637

DIAGNOSTICS

OPHTHALMICS
(see OPHTHALMIC PREPARATIONS)

OVULATION PREDICTION TEST
Clearplan Easy (Whitehall) p 434, 795

PREGNANCY TESTS
Advance Pregnancy Test (Ortho Pharmaceutical) p 417, 793
Clearblue Easy (Whitehall) p 434, 794
e.p.t. Early Pregnancy Test (Parke-Davis) p 418, 793
Fact Plus Pregnancy Test (Ortho Pharmaceutical) p 417, 793

DIAPER RASH RELIEF
(see also DERMATOLOGICALS, DERMATITIS RELIEF & DIAPER RASH RELIEF)
A and D Ointment (Schering-Plough HealthCare) p 423, 699
Aveeno Bath Oilated (Rydelle) p 422, 687
Aveeno Bath Regular (Rydelle) p 422, 687
Aveeno Moisturizing Lotion (Rydelle) p 422, 687
Balmex Baby Powder (Macsil) p 582
Balmex Emollient Lotion (Macsil) p 582
Balmex Ointment (Macsil) p 582
Borofax Ointment (Burroughs Wellcome) p 538
Caldesene Medicated Ointment (Fisons Consumer Health) p 409, 563
Caldesene Medicated Powder (Fisons Consumer Health) p 409, 563
Desitin Ointment (Pfizer Consumer) p 419, 638
Impregon Concentrate (Fleming) p 566
Keri Lotion - Original Formula (Bristol-Myers Products) p 405, 530
Keri Lotion -Silky Smooth with Vitamin E (Bristol-Myers Products) p 405, 530
Keri Lotion - Silky Smooth Fragrance Free with Vitamin E (Bristol-Myers Products) p 405, 530

DIARRHEA MEDICATIONS
Charcocaps (Requa) p 659
Diasorb Liquid (Columbia) p 408, 557
Diasorb Tablets (Columbia) p 408, 557
Donnagel Liquid and Donnagel Chewable Tablets (Wyeth-Ayerst) p 435, 786
Hyland's Diarrex Tablets (Standard Homeopathic) p 736
Imodium A-D Caplets and Liquid (McNeil Consumer Products) p 413, 583
Kaopectate Concentrated Anti-Diarrheal, Peppermint Flavor (Upjohn) p 432, 762
Kaopectate Concentrated Anti-Diarrheal, Regular Flavor (Upjohn) p 432, 762
Kaopectate Children's Chewable Tablets (Upjohn) p 432, 762
Kaopectate Children's Liquid (Upjohn) p 432, 762
Kaopectate Maximum Strength Caplets (Upjohn) p 432, 763
Loperamide Hydrochloride Caplets (Ohm Laboratories) p 416, 623
Pepto Diarrhea Control (Procter & Gamble) p 648
Pepto-Bismol Liquid & Tablets (Procter & Gamble) p 647
Maximum Strength Pepto-Bismol Liquid (Procter & Gamble) p 648
Rheaban Maximum Strength Tablets (Pfizer Consumer) p 639

DIET AIDS
(see APPETITE SUPPRESSANTS OR FOODS)

DIETARY SUPPLEMENTS
(see NUTRITIONAL SUPPLEMENTS)

DIGESTIVE AIDS
Charcocaps (Requa) p 659
DDS-Acidophilus (UAS Laboratories) p 760
Flora-Plus Capsules (Wellness International) p 772
Pepto-Bismol Liquid & Tablets (Procter & Gamble) p 647
Maximum Strength Pepto-Bismol Liquid (Procter & Gamble) p 648

DISHPAN HANDS AIDS
(see DERMATOLOGICALS, DERMATITIS RELIEF)

E

ECZEMA PREPARATIONS
(see DERMATOLOGICALS, DERMATITIS RELIEF)

ELECTROLYTES

FLUID MAINTENANCE THERAPY
Pedialyte Oral Electrolyte Maintenance Solution (Ross) p 684

FLUID REPLACEMENT THERAPY
Rehydralyte Oral Electrolyte Rehydration Solution (Ross) p 685

ENURESIS
Hyland's Bed Wetting Tablets (Standard Homeopathic) p 735
Hyland's EnurAid Tablets (Standard Homeopathic) p 737

ENZYMES & DIGESTANTS

DIGESTANTS
Dairy Ease Caplets and Tablets (Sterling Health) p 429, 430, 748
Dairy Ease Drops (Sterling Health) p 430, 748
Lactaid Caplets (Now marketed by McNeil Consumer Products Co.) (Lactaid) p 413, 575
Lactaid Drops (Now marketed by McNeil Consumer Products Co.) (Lactaid) p 413, 575
Wobenzym N (Marlyn) p 583

EXPECTORANTS
(see COLD & COUGH PREPARATIONS)

EYEWASHES
(see OPHTHALMIC PREPARATIONS)

F

FEVER BLISTER AIDS
(see HERPES TREATMENT)

FEVER PREPARATIONS
(see ANALGESICS)

FOODS

ALLERGY DIET
Ross Pediatric Nutritional Products (Ross) p 683

COMPLETE THERAPEUTIC
Ross Pediatric Nutritional Products (Ross) p 683

INFANT
(see INFANT FORMULAS)

FORMULAS
(see INFANT FORMULAS)

FUNGAL MEDICATIONS, TOPICAL
(see DERMATOLGICALS; OPHTHALMIC PREPARATIONS; VAGINAL PREPARATIONS)

G

GASTRITIS AIDS
(see ANTACIDS)

GERMICIDES/MICROBICIDES
(see ANTISEPTICS)

H

HALITOSIS PREPARATIONS
(see ORAL HYGIENE AIDS; MOUTHWASHES)

HEAD LICE RELIEF
(see ANTIPARASITICS)

HEADACHE RELIEF
(see ANALGESICS)

HEARTBURN AIDS
(see ANTACIDS & ANTIFLATULENTS)

HEMATINICS
Feosol Capsules (SmithKline Beecham Consumer) p 427, 721
Feosol Elixir (SmithKline Beecham Consumer) p 427, 721
Feosol Tablets (SmithKline Beecham Consumer) p 427, 721
Ferancee Chewable Tablets (J&J•Merck Consumer) p 409, 570
Ferancee-HP Tablets (J&J•Merck Consumer) p 410, 570
Fergon Iron Supplement Tablets (Sterling Health) p 430, 748
Ferro-Sequels (Lederle) p 411, 579
Geritol Liquid - High Potency Iron & Vitamin Tonic (SmithKline Beecham Consumer) p 723
Incremin with Iron Syrup (Lederle) p 580
Slow Fe Tablets (CIBA Consumer) p 408, 556
Stuartinic Tablets (J&J•Merck Consumer) p 410, 574
Troph-Iron Liquid (Menley & James) p 608

IRON & COMBINATIONS
Fergon Iron Supplement Tablets (Sterling Health) p 430, 748
Geritol Extend Caplets (SmithKline Beecham Consumer) p 723
Vitron-C Tablets (Fisons Consumer Health) p 566

HEMORRHOIDAL PREPARATIONS
(see ANORECTAL PRODUCTS)

HERPES TREATMENT
Anbesol Gel - Regular Strength (Whitehall) p 434, 775
Anbesol Gel - Maximum Strength (Whitehall) p 434, 775
Anbesol Liquid - Regular Strength (Whitehall) p 434, 775
Anbesol Liquid - Maximum Strength (Whitehall) p 434, 775
Chap Stick Medicated Lip Balm (Robins Consumer) p 420, 673
Herpecin-L Cold Sore Lip Balm (Campbell) p 543
Orajel Mouth-Aid for Canker and Cold Sores (Del Pharmaceuticals) p 408, 559
Zilactin Medicated Gel (Zila Pharmaceuticals) p 435, 789

HOMEOPATHIC MEDICATIONS
Bifido Factor (Natren) p 620
Hyland's Arnicaid Tablets (Standard Homeopathic) p 735
Hyland's Bed Wetting Tablets (Standard Homeopathic) p 735

Hyland's Calms Forté Tablets (Standard Homeopathic) p 735
Hyland's ClearAc Tablets (Standard Homeopathic) p 736
Hyland's Colic Tablets (Standard Homeopathic) p 736
Hyland's Cough Syrup with Honey (Standard Homeopathic) p 736
Hyland's C-Plus Cold Tablets (Standard Homeopathic) p 736
Hyland's Diarrex Tablets (Standard Homeopathic) p 736
Hyland's EnurAid Tablets (Standard Homeopathic) p 737
Hyland's Teething Tablets (Standard Homeopathic) p 737
Oscillococcinum (Boiron USA) p 404, 516
Pro-Bifidonate Powder (Natren) p 620
Pro-Bionate Powder and Capsules (Natren) p 620
Superdophilus (Natren) p 620

HYPOMAGNESEMIA
Magonate Tablets and Liquid (Fleming) p 567
Mag-Ox 400 (Blaine) p 512
Uro-Mag (Blaine) p 512

I

INFANT FORMULAS, REGULAR
LIQUID CONCENTRATE
SMA Iron Fortified Infant Formula, Concentrated, Ready-to-Feed and Powder (Wyeth-Ayerst) p 435, 787
SMA lo-iron Infant Formula, Concentrated, Ready-to-Feed, and Powder (Wyeth-Ayerst) p 435, 787
LIQUID READY-TO-FEED
SMA Iron Fortified Infant Formula, Concentrated, Ready-to-Feed and Powder (Wyeth-Ayerst) p 435, 787
SMA lo-iron Infant Formula, Concentrated, Ready-to-Feed, and Powder (Wyeth-Ayerst) p 435, 787
POWDER
SMA Iron Fortified Infant Formula, Concentrated, Ready-to-Feed and Powder (Wyeth-Ayerst) p 435, 787
SMA lo-iron Infant Formula, Concentrated, Ready-to-Feed, and Powder (Wyeth-Ayerst) p 435, 787

INFANT FORMULAS, SPECIAL PURPOSE
CORN FREE
LIQUID CONCENTRATE
Nursoy (Wyeth-Ayerst) p 435, 787
LIQUID READY-TO-FEED
Nursoy (Wyeth-Ayerst) p 435, 787
IRON SUPPLEMENT
LIQUID CONCENTRATE
Nursoy (Wyeth-Ayerst) p 435, 787
SMA Iron Fortified Infant Formula, Concentrated, Ready-to-Feed and Powder (Wyeth-Ayerst) p 435, 787
LIQUID READY-TO-FEED
Nursoy (Wyeth-Ayerst) p 435, 787
Ross Pediatric Nutritional Products (Ross) p 683
SMA Iron Fortified Infant Formula, Concentrated, Ready-to-Feed and Powder (Wyeth-Ayerst) p 435, 787
POWDER
Nursoy (Wyeth-Ayerst) p 435, 787
SMA Iron Fortified Infant Formula, Concentrated, Ready-to-Feed and Powder (Wyeth-Ayerst) p 435, 787
LACTOSE FREE
LIQUID CONCENTRATE
Nursoy (Wyeth-Ayerst) p 435, 787
LIQUID READY-TO-FEED
Nursoy (Wyeth-Ayerst) p 435, 787
POWDER
Nursoy (Wyeth-Ayerst) p 435, 787
LOW IRON
LIQUID CONCENTRATE
SMA lo-iron Infant Formula, Concentrated, Ready-to-Feed, and Powder (Wyeth-Ayerst) p 435, 787
LIQUID READY-TO-FEED
Ross Pediatric Nutritional Products (Ross) p 683
SMA lo-iron Infant Formula, Concentrated, Ready-to-Feed, and Powder (Wyeth-Ayerst) p 435, 787
POWDER
SMA lo-iron Infant Formula, Concentrated, Ready-to-Feed, and Powder (Wyeth-Ayerst) p 435, 787
MILK FREE
LIQUID CONCENTRATE
Nursoy (Wyeth-Ayerst) p 435, 787
LIQUID READY-TO-FEED
Nursoy (Wyeth-Ayerst) p 435, 787
POWDER
Nursoy (Wyeth-Ayerst) p 435, 787

INSECT BITE & STING PREPARATIONS
Americaine Topical Anesthetic First Aid Ointment (Fisons Consumer Health) p 409, 562
Americaine Topical Anesthetic Spray (Fisons Consumer Health) p 409, 562
Aveeno Anti-Itch Concentrated Lotion (Rydelle) p 422, 687
Aveeno Anti-Itch Cream (Rydelle) p 422, 687
Aveeno Bath Oilated (Rydelle) p 422, 687
Bactine Antiseptic/Anesthetic First Aid Liquid (Miles Consumer) p 415, 614
Bactine Hydrocortisone Anti-Itch Cream (Miles Consumer) p 415, 614
BiCozene Creme (Sandoz Consumer) p 422, 688
Domeboro Astringent Solution Effervescent Tablets (Miles Consumer) p 415, 616
Domeboro Astringent Solution Powder Packets (Miles Consumer) p 415, 616
Nupercainal Hemorrhoidal and Anesthetic Ointment (CIBA Consumer) p 408, 554
Nupercainal Pain Relief Cream (CIBA Consumer) p 408, 554
Rhulicream (Rydelle) p 422, 687
Rhuligel (Rydelle) p 422, 688
Rhulispray (Rydelle) p 422, 688

IRON DEFICIENCY PREPARATIONS (see HEMATINICS)

IRRIGATING SOLUTION, OPHTHALMIC (see OPHTHALMIC PREPARATIONS)

L

LAXATIVES
BULK
Citrucel Orange Flavor (SmithKline Beecham Consumer) p 426, 715
Citrucel Sugar Free Orange Flavor (SmithKline Beecham Consumer) p 426, 715
Effer-Syllium Natural Fiber Bulking Agent (J&J•Merck Consumer) p 409, 570
Fiberall Chewable Tablets, Lemon Creme Flavor (CIBA Consumer) p 552
Fiberall Fiber Wafers - Fruit & Nut (CIBA Consumer) p 407, 552
Fiberall Fiber Wafers - Oatmeal Raisin (CIBA Consumer) p 407, 552
Fiberall Powder Natural Flavor (CIBA Consumer) p 407, 553
Fiberall Powder Orange Flavor (CIBA Consumer) p 407, 553
FiberCon (Lederle) p 411, 579
Konsyl Powder (Konsyl) p 574
Konsyl-D Powder (Konsyl) p 574
Konsyl-Orange Powder (Konsyl) p 575
Maltsupex Liquid, Powder & Tablets (Wallace) p 432, 766
Metamucil Effervescent Sugar Free, Lemon-Lime Flavor (Procter & Gamble) p 645
Metamucil Effervescent Sugar Free, Orange Flavor (Procter & Gamble) p 645
Metamucil Powder, Orange Flavor (Procter & Gamble) p 645
Metamucil Powder, Regular Flavor (Procter & Gamble) p 645
Metamucil Sunrise Smooth, Citrus Flavor (Procter & Gamble) p 645
Metamucil Sunrise Smooth, Sugar Free, Citrus Flavor (Procter & Gamble) p 645
Metamucil Sunrise Smooth Powder, Orange Flavor (Procter & Gamble) p 645
Metamucil Sunrise Smooth Powder, Sugar Free, Orange Flavor (Procter & Gamble) p 645
Metamucil Wafers, Apple Crisp (Procter & Gamble) p 645
Metamucil Wafers, Cinnamon Spice (Procter & Gamble) p 645
Perdiem Fiber Granules (Rhone-Poulenc Rorer Consumer) p 420, 665
Perdiem Granules (Rhone-Poulenc Rorer Consumer) p 420, 665
Serutan Toasted Granules (Menley & James) p 414, 608
Surgeon's Choice (The Biopractic Group) p 512
Syllact Powder (Wallace) p 433, 769
COMBINATIONS
Agoral, Marshmallow Flavor (Parke-Davis) p 627
Agoral, Raspberry Flavor (Parke-Davis) p 627
Correctol Laxative Tablets (Schering-Plough HealthCare) p 425, 704
Dialose Plus Tablets (J&J•Merck Consumer) p 409, 569
Extra Gentle Ex-Lax Laxative Pills (Sandoz Consumer) p 422, 690
Feen-A-Mint Laxative Pills (Schering-Plough HealthCare) p 425, 707
Haley's M-O, Regular & Flavored (Sterling Health) p 430, 749
Nature's Remedy Natural Vegetable Laxative Tablets (SmithKline Beecham Consumer) p 427, 726
Perdiem Granules (Rhone-Poulenc Rorer Consumer) p 420, 665
Peri-Colace (Apothecon) p 403, 505
Phillips' Gelcaps (Sterling Health) p 430, 753
FECAL SOFTENERS
Colace (Apothecon) p 403, 505
Correctol Extra Gentle Stool Softener (Schering-Plough HealthCare) p 704
Correctol Laxative Tablets (Schering-Plough HealthCare) p 425, 704
Dialose Tablets (J&J•Merck Consumer) p 409, 569
Dialose Plus Tablets (J&J•Merck Consumer) p 409, 569
Doxidan Liqui-Gels (Upjohn) p 432, 761
Extra Gentle Ex-Lax Laxative Pills (Sandoz Consumer) p 422, 690
Feen-A-Mint Laxative Pills (Schering-Plough HealthCare) p 425, 707
Kasof Capsules (Roberts) p 668
Perdiem Fiber Granules (Rhone-Poulenc Rorer Consumer) p 420, 665
Perdiem Granules (Rhone-Poulenc Rorer Consumer) p 420, 665
Phillips' Gelcaps (Sterling Health) p 430, 753
Surfak Liqui-Gels (Upjohn) p 432, 764
MINERAL OIL
Haley's M-O, Regular & Flavored (Sterling Health) p 430, 749

Neo-Synephrine Maximum Strength 12 Hour Nasal Spray (Sterling Health) p 751
Neo-Synephrine Maximum Strength 12 Hour Nasal Spray Pump (Sterling Health) p 430, 751
Neo-Synephrine Nasal Sprays, Pediatric, Mild, Regular & Extra Strength (Sterling Health) p 430, 751
Nōstril 1/4% Mild Nasal Decongestant (CIBA Consumer) p 408, 553
Nōstril 1/2% Regular Nasal Decongestant (CIBA Consumer) p 408, 553
Nōstrilla Long Acting Nasal Decongestant (CIBA Consumer) p 408, 553
Privine Nasal Spray (CIBA Consumer) p 408, 555
Vicks Inhaler (Procter & Gamble) p 653
Vicks Sinex Decongestant Nasal Spray (Regular) (Procter & Gamble) p 656
Vicks Sinex Decongestant Nasal Ultra Fine Mist (Procter & Gamble) p 656
Vicks Sinex Long-Acting Decongestant Nasal Spray (Procter & Gamble) p 656
Vicks Sinex Long-Acting Decongestant Nasal Ultra Fine Mist (Procter & Gamble) p 656

NAUSEA MEDICATIONS
Dramamine Chewable Tablets (Upjohn) p 432, 761
Children's Dramamine (Upjohn) p 432, 761
Dramamine Tablets (Upjohn) p 432, 761
Dramamine II Tablets (Upjohn) p 432, 762
Emetrol (Bock Pharmacal) p 404, 516
Marezine Tablets (Burroughs Wellcome) p 406, 538
Pepto-Bismol Liquid & Tablets (Procter & Gamble) p 647
Maximum Strength Pepto-Bismol Liquid (Procter & Gamble) p 648

NUTRITIONAL SUPPLEMENTS
Allbee with C Caplets (Robins Consumer) p 671
Allbee C-800 Plus Iron Tablets (Robins Consumer) p 671
Allbee C-800 Tablets (Robins Consumer) p 671
Aloe Up (Emutech International) p 560
Beelith Tablets (Beach) p 510
Cheater's Delight (Emutech International) p 560
Ester-C Tablets, Caplets and Powder (Inter-Cal) p 568
FemIron Multivitamins and Iron (Menley & James) p 414, 604
Garfield Chewable Multivitamins - Regular (Menley & James) p 414, 604
Garfield Chewable Multivitamins Plus Extra C (Menley & James) p 414, 605
Garfield Chewable Multivitamins Plus Iron (Menley & James) p 414, 605
Garfield Chewable Multivitamins Complete with Minerals (Menley & James) p 414, 606
Geritol Complete Tablets (SmithKline Beecham Consumer) p 723
Geritol Liquid - High Potency Iron & Vitamin Tonic (SmithKline Beecham Consumer) p 723
Incremin with Iron Syrup (Lederle) p 580
Kick Start (Emutech International) p 560
Kyolic (Wakunaga) p 432, 766
Mag-Ox 400 (Blaine) p 512
MagTab SR Caplets (Niché Pharmaceuticals) p 622
Marlyn Formula 50 (Marlyn) p 583
Marlyn Formula 50 Mega Forte (Marlyn) p 583
Nutra-Lean Shake (Wellness International) p 773
Pro-Bionate Powder and Capsules (Natren) p 620
Renew (Emutech International) p 560
Sunkist Children's Chewable Multivitamins - Complete (CIBA Consumer) p 408, 556
Sunkist Children's Chewable Multivitamins - Plus Extra C (CIBA Consumer) p 408, 556
Sunkist Children's Chewable Multivitamins - Plus Iron (CIBA Consumer) p 408, 556
Sunkist Children's Chewable Multivitamins - Regular (CIBA Consumer) p 408, 556
Superdophilus (Natren) p 620
Tri-Lean Additive Drink (Wellness International) p 773
Ultra Meal (Emutech International) p 561
Uro-Mag (Blaine) p 512
Vita Fuel (Emutech International) p 561
Z-BEC Tablets (Robins Consumer) p 683

O

OBESITY PREPARATIONS (see APPETITE SUPPRESSANTS)

OPHTHALMIC PREPARATIONS

ARTIFICIAL TEARS
Celluvisc Lubricant Ophthalmic Solution (Allergan Pharmaceuticals) p 502
Tears Plus Lubricant Ophthalmic Solution (Allergan Pharmaceuticals) p 503

CLEANSERS, EXTERNAL
Almay Eyelid Cleansing Pads (Almay) p 503

DEVICES
Lavoptik Eye Cup (Lavoptik) p 793

EYEWASHES
Collyrium for Fresh Eyes (Wyeth-Ayerst) p 435, 786
Lavoptik Eye Wash (Lavoptik) p 575
Star-Optic Eye Wash (Stellar) p 428, 737

IRRIGATING SOLUTIONS
Collyrium for Fresh Eyes (Wyeth-Ayerst) p 435, 786
Lavoptik Eye Wash (Lavoptik) p 575

LUBRICANTS
Cellufresh Lubricant Ophthalmic Solution (Allergan Pharmaceuticals) p 502
Celluvisc Lubricant Ophthalmic Solution (Allergan Pharmaceuticals) p 502
Clear Eyes ACR Astringent/Lubricating Eye Redness Reliever (Ross) p 421, 683
Clear Eyes Lubricating Eye Redness Reliever (Ross) p 421, 683
Collyrium Fresh (Wyeth-Ayerst) p 435, 786
Lacri-Lube NP Lubricant Ophthalmic Ointment (Allergan Pharmaceuticals) p 502
Lacri-Lube S.O.P. Sterile Ophthalmic Ointment (Allergan Pharmaceuticals) p 502
Murine Lubricating Eye Drops (Ross) p 421, 684
Murine Plus Lubricating Redness Reliever Eye Drops (Ross) p 421, 684
Refresh P.M. Lubricant Ophthalmic Ointment (Allergan Pharmaceuticals) p 503
Tears Plus Lubricant Ophthalmic Solution (Allergan Pharmaceuticals) p 503
Visine EXTRA Eye Drops (Pfizer Consumer) p 419, 641
Viva-Drops (Vision Pharmaceuticals) p 766

SYMPATHOMIMETIC AGENTS

VASOCONSTRICTORS
Visine A.C. Eye Drops (Pfizer Consumer) p 419, 641
Visine Eye Drops (Pfizer Consumer) p 419, 641
Visine L.R. Eye Drops (Pfizer Consumer) p 419, 642

VASOCONSTRICTORS & COMBINATIONS
Clear Eyes ACR Astringent/Lubricating Eye Redness Reliever (Ross) p 421, 683
Clear Eyes Lubricating Eye Redness Reliever (Ross) p 421, 683
Collyrium Fresh (Wyeth-Ayerst) p 435, 786
Murine Plus Lubricating Redness Reliever Eye Drops (Ross) p 421, 684
Visine EXTRA Eye Drops (Pfizer Consumer) p 419, 641

ORAL HYGIENE AIDS
Cēpacol/Cēpacol Mint Mouthwash/Gargle (SmithKline Beecham Consumer) p 426, 713
Chloraseptic Liquid, Cherry, Menthol or Cool Mint (Procter & Gamble) p 643
Listerine Antiseptic (Warner-Lambert) p 433, 770
Cool Mint Listerine Antiseptic (Warner-Lambert) p 433, 770
Baby Orajel Tooth & Gum Cleanser (Del Pharmaceuticals) p 408, 559

P

PAIN RELIEVERS (see ANALGESICS)

PEDICULICIDES (see ANTIPARASITICS)

PLATELET INHIBITORS
Bayer Children's Chewable Aspirin (Sterling Health) p 429, 738
Genuine Bayer Aspirin Tablets & Caplets (Sterling Health) p 428, 738
Bayer Plus Aspirin Tablets (Sterling Health) p 429, 742
Adult Low Strength Bayer Enteric Aspirin Tablets (Sterling Health) p 429, 741
Regular Strength Bayer Enteric Aspirin Caplets (Sterling Health) p 429, 741
Norwich Aspirin (Chattem) p 546
Norwich Aspirin - Maximum Strength (Chattem) p 546
Norwich Enteric Safety Coated Aspirin (Chattem) p 546
Norwich Enteric Safety Coated Aspirin - Maximum Strength (Chattem) p 546

POISON IVY & OAK PREPARATIONS
Aveeno Anti-Itch Concentrated Lotion (Rydelle) p 422, 687
Aveeno Anti-Itch Cream (Rydelle) p 422, 687
Aveeno Bath Oilated (Rydelle) p 422, 687
Aveeno Bath Regular (Rydelle) p 422, 687
Bactine Hydrocortisone Anti-Itch Cream (Miles Consumer) p 415, 614
Benadryl Anti-Itch Cream, Regular Strength 1% and Maximum Strength 2% (Parke-Davis) p 417, 629
Caladryl Clear Lotion (Parke-Davis) p 418, 633
Caladryl Cream, Lotion, Spray (Parke-Davis) p 418, 633
Caldecort Anti-Itch Hydrocortisone Cream (Fisons Consumer Health) p 409, 563
Caldecort Anti-Itch Hydrocortisone Spray (Fisons Consumer Health) p 563
Caldecort Light Cream (Fisons Consumer Health) p 409, 563
Cortizone-5 Cream and Ointment (Thompson Medical) p 431, 757
Cortizone-5 Wipes (Thompson Medical) p 757
Cortizone-10 Cream, Ointment and Liquid (Thompson Medical) p 431, 758

Metamucil Powder, Orange Flavor (Procter & Gamble) p 645
Metamucil Powder, Regular Flavor (Procter & Gamble) p 645
Metamucil Sunrise Smooth, Citrus Flavor (Procter & Gamble) p 645
Metamucil Sunrise Smooth, Sugar Free, Citrus Flavor (Procter & Gamble) p 645
Metamucil Sunrise Smooth Powder, Orange Flavor (Procter & Gamble) p 645
Metamucil Sunrise Smooth Powder, Sugar Free, Orange Flavor (Procter & Gamble) p 645
Metamucil Wafers, Apple Crisp (Procter & Gamble) p 645
Metamucil Wafers, Cinnamon Spice (Procter & Gamble) p 645
Peri-Colace (Apothecon) p 403, 505
Z-BEC Tablets (Robins Consumer) p 683

URINARY TRACT AGENTS

ANALGESICS

Azo-Standard (PolyMedica Pharmaceuticals) p 642

V

VAGINAL PREPARATIONS

ANALGESICS, EXTERNAL

Dermarest DriCort 1% Hydrocortisone Creme (Del Pharmaceuticals) p 408, 558

ANTIFUNGALS

Mycelex-7 Vaginal Cream Antifungal (Miles Consumer) p 415, 617
Mycelex-7 Vaginal Inserts Antifungal (Miles Consumer) p 415, 617

CLEANSERS, EXTERNAL

Massengill Unscented Soft Cloth Towelette (SmithKline Beecham Consumer) p 725

CONTRACEPTIVES (see CONTRACEPTIVES)

CREAMS

Gyne-Lotrimin Vaginal Cream Antifungal (Schering-Plough HealthCare) p 425, 707
Gyne-Lotrimin Vaginal Cream with 7 Disposable Applicators (Schering-Plough HealthCare) p 425, 707
Massengill Medicated Soft Cloth Towelette (SmithKline Beecham Consumer) p 725
Monistat 7 Vaginal Cream (Ortho Pharmaceutical) p 417, 626

DOUCHES

Massengill Disposable Douches (SmithKline Beecham Consumer) p 427, 724
Massengill Liquid Concentrate (SmithKline Beecham Consumer) p 725
Massengill Medicated Disposable Douche (SmithKline Beecham Consumer) p 427, 725
Massengill Medicated Liquid Concentrate (SmithKline Beecham Consumer) p 725
Massengill Powder (SmithKline Beecham Consumer) p 724

INSERTS, SUPPOSITORIES

Encare Vaginal Contraceptive Suppositories (Thompson Medical) p 759
Gyne-Lotrimin Vaginal Inserts (Schering-Plough HealthCare) p 425, 708
Monistat 7 Vaginal Suppositories (Ortho Pharmaceutical) p 417, 626
Semicid (See 1993 Physicians' Desk Reference for picture) (Whitehall) p 783

JELLIES, OINTMENTS

Replens (Parke-Davis) p 418, 635

LUBRICANTS

Replens (Parke-Davis) p 418, 635

MOISTURIZERS

Gyne-Moistrin Vaginal Moisturizing Gel (Schering-Plough HealthCare) p 425, 708
Replens (Parke-Davis) p 418, 635

VERTIGO AGENTS

Marezine Tablets (Burroughs Wellcome) p 406, 538
Nicotinex Elixir (Fleming) p 567

VISCOELASTIC AGENTS (see OPHTHALMIC PREPARATIONS)

VITAMINS

GERIATRIC

Geritol Extend Caplets (SmithKline Beecham Consumer) p 723

INTRANASAL APPLICATION

Ener-B Vitamin B_{12} Nasal Gel Dietary Supplement (Nature's Bounty) p 416, 620

MULTIVITAMINS

Allbee with C Caplets (Robins Consumer) p 671
Allbee C-800 Tablets (Robins Consumer) p 671
Bugs Bunny Children's Chewable Vitamins (Sugar Free) (Miles Consumer) p 415, 615
Bugs Bunny With Extra C Children's Chewable Vitamins (Sugar Free) (Miles Consumer) p 415, 615
Centrum, Jr. (Children's Chewable) + Extra Calcium (Lederle) p 411, 577
Flintstones Children's Chewable Vitamins (Miles Consumer) p 415, 615
Flintstones Children's Chewable Vitamins With Extra C (Miles Consumer) p 415, 615
Garfield Chewable Multivitamins - Regular (Menley & James) p 414, 604
Garfield Chewable Multivitamins Plus Extra C (Menley & James) p 414, 605
Garfield Chewable Multivitamins Plus Iron (Menley & James) p 414, 605
Garfield Chewable Multivitamins Complete with Minerals (Menley & James) p 414, 606
One-A-Day Essential Vitamins (Miles Consumer) p 416, 618
One-A-Day Plus Extra C Vitamins (Miles Consumer) p 416, 618
One-A-Day Women's Formula Multivitamins with Calcium, Extra Iron, Zinc and Beta Carotene (Miles Consumer) p 416, 618
Sigtab Tablets (Roberts) p 420, 670
Stresstabs (Lederle) p 411, 581
Theragran Liquid (Bristol-Myers Products) p 406, 533
Theragran Tablets (Bristol-Myers Products) p 406, 533
Trophite Liquid (Menley & James) p 609
Unicap Softgel Capsules & Tablets (Upjohn) p 432, 764
Unicap Jr. Chewable Tablets (Upjohn) p 764
Zymacap Capsules (Roberts) p 670

MULTIVITAMINS WITH MINERALS

Allbee C-800 Plus Iron Tablets (Robins Consumer) p 671
Bugs Bunny Complete Children's Chewable Vitamins + Minerals with Iron and Calcium (Sugar Free) (Miles Consumer) p 415, 616
Bugs Bunny Plus Iron Children's Chewable Vitamins (Sugar Free) (Miles Consumer) p 415, 615
Centrum (Lederle) p 410, 576
Centrum, Jr. (Children's Chewable) + Extra C (Lederle) p 411, 577
Centrum, Jr. (Children's Chewable) + Extra Calcium (Lederle) p 411, 577
Centrum, Jr. (Children's Chewable) + Iron (Lederle) p 410, 579
Centrum Liquid (Lederle) p 411, 577
Centrum Silver (Lederle) p 411, 579
Femlron Multivitamins and Iron (Menley & James) p 414, 604
Flintstones Children's Chewable Vitamins Plus Iron (Miles Consumer) p 415, 615
Flintstones Complete With Calcium, Iron & Minerals Children's Chewable Vitamins (Miles Consumer) p 415, 616
Garfield Chewable Multivitamins Plus Iron (Menley & James) p 414, 605
Garfield Chewable Multivitamins Complete with Minerals (Menley & James) p 414, 606
Geritol Complete Tablets (SmithKline Beecham Consumer) p 723
Geritol Extend Caplets (SmithKline Beecham Consumer) p 723
Geritol Liquid - High Potency Iron & Vitamin Tonic (SmithKline Beecham Consumer) p 723
Gevrabon Liquid (Lederle) p 580
Gevral T Tablets (Lederle) p 580
Myadec (Parke-Davis) p 418, 635
Nutra-Lean Shake (Wellness International) p 773
One-A-Day Maximum Formula Vitamins and Minerals (Miles Consumer) p 416, 618
One-A-Day Stressgard Formula Vitamins (Miles Consumer) p 416, 618
One-A-Day Women's Formula Multivitamins with Calcium, Extra Iron, Zinc and Beta Carotene (Miles Consumer) p 416, 618
Os-Cal Fortified Tablets (SmithKline Beecham Consumer) p 428, 728
Os-Cal Plus Tablets (SmithKline Beecham Consumer) p 428, 729
Protegra Vitamin and Mineral Supplement (Lederle) p 411, 581
Sigtab-M Tablets (Roberts) p 420, 670
Stresstabs + Iron, Advanced Formula (Lederle) p 411, 581
Stresstabs + Zinc (Lederle) p 411, 581
Stuart Prenatal Tablets (Wyeth-Ayerst) p 435, 789
The Stuart Formula Tablets (J&J•Merck Consumer) p 410, 573
Sunkist Children's Chewable Multivitamins - Complete (CIBA Consumer) p 408, 556
Sunkist Children's Chewable Multivitamins - Plus Extra C (CIBA Consumer) p 408, 556
Sunkist Children's Chewable Multivitamins - Plus Iron (CIBA Consumer) p 408, 556
Sunkist Children's Chewable Multivitamins - Regular (CIBA Consumer) p 408, 556
Theragran Stress Formula (Bristol-Myers Products) p 406, 534
Theragran-M Tablets with Beta Carotene (Bristol-Myers Products) p 406, 534
Tri-Lean Additive Drink (Wellness International) p 773
Troph-Iron Liquid (Menley & James) p 608
Unicap M Tablets (Upjohn) p 432, 764
Unicap Plus Iron Vitamin Formula Tablets (Upjohn) p 765
Unicap Sr. Tablets (Upjohn) p 432, 765
Unicap T Tablets (Upjohn) p 432, 765
VitaLink II Multivitamin and Mineral Supplement (BioLink International) p 512
Z-BEC Tablets (Robins Consumer) p 683

PEDIATRIC

Bugs Bunny Children's Chewable Vitamins (Sugar Free) (Miles Consumer) p 415, 615
Bugs Bunny Complete Children's Chewable Vitamins + Minerals with Iron and Calcium (Sugar Free) (Miles Consumer) p 415, 616

SECTION 4

Active Ingredients Index

In this section the products described in the Product Information (White) Section are listed under their chemical (generic) name according to their principal ingredient(s). Products have been included under specific headings by the Publisher with the cooperation of individual manufacturers.

A

ACETAMINOPHEN

Actifed Plus Caplets (Burroughs Wellcome) p 406, 535
Actifed Plus Tablets (Burroughs Wellcome) p 406, 537
Actifed Sinus Daytime/Nighttime Caplets (Burroughs Wellcome) p 406, 535
Actifed Sinus Daytime/Nighttime Tablets (Burroughs Wellcome) p 406, 536
Allerest Headache Strength Tablets (Fisons Consumer Health) p 561
Allerest No Drowsiness Tablets (Fisons Consumer Health) p 409, 561
Allerest Sinus Pain Formula (Fisons Consumer Health) p 561
Aspirin Free Anacin Caplets (Robins Consumer) p 420, 672
Aspirin Free Anacin Gel Caplets (Robins Consumer) p 420, 672
Aspirin Free Anacin Tablets (Robins Consumer) p 420, 672
Aspirin Free Anacin P.M. Caplets (Robins Consumer) p 420, 672
Bayer Select Headache Pain Relief Formula (Sterling Health) p 429, 745
Bayer Select Menstrual Multi-Symptom Formula (Sterling Health) p 429, 745
Bayer Select Night Time Pain Relief Formula (Sterling Health) p 429, 745
Bayer Select Sinus Pain Relief Formula (Sterling Health) p 429, 745
Benadryl Allergy Sinus Headache Formula (Parke-Davis) p 417, 630
Benadryl Cold Tablets (Parke-Davis) p 417, 631
Benadryl Cold Nighttime Formula (Parke-Davis) p 418, 631
Bufferin AF Nite Time Analgesic/Sleeping Aid Caplets (Bristol-Myers Products) p 404, 518
Chlor-Trimeton Allergy-Sinus Headache Caplets (Schering-Plough HealthCare) p 424, 701
Allergy-Sinus Comtrex Multi-Symptom Allergy-Sinus Formula Tablets & Caplets (Bristol-Myers Products) p 404, 521
Cough Formula Comtrex (Bristol-Myers Products) p 404, 522
Comtrex Multi-Symptom Cold Reliever Tablets/Caplets/Liqui-Gels/Liquid (Bristol-Myers Products) p 404, 520
Comtrex Multi-Symptom Day-Night Caplet-Tablet (Bristol-Myers Products) p 404, 523
Comtrex Multi-Symptom Non-Drowsy Caplets (Bristol-Myers Products) p 404, 524
Congespirin For Children Aspirin Free Chewable Cold Tablets (Bristol-Myers Products) p 405, 525
Contac Day & Night Cold & Flu - Day Caplets (SmithKline Beecham Consumer) p 426, 715
Contac Day & Night Cold & Flu - Night Caplets (SmithKline Beecham Consumer) p 426, 716
Contac Severe Cold and Flu Formula Caplets (SmithKline Beecham Consumer) p 426, 717
Contac Severe Cold & Flu Nighttime (SmithKline Beecham Consumer) p 426, 718
Coricidin 'D' Decongestant Tablets (Schering-Plough HealthCare) p 424, 703
Coricidin Tablets (Schering-Plough HealthCare) p 424, 703
Dimetapp Cold & Flu Caplets (Robins Consumer) p 421, 675
Dristan Cold (Whitehall) p 434, 777
Dristan Juice Mix-In (Whitehall) p 434, 776
Dristan Cold, Maximum Strength Multi-symptom Formula (Whitehall) p 434, 778
Dristan Cold, Maximum Strength No Drowsiness Formula (Whitehall) p 434, 778
Drixoral Cold and Flu Extended-Release Tablets (Schering-Plough HealthCare) p 425, 705
Drixoral Sinus (Schering-Plough HealthCare) p 425, 706
Aspirin Free Excedrin Analgesic Caplets (Bristol-Myers Products) p 405, 525
Excedrin Extra-Strength Analgesic Tablets & Caplets (Bristol-Myers Products) p 405, 526
Excedrin P.M. Analgesic/Sleeping Aid Tablets, Caplets and Liquid (Bristol-Myers Products) p 405, 527
Sinus Excedrin Analgesic, Decongestant Tablets & Caplets (Bristol-Myers Products) p 405, 528
Liquiprin Infants' Drops (Menley & James) p 414, 607
Medi-Flu Caplet, Liquid (Parke-Davis) p 418, 634
Medi-Flu Without Drowsiness Caplets (Parke-Davis) p 418, 634
Maximum Strength Multi-Symptom Menstrual Formula Midol (Sterling Health) p 430, 750
Night Time Formula Midol PM (Sterling Health) p 430, 750
PMS Multi-Symptom Formula Midol (Sterling Health) p 430, 749
Regular Strength Multi-Symptom Midol Formula (Sterling Health) p 430, 749
Teen Multi-Symptom Formula Midol (Sterling Health) p 430, 750
Neopap Pediatric Suppositories (PolyMedica Pharmaceuticals) p 642
Ornex Caplets (Menley & James) p 414, 607
Maximum Strength Ornex Caplets (Menley & James) p 414, 607
Ornex Severe Cold Formula Caplets (Menley & James) p 414, 608
Multi-Symptom Pamprin Tablets and Caplets (Chattem) p 548
Maximum Pain Relief Pamprin Caplets (Chattem) p 548
Children's Panadol Chewable Tablets, Liquid, Infant's Drops (Sterling Health) p 431, 752

Mylanta Tablets (J&J•Merck Consumer) p 410, 570
Mylanta Double Strength Liquid (J&J•Merck Consumer) p 410, 571
Mylanta Double Strength Tablets (J&J•Merck Consumer) p 410, 571
Nephrox Suspension (Fleming) p 567

ALUMINUM SULFATE
Domeboro Astringent Solution Effervescent Tablets (Miles Consumer) p 415, 616
Domeboro Astringent Solution Powder Packets (Miles Consumer) p 415, 616

AMINO ACID PREPARATIONS
Marlyn Formula 50 (Marlyn) p 583
Marlyn Formula 50 Mega Forte (Marlyn) p 583

AMMONIUM ALUM
Massengill Powder (SmithKline Beecham Consumer) p 724

ARNICA MONTANA
Hyland's Arnicaid Tablets (Standard Homeopathic) p 735
Hyland's EnurAid Tablets (Standard Homeopathic) p 737

ASCORBIC ACID (see VITAMIN C)

ASPIRIN
Alka-Seltzer Effervescent Antacid and Pain Reliever (Miles Consumer) p 414, 609
Alka-Seltzer Extra Strength Effervescent Antacid and Pain Reliever (Miles Consumer) p 415, 612
Alka-Seltzer (Flavored) Effervescent Antacid and Pain Reliever (Miles Consumer) p 414, 610
Alka-Seltzer Plus Cold Medicine (Miles Consumer) p 415, 612
Alka-Seltzer Plus Cold & Cough Medicine (Miles Consumer) p 415, 613
Alka-Seltzer Plus Night-Time Cold Medicine (Miles Consumer) p 415, 612
Alka Seltzer Plus Sinus Allergy Medicine (Miles Consumer) p 415, 613
Anacin Caplets (Robins Consumer) p 420, 671
Anacin Tablets (Robins Consumer) p 420, 671
Maximum Strength Anacin Tablets (Robins Consumer) p 673
Arthritis Pain Formula, Maximum Strength Analgesic Caplets (See 1993 Physicians' Desk Reference) (Whitehall) p 775
Arthritis Strength BC Powder (Block) p 513
Ascriptin A/D Caplets (Rhone-Poulenc Rorer Consumer) p 419, 661
Extra Strength Ascriptin Caplets (Rhone-Poulenc Rorer Consumer) p 419, 660
Regular Strength Ascriptin Tablets (Rhone-Poulenc Rorer Consumer) p 419, 659
BC Powder (Block) p 514
BC Cold Powder Multi-Symptom Formula (Cold-Sinus-Allergy) (Block) p 513
BC Cold Powder Non-Drowsy Formula (Cold-Sinus) (Block) p 513
Bayer Children's Chewable Aspirin (Sterling Health) p 429, 738
Genuine Bayer Aspirin Tablets & Caplets (Sterling Health) p 428, 738
Maximum Bayer Aspirin Tablets & Caplets (Sterling Health) p 428, 740
Extended Release Bayer 8-Hour Aspirin (Sterling Health) p 429, 740
Bayer Plus Aspirin Tablets (Sterling Health) p 429, 742
Extra Strength Bayer Plus Aspirin Caplets (Sterling Health) p 429, 744
Adult Low Strength Bayer Enteric Aspirin Tablets (Sterling Health) p 429, 741
Regular Strength Bayer Enteric Aspirin Caplets (Sterling Health) p 429, 741
Arthritis Strength Bufferin Analgesic Caplets (Bristol-Myers Products) p 404, 519
Extra Strength Bufferin Analgesic Tablets (Bristol-Myers Products) p 404, 520
Bufferin Analgesic Tablets and Caplets (Bristol-Myers Products) p 404, 517
Cama Arthritis Pain Reliever (Sandoz Consumer) p 688
Ecotrin Enteric Coated Aspirin Maximum Strength Tablets and Caplets (SmithKline Beecham Consumer) p 426, 718
Ecotrin Enteric Coated Aspirin Regular Strength Tablets and Caplets (SmithKline Beecham Consumer) p 426, 718
Empirin Aspirin (Burroughs Wellcome) p 406, 538
Excedrin Extra-Strength Analgesic Tablets & Caplets (Bristol-Myers Products) p 405, 526
4-Way Cold Tablets (Bristol-Myers Products) p 529
Norwich Aspirin (Chattem) p 546
Norwich Aspirin - Maximum Strength (Chattem) p 546
Norwich Enteric Safety Coated Aspirin (Chattem) p 546
Norwich Enteric Safety Coated Aspirin - Maximum Strength (Chattem) p 546
P-A-C Analgesic Tablets (Roberts) p 420, 669
Sine-Off Sinus Medicine Tablets-Aspirin Formula (SmithKline Beecham Consumer) p 428, 731
St. Joseph Adult Chewable Aspirin (81 mg.) (Schering-Plough HealthCare) p 709
Ursinus Inlay-Tabs (Sandoz Consumer) p 696
Vanquish Analgesic Caplets (Sterling Health) p 431, 756

ASPIRIN BUFFERED
Ascriptin A/D Caplets (Rhone-Poulenc Rorer Consumer) p 419, 661
Extra Strength Ascriptin Caplets (Rhone-Poulenc Rorer Consumer) p 419, 660
Regular Strength Ascriptin Tablets (Rhone-Poulenc Rorer Consumer) p 419, 659
Extra Strength Bayer Plus Aspirin Caplets (Sterling Health) p 429, 744
Arthritis Strength Bufferin Analgesic Caplets (Bristol-Myers Products) p 404, 519
Extra Strength Bufferin Analgesic Tablets (Bristol-Myers Products) p 404, 520
Bufferin Analgesic Tablets and Caplets (Bristol-Myers Products) p 404, 517

ASPIRIN, ENTERIC COATED
Adult Low Strength Bayer Enteric Aspirin Tablets (Sterling Health) p 429, 741
Regular Strength Bayer Enteric Aspirin Caplets (Sterling Health) p 429, 741
Norwich Enteric Safety Coated Aspirin (Chattem) p 546
Norwich Enteric Safety Coated Aspirin - Maximum Strength (Chattem) p 546

ATTAPULGITE
Diasorb Liquid (Columbia) p 408, 557
Diasorb Tablets (Columbia) p 408, 557
Donnagel Liquid and Donnagel Chewable Tablets (Wyeth-Ayerst) p 435, 786
Kaopectate Concentrated Anti-Diarrheal, Peppermint Flavor (Upjohn) p 432, 762
Kaopectate Concentrated Anti-Diarrheal, Regular Flavor (Upjohn) p 432, 762
Kaopectate Children's Chewable Tablets (Upjohn) p 432, 762
Kaopectate Children's Liquid (Upjohn) p 432, 762
Kaopectate Maximum Strength Caplets (Upjohn) p 432, 763

ATTAPULGITE, ACTIVATED
Rheaban Maximum Strength Tablets (Pfizer Consumer) p 639

ATTAPULGITE, NONFIBROUS ACTIVATED
Diasorb Liquid (Columbia) p 408, 557
Diasorb Tablets (Columbia) p 408, 557

B

BACITRACIN
Bactine First Aid Antibiotic Plus Anesthetic Ointment (Miles Consumer) p 415, 614
Mycitracin Plus Pain Reliever (Upjohn) p 432, 763
Maximum Strength Mycitracin Triple Antibiotic First Aid Ointment (Upjohn) p 432, 763

BACITRACIN ZINC
Aquaphor Antibiotic Ointment (Beiersdorf) p 403, 510
Campho-Phenique Triple Antibiotic Ointment Plus Pain Reliever (Sterling Health) p 429, 747
Neosporin Ointment (Burroughs Wellcome) p 406, 538
Neosporin Plus Maximum Strength Ointment (Burroughs Wellcome) p 407, 539
Polysporin Ointment (Burroughs Wellcome) p 407, 539
Polysporin Powder (Burroughs Wellcome) p 407, 540

BALSAM PERU, SPECIAL FRACTION OF
Balmex Baby Powder (Macsil) p 582
Balmex Ointment (Macsil) p 582

BELLADONNA ALKALOIDS
Hyland's Bed Wetting Tablets (Standard Homeopathic) p 735
Hyland's EnurAid Tablets (Standard Homeopathic) p 737
Hyland's Teething Tablets (Standard Homeopathic) p 737

BENZALKONIUM CHLORIDE
Bactine Antiseptic/Anesthetic First Aid Liquid (Miles Consumer) p 415, 614
Orajel Mouth-Aid for Canker and Cold Sores (Del Pharmaceuticals) p 408, 559
Zephiran Chloride Aqueous Solution (Sanofi Winthrop Pharmaceuticals) p 697
Zephiran Chloride Spray (Sanofi Winthrop Pharmaceuticals) p 697
Zephiran Chloride Tinted Tincture (Sanofi Winthrop Pharmaceuticals) p 697

BENZETHONIUM CHLORIDE
Clinical Care Dermal Wound Cleanser (Care-Tech) p 544
Formula Magic Antibacterial Powder (Care-Tech) p 544
Orchid Fresh II Perineal/Ostomy Cleanser (Care-Tech) p 544

BENZOCAINE
Americaine Hemorrhoidal Ointment (Fisons Consumer Health) p 409, 562
Americaine Topical Anesthetic First Aid Ointment (Fisons Consumer Health) p 409, 562
Americaine Topical Anesthetic Spray (Fisons Consumer Health) p 409, 562
Baby Anbesol (Whitehall) p 434, 775

CHOLINE BITARTRATE

CHROMIUM POLYNICOTINATE

CITRIC ACID

CLEMASTINE FUMARATE

CLOTRIMAZOLE

COAL TAR

COCOA BUTTER

COD LIVER OIL

CODEINE PHOSPHATE

COLLOIDAL OATMEAL

COPPER

CYANOCOBALAMIN

Bugs Bunny Plus Iron Children's Chewable Vitamins (Sugar Free) (Miles Consumer) p 415, 615
Flintstones Children's Chewable Vitamins (Miles Consumer) p 415, 615
Flintstones Children's Chewable Vitamins With Extra C (Miles Consumer) p 415, 615
Flintstones Children's Chewable Vitamins Plus Iron (Miles Consumer) p 415, 615
Geritol Liquid - High Potency Iron & Vitamin Tonic (SmithKline Beecham Consumer) p 723
One-A-Day Essential Vitamins (Miles Consumer) p 416, 618
One-A-Day Maximum Formula Vitamins and Minerals (Miles Consumer) p 416, 618
One-A-Day Plus Extra C Vitamins (Miles Consumer) p 416, 618

CYCLIZINE HYDROCHLORIDE
Marezine Tablets (Burroughs Wellcome) p 406, 538

D

L-DESOXYEPHEDRINE
Vicks Inhaler (Procter & Gamble) p 653

DEXBROMPHENIRAMINE MALEATE
Cheracol Sinus (Roberts) p 666
Drixoral Cold and Allergy Sustained-Action Tablets (Schering-Plough HealthCare) p 425, 705
Drixoral Cold and Flu Extended-Release Tablets (Schering-Plough HealthCare) p 425, 705
Drixoral Sinus (Schering-Plough HealthCare) p 425, 706

DEXTROMETHORPHAN HYDROBROMIDE
Alka-Seltzer Plus Cold & Cough Medicine (Miles Consumer) p 415, 613
Alka-Seltzer Plus Night-Time Cold Medicine (Miles Consumer) p 415, 612
Benylin DM Pediatric Cough Formula (Parke-Davis) p 418, 632
Benylin Expectorant (Parke-Davis) p 418, 633
Cerose-DM (Wyeth-Ayerst) p 435, 785
Cheracol-D Cough Formula (Roberts) p 420, 667
Cheracol Plus Head Cold/Cough Formula (Roberts) p 420, 667
Cough Formula Comtrex (Bristol-Myers Products) p 404, 522
Comtrex Multi-Symptom Cold Reliever Tablets/Caplets/Liqui-Gels/Liquid (Bristol-Myers Products) p 404, 520
Comtrex Multi-Symptom Day-Night Caplet-Tablet (Bristol-Myers Products) p 404, 523
Comtrex Multi-Symptom Non-Drowsy Caplets (Bristol-Myers Products) p 404, 524
Contac Day & Night Cold & Flu - Day Caplets (SmithKline Beecham Consumer) p 426, 715
Contac Severe Cold and Flu Formula Caplets (SmithKline Beecham Consumer) p 426, 717
Contac Severe Cold & Flu Nighttime (SmithKline Beecham Consumer) p 426, 718
Dimetapp DM Elixir (Robins Consumer) p 421, 676
Dorcol Children's Cough Syrup (Sandoz Consumer) p 422, 689
Dristan Juice Mix-In (Whitehall) p 434, 776
Hold DM Cough Suppressant Lozenge (Menley & James) p 414, 606
Medi-Flu Caplet, Liquid (Parke-Davis) p 418, 634
Medi-Flu Without Drowsiness Caplets (Parke-Davis) p 418, 634
Novahistine DMX (SmithKline Beecham Consumer) p 427, 726
Ornex Severe Cold Formula Caplets (Menley & James) p 414, 608
Orthoxicol Cough Syrup (Roberts) p 669
PediaCare Cough-Cold Chewable Tablets (McNeil Consumer Products) p 413, 584
PediaCare Cough-Cold Liquid (McNeil Consumer Products) p 413, 584
PediaCare Night Rest Cough-Cold Liquid (McNeil Consumer Products) p 413, 584
Redacon DX Pediatric Drops (Reese Chemical) p 658
Robitussin Cough Calmers (Robins Consumer) p 680
Robitussin Maximum Strength Cough Suppressant (Robins Consumer) p 421, 680
Robitussin Maximum Strength Cough & Cold (Robins Consumer) p 421, 681
Robitussin Night Relief (Robins Consumer) p 421, 681
Robitussin Pediatric Cough & Cold Formula (Robins Consumer) p 421, 682
Robitussin Pediatric Cough Suppressant (Robins Consumer) p 421, 682
Robitussin-CF (Robins Consumer) p 421, 678
Robitussin-DM (Robins Consumer) p 421, 679
Scot-Tussin DM Cough Chasers Lozenges Sugar-Free (Scot-Tussin) p 712
Scot-Tussin DM Sugar-Free (Scot-Tussin) p 712
St. Joseph Cough Suppressant for Children (Schering-Plough HealthCare) p 711
Sudafed Cough Syrup (Burroughs Wellcome) p 407, 540
Sudafed Severe Cold Formula Caplets (Burroughs Wellcome) p 407, 542
Sudafed Severe Cold Formula Tablets (Burroughs Wellcome) p 407, 542
TheraFlu Flu, Cold and Cough Medicine (Sandoz Consumer) p 423, 691
TheraFlu Maximum Strength Nighttime Flu, Cold and Cough Medicine (Sandoz Consumer) p 423, 692
Triaminic Nite Light (Sandoz Consumer) p 423, 693
Triaminic-DM Syrup (Sandoz Consumer) p 423, 694
Triaminicol Multi-Symptom Cold and Cough Medicine (Sandoz Consumer) p 423, 695
Triaminicol Multi-Symptom Relief (Sandoz Consumer) p 423, 695
Children's Tylenol Cold Plus Cough Multi Symptom Liquid Formula (McNeil Consumer Products) p 412, 591
Tylenol Cold & Flu Hot Medication, Packets (McNeil Consumer Products) p 412, 593
Tylenol Cold & Flu No Drowsiness Hot Medication, Packets (McNeil Consumer Products) p 412, 596
Tylenol Cold Multi Symptom Medication Caplets and Tablets (McNeil Consumer Products) p 412, 594
Tylenol Cold Medication No Drowsiness Formula Gelcaps and Caplets (McNeil Consumer Products) p 412, 595
Tylenol Cold Night Time Medication Liquid (McNeil Consumer Products) p 412, 597
Tylenol Cough Medication Maximum Strength Liquid (McNeil Consumer Products) p 412, 598
Tylenol Cough Medication Maximum Strength Liquid with Decongestant (McNeil Consumer Products) p 412, 599
Vicks Children's NyQuil Nighttime Cold/Cough Medicine (Procter & Gamble) p 649
Vicks DayQuil (Procter & Gamble) p 651
Vicks DayQuil LiquiCaps (Procter & Gamble) p 651
Vicks Formula 44 Cough Medicine (Procter & Gamble) p 651
Vicks Formula 44D Cough & Decongestant Medicine (Procter & Gamble) p 652
Vicks Formula 44E Cough & Expectorant Medicine (Procter & Gamble) p 652
Vicks Formula 44M Multi-Symptom Cough & Cold Medicine (Procter & Gamble) p 652
Vicks NyQuil LiquiCaps Nighttime Cold/Flu Medicine (Procter & Gamble) p 653
Vicks NyQuil Nighttime Cold/Flu Medicine - Regular & Cherry Flavor (Procter & Gamble) p 653
Vicks Pediatric Formula 44 Cough Medicine (Procter & Gamble) p 654
Vicks Pediatric Formula 44d Cough & Decongestant Medicine (Procter & Gamble) p 654
Vicks Pediatric Formula 44e Cough & Expectorant Medicine (Procter & Gamble) p 655
Vicks Pediatric Formula 44m Multi-Symptom Cough & Cold Medicine (Procter & Gamble) p 655

DEXTROMETHORPHAN POLISTIREX
Delsym Cough Formula (Fisons Corporation) p 566

DEXTROSE
Emetrol (Bock Pharmacal) p 404, 516

DIBUCAINE
Nupercainal Hemorrhoidal and Anesthetic Ointment (CIBA Consumer) p 408, 554
Nupercainal Pain Relief Cream (CIBA Consumer) p 408, 554

DIHYDROXYALUMINUM SODIUM CARBONATE
Rolaids Antacid Tablets (Warner-Lambert) p 433, 770

DIMENHYDRINATE
Dramamine Chewable Tablets (Upjohn) p 432, 761
Children's Dramamine (Upjohn) p 432, 761
Dramamine Tablets (Upjohn) p 432, 761

DIMETHICONE
Almay Therapeutic Body Treatment (Almay) p 504
Vaseline Intensive Care Lotion Extra Strength (Chesebrough-Pond's) p 549

DIOCTYL SODIUM SULFOSUCCINATE (see DOCUSATE SODIUM)

DIPERODON HYDROCHLORIDE
Bactine First Aid Antibiotic Plus Anesthetic Ointment (Miles Consumer) p 415, 614

DIPHENHYDRAMINE CITRATE
Bufferin AF Nite Time Analgesic/Sleeping Aid Caplets (Bristol-Myers Products) p 404, 518
Excedrin P.M. Analgesic/Sleeping Aid Tablets, Caplets and Liquid (Bristol-Myers Products) p 405, 527

DIPHENHYDRAMINE HYDROCHLORIDE
Actifed Sinus Daytime/Nighttime Caplets (Burroughs Wellcome) p 406, 535
Actifed Sinus Daytime/Nighttime Tablets (Burroughs Wellcome) p 406, 536

Dermarest DriCort 1% Hydrocortisone Creme (Del Pharmaceuticals) p 408, 558

I

IBUPROFEN
Advil Cold and Sinus (formerly CoAdvil) (Whitehall) p 433, 774
Advil Ibuprofen Caplets and Tablets (Whitehall) p 433, 774
Bayer Select Ibuprofen Pain Relief Formula (Sterling Health) p 429, 744
Cramp End Tablets (Ohm Laboratories) p 416, 623
Dimetapp Sinus Caplets (Robins Consumer) p 421, 677
Dristan Sinus (Whitehall) p 434, 779
Haltran Tablets (Roberts) p 420, 668
Ibuprohm Ibuprofen Caplets (Ohm Laboratories) p 416, 623
Ibuprohm Ibuprofen Tablets (Ohm Laboratories) p 416, 623
Cramp Relief Formula Midol IB (Sterling Health) p 430, 749
Motrin IB Caplets and Tablets (Upjohn) p 432, 763
Nuprin Ibuprofen/Analgesic Tablets & Caplets (Bristol-Myers Products) p 405, 531

ICHTHAMMOL
PRID Salve (Walker Pharmacal) p 766

IODINE
One-A-Day Maximum Formula Vitamins and Minerals (Miles Consumer) p 416, 618
Stuart Prenatal Tablets (Wyeth-Ayerst) p 435, 789
The Stuart Formula Tablets (J&J•Merck Consumer) p 410, 573

IPECAC
Hyland's Cough Syrup with Honey (Standard Homeopathic) p 736

IRON POLYSACCHARIDE COMPLEX (see POLYSACCHARIDE IRON COMPLEX)

ISOTONIC SOLUTION
Lavoptik Eye Wash (Lavoptik) p 575

L

LACTASE (BETA-D-GALACTOSIDASE)
Dairy Ease Caplets and Tablets (Sterling Health) p 429, 430, 748
Dairy Ease Drops (Sterling Health) p 430, 748
Lactaid Caplets (Now marketed by McNeil Consumer Products Co.) (Lactaid) p 413, 575
Lactaid Drops (Now marketed by McNeil Consumer Products Co.) (Lactaid) p 413, 575

LACTIC ACID
Massengill Liquid Concentrate (SmithKline Beecham Consumer) p 725
Massengill Unscented Soft Cloth Towelette (SmithKline Beecham Consumer) p 725

LACTOBACILLUS ACIDOPHILUS
DDS-Acidophilus (UAS Laboratories) p 760
Flora-Plus Capsules (Wellness International) p 772
Pro-Bionate Powder and Capsules (Natren) p 620
Superdophilus (Natren) p 620

LACTOBACILLUS BIFIDUS
Flora-Plus Capsules (Wellness International) p 772

LACTOBACILLUS BULGARICUS
Flora-Plus Capsules (Wellness International) p 772

LANOLIN
A and D Ointment (Schering-Plough HealthCare) p 423, 699
Borofax Ointment (Burroughs Wellcome) p 538
Eucerin Dry Skin Care Lotion (Fragrance-free) (Beiersdorf) p 404, 511

LANOLIN OIL
Alpha Keri Moisture Rich Body Oil (Bristol-Myers Products) p 405, 517
Balmex Emollient Lotion (Macsil) p 582

LEVULOSE
Emetrol (Bock Pharmacal) p 404, 516

LIDOCAINE
Campho-Phenique Triple Antibiotic Ointment Plus Pain Reliever (Sterling Health) p 429, 747
DermaFlex Topical Anesthetic Gel Coating (Zila Pharmaceuticals) p 435, 789
Mycitracin Plus Pain Reliever (Upjohn) p 432, 763
Neosporin Plus Maximum Strength Cream (Burroughs Wellcome) p 406, 539
Neosporin Plus Maximum Strength Ointment (Burroughs Wellcome) p 407, 539
Water-Jel Burn Jel (Water-Jel Technologies) p 772
Xylocaine 2.5% Ointment (Astra) p 403, 507
Zilactin-L Liquid (Zila Pharmaceuticals) p 435, 789

LIDOCAINE HYDROCHLORIDE
Bactine Antiseptic/Anesthetic First Aid Liquid (Miles Consumer) p 415, 614
Campho-Phenique Triple Antibiotic Ointment Plus Pain Reliever (Sterling Health) p 429, 747

LIVE YEAST CELL DERIVATIVE
Preparation H Hemorrhoidal Cream (Whitehall) p 434, 780
Preparation H Hemorrhoidal Ointment (Whitehall) p 434, 780
Preparation H Hemorrhoidal Suppositories (Whitehall) p 434, 780
Wyanoids Relief Factor Hemorrhoidal Suppositories (Wyeth-Ayerst) p 435, 789

LOPERAMIDE HYDROCHLORIDE
Imodium A-D Caplets and Liquid (McNeil Consumer Products) p 413, 583
Loperamide Hydrochloride Caplets (Ohm Laboratories) p 416, 623
Pepto Diarrhea Control (Procter & Gamble) p 648

LYSINE
Incremin with Iron Syrup (Lederle) p 580

M

MAGALDRATE
Riopan Suspension (Whitehall) p 782
Riopan Plus Suspension (Whitehall) p 782
Riopan Plus 2 Suspension (Whitehall) p 434, 782

MAGNESIUM CARBONATE
Gaviscon Extra Strength Relief Formula Antacid Tablets (SmithKline Beecham Consumer) p 427, 722
Gaviscon Extra Strength Relief Formula Liquid Antacid (SmithKline Beecham Consumer) p 427, 722
Gaviscon Liquid Antacid (SmithKline Beecham Consumer) p 427, 722
Maalox HRF Heartburn Relief Formula Suspension (Rhone-Poulenc Rorer Consumer) p 419, 662
Maalox HRF Heartburn Relief Formula Antacid Tablets (Rhone-Poulenc Rorer Consumer) p 419, 662
Marblen Suspension Peach/Apricot (Fleming) p 567
Marblen Suspension Unflavored (Fleming) p 567
Marblen Tablets (Fleming) p 567
Mylanta Gelcaps Antacid (J&J•Merck Consumer) p 410, 573

MAGNESIUM CHLORIDE
Chlor-3 Condiment (Fleming) p 566

MAGNESIUM GLUCONATE
Magonate Tablets and Liquid (Fleming) p 567

MAGNESIUM HYDROXIDE
Aludrox Oral Suspension (Wyeth-Ayerst) p 435, 784
Ascriptin A/D Caplets (Rhone-Poulenc Rorer Consumer) p 419, 661
Extra Strength Ascriptin Caplets (Rhone-Poulenc Rorer Consumer) p 419, 660
Regular Strength Ascriptin Tablets (Rhone-Poulenc Rorer Consumer) p 419, 659
Di-Gel Antacid/Anti-Gas (Schering-Plough HealthCare) p 425, 704
Gelusil Liquid & Tablets (Parke-Davis) p 418, 634
Haley's M-O, Regular & Flavored (Sterling Health) p 430, 749
Maalox Suspension (Rhone-Poulenc Rorer Consumer) p 420, 663
Maalox Plus Tablets (Rhone-Poulenc Rorer Consumer) p 420, 663
Extra Strength Maalox Plus Suspension (Rhone-Poulenc Rorer Consumer) p 420, 664
Extra Strength Maalox Plus Tablets (Rhone-Poulenc Rorer Consumer) p 420, 664
Mylanta Liquid (J&J•Merck Consumer) p 410, 570
Mylanta Tablets (J&J•Merck Consumer) p 410, 570
Mylanta Double Strength Liquid (J&J•Merck Consumer) p 410, 571
Mylanta Double Strength Tablets (J&J•Merck Consumer) p 410, 571
Phillips' Chewable Tablets (Sterling Health) p 431, 754
Concentrated Phillips' Milk of Magnesia (Sterling Health) p 430, 754
Phillips' Milk of Magnesia Liquid (Sterling Health) p 430, 753
Tempo Soft Antacid with Antigas Action (Thompson Medical) p 431, 760
WinGel Liquid (Sterling Health) p 757

MAGNESIUM LACTATE
CalLink Calcium and Magnesium Complex (BioLink International) p 512
MagTab SR Caplets (Niché Pharmaceuticals) p 622

MAGNESIUM OXIDE
Beelith Tablets (Beach) p 510
Bufferin Analgesic Tablets and Caplets (Bristol-Myers Products) p 404, 517
Cama Arthritis Pain Reliever (Sandoz Consumer) p 688
Mag-Ox 400 (Blaine) p 512
Uro-Mag (Blaine) p 512

MAGNESIUM SALICYLATE
Doan's - Extra-Strength Analgesic (CIBA Consumer) p 407, 550
Extra Strength Doan's P.M. (CIBA Consumer) p 407, 550
Doan's - Regular Strength Analgesic (CIBA Consumer) p 407, 551
Mobigesic Analgesic Tablets (Ascher) p 403, 506
Maximum Pain Relief Pamprin Caplets (Chattem) p 548

MAGNESIUM TRISILICATE

Gaviscon Antacid Tablets (SmithKline Beecham Consumer) p 427, 722
Gaviscon-2 Antacid Tablets (SmithKline Beecham Consumer) p 427, 723

MALT SOUP EXTRACT

Maltsupex Liquid, Powder & Tablets (Wallace) p 432, 766

MECLIZINE HYDROCHLORIDE

Bonine Tablets (Pfizer Consumer) p 638
Dramamine II Tablets (Upjohn) p 432, 762

MENTHOL

Almay Anti-Itch Lotion (Almay) p 503
Aurum Analgesic Lotion (Au Pharmaceuticals) p 507
Ben-Gay External Analgesic Products (Pfizer Consumer) p 638
Cēpacol Dry Throat Lozenges, Cherry Flavor (SmithKline Beecham Consumer) p 426, 713
Cēpacol Dry Throat Lozenges, Honey-Lemon Flavor (SmithKline Beecham Consumer) p 426, 713
Cēpacol Dry Throat Lozenges, Menthol-Eucalyptus Flavor (SmithKline Beecham Consumer) p 426, 713
Cēpastat Cherry Flavor Sore Throat Lozenges (SmithKline Beecham Consumer) p 426, 714
Cēpastat Extra Strength Sore Throat Lozenges (SmithKline Beecham Consumer) p 426, 714
Chap Stick Medicated Lip Balm (Robins Consumer) p 420, 673
Chloraseptic Lozenges, Cherry, Cool Mint or Menthol (Procter & Gamble) p 644
Eucalyptamint 100% All Natural Ointment (CIBA Consumer) p 407, 552
Eucalyptamint Muscle Pain Relief Formula (CIBA Consumer) p 407, 552
Feminine Gold Analgesic Lotion (Au Pharmaceuticals) p 507
Flex-all 454 Pain Relieving Gel (Chattem) p 545
Halls Mentho-Lyptus Cough Suppressant Tablets (Warner-Lambert) p 433, 769
Halls Plus Cough Suppressant Tablets (Warner-Lambert) p 433, 769
Icy Hot Balm (Chattem) p 545
Icy Hot Cream (Chattem) p 545
Icy Hot Stick (Chattem) p 545
Listerine Antiseptic (Warner-Lambert) p 433, 770
Cool Mint Listerine Antiseptic (Warner-Lambert) p 433, 770
N'ICE Medicated Sugarless Sore Throat and Cough Lozenges (SmithKline Beecham Consumer) p 726
Rhuligel (Rydelle) p 422, 688
Robitussin Cough Drops (Robins Consumer) p 421, 680
Soothers Throat Drops (Warner-Lambert) p 433, 771
Sportscreme External Analgesic Rub Ice (Thompson Medical) p 431, 760
Theragold Analgesic Lotion (Au Pharmaceuticals) p 507
Therapeutic Gold Analgesic Lotion (Au Pharmaceuticals) p 507
Therapeutic Mineral Ice, Pain Relieving Gel (Bristol-Myers Products) p 405, 534
Therapeutic Mineral Ice Exercise Formula, Pain Relieving Gel (Bristol-Myers Products) p 406, 534
Vicks Cough Drops (Procter & Gamble) p 650
Extra Strength Vicks Cough Drops (Procter & Gamble) p 651
Vicks VapoRub (Procter & Gamble) p 656
Vicks VapoSteam (Procter & Gamble) p 657

MENTHYL ANTHRANILATE

Neutrogena Sunblock SPF 15 (Neutrogena) p 416, 621
Neutrogena Sunblock SPF 30 (Neutrogena) p 416, 621

METHIONINE

Geritol Liquid - High Potency Iron & Vitamin Tonic (SmithKline Beecham Consumer) p 723

METHYL SALICYLATE

Aurum Analgesic Lotion (Au Pharmaceuticals) p 507
Ben-Gay External Analgesic Products (Pfizer Consumer) p 638
Icy Hot Balm (Chattem) p 545
Icy Hot Cream (Chattem) p 545
Icy Hot Stick (Chattem) p 545
Listerine Antiseptic (Warner-Lambert) p 433, 770
Cool Mint Listerine Antiseptic (Warner-Lambert) p 433, 770
Theragold Analgesic Lotion (Au Pharmaceuticals) p 507
Therapeutic Gold Analgesic Lotion (Au Pharmaceuticals) p 507

METHYLCELLULOSE

Citrucel Orange Flavor (SmithKline Beecham Consumer) p 426, 715
Citrucel Sugar Free Orange Flavor (SmithKline Beecham Consumer) p 426, 715

MICONAZOLE NITRATE

Micatin Antifungal Cream (Ortho Pharmaceutical) p 417, 626
Micatin Antifungal Odor Control Spray Powder (Ortho Pharmaceutical) p 417, 626
Micatin Antifungal Powder (Ortho Pharmaceutical) p 417, 626
Micatin Antifungal Spray Liquid (Ortho Pharmaceutical) p 417, 626
Micatin Antifungal Spray Powder (Ortho Pharmaceutical) p 417, 626
Micatin Jock Itch Cream (Ortho Pharmaceutical) p 626
Micatin Jock Itch Spray Powder (Ortho Pharmaceutical) p 626
Monistat 7 Vaginal Cream (Ortho Pharmaceutical) p 417, 626
Monistat 7 Vaginal Suppositories (Ortho Pharmaceutical) p 417, 626

MILK, LACTASE REDUCED

Dairy Ease Real Milk (Sterling Health) p 430, 748

MILK OF MAGNESIA

Phillips' Chewable Tablets (Sterling Health) p 431, 754
Concentrated Phillips' Milk of Magnesia (Sterling Health) p 430, 754
Phillips' Milk of Magnesia Liquid (Sterling Health) p 430, 753

MINERAL OIL

Agoral, Marshmallow Flavor (Parke-Davis) p 627
Agoral, Raspberry Flavor (Parke-Davis) p 627
Anusol Ointment (Parke-Davis) p 417, 628
Aquaphor Healing Ointment (Beiersdorf) p 403, 511
Aquaphor Healing Ointment, Original Formula (Beiersdorf) p 403, 510
Eucerin Dry Skin Care Lotion (Fragrance-free) (Beiersdorf) p 404, 511
Eucerin Plus Moisturizing Lotion (Beiersdorf) p 404, 512
Haley's M-O, Regular & Flavored (Sterling Health) p 430, 749
Keri Lotion - Original Formula (Bristol-Myers Products) p 405, 530
Lacri-Lube NP Lubricant Ophthalmic Ointment (Allergan Pharmaceuticals) p 502
Lacri-Lube S.O.P. Sterile Ophthalmic Ointment (Allergan Pharmaceuticals) p 502
Lubriderm Bath Oil (Warner-Lambert) p 770
Nephrox Suspension (Fleming) p 567
P & S Liquid (Baker Cummins Dermatologicals) p 403, 508
Refresh P.M. Lubricant Ophthalmic Ointment (Allergan Pharmaceuticals) p 503
Replens (Parke-Davis) p 418, 635
Ultra Mide 25 (Baker Cummins Dermatologicals) p 403, 509

MINERAL WAX

Aquaphor Healing Ointment (Beiersdorf) p 403, 511
Aquaphor Healing Ointment, Original Formula (Beiersdorf) p 403, 510

MONOCLONAL ANTIBODY

Clearblue Easy (Whitehall) p 434, 794

MULTIMINERALS
(see VITAMINS WITH MINERALS)

MULTIVITAMINS
(see VITAMINS, MULTIPLE)

MULTIVITAMINS WITH MINERALS
(see VITAMINS WITH MINERALS)

N

NAPHAZOLINE HYDROCHLORIDE

Clear Eyes ACR Astringent/Lubricating Eye Redness Reliever (Ross) p 421, 683
Clear Eyes Lubricating Eye Redness Reliever (Ross) p 421, 683
4-Way Fast Acting Nasal Spray (regular & mentholated) & Metered Spray Pump (regular) (Bristol-Myers Products) p 405, 529
Privine Nasal Solution and Drops (CIBA Consumer) p 408, 555
Privine Nasal Spray (CIBA Consumer) p 408, 555

NEOMYCIN SULFATE

Bactine First Aid Antibiotic Plus Anesthetic Ointment (Miles Consumer) p 415, 614
Campho-Phenique Triple Antibiotic Ointment Plus Pain Reliever (Sterling Health) p 429, 747
Mycitracin Plus Pain Reliever (Upjohn) p 432, 763
Maximum Strength Mycitracin Triple Antibiotic First Aid Ointment (Upjohn) p 432, 763
Neosporin Ointment (Burroughs Wellcome) p 406, 538
Neosporin Plus Maximum Strength Cream (Burroughs Wellcome) p 406, 539
Neosporin Plus Maximum Strength Ointment (Burroughs Wellcome) p 407, 539

NIACIN

Allbee with C Caplets (Robins Consumer) p 671
Allbee C-800 Plus Iron Tablets (Robins Consumer) p 671
Allbee C-800 Tablets (Robins Consumer) p 671
Bugs Bunny Children's Chewable Vitamins (Sugar Free) (Miles Consumer) p 415, 615
Bugs Bunny With Extra C Children's Chewable Vitamins (Sugar Free) (Miles Consumer) p 415, 615
Bugs Bunny Plus Iron Children's Chewable Vitamins (Sugar Free) (Miles Consumer) p 415, 615
Flintstones Children's Chewable Vitamins (Miles Consumer) p 415, 615
Flintstones Children's Chewable Vitamins With Extra C (Miles Consumer) p 415, 615

PETROLATUM
A and D Ointment (Schering-Plough HealthCare) p 423, 699
Aquaphor Healing Ointment (Beiersdorf) p 403, 511
Aquaphor Healing Ointment, Original Formula (Beiersdorf) p 403, 510
Caldesene Medicated Ointment (Fisons Consumer Health) p 409, 563
Chap Stick Lip Balm (Robins Consumer) p 420, 673
Chap Stick Medicated Lip Balm (Robins Consumer) p 420, 673
Chap Stick Sunblock 15 Lip Balm (Robins Consumer) p 420, 674
Chap Stick Petroleum Jelly Plus (Robins Consumer) p 420, 674
Chap Stick Petroleum Jelly Plus with Sunblock 15 (Robins Consumer) p 420, 674
Eucerin Dry Skin Care Creme (Beiersdorf) p 404, 511
Keri Lotion -Silky Smooth with Vitamin E (Bristol-Myers Products) p 405, 530
Keri Lotion - Silky Smooth Fragrance Free with Vitamin E (Bristol-Myers Products) p 405, 530
Lacri-Lube NP Lubricant Ophthalmic Ointment (Allergan Pharmaceuticals) p 502
Lacri-Lube S.O.P. Sterile Ophthalmic Ointment (Allergan Pharmaceuticals) p 502
Neutrogena Norwegian Formula Emulsion (Neutrogena) p 416, 621
Preparation H Hemorrhoidal Cream (Whitehall) p 434, 780
Preparation H Hemorrhoidal Ointment (Whitehall) p 434, 780
Refresh P.M. Lubricant Ophthalmic Ointment (Allergan Pharmaceuticals) p 503

PETROLATUM, WHITE
Vaseline Pure Petroleum Jelly Skin Protectant (Chesebrough-Pond's) p 548

PHENAZOPYRIDINE HYDROCHLORIDE
Azo-Standard (PolyMedica Pharmaceuticals) p 642

PHENIRAMINE MALEATE
Dristan Nasal Spray, Regular (Whitehall) p 777
Dristan Nasal Spray, Menthol (Whitehall) p 777

PHENOBARBITAL
Bronkolixir (Sanofi Winthrop Pharmaceuticals) p 696
Bronkotabs Tablets (Sanofi Winthrop Pharmaceuticals) p 696

PHENOL
Anbesol Gel - Regular Strength (Whitehall) p 434, 775
Anbesol Liquid - Regular Strength (Whitehall) p 434, 775
Campho-Phenique Cold Sore Gel (Sterling Health) p 429, 747
Campho-Phenique Liquid (Sterling Health) p 429, 747
Cēpastat Cherry Flavor Sore Throat Lozenges (SmithKline Beecham Consumer) p 426, 714
Cēpastat Extra Strength Sore Throat Lozenges (SmithKline Beecham Consumer) p 426, 714
Chap Stick Medicated Lip Balm (Robins Consumer) p 420, 673
Cheracol Sore Throat Spray (Roberts) p 667
Vicks Children's Chloraseptic Spray (Procter & Gamble) p 643
Chloraseptic Liquid, Cherry, Menthol or Cool Mint (Procter & Gamble) p 643
PRID Salve (Walker Pharmacal) p 766

PHENOLPHTHALEIN
Agoral, Marshmallow Flavor (Parke-Davis) p 627
Agoral, Raspberry Flavor (Parke-Davis) p 627
Correctol Laxative Tablets (Schering-Plough HealthCare) p 425, 704
Dialose Plus Tablets (J&J•Merck Consumer) p 409, 569
Doxidan Liqui-Gels (Upjohn) p 432, 761
Ex-Lax Chocolated Laxative Tablets (Sandoz Consumer) p 422, 690
Extra Gentle Ex-Lax Laxative Pills (Sandoz Consumer) p 422, 690
Maximum Relief Formula Ex-Lax Laxative Pills (Sandoz Consumer) p 422, 690
Regular Strength Ex-Lax Laxative Pills (Sandoz Consumer) p 422, 690
Feen-A-Mint Gum (Schering-Plough HealthCare) p 425, 707
Feen-A-Mint Laxative Pills (Schering-Plough HealthCare) p 425, 707
Phillips' Gelcaps (Sterling Health) p 430, 753

2-PHENYLBENZIMIDAZOLE-5-SULFONIC ACID
Eucerin Dry Skin Care Daily Facial Lotion SPF 20 (Beiersdorf) p 404, 511
Oil of Olay Daily UV Protectant SPF 15 Beauty Fluid-Original and Fragrance Free (Olay Co. Inc.) (Procter & Gamble) p 647
Oil of Olay Daily UV Protectant SPF 15 Moisture Replenishing Cream-Original and Fragrance Free (Olay Co. Inc.) (Procter & Gamble) p 647

PHENYLEPHRINE HYDROCHLORIDE
Alconephrin Nasal Decongestant (PolyMedica Pharmaceuticals) p 642
Anusol Hemorrhoidal Suppositories (Parke-Davis) p 417, 628
Cerose-DM (Wyeth-Ayerst) p 435, 785
Congespirin For Children Aspirin Free Chewable Cold Tablets (Bristol-Myers Products) p 405, 525
Dristan Cold (Whitehall) p 434, 777
Dristan Nasal Spray, Regular (Whitehall) p 777
Dristan Nasal Spray, Menthol (Whitehall) p 777
4-Way Fast Acting Nasal Spray (regular & mentholated) & Metered Spray Pump (regular) (Bristol-Myers Products) p 405, 529
Neo-Synephrine Nasal Drops, Pediatric, Mild, Regular & Extra Strength (Sterling Health) p 430, 751
Neo-Synephrine Nasal Sprays, Pediatric, Mild, Regular & Extra Strength (Sterling Health) p 430, 751
Nōstril 1/4% Mild Nasal Decongestant (CIBA Consumer) p 408, 553
Nōstril 1/2% Regular Nasal Decongestant (CIBA Consumer) p 408, 553
Novahistine Elixir (SmithKline Beecham Consumer) p 427, 727
Vicks Sinex Decongestant Nasal Spray (Regular) (Procter & Gamble) p 656
Vicks Sinex Decongestant Nasal Ultra Fine Mist (Procter & Gamble) p 656

PHENYLPROPANOLAMINE BITARTRATE
Alka-Seltzer Plus Cold Medicine (Miles Consumer) p 415, 612
Alka-Seltzer Plus Cold & Cough Medicine (Miles Consumer) p 415, 613
Alka-Seltzer Plus Night-Time Cold Medicine (Miles Consumer) p 415, 612
Alka Seltzer Plus Sinus Allergy Medicine (Miles Consumer) p 415, 613

PHENYLPROPANOLAMINE HYDROCHLORIDE
A.R.M. Allergy Relief Medicine Caplets (Menley & James) p 414, 601
Acutrim 16 Hour Steady Control Appetite Suppressant (CIBA Consumer) p 407, 550
Acutrim Late Day Strength Appetite Suppressant (CIBA Consumer) p 407, 550
Acutrim II Maximum Strength Appetite Suppressant (CIBA Consumer) p 407, 550
Allerest Children's Chewable Tablets (Fisons Consumer Health) p 561
Allerest 12 Hour Caplets (Fisons Consumer Health) p 561
BC Cold Powder Multi-Symptom Formula (Cold-Sinus-Allergy) (Block) p 513
BC Cold Powder Non-Drowsy Formula (Cold-Sinus) (Block) p 513
Cheracol Plus Head Cold/Cough Formula (Roberts) p 420, 667
Chlor-Trimeton Allergy-Sinus Headache Caplets (Schering-Plough HealthCare) p 424, 701
Contac Continuous Action Decongestant/Antihistamine Capsules (SmithKline Beecham Consumer) p 426, 717
Contac Maximum Strength Continuous Action Decongestant/Antihistamine Caplets (SmithKline Beecham Consumer) p 426, 716
Contac Severe Cold and Flu Formula Caplets (SmithKline Beecham Consumer) p 426, 717
Coricidin 'D' Decongestant Tablets (Schering-Plough HealthCare) p 424, 703
Dexatrim Capsules, Caplets, Tablets (Thompson Medical) p 758
Dexatrim Maximum Strength Caffeine-Free Caplets (Thompson Medical) p 758
Dexatrim Maximum Strength Caffeine-Free Capsules (Thompson Medical) p 758
Dexatrim Maximum Strength Extended Duration Time Tablets (Thompson Medical) p 758
Dexatrim Maximum Strength Plus Vitamin C/Caffeine-free Caplets (Thompson Medical) p 431, 758
Dexatrim Maximum Strength Plus Vitamin C/Caffeine-free Capsules (Thompson Medical) p 431, 758
Dimetapp Elixir (Robins Consumer) p 421, 676
Dimetapp Extentabs (Robins Consumer) p 421, 677
Dimetapp Liqui-Gels (Robins Consumer) p 421, 678
Dimetapp Tablets (Robins Consumer) p 421, 678
Dimetapp Cold & Allergy Chewable Tablets (Robins Consumer) p 421, 674
Dimetapp Cold & Flu Caplets (Robins Consumer) p 421, 675
Dimetapp DM Elixir (Robins Consumer) p 421, 676
4-Way Cold Tablets (Bristol-Myers Products) p 529
Orthoxicol Cough Syrup (Roberts) p 669
Pyrroxate Capsules (Roberts) p 420, 669
Redacon DX Pediatric Drops (Reese Chemical) p 658
Robitussin-CF (Robins Consumer) p 421, 678
Sine-Off Sinus Medicine Tablets-Aspirin Formula (SmithKline Beecham Consumer) p 428, 731
St. Joseph Cold Tablets for Children (Schering-Plough HealthCare) p 710
Tavist-D 12 Hour Relief Medicine (Sandoz Consumer) p 423, 691
Triaminic Allergy Medicine (Sandoz Consumer) p 692
Triaminic Chewable Tablets For Children (Sandoz Consumer) p 692
Triaminic Cold Medicine (Sandoz Consumer) p 423, 693

Maximum Strength Multi-Symptom Menstrual Formula Midol (Sterling Health) p 430, 750
PMS Multi-Symptom Formula Midol (Sterling Health) p 430, 749
Regular Strength Multi-Symptom Midol Formula (Sterling Health) p 430, 749
Multi-Symptom Pamprin Tablets and Caplets (Chattem) p 548
Prēmsyn PMS (Chattem) p 548
Robitussin Night Relief (Robins Consumer) p 421, 681

PYRITHIONE ZINC

Head & Shoulders Antidandruff Shampoo (Procter & Gamble) p 644
Head & Shoulders Antidandruff Shampoo 2-in-1 plus Conditioner (Procter & Gamble) p 644
Head & Shoulders Dry Scalp Shampoo (Procter & Gamble) p 644
Head & Shoulders Dry Scalp Shampoo 2-in-1 plus Conditioner (Procter & Gamble) p 644
X-Seb Shampoo (Baker Cummins Dermatologicals) p 403, 509
X-Seb Plus Conditioning Shampoo (Baker Cummins Dermatologicals) p 403, 509
Zincon Dandruff Shampoo (Lederle) p 411, 582

Q

QUININE SULFATE

Legatrin Tablets (Columbia) p 408, 557
Q-vel Muscle Relaxant Pain Reliever (CIBA Consumer) p 408, 555

R

RACEPINEPHRINE HYDROCHLORIDE

AsthmaNefrin Solution "A" Bronchodilator (Menley & James) p 603

RESORCINOL

Acnomel Acne Medication Cream (Menley & James) p 414, 602
BiCozene Creme (Sandoz Consumer) p 422, 688

RETINYL PALMITATE

Aqua-A Cream (Baker Cummins Dermatologicals) p 508

RHUS AROMATICA

Hyland's Bed Wetting Tablets (Standard Homeopathic) p 735

RIBOFLAVIN
(see VITAMIN B_2)

RICE SYRUP SOLIDS

Ricelyte Oral Electrolyte Maintenance Solution Made With Rice Syrup Solids (Mead Johnson Nutritionals) p 601

S

SALICYLAMIDE

Arthritis Strength BC Powder (Block) p 513
BC Powder (Block) p 514

SALICYLIC ACID

Almay Therapeutic Shampoo (Almay) p 504
Compound W Gel (See 1993 Physicians' Desk Reference) (Whitehall) p 775
Compound W Liquid (See 1993 Physicians' Desk Reference) (Whitehall) p 775
DuoFilm Liquid (Schering-Plough HealthCare) p 425, 706
DuoFilm Patch (Schering-Plough HealthCare) p 425, 707
DuoPlant Gel (Schering-Plough HealthCare) p 425, 707
MG 217 Medicated Tar-Free Shampoo (Triton Consumer) p 760
Neutrogena T/Sal Therapeutic Shampoo (Neutrogena) p 416, 622
Oxy Medicated Cleanser (SmithKline Beecham Consumer) p 729
Oxy Medicated Pads - Regular, Sensitive Skin, and Maximum Strength (SmithKline Beecham Consumer) p 730
Oxy Night Watch Nighttime Acne Medication-Maximum Strength and Sensitive Skin Formulas (SmithKline Beecham Consumer) p 730
P & S Shampoo (Baker Cummins Dermatologicals) p 403, 509
Stri-Dex Dual Textured Maximum Strength Pads (Sterling Health) p 431, 756
Stri-Dex Dual Textured Regular Strength Pads (Sterling Health) p 431, 756
Stri-Dex Dual Textured Sensitive Skin Pads (Sterling Health) p 756
Stri-Dex Single Textured Maximum Strength Pads (Sterling Health) p 431, 756
Stri-Dex Super Scrub Pads-Oil Fighting Formula (Sterling Health) p 431, 756
Wart-Off Wart Remover (Pfizer Consumer) p 642

SALINE SOLUTION

Dristan Saline Spray (Whitehall) p 434, 779

SELENIUM SULFIDE

Head & Shoulders Intensive Treatment Dandruff Shampoo (Procter & Gamble) p 645
Head & Shoulders Intensive Treatment Dandruff Shampoo 2-in-1 plus Conditioner (Procter & Gamble) p 645
Selsun Blue Dandruff Shampoo (Ross) p 421, 685
Selsun Blue Dandruff Shampoo Medicated Treatment Formula (Ross) p 421, 685
Selsun Blue Extra Conditioning Formula Dandruff Shampoo (Ross) p 421, 685
Selsun Gold for Women Dandruff Shampoo (Ross) p 422, 686

SENNA CONCENTRATES

Ex-Lax Gentle Nature Laxative Pills (Sandoz Consumer) p 422, 690
Perdiem Granules (Rhone-Poulenc Rorer Consumer) p 420, 665

SHARK LIVER OIL

Preparation H Hemorrhoidal Cream (Whitehall) p 434, 780
Preparation H Hemorrhoidal Ointment (Whitehall) p 434, 780
Preparation H Hemorrhoidal Suppositories (Whitehall) p 434, 780
Wyanoids Relief Factor Hemorrhoidal Suppositories (Wyeth-Ayerst) p 435, 789

SIMETHICONE

Colicon Drops (Reese Chemical) p 658
Di-Gel Antacid/Anti-Gas (Schering-Plough HealthCare) p 425, 704
Gas-X Chewable Tablets (Sandoz Consumer) p 422, 690
Extra Strength Gas-X Chewable Tablets (Sandoz Consumer) p 423, 690
Gelusil Liquid & Tablets (Parke-Davis) p 418, 634
Maalox Plus Tablets (Rhone-Poulenc Rorer Consumer) p 420, 663
Extra Strength Maalox Plus Suspension (Rhone-Poulenc Rorer Consumer) p 420, 664
Extra Strength Maalox Plus Tablets (Rhone-Poulenc Rorer Consumer) p 420, 664
Mylanta Gas Tablets-40 mg (J&J•Merck Consumer) p 410, 572
Mylanta Gas Tablets-80 mg (J&J•Merck Consumer) p 410, 573
Maximum Strength Mylanta Gas Tablets-125 mg (J&J•Merck Consumer) p 410, 573
Mylanta Liquid (J&J•Merck Consumer) p 410, 570
Mylanta Tablets (J&J•Merck Consumer) p 410, 570
Mylanta Double Strength Liquid (J&J•Merck Consumer) p 410, 571
Mylanta Double Strength Tablets (J&J•Merck Consumer) p 410, 571
Mylicon Drops (J&J•Merck Consumer) p 410, 572
Baby Orajel Tooth & Gum Cleanser (Del Pharmaceuticals) p 408, 559
Phazyme Drops (Reed & Carnrick) p 419, 658
Phazyme Tablets (Reed & Carnrick) p 419, 657
Phazyme-125 Softgels Maximum Strength (Reed & Carnrick) p 419, 658
Phazyme-95 Tablets (Reed & Carnrick) p 419, 657
Riopan Plus Suspension (Whitehall) p 782
Riopan Plus 2 Suspension (Whitehall) p 434, 782
Extra Strength Rolaids Antacid Plus Anti-Gas Tablets (Warner-Lambert) p 433, 771
Tempo Soft Antacid with Antigas Action (Thompson Medical) p 431, 760
Tums Anti-gas/Antacid Formula Tablets, Assorted Fruit (SmithKline Beecham Consumer) p 428, 734

SODIUM ASCORBATE

Hyland's Vitamin C for Children (Standard Homeopathic) p 737

SODIUM BICARBONATE

Alka-Seltzer Effervescent Antacid (Miles Consumer) p 415, 611
Alka-Seltzer Effervescent Antacid and Pain Reliever (Miles Consumer) p 414, 609
Alka-Seltzer Extra Strength Effervescent Antacid and Pain Reliever (Miles Consumer) p 415, 612
Alka-Seltzer (Flavored) Effervescent Antacid and Pain Reliever (Miles Consumer) p 414, 610
Arm & Hammer Pure Baking Soda (Church & Dwight) p 549
Citrocarbonate Antacid (Roberts) p 668
Massengill Liquid Concentrate (SmithKline Beecham Consumer) p 725

SODIUM BORATE

Collyrium for Fresh Eyes (Wyeth-Ayerst) p 435, 786
Collyrium Fresh (Wyeth-Ayerst) p 435, 786

SODIUM CARBOXYMETHYLCELLULOSE

Salivart Saliva Substitute (Gebauer) p 567

SODIUM CHLORIDE

Afrin Saline Mist (Schering-Plough HealthCare) p 424, 700
Ayr Saline Nasal Drops (Ascher) p 403, 506
Ayr Saline Nasal Mist (Ascher) p 403, 506
Broncho Saline (Blairex Laboratories) p 513
Chlor-3 Condiment (Fleming) p 566
Nasal Moist (Blairex Laboratories) p 513
NāSal Moisturizer AF Nasal Spray (Sterling Health) p 430, 751
NāSal Moisturizer AF Nasal Drops (Sterling Health) p 430, 751
Ocean Mist (Fleming) p 567
Salinex Nasal Mist and Drops (Muro) p 619
Star-Optic Eye Wash (Stellar) p 428, 737

VITAMIN E

VITAMIN K

VITAMINS WITH IRON

VITAMINS WITH MINERALS

VITAMINS, MULTIPLE

W

WHEY PROTEIN ISOLATE

WHITE PETROLATUM (see PETROLATUM)

WITCH HAZEL
Tucks Cream (Parke-Davis) p 637
Tucks Premoistened Pads (Parke-Davis) p 419, 637
Tucks Take-Alongs (Parke-Davis) p 637

WOOL WAX ALCOHOL
Eucerin Dry Skin Care Creme (Beiersdorf) p 404, 511

X

XYLOMETAZOLINE HYDROCHLORIDE
Otrivin Nasal Drops (CIBA Consumer) p 408, 554
Otrivin Pediatric Nasal Drops (CIBA Consumer) p 408, 554

Z

ZINC
One-A-Day Maximum Formula Vitamins and Minerals (Miles Consumer) p 416, 618
One-A-Day Stressgard Formula Vitamins (Miles Consumer) p 416, 618
One-A-Day Women's Formula Multivitamins with Calcium, Extra Iron, Zinc and Beta Carotene (Miles Consumer) p 416, 618
Stuart Prenatal Tablets (Wyeth-Ayerst) p 435, 789

ZINC CHLORIDE
Orajel Mouth-Aid for Canker and Cold Sores (Del Pharmaceuticals) p 408, 559

ZINC OXIDE
Anusol Ointment (Parke-Davis) p 417, 628
Balmex Baby Powder (Macsil) p 582
Balmex Ointment (Macsil) p 582
Caladryl Clear Lotion (Parke-Davis) p 418, 633
Caldesene Medicated Ointment (Fisons Consumer Health) p 409, 563
Desitin Ointment (Pfizer Consumer) p 419, 638
Nupercainal Suppositories (CIBA Consumer) p 408, 554
Pazo Hemorrhoid Ointment & Suppositories (Bristol-Myers Products) p 405, 531
Tronolane Hemorrhoidal Suppositories (Ross) p 422, 686

ZINC PYRITHIONE (see PYRITHIONE ZINC)

ZINC SULFATE
Clear Eyes ACR Astringent/Lubricating Eye Redness Reliever (Ross) p 421, 683
Visine A.C. Eye Drops (Pfizer Consumer) p 419, 641
Z-BEC Tablets (Robins Consumer) p 683

ZINC UNDECYLENATE
Cruex Antifungal Cream (Fisons Consumer Health) p 409, 563
Cruex Antifungal Spray Powder (Fisons Consumer Health) p 409, 563
Desenex Antifungal Cream (Fisons Consumer Health) p 564
Desenex Antifungal Ointment (Fisons Consumer Health) p 409, 564
Desenex Antifungal Powder (Fisons Consumer Health) p 409, 564
Desenex Antifungal Spray Powder (Fisons Consumer Health) p 409, 564

SECTION 5

Product Identification Section

This section is designed to help you identify products and their packaging.

Participating manufacturers have included selected products in full color. Where capsules and tablets are included they are shown in actual size. Packages generally are reduced in size.

Where other dosage forms are available, the product name is preceded by the † symbol. For more information, refer to the product's description in the PRODUCT INFORMATION SECTION or check directly with the manufacturer.

While every effort has been made to reproduce products faithfully, this section should be considered only as a quick-reference identification aid.

INDEX BY MANUFACTURER

APOTHECON

p. 505

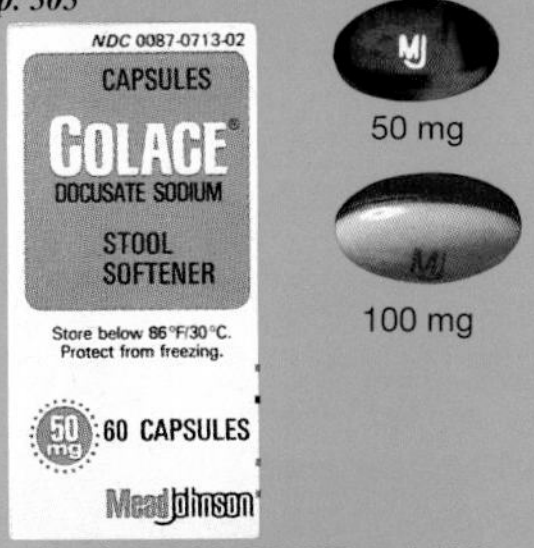
NDC 0087-0713-02
CAPSULES
COLACE
DOCUSATE SODIUM
STOOL SOFTENER
Store below 86°F/30°C. Protect from freezing.
60 CAPSULES
Mead Johnson
50 mg
100 mg

Bottles of 30, 60, 250 and 1000
Stool Softener

†COLACE®
(docusate sodium)

B. F. Ascher & Co., Inc.
p. 506

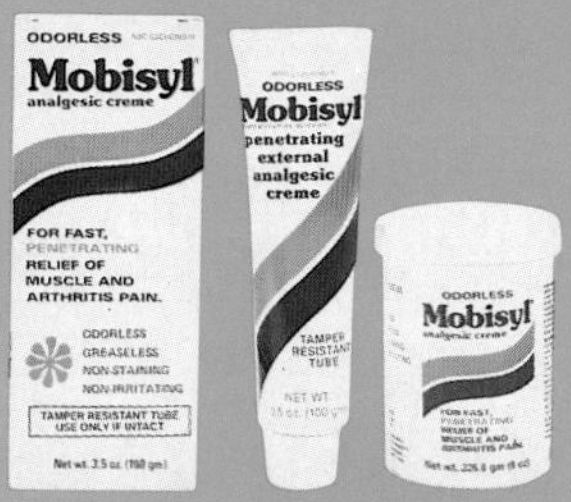

Also Available: 1.25 oz

MOBISYL®
ANALGESIC CREME
FOR FAST, PENETRATING RELIEF OF MUSCLE AND ARTHRITIS PAIN.

For more detailed information on products illustrated in this section, consult the Product Information Section or manufacturers may be contacted directly.

Baker Cummins Dermatological, Inc.
p. 509

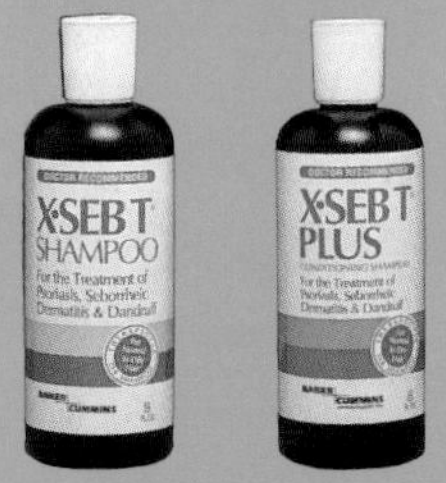
X-SEB T
SHAMPOO
X-SEB T
PLUS

X • SEB T® and X • SEB T® PLUS
SHAMPOO

Apothecon
p. 505

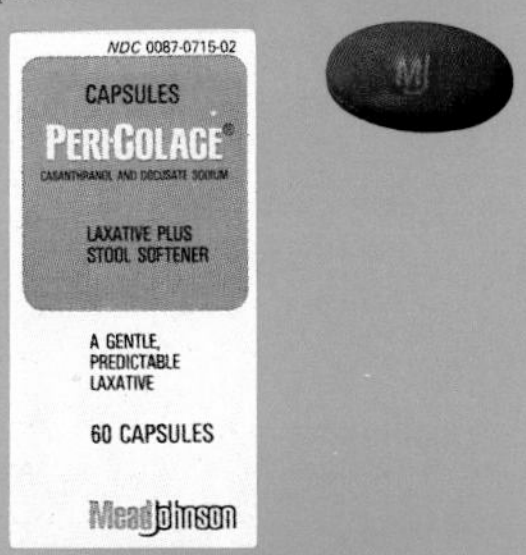
NDC 0087-0715-02
CAPSULES
PERI-COLACE
LAXATIVE PLUS STOOL SOFTENER
A GENTLE, PREDICTABLE LAXATIVE
60 CAPSULES
Mead Johnson

Bottles of 30, 60, 250 and 1000
Laxative and Stool Softener

†PERI-COLACE®
(casanthranol and docusate sodium)

B. F. Ascher & Co., Inc.
p. 506

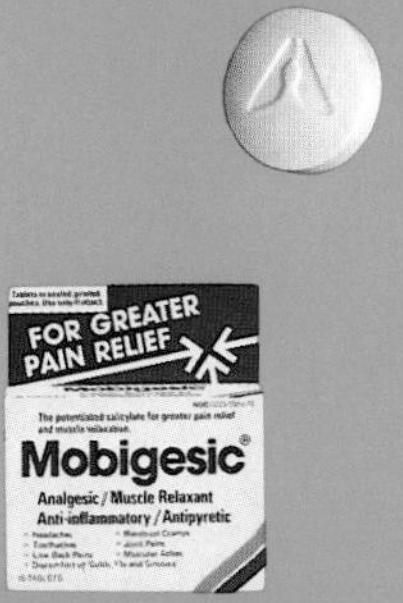
FOR GREATER PAIN RELIEF
Mobigesic
Analgesic / Muscle Relaxant
Anti-inflammatory / Antipyretic

Available: 18's, 50's & 100's

MOBIGESIC®
ANALGESIC TABLETS

BAKER CUMMINS

Dermatological, Inc.
p. 508

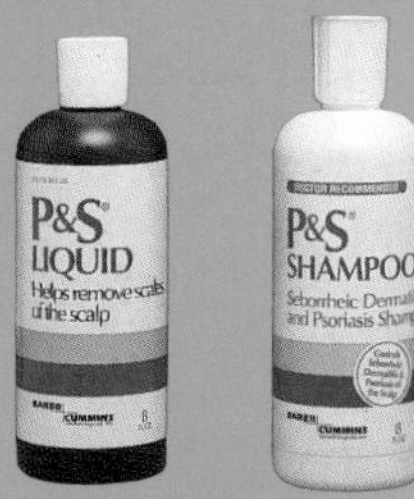
P&S
LIQUID
Helps remove scales of the scalp
P&S
SHAMPOO

P & S®
LIQUID and SHAMPOO

Baker Cummins Dermatological, Inc.
p. 508

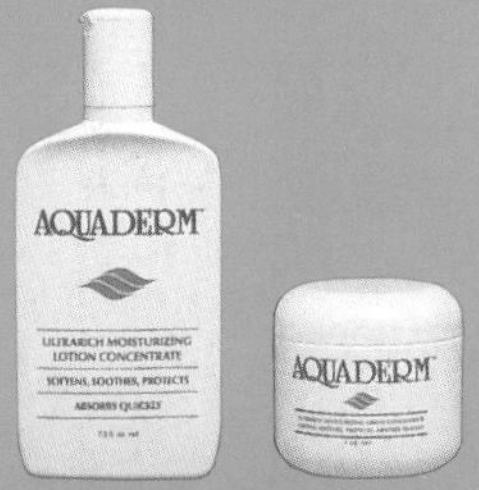
AQUADERM
AQUADERM

AQUADERM®
LOTION and CREAM

ASCHER

p. 506

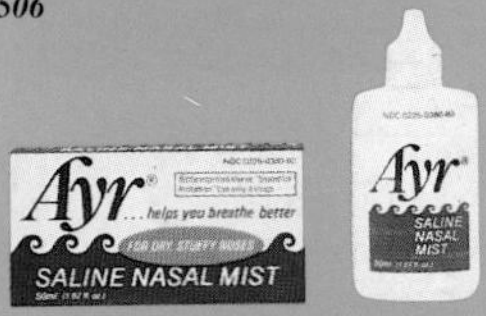
Ayr
SALINE NASAL MIST

AYR® SALINE NASAL MIST

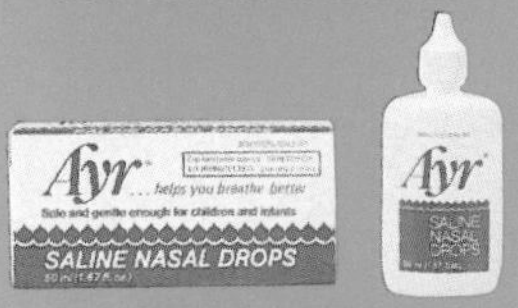
Ayr
SALINE NASAL DROPS

AYR® SALINE NASAL DROPS

B. F. Ascher & Co., Inc.
p. 506

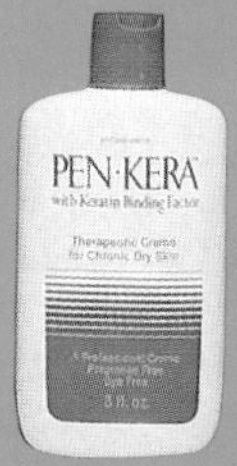
PEN•KERA

Available in 8 oz bottle

PEN•KERA®

Therapeutic Creme
for Chronic Dry Skin

Baker Cummins Dermatological, Inc.
p. 509

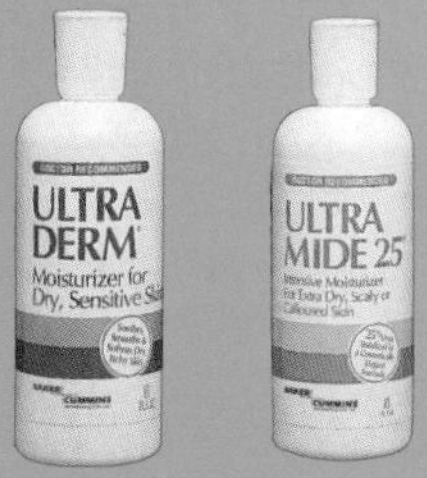
ULTRA DERM
Moisturizer for Dry, Sensitive Skin
ULTRA MIDE 25

ULTRA DERM® and ULTRA MIDE 25®
MOISTURIZER

BEIERSDORF

p. 510

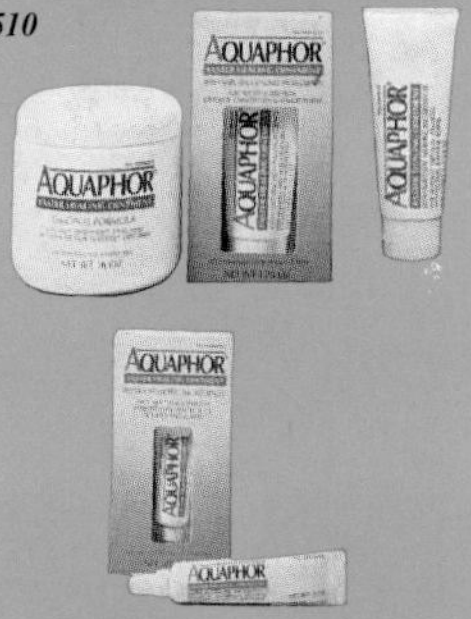

AQUAPHOR®
Healing Ointments
For dry skin, minor cuts and burns

B. F. Ascher & Co., Inc.
p. 506

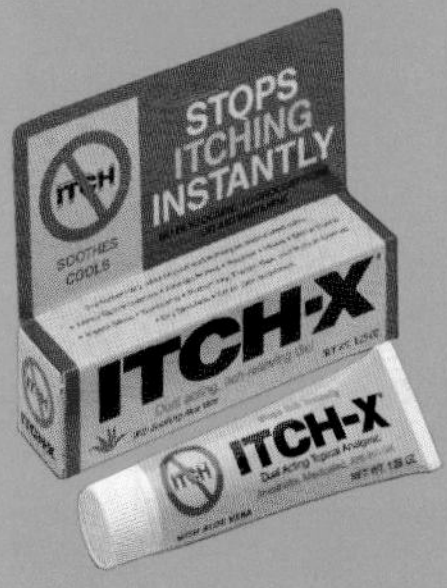
STOPS ITCHING INSTANTLY
ITCH-X
ITCH-X

Available in 35.4 g (1.25 oz) tube

ITCH-X® GEL
(benzyl alcohol 10% & pramoxine hydrochloride 1%)

ASTRA

p. 507

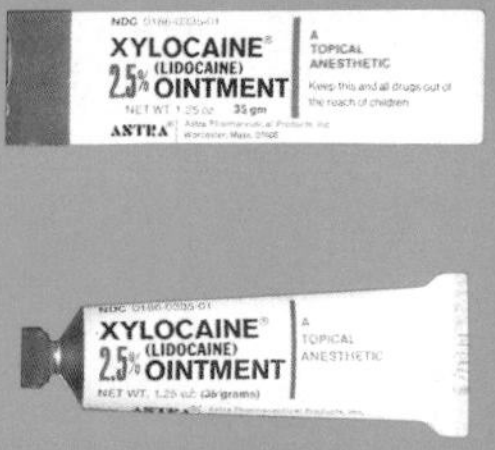

Available in 35g Tube

XYLOCAINE® 2.5% OINTMENT
(lidocaine)

Baker Cummins Dermatological, Inc.
p. 509

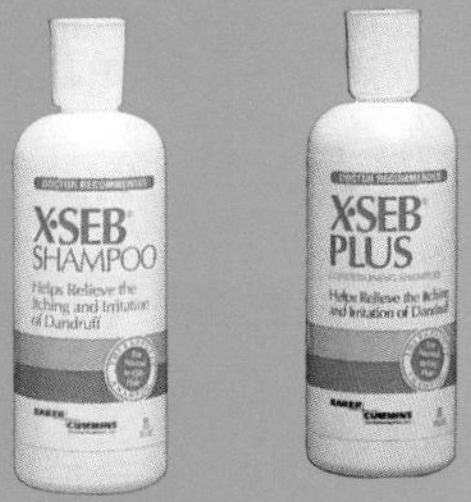
X-SEB
SHAMPOO
X-SEB
PLUS

X • SEB® and X • SEB® PLUS
SHAMPOO

While every effort has been made to reproduce products faithfully, this section is to be considered a Quick-Reference identification aid.

Beiersdorf *p. 511*

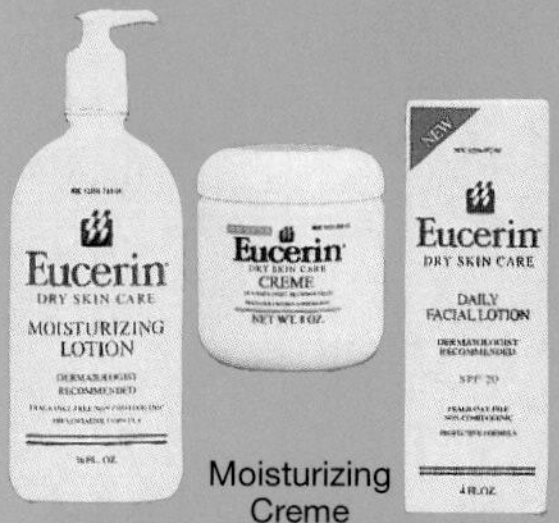

Moisturizing Creme

Moisturizing Lotion

Daily Facial Lotion

EUCERIN®
Fragrance-Free Dry
Skin Care

Beiersdorf *p. 511*

Moisturizing Lotion

Cleansing Lotion

Cleansing Bar

EUCERIN®
Fragrance-Free Dry
Skin Care

BOCK PHARMACAL

p. 516

Original Lemon Mint

Cherry

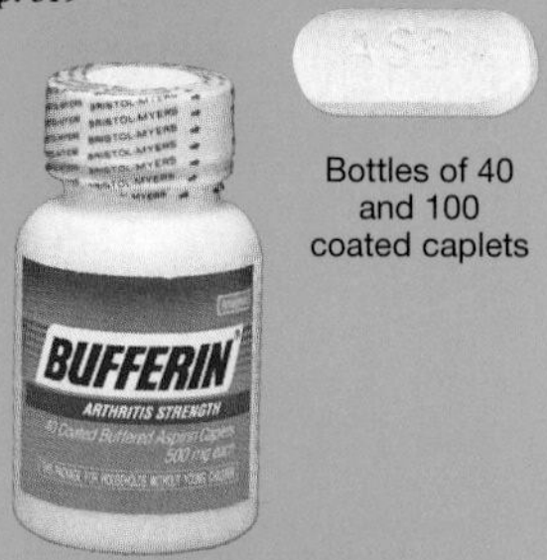

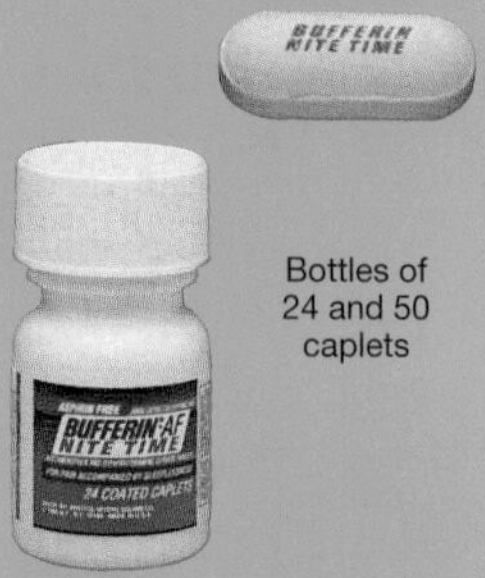

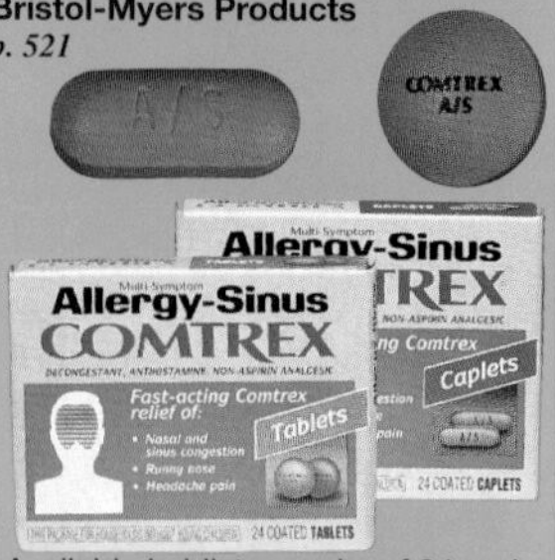

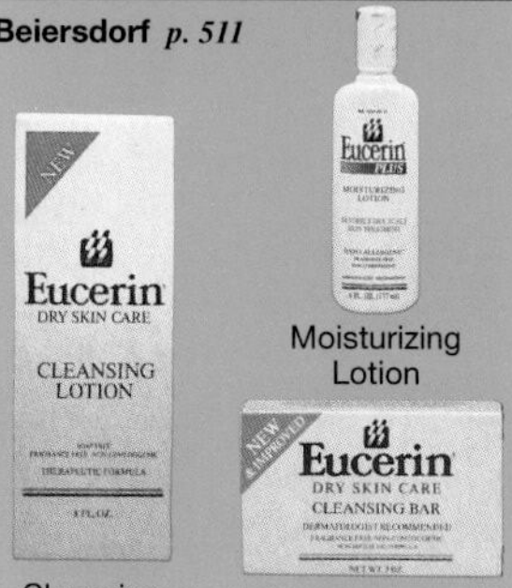

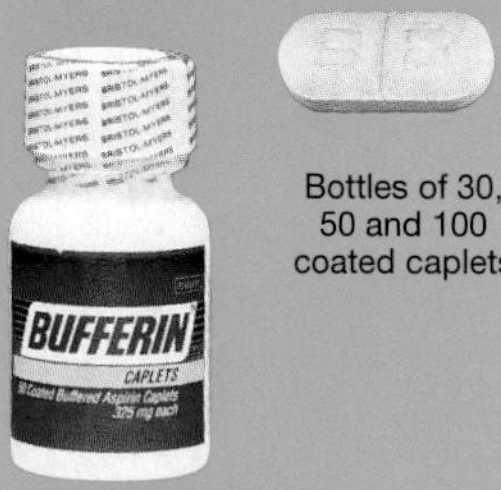

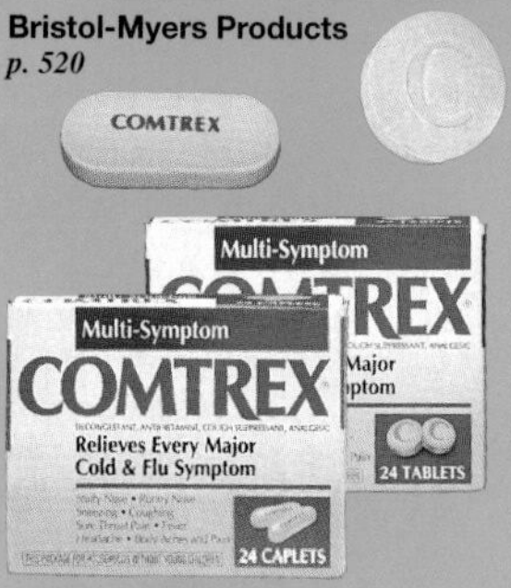

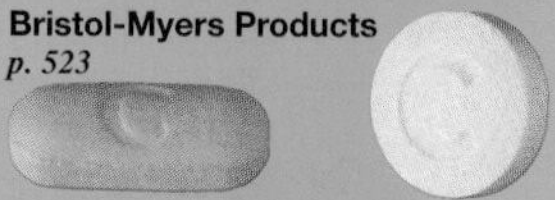

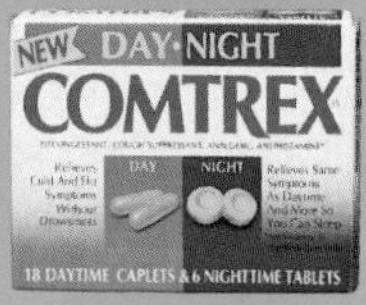

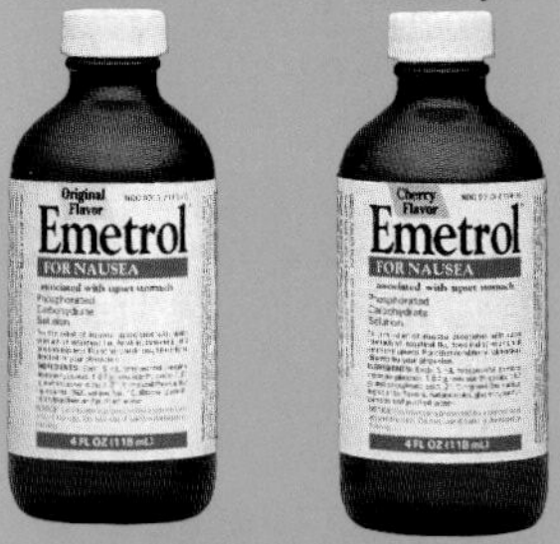

Emetrol®
(phosphorated carbohydrate solution)

BOIRON

p. 516

SYMPTOMS OF FLU

oscillococcinum

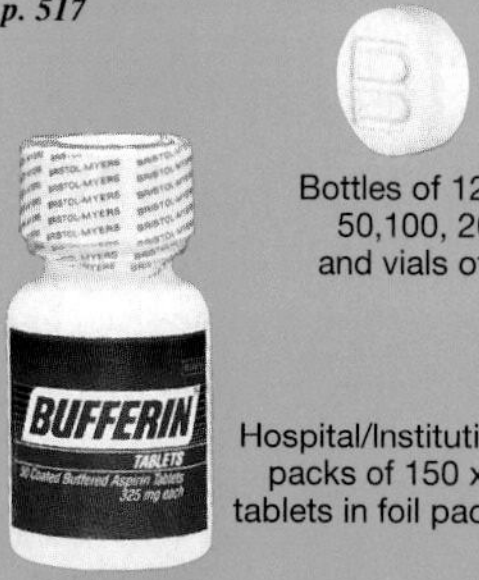

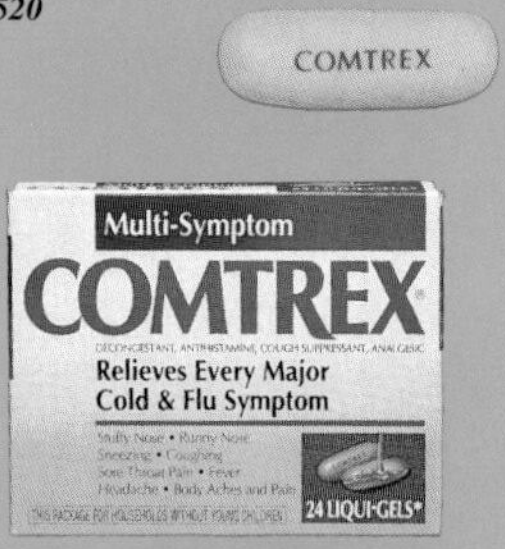

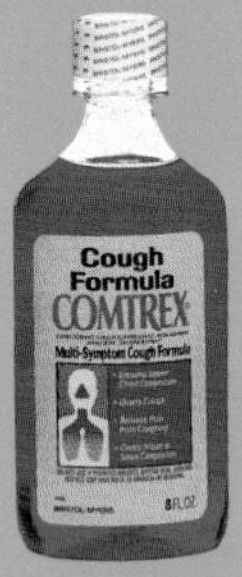

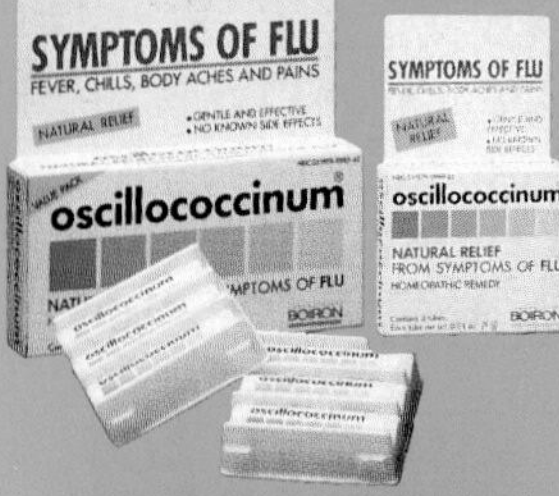

OSCILLOCOCCINUM®
Homeopathic remedy for the natural
relief of flu-like symptoms.
Now also available in new family
value pak. (6 doses)

Bristol-Myers Products

p. 519

Bottles of 40
and 100
coated caplets

ARTHRITIS STRENGTH
BUFFERIN® CAPLET
(buffered aspirin)

Bristol-Myers Products
p. 517

Bottles of 30,
50 and 100
coated caplets

BUFFERIN® CAPLET
(buffered aspirin)

Bristol-Myers Products
p. 517

Bottles of 12, 30,
50,100, 200
and vials of 10

Hospital/Institutional
packs of 150 x 2
tablets in foil packets

BUFFERIN® TABLET
(buffered aspirin)

Bristol-Myers Products
p. 520

Bottles of 30,
50 and 100
coated tablets

EXTRA STRENGTH
BUFFERIN® TABLET
(buffered aspirin)

Bristol-Myers Products
p. 518

Bottles of
24 and 50
caplets

BUFFERIN® A/F NITE TIME
Analgesic/Sleeping Aid Caplets
(acetaminophen and diphenhydramine citrate)

Bristol-Myers Products
p. 520

Multi-Symptom
COMTREX®
Relieves Every Major
Cold & Flu Symptom

Caplets: Blister packs of 24 and
bottles of 50. Tablets: Blister packs
of 24, bottles of 50, vials of 10.

COMTREX®
CAPLETS AND TABLETS

Bristol-Myers Products
p. 520

Multi-Symptom
COMTREX
Relieves Every Major
Cold & Flu Symptom

Blister packs of 24 and 50

COMTREX®
LIQUI-GELS

Bristol-Myers Products
p. 524

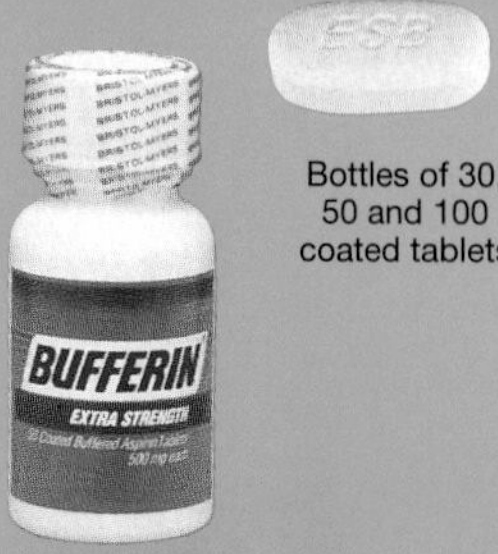

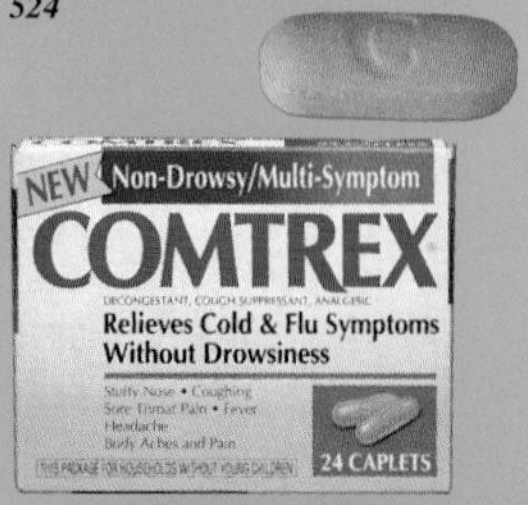

NEW Non-Drowsy/Multi-Symptom
COMTREX
Relieves Cold & Flu Symptoms
Without Drowsiness

Blister packs of 24 and bottles of 50

NON-DROWSY COMTREX®
Multi-Symptom
Cold Reliever Caplets
(acetaminophen, pseudoephedrine HCl,
dextromethorphan HBr)

Bristol-Myers Products
p. 521

Allergy-Sinus COMTREX
Fast-acting Comtrex
relief of:

Available in blister packs of 24 and
bottles of 50

COMTREX® A/S MULTI-SYMPTOM
CAPLETS AND TABLETS
ALLERGY-SINUS FORMULA
(acetaminophen, pseudoephedrine,
chlorpheniramine)

Bristol-Myers Products
p. 523

Day

Night

Multi-Symptom Cold Reliever

NEW **DAY-NIGHT**
COMTREX

Blister packs of 24
DAY-NIGHT COMTREX®
Caplets: (acetaminophen, pseudoephedrine HCl, dextromethorphan HBr)
Tablets: (acetaminophen, pseudoephedrine HCl, dextromethorphan HBr,
chlorpheniramine maleate)

Bristol-Myers Products
p. 522

Cough
Formula
COMTREX

Bottles of
4 & 8
oz.

COUGH FORMULA
COMTREX®

Bristol-Myers Products
p. 520

Bottles of
6 oz.

Liquid
COMTREX

COMTREX® LIQUID

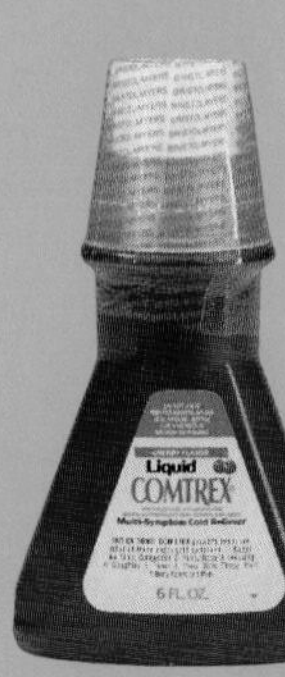

Bristol-Myers Products
p. 525

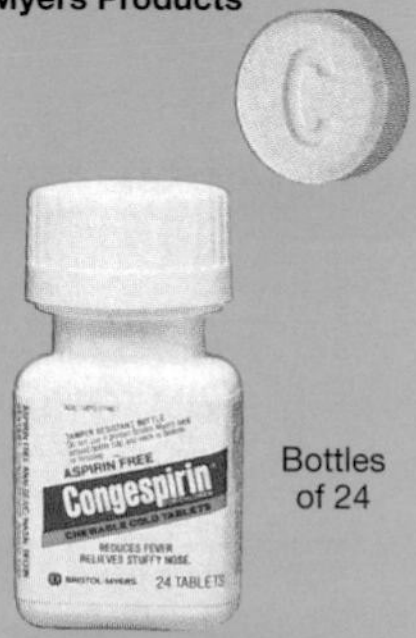

Bottles of 24

ASPIRIN FREE CONGESPIRIN®
(acetaminophen 81 mg., phenylephrine 1.25 mg.)

Bristol-Myers Products
p. 527

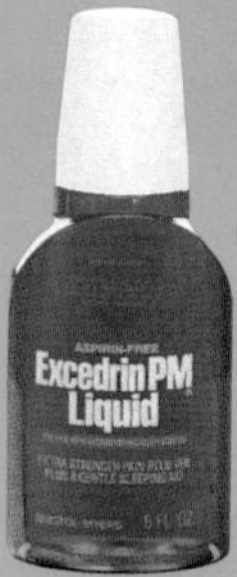

Bottles of 6 oz.

EXCEDRIN P.M.®
LIQUID

Bristol-Myers Products
p. 530

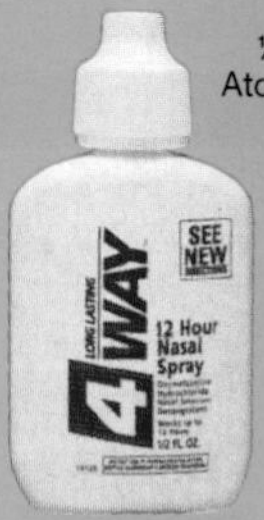

½ oz. Atomizers

4-WAY® LONG ACTING NASAL SPRAY
(oxymetazoline hydrochloride 0.05%)

Bristol-Myers Products
p. 530

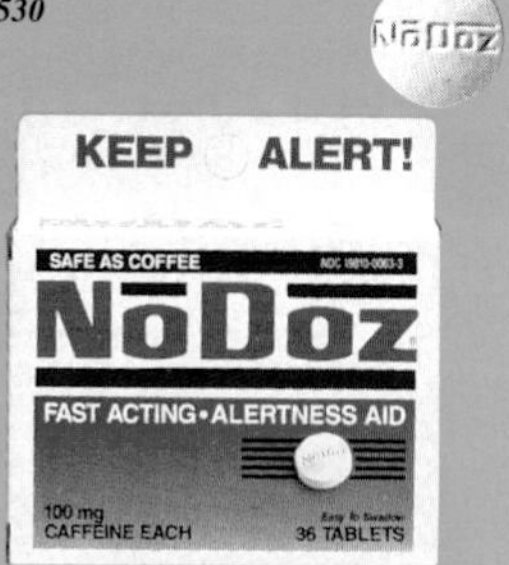

Blister packs of 16 and 36, bottles of 60 and vials of 15

NO-DOZ® TABLETS
(caffeine)

Bristol-Myers Products
p. 526

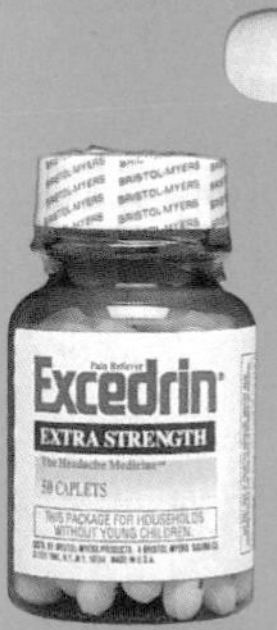

Bottles of 24, 50 and 100

EXCEDRIN® CAPLETS
Aspirin/Acetaminophen/Caffeine

Bristol-Myers Products
p. 525

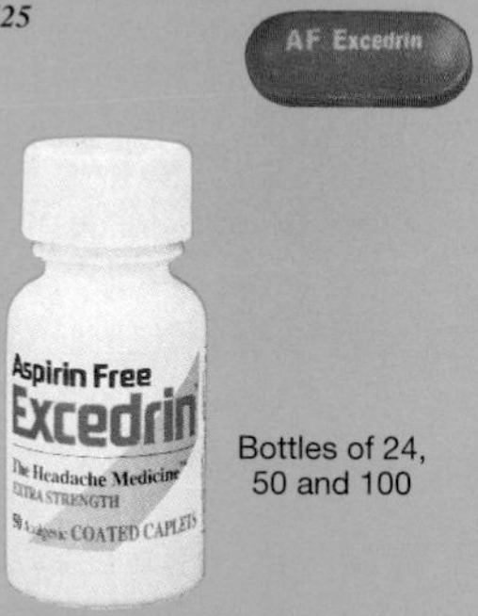

Bottles of 24, 50 and 100

ASPIRIN FREE
EXCEDRIN® CAPLETS
(acetaminophen/caffeine)

Bristol-Myers Products
p. 517

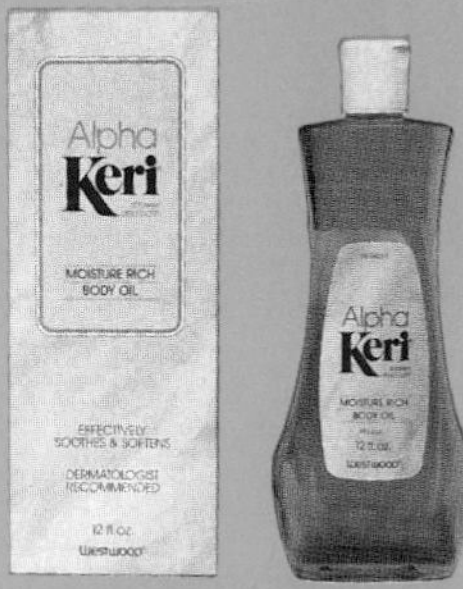

4, 8, 12 and 16 oz.

ALPHA KERI®
Shower and Bath Products

Bristol-Myers Products
p. 531

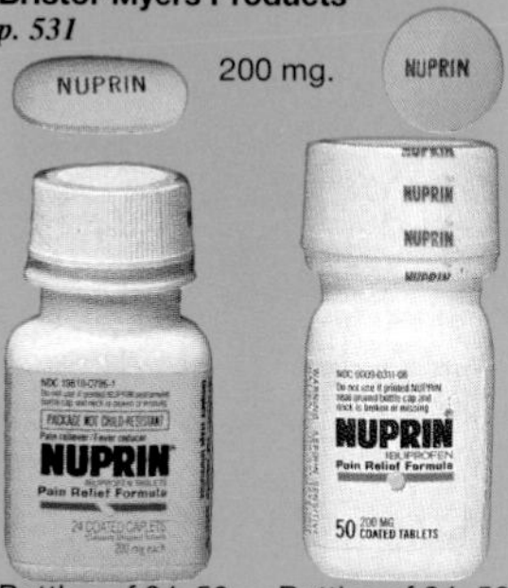

200 mg.

Bottles of 24, 50 and 100 caplets

Bottles of 24, 50, 100, 150 and vials of 10

NUPRIN® CAPLET & TABLET
(ibuprofen)

Bristol-Myers Products
p. 526

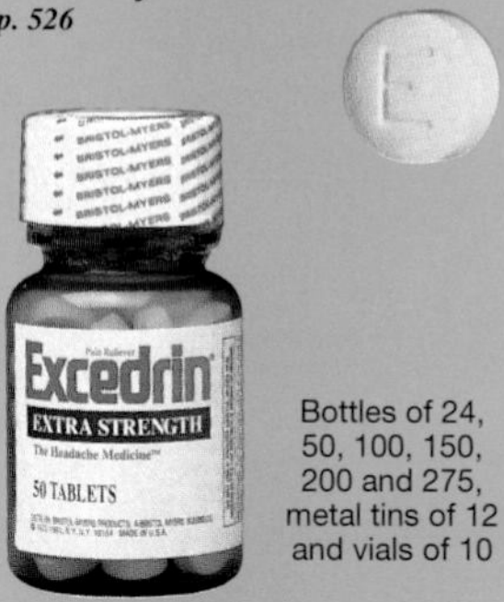

Bottles of 24, 50, 100, 150, 200 and 275, metal tins of 12 and vials of 10

EXCEDRIN® TABLETS
Aspirin/Acetaminophen/Caffeine

Bristol-Myers Products
p. 528

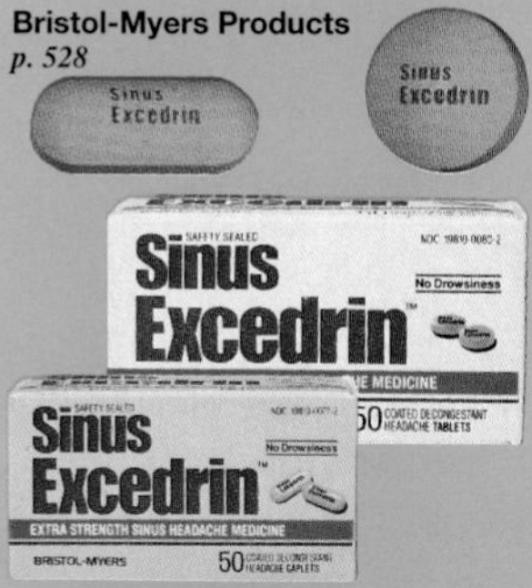

Available in blister packs of 24 and bottles of 50 caplets and tablets

SINUS EXCEDRIN®
CAPLETS & TABLETS
(acetaminophen, pseudoephedrine)

Bristol-Myers Products
p. 530

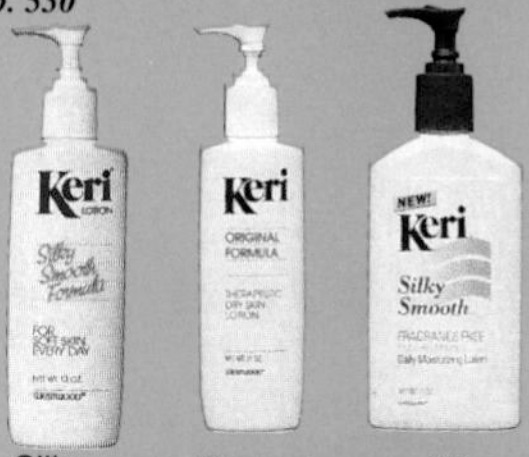

Silky Smooth

Original Formula

Silky Smooth Fragrance Free

6.5, 11 and 15 oz.
20 oz. size for Original Formula only

KERI® LOTION
For Dry Skin Care

Bristol-Myers Products
p. 531

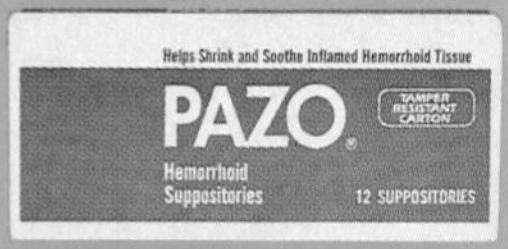

Boxes of 12 suppositories

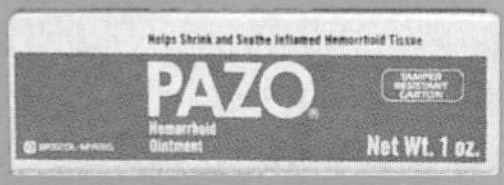

Tubes of 1 oz.

PAZO®
Hemorrhoid Ointment and Suppositories

Bristol-Myers Products
p. 527

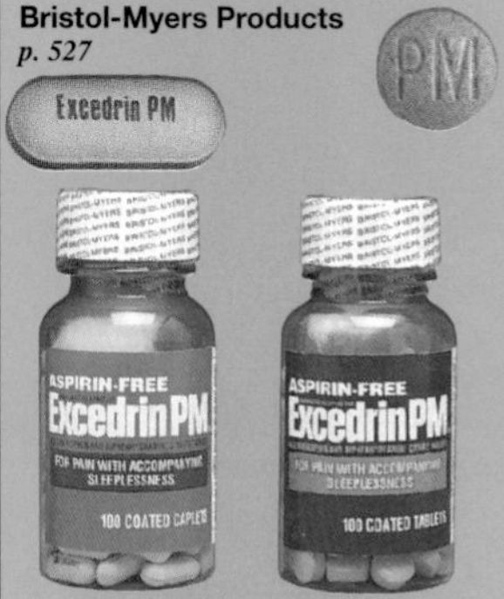

Bottles of 10, 30, 50 and 80 and vials of 10

EXCEDRIN P.M.®

Bristol-Myers Products
p. 529

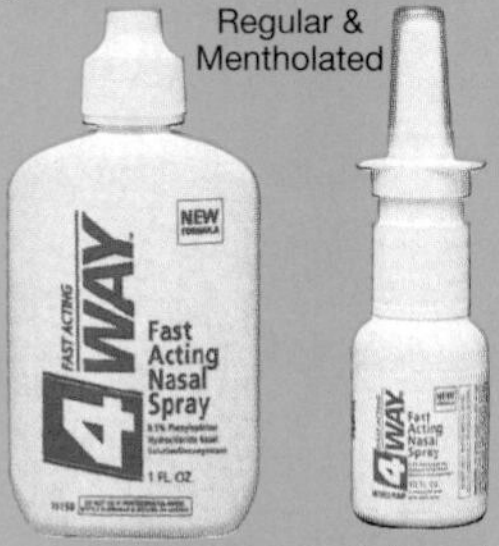

Regular & Mentholated

Atomizers of ½ and 1 oz.

Available in ½ oz. metered spray pump

4-WAY® FAST ACTING
NASAL SPRAY

Bristol-Myers Products
p. 531

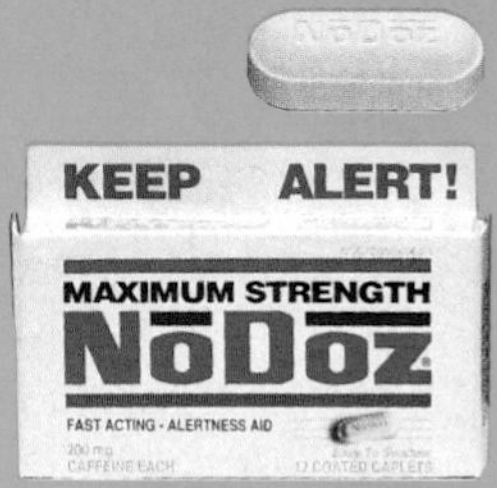

Blister packs of 12

NO DOZ® MAXIMUM
STRENGTH CAPLETS
(caffeine)

Bristol-Myers Products
p. 534

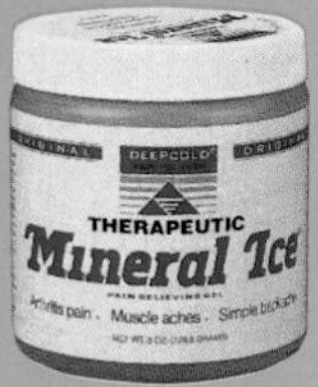

Available in:
3.5 oz., 8 oz. and 16 oz.

THERAPEUTIC
MINERAL ICE™
Pain Relieving Gel

Bristol-Myers Products
p. 534

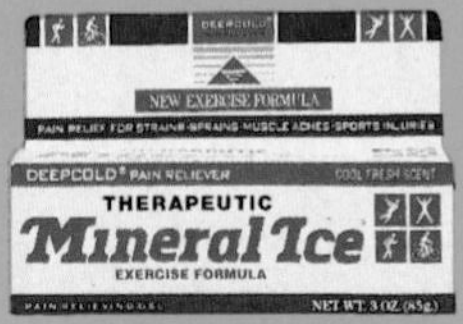

Tubes of 3 oz.

THERAPEUTIC MINERAL ICE® EXERCISE FORMULA

Pain Relieving Gel

Bristol-Myers Products
p. 533

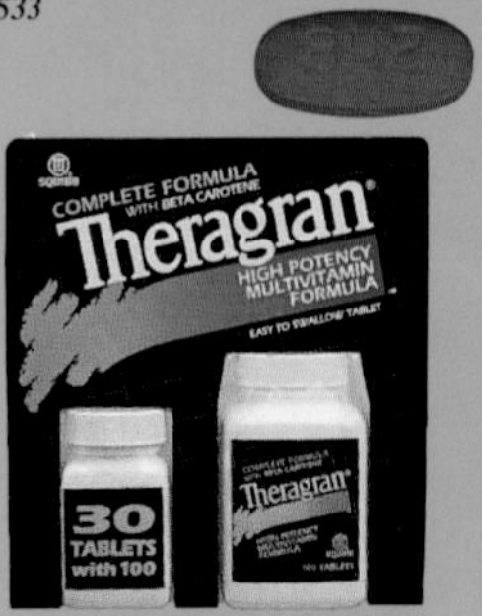

COMPLETE FORMULA THERAGRAN®
High Potency Multivitamin Formula

Burroughs Wellcome
p. 536

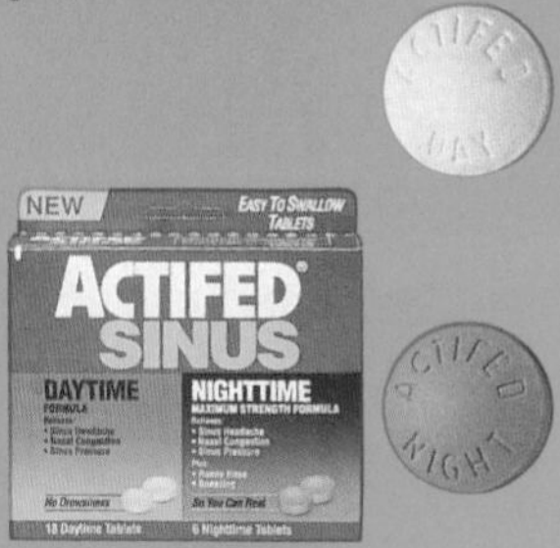

ACTIFED® SINUS DAYTIME/NIGHTTIME TABLETS

Burroughs Wellcome
p. 538

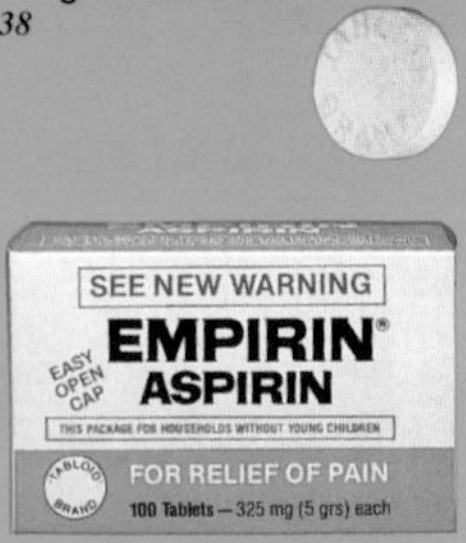

100

Also available in 50s

EMPIRIN® ASPIRIN TABLETS

Bristol-Myers Products
p. 533

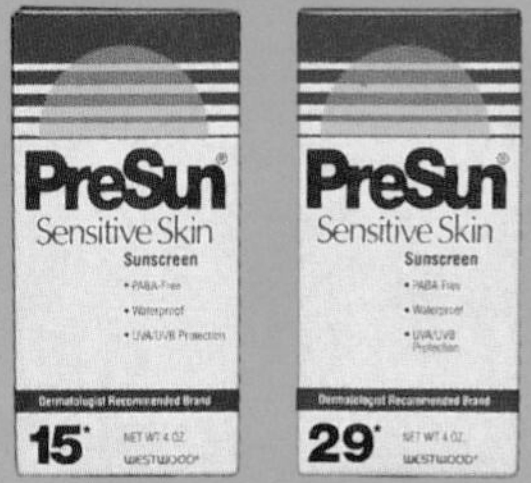

Sensitive Skin Sunscreen 15 | Sensitive Skin Sunscreen 29

4 oz.

PRESUN®
Creamy, Lotion, Facial, Sensitive Skin and Stick Formulas

Bristol-Myers Products
p. 534

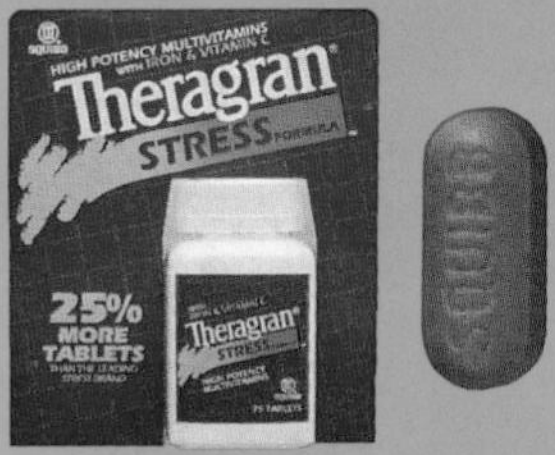

THERAGRAN® STRESS FORMULA
High Potency Multivitamin Formula with Iron and Biotin

Burroughs Wellcome
p. 537

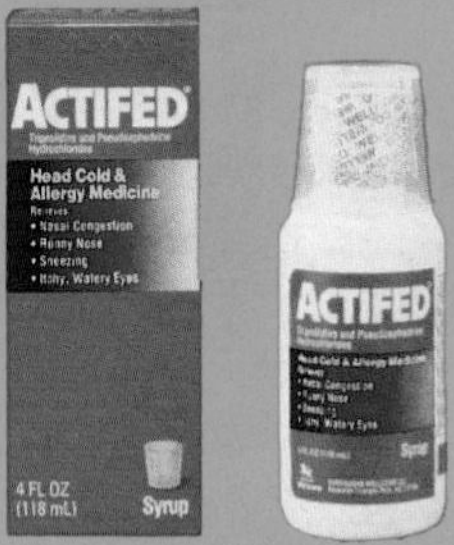

4 fl. oz.

Also available in pints

ACTIFED® SYRUP

Burroughs Wellcome
p. 538

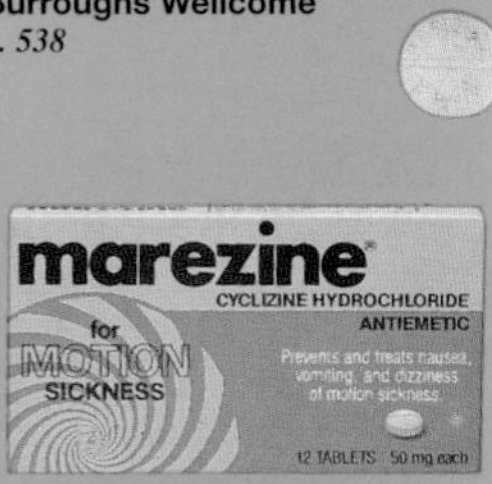

12

Also available in 100s

MAREZINE® TABLETS

Bristol-Myers Products
p. 532

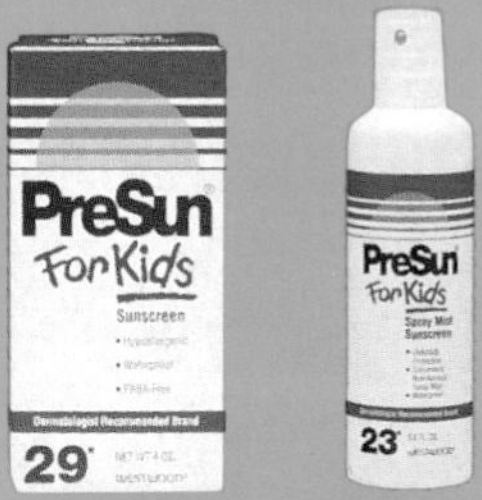

4 oz. | 3.5 oz.

PRESUN® FOR KIDS

Bristol-Myers Products
p. 533

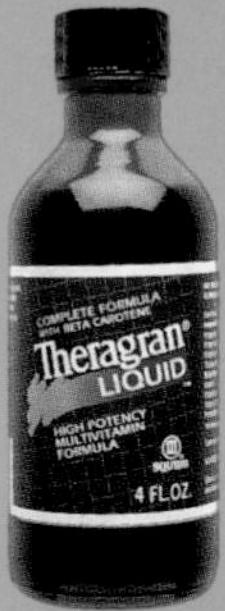

THERAGRAN® LIQUID
High Potency Liquid Vitamin Supplement

Burroughs Wellcome
p. 537

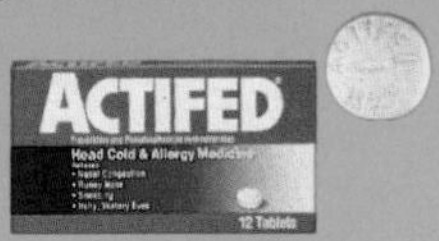

12

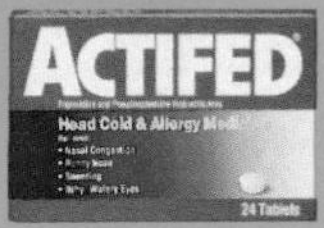

24

Also available in 48s and in bottles of 100

ACTIFED® TABLETS

Burroughs Wellcome
p. 538

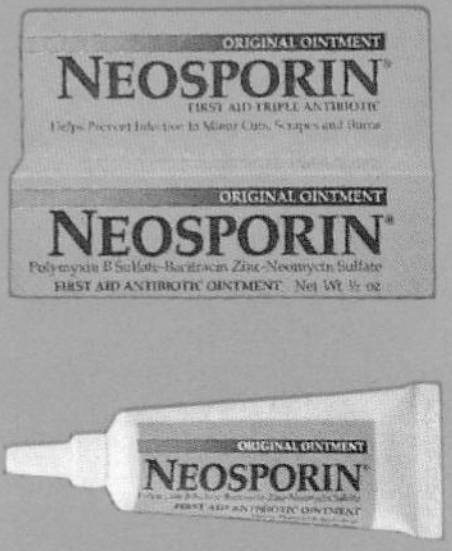

Available in ½ and 1 oz. tubes

NEOSPORIN® FIRST AID ANTIBIOTIC OINTMENT

Bristol-Myers Products
p. 534

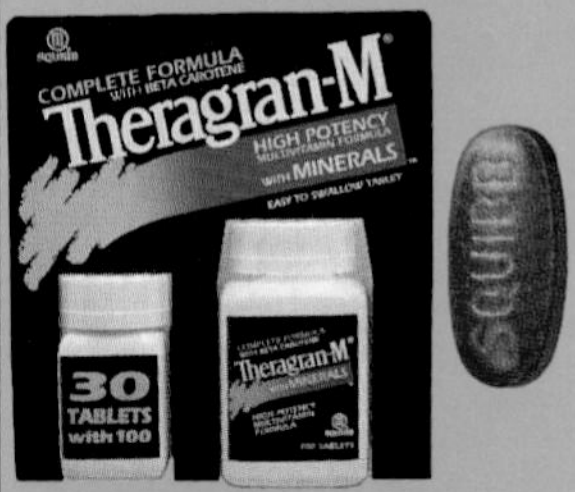

COMPLETE FORMULA THERAGRAN-M®
High Potency Multivitamin Formula with Minerals

BURROUGHS WELLCOME

p. 535

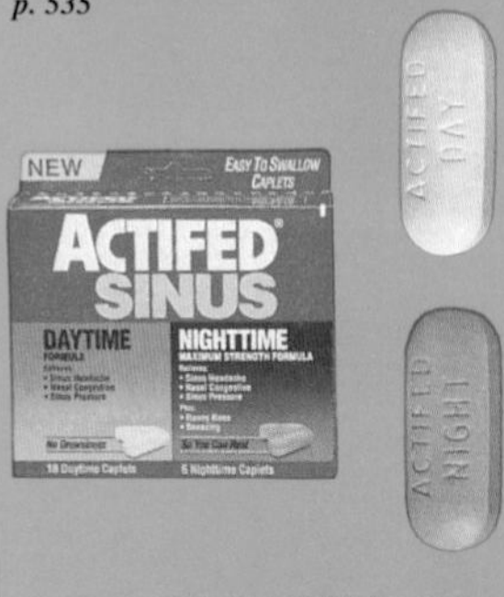

ACTIFED® SINUS DAYTIME/NIGHTTIME CAPLETS

Burroughs Wellcome
p. 535

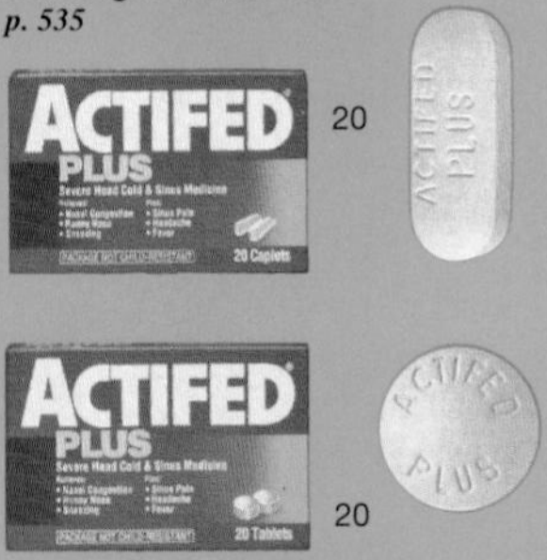

20

20

Also available in 40s

ACTIFED® PLUS CAPLETS & TABLETS

Burroughs Wellcome
p. 539

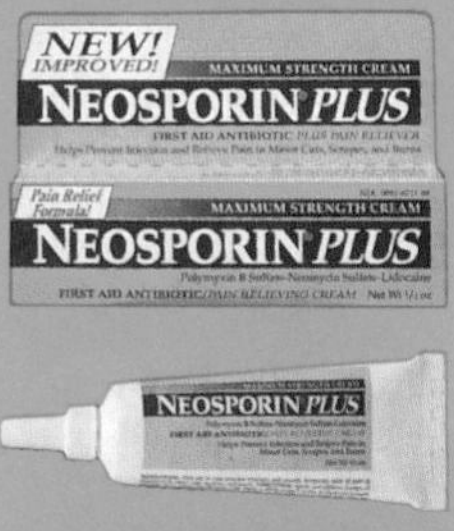

Available in ½ oz. tubes

MAXIMUM STRENGTH NEOSPORIN® PLUS CREAM

Burroughs Wellcome
p. 539

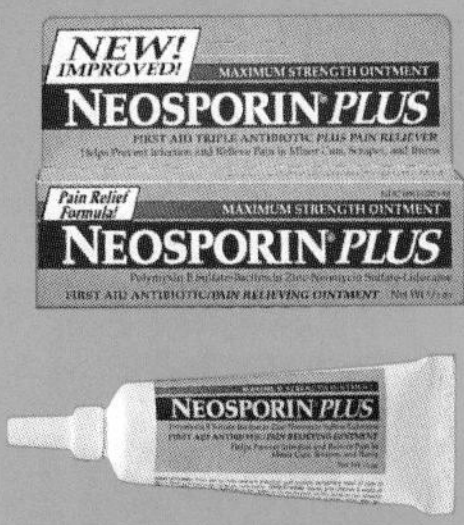

Available in ½ and 1 oz. tubes

MAXIMUM STRENGTH NEOSPORIN® PLUS OINTMENT

Burroughs Wellcome
p. 541

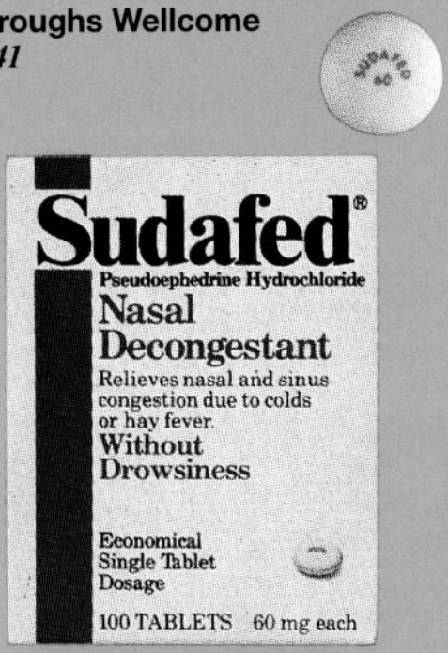

100

SUDAFED® 60 mg TABLETS

Burroughs Wellcome
p. 542

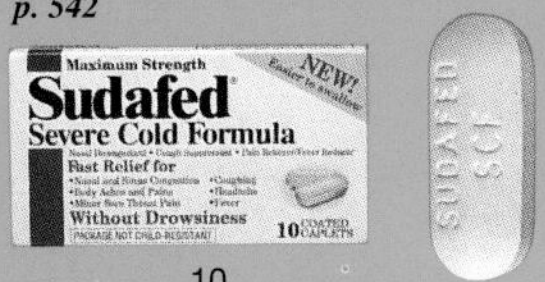

10

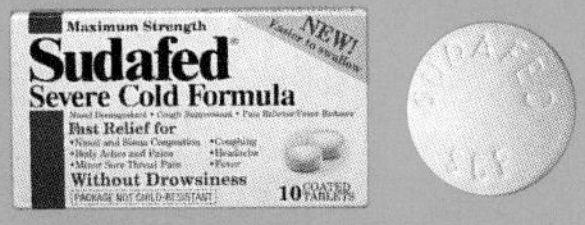

10

Also available in 20s

SUDAFED® SEVERE COLD FORMULA CAPLETS & TABLETS

Ciba Consumer *p. 550*

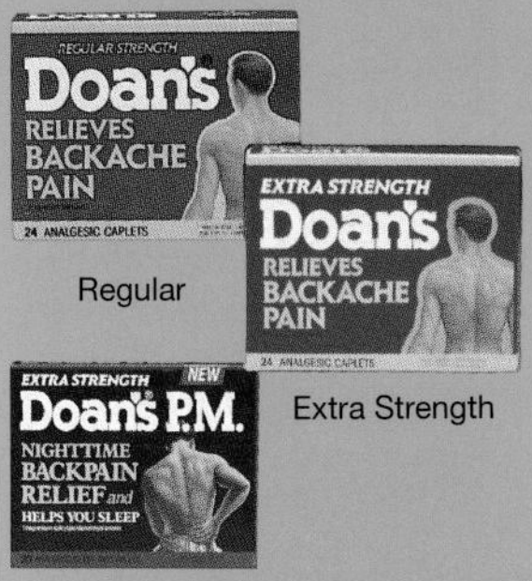

Regular

Extra Strength

Nighttime

DOAN'S® & DOAN'S® P.M.
Backache Analgesic
Relieves Back Pain

Burroughs Wellcome
p. 539

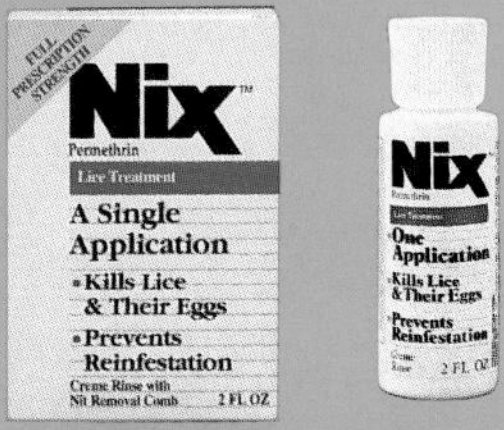

2 fl. oz.

Also available: 2-bottle family pack

NIX®
LICE TREATMENT
CREME RINSE

Burroughs Wellcome
p. 543

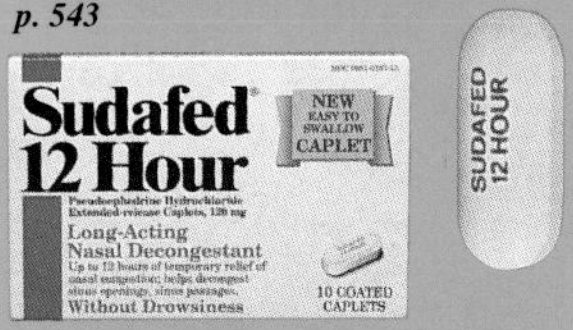

10

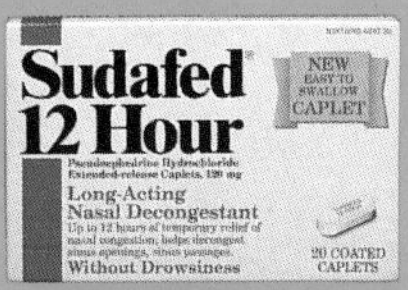

20

SUDAFED® 12 HOUR CAPLETS

Burroughs Wellcome
p. 542

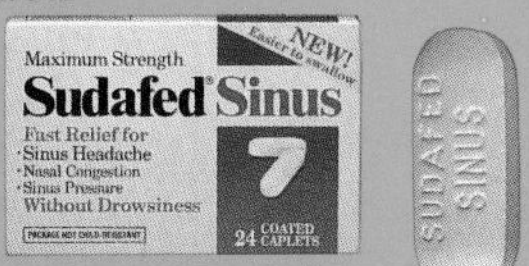

24

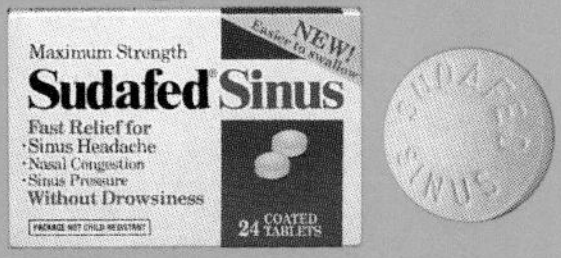

24

Also available in 48s

SUDAFED® SINUS CAPLETS & TABLETS

Ciba Consumer *p. 551*

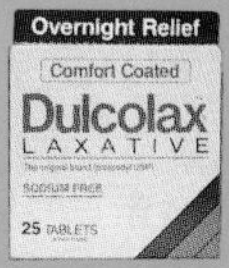

Tablets

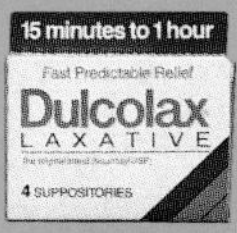

Suppositories

DULCOLAX® LAXATIVE
Tablets & Suppositories
(bisacodyl USP)

Burroughs Wellcome
p. 539

Powder, 0.35 oz. (10 g)

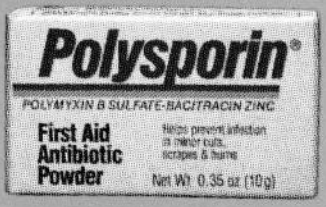

Ointment, ½ oz. and 1 oz.

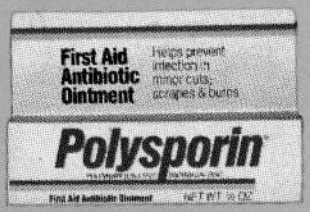

POLYSPORIN®
FIRST AID ANTIBIOTIC
POWDER & OINTMENT

Burroughs Wellcome
p. 540

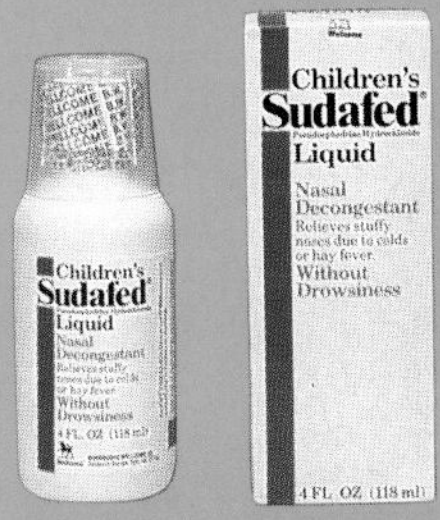

4 fl. oz.

CHILDREN'S SUDAFED® LIQUID

Burroughs Wellcome
p. 541

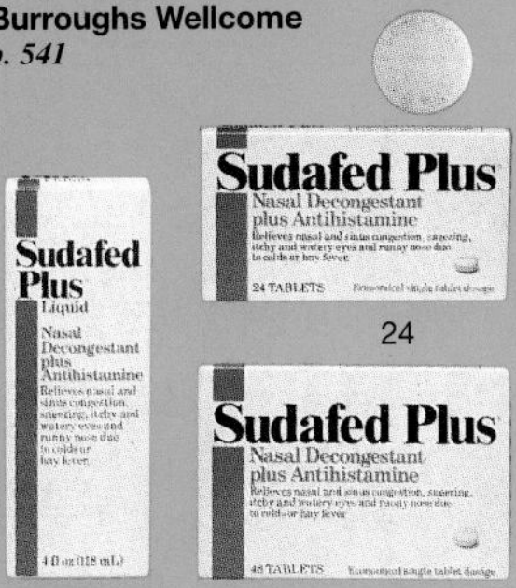

24

4 fl. oz.

48

SUDAFED® PLUS LIQUID & TABLETS

Ciba Consumer *p. 552*

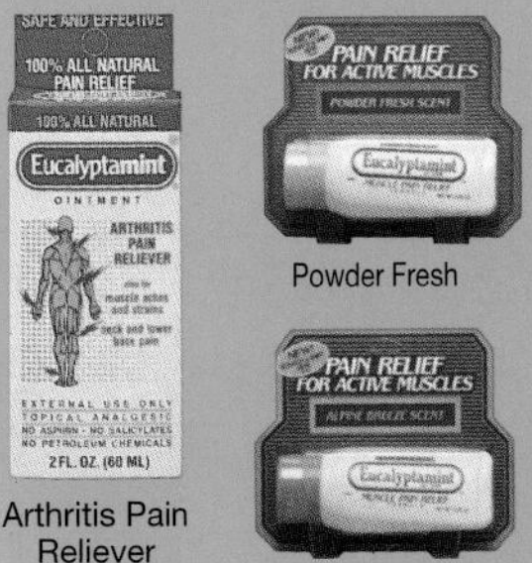

Powder Fresh

Arthritis Pain Reliever
2 oz., 4 oz.
Ointment

Alpine Breeze
Muscle Pain Relief Formula
2.25 oz. Gel Cream

EUCALYPTAMINT®
External Analgesics

Burroughs Wellcome
p. 540

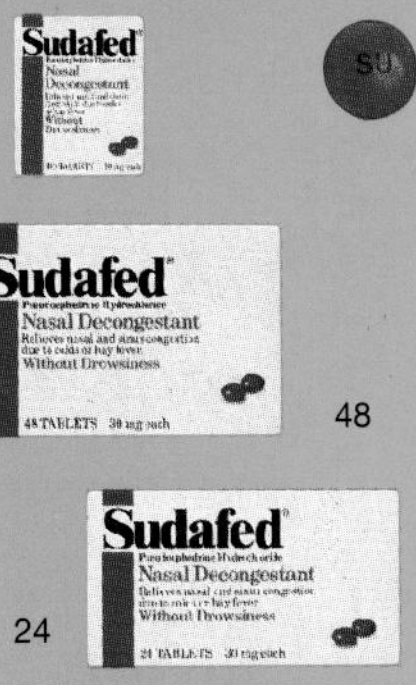

100

48

24

SUDAFED® 30 mg TABLETS

Burroughs Wellcome
p. 540

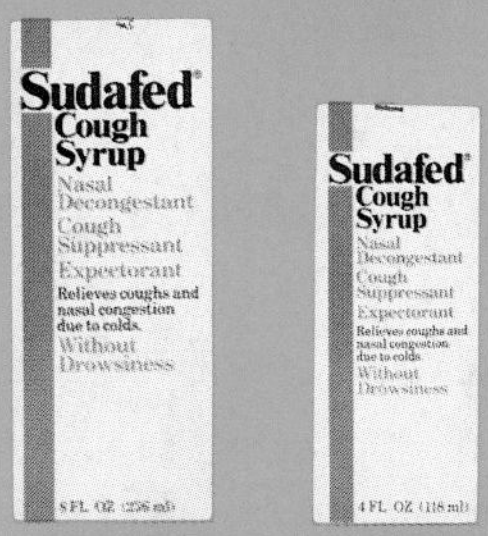

8 fl. oz.

4 fl. oz.

SUDAFED® COUGH SYRUP

CIBA CONSUMER

p. 550

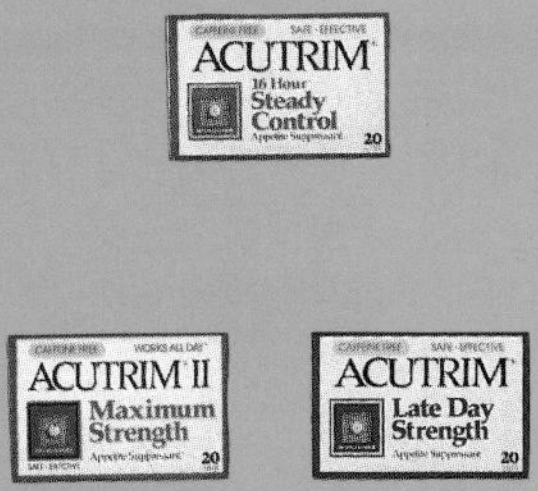

ACUTRIM®
Appetite Suppressants
Caffeine Free/Works All Day

Ciba Consumer *p. 552*

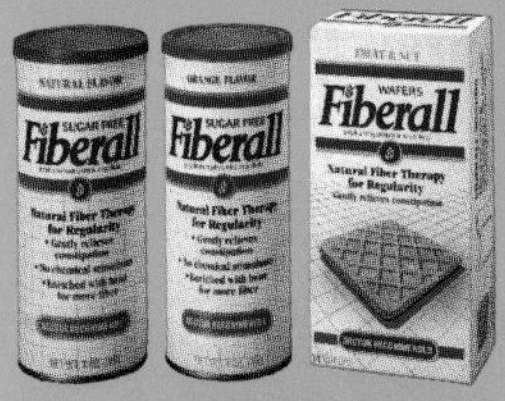

FIBERALL
Natural Fiber Therapy
for Regularity

Available in:
Powders: 10 and 15 oz. Natural, Orange
Wafers: 14 Fruit & Nut, Oatmeal Raisin
Tablets: 18

Ciba Consumer *p. 553*

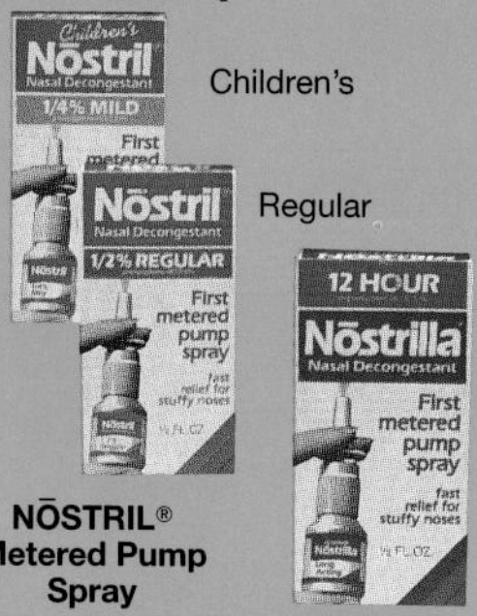

Children's

Regular

NŌSTRIL®
Metered Pump Spray

NŌSTRILLA™
12 Hour
Metered Pump Spray

Ciba Consumer *p. 555*

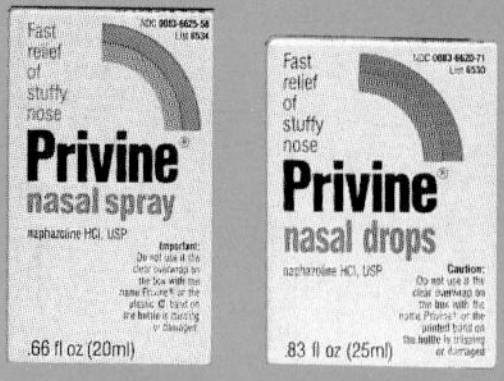

Nasal Spray

Nasal Drops

PRIVINE®
Nasal Drops & Spray

Ciba Consumer *p. 557*

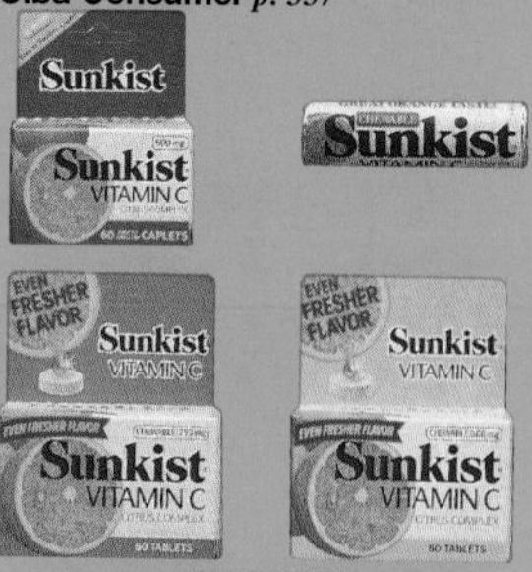

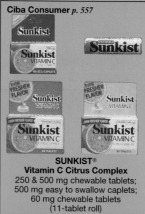

SUNKIST®
Vitamin C Citrus Complex
250 & 500 mg chewable tablets;
500 mg easy to swallow caplets;
60 mg chewable tablets
(11-tablet roll)

DEL PHARMACEUTICALS

p. 558

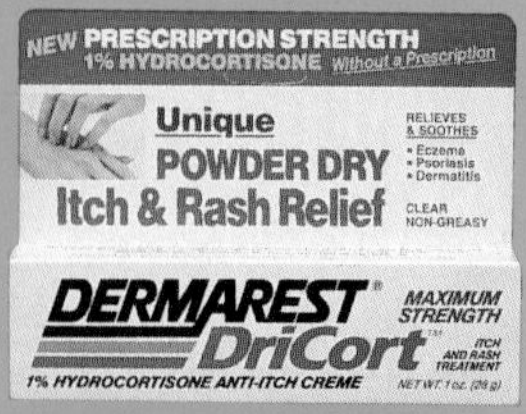

DERMAREST® DRICORT™
1.0% Hydrocortisone Anti-Itch Creme

Ciba Consumer *p. 554*

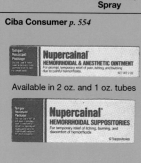

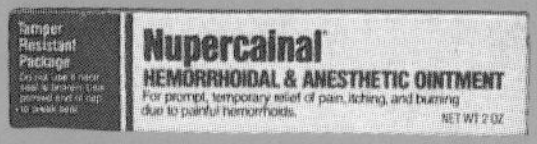

Available in 2 oz. and 1 oz. tubes

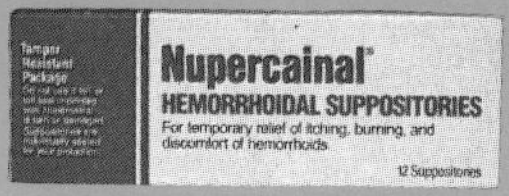

Available in boxes of
12 and 24 suppositories

NUPERCAINAL®
Hemorrhoidal & Anesthetic Ointment & Suppositories

Ciba Consumer *p. 555*

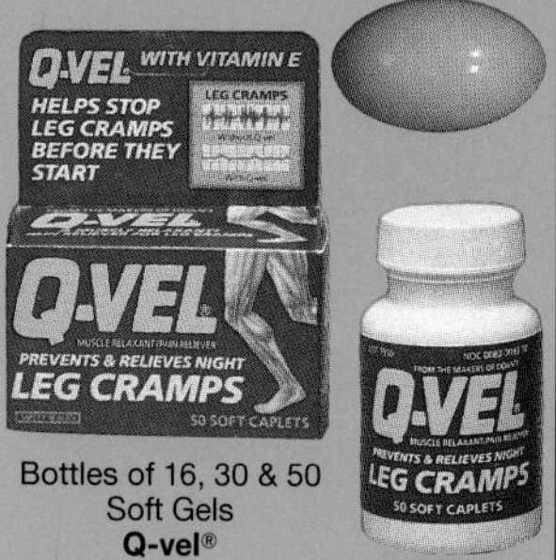

Bottles of 16, 30 & 50
Soft Gels
Q-vel®
Muscle Relaxant
Pain Reliever

COLUMBIA

p. 557

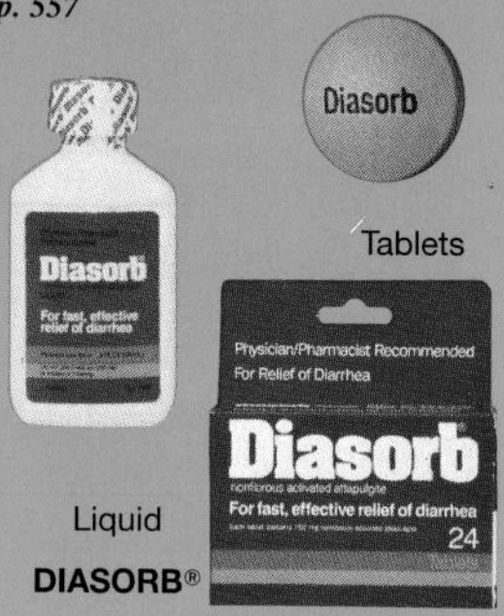

Tablets

Liquid

DIASORB®

Activated Nonfibrous Attapulgite
ANTI-DIARRHEAL

Del Pharmaceuticals
p. 558

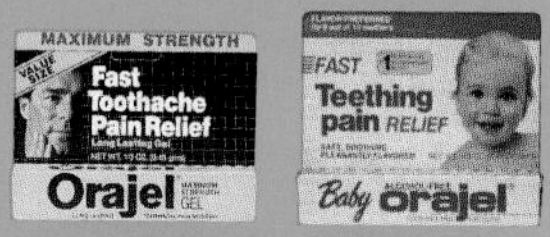

ORAJEL®
MAXIMUM STRENGTH

BABY ORAJEL®
Teething Medicine

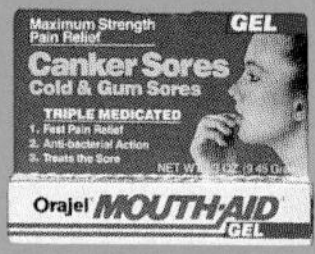

ORAJEL®
MOUTH-AID

Ciba Consumer *p. 554*

1½ oz.

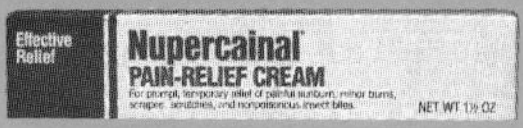

Prompt, temporary relief of painful sunburn, minor burns, scrapes, scratches, and nonpoisonous insect bites.

NUPERCAINAL®
Pain-Relief Cream

Ciba Consumer *p. 556*

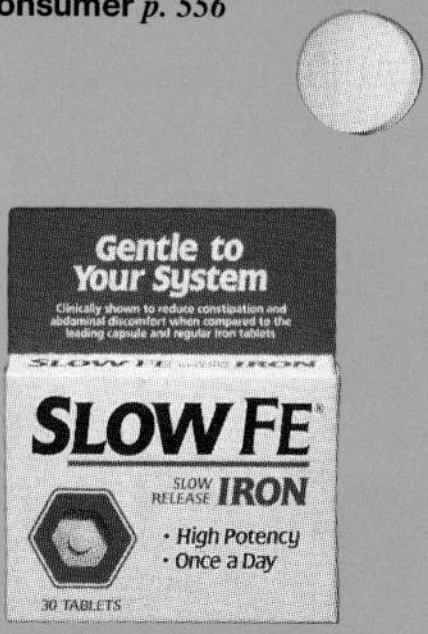

Available in packages of
30, 60 & 100 tablets
SLOW FE®
Slow Release Iron

Columbia
p. 557

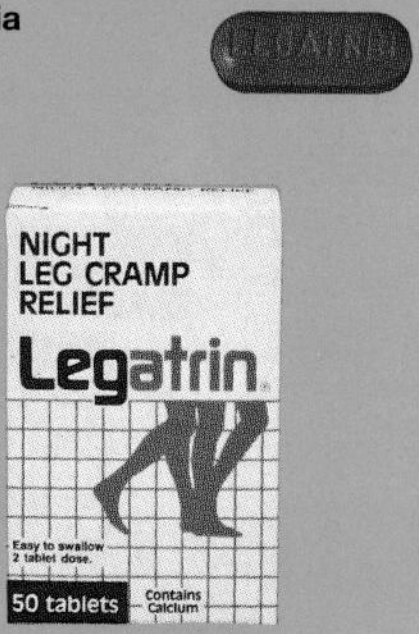
NIGHT LEG CRAMP RELIEF
Legatrin
50 tablets

Available in Packages of 30
and 50 Tablets
LEGATRIN®
Night leg cramp relief

Del Pharmaceuticals
p. 559

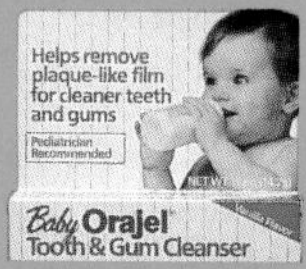

Vanilla Flavor

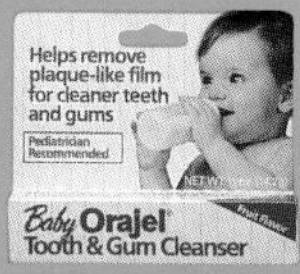

Fruit Flavor

BABY ORAJEL®
TOOTH & GUM CLEANSER

Ciba Consumer *p. 554*

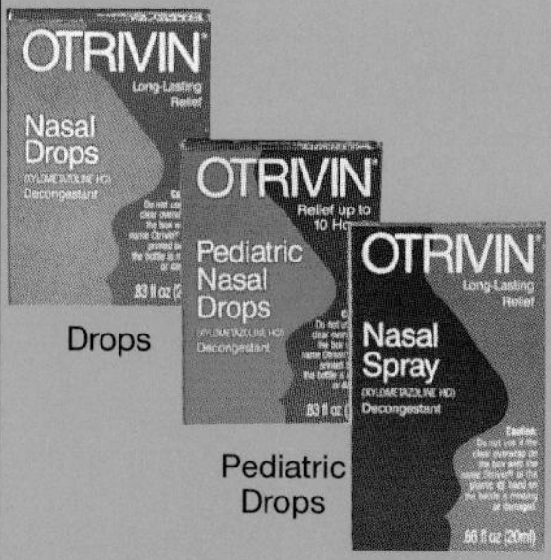

Drops

Pediatric Drops

Nasal Spray

OTRIVIN®
Nasal Decongestant

Ciba Consumer *p. 556*

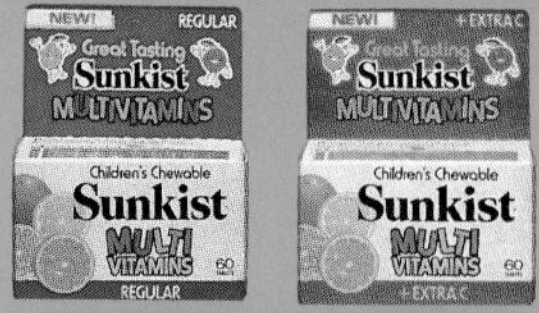

Regular

+ Extra C

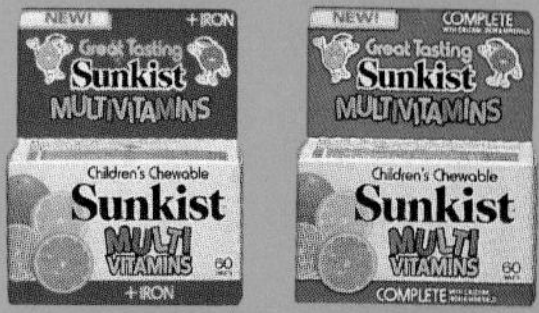

+ Iron

Complete

SUNKIST®
Children's Multivitamins

Copley Pharmaceutical

p. 558

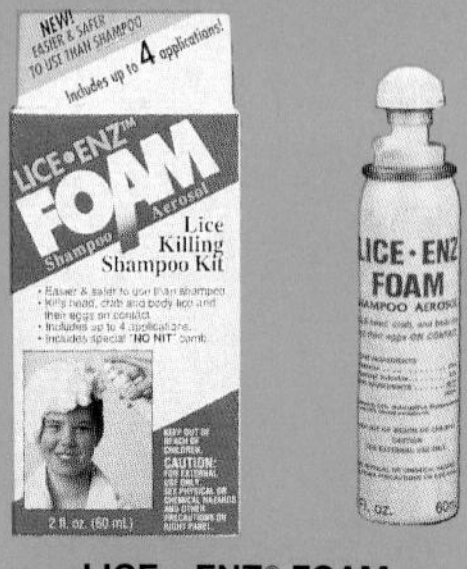

LICE • ENZ® FOAM
Pediculicide Mousse
Easy to use—child friendly

Del Pharmaceuticals
p. 559

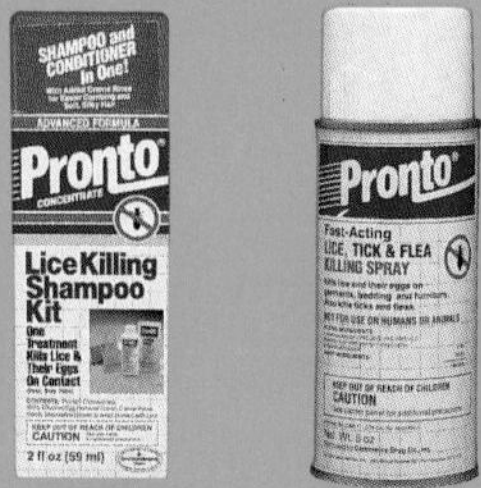

LiceKilling Shampoo Kit

LiceKilling Spray

PRONTO®

EFFCON LABORATORIES

p. 560

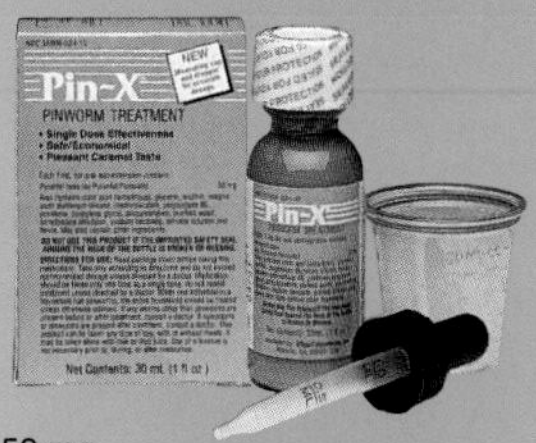

50 mg.

Pin-X®
(Pyrantel Pamoate)

Fisons
p. 563

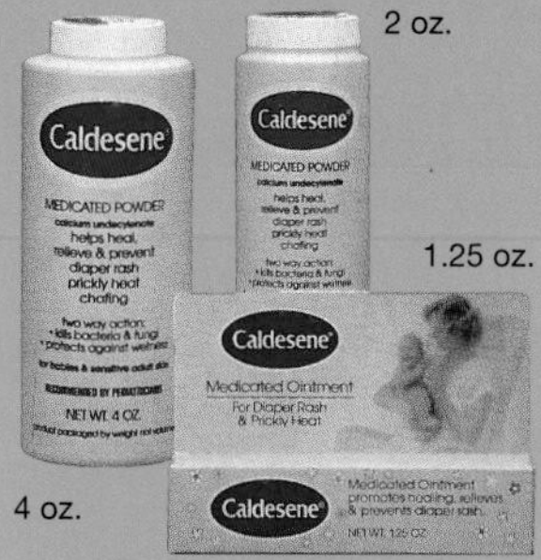

2 oz.
1.25 oz.
4 oz.

CALDESENE®
MEDICATED POWDER and OINTMENT

Fisons
p. 564

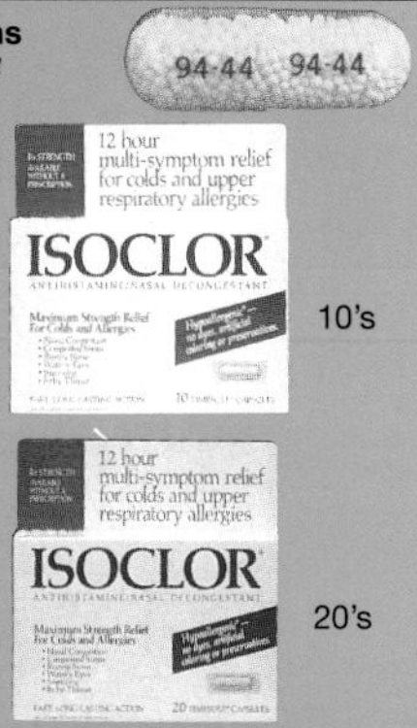

10's
20's

ISOCLOR® TIMESULE® CAPSULES
Nasal Decongestant/Antihistamine

J&J-MERCK

p. 569

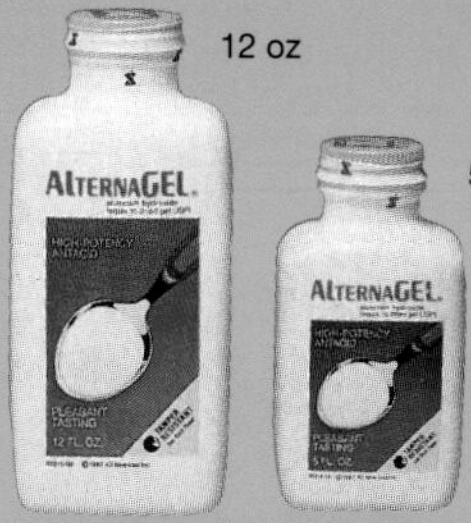
ALTERNAGEL
ALTERNAGEL

12 oz
5 oz

ALternaGEL®
High Potency Aluminum Hydroxide
Antacid

FISONS

p. 561

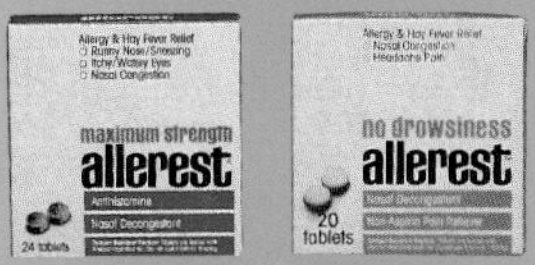

24 tablets — 20 tablets

MAXIMUM STRENGTH ALLEREST® TABLETS

NO DROWSINESS ALLEREST® TABLETS

Allergy & Hay Fever Relief

Fisons
p. 563

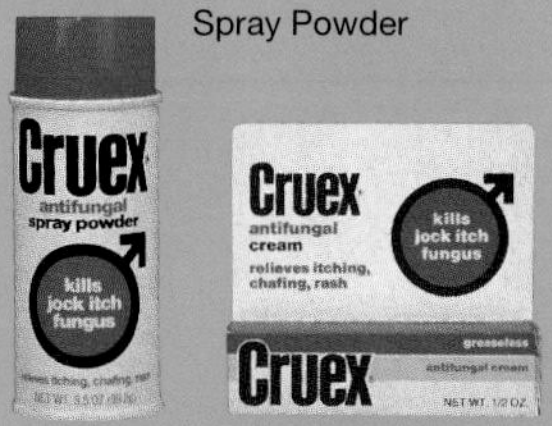

Spray Powder

Cream

CRUEX®
Antifungal Spray Powder & Cream
Relieves Itching, Chafing, Rash

Fisons
p. 565

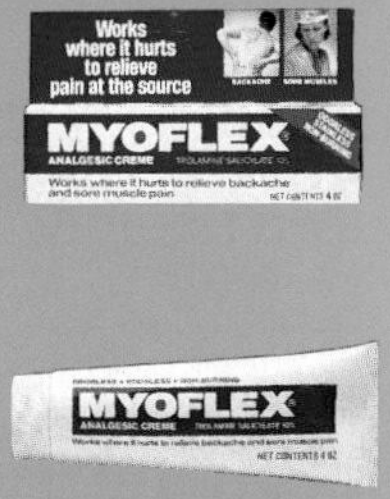

Available in 2 oz. and 4 oz. tubes,
8 oz. and 16 oz. jars

MYOFLEX®
Analgesic Cream
(trolamine salicylate)

J&J-Merck
p. 569

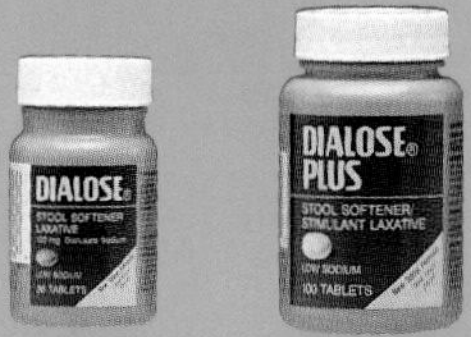
DIALOSE
DIALOSE PLUS

Bottles of 36 & 100 tablets

DIALOSE®
(docusate sodium, 100 mg)

DIALOSE® PLUS
(docusate sodium, 100 mg
yellow phenolphthalein, 65 mg)

Fisons
p. 562

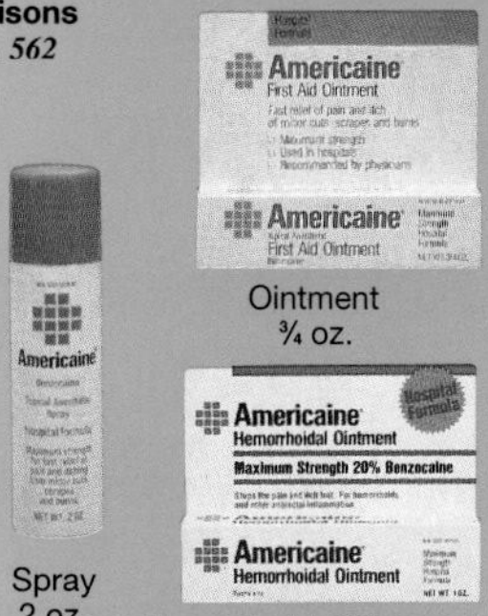

Ointment
¾ oz.

Spray
2 oz.

Hemorrhoidal Ointment
1 oz.

AMERICAINE®
(benzocaine)

Fisons
p. 564

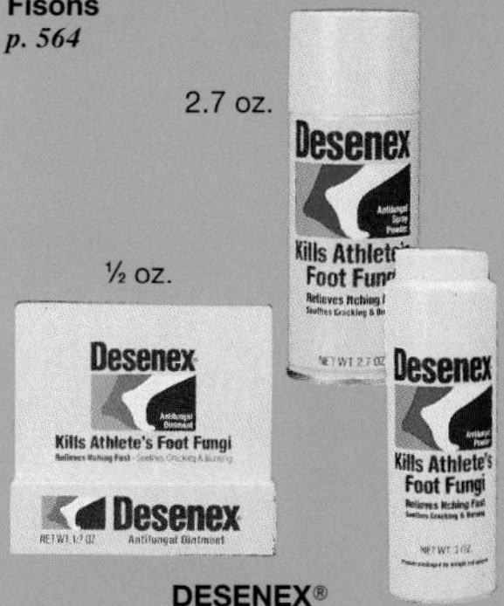

2.7 oz.
½ oz.

DESENEX®
Spray Powder, Powder, Cream & Ointment
Relieves Symptoms of Athlete's Foot

Fisons
p. 565

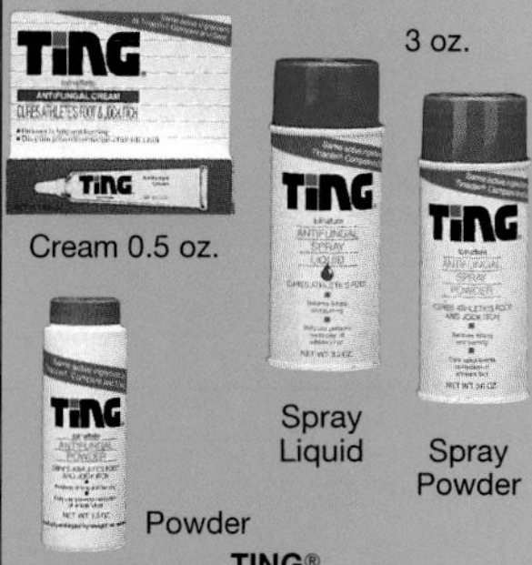
TING
TING
TING
TING
TING

3 oz.
Cream 0.5 oz.
Spray Liquid
Spray Powder
Powder

TING®
(tolnaftate)
For Athlete's Foot & Jock Itch

J&J-Merck
p. 570

Available in 9 oz and 16 oz bottles

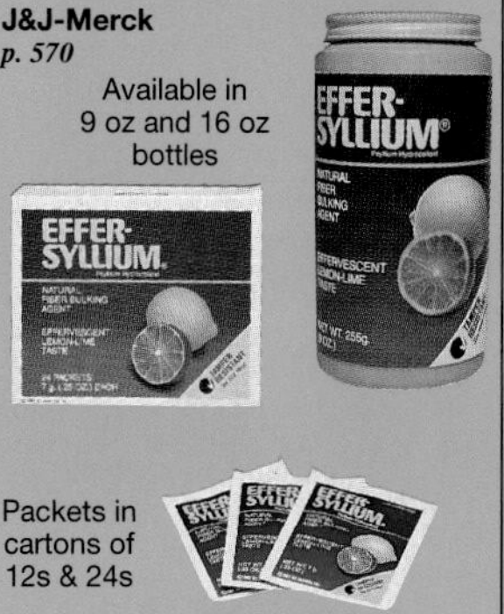
EFFER-SYLLIUM
EFFER-SYLLIUM

Packets in cartons of 12s & 24s

EFFER-SYLLIUM®
Natural Fiber Bulking Agent

Fisons
p. 563

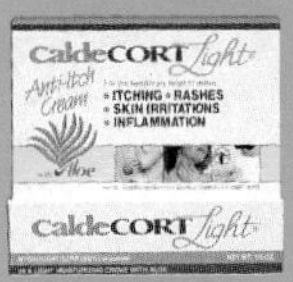

½ oz.

CALDECORT Light® —½% Cream

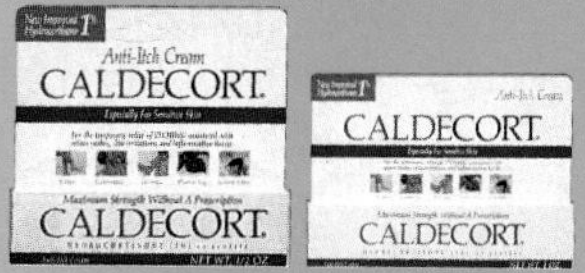

½ oz. — 1 oz.

CALDECORT® —1% Cream
(hydrocortisone acetate)

Fisons
p. 564

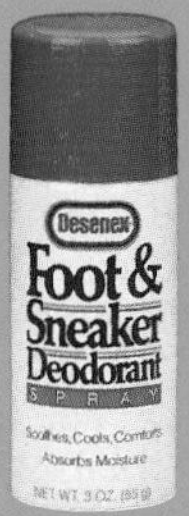
Desenex
Foot & Sneaker Deodorant
SPRAY

3 oz.

DESENEX®
FOOT & SNEAKER DEODORANT
Soothes, Cools, Comforts & Absorbs Moisture

JOHNSON & JOHNSON

Consumer Products
p. 568

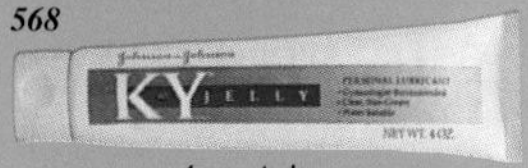
K-Y JELLY

4 oz. tube

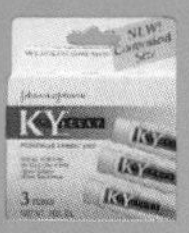

3-pack carton

Available in 2 and 4 oz. tubes and convenient sized 3-packs

K-Y® BRAND **JELLY PERSONAL LUBRICANT**
Water soluble for general lubricating needs

J&J-Merck
p. 570

(layered tablet)

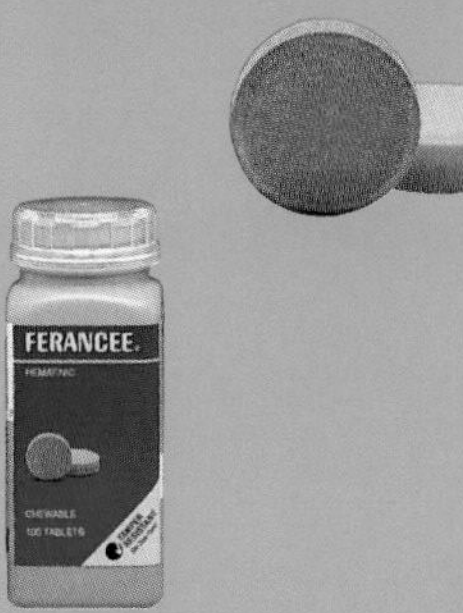
FERANCEE

FERANCEE® Chewable Tablets
Hematinic (iron 67 mg, vitamin C 150 mg)

J&J-Merck
p. 570

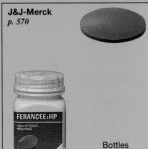

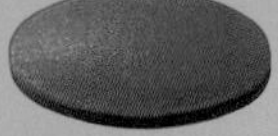
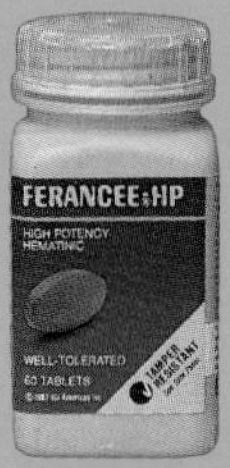

Bottles of 60 tablets

FERANCEE®-HP
High Potency Hematinic

J&J-Merck
p. 570

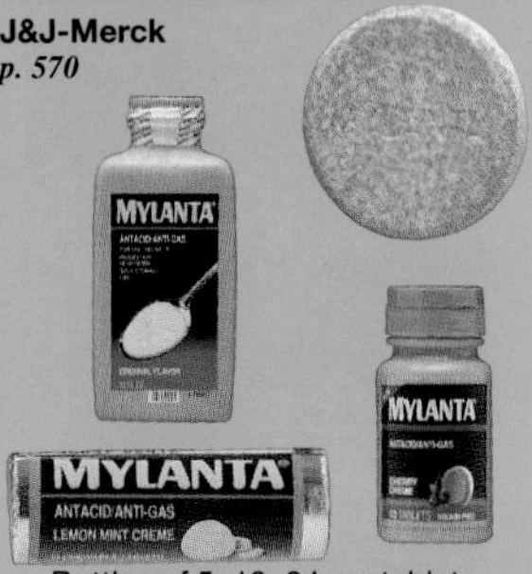

Bottles of 5, 12, 24 oz; tablets in 48 & 100 count bottles; 12 tablet rollpack
MYLANTA® LIQUID & TABLETS
(aluminum hydroxide 200 mg, and magnesium hydroxide 200 mg; simethicone 20 mg)

J&J-Merck
p. 571

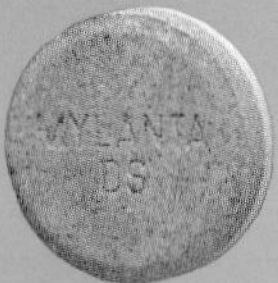

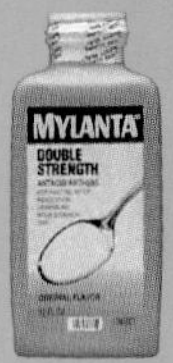

5, 12 & 24 oz liquid

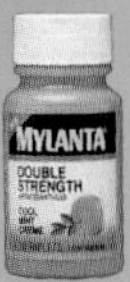

Bottles of 30 & 60 tablets & 8 tablet rollpacks
MYLANTA® DOUBLE STRENGTH LIQUID & TABLETS
(aluminum hydroxide, 400 mg; magnesium hydroxide, 400 mg; simethicone, 40 mg)

J&J-Merck
p. 572

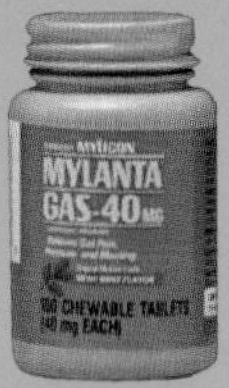

Antiflatulent
Bottles of 100 tablets

MYLANTA® GAS-40 MG
(simethicone, 40 mg)

J&J-Merck
p. 573

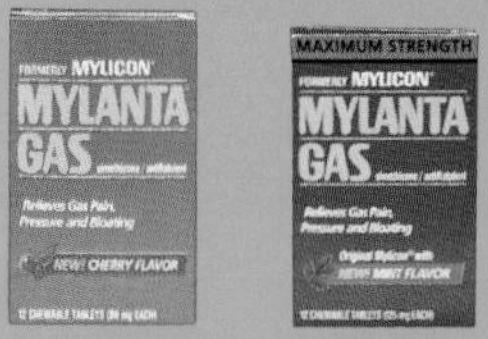

Bottles of 100 12 & 48 tablet Convenience Packs	12 & 60 tablet Convenience Packs
MYLANTA® GAS	**MAXIMUM STRENGTH MYLANTA® GAS**
(simethicone, 80 mg)	(simethicone, 125 mg)

J&J-Merck
p. 573

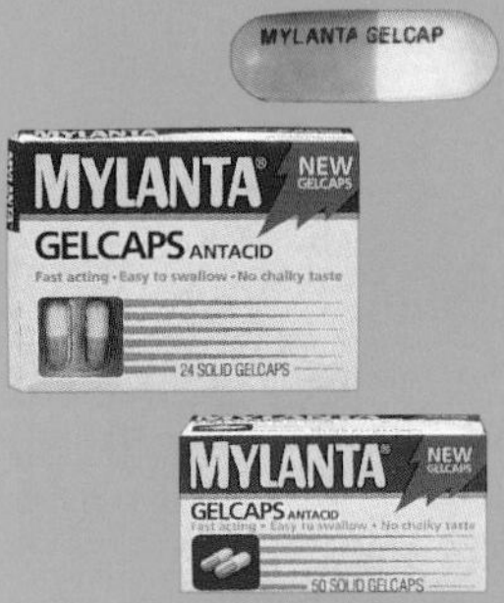

MYLANTA® GELCAPS Antacid
(calcium carbonate 311 mg, magnesium carbonate 232 mg)

J&J-Merck
p. 572

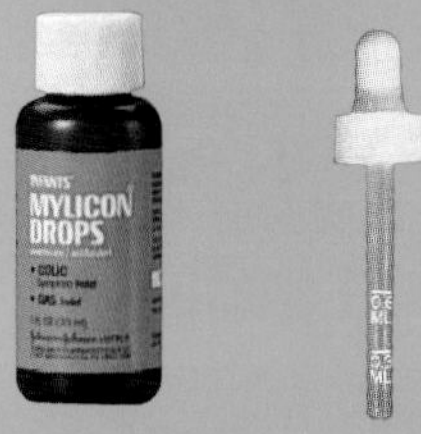

Available in 0.5 oz and 1.0 oz bottles

INFANT'S MYLICON® DROPS
(simethicone, 40 mg per 6 mL dropper)

J&J-Merck
p. 573

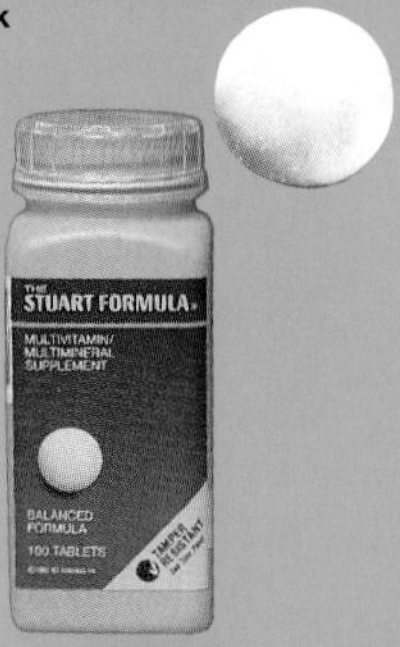

Bottles of 100 and 250 tablets

STUART FORMULA® TABLETS
Multivitamin/Multimineral Supplement

J&J-Merck
p. 574

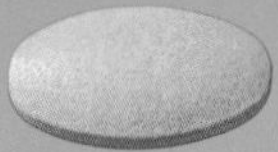
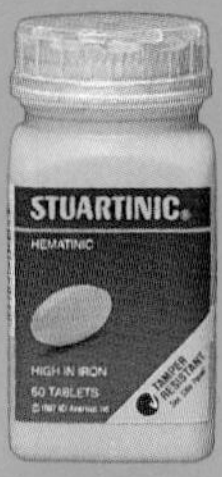

Bottles of 60 tablets

STUARTINIC®
Hematinic

For more detailed information on products illustrated in this section, consult the Product Information Section or manufacturers may be contacted directly.

LEDERLE

LEDERMARK®
Product Identification Code

Many Lederle tablets and capsules bear an identification code, and these codes are listed with each product pictured. A current listing appears in the Product Information Section of the 1993 Physicians' Desk Reference.

Lederle
p. 576

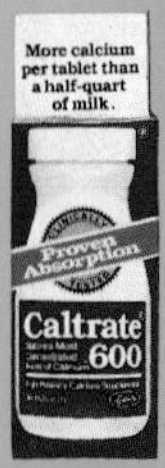

C600

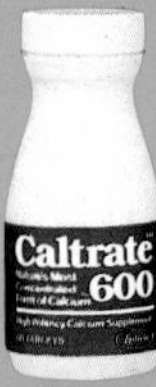

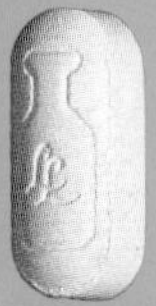

Bottles of 60

CALTRATE® 600
High Potency Calcium Supplement

Lederle
p. 576

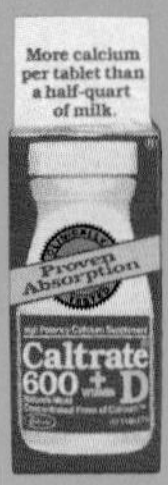

C40

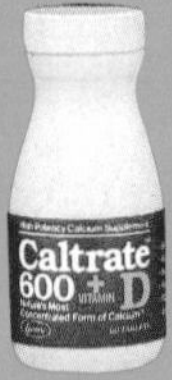

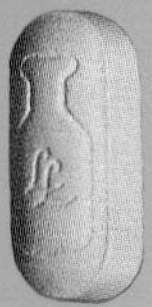

Bottles of 60

CALTRATE® 600+D
High Potency Calcium Supplement

Lederle
p. 576

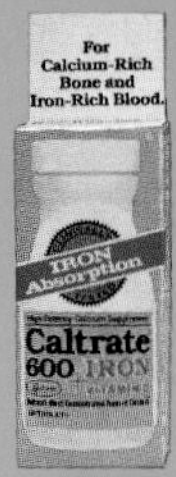

C45

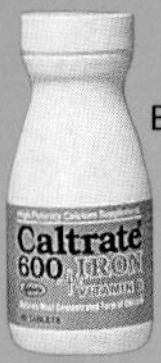

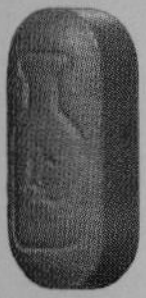

Bottles of 60

CALTRATE® 600+IRON+ VITAMIN D
High Potency Calcium Supplement

Lederle
p. 576

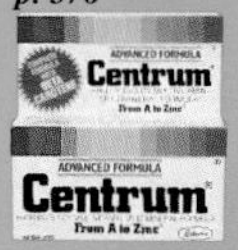

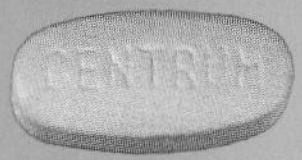

Bottles of 100 + 30
Bottles of 60

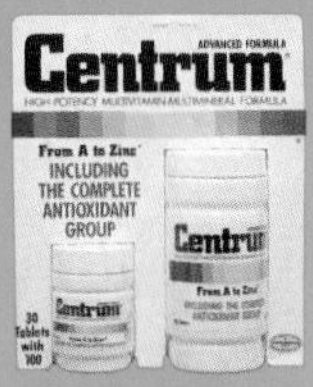

CENTRUM®
High Potency Multivitamin/ Multimineral Formula

Lederle
p. 579

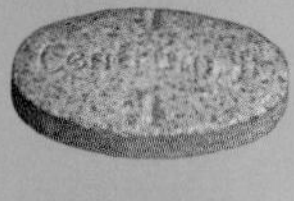

C2

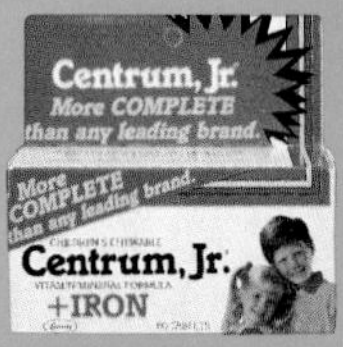

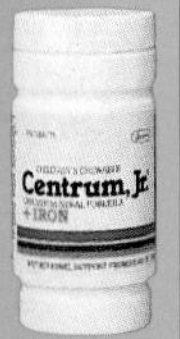

60 tablets

CENTRUM, JR.® + Iron
Children's Chewable Vitamin/Mineral Formula

Lederle
p. 577

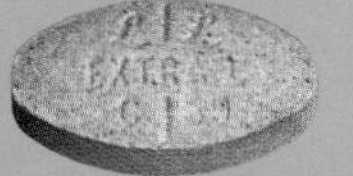

C39

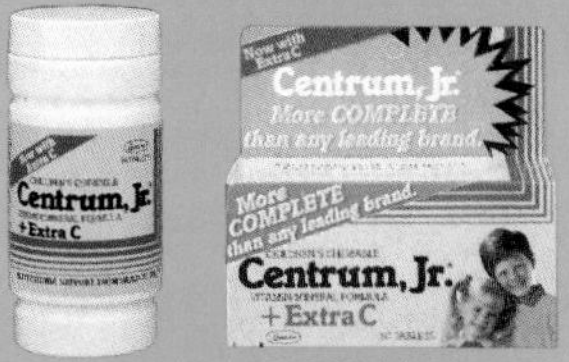

60 tablets

CENTRUM, JR.® + Extra C
Children's Chewable
Vitamin/Mineral Formula

Lederle
p. 579

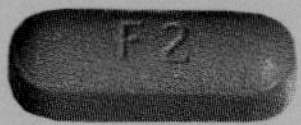

F2

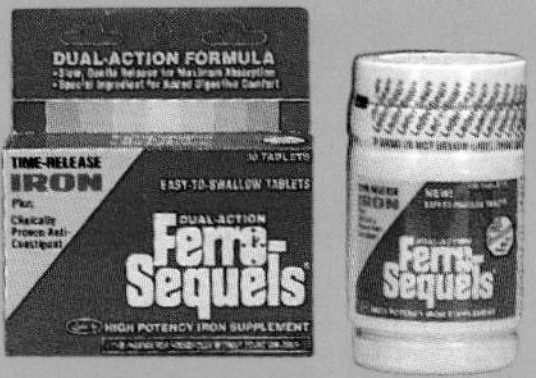

Available in blister packs of 30 and bottles of 30 and 100

FERRO-SEQUELS®
High Potency Iron Supplement
with Proven Anti-Constipant

Lederle
p. 581

S2

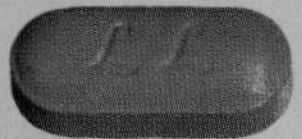

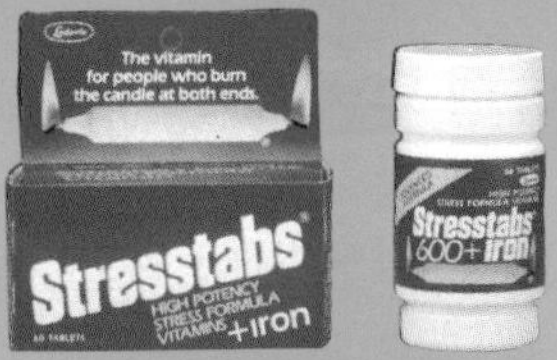

Bottles of 60

Advanced Formula
STRESSTABS®
with IRON

High Potency Stress Formula
Vitamins

Lever Brothers
p. 582

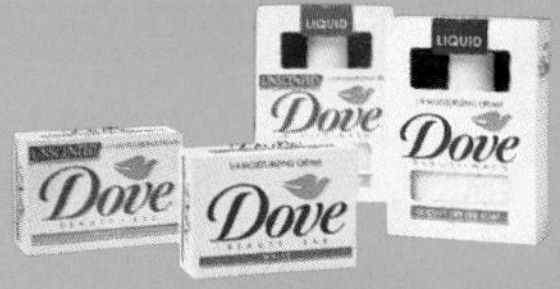

DOVE® BAR & LIQUID DOVE®
BEAUTY WASH

Lederle
p. 577

C60

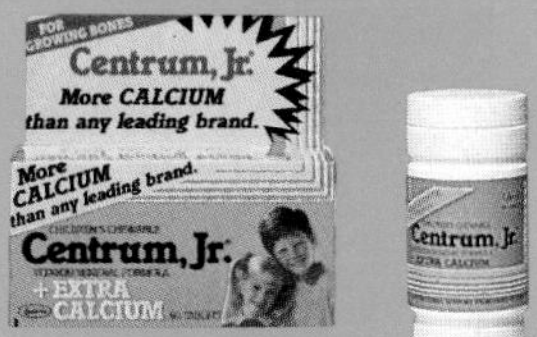

60 tablets

CENTRUM, JR.® + Extra Calcium
Children's Chewable
Vitamin/Mineral Formula

Lederle
p. 579

F66**

Available in boxes of 36 and 60 and bottles of 90

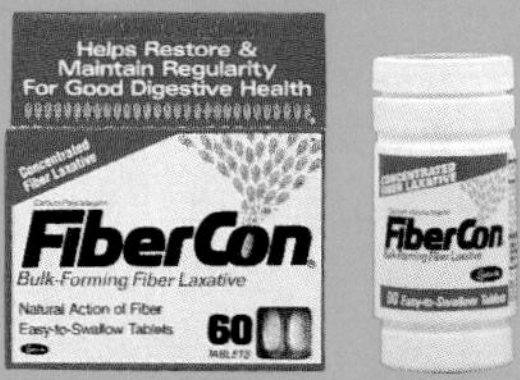

FIBERCON®
(calcium polycarbophil)

Lederle
p. 581

S3

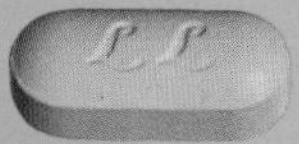

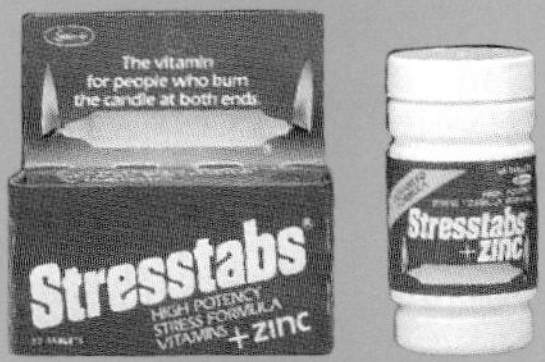

Bottles of 60

Advanced Formula
STRESSTABS®
with ZINC

High Potency Stress Formula
Vitamins

McNEIL CONSUMER

p. 587

325 mg.

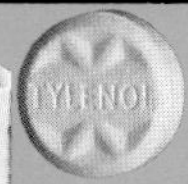

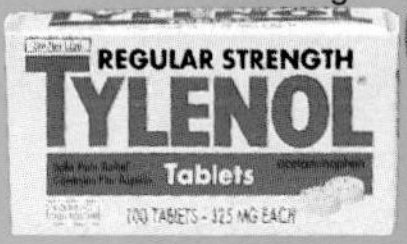

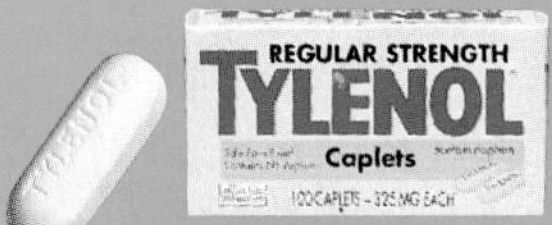

Tablets and Caplets
Available in 24's, 50's, 100's and 200's.

REGULAR STRENGTH TYLENOL®
acetaminophen Tablets and Caplets

Lederle
p. 577

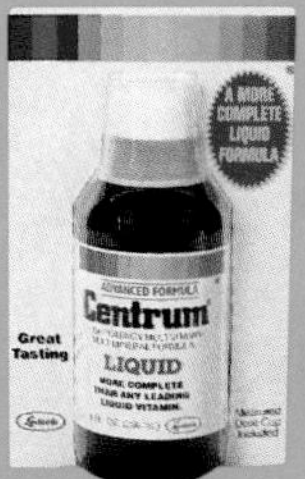

CENTRUM® LIQUID
High Potency
Multivitamin/Multimineral
Formula

Lederle
p. 581

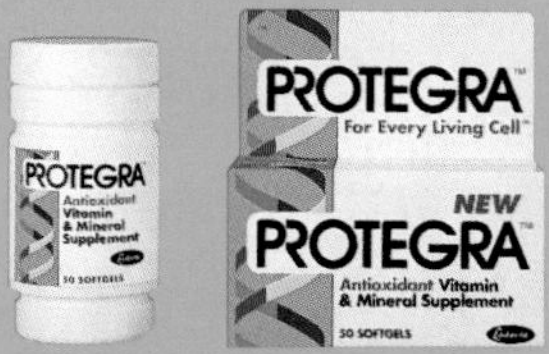

Bottle of 50 Softgels

PROTEGRA™
Antioxidant Vitamin & Mineral
Supplement

Lederle
p. 582

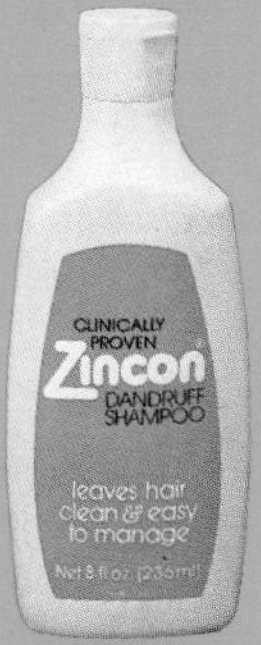

Bottles of 4 fl. oz. and 8 fl. oz.

ZINCON®
Pyrithione Zinc 1%
Dandruff Shampoo

McNeil Consumer
p. 588

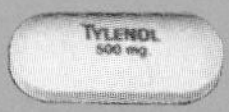

500 mg.

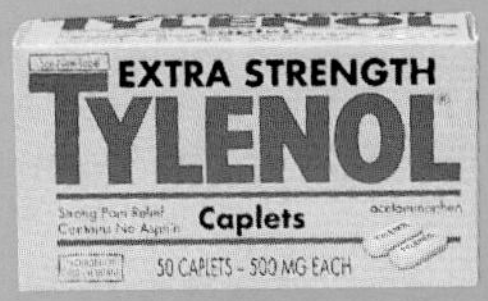

Caplets available in tamper-resistant vials of 10 and bottles of 24, 50, 100, 175 and 250.

EXTRA STRENGTH TYLENOL®
acetaminophen
Caplets

Lederle
p. 579

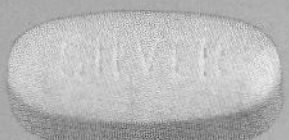

CS11

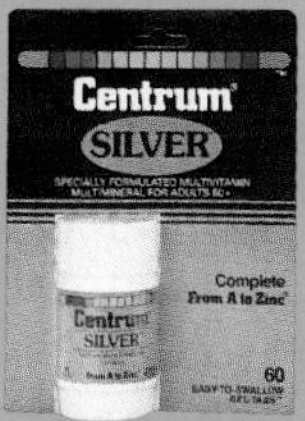

Bottles of 60 and 100

CENTRUM SILVER®
Specially Formulated
Multivitamin/Multimineral
For adults 50+

Lederle
p. 581

S1

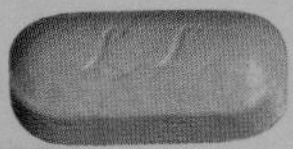

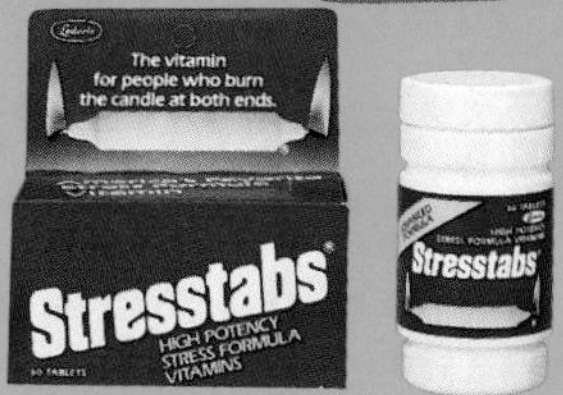

Bottles of 60

Advanced Formula
STRESSTABS®

High Potency Stress Formula
Vitamins

LEVER BROTHERS

p. 582

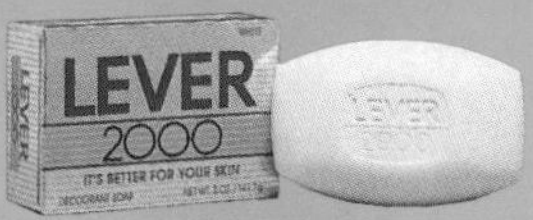

LEVER 2000®
Antibacterial/Deodorant Soap

McNeil Consumer
p. 588

500 mg.

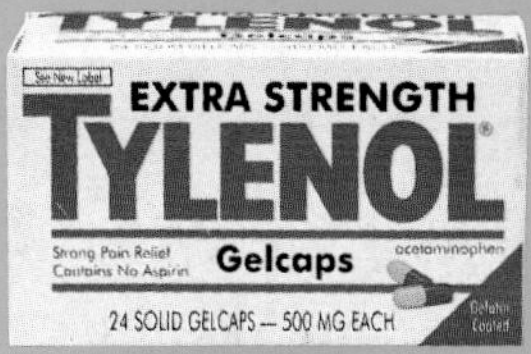

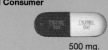

Gelcaps available in tamper-resistant bottles of 24, 50, 100 and 150.

EXTRA STRENGTH TYLENOL®
acetaminophen
GELCAPS®

McNeil Consumer
p. 588

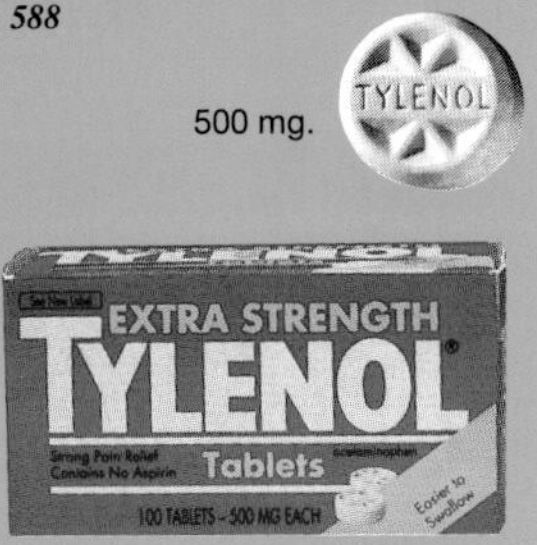

Tablets available in tamper-resistant vials of 10 and bottles of 30, 60, 100 and 200. Liquid: 8 fl. oz.

EXTRA STRENGTH TYLENOL®
acetaminophen
Tablets & Liquid

McNeil Consumer
p. 591

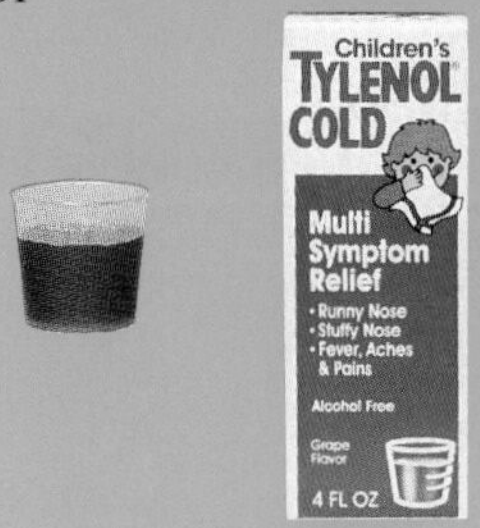

Available in 4 fl. oz. bottle with child-resistant safety cap and convenient dosage cup.

CHILDREN'S TYLENOL® COLD
Multi-Symptom Formula

McNeil Consumer
p. 595

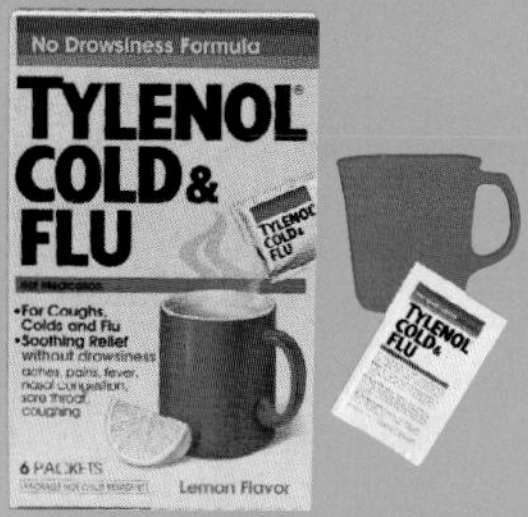

Available in cartons of 6 or 12 individual packets.

TYLENOL® COLD & FLU
Hot Liquid Medication
No Drowsiness Formula

McNeil Consumer
p. 597

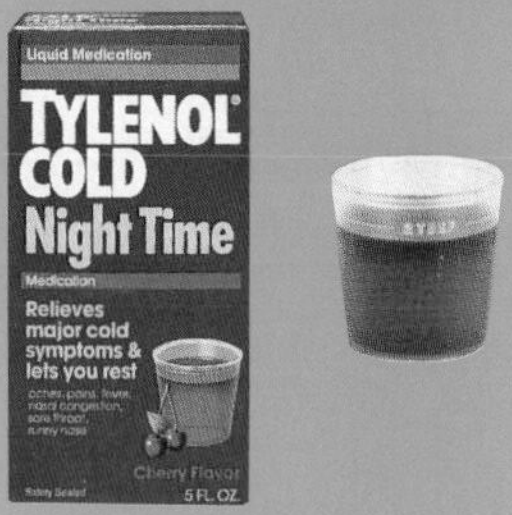

Available in 5 fl. oz. bottle with child-resistant safety cap and convenient dosage cup enclosed.

TYLENOL® COLD NIGHT TIME
Liquid Medication

McNeil Consumer
p. 586

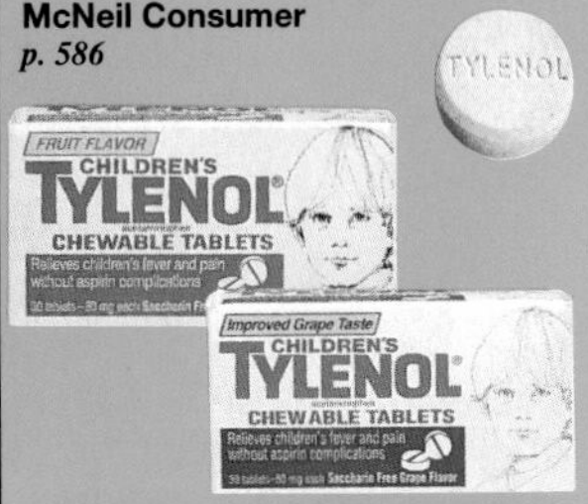

Fruit flavor: available in bottles of 30 with child-resistant safety cap and blister-packs of 48.

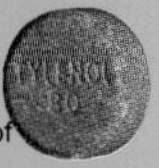

Grape flavor: available in bottles of 30 with child-resistant safety cap.

CHILDREN'S TYLENOL®
acetaminophen
80 mg. Chewable Tablets

McNeil Consumer
p. 591

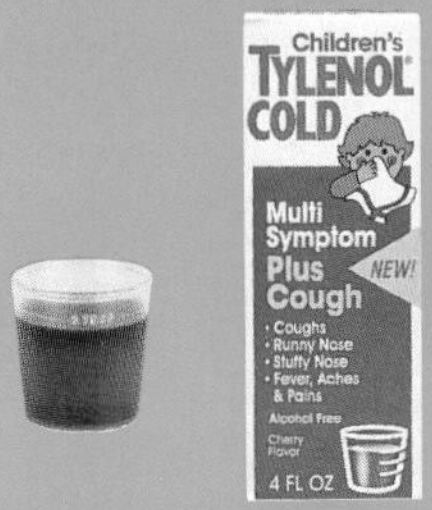

Available in 4 fl. oz. bottle with child-resistant safety cap and convenient dosage cup.

CHILDREN'S TYLENOL® COLD
Multi-Symptom Plus Cough Formula

McNeil Consumer
p. 596

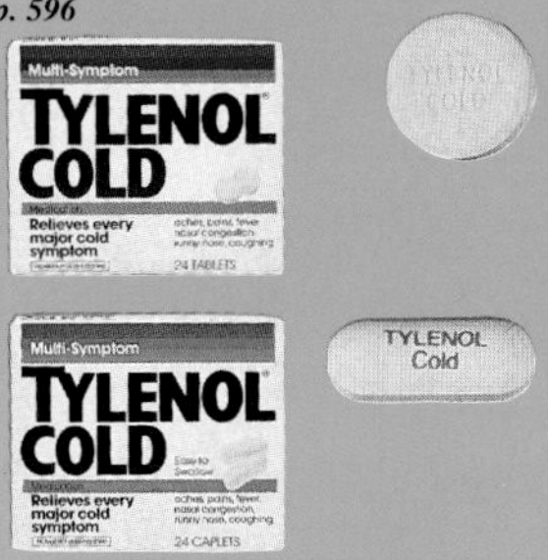

Available in blister-packs of 24 and bottles of 50.

TYLENOL® COLD
Medication
Tablets and Caplets

McNeil Consumer
p. 598

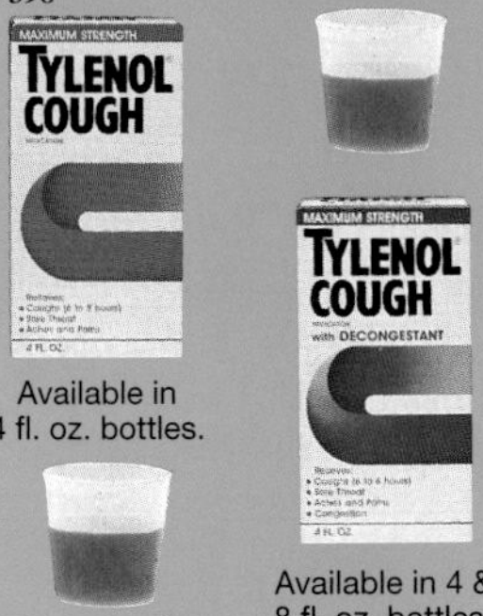

Available in 4 fl. oz. bottles.

Available in 4 & 8 fl. oz. bottles.

MAXIMUM STRENGTH
TYLENOL® COUGH

McNeil Consumer
p. 586

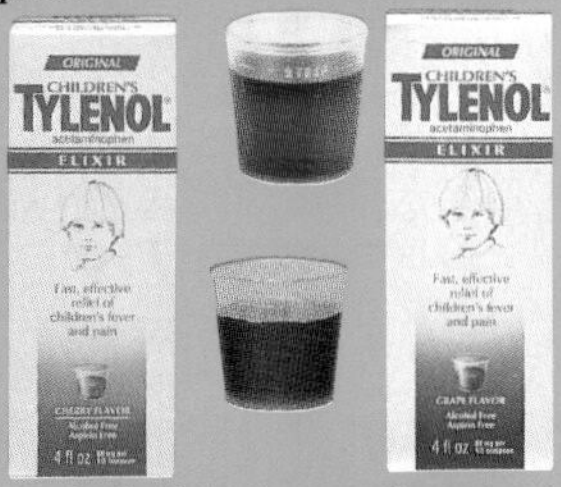

Available in cherry and grape flavors in 2 and 4 fl. oz. bottles with child-resistant safety cap and convenient dosage cup.

CHILDREN'S TYLENOL®
acetaminophen
Alcohol Free Elixir

McNeil Consumer
p. 586

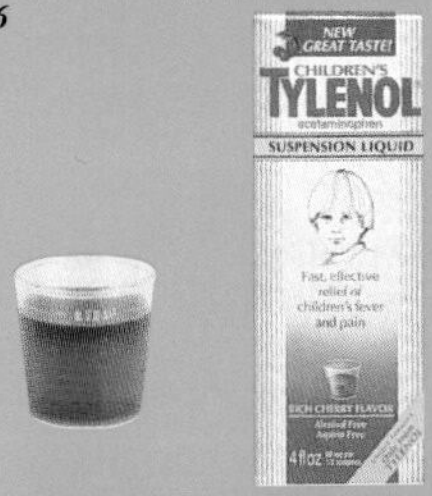

Available in rich cherry flavor in 2 and 4 fl. oz. bottles with child-resistant safety cap and convenient dosage cup.

CHILDREN'S TYLENOL®
SUSPENSION LIQUID
Alcohol Free Suspension Liquid

McNeil Consumer
p. 594

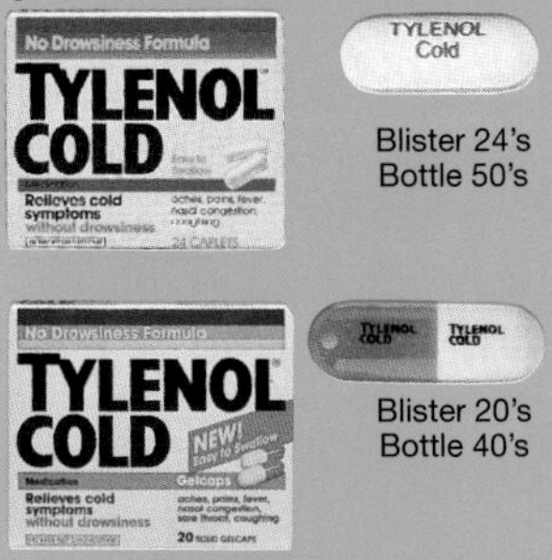

Blister 24's
Bottle 50's

Blister 20's
Bottle 40's

TYLENOL® COLD
Medication
No Drowsiness Formula
Caplets and Gelcaps

McNeil Consumer
p. 589

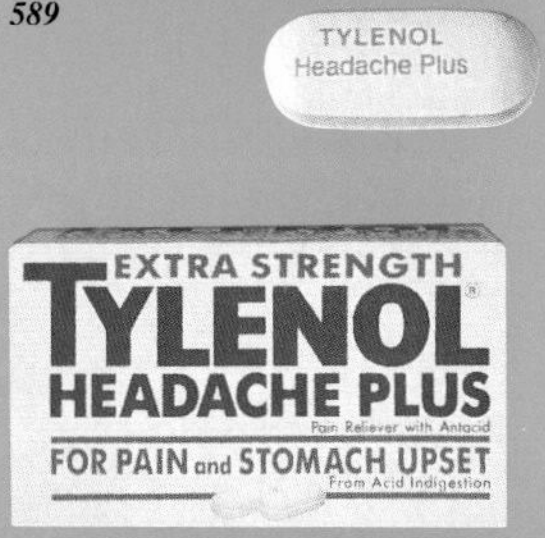

Caplets available in 24's, 50's and 100's.

TYLENOL® HEADACHE PLUS

McNeil Consumer
p. 591

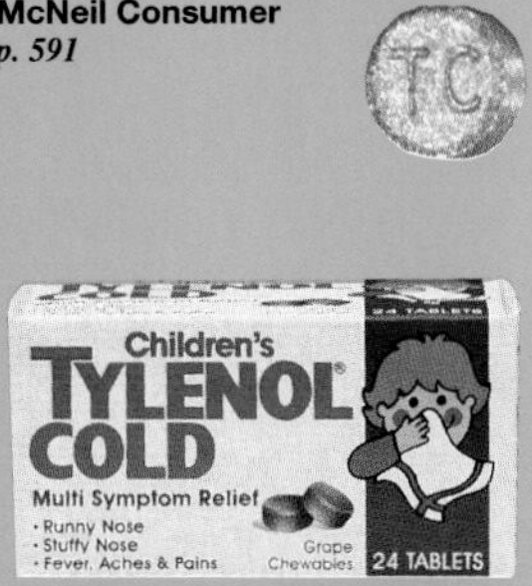

Available in bottles of 24 chewable tablets with child-resistant safety cap.

CHILDREN'S TYLENOL® COLD
Chewable Cold Tablets

McNeil Consumer
p. 593

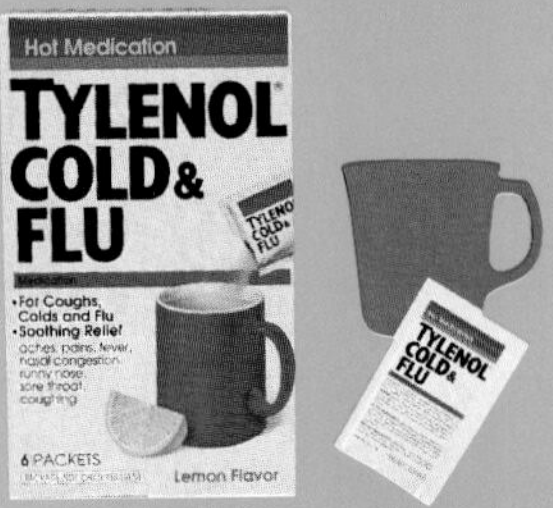

Available in cartons of 6 or 12 individual packets.

TYLENOL® COLD & FLU
Hot Liquid Medication

McNeil Consumer
p. 592

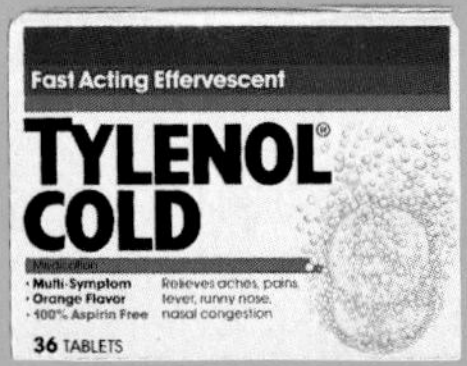

Available in cartons of 20.

TYLENOL® COLD MEDICATION
Effervescent Formula

While every effort has been made to reproduce products faithfully, this section is to be considered a Quick-Reference identification aid.

McNeil Consumer
p. 586

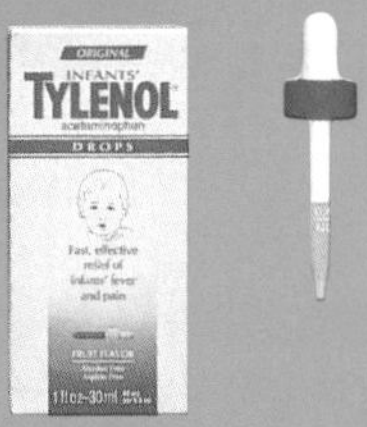

Available in ½ and 1 fl. oz. bottle with child-resistant safety cap and calibrated dropper.

INFANTS' TYLENOL®
acetaminophen
Alcohol Free Drops

McNeil Consumer
p. 586

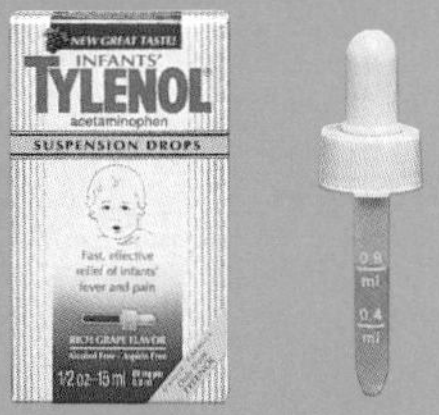

Available in ½ oz. bottle with child-resistant safety cap and calibrated dropper. Rich Grape Flavor.

INFANTS' TYLENOL® SUSPENSION DROPS
Alcohol Free Suspension

McNeil Consumer
p. 587

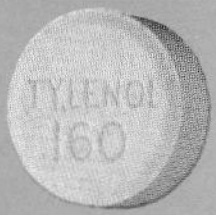

Fruit Flavored Chewable

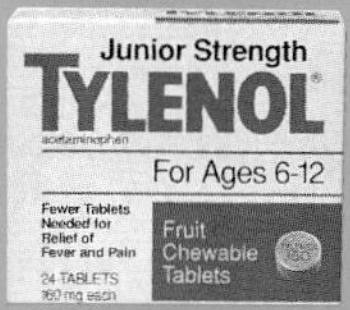

JUNIOR STRENGTH FRUIT FLAVORED CHEWABLE TYLENOL® TABLETS

Available in blister pack of 24.

McNeil Consumer
p. 587

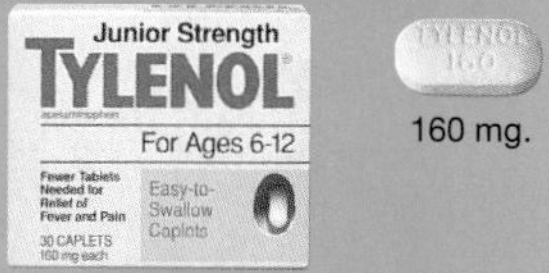

160 mg.

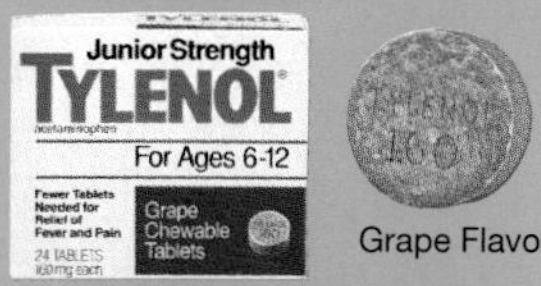

Grape Flavor

JUNIOR STRENGTH TYLENOL®
acetaminophen

Swallowable Caplets: Blister pack of 30.
Chewable Tablets: Blister pack of 24.

McNeil Consumer
p. 590

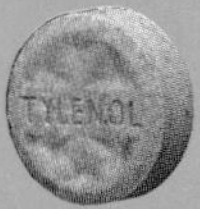

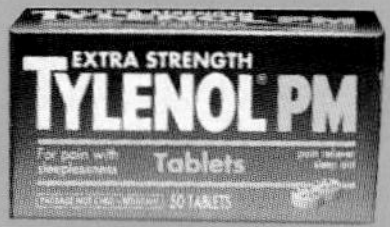

Tablets available in tamper-resistant bottles of 24 and 50.

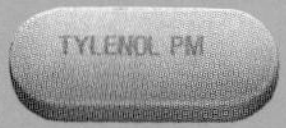

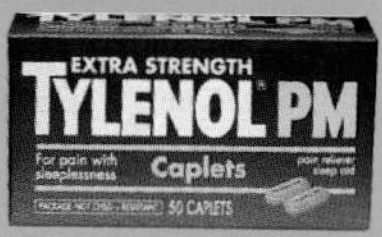

Caplets available in tamper-resistant bottles of 24 and 50.

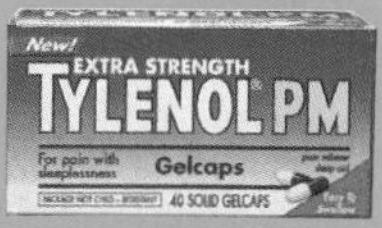

Gelcaps available in tamper-resistant bottles of 20 and 40.

TYLENOL® PM

McNeil Consumer
p. 600

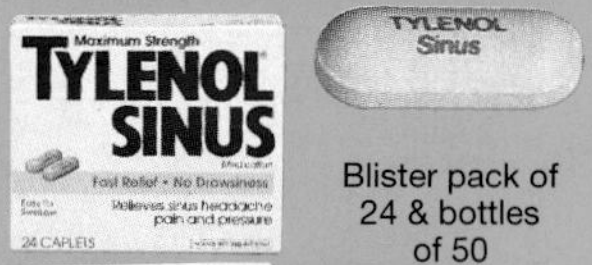

Blister pack of 24 & bottles of 50

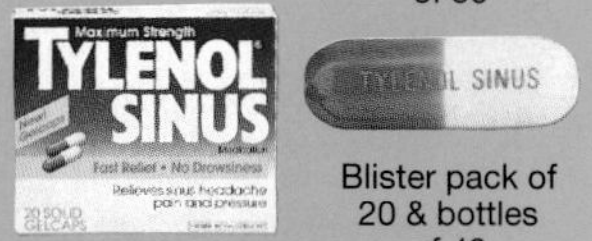

Blister pack of 20 & bottles of 40

Also available in tablet form.

MAXIMUM-STRENGTH TYLENOL® SINUS MEDICATION

McNeil Consumer
p. 598

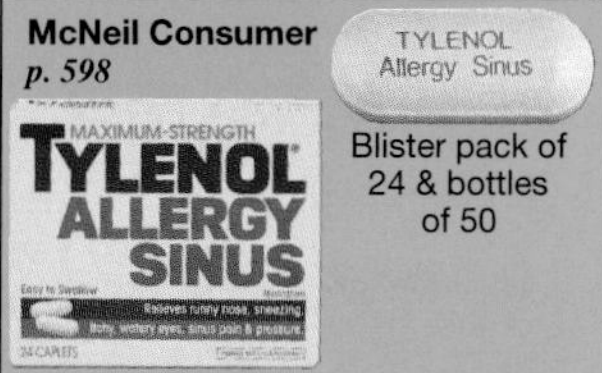

Blister pack of 24 & bottles of 50

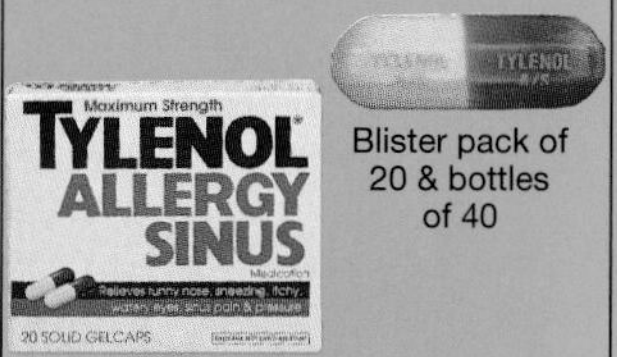

Blister pack of 20 & bottles of 40

MAXIMUM-STRENGTH TYLENOL® ALLERGY SINUS MEDICATION

McNeil Consumer
p. 583

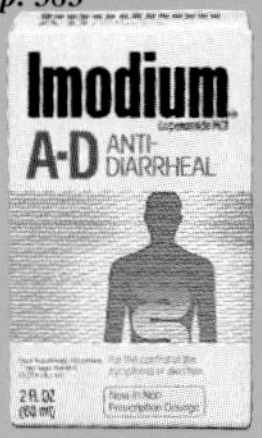

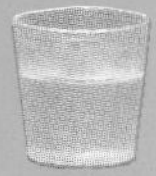

Available in 2, 3 and 4 fl. oz. bottles with a convenient dosage cup, and caplets in 6's, 12's and 18's.

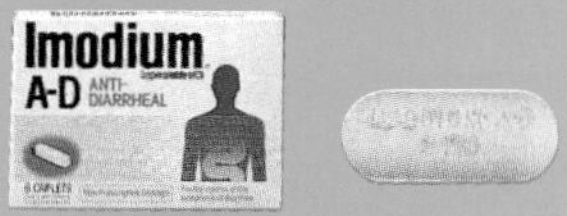

IMODIUM® A-D
loperamide HCl
ANTI-DIARRHEAL

Lactaid Inc. Marketed by McNeil Consumer Products
p. 575

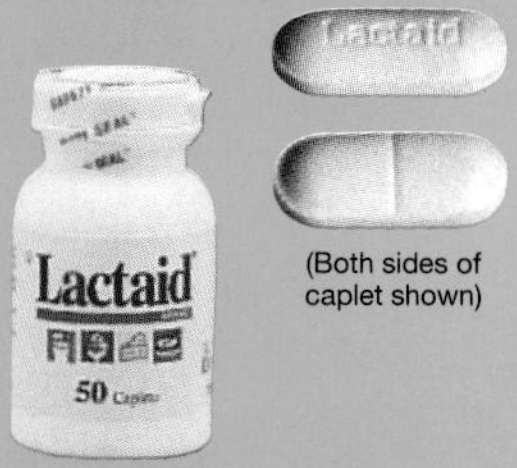

(Both sides of caplet shown)

LACTAID® CAPLETS
(lactase enzyme caplets)

Lactaid Inc. Marketed by McNeil Consumer Products

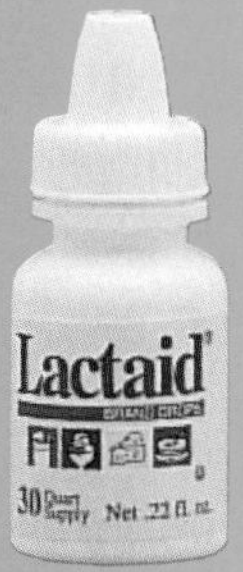

LACTAID® DROPS
(lactase enzyme)

McNeil Consumer
p. 584

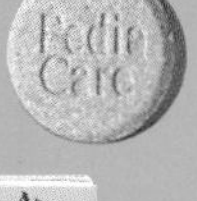
Pedia
Care

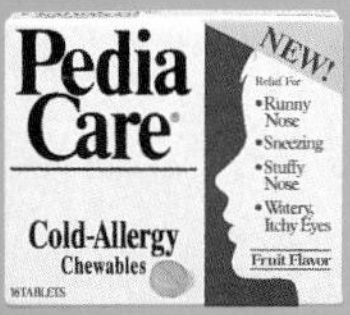
NEW!
Pedia
Care
Cold-Allergy
Chewables

Blister packs of 16 chewable tablets.

PEDIACARE®
Cold-Allergy Chewable Tablets

McNeil Consumer
p. 584

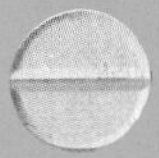

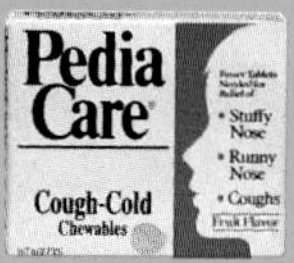
Pedia
Care
Cough-Cold
Chewables

Blister packs of 16 chewable tablets.

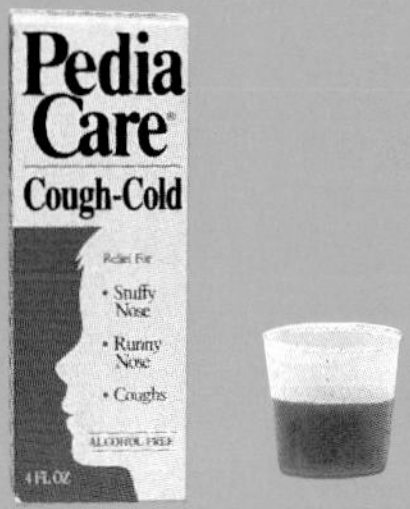

4 fl. oz. bottle with convenient dosage cup.

Available in 4 fl. oz. bottle with child-resistant safety cap and convenient dosage cup.

PEDIACARE®
Cough-Cold Formula

McNeil Consumer
p. 584

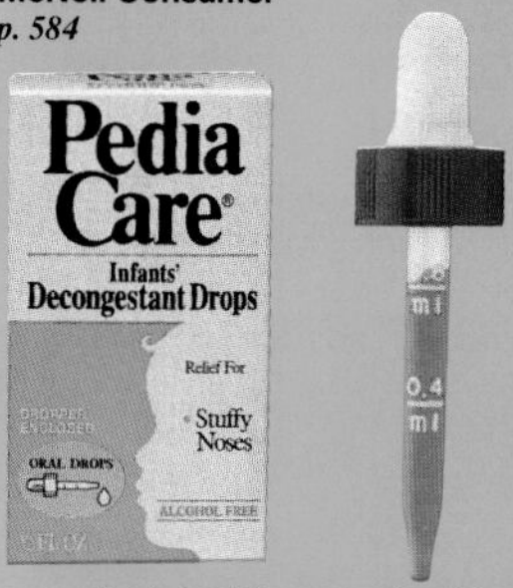
Pedia
Care
Infants'
Decongestant Drops

Available in ½ fl. oz. bottle with child-resistant safety cap and calibrated dropper.

PEDIACARE®
Oral Decongestant Drops

McNeil Consumer
p. 584

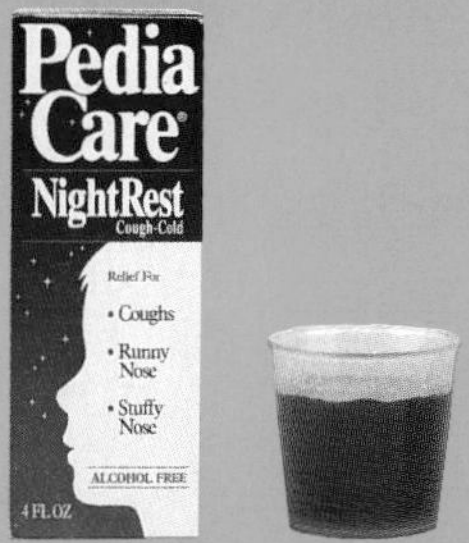

Available in 4 fl. oz. bottle with child-resistant safety cap and convenient dosage cup.

PEDIACARE® NIGHTREST
Cough-Cold Formula

McNeil Consumer
p. 585

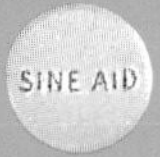

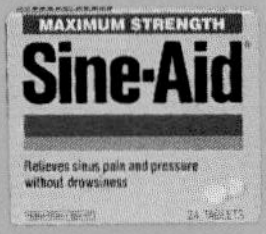

Blister packs of 24 & bottles of 50 tablets.

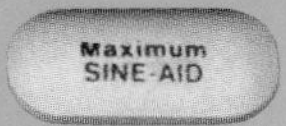

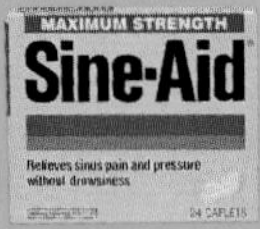

Blister packs of 24 & bottles of 50 caplets.

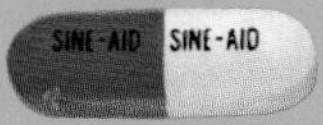

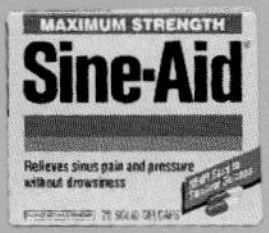

Blister packs of 20 & bottles of 40 gelcaps.

MAXIMUM-STRENGTH SINE-AID®
Relieves sinus headache and pressure

MENLEY & JAMES

p. 602

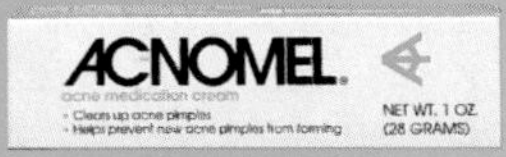

1 oz. tube

ACNOMEL®
ACNE MEDICATION CREAM
(resorcinol, sulfur)

Menley & James
p. 601

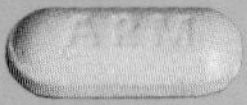

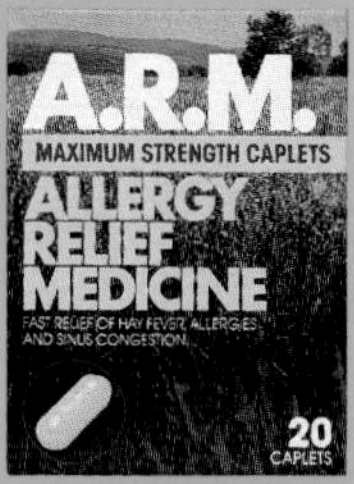

Packages of 20 and 40 caplets
A.R.M.® ALLERGY RELIEF MEDICINE
(chlorpheniramine maleate, phenylpropanolamine HCl)

Menley & James
p. 602

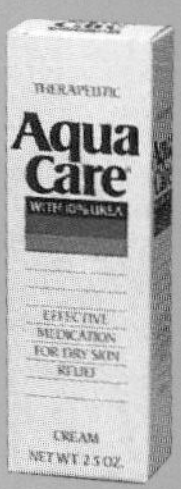

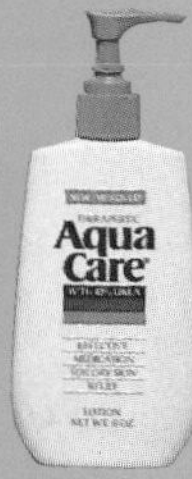

2.5 oz. tube 8 oz. bottle

AQUA CARE® CREAM AND LOTION with 10% Urea

Menley & James
p. 603

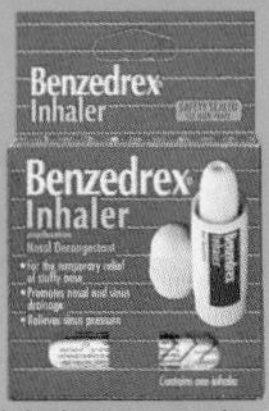

1 inhaler per package
BENZEDREX® INHALER
(propylhexedrine)

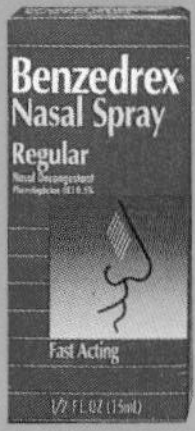

BENZEDREX® NASAL SPRAY REGULAR
(phenylephrine HCl)

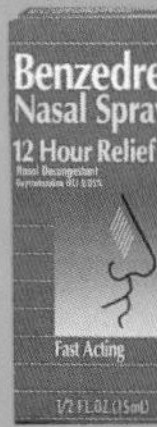

BENZEDREX® NASAL SPRAY 12 HOUR RELIEF
(oxymetazoline HCl)

Menley & James
p. 604

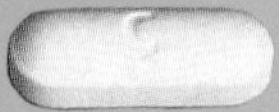

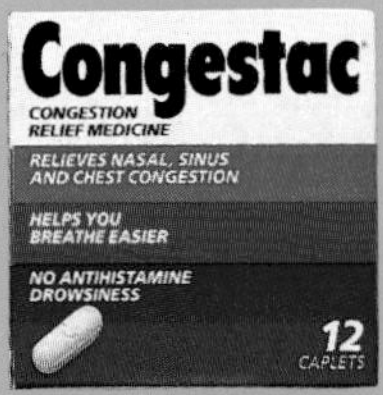

Packages of 12 and 24 caplets

CONGESTAC®
Congestion Relief Medicine
Decongestant/Expectorant

Menley & James
p. 604

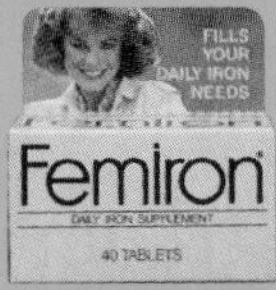

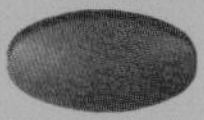

FEMIRON® REGULAR
Bottles of 40 and 120

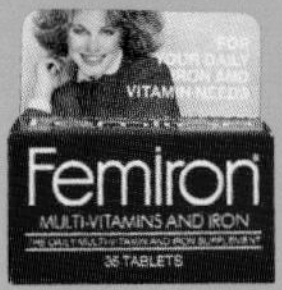

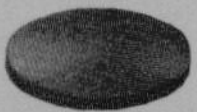

FEMIRON® WITH VITAMINS
Bottles of 35, 60 and 90

Menley & James
p. 604

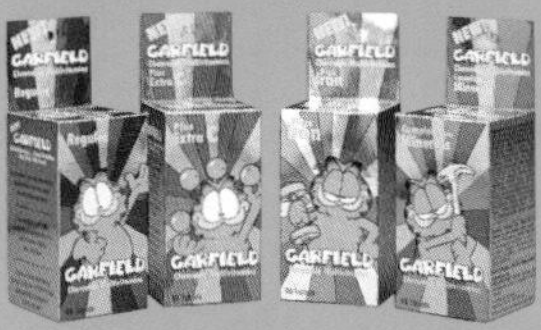

GARFIELD CHILDREN'S CHEWABLE MULTIVITAMINS

Available in: Regular, Plus Extra C, Plus Iron and Complete with Minerals

GARFIELD: ©1978 United Feature Syndicate, Inc.

Menley & James
p. 606

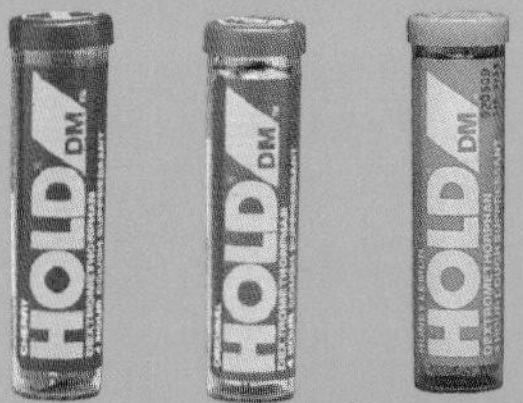

Cherry Original HoneyLemon

Each contains 10 lozenges

HOLD®
Cough Suppressant
Lozenges with Dextromethorphan

Menley & James
p. 607

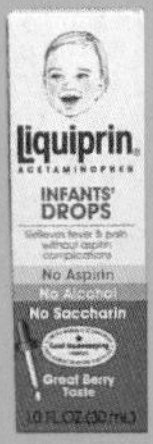

1 fl. oz. Berry Flavored
No Aspirin No Alcohol No Saccharin
Child-Resistant Safety Cap

LIQUIPRIN®
Acetaminophen

Menley & James
p. 607

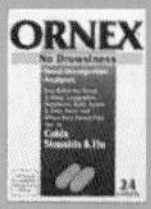
ORNEX

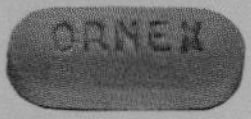
ORNEX

Regular Strength

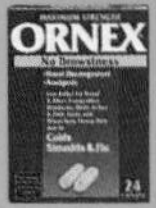

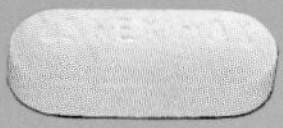

Maximum Strength

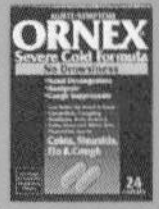

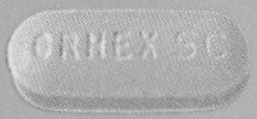

Severe Cold Formula

ORNEX® CAPLETS
Decongestant/Analgesic

Menley & James
p. 608

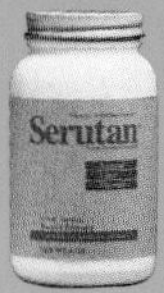

6 oz.

Toasted Granules

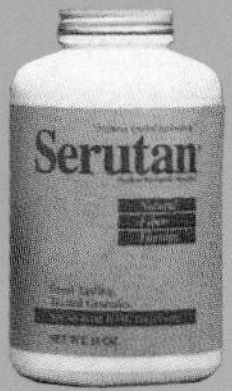

18 oz.

SERUTAN®
Natural Fiber
Therapy For Regularity (psyllium)

Available in:
Toasted Granules—6 and 18 oz.
Regular Powder—7, 14 and 21 oz.
Fruit Flavored Powder—6, 12 and 18 oz.

MILES INC.

Consumer Healthcare Products
p. 609

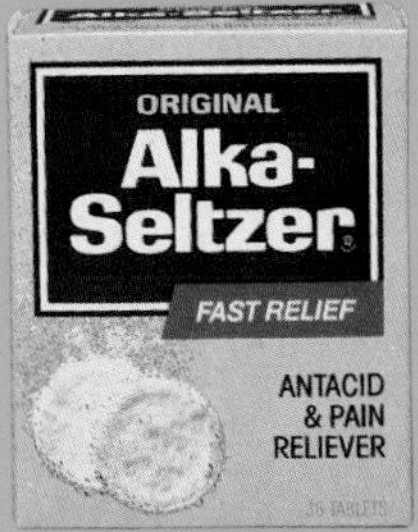
ORIGINAL
Alka-Seltzer
FAST RELIEF
ANTACID & PAIN RELIEVER

ALKA-SELTZER®
EFFERVESCENT
ANTACID & PAIN RELIEVER

Miles Inc.
Consumer Healthcare Products
p. 610

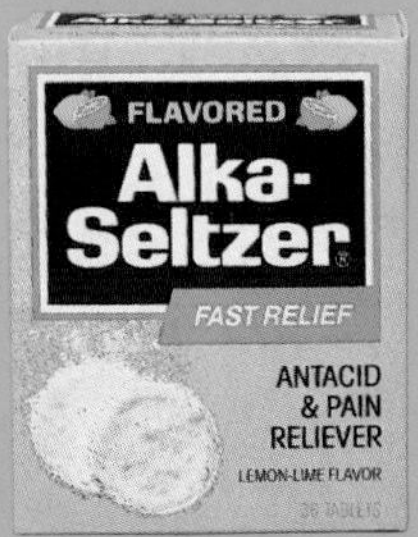
FLAVORED
Alka-Seltzer
FAST RELIEF
ANTACID & PAIN RELIEVER
LEMON-LIME FLAVOR

ALKA-SELTZER®
FLAVORED EFFERVESCENT
ANTACID & PAIN RELIEVER

Miles Inc.
Consumer Healthcare Products
p. 611

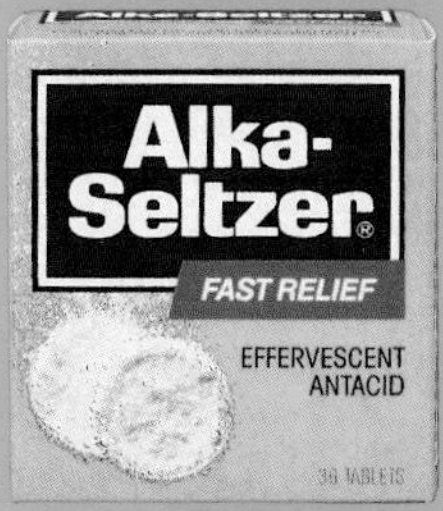

ALKA-SELTZER® EFFERVESCENT ANTACID

Miles Inc.
Consumer Healthcare Products
p. 612

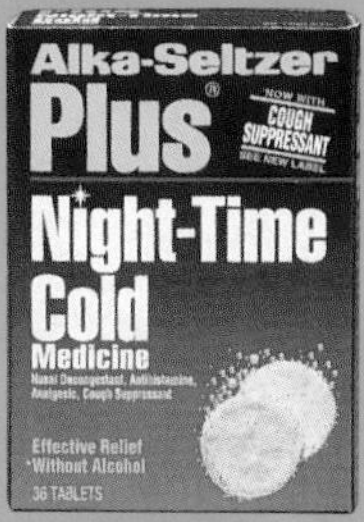

ALKA-SELTZER PLUS® NIGHT-TIME COLD MEDICINE NASAL DECONGESTANT ANTIHISTAMINE ANALGESIC COUGH SUPPRESSANT

Miles Inc.
Consumer Healthcare Products
p. 614

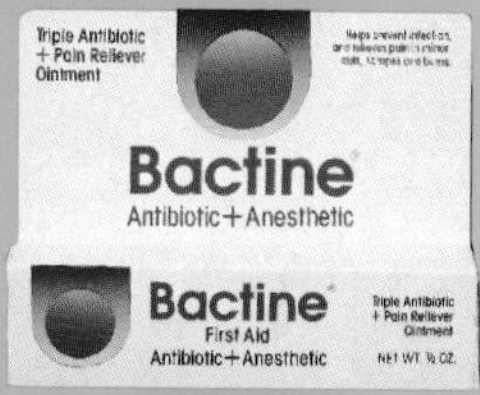

BACTINE® FIRST AID ANTIBIOTIC OINTMENT

Miles Inc.
Consumer Healthcare Products
p. 616

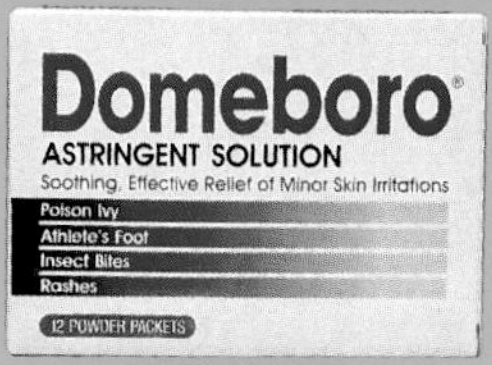

DOMEBORO® ASTRINGENT SOLUTION

Miles Inc.
Consumer Healthcare Products
p. 612

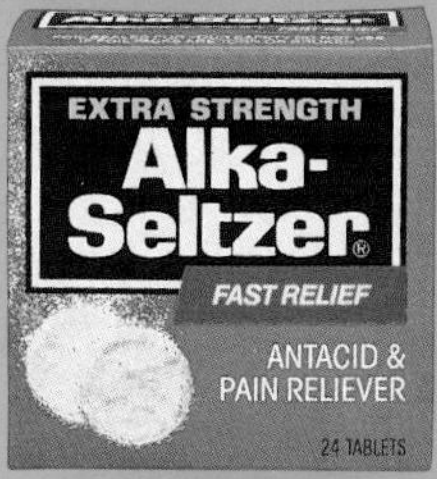

ALKA-SELTZER® EXTRA STRENGTH EFFERVESCENT ANTACID & PAIN RELIEVER

Miles Inc.
Consumer Healthcare Products
p. 613

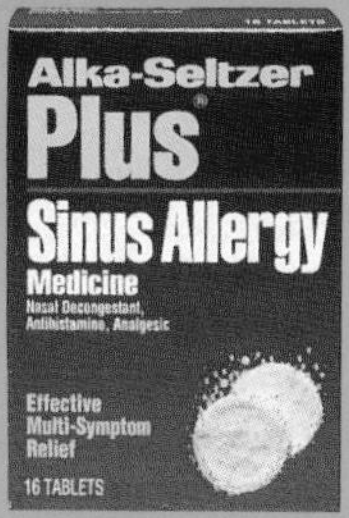

ALKA-SELTZER PLUS® SINUS ALLERGY MEDICINE NASAL DECONGESTANT ANTIHISTAMINE ANALGESIC

Miles Inc.
Consumer Healthcare Products
p. 614

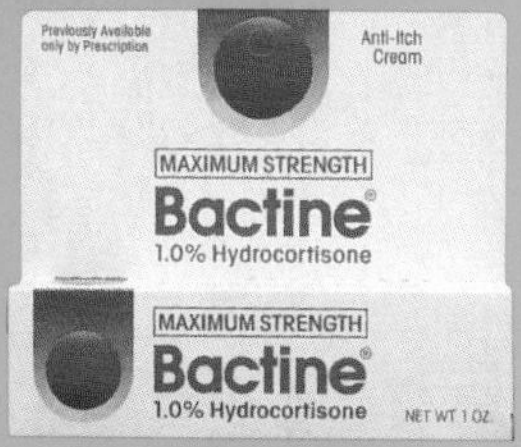

BACTINE® HYDROCORTISONE (1.0%) ANTI-ITCH CREAM

Miles Inc.
Consumer Healthcare Products
p. 615

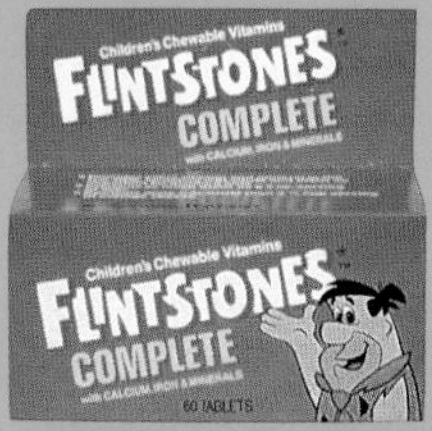

FLINTSTONES™ BRAND COMPLETE CHILDREN'S CHEWABLE VITAMINS WITH IRON, CALCIUM & MINERALS

Miles Inc.
Consumer Healthcare Products
p. 612

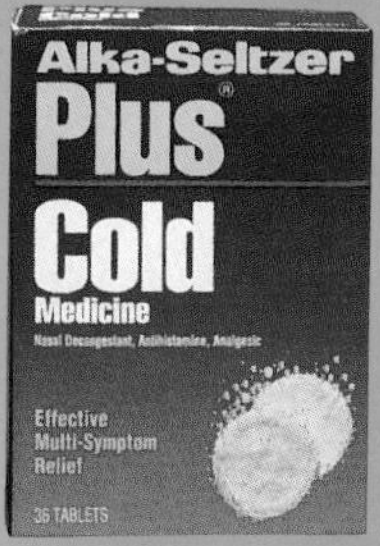

ALKA-SELTZER PLUS® COLD MEDICINE NASAL DECONGESTANT ANTIHISTAMINE ANALGESIC

Miles Inc.
Consumer Healthcare Products
p. 609

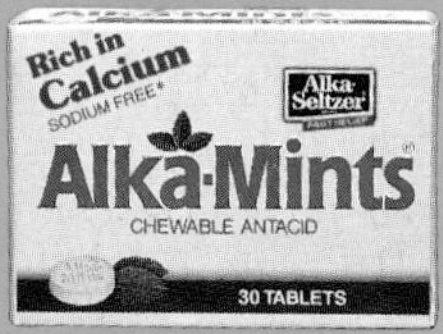

ALKA-MINTS® CHEWABLE ANTACID
(Calcium Carbonate 850 mg)

Miles Inc.
Consumer Healthcare Products
p. 615

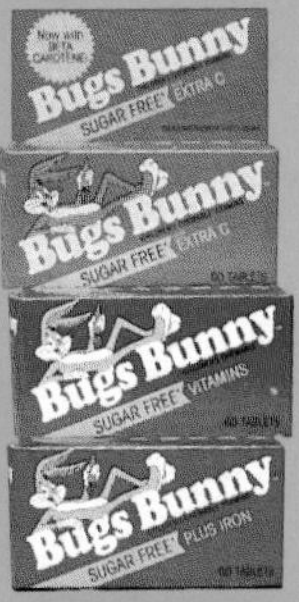

BUGS BUNNY™ BRAND SUGAR FREE CHILDREN'S CHEWABLE VITAMINS WITH EXTRA C, REGULAR, AND PLUS IRON

Miles Inc.
Consumer Healthcare Products
p. 615

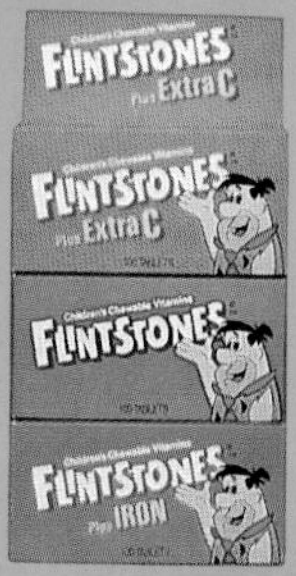

FLINTSTONES™ BRAND CHILDREN'S CHEWABLE VITAMINS WITH EXTRA C, REGULAR, AND PLUS IRON

Miles Inc.
Consumer Healthcare Products
p. 613

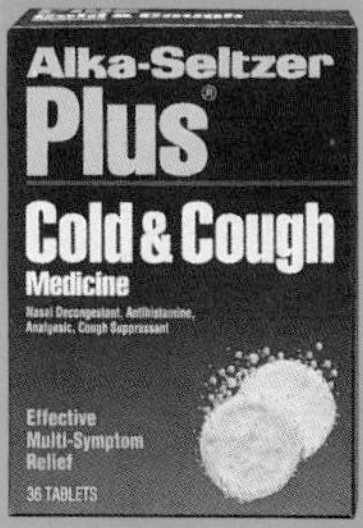

ALKA-SELTZER PLUS® COLD & COUGH MEDICINE NASAL DECONGESTANT ANTIHISTAMINE ANALGESIC COUGH SUPPRESSANT

Miles Inc.
Consumer Healthcare Products
p. 614

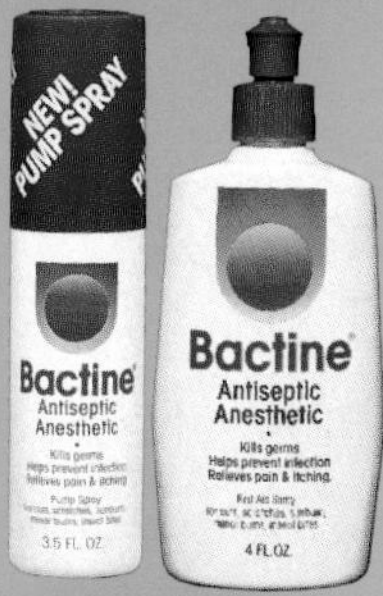

BACTINE® ANTISEPTIC • ANESTHETIC FIRST AID SPRAY
Liquid

Miles Inc.
Consumer Healthcare Products
p. 615

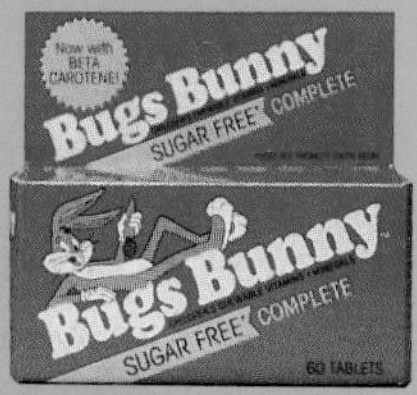

BUGS BUNNY™ BRAND SUGAR FREE CHILDREN'S CHEWABLE VITAMINS + MINERALS

Miles Inc.
Consumer Healthcare Products
p. 617

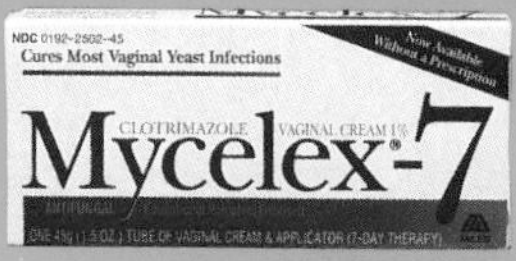

Also available:
Mycelex-7 Vaginal Inserts 100 mg

MYCELEX-7® CLOTRIMAZOLE (ANTIFUNGAL) VAGINAL CREAM 1%

Miles Inc.
Consumer Healthcare Products
p. 617

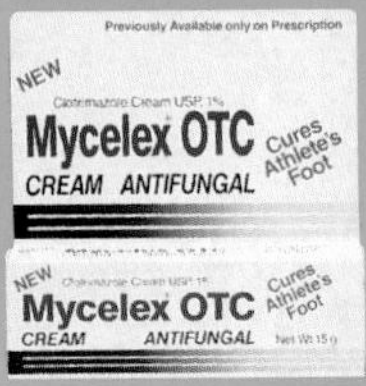

Cream
Also available:
Mycelex OTC Solution

MYCELEX® OTC ANTIFUNGAL

Cures Athlete's Foot

Miles Inc.
Consumer Healthcare Products
p. 616

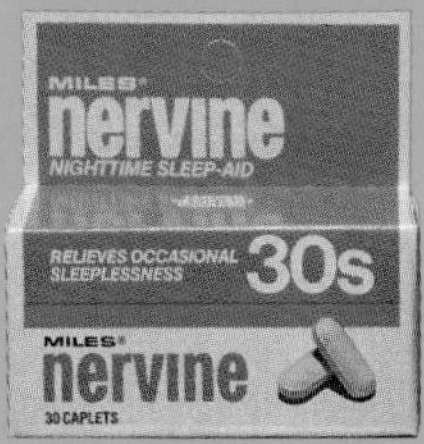

MILES® NERVINE NIGHTTIME SLEEP-AID
(Diphenhydramine HCl 25 mg)

Miles Inc.
Consumer Healthcare Products
p. 618

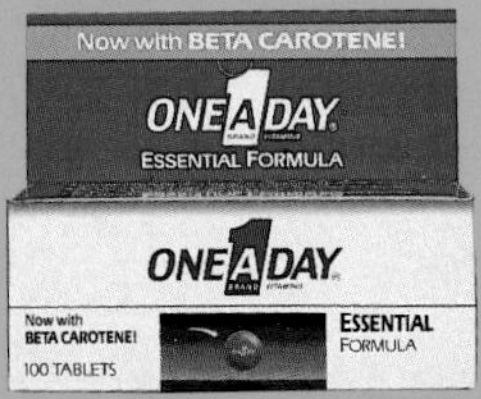

ONE A DAY® BRAND ESSENTIAL VITAMINS

Miles Inc.
Consumer Healthcare Products
p. 618

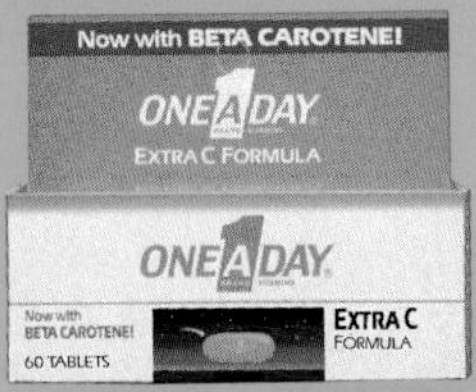

ONE A DAY® BRAND PLUS EXTRA C VITAMINS
11 essential vitamins
with high potency
300 mg Vitamin C

Miles Inc.
Consumer Healthcare Products
p. 618

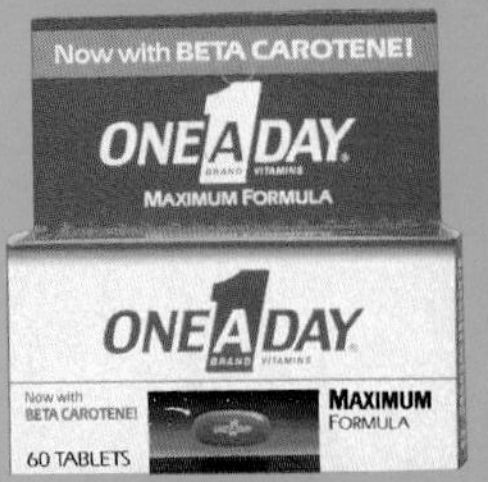

ONE A DAY® BRAND MAXIMUM FORMULA THE MOST COMPLETE ONE A DAY® BRAND

Miles Inc.
Consumer Healthcare Products
p. 618

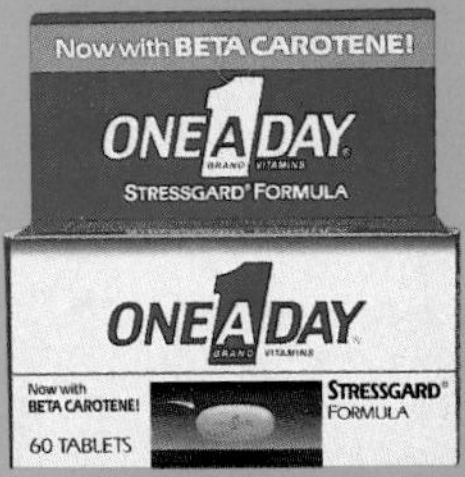

STRESSGARD® MULTIVITAMIN/MULTIMINERAL SUPPLEMENT

Miles Inc.
Consumer Healthcare Products
p. 618

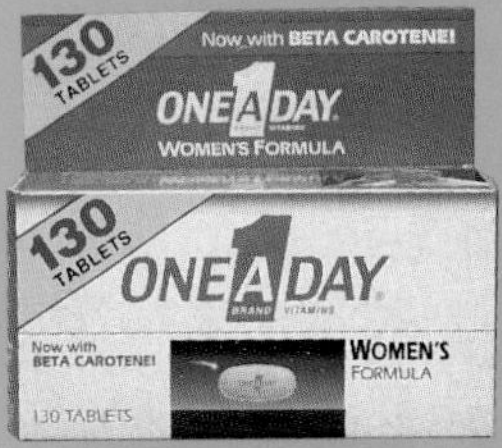

ONE-A-DAY® WOMEN'S FORMULA Multivitamin for Women with Extra Iron and Calcium

NATURE'S BOUNTY

p. 620

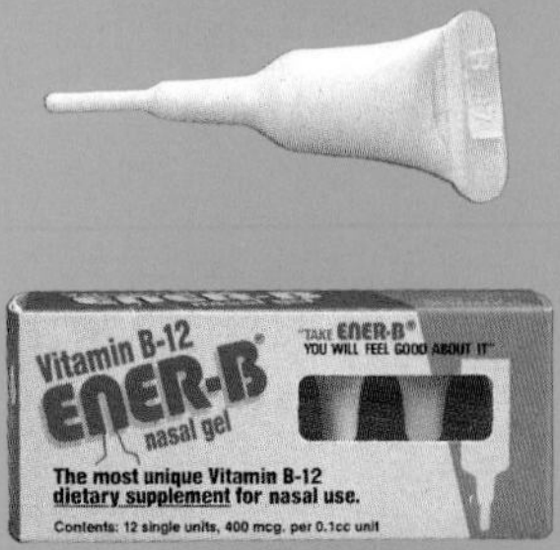

ENER-B®
Vitamin B-12 Nasal Gel

NEUTROGENA

p. 620

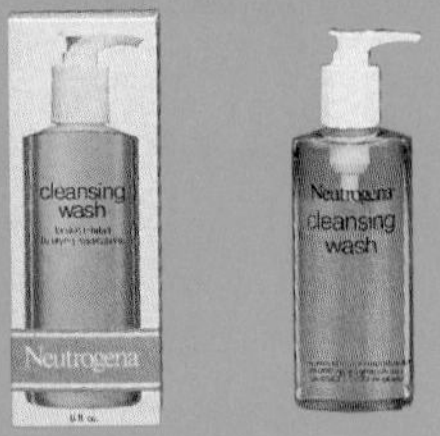

6 fl. oz.

NEUTROGENA® CLEANSING WASH

Especially formulated for skin irritated by drying medications.

Neutrogena *p. 621*

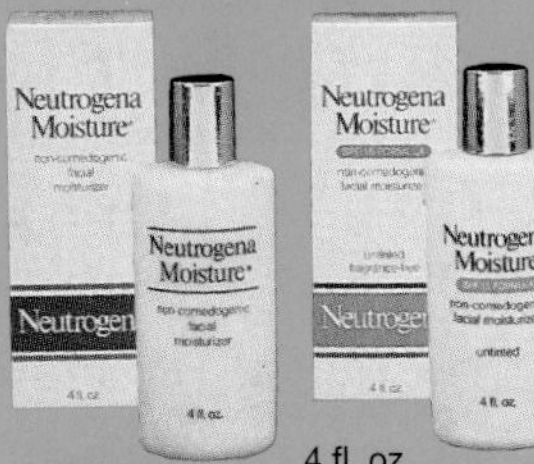

4 fl. oz.

NEUTROGENA MOISTURE® and NEUTROGENA MOISTURE® SPF 15 Formula Untinted**

Non-Comedogenic Facial Moisturizer
**Also available in Sheer Tint

Neutrogena *p. 621*

5.25 fl. oz. 2 oz.

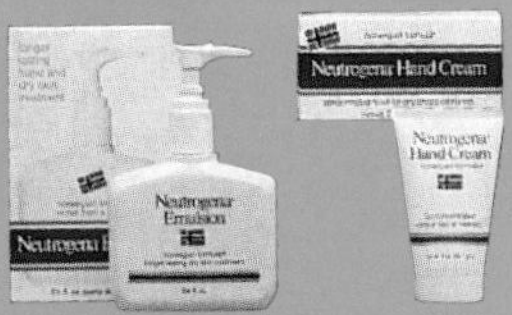

NEUTROGENA® NORWEGIAN FORMULA® EMULSION AND HAND CREAM

Glycerin-enriched hand and body moisturizers. Available fragrance-free.

Neutrogena *p. 621*

2¼ oz.

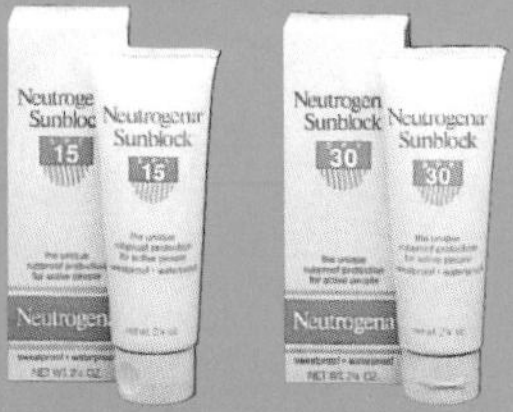

SPF 15 SPF 30

NEUTROGENA® SUNBLOCK
Ideal for the Active Patient
Rubproof—Sweatproof
Waterproof—Paba-free

Neutrogena *p. 622*

4.4 fl. oz. 4.5 fl. oz.

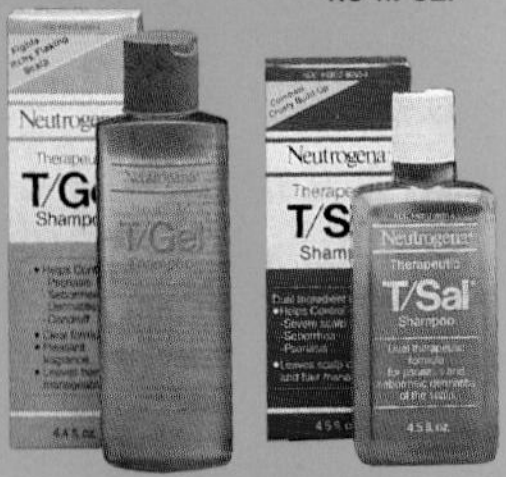

NEUTROGENA® T/GEL® AND NEUTROGENA® T/SAL® SHAMPOOS
For relief of symptoms associated with psoriasis and seborrheic dermatitis.

OHM LABORATORIES

p. 623

200 mg.

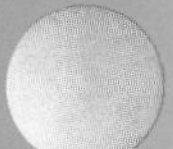

12 coated tablets

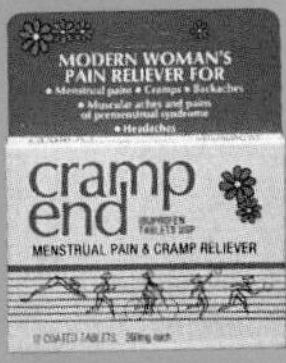

CRAMP END
(ibuprofen tablets USP)
Menstrual Pain & Cramp Reliever

Ohm Laboratories *p. 623*

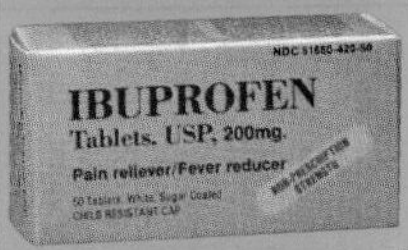

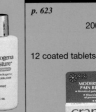

200 mg.

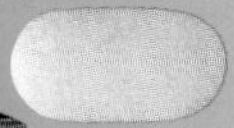

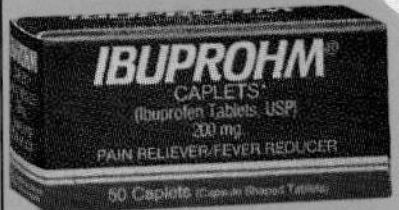

200 mg.

Tablets and Caplets available in bottles of 24, 50 and 100

IBUPROFEN TABLETS
IBUPROHM CAPLETS

Ohm Laboratories *p. 623*

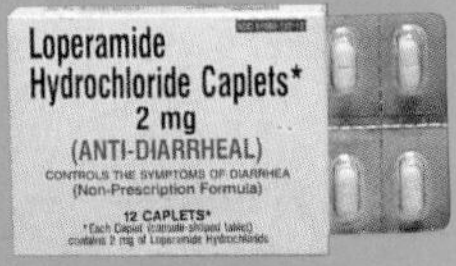

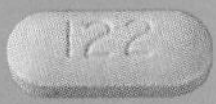

LOPERAMIDE HYDROCHLORIDE CAPLETS
(anti-diarrheal)

ORTHO

Ortho—Advanced Care Prods.
p. 793

Available in Single and Double Kits

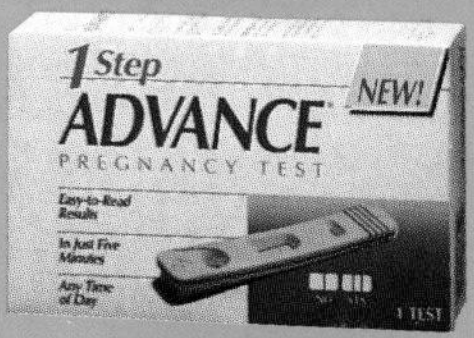

Use any time of day, as early as the first day of a missed period.

ADVANCE®
Pregnancy Test
"One Step: After urine collection"

Ortho—Advanced Care Prods.
p. 624

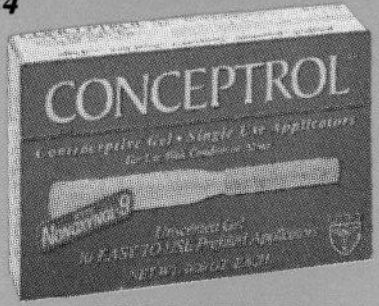

CONCEPTROL®
Contraceptive Gel
Single Use Contraceptive
[nonoxynol-9, 4% (100 mg/ea)]

For use with condom or alone.

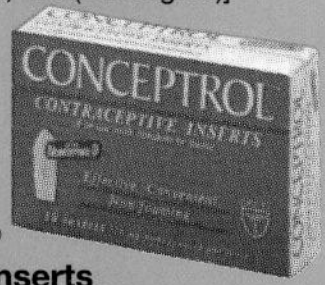

CONCEPTROL®
Contraceptive Inserts
[nonoxynol-9, 8.34% (150 mg/ea)]

Ortho—Advanced Care Prods.
p. 624

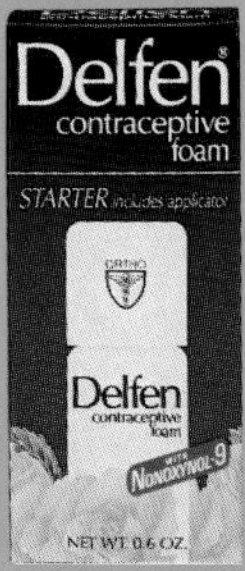

Starter (0.60 oz. vial w/applicator package)
Refill (1.40 oz. vial only packages)

DELFEN® Contraceptive Foam
[nonoxynol-9, 12.5% (100 mg/app)]

Ortho—Advanced Care Prods.
p. 793

Available in Single and Double Kits

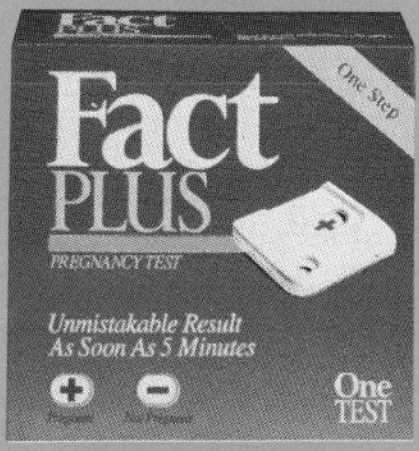

Unmistakable +/– Result

FACT PLUS®
Pregnancy Test
"One Step: After urine collection"

Ortho—Advanced Care Prods.
p. 625

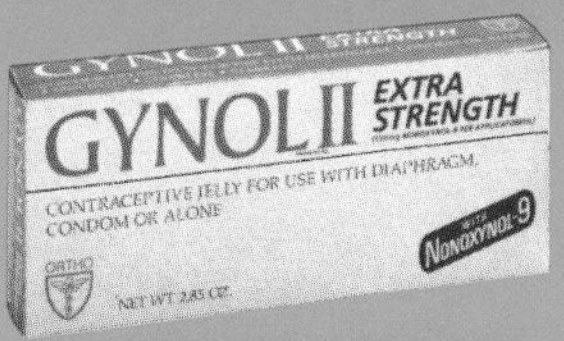

Contraceptive Jelly.
For use with condom, diaphragm or alone.

GYNOL II™
Extra Strength
[nonoxynol-9, 2% (100 mg/app)]

Ortho—Advanced Care Prods.
p. 625

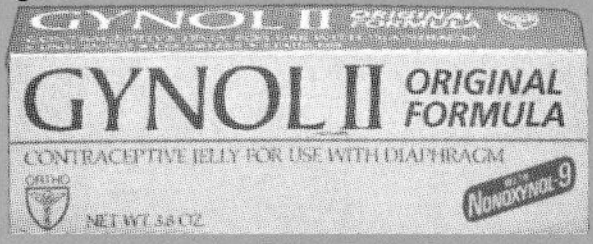

GYNOL II® ORIGINAL FORMULA
Contraceptive Jelly
[nonoxynol-9, 2% (100 mg/app)]

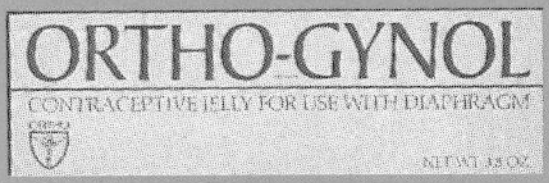

ORTHO-GYNOL®
Contraceptive Jelly
[diisobutylphenoxypolyethoxyethanol, 1% (80 mg/app)]

Ortho—Advanced Care Prods.
p. 626

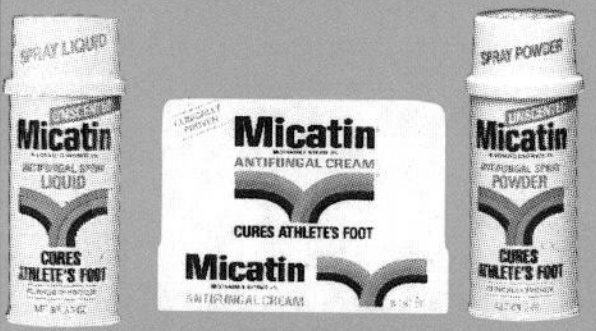

Spray Liquid (3.5 oz.)

Cream (½ oz. and 1 oz.)

Spray Powder and Spray Deodorant Powder with Odor Control (3.0 oz.)

MICATIN® Antifungal
For Athlete's Foot
(miconazole nitrate, 2%)

Ortho—Advanced Care Prods.
p. 626

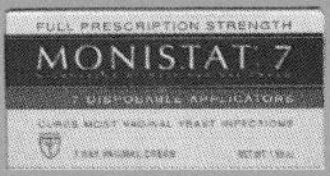

Cream: 2% (100 mg per dose)
Available with 7 disposable cardboard applicators, or one reusable plastic applicator.

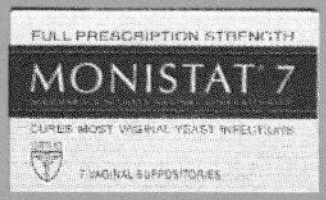

Suppositories: 100 mg each suppository

MONISTAT® 7
(miconazole nitrate vaginal cream and suppositories)

PARKE-DAVIS

p. 628

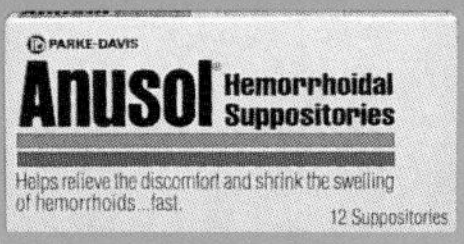

Available in boxes of 12, 24 and 48

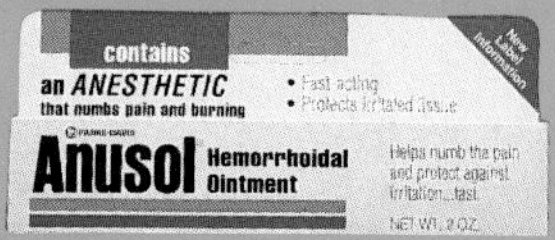

Available in 1 Oz. and 2 Oz. Tubes

ANUSOL®
Suppositories and Ointment

Parke-Davis
p. 628

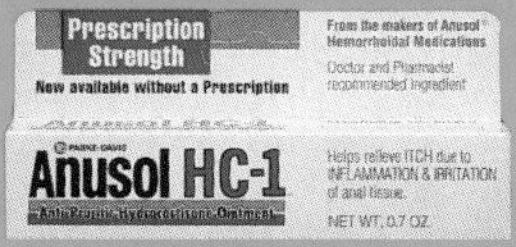

ANUSOL HC-1™
Anti-Pruritic Hydrocortisone Ointment

Parke-Davis
p. 629

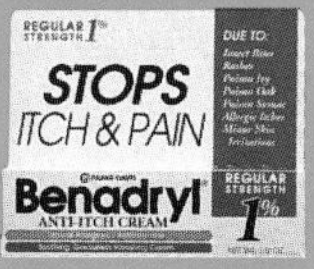

1% Regular Strength

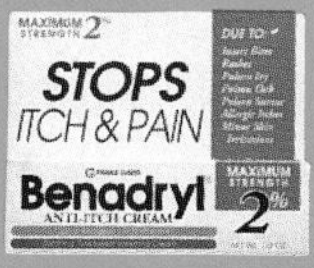

2% Maximum Strength

BENADRYL®
Cream
Topical Antihistamine

Parke-Davis
p. 629

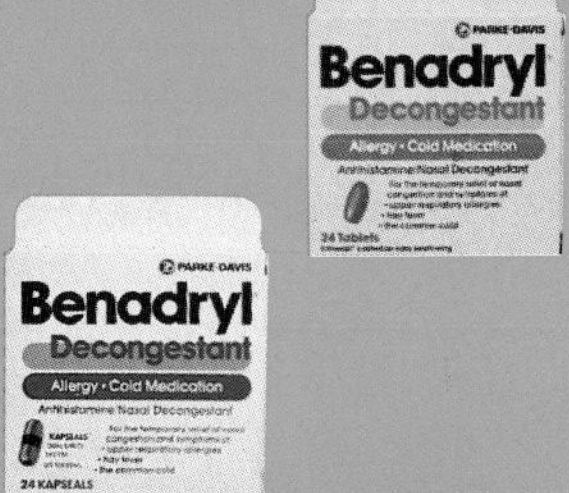

Available in boxes of 24

BENADRYL®
Decongestant

Parke-Davis
p. 632

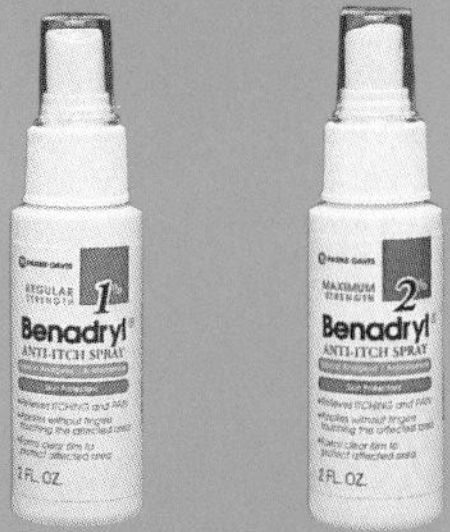

Regular Strength

Maximum Strength

BENADRYL®
Spray
Topical Antihistamine

Parke-Davis
p. 630

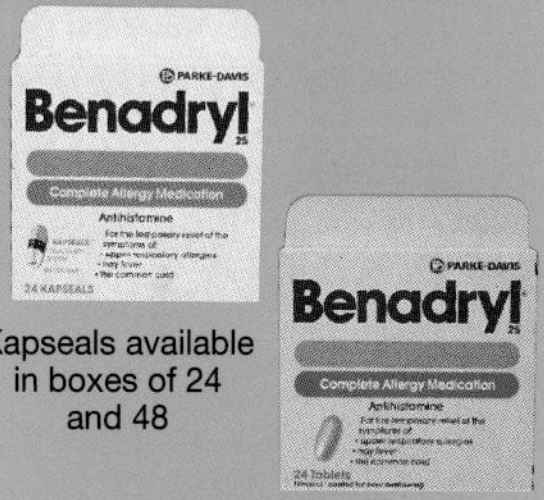

Kapseals available in boxes of 24 and 48

Tablets available in boxes of 24 and bottles of 100

BENADRYL® 25

Parke-Davis
p. 630

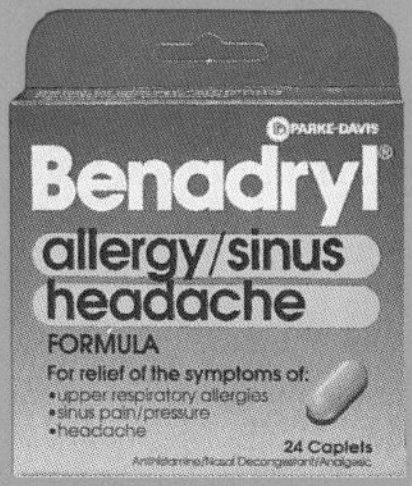

Available in boxes of 24

BENADRYL®
Allergy/Sinus/Headache

Parke-Davis
p. 631

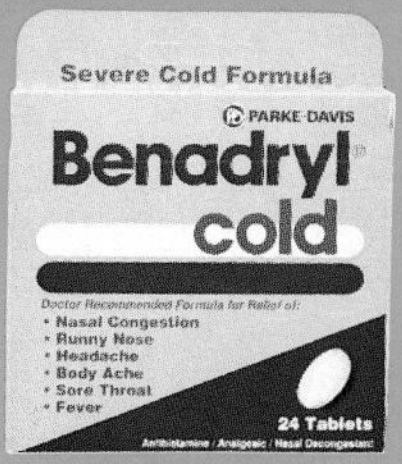

Available in boxes of 24 and 48

BENADRYL® COLD
Decongestant/Analgesic/ Antihistamine

Parke-Davis
p. 631

Honey-Lemon Flavor

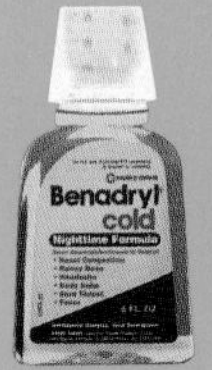

Available in 6 Fl. Oz. Bottles

BENADRYL® COLD NIGHTTIME FORMULA

Parke-Davis
p. 633

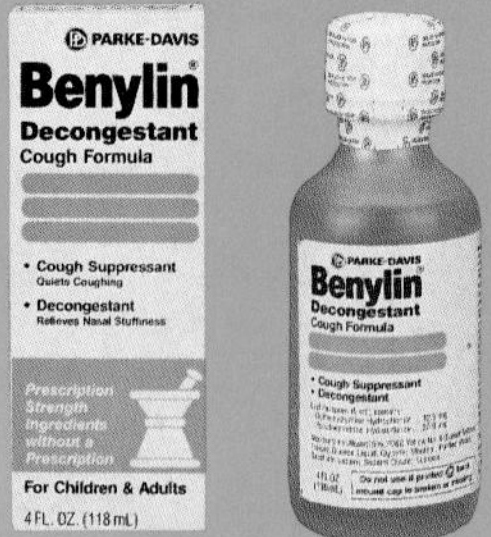

Available in 4 Oz. Bottles

BENYLIN® Decongestant Cough Formula

Parke-Davis
p. 793

1 test kit

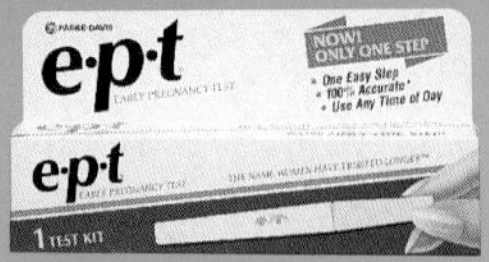

2 test kits

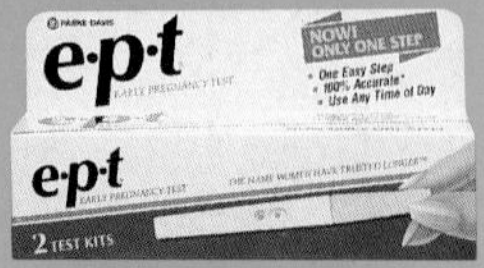

e•p•t® One Step. Easy to read. Accurate results.

e•p•t® STICK TEST Early Pregnancy Test

Parke-Davis
p. 635

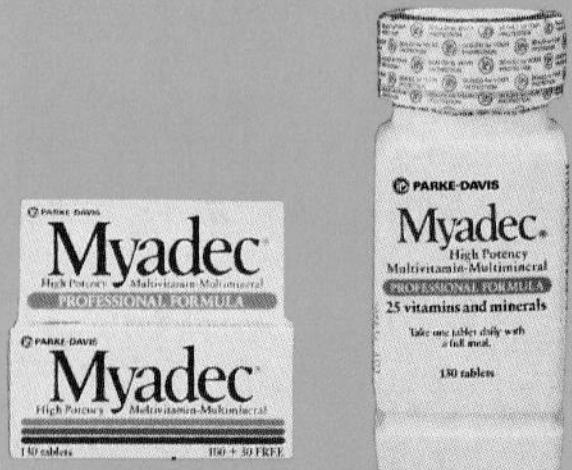

Available in bottles of 130 Tablets

MYADEC® Multivitamin-Multimineral Supplement

Parke-Davis
p. 629

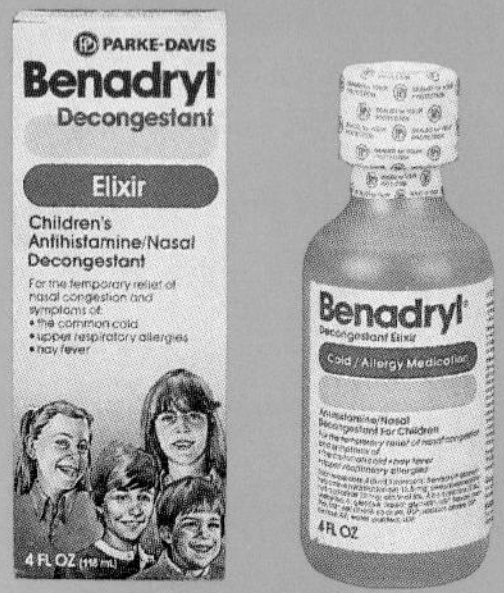

Available in 4 Oz. Bottles

BENADRYL® Decongestant Elixir

Parke-Davis
p. 632

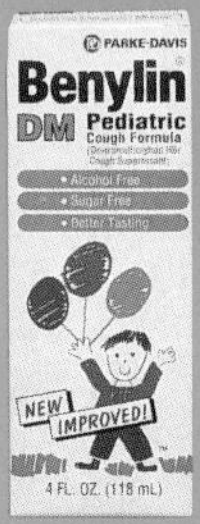

Available in 4 Oz. Bottles

BENYLIN® DM Pediatric Cough Formula

Parke-Davis
p. 634

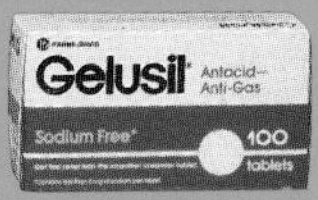

100 tablets

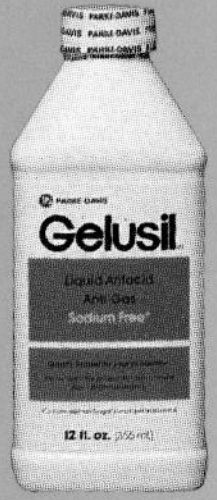

GELUSIL® Antacid-Anti-gas Sodium Free

12 Fl. Oz.

Parke-Davis
p. 635

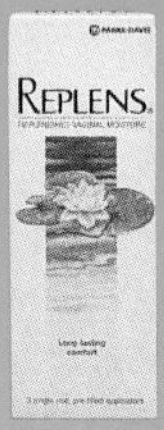

Available in boxes of 3 and 8 single-use applicators.

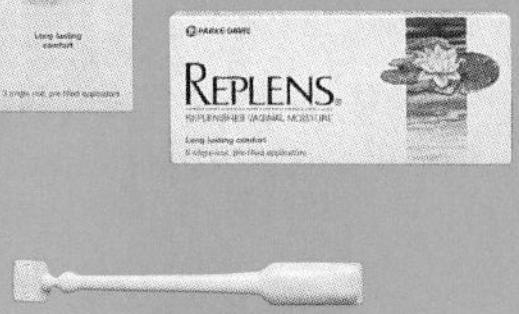

REPLENS® Vaginal Moisturizer

Parke-Davis
p. 630

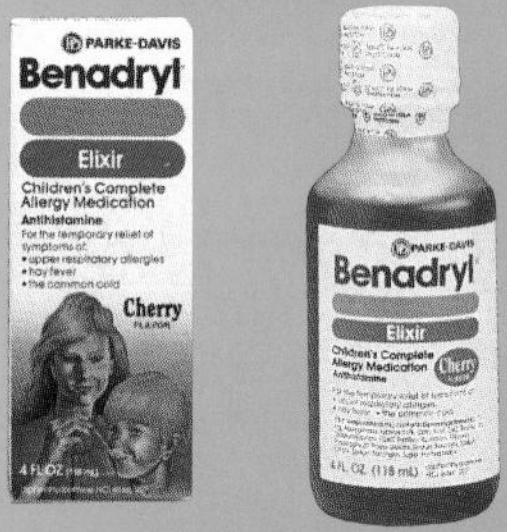

Available in 4 Oz. and 8 Oz. Bottles

BENADRYL® Elixir

Parke-Davis
p. 633

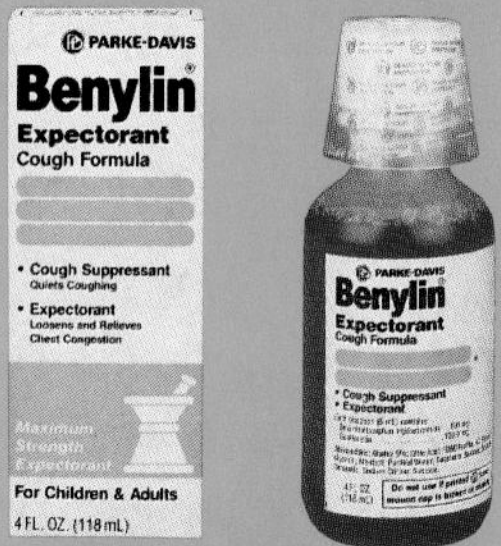

Available in 4 Oz. and 8 Oz. Bottles

BENYLIN® EXPECTORANT

Parke-Davis
p. 634

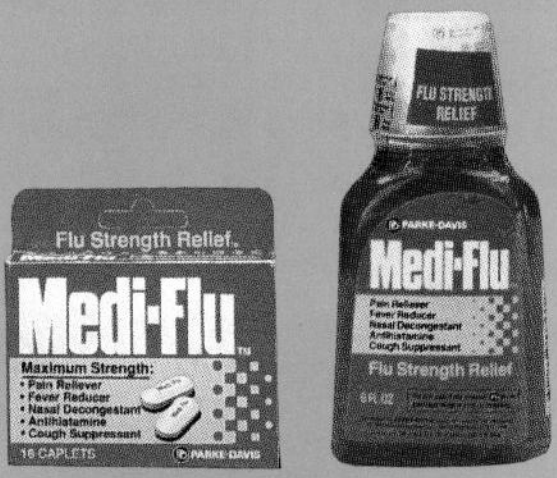

16 Caplets

6 Fl. Oz.

FLU STRENGTH RELIEF™ MEDI-FLU®

Parke-Davis
p. 635

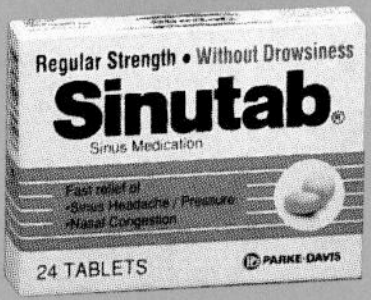

SINUTAB® SINUS MEDICATION

Regular Strength Without Drowsiness Formula

Parke-Davis
p. 632

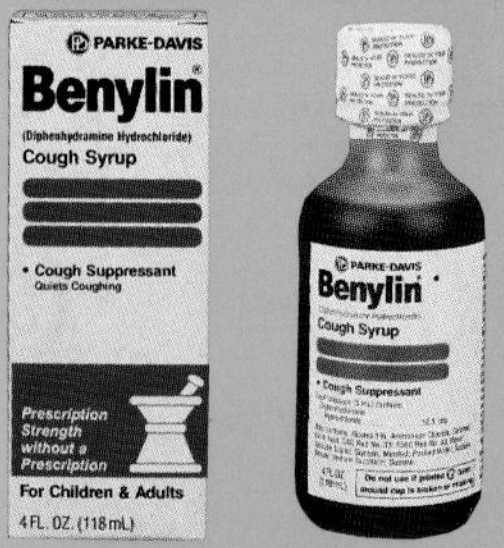

Available in 4 Oz. and 8 Oz. Bottles

BENYLIN® Cough Syrup

Parke-Davis
p. 633

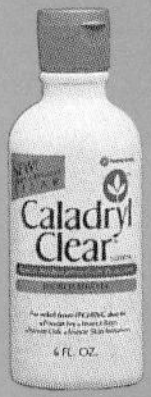

Lotion

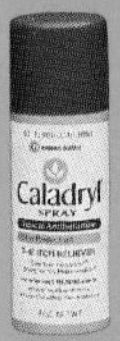

Spray

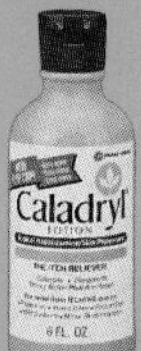

Lotion

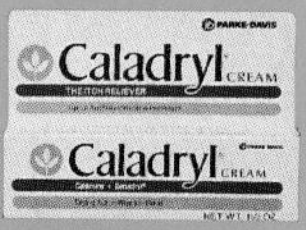

Cream

For relief from itching due to: Poison Ivy, Insect Bites, Poison Oak, Skin Irritation

CALADRYL® Topical Antihistamine/Skin Protectant

Parke-Davis
p. 634

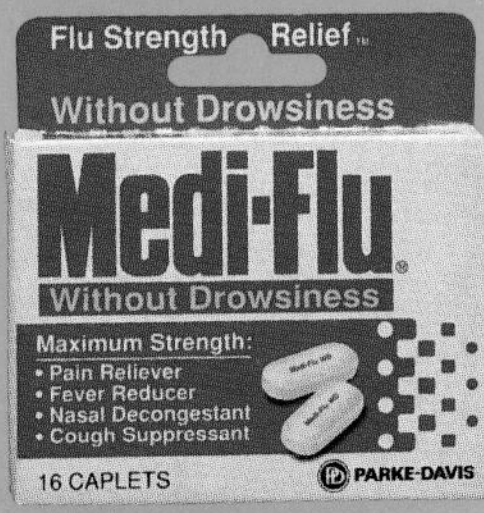

16 Caplets

MEDI-FLU® Flu Strength Relief Without Drowsiness

Parke-Davis
p. 636

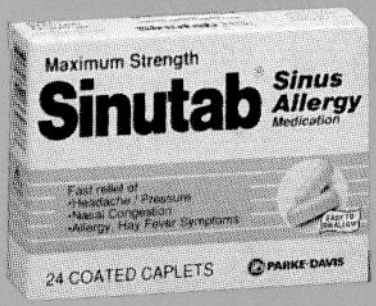

SINUTAB® SINUS ALLERGY MEDICATION

Maximum Strength Formula

Available in Caplets or Tablets

Parke-Davis
p. 636

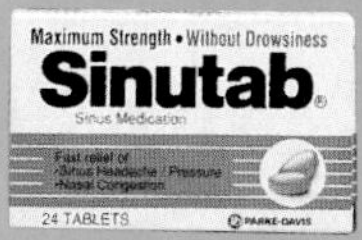

SINUTAB®
SINUS MEDICATION

Maximum Strength
Without Drowsiness
Formula

Available in Caplets or Tablets

REED & CARNRICK

p. 657

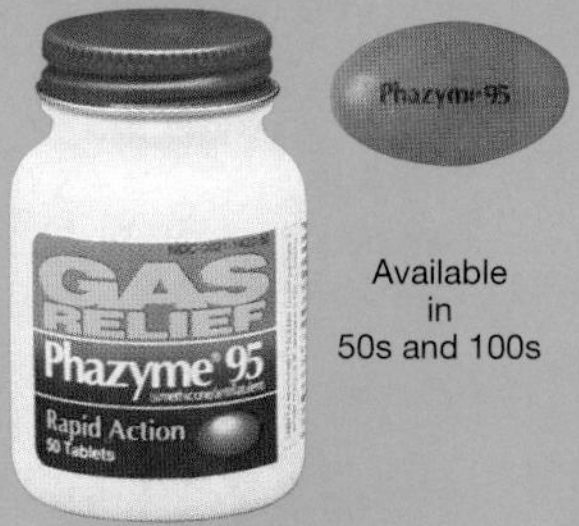

Available in 50s and 100s

PHAZYME® 95
An antiflatulent to alleviate or relieve the symptoms of gas.

Reed & Carnrick
p. 658

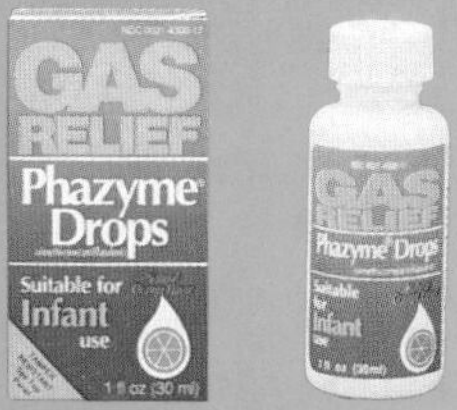

Available in 1 oz. and ½ oz. bottles

PHAZYME® DROPS
A liquid antiflatulent suitable for relieving infant gas symptoms and for those who prefer liquid dosage forms

Rhône-Poulenc Rorer
Consumer Div.
p. 661

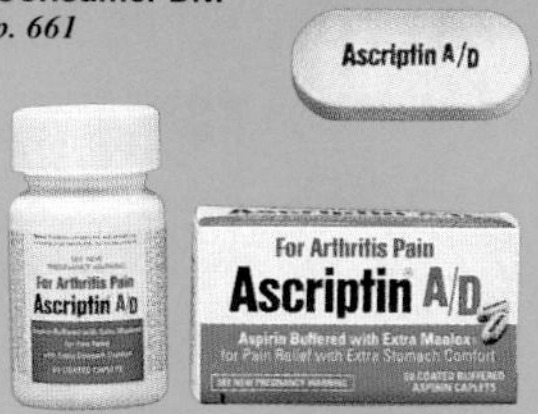

Bottles of 60, 100, 225 & 500 Caplets

FOR ARTHRITIS PAIN
ASCRIPTIN® A/D
aspirin (325 mg) buffered with Maalox (alumina-magnesia) and calcium carbonate

Parke-Davis
p. 637

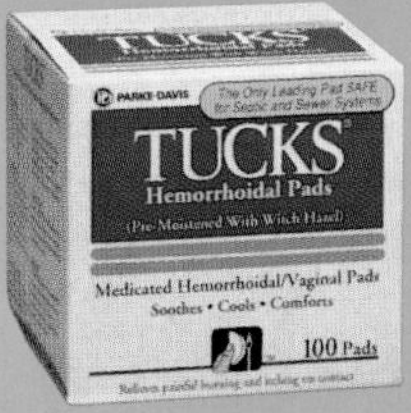

40 pads

Also available in 100 pad packages

TUCKS®
Pre-Moistened Pads

Reed & Carnrick
p. 657

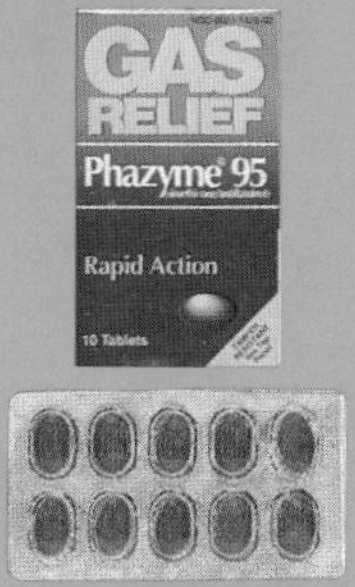

PHAZYME® 95
Consumer 10 Packs
An antiflatulent to alleviate or relieve the symptoms of gas.

REESE CHEMICAL CO.

p. 658

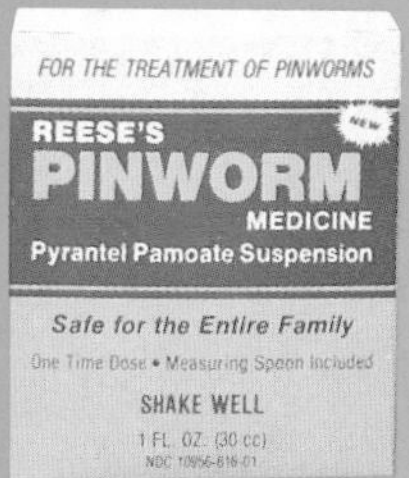
FOR THE TREATMENT OF PINWORMS
REESE'S
PINWORM
MEDICINE
Pyrantel Pamoate Suspension
Safe for the Entire Family
SHAKE WELL

Now available: 1 fl. oz. w/measuring spoon or caplets strip packed in 24's.

REESE'S PINWORM MEDICINE
With English and Spanish directions

Rhône-Poulenc Rorer
Consumer Div.
p. 662

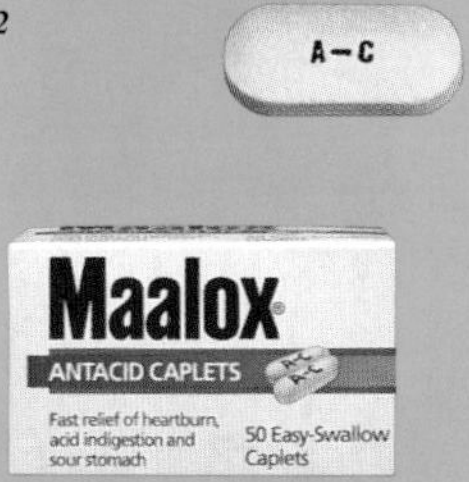

Blister Packs of 24's
Bottles of 50's

MAALOX® ANTACID CAPLET
calcium carbonate (1000 mg)

PFIZER

Consumer Health Care *p. 638*

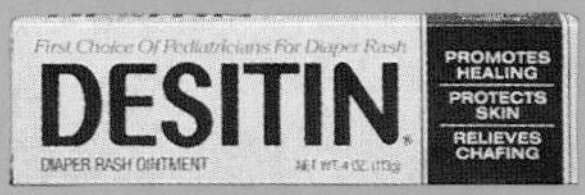

DESITIN®
Diaper Rash Ointment

Reed & Carnrick
p. 658

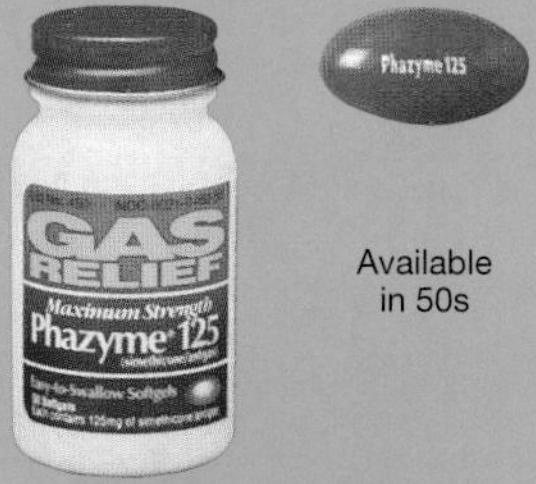

Available in 50s

MAXIMUM STRENGTH
PHAZYME® 125
An antiflatulent to alleviate or relieve the symptoms of gas. Softgel capsule for ease of swallowing.

RHÔNE-POULENC RORER

Consumer Div.
p. 659

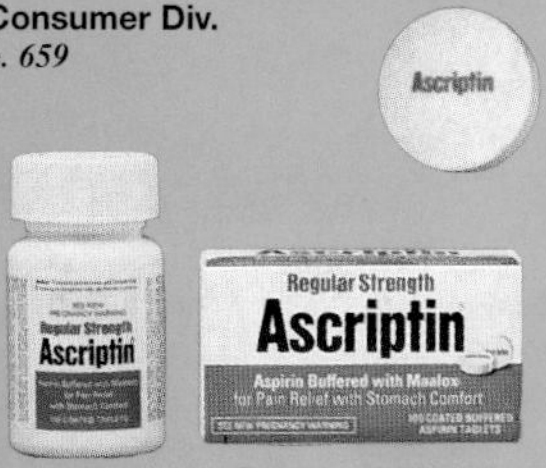

Bottles of 60, 100, 160, 225 & 500 Tablets

REGULAR STRENGTH
ASCRIPTIN®
aspirin (325 mg) buffered with Maalox (alumina-magnesia) and calcium carbonate

Rhône-Poulenc Rorer
Consumer Div.
p. 662

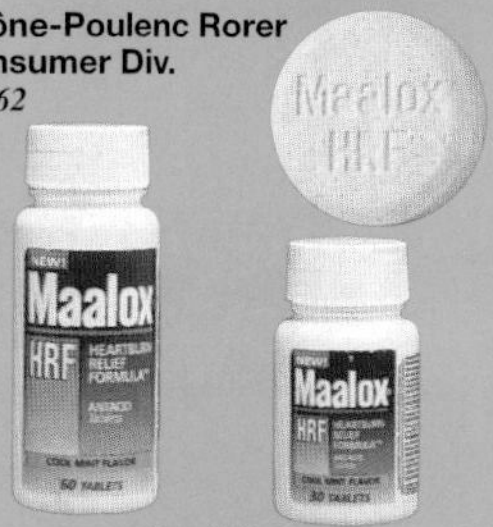

Cool Mint
Bottles of 30 and 60 tablets

MAALOX® HRF
Heartburn Relief Formula™
aluminum hydroxide-magnesium carbonate codried gel 180 mg, magnesium carbonate USP 160 mg

Consumer Health Care *p. 641*

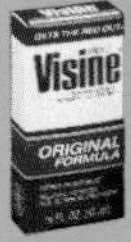

Original Formula

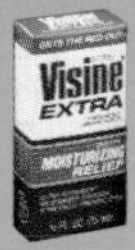

With Moisturizing Relief

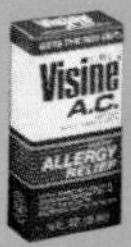

With Allergy Relief

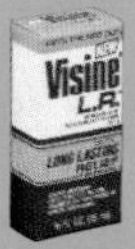

With Long Lasting Relief

VISINE® Redness Reliever
Eye Drops

Reed & Carnrick
p. 658

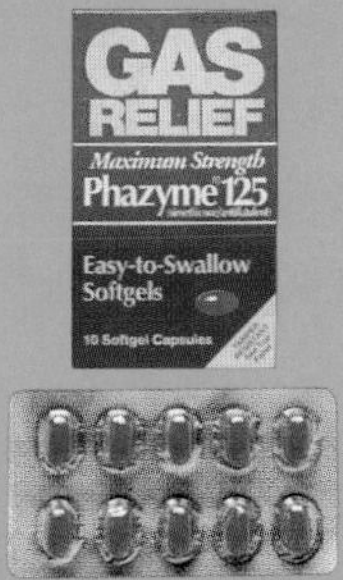

MAXIMUM STRENGTH
PHAZYME® 125
Consumer 10 Packs
An antiflatulent to alleviate or relieve the symptoms of gas.

Rhône-Poulenc Rorer
Consumer Div.
p. 660

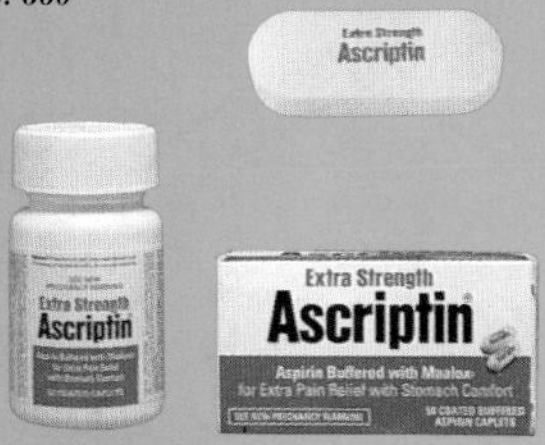

Bottles of 36, 50 & 85 Caplets

EXTRA STRENGTH
ASCRIPTIN®
aspirin (500 mg) buffered with Maalox (alumina-magnesia) and calcium carbonate

Rhône-Poulenc Rorer
Consumer Div.
p. 662

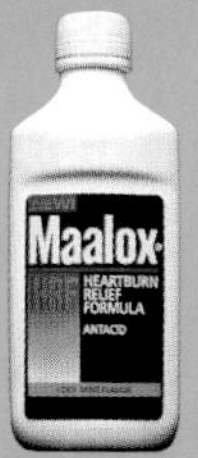

12 oz.
Cool Mint Flavor

MAALOX® HRF
Heartburn Relief Formula™
aluminum hydroxide-magnesium carbonate codried gel 280 mg, magnesium carbonate USP 350 mg

Rhône-Poulenc Rorer Consumer Div.
p. 663

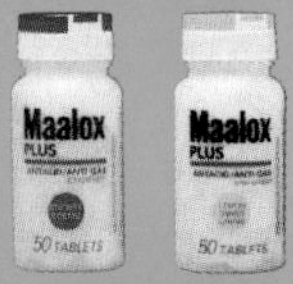

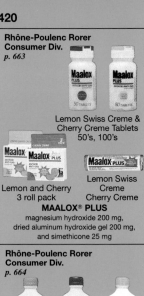

Lemon Swiss Creme & Cherry Creme Tablets
50's, 100's

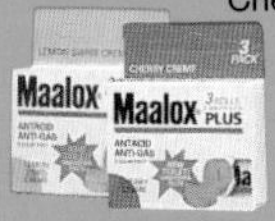

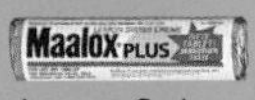

Lemon and Cherry
3 roll pack

Lemon Swiss Creme
Cherry Creme

MAALOX® PLUS
magnesium hydroxide 200 mg,
dried aluminum hydroxide gel 200 mg,
and simethicone 25 mg

Rhône-Poulenc Rorer Consumer Div.
p. 665

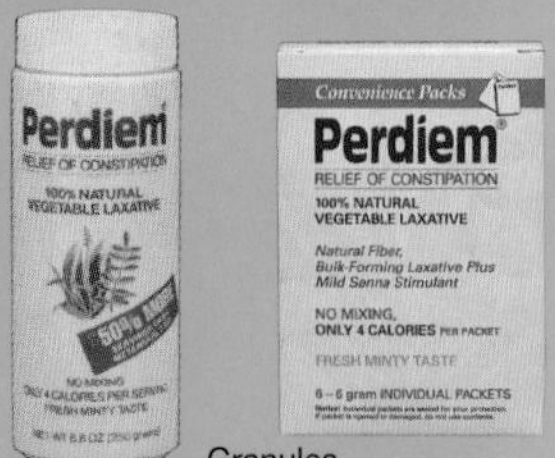

Granules
100 gm and 250 gm
6—6gm packets and 20—6gm packets
PERDIEM®
100% Natural Vegetable Laxative
82 percent psyllium (Plantago Hydrocolloid)
18 percent senna (Cassia Pod Concentrate)

Roberts Pharmaceutical
p. 669

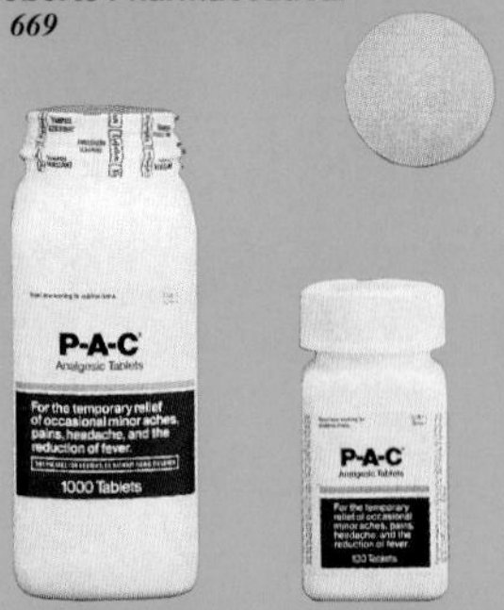

1,000 tablets
100 tablets

P-A-C®
Analgesic Tablets

A. H. Robins
p. 672

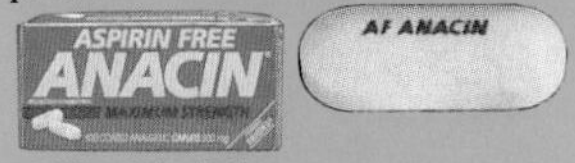

30's, 60's, 100's

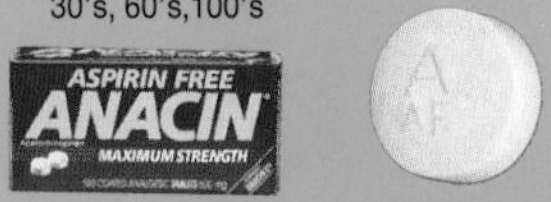

12's, 30's, 60's, 100's (reverse: "500")

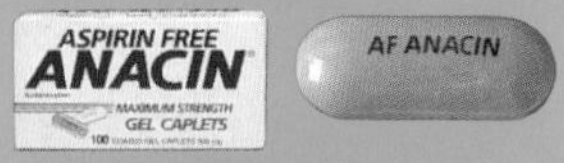

24's, 50's, 100's

ASPIRIN FREE ANACIN®
Acetaminophen Tablets,
Caplets and Gelcaplets

Rhône-Poulenc Rorer Consumer Div.
p. 664

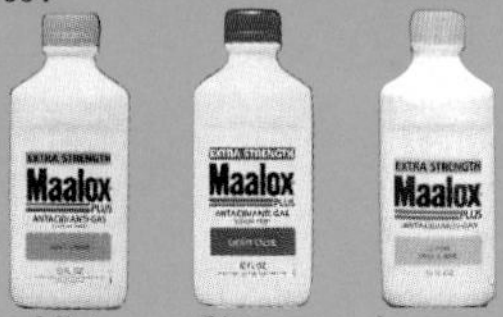

Mint Creme
Cherry Creme
Lemon Swiss Creme

12 oz. suspension
Lemon Swiss Creme 26 oz.
Cherry Creme 26 oz.
Mint Creme 26 oz.

EXTRA STRENGTH MAALOX® PLUS
magnesium hydroxide 450 mg,
aluminum hydroxide 500 mg,
and simethicone 40 mg

Rhône-Poulenc Rorer Consumer Div.
p. 665

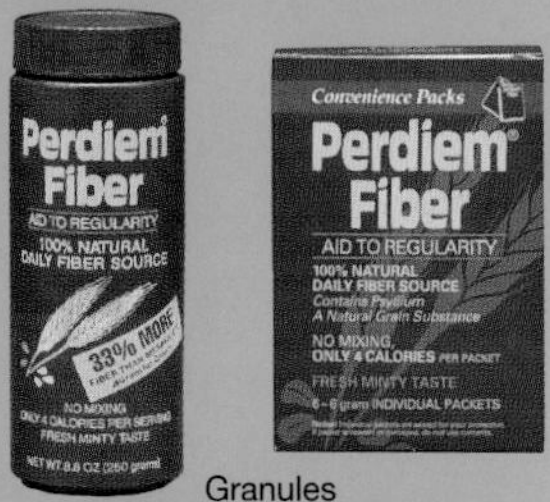

Granules
100 gm and 250 gm
6—6gm packets and 20—6gm packets
PERDIEM® FIBER
100% Natural Daily Fiber Source
100% Psyllium (Plantago Hydrocolloid)

Roberts Pharmaceutical
p. 669

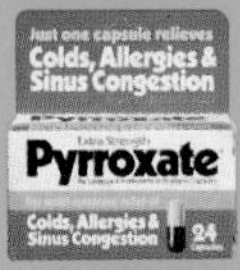

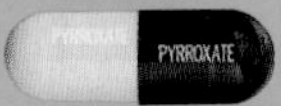

Bottles of 24 and 500 tablets

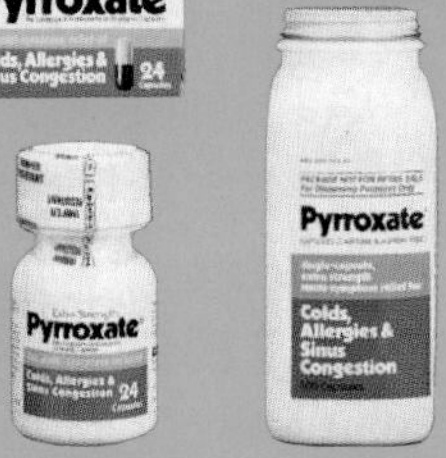

PYRROXATE® Capsules
Nasal Decongestant/Antihistamine/
Analgesic

A. H. Robins
p. 672

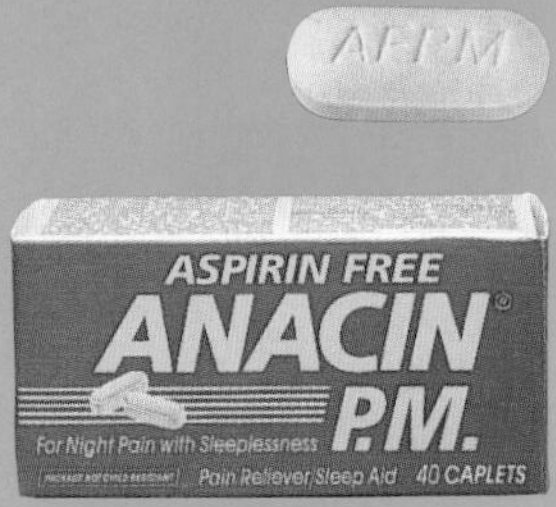

20's, 40's

ASPIRIN FREE ANACIN® P.M.

Rhône-Poulenc Rorer Consumer Div.
p. 664

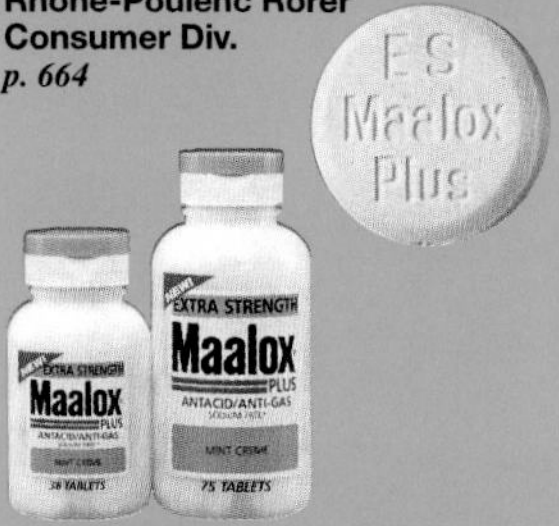

Mint Creme Tablets
38's, 75's

EXTRA STRENGTH MAALOX® PLUS TABLETS
magnesium hydroxide 350 mg,
dried aluminum hydroxide gel 350 mg
and simethicone 30 mg

ROBERTS

p. 667

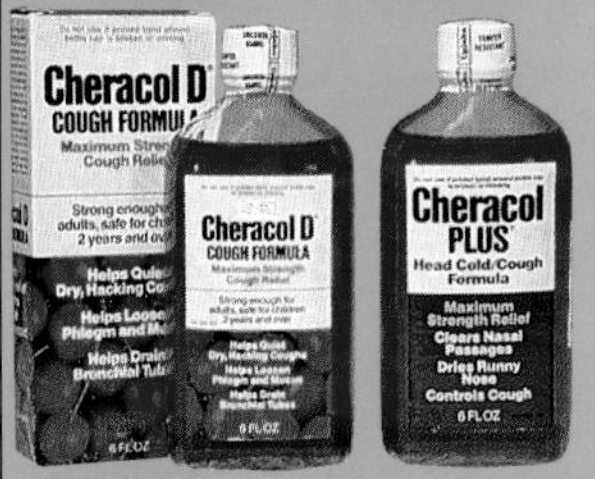

2 oz, 4 oz,
6 oz
CHERACOL D®
Cough Formula

4 oz, 6 oz
CHERACOL PLUS®
Head Cold/Cough
Formula

Roberts Pharmaceutical
p. 670

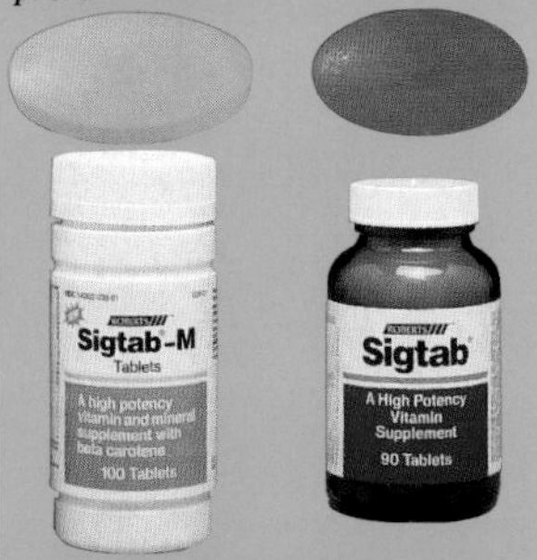

Bottle of 100 tablets
Bottles of 90 and 500 tablets

SIGTAB® and SIGTAB-M®
High Potency Vitamin Supplement

A. H. Robins
p. 673

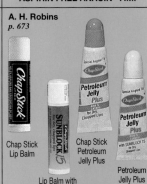

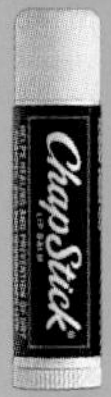

Chap Stick
Lip Balm

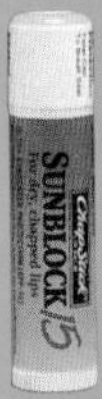

Lip Balm with
Sunblock 15

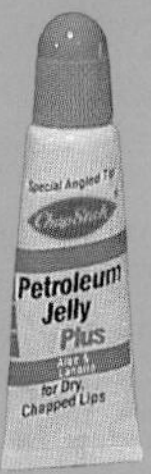

Chap Stick
Petroleum
Jelly Plus

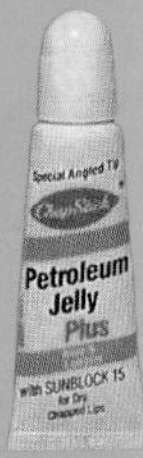

Petroleum
Jelly Plus
with
Sunblock 15

CHAP STICK®

Rhône-Poulenc Rorer Consumer Div.
p. 663

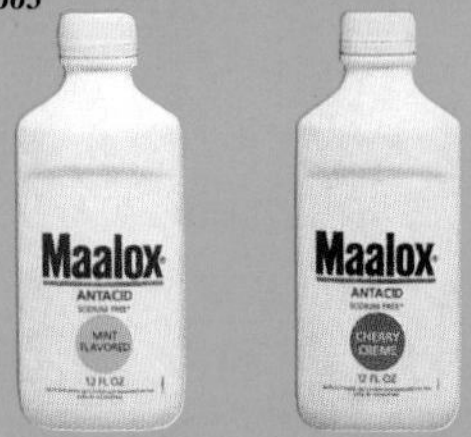

Mint Flavor
Cherry Creme

12 oz. suspension
Mint Flavored 26 oz.
Cherry Creme 26 oz.
MAALOX® SUSPENSION
magnesium hydroxide 200 mg,
aluminum hydroxide 225 mg

Roberts Pharmaceutical
p. 668

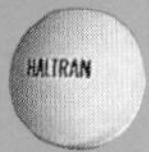

200 mg

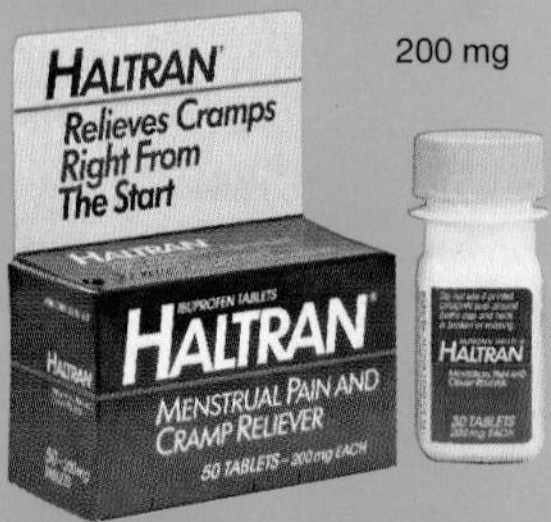

Bottles of 30

HALTRAN® Tablets
(ibuprofen tablets, USP)

A. H. ROBINS

p. 671

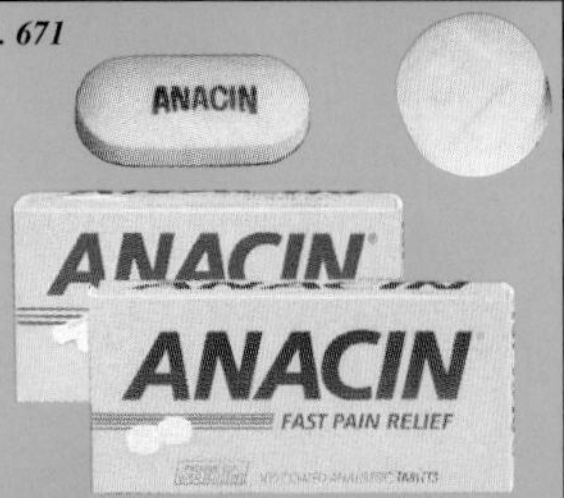

Coated Tablets in Tins of 12 and
Bottles of 30, 50, 100, 200 and 300.
Coated Caplets in Bottles of
30, 50 and 100.

ANACIN®
Analgesic Tablets and Caplets

A. H. Robins
p. 673

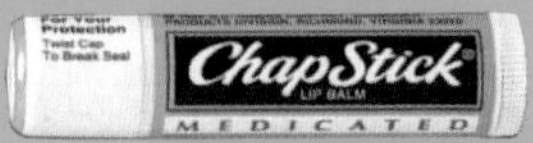

Stick

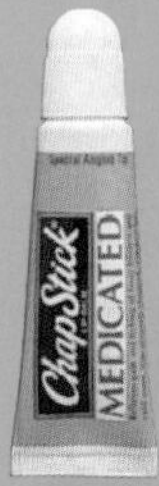

Tube

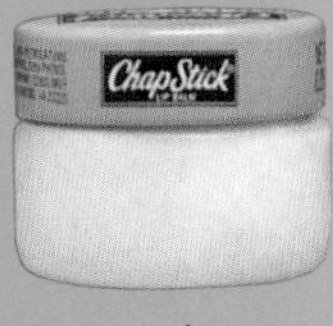

Jar

Medicated CHAP STICK®

A. H. Robins
p. 674

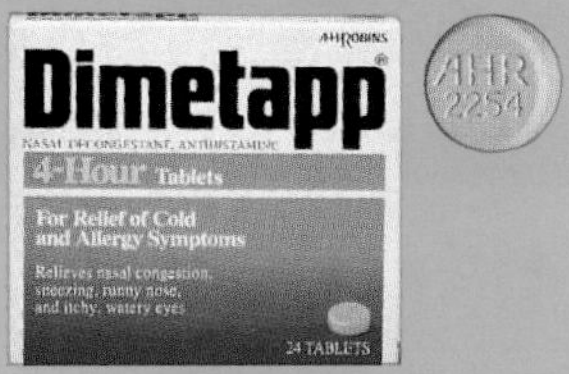

24's
DIMETAPP® TABLETS

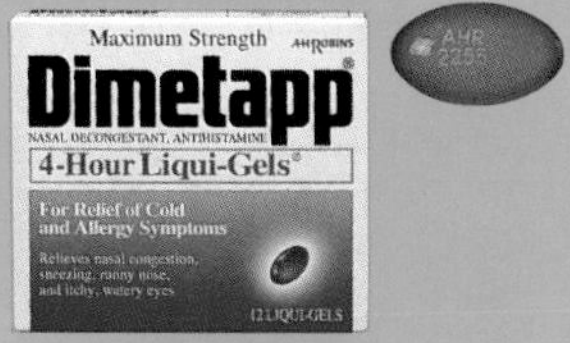

12's, 24's
DIMETAPP® LIQUI-GELS

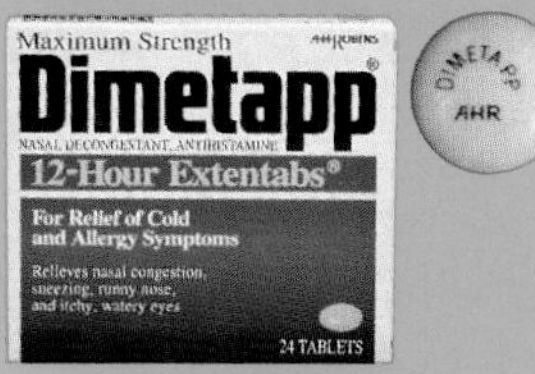

12's, 24's, 48's, 100's, 500's
DIMETAPP EXTENTABS®

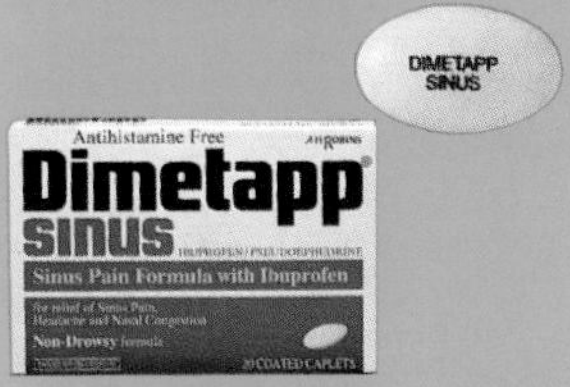

20's, 40's
DIMETAPP® SINUS CAPLETS

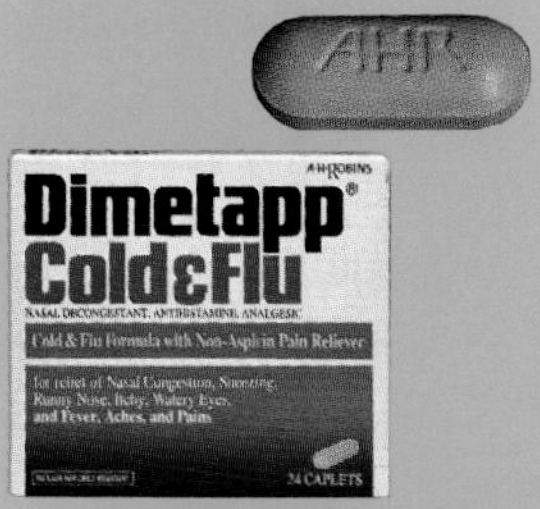

24's, 48's
DIMETAPP®
COLD AND FLU CAPLETS

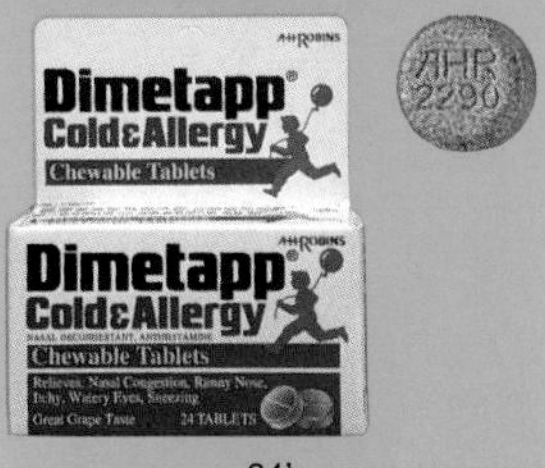

24's
DIMETAPP® COLD & ALLERGY
Children's Chewables

A. H. Robins
p. 676

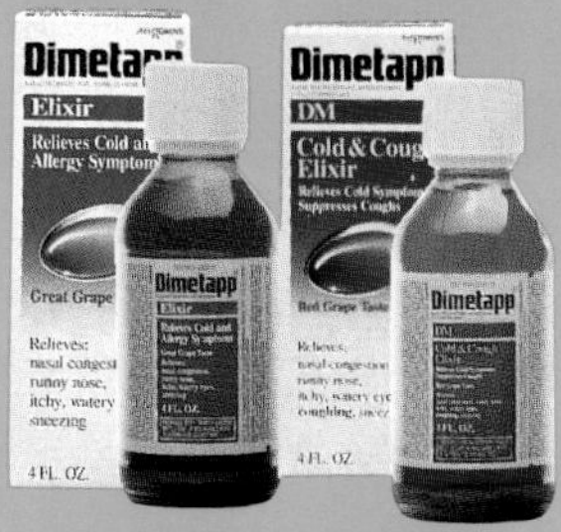

4 oz., 8 oz., 12 oz., 16 oz., 128 oz.
DIMETAPP® ELIXIR

4 oz., 8 oz., 12 oz.
DIMETAPP® DM COLD & COUGH ELIXIR

A. H. Robins
p. 680

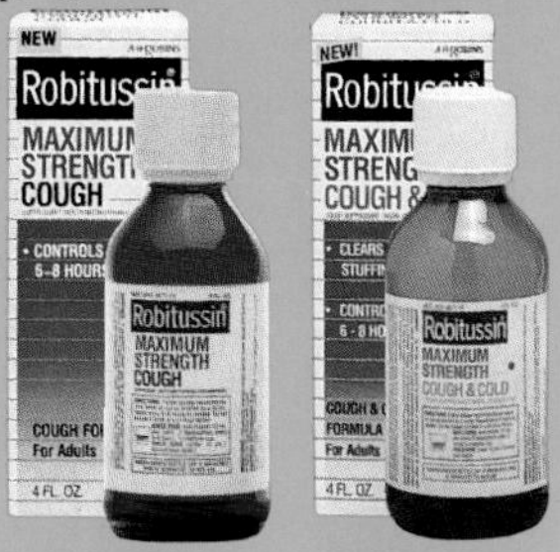

4 oz., 8 oz.
Cough Suppressant

4 oz., 8 oz.
Cough & Cold

ROBITUSSIN®
MAXIMUM STRENGTH FORMULAS

A. H. Robins
p. 682

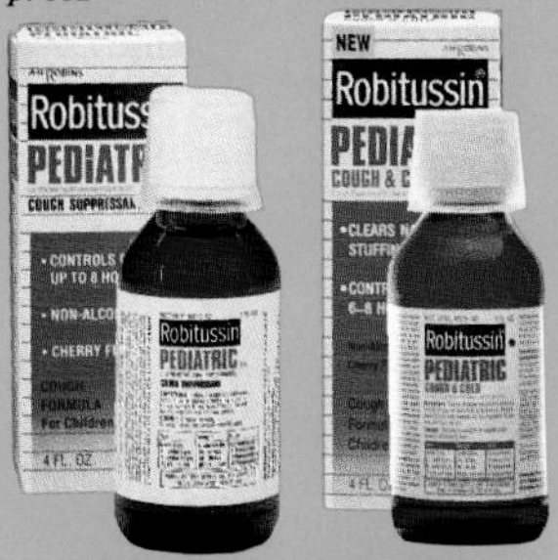

4 oz., 8 oz.
Cough Suppressant

4 oz., 8 oz.
Cough & Cold

ROBITUSSIN®
PEDIATRIC FORMULAS

A. H. Robins
p. 680

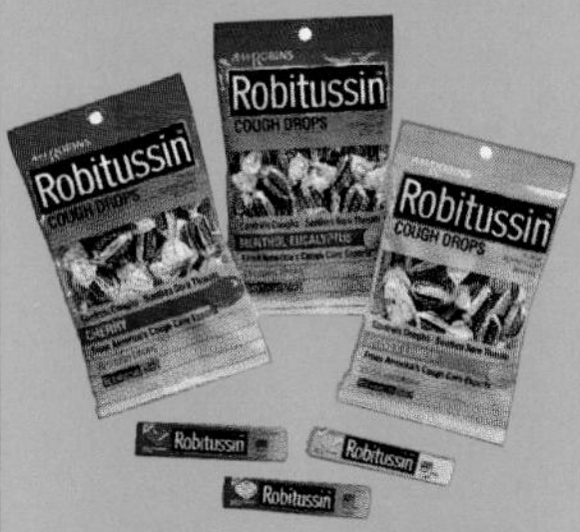

Available in packages of 25 and sticks of 9

ROBITUSSIN®
Cough Drops

A. H. Robins
p. 678

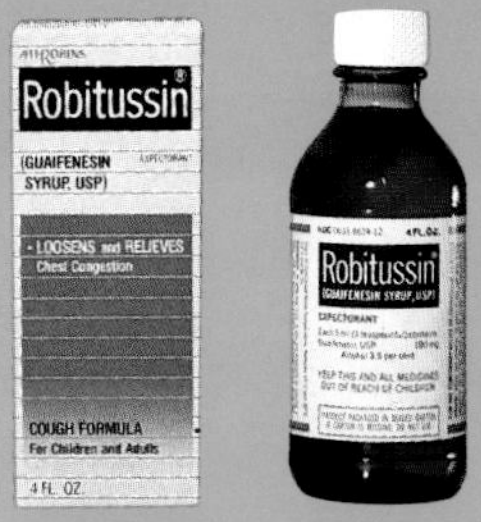

4 oz., 8 oz., 16 oz., 128 oz.

ROBITUSSIN® SYRUP

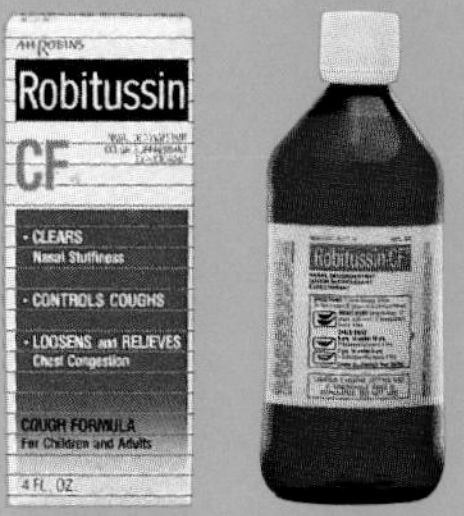

4 oz., 8 oz., 12 oz., 16 oz.

ROBITUSSIN®-CF SYRUP

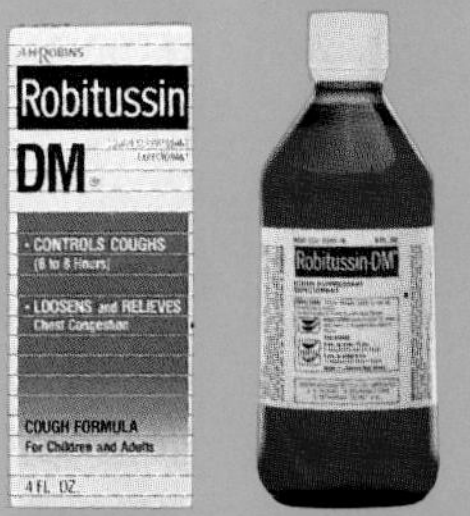

4 oz., 8 oz., 12 oz., 16 oz., 128 oz.

ROBITUSSIN®-DM SYRUP

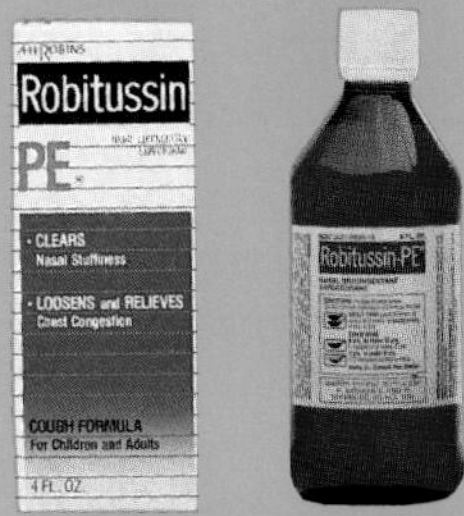

4 oz., 8 oz., 16 oz.

ROBITUSSIN®-PE SYRUP

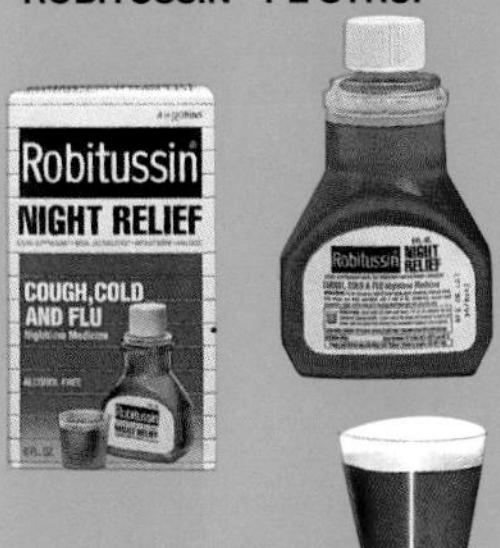

6 oz., 10 oz.

ROBITUSSIN NIGHT RELIEF®

ROSS

p. 683

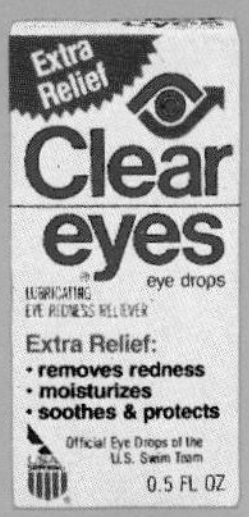

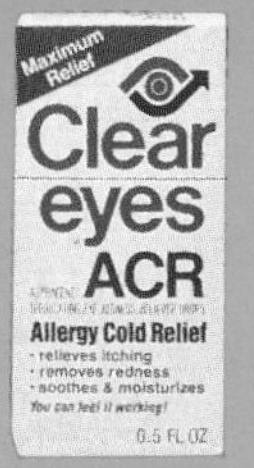

CLEAR EYES®
Lubricating Eye Redness Reliever

CLEAR EYES® ACR
Astringent/Lubricating Eye Redness Reliever Drops

Ross *p. 684*

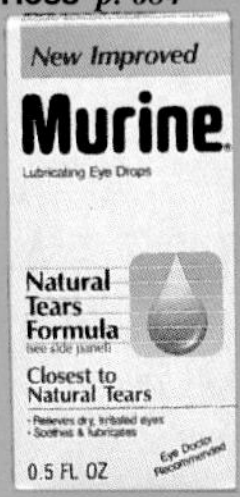

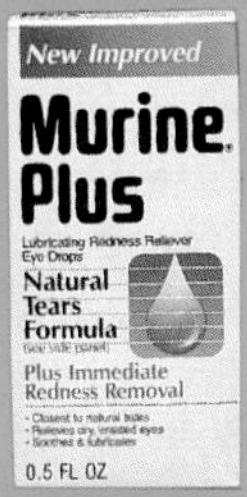

MURINE®
Lubricating Eye Drops

MURINE® PLUS
Lubricating Redness Reliever Eye Drops

Natural Tears Formula
Closest to Natural Tears
Available in:
0.5 and 1.0 Fl. Oz.

Ross *p. 684*

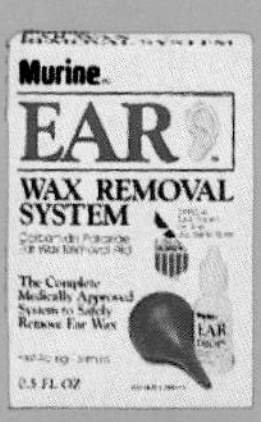

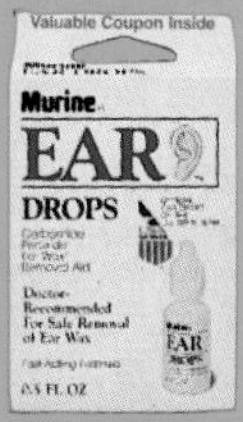

0.5 Fl. Oz.
MURINE® EAR WAX REMOVAL SYSTEM

0.5 Fl. Oz.
MURINE® EAR DROPS

Ross *p. 685*

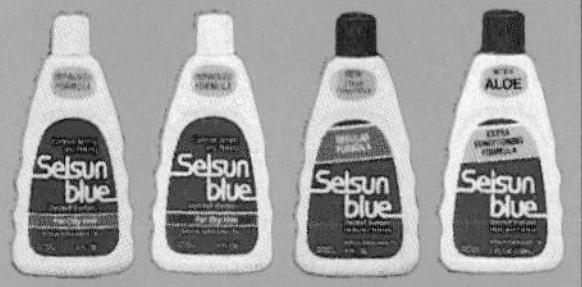

For Oily Hair | For Dry Hair | For Regular Hair | For All Hair Types

4 Fl. Oz.

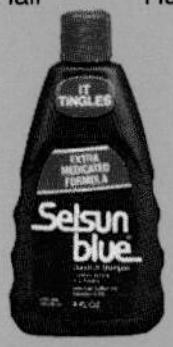

Medicated Treatment For All Hair Types

SELSUN BLUE®
Dandruff Shampoo

Also available in 7 and 11 Fl. Oz.

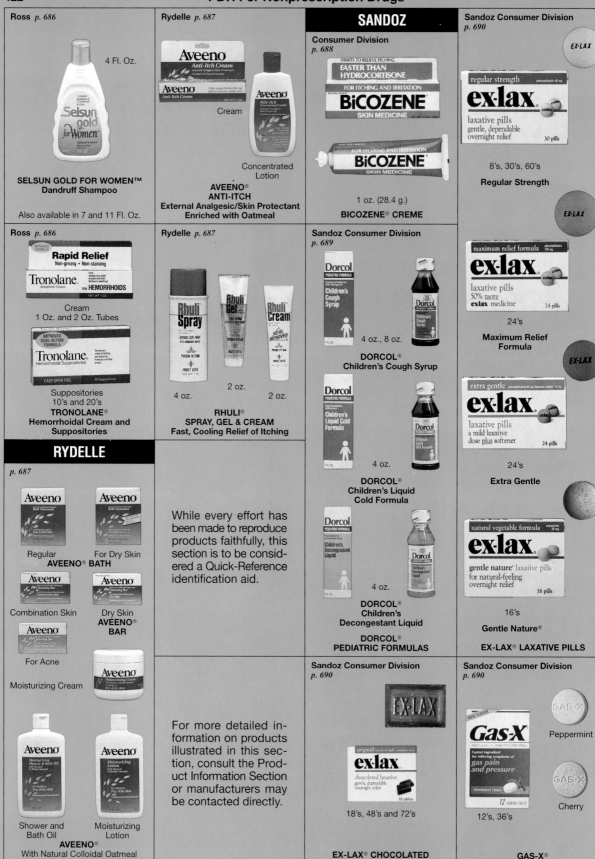

Ross *p. 686*

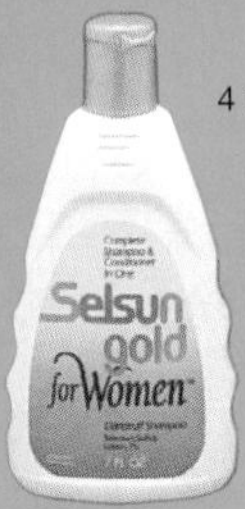

4 Fl. Oz.

SELSUN GOLD FOR WOMEN™
Dandruff Shampoo

Also available in 7 and 11 Fl. Oz.

Rydelle *p. 687*

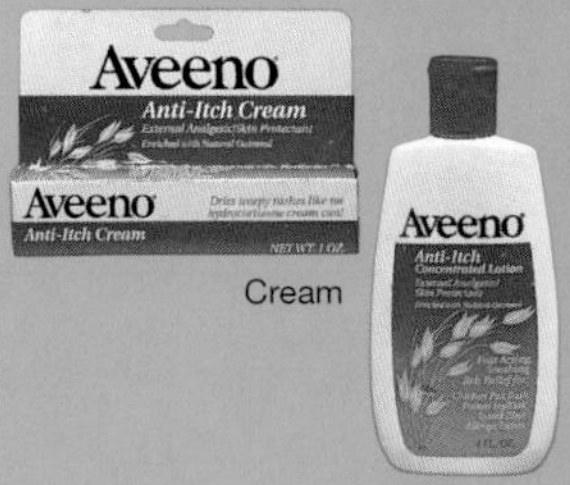

Cream

Concentrated Lotion

AVEENO®
ANTI-ITCH
External Analgesic/Skin Protectant
Enriched with Oatmeal

SANDOZ

Consumer Division
p. 688

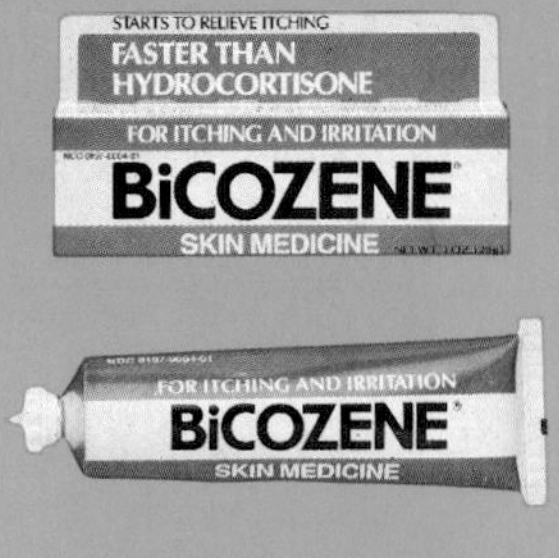
STARTS TO RELIEVE ITCHING
FASTER THAN
HYDROCORTISONE
FOR ITCHING AND IRRITATION
BiCOZENE
SKIN MEDICINE
FOR ITCHING AND IRRITATION
BiCOZENE
SKIN MEDICINE

1 oz. (28.4 g.)

BICOZENE® CREME

Sandoz Consumer Division
p. 690

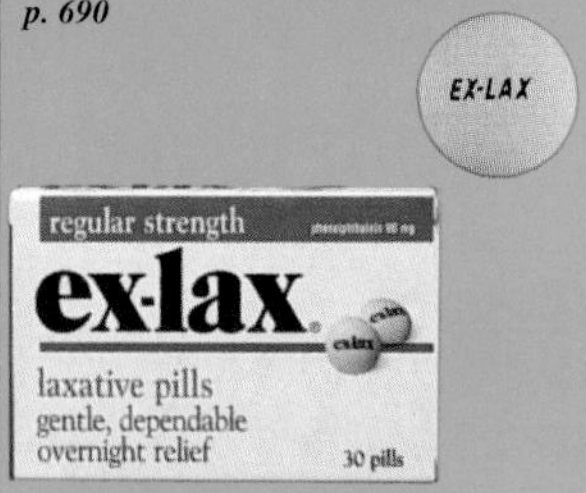
EX-LAX
regular strength
ex-lax
laxative pills
gentle, dependable
overnight relief
30 pills

8's, 30's, 60's

Regular Strength

Ross *p. 686*

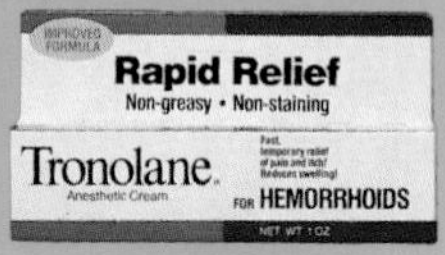
IMPROVED FORMULA
Rapid Relief
Non-greasy • Non-staining
Tronolane
Anesthetic Cream
FOR HEMORRHOIDS

Cream
1 Oz. and 2 Oz. Tubes

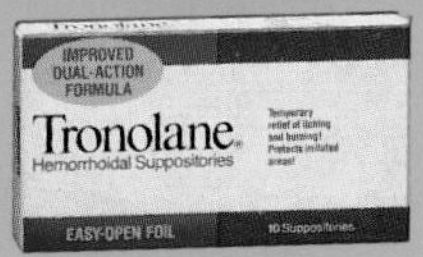

Suppositories
10's and 20's

TRONOLANE®
Hemorrhoidal Cream and Suppositories

Rydelle *p. 687*

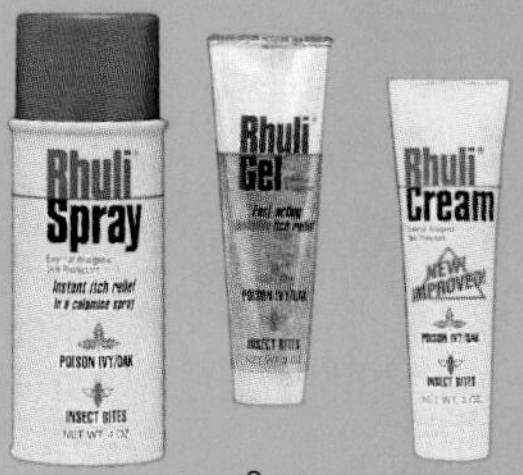

4 oz. 2 oz. 2 oz.

RHULI®
SPRAY, GEL & CREAM
Fast, Cooling Relief of Itching

Sandoz Consumer Division
p. 689

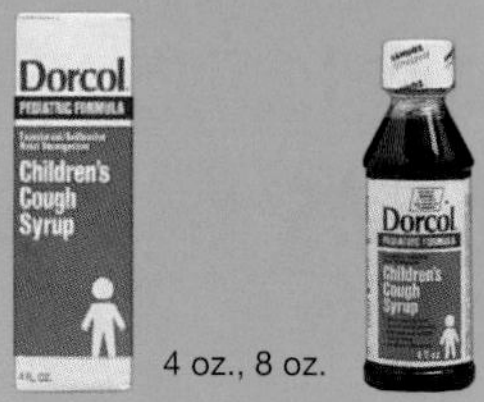
Dorcol
PEDIATRIC FORMULA
Children's Cough Syrup
Dorcol

4 oz., 8 oz.

DORCOL®
Children's Cough Syrup

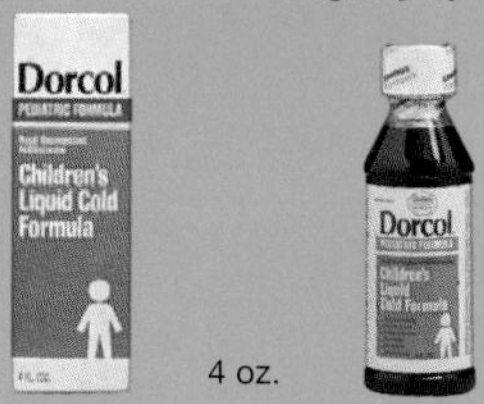
Dorcol
PEDIATRIC FORMULA
Children's Liquid Cold Formula
Dorcol

4 oz.

DORCOL®
Children's Liquid Cold Formula

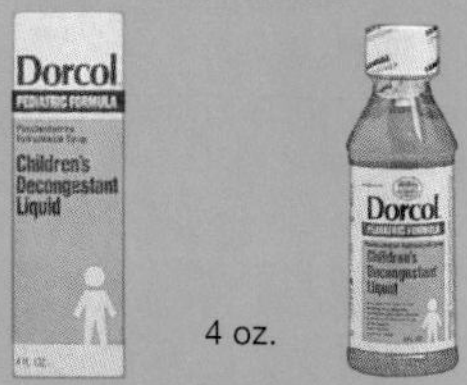
Dorcol
PEDIATRIC FORMULA
Children's Decongestant Liquid
Dorcol

4 oz.

DORCOL®
Children's Decongestant Liquid

DORCOL®
PEDIATRIC FORMULAS

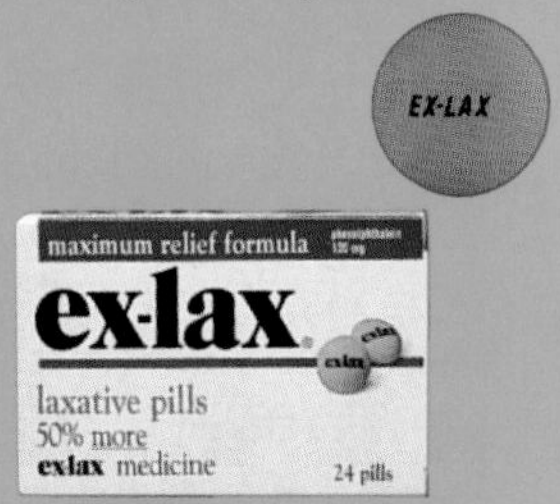
EX-LAX
maximum relief formula
ex-lax
laxative pills
50% more
ex-lax medicine
24 pills

24's

Maximum Relief Formula

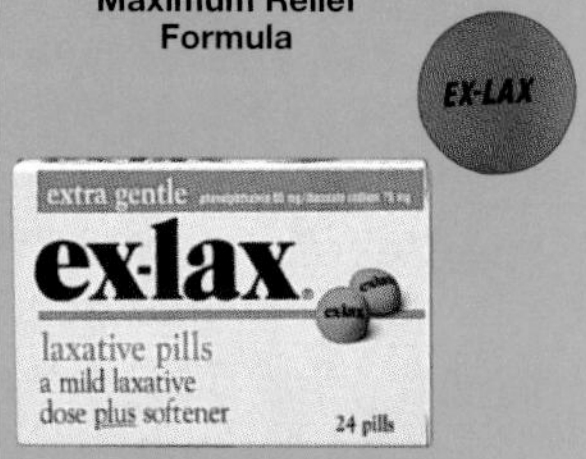
EX-LAX
extra gentle
ex-lax
laxative pills
a mild laxative
dose plus softener
24 pills

24's

Extra Gentle

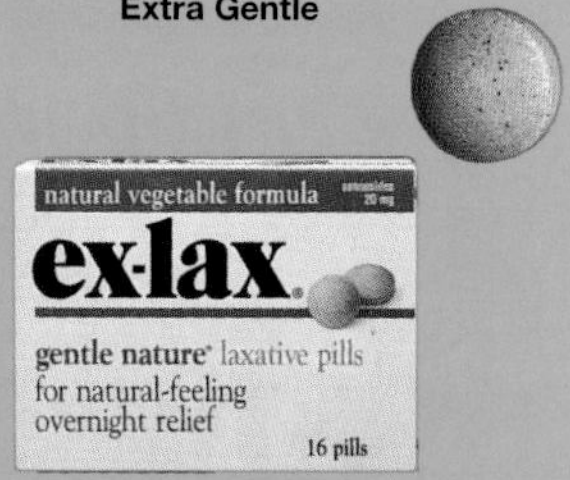
natural vegetable formula
ex-lax
gentle nature laxative pills
for natural-feeling
overnight relief
16 pills

16's

Gentle Nature®

EX-LAX® LAXATIVE PILLS

RYDELLE

p. 687

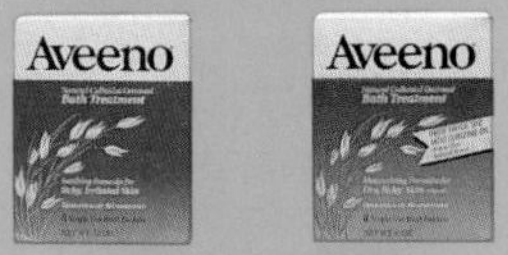
Aveeno
Aveeno

Regular For Dry Skin
AVEENO® BATH

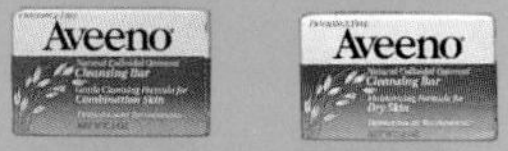
Aveeno
Aveeno

Combination Skin Dry Skin
AVEENO® BAR

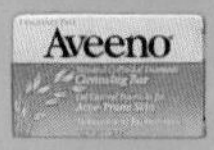
Aveeno

For Acne

Moisturizing Cream

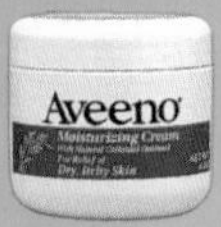
Aveeno
Moisturizing Cream

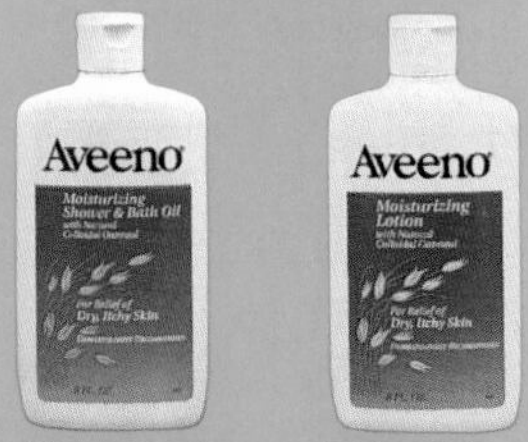
Aveeno
Moisturizing Shower & Bath Oil
Aveeno
Moisturizing Lotion

Shower and Bath Oil Moisturizing Lotion
AVEENO®
With Natural Colloidal Oatmeal
For the Relief of Dry, Itchy Skin

While every effort has been made to reproduce products faithfully, this section is to be considered a Quick-Reference identification aid.

For more detailed information on products illustrated in this section, consult the Product Information Section or manufacturers may be contacted directly.

Sandoz Consumer Division
p. 690

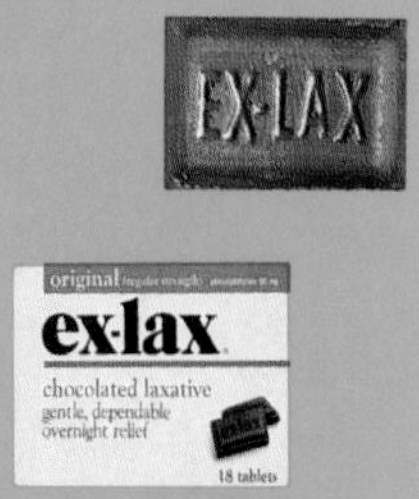

18's, 48's and 72's

EX-LAX® CHOCOLATED LAXATIVE TABLETS

Sandoz Consumer Division
p. 690

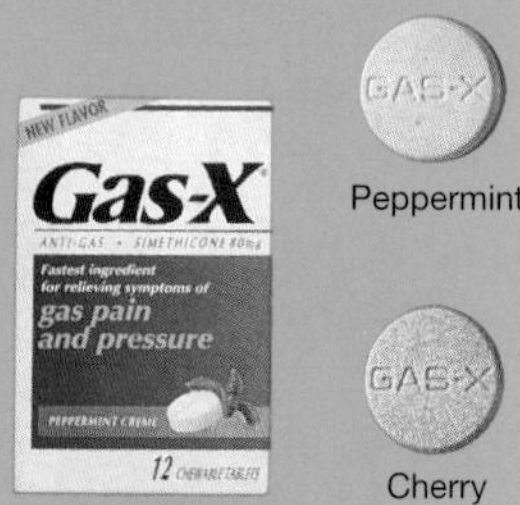
GAS-X
NEW FLAVOR
Gas-X
Fastest ingredient for relieving symptoms of
gas pain and pressure
12
GAS-X

Peppermint

Cherry

12's, 36's

GAS-X®
(80 mg. simethicone)

Sandoz Consumer Division
p. 690

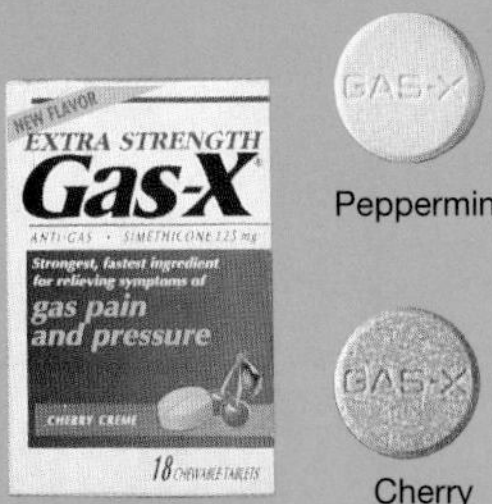

Peppermint

Cherry

18's, 48's

EXTRA-STRENGTH GAS-X®
(125 mg. simethicone)

Sandoz Consumer Division
p. 691

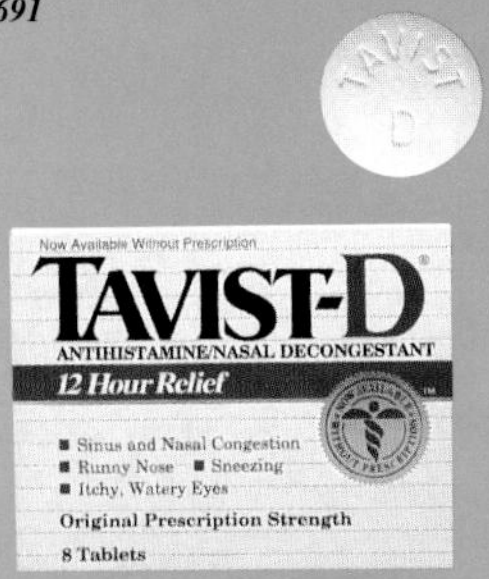
TAVIST-D
ANTIHISTAMINE/NASAL DECONGESTANT
12 Hour Relief
Original Prescription Strength
8 Tablets

8's, 16's

TAVIST-D

Sandoz Consumer Division
p. 694

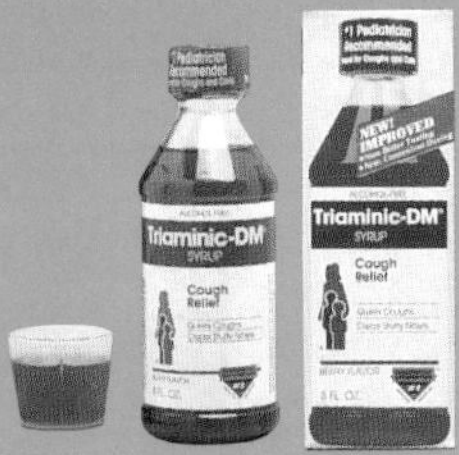

4 oz., 8 oz.

TRIAMINIC-DM®
COUGH RELIEF

Sandoz Consumer Division
p. 695

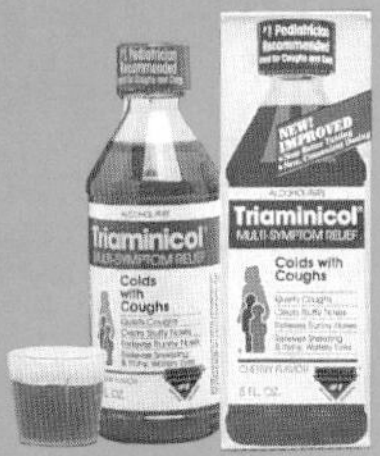

4 oz., 8 oz.

TRIAMINICOL®
MULTI-SYMPTOM
RELIEF

Sandoz Consumer Division
p. 691

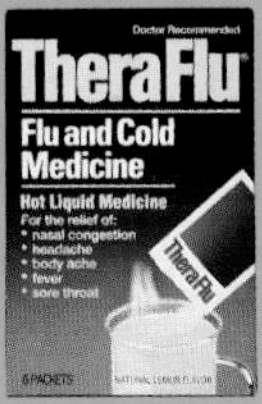

6's and 12's
Flu and Cold Medicine

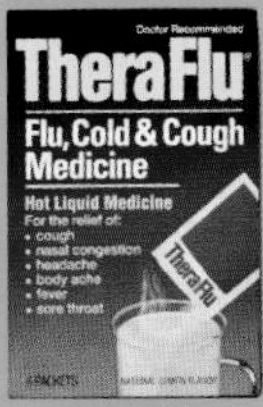

6's and 12's
Flu, Cold & Cough Medicine

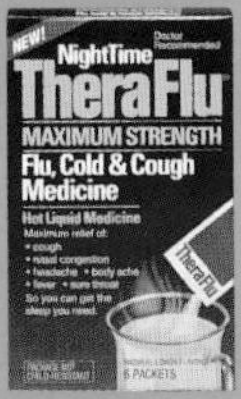

6's and 12's
Maximum Strength Nighttime
Flu, Cold & Cough Medicine
THERAFLU®

Sandoz Consumer Division
p. 693

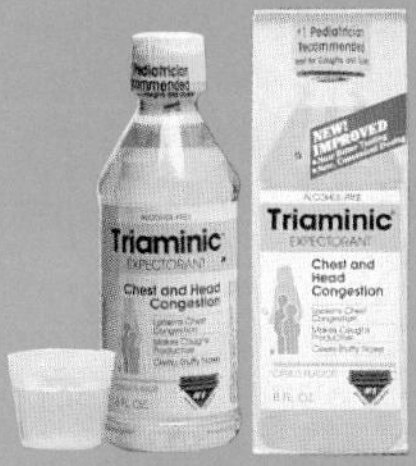

4 oz., 8 oz.

TRIAMINIC®
EXPECTORANT

Sandoz Consumer Division
p. 695

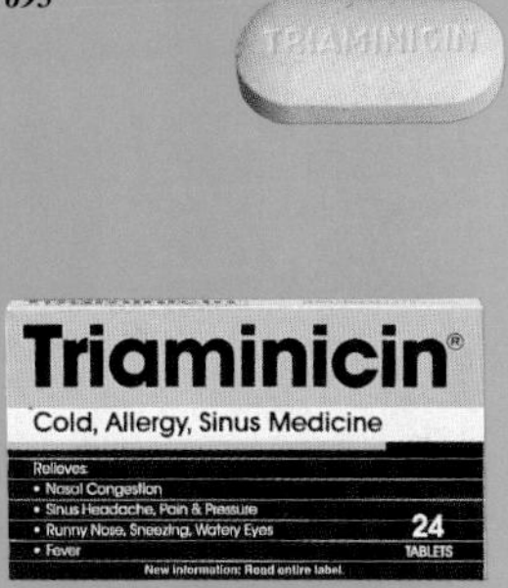
TRIAMINICIN
Triaminicin
Cold, Allergy, Sinus Medicine
24 TABLETS

12's, 24's, 48's, 100's

TRIAMINICIN®
TABLETS

Schering-Plough HealthCare

p. 699

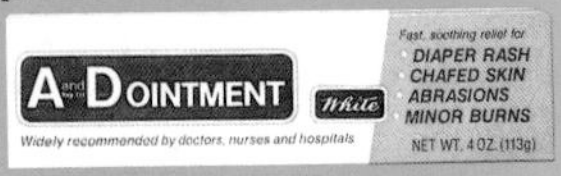
A and D OINTMENT
DIAPER RASH
CHAFED SKIN
ABRASIONS
MINOR BURNS

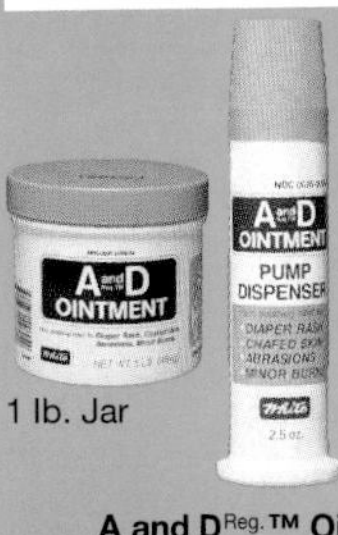

Pump
Dispenser

1 lb. Jar

A and D[Reg. TM] Ointment

Sandoz Consumer Division
p. 693

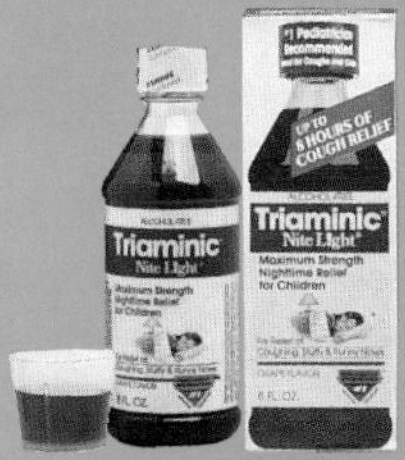

4 oz., 8 oz.

TRIAMINIC® NITE LIGHT®

Sandoz Consumer Division
p. 693

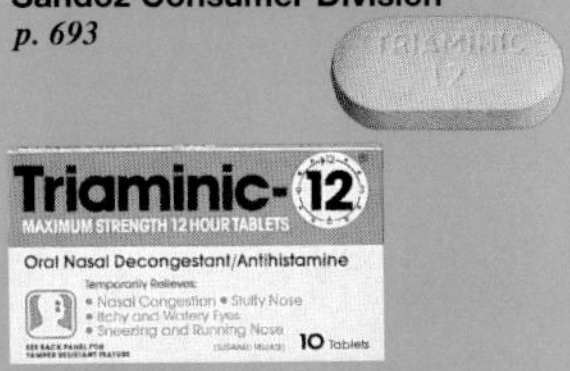
Triaminic-12
MAXIMUM STRENGTH 12 HOUR TABLETS
Oral Nasal Decongestant/Antihistamine
10 Tablets

10's, 20's

TRIAMINIC-12®
TABLETS
(Sustained Release)

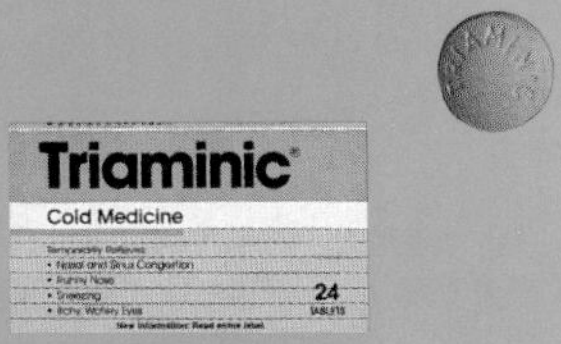
Triaminic
Cold Medicine
24

24's

TRIAMINIC®
COLD TABLETS

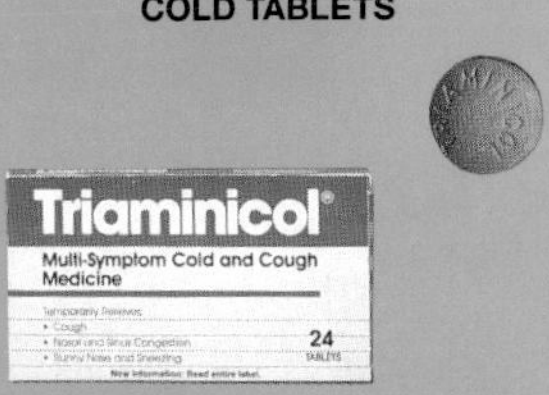
Triaminicol
Multi-Symptom Cold and Cough Medicine
24

24's

TRIAMINICOL®
MULTI-SYMPTOM COLD TABLETS

Schering-Plough HealthCare
p. 699

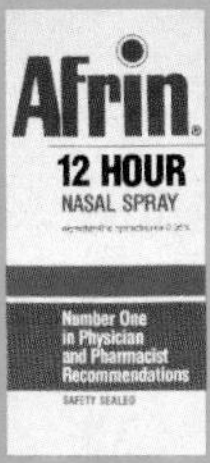
Afrin
12 HOUR
NASAL SPRAY

Safety Sealed

AFRIN®
NASAL SPRAY
0.05%

(oxymetazoline hydrochloride, USP)

Sandoz Consumer Division
p. 691

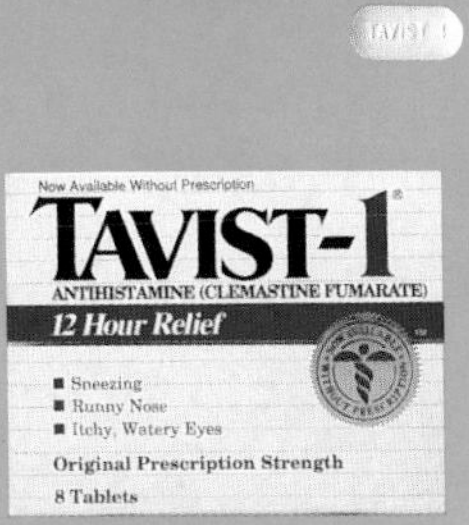
TAVIST-1
ANTIHISTAMINE (CLEMASTINE FUMARATE)
12 Hour Relief
Original Prescription Strength
8 Tablets

8's, 16's

TAVIST-1

Sandoz Consumer Division
p. 694

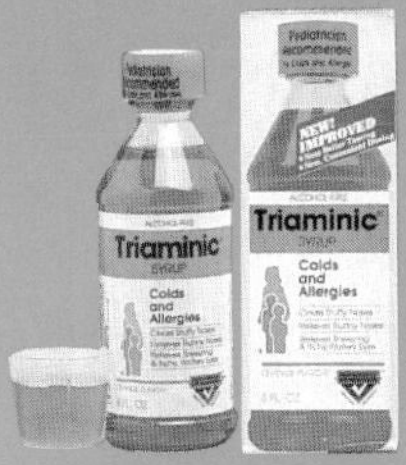

4 oz., 8 oz.

TRIAMINIC® Syrup

Schering-Plough HealthCare
p. 699

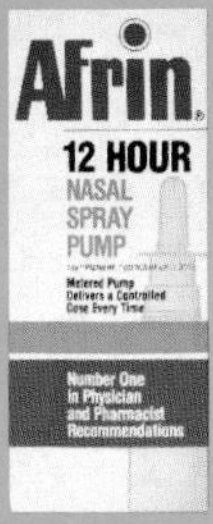
Afrin
12 HOUR
NASAL SPRAY PUMP

Safety Sealed

AFRIN® NASAL SPRAY PUMP
(oxymetazoline hydrochloride 0.05%)

Schering-Plough HealthCare
p. 699

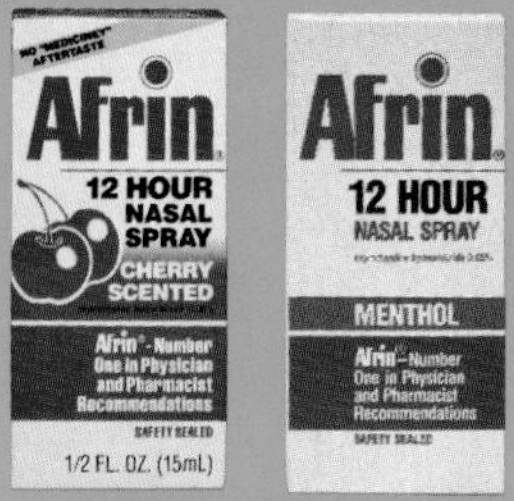

Safety Sealed

AFRIN® CHERRY SCENTED NASAL SPRAY 0.05%

AFRIN® MENTHOL NASAL SPRAY 0.05%

(oxymetazoline hydrochloride, USP)

Schering-Plough HealthCare
p. 700

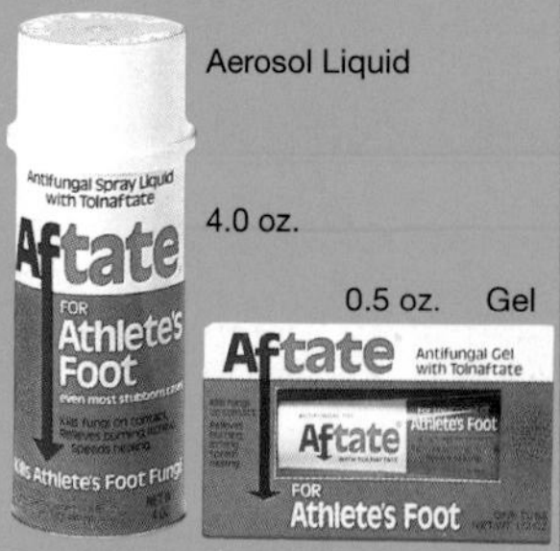

Aerosol Liquid

4.0 oz.

0.5 oz. Gel

Also available in 3.5 oz. spray powder and 2.25 oz. shaker powder.

AFTATE® FOR ATHLETE'S FOOT

(tolnaftate 1%)

Schering-Plough HealthCare
p. 701

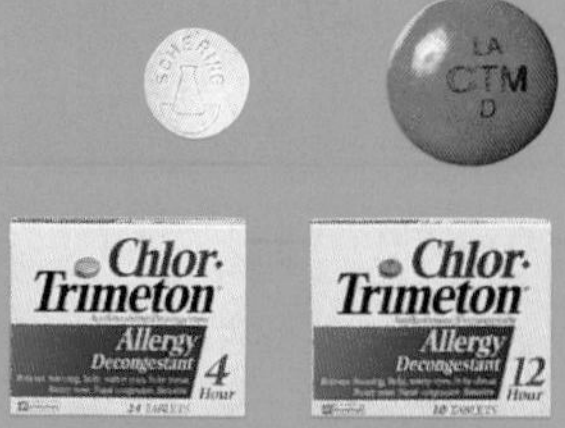

CHLOR-TRIMETON® ALLERGY DECONGESTANT TABLETS

4 Hour (4 mg chlorpheniramine maleate, 60 mg pseudoephedrine sulfate)
12 Hour (8 mg chlorpheniramine maleate, 120 mg pseudoephedrine sulfate)

Schering-Plough HealthCare
p. 702

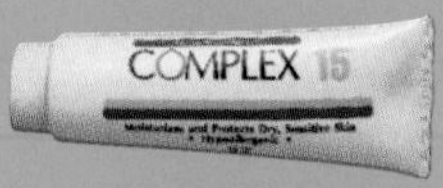

Face Cream

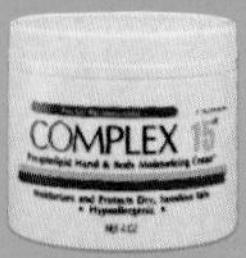

Cream

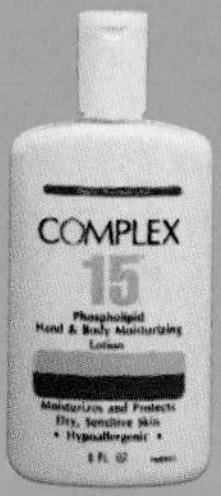

Lotion

COMPLEX 15® Phospholipid Hand and Body Moisturizer

Schering-Plough HealthCare
p. 699

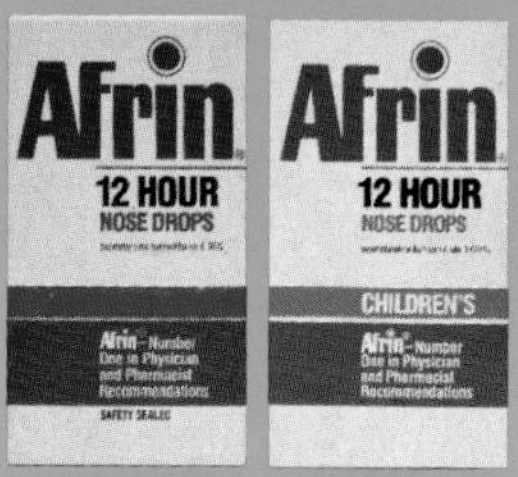

Safety Sealed

Nose Drops 0.05%

Children's Strength Nose Drops 0.025%

AFRIN® NOSE DROPS

(oxymetazoline hydrochloride)

Schering-Plough HealthCare
p. 700

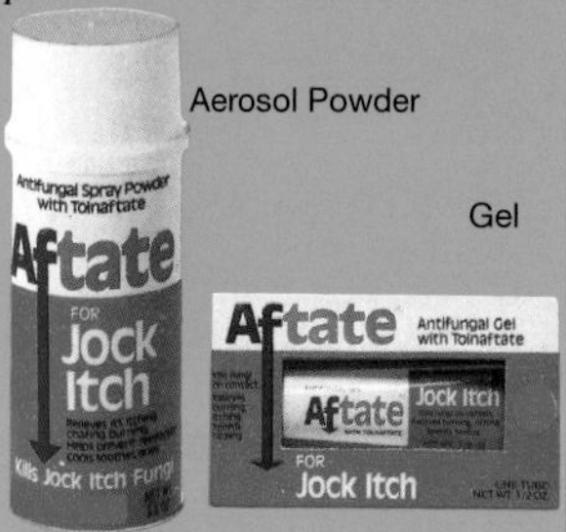

Aerosol Powder

Gel

3.5 oz. 0.5 oz.

Also available in 1.5 oz. shaker powder.

AFTATE® FOR JOCK ITCH

(tolnaftate 1%)

Schering-Plough HealthCare
p. 701

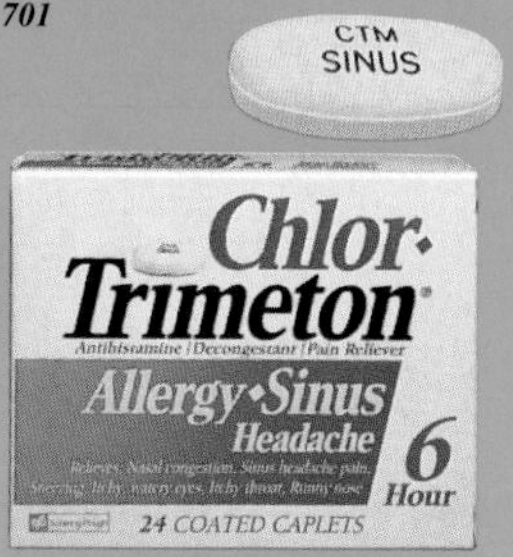

CHLOR-TRIMETON® ALLERGY/SINUS HEADACHE

(2 mg chlorpheniramine maleate, 12.5 mg phenylpropanolamine HCl, and 500 mg acetaminophen)

Schering-Plough HealthCare
p. 700

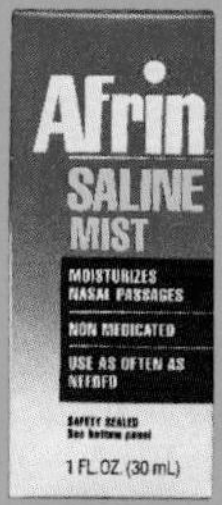

Safety Sealed

AFRIN® SALINE MIST

Schering-Plough HealthCare
p. 700

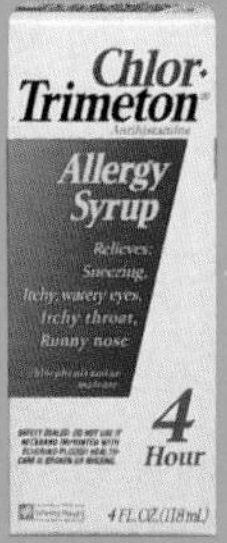

CHLOR-TRIMETON® ALLERGY SYRUP

(2 mg chlorpheniramine maleate)

Schering-Plough HealthCare
p. 702

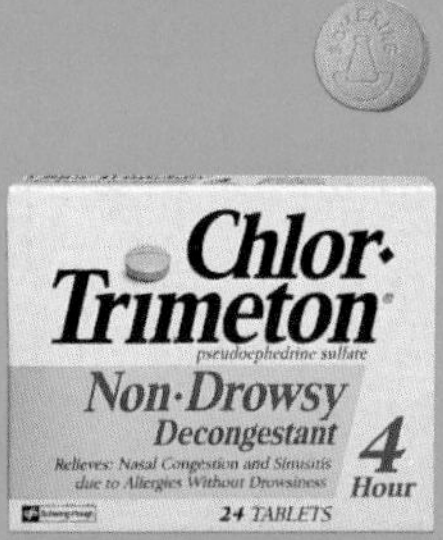

CHLOR-TRIMETON® NON-DROWSY DECONGESTANT TABLETS

(60 mg pseudoephedrine sulfate)

Schering-Plough HealthCare
p. 703

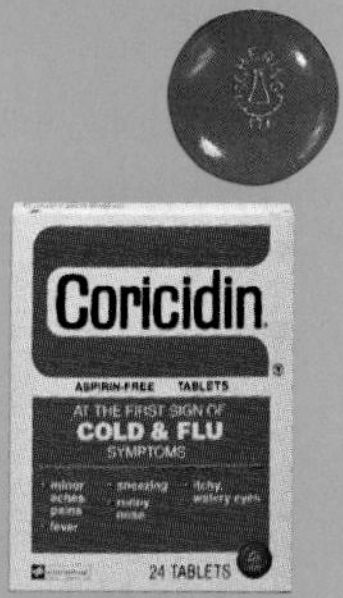

CORICIDIN® TABLETS

(2 mg chlorpheniramine maleate and 325 mg acetaminophen)

Schering-Plough HealthCare
p. 700

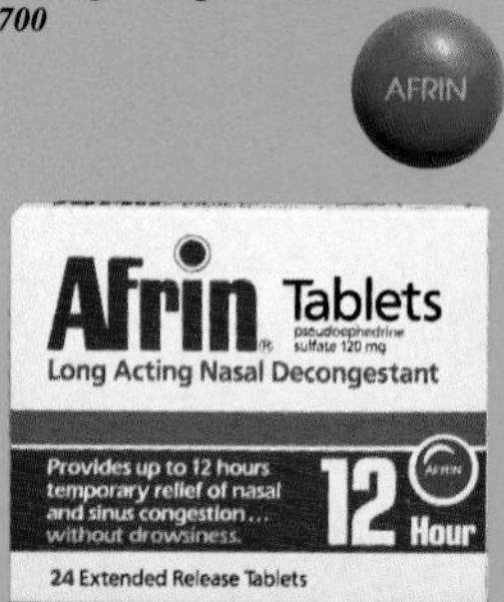

AFRIN® EXTENDED RELEASE TABLETS

(pseudoephedrine sulfate)

Schering-Plough HealthCare
p. 700

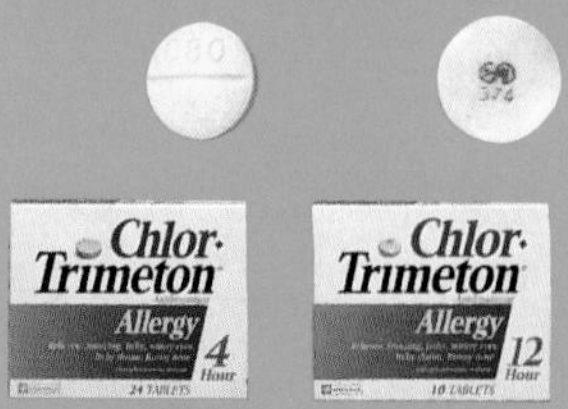

CHLOR-TRIMETON® ALLERGY TABLETS

4 Hour (4 mg chlorpheniramine maleate)
12 Hour (12 mg chlorpheniramine maleate)

Schering-Plough HealthCare
p. 702

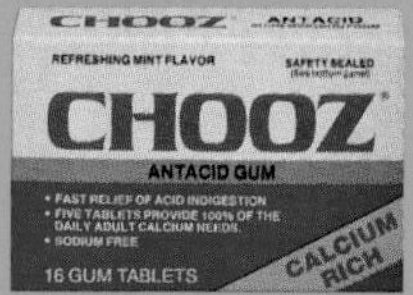

16 Gum Tablets

CHOOZ® ANTACID GUM

(Calcium Carbonate)

Schering-Plough HealthCare
p. 703

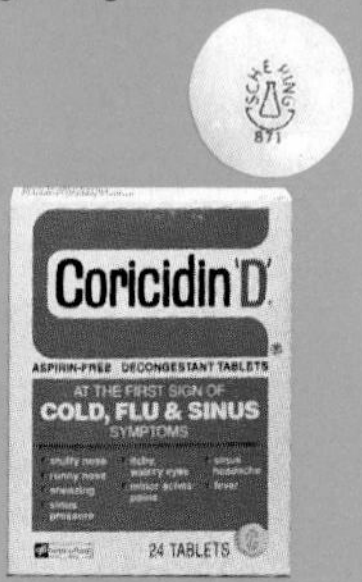

CORICIDIN 'D'® DECONGESTANT TABLETS

(2 mg chlorpheniramine maleate, 12.5 mg phenylpropanolamine HCl, and 325 mg acetaminophen)

Schering-Plough HealthCare
p. 704

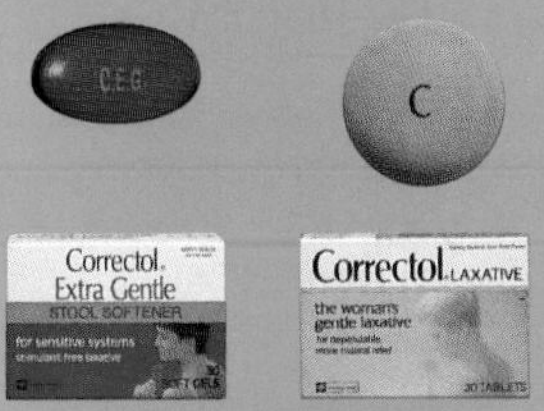

CORRECTOL® LAXATIVE AND EXTRA GENTLE STOOL SOFTENER

(Tablet contains 100 mg docusate sodium and 65 mg yellow phenolphthalein)

(Soft Gel contains 100 mg docusate sodium)

Schering-Plough HealthCare
p. 705

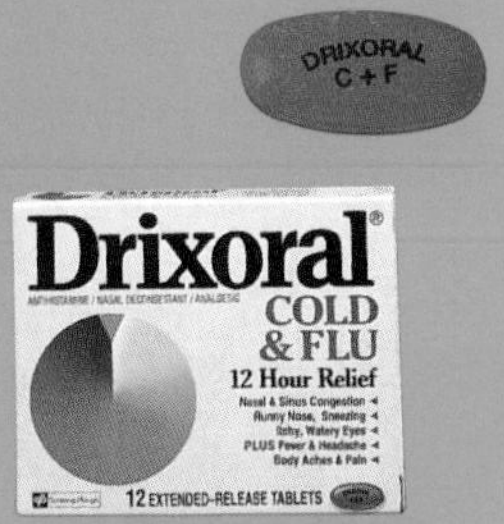

DRIXORAL® COLD & FLU EXTENDED-RELEASE TABLETS

(60 mg pseudoephedrine sulfate, 3 mg dexbrompheniramine maleate and 500 mg acetaminophen)

Schering-Plough HealthCare
p. 707

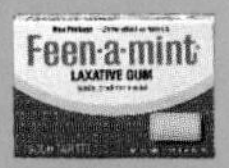

Laxative Gum

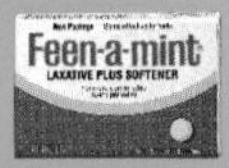

Laxative plus Softener

FEEN-A-MINT® LAXATIVE

Gum contains: 97.2 mg phenolphthalein. Pills contain: 100 mg docusate sodium and 65 mg phenolphthalein.

Schering-Plough HealthCare

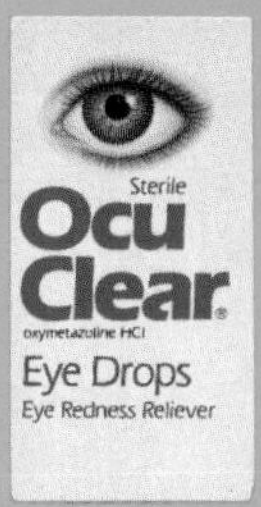

Safety Sealed

OCUCLEAR® EYE DROPS

(oxymetazoline HCl 0.025%)

Schering-Plough HealthCare
p. 704

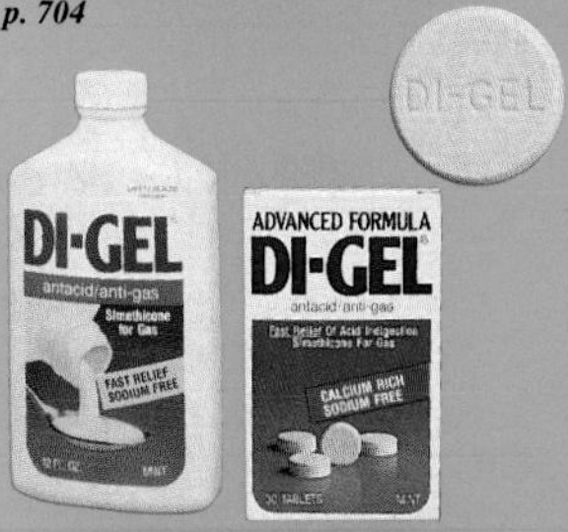

Liquid Tablets

Mint and Lemon/Orange flavors, 6 fl. oz. and 12 fl. oz. liquid plus 30 and 90 tablet sizes.

DI-GEL®

Schering-Plough HealthCare
p. 706

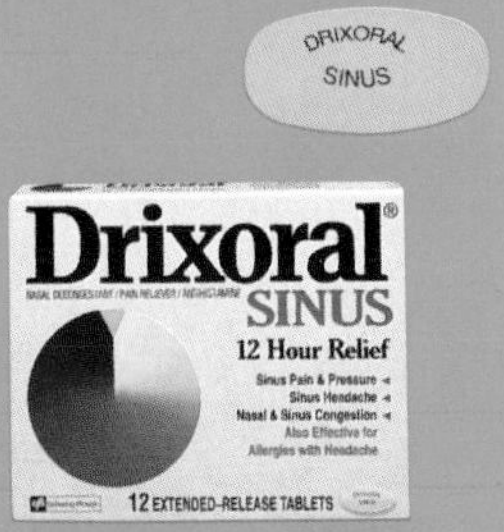

DRIXORAL® SINUS EXTENDED-RELEASE TABLETS

(60 mg pseudoephedrine sulfate, 3 mg dexbrompheniramine maleate, 500 mg acetaminophen)

Schering-Plough HealthCare
p. 707

Cream

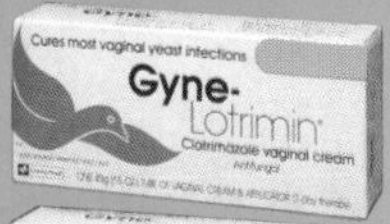

Inserts

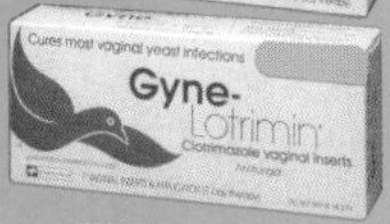

Disposables

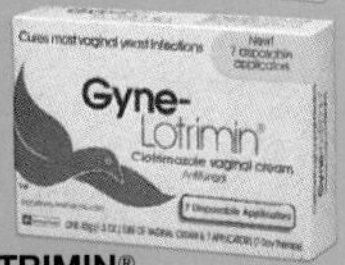

GYNE-LOTRIMIN® Clotrimazole Vaginal Antifungal

Schering-Plough HealthCare
p. 711

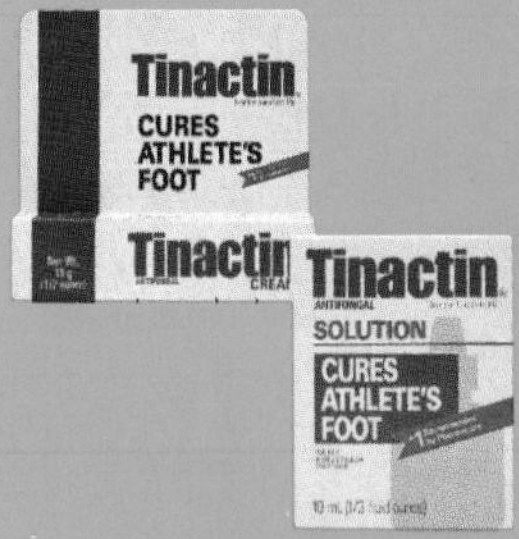

TINACTIN® CREAM AND SOLUTION

(tolnaftate 1%)

Schering-Plough HealthCare
p. 705

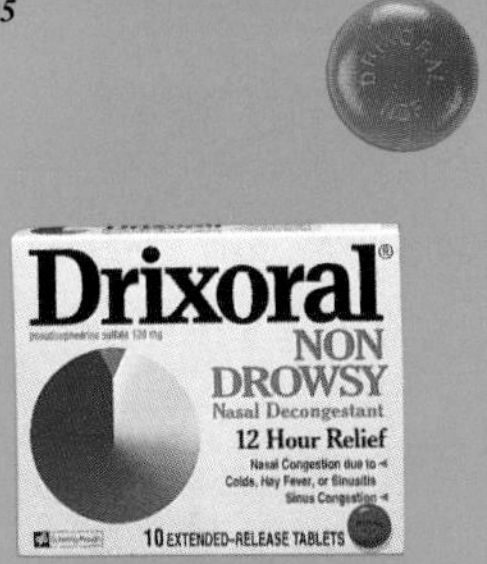

DRIXORAL® NON-DROWSY EXTENDED-RELEASE TABLETS

(120 mg pseudoephedrine sulfate)

Schering-Plough HealthCare
p. 706

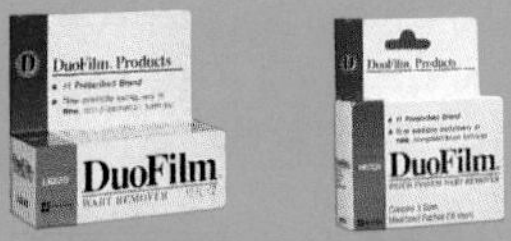

DuoFilm Wart Remover

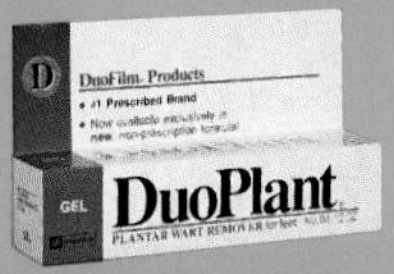

DuoPlant Plantar Wart Remover for Feet

DUOFILM®/DUOPLANT®

Schering-Plough HealthCare
p. 708

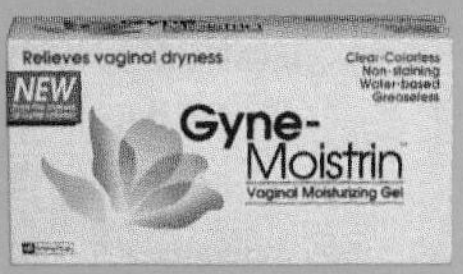

Available in 1.5 and 2.5 oz. sizes

GYNE-MOISTRIN™ Vaginal Moisturizing Gel Relieves vaginal dryness

Schering-Plough HealthCare
p. 711

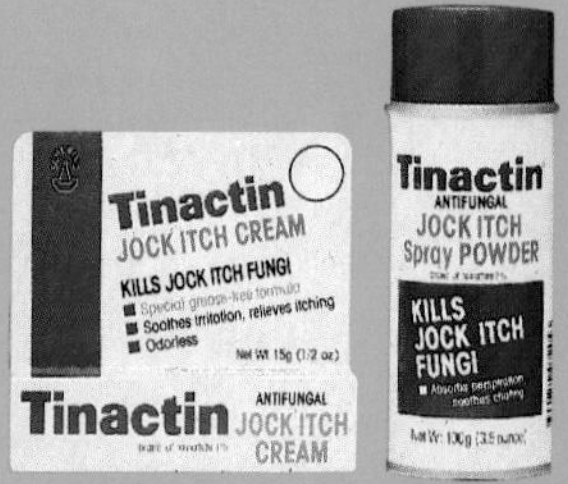

TINACTIN® JOCK ITCH CREAM AND SPRAY POWDER

(tolnaftate 1%)

Schering-Plough HealthCare
p. 705

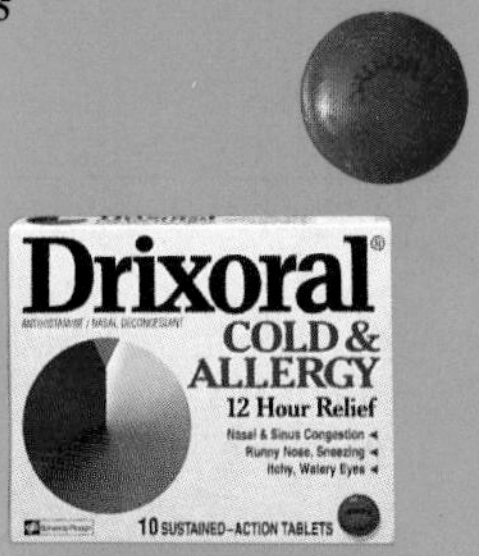

DRIXORAL® COLD & ALLERGY SUSTAINED-ACTION TABLETS

(6 mg dexbrompheniramine maleate and 120 mg pseudoephedrine sulfate)

Schering-Plough HealthCare
p. 707

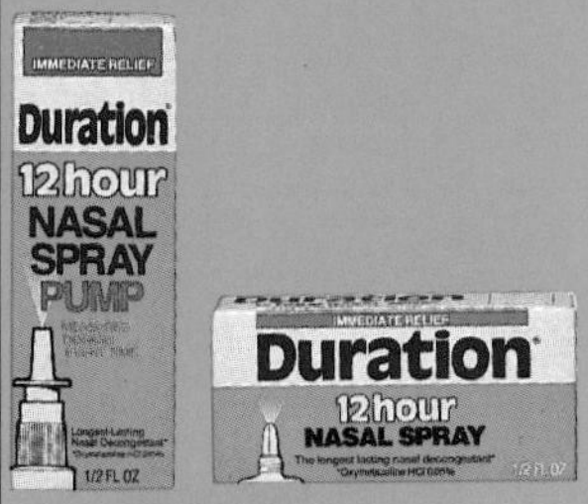

Available in ½ oz., 1 oz. and ½ oz. measured dosage pump spray.

(oxymetazoline HCl)

DURATION® NASAL SPRAY

Schering-Plough HealthCare
p. 708

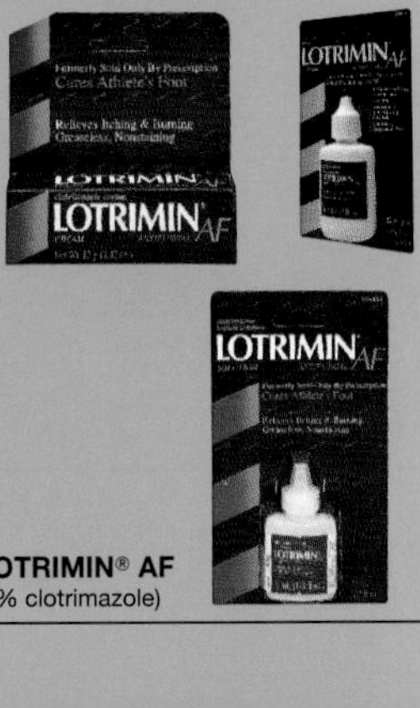

LOTRIMIN® AF

(1% clotrimazole)

Schering-Plough HealthCare
p. 711

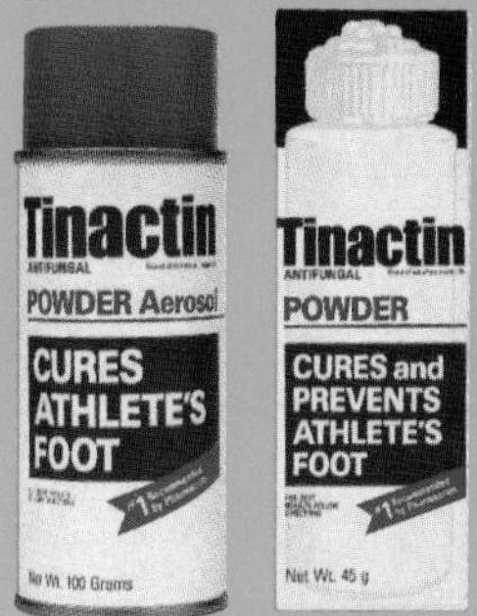

TINACTIN® POWDER AEROSOL AND POWDER

(tolnaftate 1%)

Schering-Plough HealthCare
p. 711

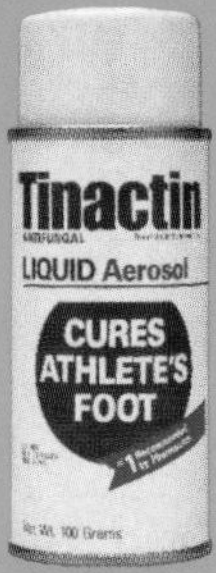

TINACTIN®
LIQUID AEROSOL
(tolnaftate 1%)

SmithKline Beecham Consumer Brands
p. 714

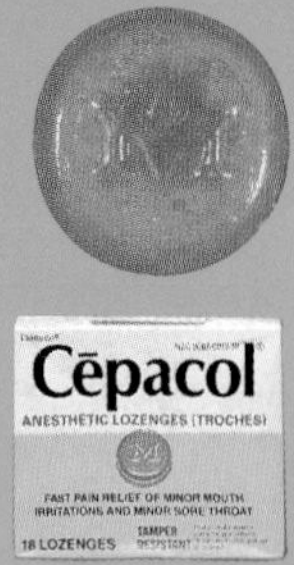

18 lozenges per package

CĒPACOL® ANESTHETIC LOZENGES
(Troches)

SmithKline Beecham Consumer Brands
p. 715

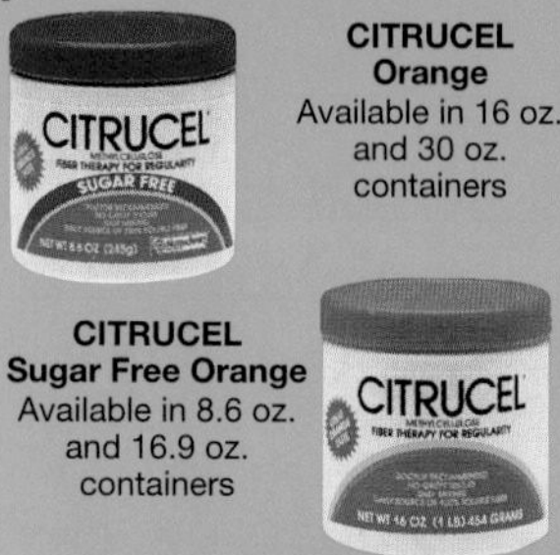

CITRUCEL
Orange
Available in 16 oz. and 30 oz. containers

CITRUCEL
Sugar Free Orange
Available in 8.6 oz. and 16.9 oz. containers

CITRUCEL®
Fiber Therapy for Regularity

SmithKline Beecham Consumer Brands
p. 717

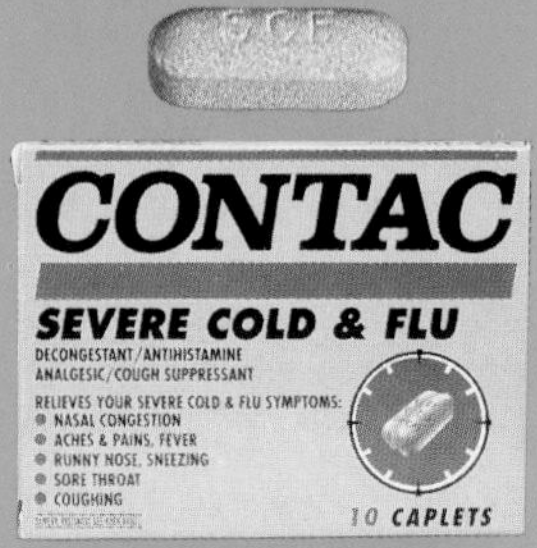

Packages of 10, 20 and 40 caplets

CONTAC®
SEVERE COLD FORMULA

SMITHKLINE BEECHAM

Consumer Brands
p. 712

Special Comb Included

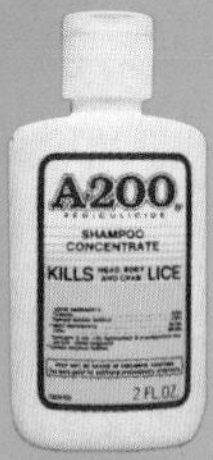

4 fl. oz.

A-200™
Pediculicide
Shampoo

Also available:
A-200 Shampoo 2 fl. oz.
A-200 Gel Concentrate, 1 oz.

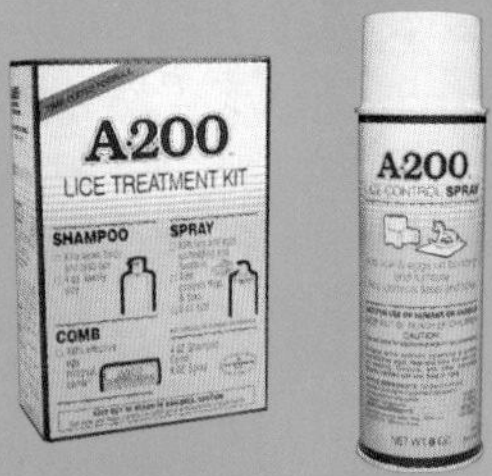

A-200®
Lice Treatment Kit
includes
Shampoo, Spray & Comb

6 fl. oz.

A-200®
Spray

SmithKline Beecham Consumer Brands
p. 713

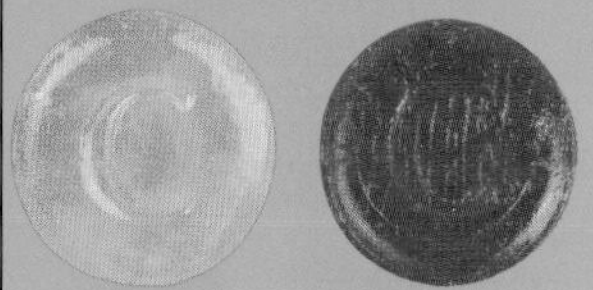

18 lozenges per package

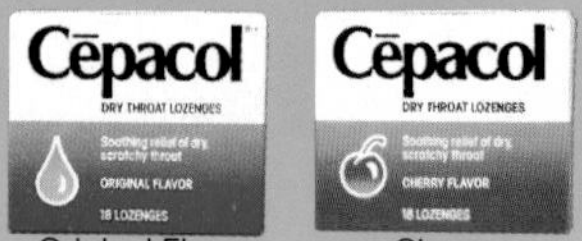

Original Flavor Cherry

CĒPACOL®
DRY THROAT LOZENGES

SmithKline Beecham Consumer Brands
p. 715

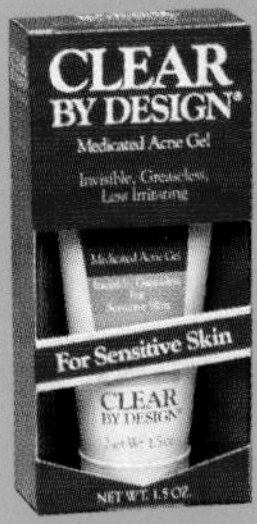

1.5 oz. tube

CLEAR BY DESIGN®
Medicated Acne Gel
(benzoyl peroxide 2.5%)

SmithKline Beecham Consumer Brands
p. 718

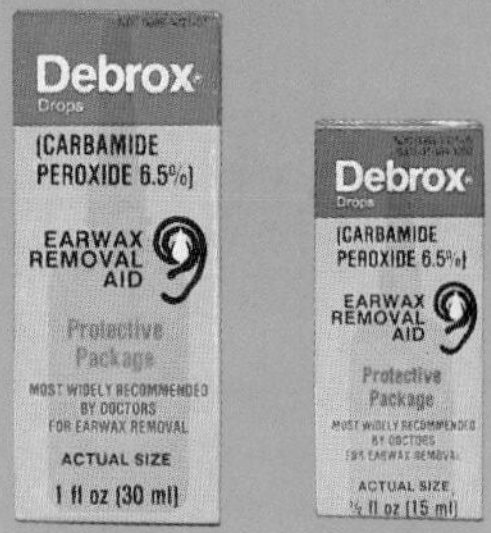

1 fl. oz. ½ fl. oz.

DEBROX®
Drops

SmithKline Beecham Consumer Brands
p. 713

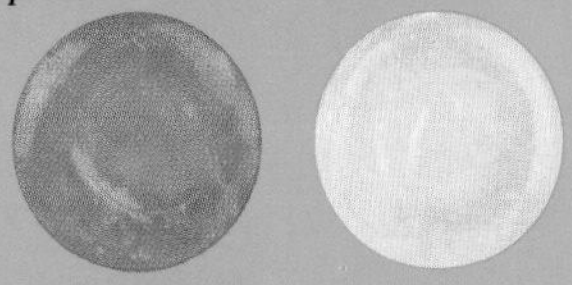

18 lozenges per package

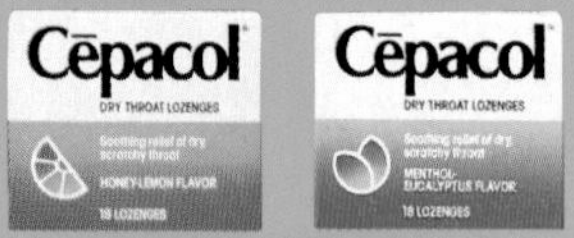

Honey-Lemon Menthol-Eucalyptus

CĒPACOL®
DRY THROAT LOZENGES

SmithKline Beecham Consumer Brands
p. 717

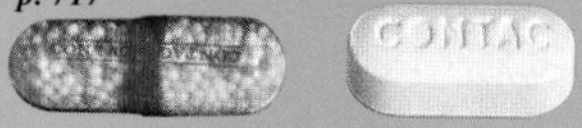

Packages of 10, 20 and 40 capsules and caplets

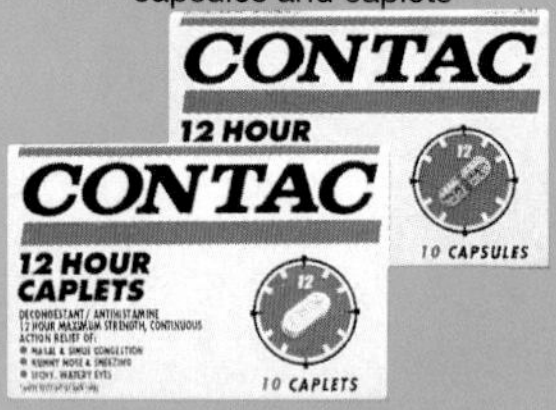

CONTAC®
CONTINUOUS ACTION NASAL DECONGESTANT ANTIHISTAMINE CAPLETS & CAPSULES

SmithKline Beecham Consumer Brands
p. 718

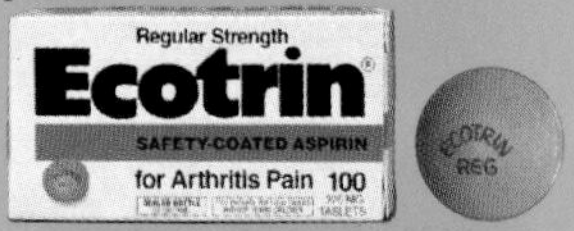

Tablets in bottles of 100, 250, 500 and 1000

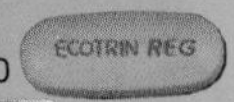

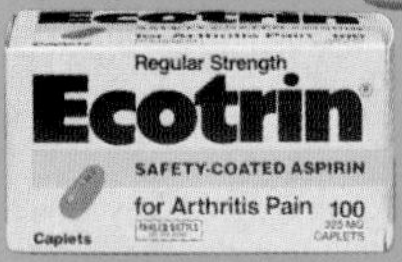

Caplets in bottles of 100
REGULAR STRENGTH
ECOTRIN® TABLETS AND CAPLETS
Enteric coated 5 gr. aspirin

SmithKline Beecham Consumer Brands
p. 713

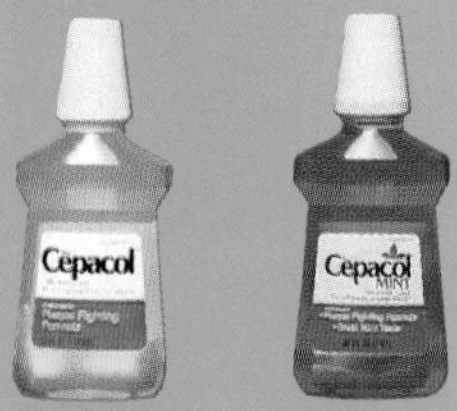

Cēpacol Gold **Cēpacol MInt**

Available in 4, 12, 18, 24 and 32 fl. oz. bottles

CĒPACOL®
Mouthwash/Gargle

SmithKline Beecham Consumer Brands
p. 714

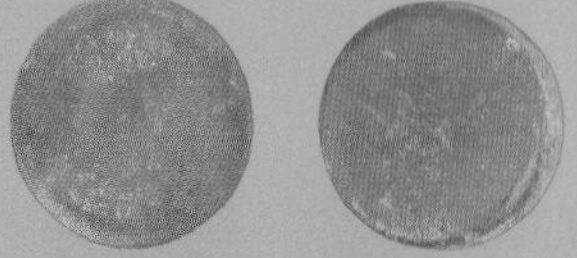

18 lozenges per package

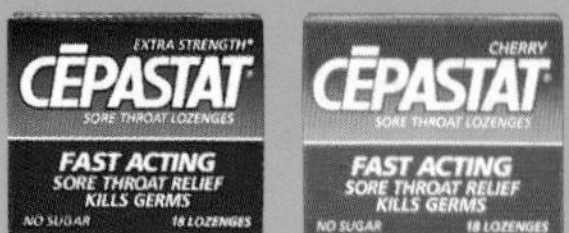

Extra Strength Cherry

CĒPASTAT®
SORE THROAT LOZENGES

SmithKline Beecham Consumer Brands
p. 715

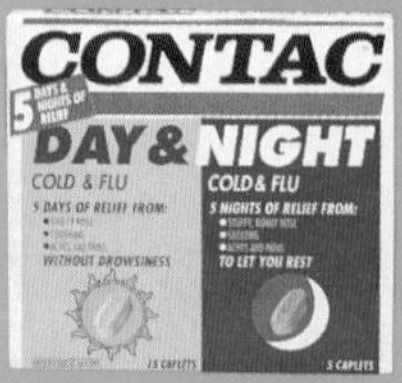

CONTAC®
DAY & NIGHT COLD & FLU

SmithKline Beecham Consumer Brands

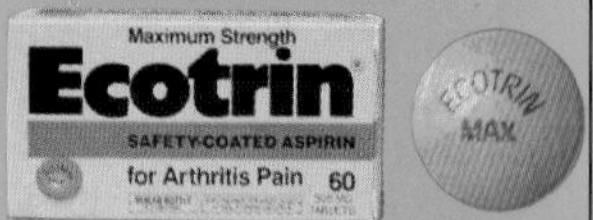

Tablets in bottles of 60, 150, and 300

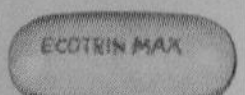

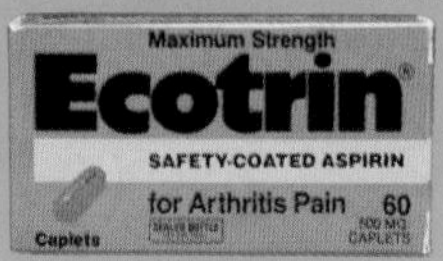

Caplets in bottles of 60
MAXIMUM STRENGTH
ECOTRIN® TABLETS AND CAPLETS
Enteric coated 7.7 gr. aspirin

SmithKline Beecham Consumer Brands
p. 721

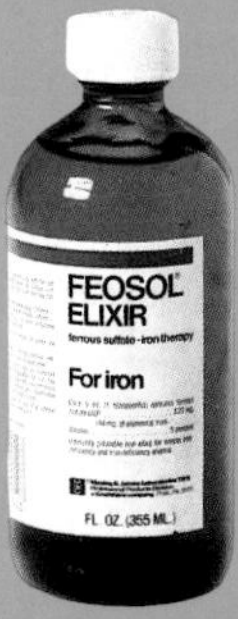

16 oz. bottle
FEOSOL® ELIXIR
(ferrous sulfate USP)

SmithKline Beecham Consumer Brands
p. 722

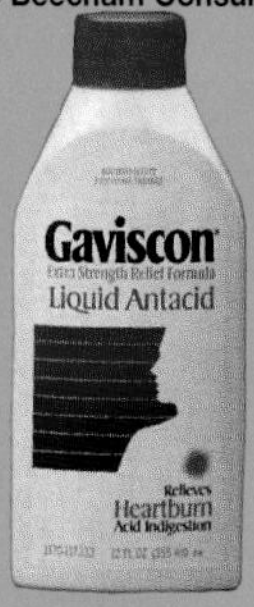

12 fl. oz.
GAVISCON®
Extra Strength
Relief Formula
Liquid Antacid

SmithKline Beecham Consumer Brands
p. 724

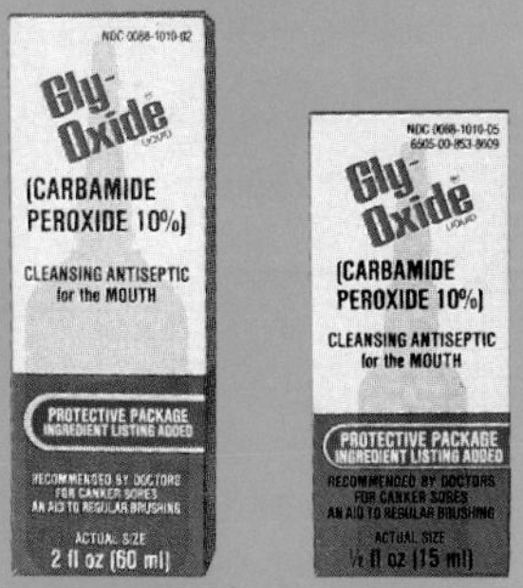

2 fl. oz. ½ fl. oz.
GLY-OXIDE® Liquid

SmithKline Beecham Consumer Brands
p. 728

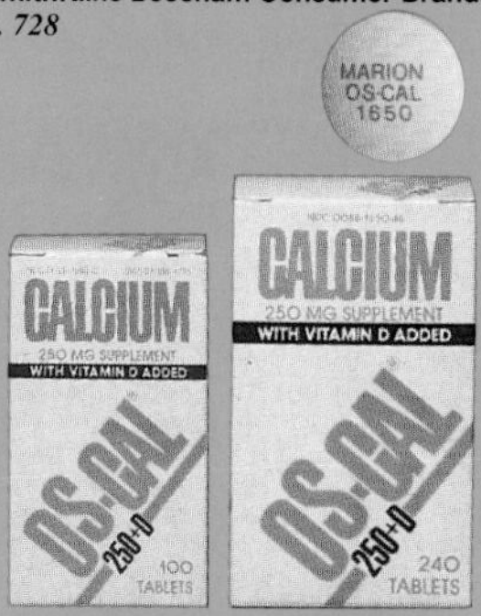

Bottles of 100 and 240 tablets
OS-CAL® 250+D Tablets
(calcium with vitamin D)

SmithKline Beecham Consumer Brands
p. 721

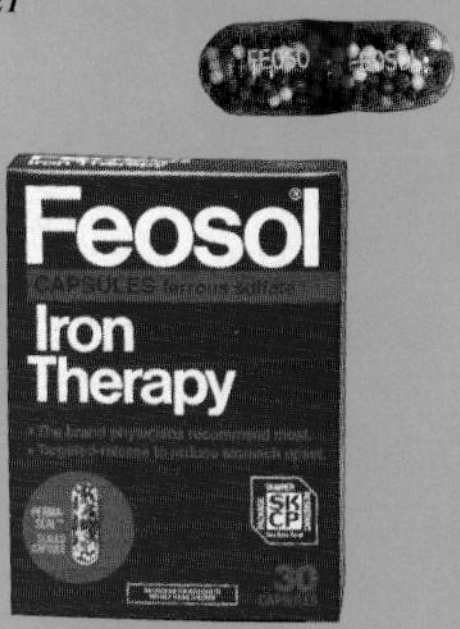

Packages of 30 and
60 capsules
FEOSOL® CAPSULES
(ferrous sulfate USP)

SmithKline Beecham Consumer Brands
p. 722

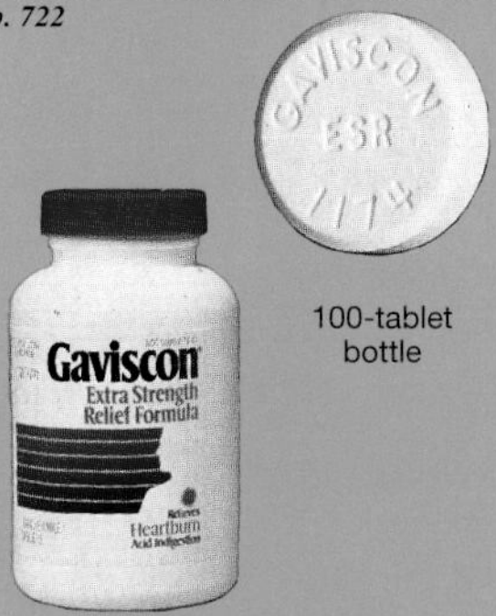

100-tablet
bottle

GAVISCON®
Extra Strength
Relief Formula Antacid Tablets

SmithKline Beecham Consumer Brands
p. 725

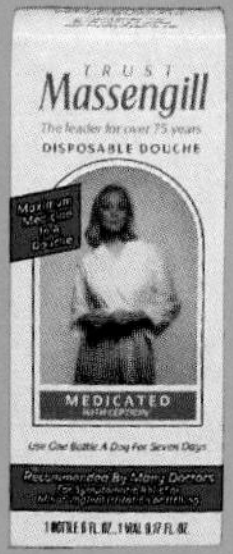

Available in single or twin packs

MASSENGILL® Medicated
Disposable Douche
With Povidone-iodine

SmithKline Beecham Consumer Brands
p. 728

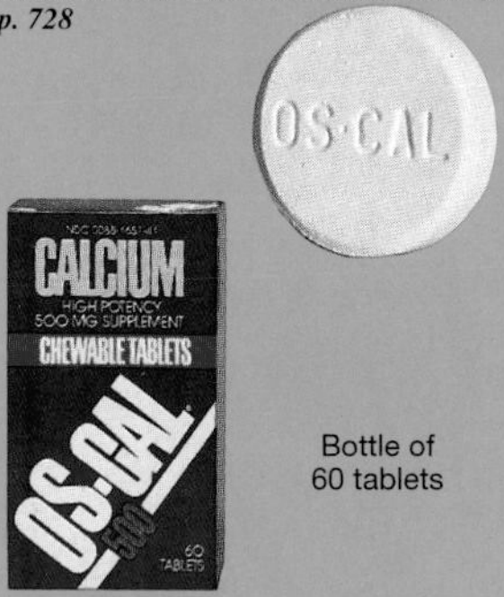

Bottle of
60 tablets

OS-CAL® 500
Chewable Tablets

SmithKline Beecham Consumer Brands
p. 721

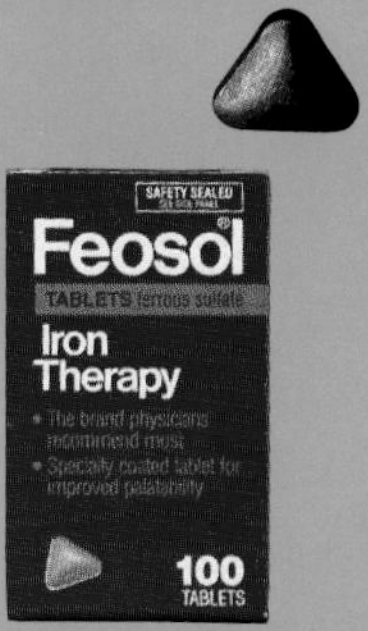

In 100 and 1000 tablet bottles

FEOSOL® TABLETS
(ferrous sulfate USP)

SmithKline Beecham Consumer Brands
p. 722

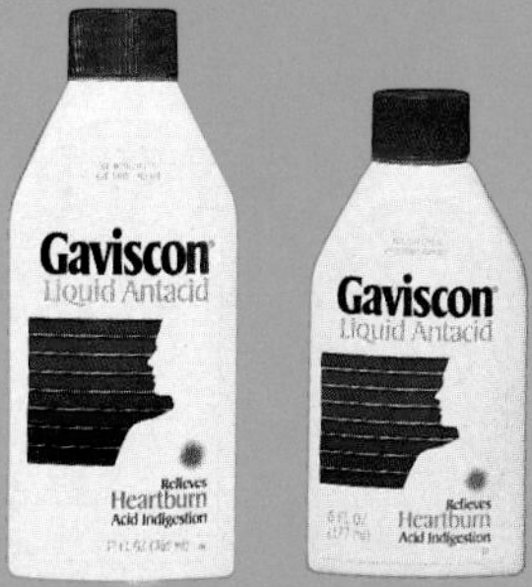

12 fl. oz. 6 fl .oz.

GAVISCON®
Liquid Antacid

SmithKline Beecham Consumer Brands
p. 726

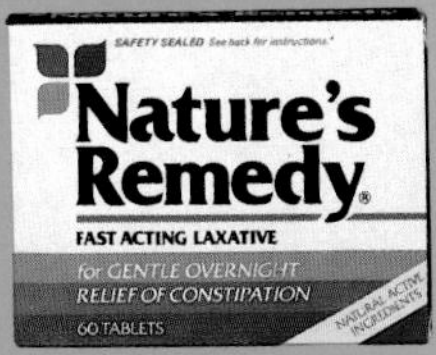

60 tablets
NATURE'S REMEDY®
LAXATIVE TABLETS
Also available:
Box 12s and 30s

SmithKline Beecham Consumer Brands
p. 728

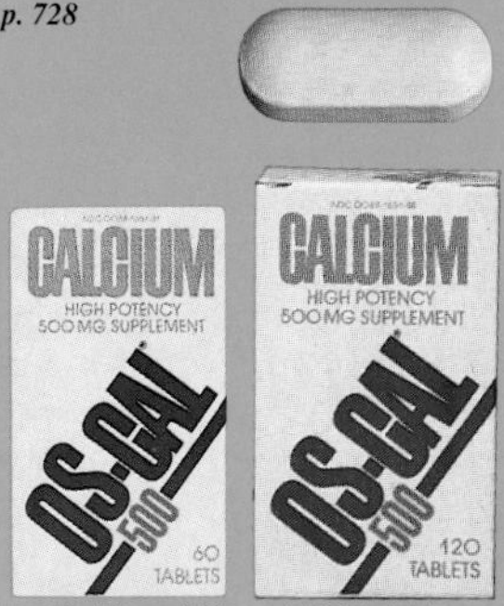

Bottles of 60 and 120 tablets

OS-CAL® 500
Tablets

SmithKline Beecham Consumer Brands
p. 722

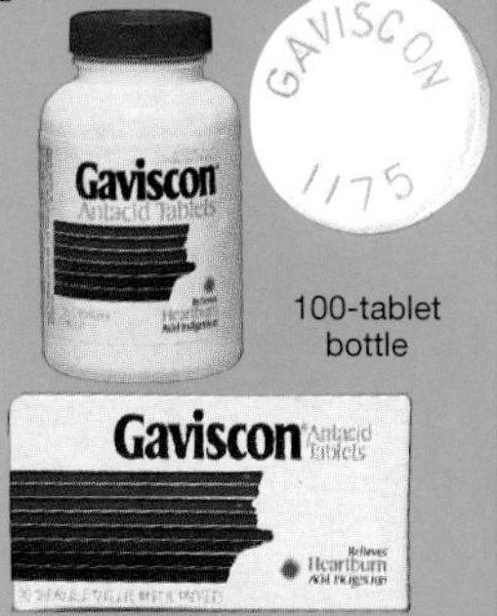

100-tablet
bottle

30-tablet box (foil-wrapped 2s)
GAVISCON®
Antacid Tablets

SmithKline Beecham Consumer Brands
p. 723

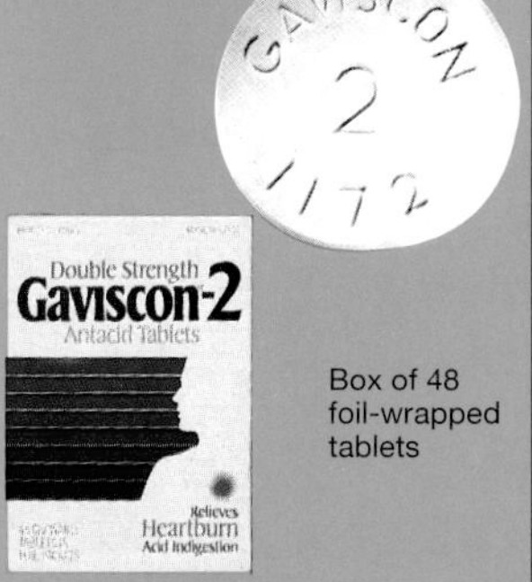

Box of 48
foil-wrapped
tablets

GAVISCON®-2
Antacid Tablets

SmithKline Beecham Consumer Brands
p. 726

Novahistine DMX
Cough/Cold Formula &
Decongestant

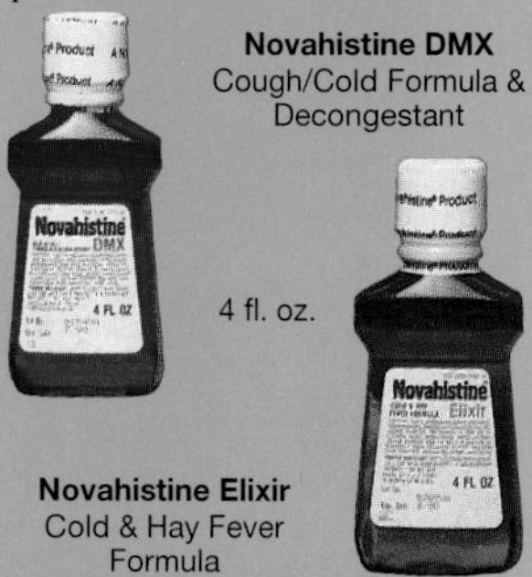

4 fl. oz.

Novahistine Elixir
Cold & Hay Fever
Formula

NOVAHISTINE® DMX & ELIXIR
Cough/Cold
Products

SmithKline Beecham Consumer Brands
p. 728

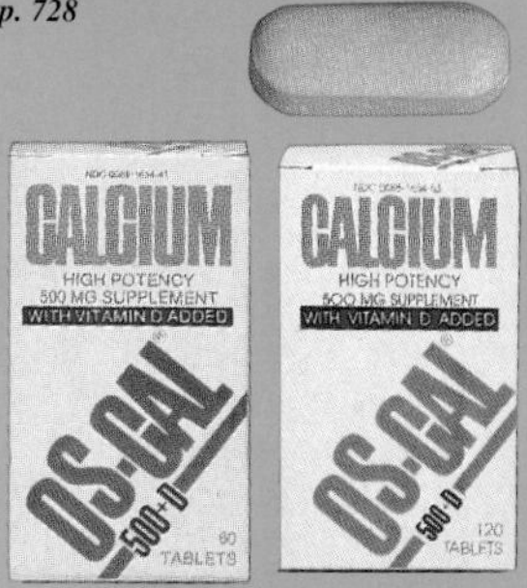

Bottle of 60 tablets
OS-CAL® 500+D
Tablets
(calcium with vitamin D)

SmithKline Beecham Consumer Brands *p. 728*

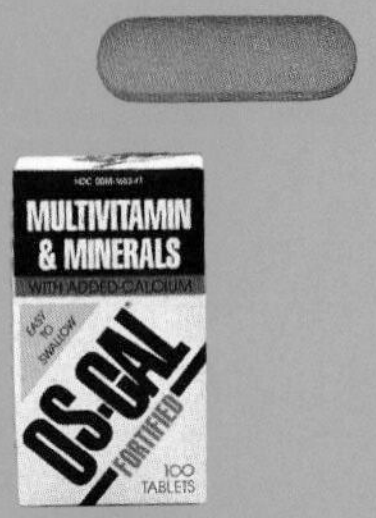

Bottles of 100 tablets

OS-CAL® Fortified Multivitamin and Minerals With Added Calcium

SmithKline Beecham Consumer Brands *p. 731*

24 caplet package

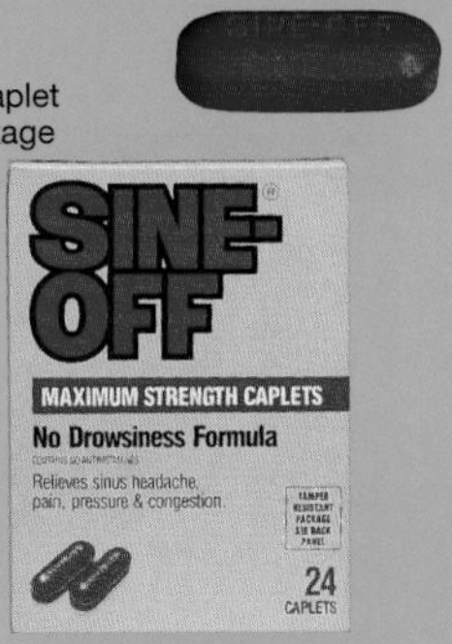
SINE-OFF
MAXIMUM STRENGTH CAPLETS
No Drowsiness Formula
Relieves sinus headache, pain, pressure & congestion
24 CAPLETS

SINE-OFF® MAXIMUM STRENGTH NO DROWSINESS FORMULA CAPLETS

SmithKline Beecham Consumer Brands *p. 734*

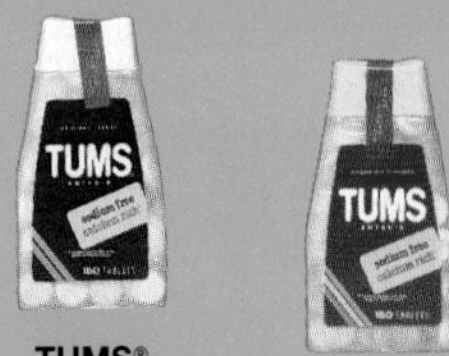

TUMS® Peppermint

TUMS® Assorted Flavors

Stellar *p. 737*

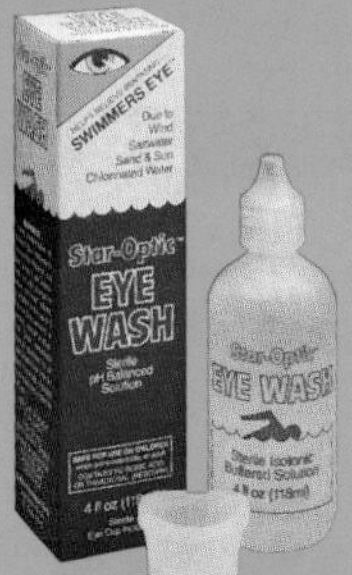

4 fl. oz. (118 ml) with sterile eye cup

STAR-OPTIC® EYE WASH

SmithKline Beecham Consumer Brands *p. 729*

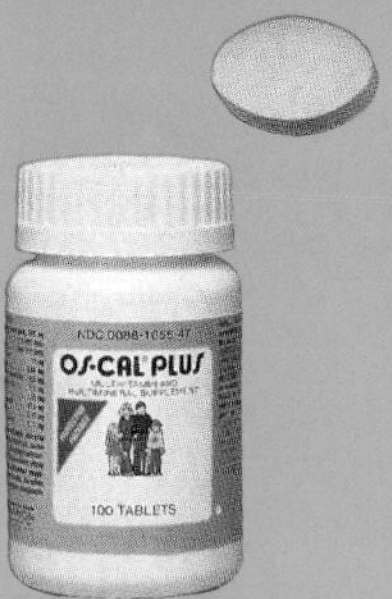

Bottles of 100 tablets

OS-CAL® PLUS Multivitamin and Multimineral Supplement

SmithKline Beecham Consumer Brands *p. 732*

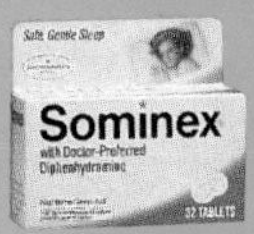
Sominex

Regular Formula in Tablets and Single-dose Caplets

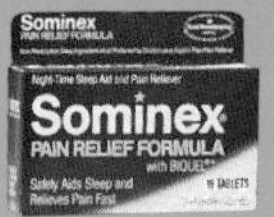
Sominex
PAIN RELIEF FORMULA

Pain Relief Formula

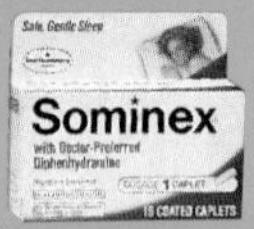
Sominex

SOMINEX® Night-Time Sleep Aids

SmithKline Beecham Consumer Brands *p. 734*

60 Tablets

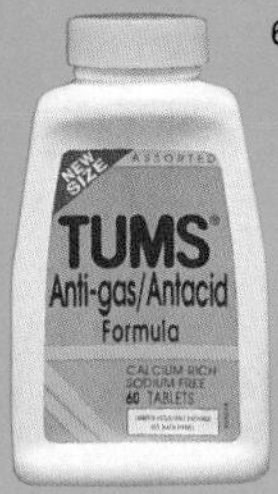

TUMS® Anti-gas/Antiacid Formula

Assorted Flavors

STERLING HEALTH

p. 738

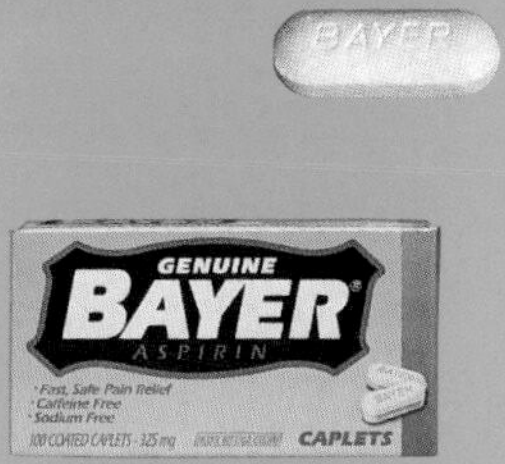
BAYER
GENUINE
BAYER
ASPIRIN
CAPLETS

Caplets available in bottles of 50, 100 and 200

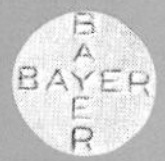
BAYER

325 mg.

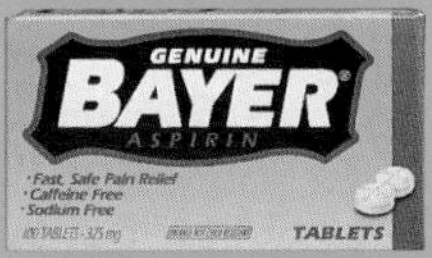

Available in packs of 12 tablets and bottles of 24, 50, 100, 200, 300 and 365

Genuine BAYER® ASPIRIN Toleraid® Micro-Thin Coating Sodium Free • Caffeine Free

SmithKline Beecham Consumer Brands *p. 729*

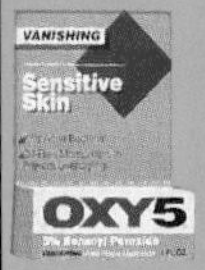
Sensitive Skin
OXY5

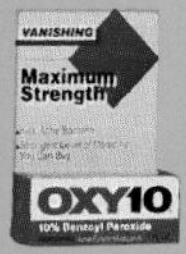
Maximum Strength
OXY10

OXY-5®

OXY-10®

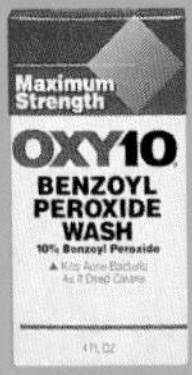
Maximum Strength
OXY10
BENZOYL PEROXIDE WASH

OXY10® BENZOYL PEROXIDE WASH

SmithKline Beecham Consumer Brands *p. 733*

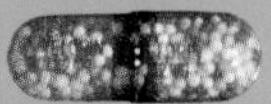

Packages of 12, 24 and 48 capsules

12 mg.

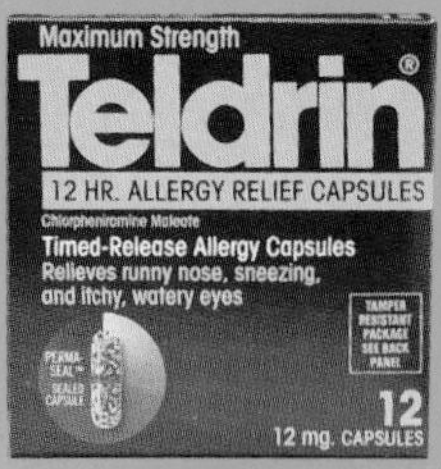
Maximum Strength
Teldrin
12 HR. ALLERGY RELIEF CAPSULES
Timed-Release Allergy Capsules
Relieves runny nose, sneezing, and itchy, watery eyes
12
12 mg. CAPSULES

TELDRIN® TIMED-RELEASE CAPSULES
(chlorpheniramine maleate)

SmithKline Beecham Consumer Brands *p. 734*

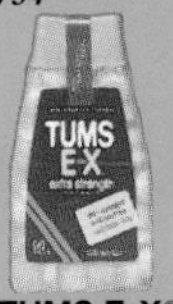
TUMS
E-X

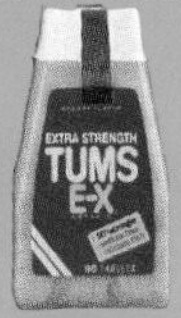

TUMS E-X® Wintergreen

TUMS E-X® Cherry

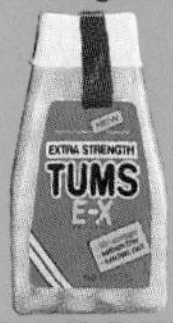

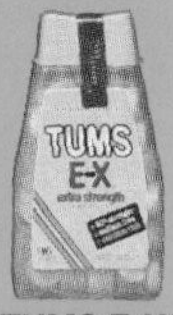

TUMS E-X® Peppermint

TUMS E-X® Assorted Flavors

SmithKline Beecham Consumer Brands *p. 731*

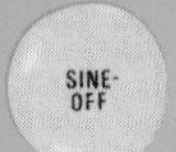
SINE-OFF

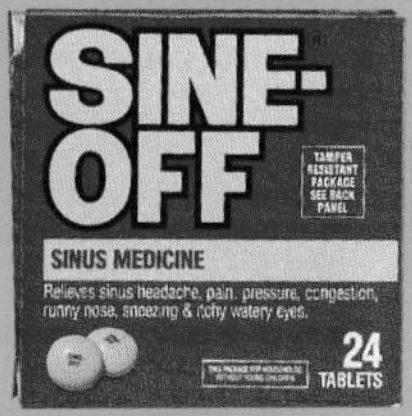
SINE-OFF
SINUS MEDICINE
Relieves sinus headache, pain, pressure, congestion, runny nose, sneezing & itchy watery eyes.
24 TABLETS

Packages of 24, 48, and 100 tablets

SINE-OFF® REGULAR STRENGTH ASPIRIN FORMULA

SmithKline Beecham Consumer Brands *p. 734*

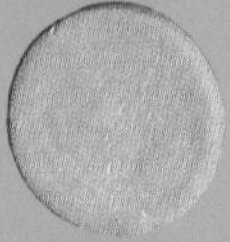

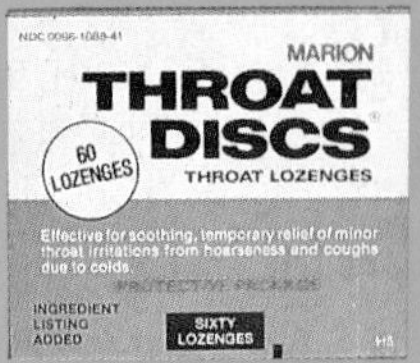
MARION
THROAT DISCS
60 LOZENGES
THROAT LOZENGES
SIXTY LOZENGES

Box of 60 lozenges

THROAT DISCS® Throat Lozenges

STELLAR

p. 737

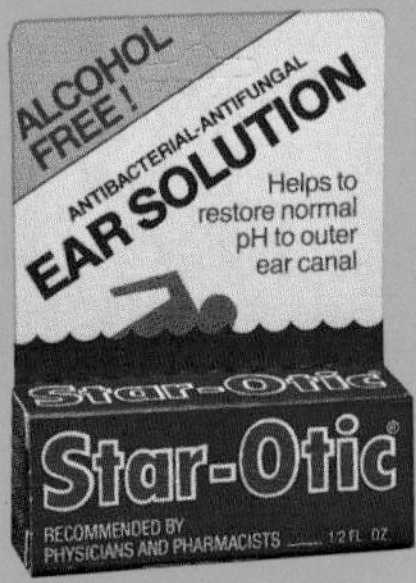
ALCOHOL FREE!
ANTIBACTERIAL-ANTIFUNGAL
EAR SOLUTION
Helps to restore normal pH to outer ear canal
Star-Otic
Star-Otic
RECOMMENDED BY PHYSICIANS AND PHARMACISTS

STAR-OTIC® EAR SOLUTION
Antibacterial • Antifungal

Sterling Health *p. 740*

500

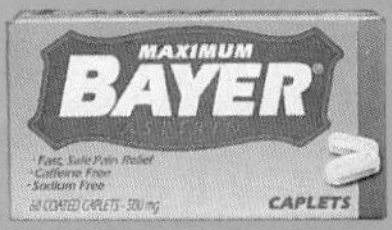

Available in bottles of 30 and 60

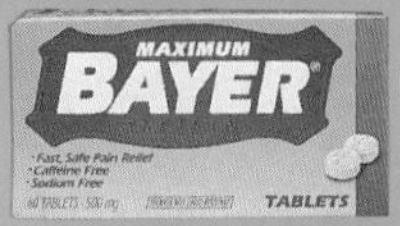

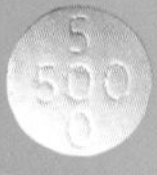

500 mg.

Available in boxes of 30, 60 and 100 tablets

Maximum BAYER® ASPIRIN Toleraid® Micro-Thin Coating Sodium Free • Caffeine Free

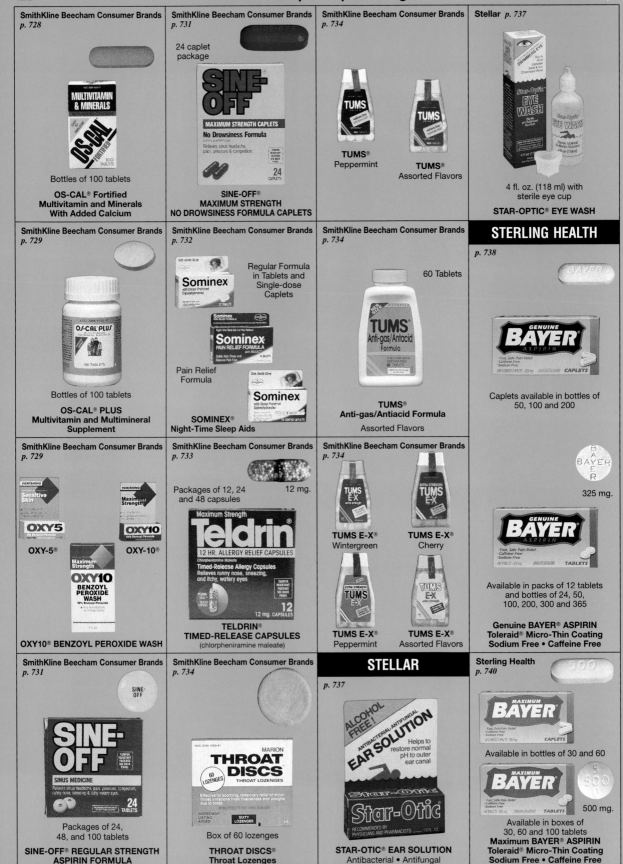

Sterling Health
p. 740

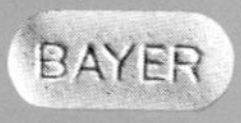

650 mg.

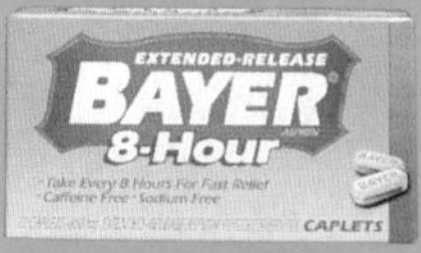

Available in bottles of
72 and 125 caplets

8-Hour BAYER®
Extended-Release Aspirin
Sodium Free • Caffeine Free

Sterling Health
p. 744

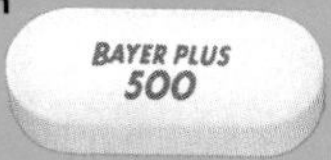

500 mg.

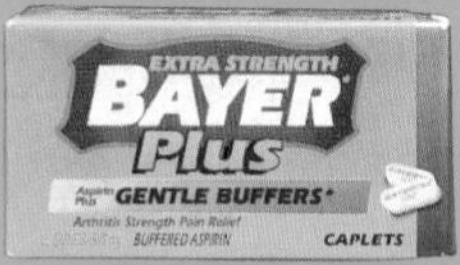

Available in bottles of
30 and 60 caplets

EXTRA STRENGTH
BAYER® PLUS
Aspirin Plus Gentle Buffers
Extra Strength Pain Relief
Plus Stomach Protection.

Sterling Health
p. 745

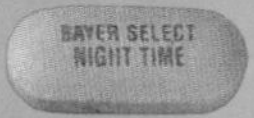

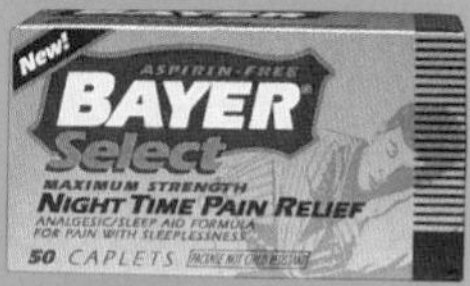

Available in bottles of
24 and 50 caplets

BAYER® SELECT™
NIGHT TIME PAIN RELIEF
Aspirin-Free • Maximum Strength

Sterling Health
p. 747

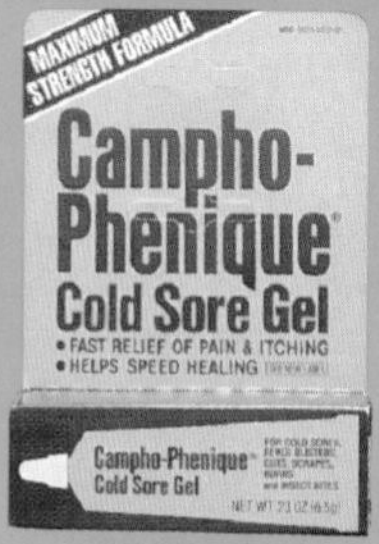

CAMPHO-PHENIQUE®
Cold Sore Gel
.23 oz and .5 oz

Sterling Health
p. 741

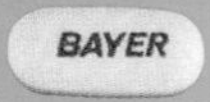

325 mg.

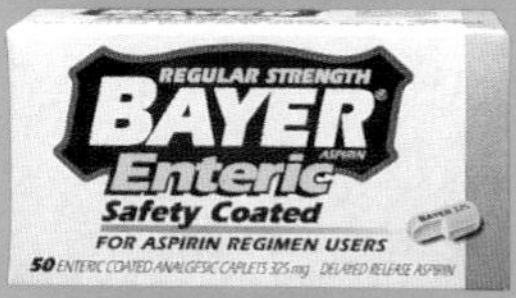

Available in bottles of
50 and 100 caplets

Regular Strength BAYER® ENTERIC
Delayed Release Enteric Aspirin
Sodium Free • Caffeine Free

Sterling Health
p. 738

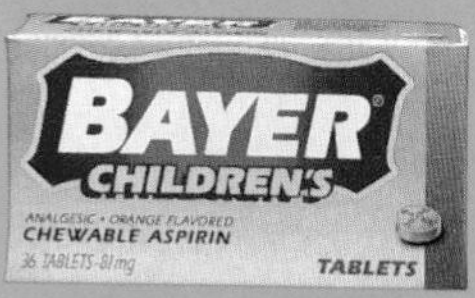

Available in bottles
of 36 tablets

BAYER® CHILDREN'S
CHEWABLE ASPIRIN

Sterling Health
p. 744

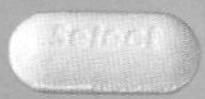

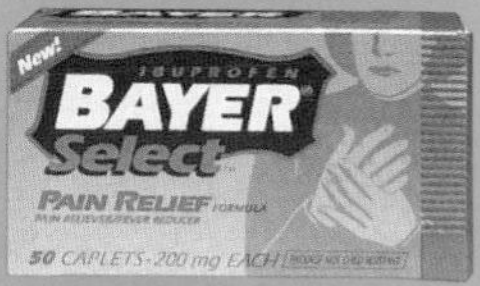

Available in bottles of
24, 50 and 100 caplets

BAYER® SELECT™ PAIN RELIEF
Aspirin-Free • Maximum Strength

Sterling Health
p. 747

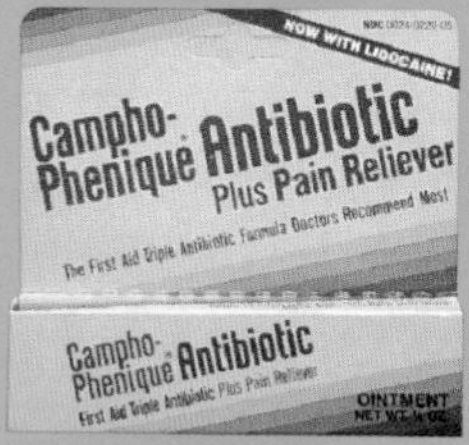

Available in .5 oz tubes

CAMPHO-PHENIQUE®
First Aid Triple Antibiotic Plus
Pain Reliever Ointment

Sterling Health
p. 741

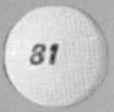

81 mg.

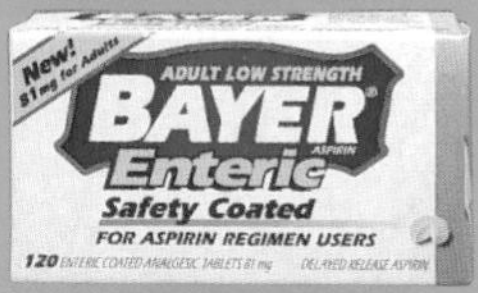

Available in bottles of
120 tablets

ADULT LOW STRENGTH
BAYER® ENTERIC
Delayed Release Enteric Aspirin

Sterling Health
p. 745

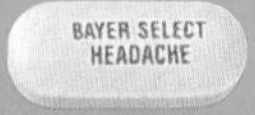

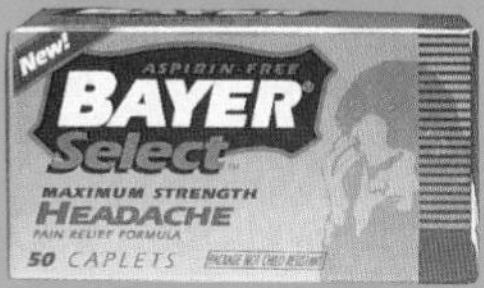

Available in bottles of
24, 50 and 100 caplets

BAYER® SELECT™ HEADACHE
Aspirin-Free • Maximum Strength

Sterling Health
p. 745

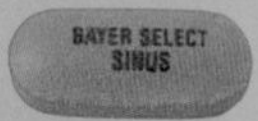

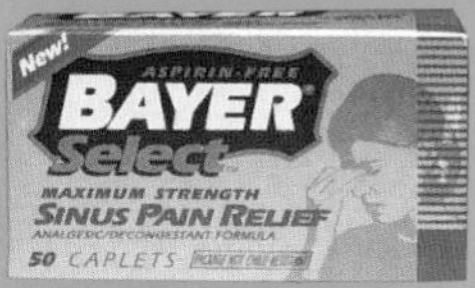

Available in bottles of
24 and 50 caplets

BAYER® SELECT™
SINUS PAIN RELIEF
Aspirin-Free • Maximum Strength

Sterling Health
p. 747

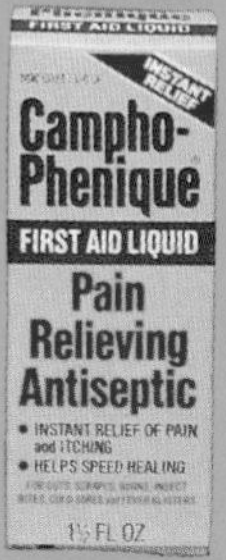

CAMPHO-PHENIQUE®
First Aid Liquid
.75 oz, 1.5 oz, 4 oz

Sterling Health
p. 742

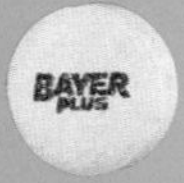

325 mg.

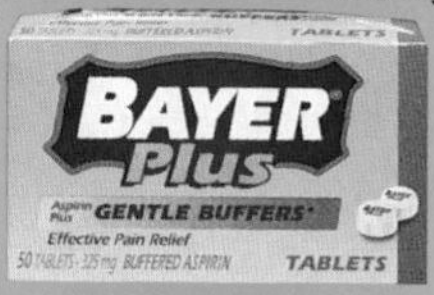

Available in bottles of 24,
50 and 100 tablets

BAYER® PLUS
Aspirin Plus Gentle Buffers
Effective Pain Relief Plus
Stomach Protection. Coated
For Easy Swallowing.

Sterling Health
p. 745

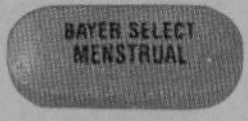

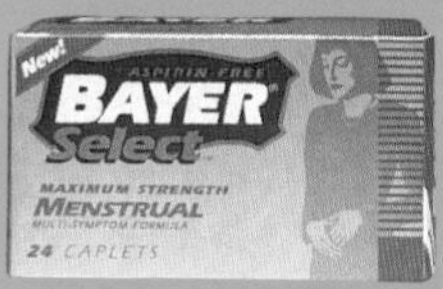

Available in bottles of
24 and 50 caplets

BAYER® SELECT™ MENSTRUAL
Aspirin-Free • Maximum Strength

Sterling Health
p. 746

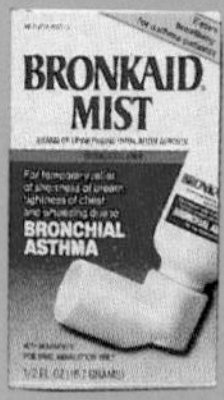

Available in 15 cc
Inhaler Units and
15 cc and 22.5 cc
Refills

Available in
packages of 24
and 60 tablets

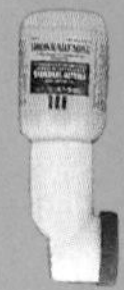

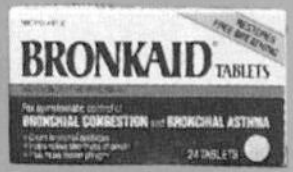

BRONKAID®
Mist and Tablets
Asthma Remedy

Sterling Health
p. 748

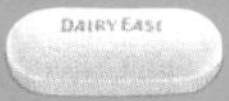

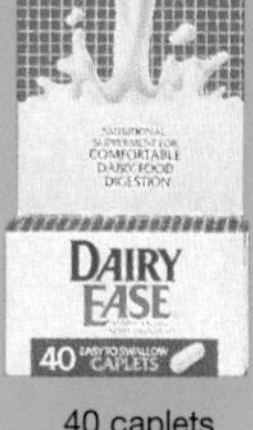

40 caplets
DAIRY EASE®
CAPLETS
(lactase enzyme)

Sterling Health
p. 748

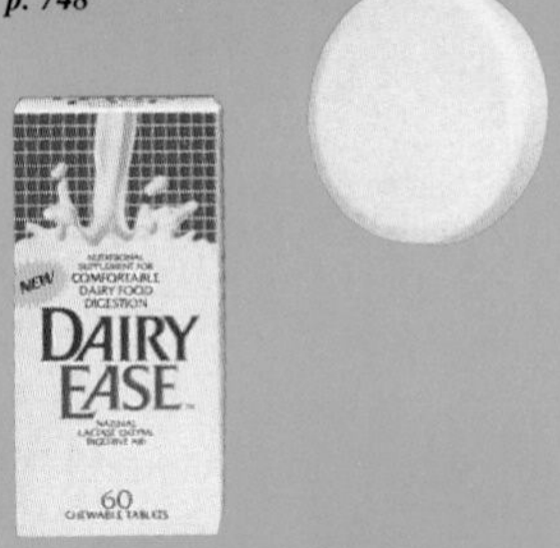

Available: 12, 36, 60, 100 count

DAIRY EASE® CHEWABLE TABLETS
(lactase enzyme)

Sterling Health
p. 749

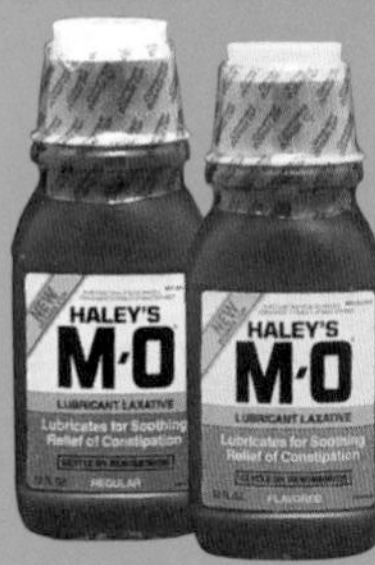

Available in regular 12 oz and flavored 12 oz and 26 oz plastic bottles

HALEY'S M-O®

Sterling Health
p. 750

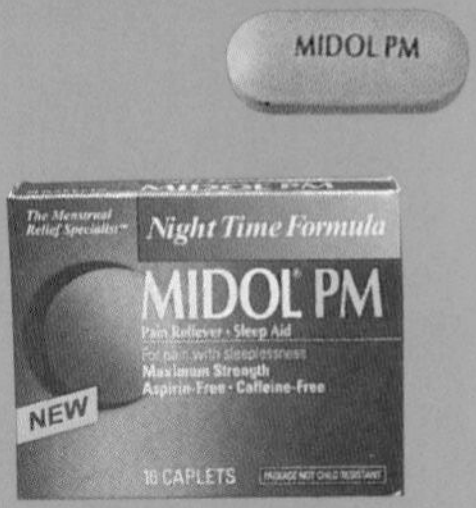

Available in packages of 16 and 32 caplets

MIDOL® PM

Sterling Health
p. 751

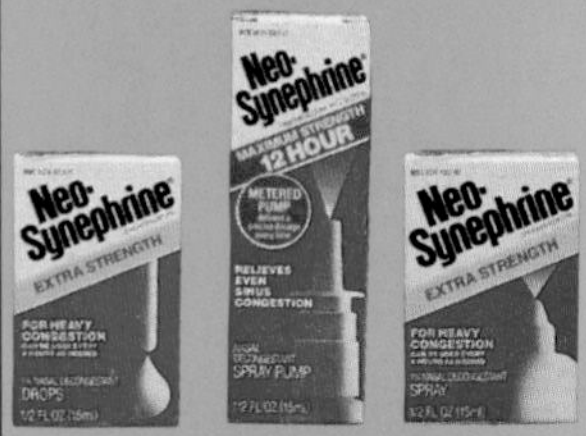

NEO-SYNEPHRINE®
Nasal Decongestant

Spray, Spray Pump or Drops

Sterling Health
p. 748

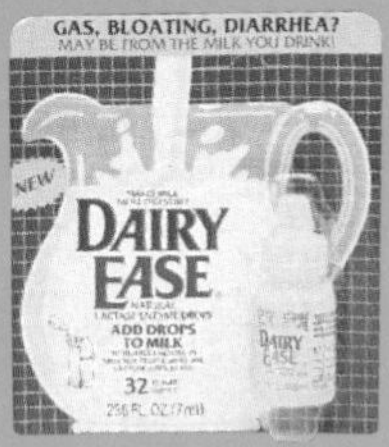

32 quart supply

DAIRY EASE® DROPS
(lactase enzyme)

Sterling Health
p. 749

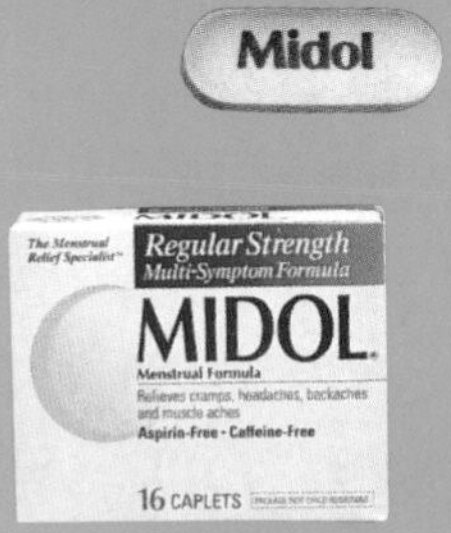

Available in packages of 16 and 32 caplets

MIDOL®

Sterling Health
p. 749

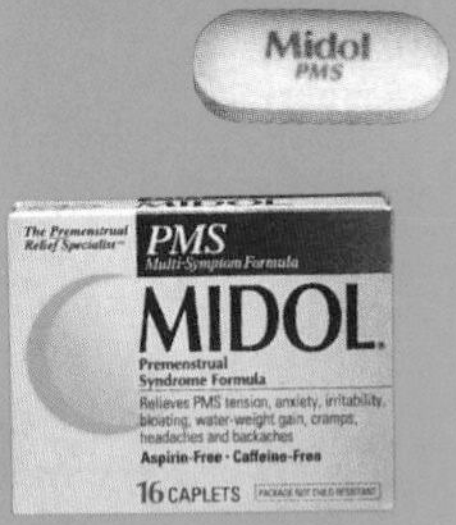

Available in bottles of 8, 16 and 32 caplets

MIDOL® PMS MAXIMUM STRENGTH

Sterling Health
p. 753

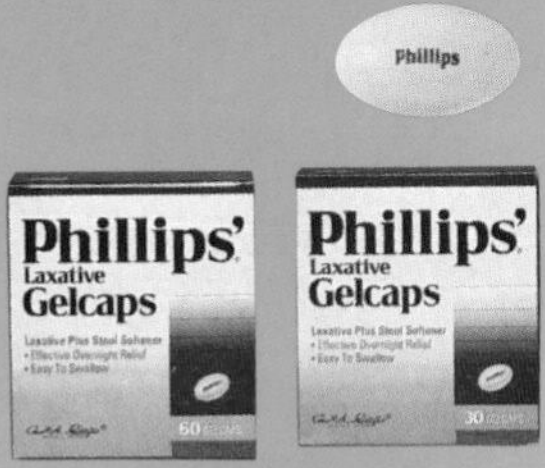

60 gelcaps 30 gelcaps

PHILLIPS'® GELCAPS
Laxative Plus Stool Softener

Sterling Health
p. 748

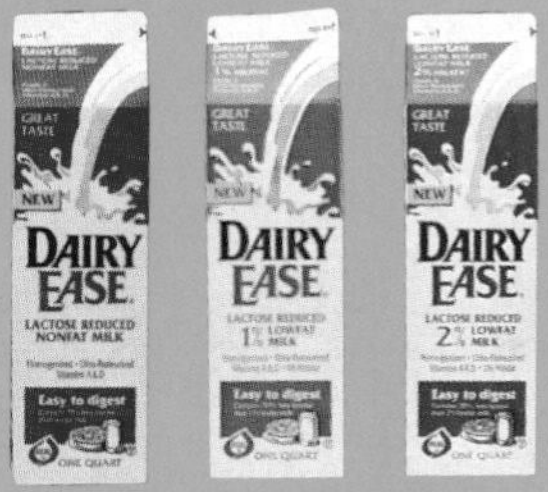

Available: 1%, 2%, Nonfat

DAIRY EASE® REAL MILK
(lactose reduced milk)

Sterling Health
p. 749

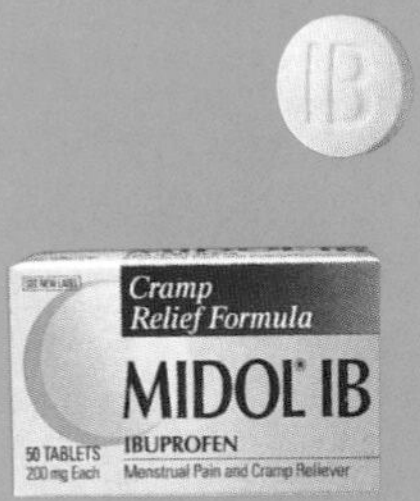
IB
Cramp Relief Formula
MIDOL IB
IBUPROFEN

Available in packages of 24 and 50 caplets

MIDOL® IB

Sterling Health
p. 750

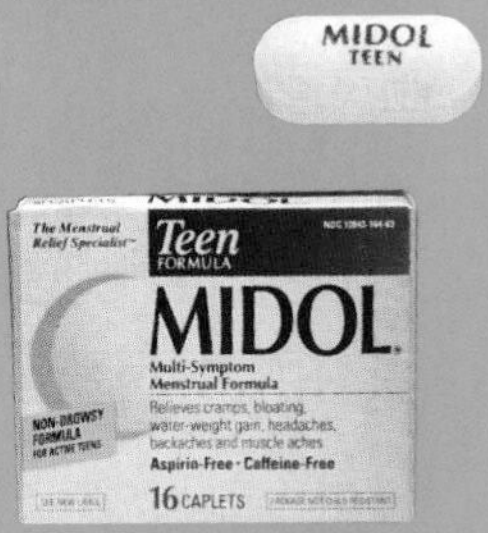

Available in packages of 16 and 32 caplets

TEEN FORMULA MIDOL®

Sterling Health
p. 753

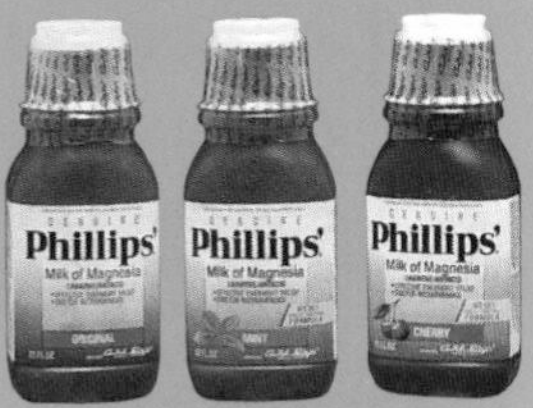

Available in original, mint, and cherry flavors
4 oz, 12 oz, and 16 oz plastic bottles

PHILLIPS'® MILK OF MAGNESIA

Sterling Health
p. 748

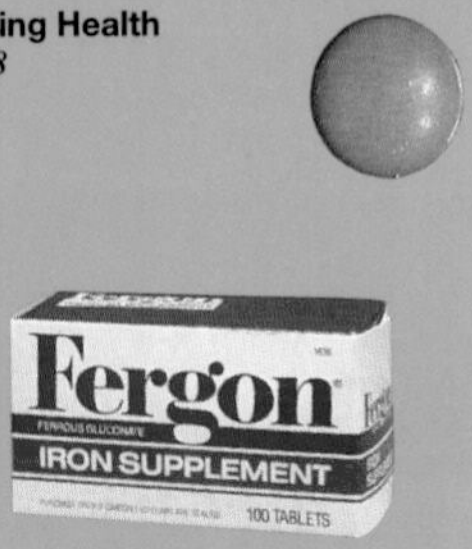
Fergon
IRON SUPPLEMENT
100 TABLETS

Available in 100 count container

FERGON®
Ferrous Gluconate Iron Supplement

Sterling Health
p. 750

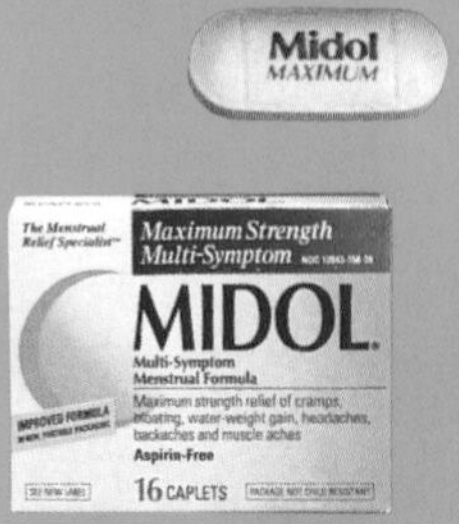

Available in packages of 8, 16 and 32 caplets

MIDOL® MAXIMUM STRENGTH

Sterling Health
p. 751

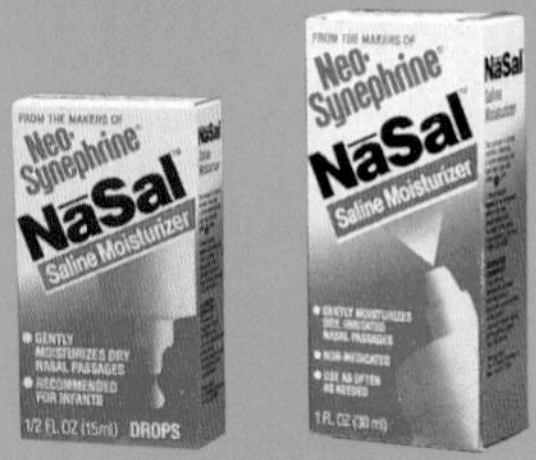

15 ml 30 ml

NāSal™
Nasal Moisturizer
Spray and Drops

Sterling Health
p. 754

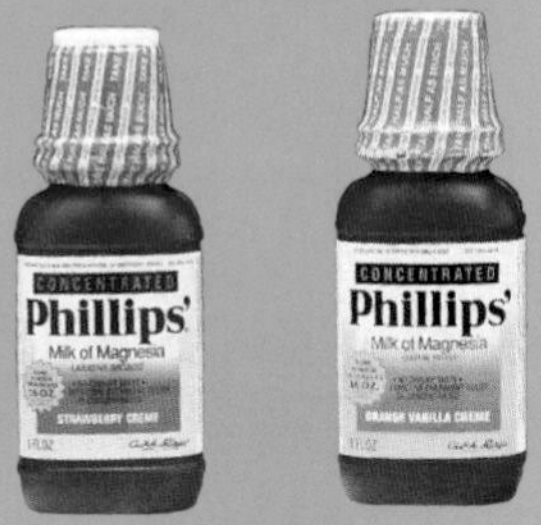

Strawberry Creme and Orange Vanilla Creme 8 oz bottles

CONCENTRATED PHILLIPS'® MILK OF MAGNESIA

Sterling Health
p. 754

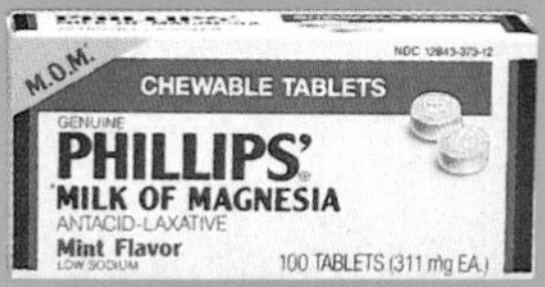

PHILLIPS'® MILK OF MAGNESIA TABLETS
Available in mint flavored chewable tablets in bottles of 100 and 200

Sterling Health
p. 755

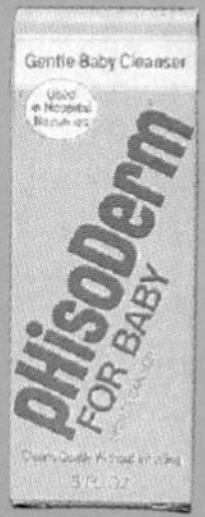

Skin cleanser available in 5 oz and 9 oz bottles

pHisoDerm® for Baby

Sterling Health
p. 756

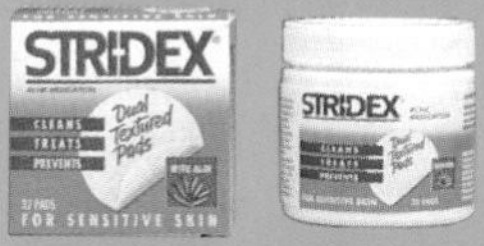

Sensitive Skin Pads with Aloe

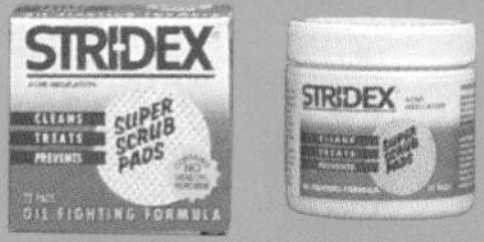

Super Scrub Pads
Oil Fighting Formula

Both available in 32 pad containers
STRI-DEX®

Thompson Medical Company, Inc.
p. 758

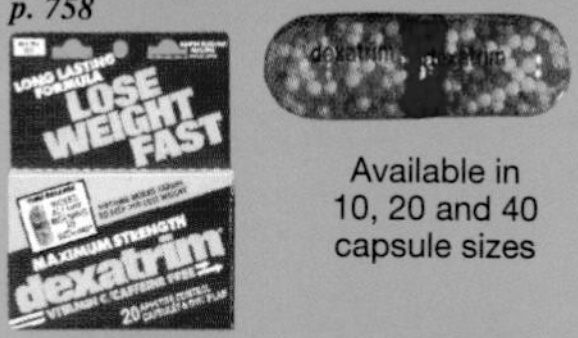

Available in 10, 20 and 40 capsule sizes

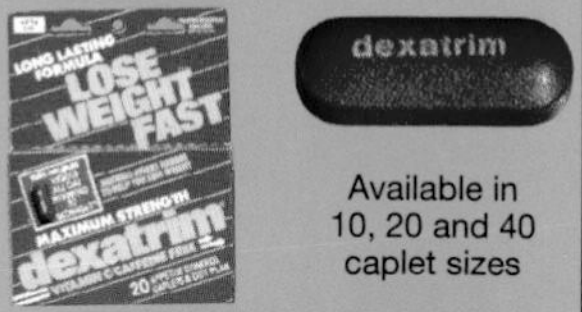

Available in 10, 20 and 40 caplet sizes

MAXIMUM STRENGTH DEXATRIM®
Capsules & Caplets
Plus Vitamin C

Sterling Health
p. 752

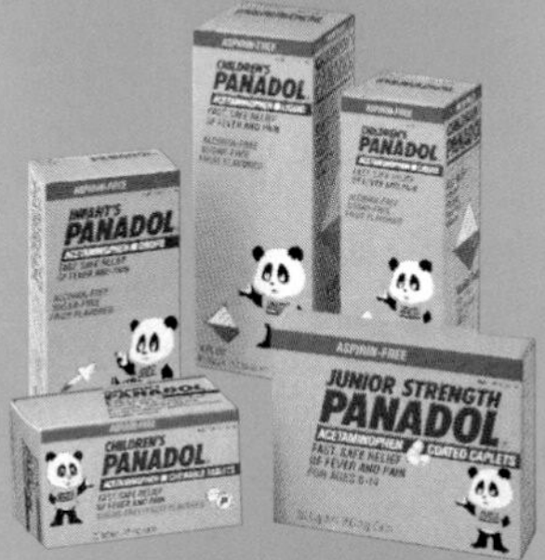

CHILDREN'S PANADOL®
Chewable Tablets, Caplets, Liquid and Drops
Acetaminophen

Sterling Health
p. 755

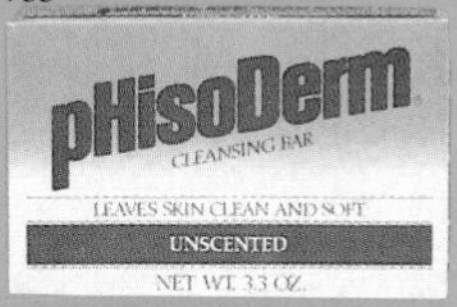

Unscented 3.3 oz

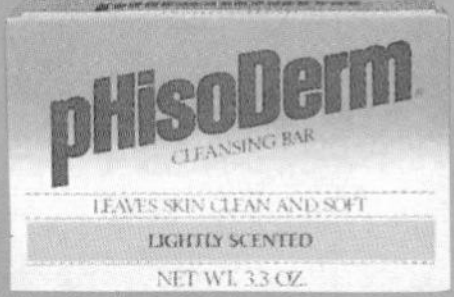

Lightly Scented 3.3 oz

pHisoDerm®
CLEANSING BAR

Sterling Health
p. 756

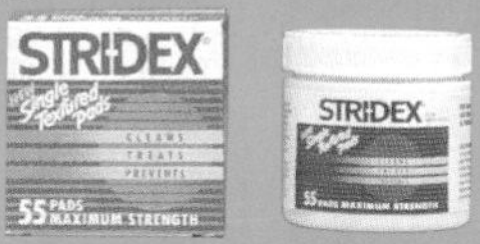

Single Textured
Maximum Strength Pads
55 pads in container

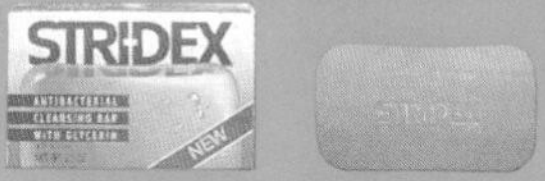

Anti-Bacterial Cleansing Bar with Glycerin 3.5 oz
STRI-DEX®

Thompson Medical Company, Inc.
p. 759

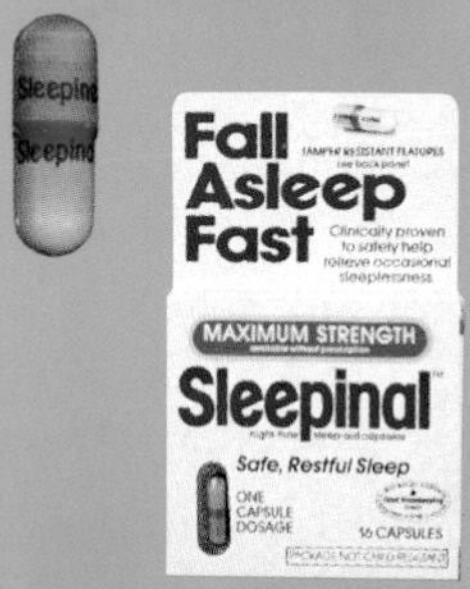

Available in 16 and 32 capsule sizes

SLEEPINAL™
(diphenhydramine HCl 50 mg.)

Sterling Health
p. 753

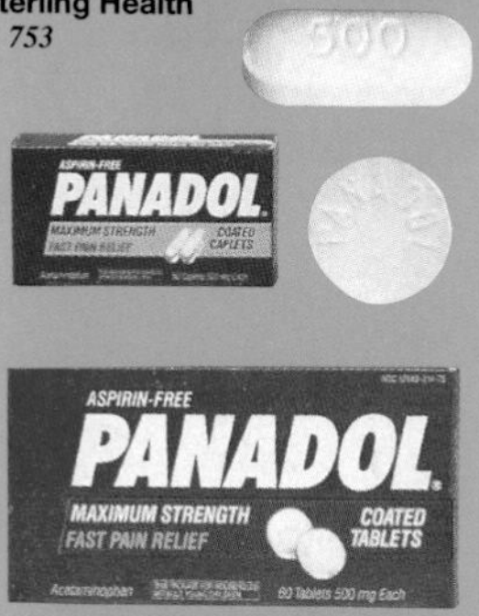

MAXIMUM STRENGTH PANADOL®
Coated Caplets and Tablets
Acetaminophen

Sterling Health
p. 755

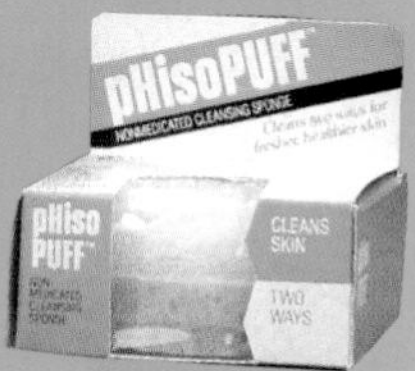

pHisoPUFF®
Exfoliating Sponge

Sterling Health
p. 756

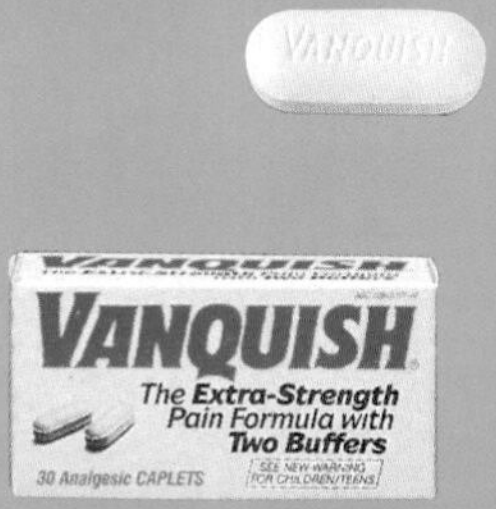

Available in packages of 30, 60 and 100 caplets

VANQUISH®
Extra-Strength Pain Formula with Two Buffers

Thompson Medical Company, Inc.
p. 760

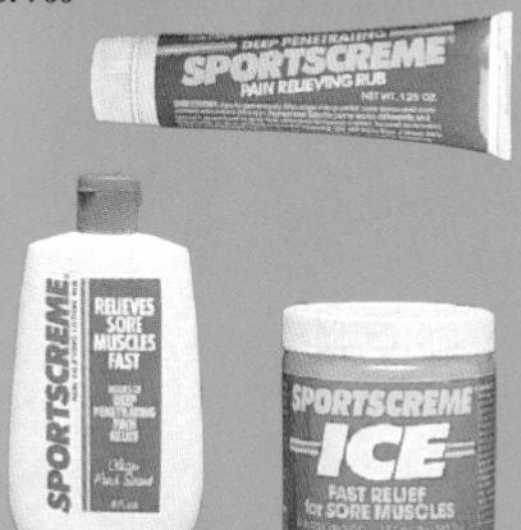

Available in 1¼ oz., 3 oz. and 5 oz. cream; 6 oz. lotion; 8 oz. ice

SPORTSCREME®
External Analgesic

Sterling Health
p. 754

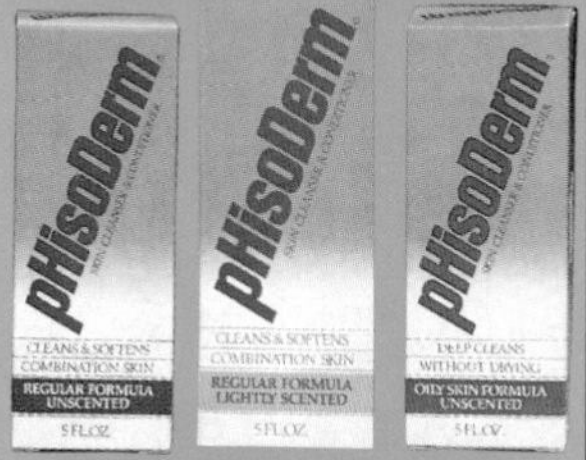

Regular Unscented | Regular Lightly Scented | Oily Skin Unscented

5 oz, 9 oz, 16 oz bottles | 5 oz, 16 oz bottles

pHisoDerm®

Sterling Health
p. 756

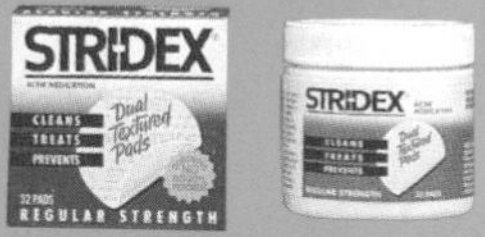

Regular Strength Pads

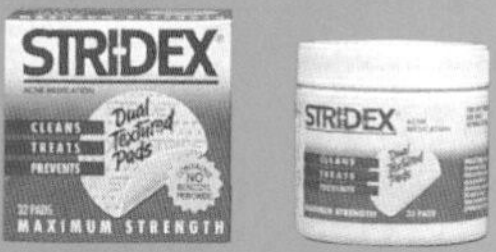

Maximum Strength Pads

Available in 32 and 50 pad containers
STRI-DEX®

THOMPSON MEDICAL

p. 758

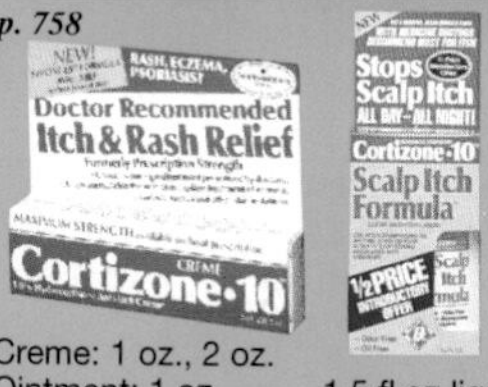

Creme: 1 oz., 2 oz.
Ointment: 1 oz.
1.5 fl.oz.liquid

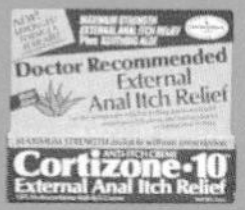

Cream with Aloe: 1 oz.
CORTIZONE-10™
(hydrocortisone 1%)

Thompson Medical Company, Inc.
p. 760

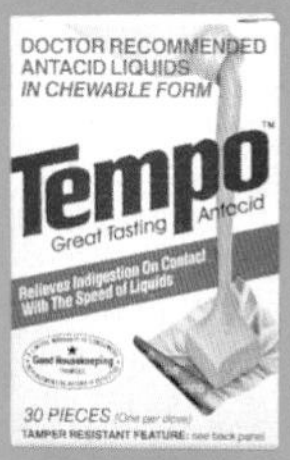

Available in 10, 30 and 60 tablet sizes

TEMPO®
Soft Antacid

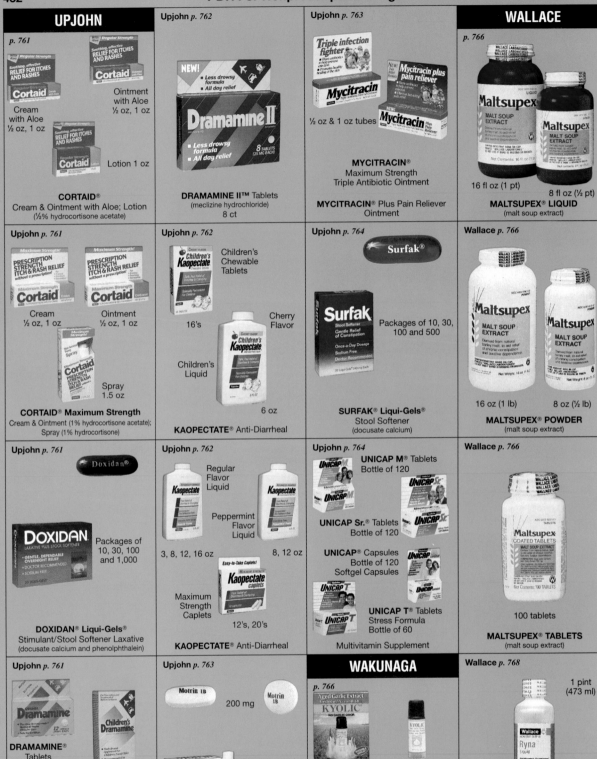

UPJOHN

p. 761

CORTAID®
Cream & Ointment with Aloe; Lotion
(½% hydrocortisone acetate)

Cream with Aloe
½ oz, 1 oz

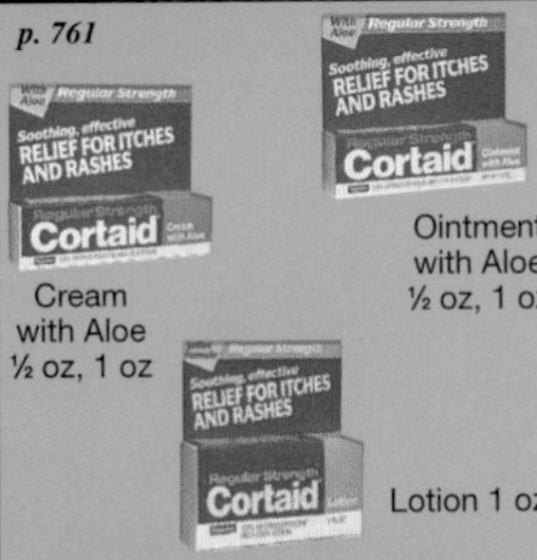

Ointment with Aloe
½ oz, 1 oz

Lotion 1 oz

Upjohn p. 761

CORTAID® Maximum Strength
Cream & Ointment (1% hydrocortisone acetate);
Spray (1% hydrocortisone)

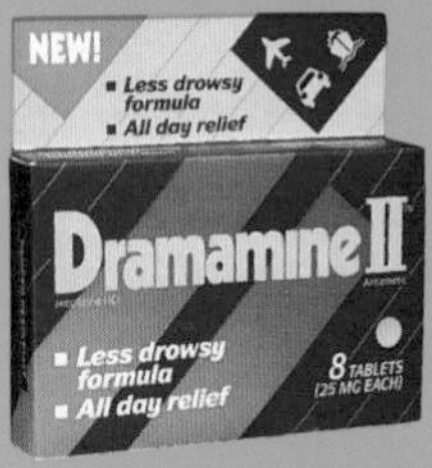

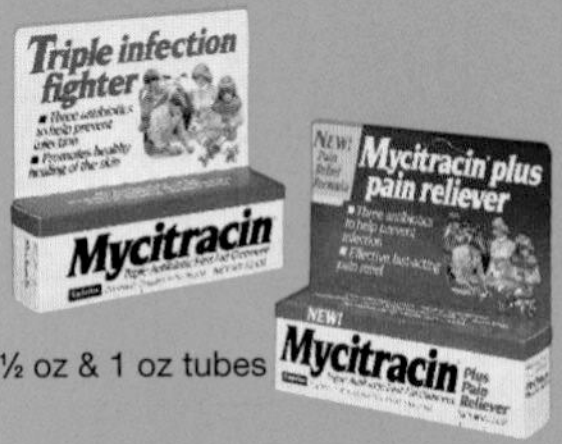

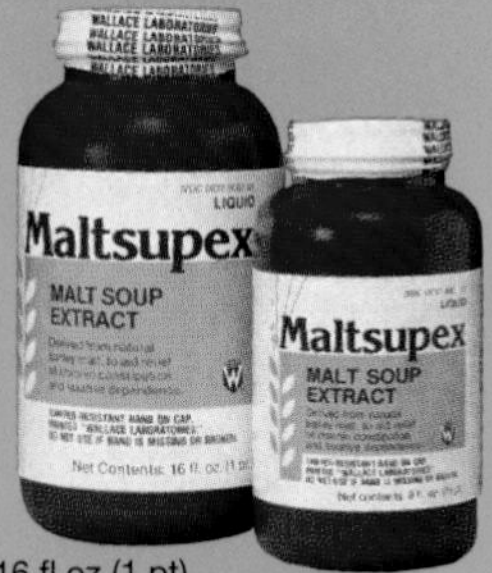

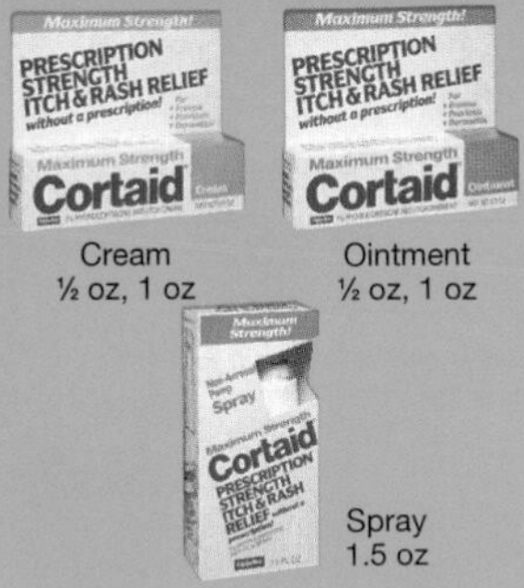

Cream
½ oz, 1 oz

Ointment
½ oz, 1 oz

Spray
1.5 oz

Upjohn p. 761

DOXIDAN® Liqui-Gels®
Stimulant/Stool Softener Laxative
(docusate calcium and phenolphthalein)

Packages of 10, 30, 100 and 1,000

Upjohn p. 761

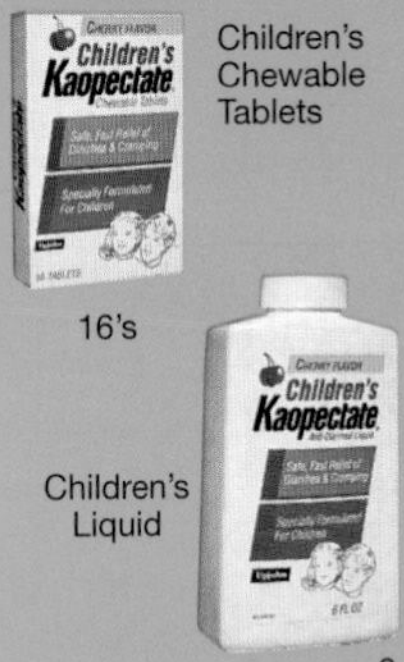

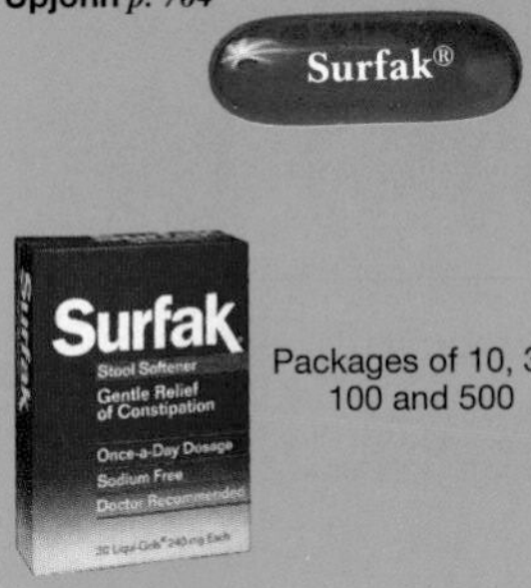

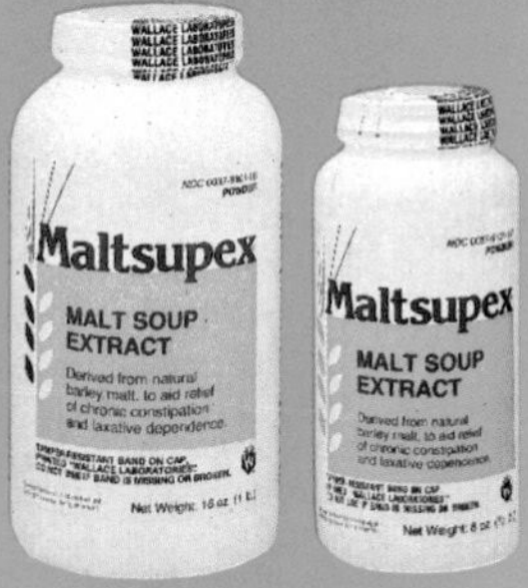

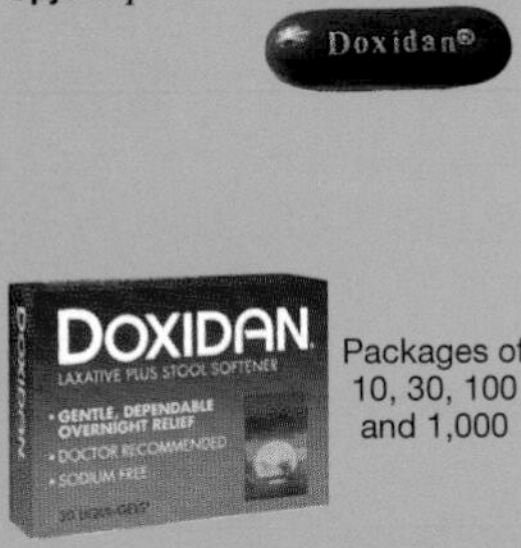

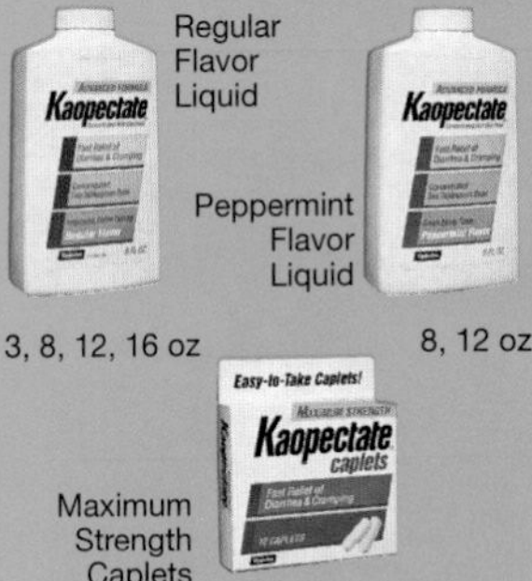

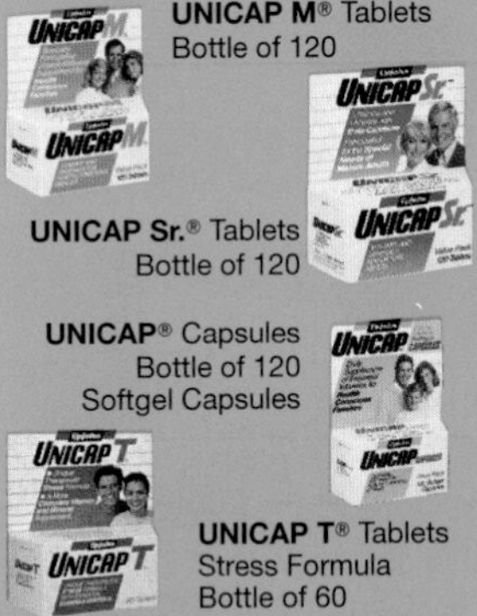

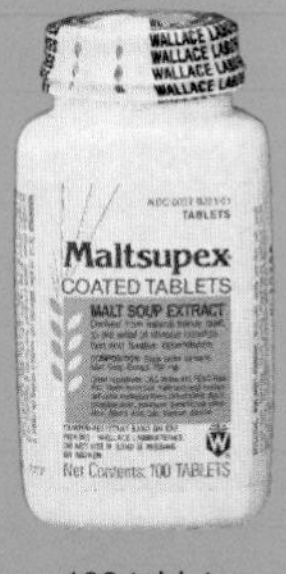

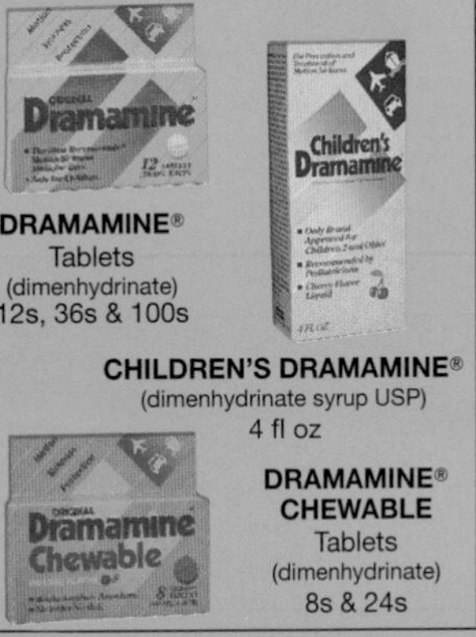

DRAMAMINE®
Tablets
(dimenhydrinate)
12s, 36s & 100s

CHILDREN'S DRAMAMINE®
(dimenhydrinate syrup USP)
4 fl oz

DRAMAMINE® CHEWABLE
Tablets
(dimenhydrinate)
8s & 24s

Upjohn p. 762

DRAMAMINE II™ Tablets
(meclizine hydrochloride)
8 ct

NEW!
- Less drowsy formula
- All day relief

Upjohn p. 762

Children's Chewable Tablets
16's

Cherry Flavor

Children's Liquid
6 oz

KAOPECTATE® Anti-Diarrheal

Upjohn p. 762

Regular Flavor Liquid
3, 8, 12, 16 oz

Peppermint Flavor Liquid
8, 12 oz

Maximum Strength Caplets
12's, 20's

KAOPECTATE® Anti-Diarrheal

Upjohn p. 763

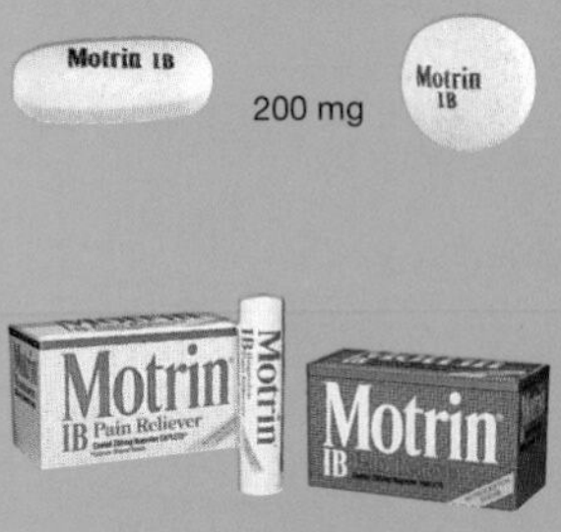

200 mg

MOTRIN® IB
Caplets and Tablets
(ibuprofen, USP)
Bottles of 24, 50,100 and 165;
Convenience pack (vial) of 8

Upjohn p. 763

½ oz & 1 oz tubes

MYCITRACIN®
Maximum Strength
Triple Antibiotic Ointment

MYCITRACIN® Plus Pain Reliever
Ointment

Triple infection fighter

Upjohn p. 764

Surfak®

Packages of 10, 30, 100 and 500

SURFAK® Liqui-Gels®
Stool Softener
(docusate calcium)

Upjohn p. 764

UNICAP M® Tablets
Bottle of 120

UNICAP Sr.® Tablets
Bottle of 120

UNICAP® Capsules
Bottle of 120
Softgel Capsules

UNICAP T® Tablets
Stress Formula
Bottle of 60

Multivitamin Supplement

WAKUNAGA

p. 766

KYOLIC®
Aged Garlic Extract™
with B, and B₁₂

KYOLIC®
Aged Garlic Extract™
Super Formula
101-Capsules

WALLACE

p. 766

16 fl oz (1 pt)

8 fl oz (½ pt)

MALTSUPEX® LIQUID
(malt soup extract)

Wallace p. 766

16 oz (1 lb)

8 oz (½ lb)

MALTSUPEX® POWDER
(malt soup extract)

Wallace p. 766

100 tablets

MALTSUPEX® TABLETS
(malt soup extract)

Wallace p. 768

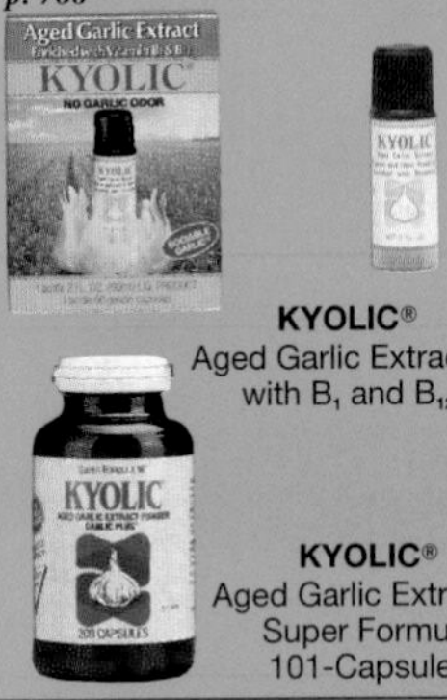

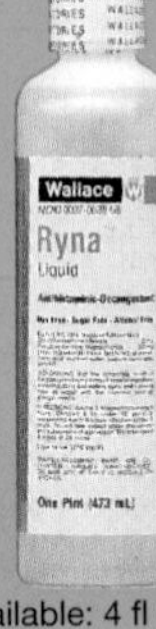

1 pint
(473 ml)

Also available: 4 fl oz (118 ml)

RYNA® LIQUID
(antihistamine-decongestant)

Wallace *p. 768*

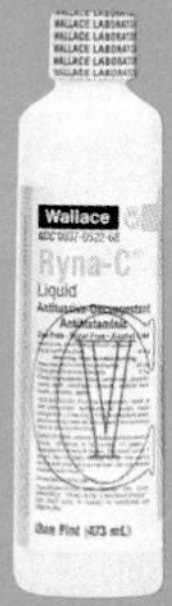

1 pint (473 ml)

Also available: 4 fl oz (118 ml)

RYNA-C® LIQUID
(antitussive-antihistamine-decongestant)

Warner-Lambert Co. *p. 769*

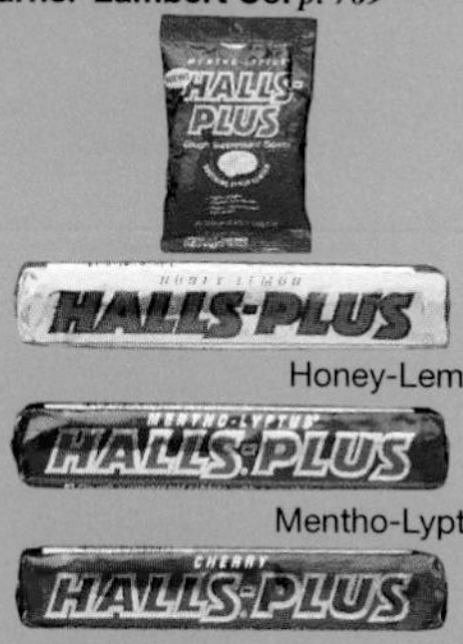
HALLS PLUS
HALLS-PLUS
HALLS-PLUS
HALLS-PLUS

Honey-Lemon

Mentho-Lyptus

Cherry

HALLS® PLUS
Cough Suppressant Tablets
Soothing Syrup Center

Warner-Lambert Co. *p.770*

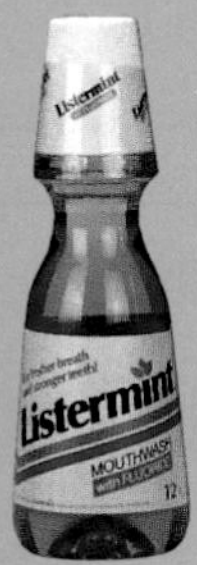

LISTERMINT® with FLUORIDE
Anticavity Dental Rinse & Mouthwash

Warner-Lambert Co. *p. 771*

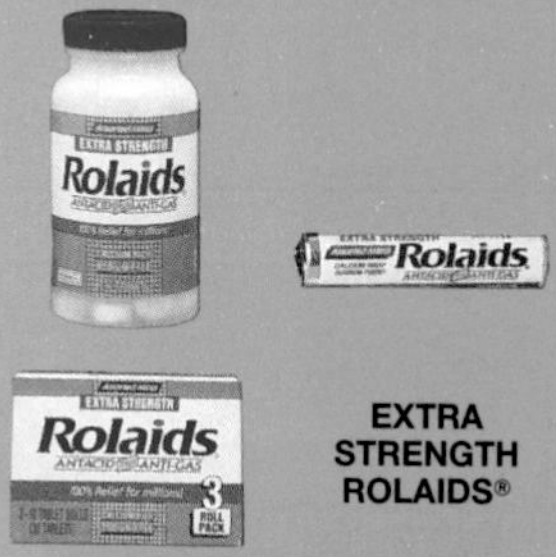

EXTRA STRENGTH ROLAIDS®

Extra Strength Calcium, Sodium Free Relief from Heartburn, Sour Stomach or Acid Indigestion and Upset Stomach Associated with these Symptoms

Wallace *p. 768*

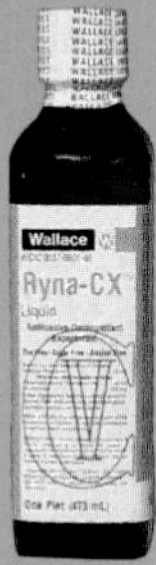

1 pint (473 ml)

Also available: 4 fl oz (118 ml)

RYNA-CX® LIQUID
(antitussive-decongestant-expectorant)

Warner-Lambert Co. *p. 769*

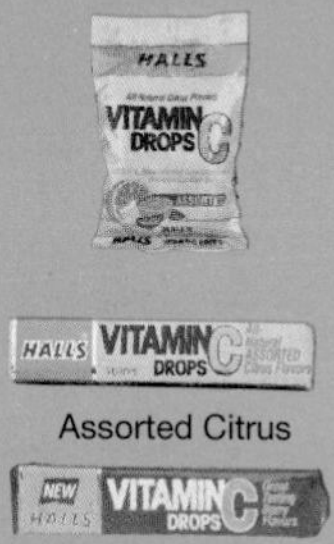

Assorted Citrus

Assorted Berry

HALLS® VITAMIN C DROPS

Warner-Lambert Co. *p. 770*

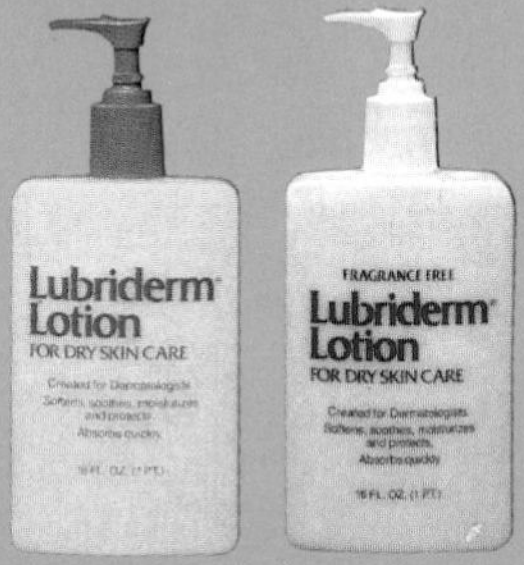
Lubriderm Lotion
FOR DRY SKIN CARE
FRAGRANCE FREE
Lubriderm Lotion
FOR DRY SKIN CARE

Scented Unscented

LUBRIDERM® LOTION
For Dry Skin Care

Warner-Lambert Co. *p. 771*

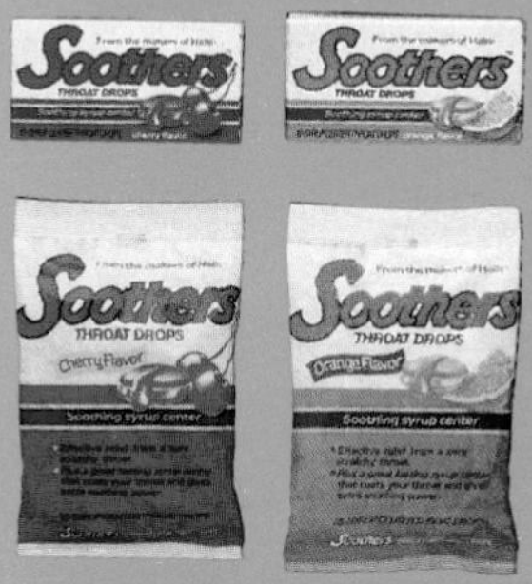

From the Makers of Hall's
SOOTHERS THROAT DROPS®

Wallace *p. 769*

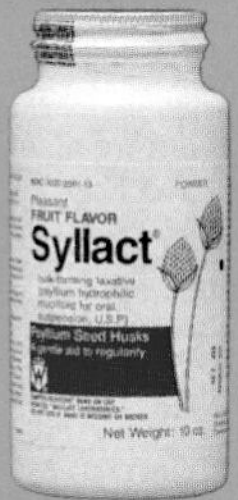

SYLLACT®
(powdered psyllium seed husks)

Warner-Lambert Co. *p. 770*

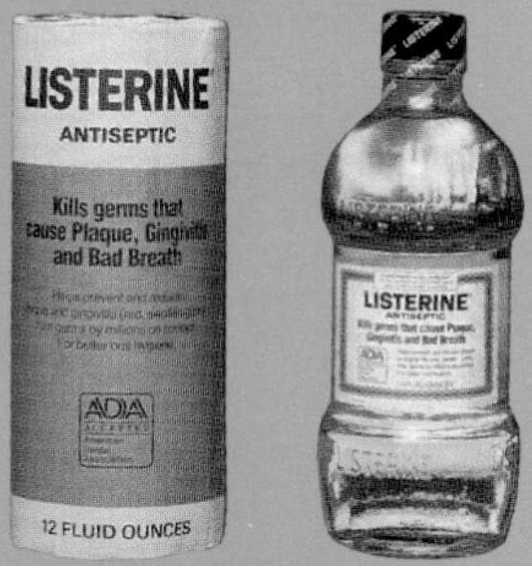
LISTERINE
ANTISEPTIC
Kills germs that cause Plaque, Gingivitis and Bad Breath
12 FLUID OUNCES
LISTERINE

LISTERINE® ANTISEPTIC

Warner-Lambert Co. *p. 770*

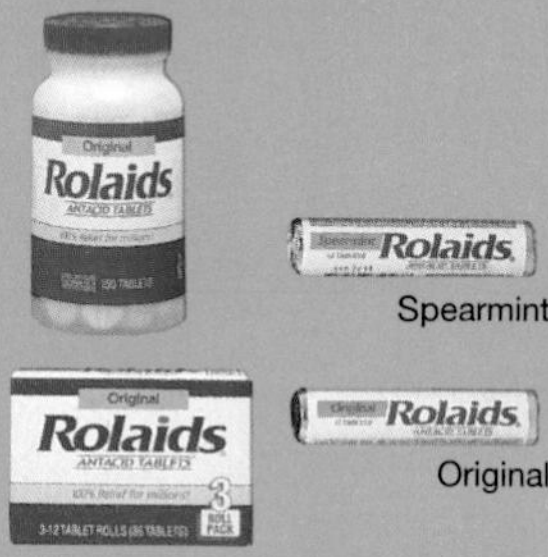

Spearmint

Original

ROLAIDS®
Fast, Safe, Lasting Relief from Heartburn, Sour Stomach or Acid Indigestion and Upset Stomach Associated with these Symptoms

WHITEHALL

p. 774

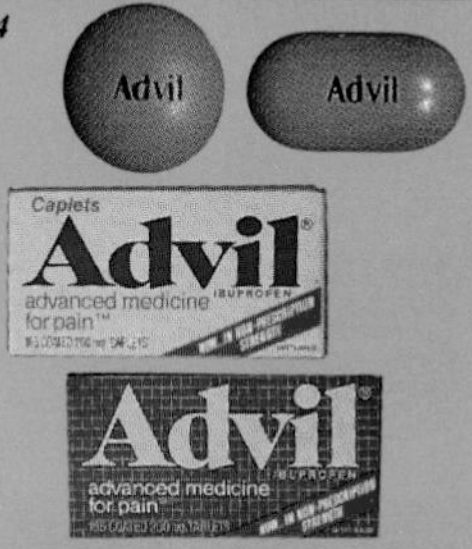
Advil
Advil
Caplets
Advil
IBUPROFEN
advanced medicine for pain
Advil
advanced medicine for pain

Coated Tablets in Bottles of 24, 50, 100, 165 and 250. Coated Caplets in Bottles of 24, 50, 100, 165 and 250.
ADVIL®
Ibuprofen Tablets and Caplets, USP

WARNER-LAMBERT CO.

p. 769

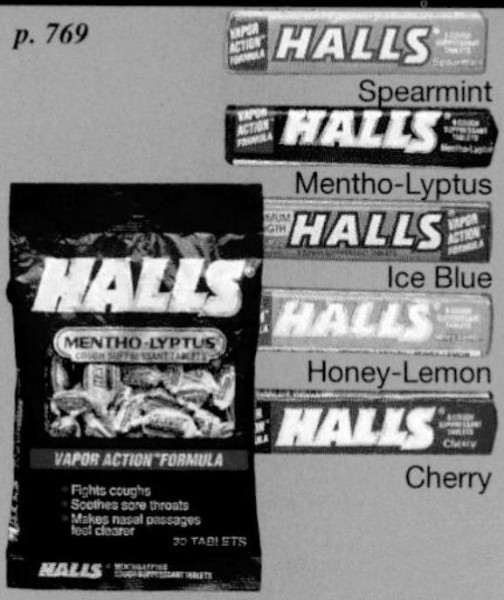
HALLS
HALLS
HALLS
HALLS
HALLS
HALLS
MENTHO-LYPTUS
VAPOR ACTION FORMULA

Spearmint

Mentho-Lyptus

Ice Blue

Honey-Lemon

Cherry

HALLS® MENTHO-LYPTUS
Cough Suppressant Tablets

Warner-Lambert Co. *p. 770*

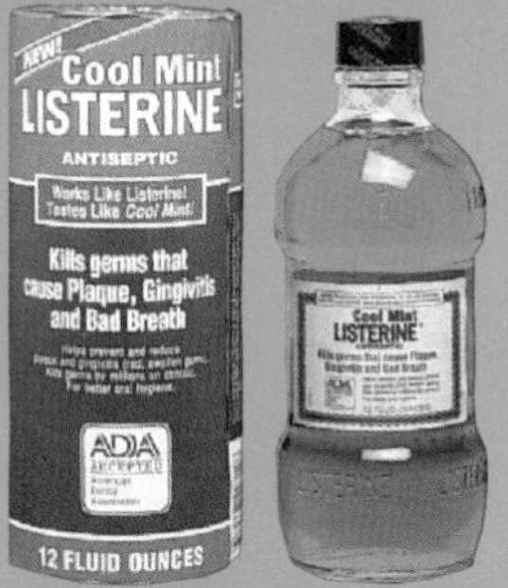
NEW!
Cool Mint
LISTERINE
ANTISEPTIC
Kills germs that cause Plaque, Gingivitis and Bad Breath
12 FLUID OUNCES

COOL MINT
LISTERINE™ ANTISEPTIC

Warner-Lambert Co. *p. 771*

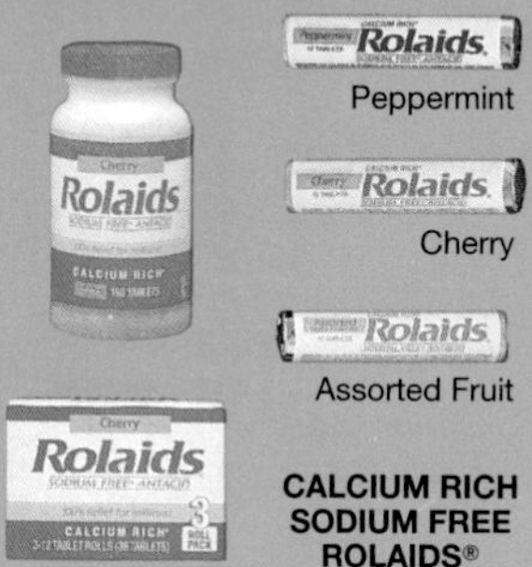
Rolaids
Rolaids
Rolaids
Rolaids
Rolaids

Peppermint

Cherry

Assorted Fruit

CALCIUM RICH SODIUM FREE ROLAIDS®

Calcium Rich, Sodium Free Relief from Heartburn, Sour Stomach or Acid Indigestion and Upset Stomach Associated with these Symptoms

Whitehall
p. 774

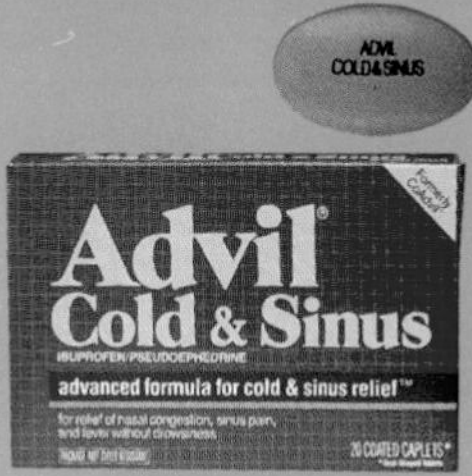

Coated Caplets in Packages of 20 and Bottles of 40.

ADVIL® COLD & SINUS
Ibuprofen/Pseudoephedrine Caplets

Whitehall
p. 775

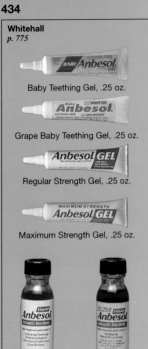

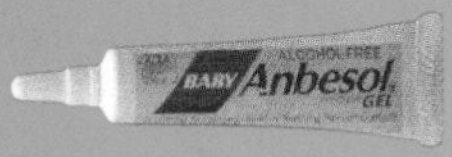

Baby Teething Gel, .25 oz.

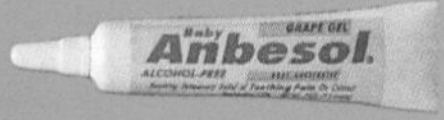

Grape Baby Teething Gel, .25 oz.

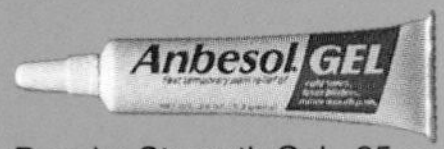

Regular Strength Gel, .25 oz.

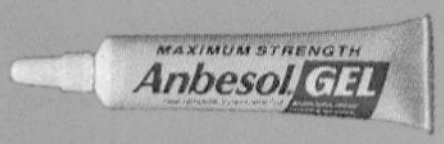

Maximum Strength Gel, .25 oz.

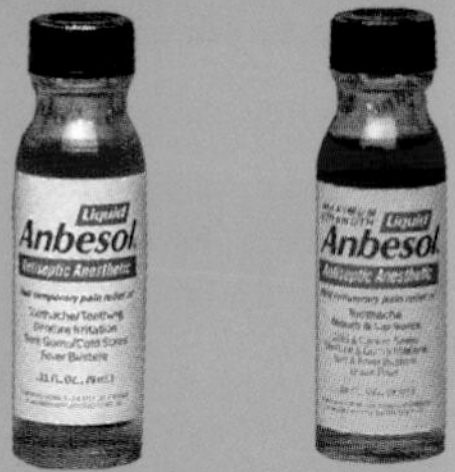

Regular Strength Liquid, .31 oz., .74 oz. | Maximum Strength Liquid, .31 oz.

ANBESOL®
Anesthetic for Oral Topical Pain Relief

Whitehall
p. 795

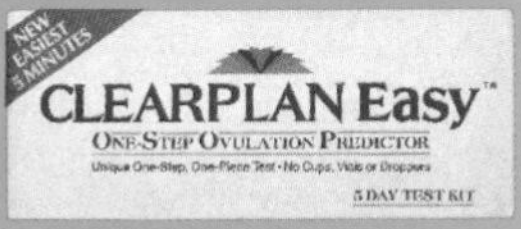

CLEARPLAN EASY™
One-Step Ovulation Predictor

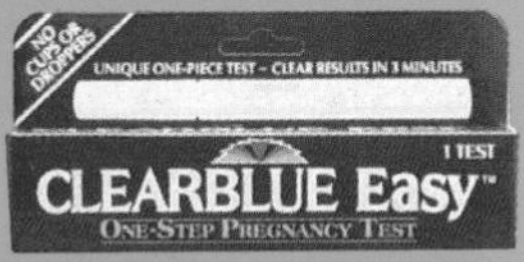

CLEARBLUE EASY™
One-Step Pregnancy Test

Whitehall
p. 776

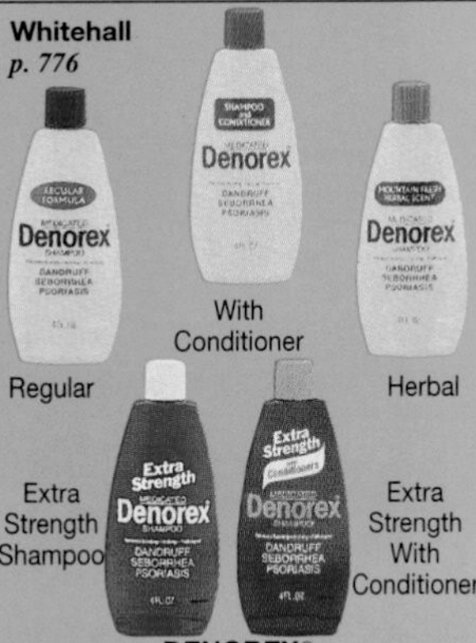

Regular | With Conditioner | Herbal | Extra Strength Shampoo | Extra Strength With Conditioner

DENOREX®
Medicated Shampoo

Whitehall
p. 776

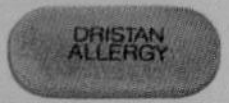

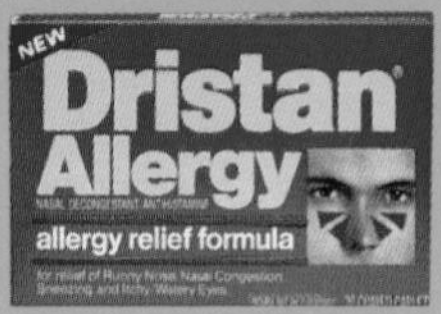

20's, 40's

DRISTAN® ALLERGY

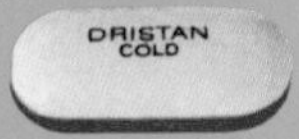

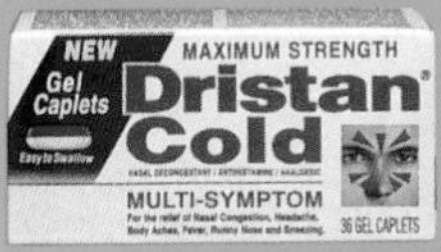

16's, 36's

MAXIMUM STRENGTH DRISTAN® COLD MULTI-SYMPTOM FORMULA

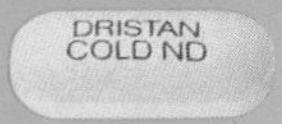

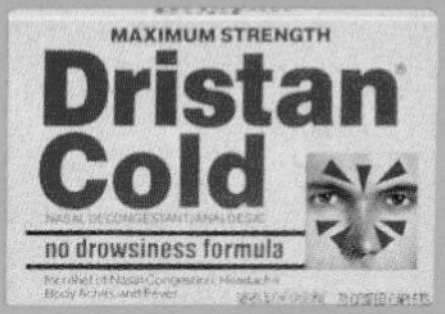

20's, 40's

MAXIMUM STRENGTH DRISTAN® COLD NO DROWSINESS FORMULA

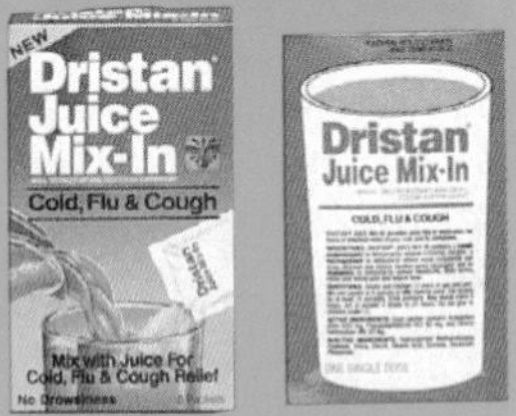

5's, 10's

DRISTAN® JUICE MIX-IN

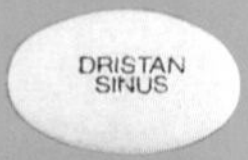

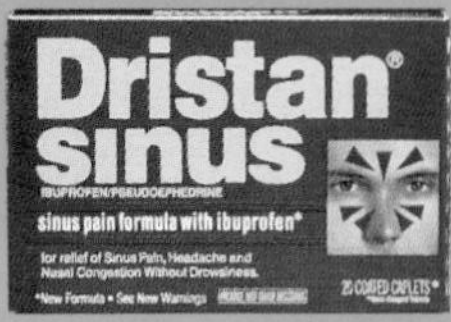

20's, 40's

DRISTAN® SINUS

Whitehall
p. 779

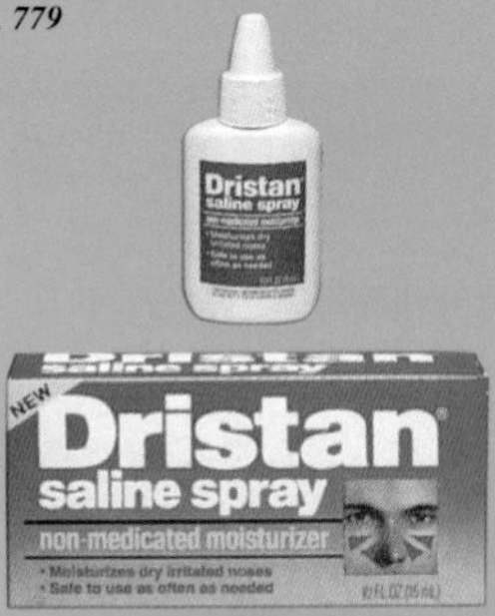

DRISTAN®
SALINE SPRAY
Non-Medicated Moisturizer

Whitehall
p. 780

Ointment
1 oz. and 2 oz. Tubes

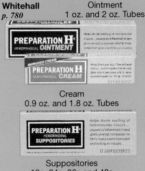

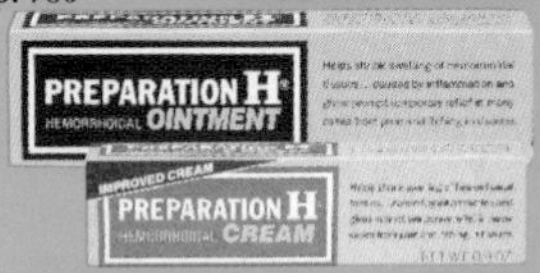

Cream
0.9 oz. and 1.8 oz. Tubes

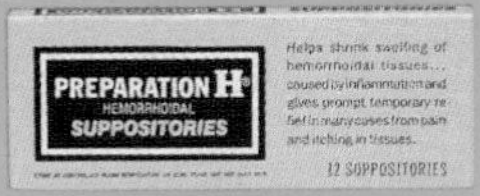

Suppositories
12s, 24s, 36s and 48s

PREPARATION H®
Hemorrhoidal Ointment, Cream and Suppositories

Whitehall
p. 780

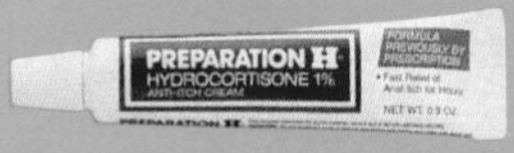

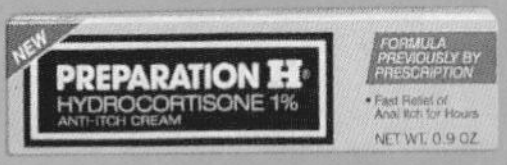

PREPARATION H®
HYDROCORTISONE 1%

Whitehall
p. 780

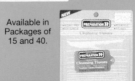

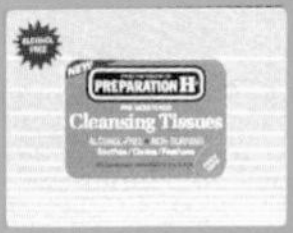

Available in Packages of 15 and 40.

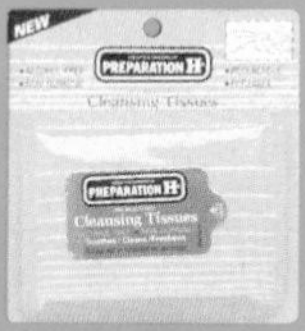

PREPARATION H®
CLEANSING TISSUES
Pre-moistened Alcohol-free
Non-burning

Whitehall
p. 781

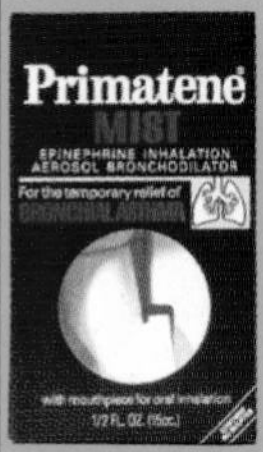

Available in 15mL Inhaler Unit, 10mL Suspension, 15mL and 22.5mL Refills.

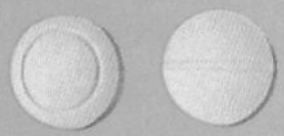

Front | Back

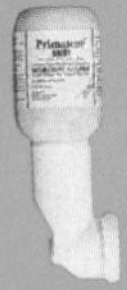

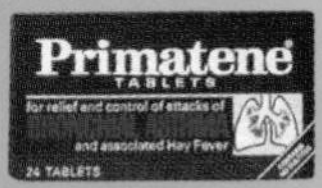

24's, 60's

PRIMATENE® MIST and TABLETS

Whitehall
p. 782

Available in 12 oz. Suspension.

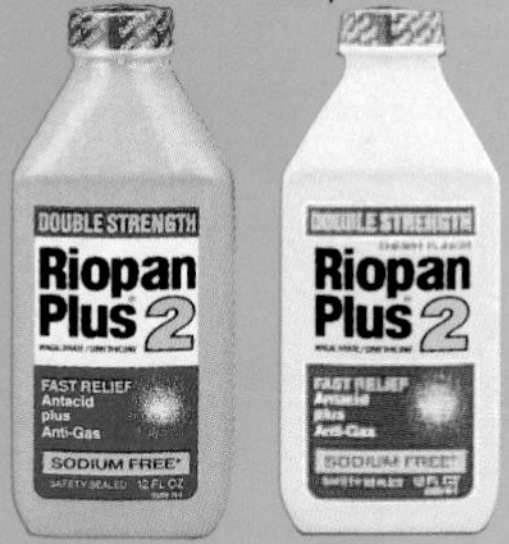

Mint | Cherry

RIOPAN PLUS® 2
High-Potency Antacid plus Anti-Gas
(magaldrate and simethicone)

Whitehall
p. 783

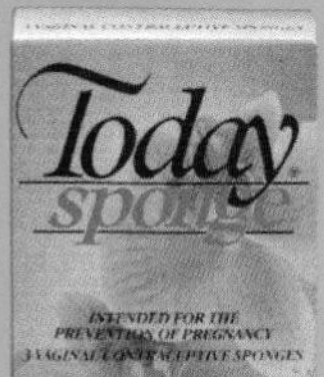

Available in Packages of 3, 6 and 12.

(Shown smaller than actual size)

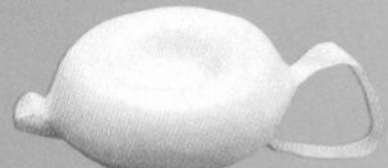

TODAY®
Vaginal Contraceptive Sponge

While every effort has been made to reproduce products faithfully, this section is to be considered a Quick-Reference identification aid.

WYETH-AYERST

Tamper-Resistant/Evident Packaging

Statements alerting consumers to the specific type of Tamper-Resistant/Evident Packaging appear on the bottle labels and cartons of all over-the-counter products of Wyeth-Ayerst. This includes plastic cap seals on bottles, individually wrapped tablets or suppositories, and sealed cartons. This packaging has been developed to better protect the consumer.

Wyeth-Ayerst
p. 785

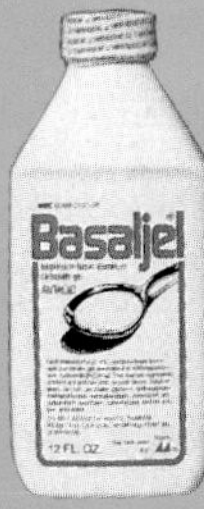

12 Fl. Oz.

BASALJEL®
SUSPENSION
Antacid

Wyeth-Ayerst
p. 786

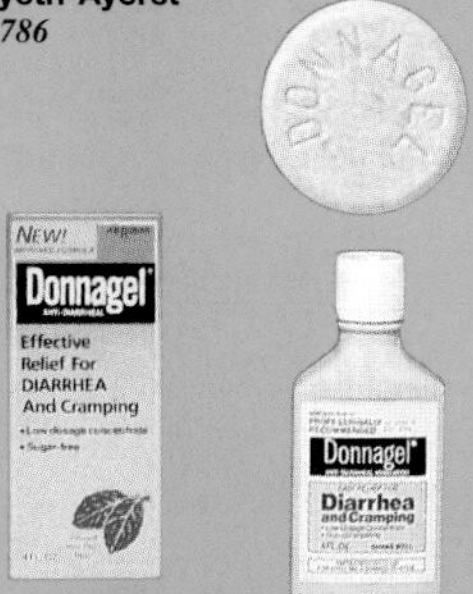

Available in bottles of 4 Fl. Oz., 8 Fl. Oz. and 16 Fl. Oz. and chewable tablets in cartons of 18

DONNAGEL®

Wyeth-Ayerst
p. 789

12 Suppositories

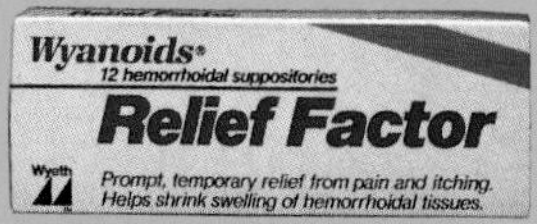

Also available in boxes of 24

WYANOIDS®
RELIEF FACTOR
Hemorrhoidal Suppositories

Wyeth-Ayerst
p. 784

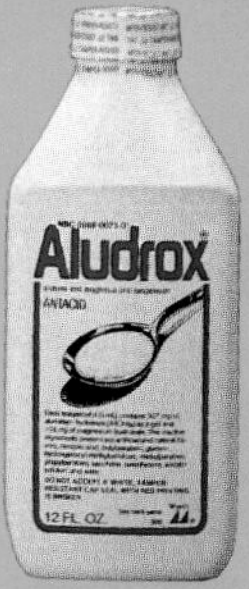

12 Fl. Oz.

ALUDROX® SUSPENSION
Antacid

Wyeth-Ayerst
p. 785

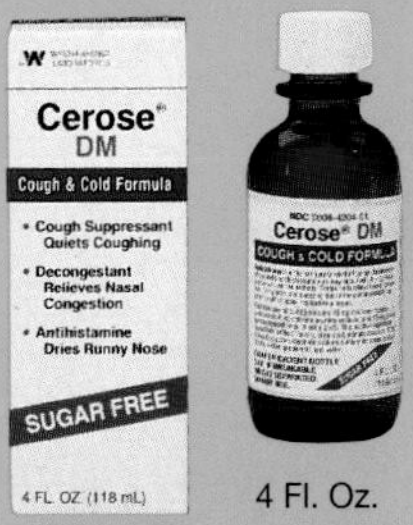

4 Fl. Oz.

CEROSE-DM®
Cough/Cold Formula
with Dextromethorphan
Also available in 1-pint bottles

Wyeth-Ayerst
p. 787

Also available in Ready-to-Feed Liquid and Powder

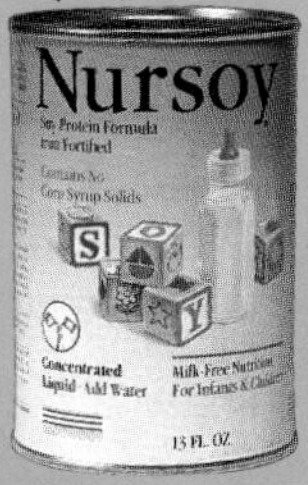

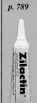

13 Fl. Oz.

Iron Fortified

NURSOY®
SOY PROTEIN ISOLATE FORMULA
Concentrated Liquid

ZILA

p. 789

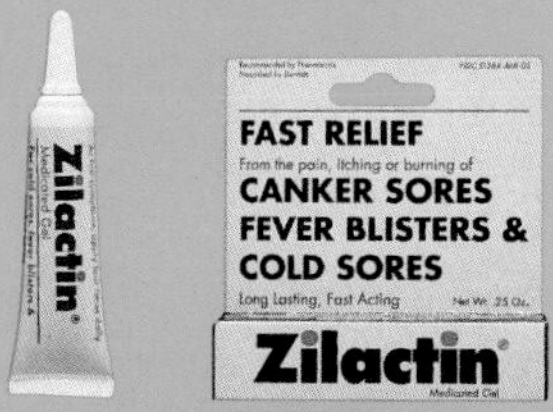
Zilactin
FAST RELIEF
From the pain, itching or burning of
CANKER SORES
FEVER BLISTERS &
COLD SORES
Long Lasting, Fast Acting
Zilactin
Medicated Gel

.25 oz Tube
Zilactin® Medicated Gel

Also from Zila: Zilactin-L® Liquid Treats cold sores and fever blisters before they break out

Wyeth-Ayerst
p. 784

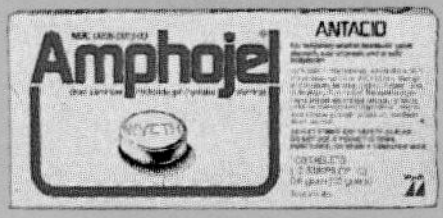
Amphojel
ANTACID

100 tablets

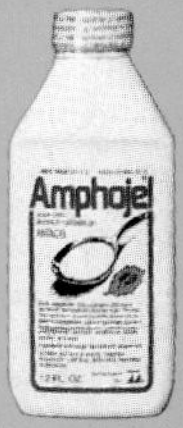

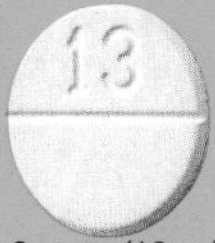

0.6 gram (10 gr.)

AMPHOJEL® TABLETS
and
SUSPENSION
Antacid

12 Fl. Oz.
Also available in 0.3 gram (5 gr.) tablets

Wyeth-Ayerst
p. 786

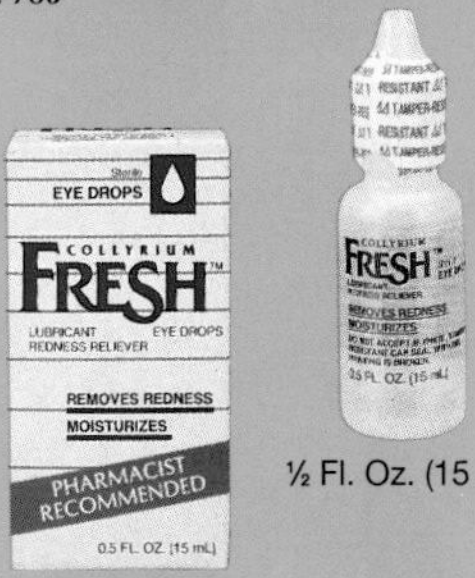

½ Fl. Oz. (15 ml)

COLLYRIUM FRESH™
Eye drops with tetrahydrozoline HCl plus glycerin

Wyeth-Ayerst
p. 787

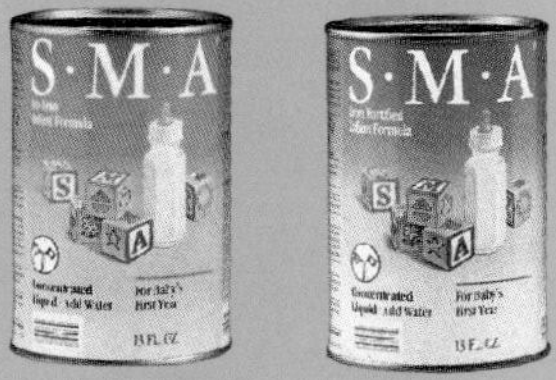

Lo-Iron

Iron Fortified

13 Fl. Oz.

Also available in Ready-to-Feed Liquid and Powder

S • M • A® INFANT FORMULA
Concentrated Liquid

Zila
p. 789

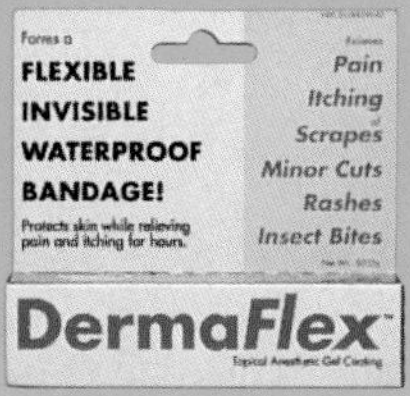
FLEXIBLE
INVISIBLE
WATERPROOF
BANDAGE!
Pain
Itching
Scrapes
Minor Cuts
Rashes
Insect Bites
DermaFlex

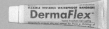

.5 oz Tube
DermaFlex® Topical Anesthetic Gel Coating

Wyeth-Ayerst
p. 785

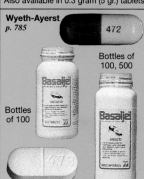

472

Bottles of 100, 500

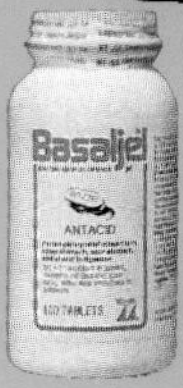

Bottles of 100

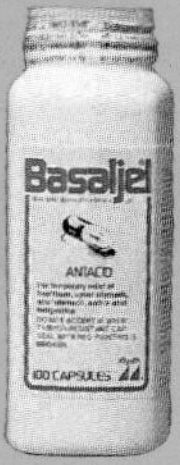

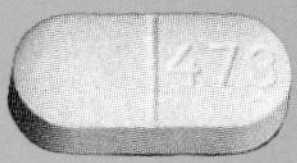

BASALJEL®
TABLETS and CAPSULES
Antacid

Wyeth-Ayerst
p. 786

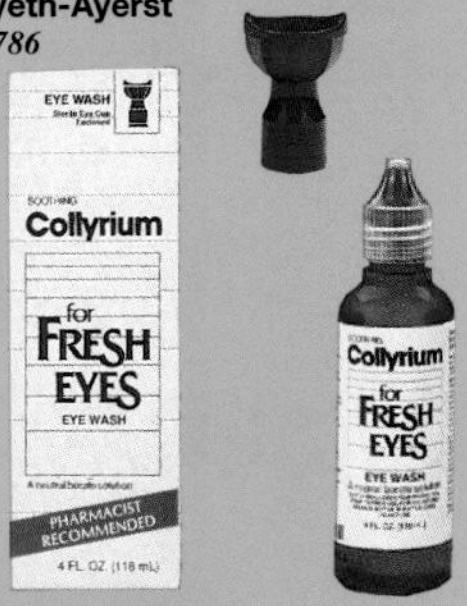

Eye Wash 4 Fl. Oz. (118 ml) with separate eyecup bottle cap.

COLLYRIUM for FRESH EYES
Eye Wash

Wyeth-Ayerst
p. 789

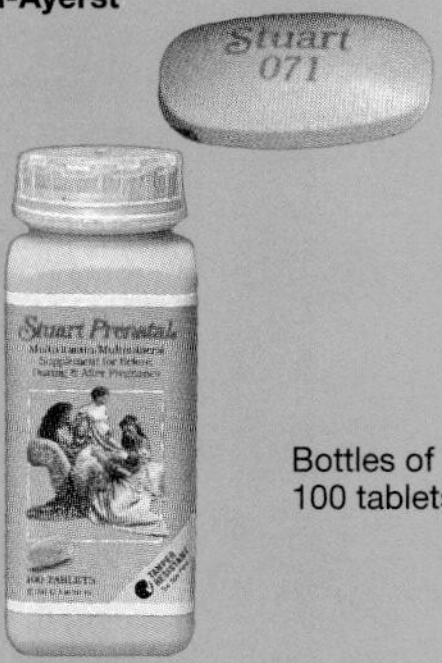

Bottles of 100 tablets

STUART PRENATAL® TABLETS
Multivitamin/Multimineral Supplement for pregnant or lactating women

For more detailed information on products illustrated in this section, consult the Product Information Section or manufacturers may be contacted directly.

MEDICAL ECONOMICS DATA

SECTION 6

Product Information Section

This section is made possible through the courtesy of the manufacturers whose products appear on the following pages. The information concerning each product has been prepared, edited and approved by the manufacturer.

Products described in this edition comply with labeling regulations. Copy may include all the essential information necessary for informed usage such as active ingredients, indications, actions, warnings, drug interactions, precautions, symptoms and treatment of oral overdosage, dosage and administration, professional labeling, and how supplied. In some cases additional information has been supplied to complement the foregoing. The Publisher has emphasized to manufacturers the necessity of describing products comprehensively so that all information essential for intelligent and informed use is available. In organizing and presenting the material in this edition the Publisher is providing all the information made available by manufacturers.

In presenting the following material to the medical profession, the Publisher is not necessarily advocating the use of any product.

Allergan Pharmaceuticals
A Division of Allergan, Inc.
2525 DUPONT DRIVE
P.O. BOX 19534
IRVINE, CA 92713-9534

CELLUFRESH™
(carboxymethylcellulose sodium) 0.5%
Lubricant Ophthalmic Solution

Description: Cellufresh™ solution is a preservative-free ophthalmic lubricant formulated for the patient who may need relief from dryness or minor irritation of the eye that may be caused by exposure to wind, sun, or heat.
The special lubricating formula was designed to supplement the natural balance of essential ions found in your own tears.
The active ingredient combines with your own tears to provide comforting relief from the burning and irritation associated with a dry eye through proper lubrication.
Preservative-free to avoid the risk of preservative-induced irritation.

Contains: Active: Carboxymethylcellulose sodium 0.5%. **Inactives:** calcium chloride, magnesium chloride, potassium chloride, purified water, sodium chloride, and sodium lactate. May also contain hydrochloric acid or sodium hydroxide to adjust pH.

FDA APPROVED USES

Indications: FOR USE AS A LUBRICANT TO PREVENT FURTHER IRRITATION OR TO RELIEVE DRYNESS OF THE EYE.

Warnings: To avoid contamination, do not touch tip of container to any surface. Do not reuse. Once opened, discard. If you experience eye pain, changes in vision, continued redness or irritation of the eye, or if the condition worsens or persists for more than 72 hours, discontinue use and consult a doctor. If solution changes color or becomes cloudy, do not use. Keep this and all drugs out of the reach of children. In case of accidental ingestion, seek professional assistance or contact a Poison Control Center immediately.

Directions: Instill 1 or 2 drops in the affected eye(s) as needed.

Note: Do not touch unit-dose tip to eye.

How Supplied: Solution is supplied in sterile, preservative-free, disposable, single-use containers of 0.01 fluid ounce each in the following size:
30 SINGLE-USE CONTAINERS—
NDC 0023-5487-30.

CELLUVISC®
(carboxymethylcellulose sodium) 1%
Lubricant Ophthalmic Solution

Celluvisc® Ophthalmic Solution is a preservative-free ophthalmic lubricant formulated specifically for the patient who needs frequent relief from dryness of the eye:

- Special lubricating formula was designed to supplement the natural balance of essential ions found in your tears.
- Preservative-free for no preservative-induced irritation.
- Single, unit-dose containers for greater convenience.

Contains: Active: Carboxymethylcellulose sodium 1%. **Inactives:** calcium chloride, potassium chloride, purified water, sodium chloride, and sodium lactate.

FDA APPROVED USES

Indications: FOR USE AS A LUBRICANT TO PREVENT FURTHER IRRITATION OR TO RELIEVE DRYNESS OF THE EYE.

Warnings: To avoid contamination, do not touch tip of container to any surface. Do not reuse. Once opened, discard. If you experience eye pain, changes in vision, continued redness or irritation of the eye, or if the condition worsens or persists for more than 72 hours, discontinue use and consult a doctor. If solution changes color or becomes cloudy, do not use. Keep this and all drugs out of the reach of children. In case of accidental ingestion, seek professional assistance or contact a Poison Control Center immediately.

Directions: Instill 1 or 2 drops in the affected eye(s) as needed.

NOTE: Do not touch unit-dose tip to eye. Celluvisc may cause temporary blurring due to its viscosity.

How Supplied: Celluvisc® (carboxymethylcellulose sodium) 1% Lubricant Ophthalmic Solution is supplied in sterile, preservative-free, disposable, single-use containers of 0.01 fluid ounce each, in the following size:

30 SINGLE-USE CONTAINERS—
NDC 0023-4554-30

LACRI-LUBE® S.O.P.®
(white petrolatum 56.8%, mineral oil 42.5%)
Lubricant Ophthalmic Ointment

Contains: Actives: white petrolatum 56.8%, mineral oil 42.5%. **Inactives:** chlorobutanol (chloral deriv.) 0.5% and lanolin alcohols.

FDA APPROVED USES

Indications: FOR USE AS A LUBRICANT TO PREVENT FURTHER IRRITATION OR TO RELIEVE DRYNESS OF THE EYE.

Warnings: To avoid contamination, do not touch tip of container to any surface. Replace cap after using either the 3.5 g or 7.0 g tube. If you are using the unit-dose product, do not reuse it after it has been opened. Once the unit-dose is opened, it should be discarded. If you experience eye pain, changes in vision, continued redness or irritation of the eye, or if the condition worsens or persists for more than 72 hours, discontinue use and consult a doctor. Keep this and all drugs out of the reach of children. In case of accidental ingestion, seek professional assistance or contact a Poison Control Center immediately.

Directions: Pull down the lower lid of the affected eye and apply a small amount (one-fourth inch) of ointment to the inside of the eyelid.

How Supplied: Lacri-Lube® S.O.P.® (white petrolatum 56.8%, mineral oil 42.5%) Lubricant Ophthalmic Ointment is supplied in sterile, disposable unit-dose containers of 0.7 g each and sterile, ophthalmic ointment tubes as follows:
24 UNIT-DOSE CONTAINERS—
NDC 0023-0312-01
3.5 g TUBE—NDC 0023-0312-04
7.0 g TUBE—NDC 0023-0312-07

LACRI-LUBE® NP
(white petrolatum 57.3%, mineral oil 42.5%)
Lubricant Ophthalmic Ointment

Contains:
Actives:
white petrolatum 57.3%
mineral oil 42.5%
Inactive: lanolin alcohols.

FDA APPROVED USES

Indications: FOR USE AS A LUBRICANT TO PREVENT FURTHER IRRITATION OR TO RELIEVE DRYNESS OF THE EYE.

Warnings: To avoid contamination, do not touch tip of container to any surface. Do not reuse. Once the product is opened, discard. If you experience eye pain, changes in vision, continued redness or irritation of the eye, or if the condition worsens or persists for more than 72 hours, discontinue use and consult a doctor. Keep this and all drugs out of the reach of children. In case of accidental ingestion, seek professional assistance or contact a Poison Control Center immediately.

Directions: Pull down the lower lid of the affected eye and apply a small amount (one-fourth inch) of ointment to the inside of the eyelid.

Note: Do not touch unit-dose tip to eye.

How Supplied: Lacri-Lube® NP (white petrolatum 57.3%, mineral oil 42.5%) Lubricant Ophthalmic Ointment is supplied in sterile, preservative-free, disposable, single-use containers of 0.025 oz (0.7 g) each, in the following size:

SINGLE-USE CONTAINERS—
NDC 0023-0240-01

REFRESH® P.M.
(white petrolatum 56.8%, mineral oil 41.5%)
Lubricant Ophthalmic Ointment

Contains: Actives : white petrolatum 56.8%, mineral oil 41.5%. **Inactives:** lanolin alcohols, purified water and sodium chloride.

FDA APPROVED USES

Indications: FOR USE AS A LUBRICANT TO PREVENT FURTHER IRRITATION OR TO RELIEVE DRYNESS OF THE EYE.

Warnings: To avoid contamination, do not touch tip of container to any surface. Replace cap after using. If you experience eye pain, changes in vision, continued redness or irritation of the eye, or if the condition worsens or persists for more than 72 hours, discontinue use and consult a doctor. Keep this and all drugs out of the reach of children. In case of accidental ingestion, seek professional assistance or contact a Poison Control Center immediately.

Directions: Pull down the lower lid of the affected eye and apply a small amount (one-fourth inch) of ointment to the inside of the eyelid.

Note: Store away from heat. Protect from freezing.

How Supplied: Refresh® P.M. (white petrolatum 56.8%, mineral oil 41.5%) Lubricant Ophthalmic Ointment is supplied in sterile, preservative-free, ophthalmic ointment tubes in the following size:

3.5 g—NDC 0023-0667-04

TEARS PLUS®
(polyvinyl alcohol 1.4%, povidone 0.6%)
Lubricant Ophthalmic Solution

Contains: Actives: Polyvinyl alcohol 1.4% and povidone 0.6%. **Inactives:** chlorobutanol (chloral deriv.) 0.5%, purified water and sodium chloride. May also contain hydrochloric acid or sodium hydroxide to adjust pH.

FDA APPROVED USES

Indications: FOR USE AS A LUBRICANT TO PREVENT FURTHER IRRITATION OR TO RELIEVE DRYNESS OF THE EYE.

Warnings: To avoid contamination, do not touch tip of container to any surface. Replace cap after using. If you experience eye pain, changes in vision, continued redness or irritation of the eye, or if the condition worsens or persists for more than 72 hours, discontinue use and consult a doctor. If solution changes color or becomes cloudy, do not use. Keep this and all drugs out of the reach of children. In case of accidental ingestion, seek professional assistance or contact a Poison Control Center immediately.

Directions: Instill 1 or 2 drops in the affected eye(s) as needed.

Note: Not for use while wearing soft contact lenses.

How Supplied: Tears Plus® (polyvinyl alcohol 1.4%, povidone 0.6%) Lubricant Ophthalmic Solution is supplied in sterile, plastic dropper bottles in the following sizes:

½ fl oz—NDC 11980-165-15
1 fl oz—NDC 11980-165-30

Almay, Inc.
625 MADISON AVENUE
NEW YORK, NY 10022

Brief Overview:

- Hypo-Allergenic
- Clinically, Dermatologist and Allergy Tested
- 100% Fragrance Free
- Non-Comedogenic

ANTI-ITCH LOTION
Relieves Itching

Active Ingredients: Pramoxine HCl 1%, Menthol 0.2%

Ingredients: Water, Petrolatum, Glyceryl Stearate, Glycerin, PEG-40 Stearate, Mineral Oil, Steareth-20, Ceteth-20, Cetyl Alcohol, PEG-150 Stearate, Magnesium Aluminum Silicate, Hydroxypropyl Methylcellulose, Benzyl Alcohol.

Indications: Relieves itching with or without associated dermatosis such as hives, rashes, poison ivy or insect bites. Alternative to potentially sensitizing benzocaine or diphenhydramine with both immediate and prolonged effects.

Warnings: For external use only. Avoid contact with eyes. If condition does not improve or recurs within 7 days discontinue use and consult your physician. Keep out of reach of children.

Administration: Apply liberally to affected areas several times daily as needed or as directed by your physician or pharmacist.

How Supplied: 2 fl. oz./59 ml.

EYELID CLEANSING PADS
Mild Cleanser for Blepharitis

Ingredients: Water, Poloxamer 184, Butylene Glycol, Disodium Lauroamphodiacetate, Sodium Trideceth Sulfate, Hexylene Glycol, Phenoxyethanol, Citric Acid, Benzyl Alcohol.

Indications: Removes scaling, crusting and debris associated with blepharitis such as occurs with seborrhea. Extremely mild formula dispensed as individually wrapped textured pads for maximum hygiene.

Administration: Remove one pad from packette. Wipe eye area and lashes gently and discard pad. Rinse with warm water. Use second pad for other eye area and rinse. Cleanse eye area once daily, or as directed by your physician or pharmacist.

How Supplied: 30 Packettes (60 Pads)

HYDROCORTISONE ANTIPRURITIC CREAM
Relieves Itching Associated with Inflammation and Rashes

Active Ingredient: Hydrocortisone Acetate

Other Ingredients: Water, Light Mineral Oil, Glyceryl Stearate, Glycerin, Polysorbate 60, Sorbitan Stearate, Aloe Vera Gel, Methylparaben, Propylparaben.

Indications: Relieves itching associated with inflammation and rashes such as occur with eczema and psoriasis. Lotion vehicle in large 4 oz. container allowing economical use over wide body area.

Warnings: For external use only. Avoid contact with eyes. If condition does not improve or recurs within 7 days discontinue use. Do not use any other hydrocortisone product and consult your physician. Do not use for diaper rash. Keep this and all drugs out of reach of children. In case of accidental ingestion seek professional assistance or contact a poison control center immediately. Store at room temperature.

Administration: Apply to affected areas not more than 3 or 4 times daily, or as directed by your physician or pharmacist. Consult a physician before using on children under age 2.

How Supplied: Net Wt. 1 oz./28 g.

HYDROCORTISONE ANTIPRURITIC LOTION
Relieves Itching Associated with Inflammation and Rashes

Active Ingredient: Hydrocortisone Acetate

Continued on next page

Almay—Cont.

Other Ingredients: Water, Mineral Oil, Glycerin, Glyceryl Stearate, Steareth-20, Petrolatum, Peg-150 Stearate, Stearyl Alcohol, Ceteth-20, Dimethicone, Carbomer, Menthol, Triethanolamine, Benzyl Alcohol.

Indications: Relieves itching associated with inflammation and rashes such as occur with eczema and psoriasis. Lotion vehicle in large 4 oz. container allowing economical use over wide body area.

Warnings: For external use only. Avoid contact with eyes. If condition does not improve or recurs within 7 days discontinue use. Do not use any other hydrocortisone product and consult your physician. Do not use for diaper rash. Keep this and all drugs out of reach of children. In case of accidental ingestion seek professional assistance or contact a poison control center immediately. Store at room temperature.

Administration: Apply to affected areas not more than 3 or 4 times daily, or as directed by your physician or pharmacist. Consult a physician before using on children under age 2.

How Supplied: Net Wt. 4 fl. oz./ 118 ml.

PROTECTIVE EYE TREATMENT SPF 12
Moisturizer and Protectant for Sensitive Skin

Active Ingredients: Titanium Dioxide, Allantoin

Other Ingredients: Glycerin, Water, Propylene Glycol, Dicaprylate/Dicaprate, Butylene Glycol, Safflower Oil, Hydrogenated Coco-Glycerides, Stearyl Alcohol, Cetyl Alcohol, Steareth-20, PEG-20 Methyl Glucose Sesquistearate, Sodium PCA, Barium Sulfate, Petrolatum, Ascorbyl Palmitate, Retinyl Palmitate, Tocopheryl Acetate, Glyceryl Stearate, Xanthan Gum, Magnesium Aluminum Silicate, Nonoxynyl Hydroxyethycellulose, Talc, PEG-16, Soya Sterol, Methyl Glucose Sesquistearate, Citric Acid, Disodium EDTA, Iron Oxides.

Indications: Protect and moisturize sun-sensitive, extremely dry or irritated skin in the delicate eye area. Skin subject to potentially irritating treatments such as Retin-A®. Preservative-free with non-chemical sunscreen.

Warnings: For external use only. Avoid contact with eyes. If condition worsens or does not improve within 7 days, consult a physician. Keep out of reach of children.

Administration: Apply liberally at least once daily, or as directed by your physician or pharmacist.

How Supplied: 1 oz./28 g.
Retin-A® is a registered trademark of Ortho Pharmaceuticals.

PROTECTIVE FACE CREAM SPF 15
Heals, Protects, and Moisturizes Dry, Sensitive Skin

Active Ingredients: Titanium Dioxide, Ethylhexyl *p*-Methoxycinnamate, Allantoin

Other Ingredients: Glycerin, Water, Butylene Glycol, Propylene Glycol, Dicaprylate/Dicaprate, Safflower Oil, Stearyl Alcohol, Cetyl Alcohol, Hydrogenated Coco-glycerides, Steareth-20, PEG-20 Methyl Glucose Sesquistearate, Barium Sulfate, Petrolatum, Sodium PCA, Glyceryl Stearate, Methyl Glucose Sesquistearate, Retinyl Palmitate, Ascorbyl Palmitate, Tocopheryl Acetate, Nonoxynyl Hydroxyethycellulose, Talc, PEG-16 Soya Sterol, Xanthan Gum, Magnesium Aluminum Silicate, Citric Acid, Disodium EDTA, Iron Oxides.

Indications: Protects and moisturizes sun-sensitive, extremely dry or irritated skin. Skin subject to potentially irritating treatments such as Retin-A®. Preservative-free with minimal level of chemical sunscreen to provide SPF 15 broad-spectrum UVA/UVB protection.

Warnings: For external use only. Avoid contact with eyes. If condition worsens or does not improve within 7 days consult a physician. Keep out of reach of children.

Administration: Apply liberally to moist skin on face and throat as needed, or as directed by your physician or pharmacist.

How Supplied: 2 oz./56 g.
Retin-A® is a registered trademark of Ortho Pharmaceuticals.

THERAPEUTIC BODY TREATMENT
Relieves Severely Dry, Flaking and Cracked Skin

Active Ingredient: Dimethicone

Other Ingredients: Water, Methoxypropylgluconamide (Hydrodextrol), Cyclomethicone, Glycerin, Butylene Glycol, Propylene Glycol, Dicaprylate/Dicaprate, Mineral Oil, Cetyl Alcohol, Stearyl Alcohol, Tocopherol, Magnesium Ascorbate Phosphate, Citric Acid, Glyceryl Stearate SE, Steareth-20, Steareth-2, Xanthan Gum, Magnesium Aluminum Silicate, Disodium EDTA, Methylparaben, Ethylparaben, Imidazolidinyl Urea.

Indications: Moderate to severe flaking of dry skin such as found in xerosis, asteosis or ichthyosis. Patented formula contains Hydrodextrol (methoxypropylgluconamide), which is comparable to alpha-hydroxy acids to normalize skin surface.

Warnings: For external use only. Avoid contact with eyes. If condition worsens or does not improve within 7 days consult a physician. Keep out of reach of children.

Administration: Apply liberally at least once daily as needed or as directed by your physician or pharmacist.

How Supplied: 8 fl. oz./236 ml.

THERAPEUTIC FACE LOTION
Relieves Severely Dry, Flaking and Cracked Skin

Active Ingredient: Allantoin

Other Ingredients: Water, Methoxypropylgluconamide (Hydrodextrol), Cyclomethicone, Glycerin, Butylene Glycol, Propylene Glycol, Dicaprylate/Dicaprate, Mineral Oil, Tocopherol, Magnesium Ascorbate Phosphate, Citric Acid, Glyceryl Stearate SE, Cetyl Alcohol, Stearyl Alcohol, Steareth-20, Steareth-2, Xanthan Gum, Magnesium Aluminum Silicate, Disodium EDTA, Methylparaben, Ethylparaben, Imidazolidinyl, Urea, FD&C Red No. 40, Titanium Dioxide.

Indications: Moderate to severe flaking of dry skin such as found in xerosis, asteosis or ichthyosis. Patented formula contains Hydrodextrol (methoxypropylgluconamide), which is comparable to alpha-hydroxy acids to normalize skin surface.

Warnings: For external use only. Avoid contact with eyes. If condition worsens or does not improve within 7 days, consult a physician. Keep out of reach of children.

Administration: Apply liberally at least once daily as needed or as directed by your physician or pharmacist.

How Supplied: 4 fl. oz./118 ml.

THERAPEUTIC SHAMPOO
Reduces Flaking and Scaling

Active Ingredient: Salicylic Acid

Other Ingredients: Water, Sodium C14-16 Olefin Sulfonate, Lauramidopropyl Betaine, Sodium Citrate, Stearyltrimonium Hydroxyethyl Hydrolyzed Protein, Sodium Chloride, Lauramide DEA, PPG-5 Ceteth-10 Phosphate, Menthol, Lactic Acid, Tetrasodium EDTA, Triethanolamine, Methylparaben, Propylparaben, Diazolidinyl Urea.

Indications: Scalp scaling, flaking and itching associated with psoriasis, seborrheic dermatitis and dandruff. Combination of ingredients which debrides scalp but leaves hair manageable.

Warnings: For external use only. Avoid contact with eyes. If contact occurs rinse eyes thoroughly with water. If condition worsens or does not improve after regular use of this product as directed, consult a physician. Keep out of reach of children.

Administration: Wet hair thoroughly; massage liberally into scalp. Leave lather on scalp for 5 minutes. Rinse. For best results, use daily until condition clears, then twice a week or as directed by your physician or pharmacist.

How Supplied: 8 fl. oz./236 ml.

Apothecon
A Bristol-Myers Squibb Company
POB 4500
PRINCETON, NJ 08543-4500

COLACE®
[*kōlās*]
docusate sodium, Apothecon
capsules • syrup • liquid (drops)

Description: Colace (docusate sodium) is a stool softener.
Colace Capsules, 50 mg, contain the following inactive ingredients: citric acid, D&C Red No. 33, FD&C Red No. 40, nonporcine gelatin, edible ink, polyethylene glycol, propylene glycol, and purified water.
Colace Capsules, 100 mg, contain the following inactive ingredients: citric acid, D&C Red No. 33, FD&C Red No. 40, FD&C Yellow No. 6, nonporcine gelatin, edible ink, polyethylene glycol, propylene glycol, titanium dioxide, and purified water.
Colace Liquid, 1%, contains the following inactive ingredients: citric acid, D&C Red No. 33, methylparaben, poloxamer, polyethylene glycol, propylene glycol, propylparaben, sodium citrate, vanillin, and purified water.
Colace Syrup, 20 mg/5 mL, contains the following inactive ingredients: alcohol (not more than 1%), citric acid, D&C Red No. 33, FD&C Red No. 40, flavor (natural), menthol, methylparaben, peppermint oil, poloxamer, polyethylene glycol, propylparaben, sodium citrate, sucrose, and purified water.

Actions and Uses: Colace, a surface-active agent, helps to keep stools soft for easy, natural passage and is not a laxative, thus, not habit forming. Useful in constipation due to hard stools, in painful anorectal conditions, in cardiac and other conditions in which maximum ease of passage is desirable to avoid difficult or painful defecation, and when peristaltic stimulants are contraindicated.
Note: When peristaltic stimulation is needed due to inadequate bowel motility, see Peri-Colace® (laxative and stool softener).

Contraindications: There are no known contraindications to Colace.

Warning: As with any drug, if you are pregnant or nursing a baby, seek the advice of a health professional before using this product.

Side Effects: The incidence of side effects—none of a serious nature—is exceedingly small. Bitter taste, throat irritation, and nausea (primarily associated with the use of the syrup and liquid) are the main side effects reported. Rash has occurred.

Administration and Dosage: *Orally*—Suggested daily Dosage: *Adults and older children:* 50 to 200 mg *Children 6 to 12:* 40 to 120 mg *Children 3 to 6:* 20 to 60 mg. *Infants and children under 3:* 10 to 40 mg. The higher doses are recommended for initial therapy. Dosage should be adjusted to individual response. The effect on stools is usually apparent 1 to 3 days after the first dose. Give Colace liquid in half a glass of milk or fruit juice or in infant formula, to mask bitter taste. *In enemas*—Add 50 to 100 mg Colace (5 to 10 mL Colace liquid) to a retention or flushing enema.

How Supplied: Colace capsules, 50 mg
NDC 0087-0713-01 Bottles of 30
NDC 0087-0713-02 Bottles of 60
NDC 0087-0713-03 Bottles of 250
NDC 0087-0713-05 Bottles of 1000
NDC 0087-0713-07 Cartons of 100 single unit packs
Colace capsules, 100 mg
NDC 0087-0714-01 Bottles of 30
NDC 0087-0714-02 Bottles of 60
NDC 0087-0714-03 Bottles of 250
NDC 0087-0714-05 Bottles of 1000
NDC 0087-0714-07 Cartons of 100 single unit packs
Note: Colace capsules should be stored at controlled room temperature (59°–86°F or 15°–30°C)
Colace liquid, 1% solution; 10 mg/mL (with calibrated dropper)
NDC 0087-0717-04 Bottles of 16 fl oz
NDC 0087-0717-02 Bottles of 30 mL
NSN 6505-00-045-7786 Bottles of 30 mL (M)
Colace syrup, 20 mg/5-mL teaspoon; contains not more than 1% alcohol
NDC 0087-0720-01 Bottles of 8 fl oz
NDC 0087-0720-02 Bottles of 16 fl oz

Shown in Product Identification Section, page 403

PERI-COLACE® capsules • syrup (casanthranol and docusate sodium)

Description: Peri-Colace is a combination of the mild stimulant laxative casanthranol, and the stool-softener Colace® (docusate sodium). Each capsule contains 30 mg of casanthranol and 100 mg of Colace; the syrup contains 30 mg of casanthranol and 60 mg of Colace per 15-mL tablespoon (10 mg of casanthranol and 20 mg of Colace per 5-mL teaspoon) and 10% alcohol.
Peri-Colace Capsules contain the following inactive ingredients: D&C Red No. 33, FD&C Red No. 40, nonporcine gelatin, edible ink, polyethylene glycol, propylene glycol, titanium dioxide, and purified water.
Peri-Colace Syrup contains the following inactive ingredients: alcohol (10% v/v), citric acid, flavors, methyl salicylate, methylparaben, poloxamer, polyethylene glycol, propylparaben, sodium citrate, sorbitol solution, sucrose, and purified water.

Action and Uses: Peri-Colace provides gentle peristaltic stimulation and helps to keep stools soft for easier passage. Bowel movement is induced gently—usually overnight or in 8 to 12 hours. Nausea, griping, abnormally loose stools, and constipation rebound are minimized. Useful in management of chronic or temporary constipation.
Note: To prevent hard stools when laxative stimulation is not needed or undesirable, see Colace (stool softener).

Warnings: Do not use when abdominal pain, nausea, or vomiting are present. Frequent or prolonged use of this preparation may result in dependence on laxatives.
As with any drug, if you are pregnant or nursing a baby, seek the advice of a health professional before using this product.

Side Effects: The incidence of side effects—none of a serious nature—is exceedingly small. Nausea, abdominal cramping or discomfort, diarrhea, and rash are the main side effects reported.

Administration and Dosage:
Adults—1 or 2 capsules, or 1 or 2 tablespoons syrup at bedtime, or as indicated. In severe cases, dosage may be increased to 2 capsules or 2 tablespoons twice daily, or 3 capsules at bedtime. *Children*—1 to 3 teaspoons of syrup at bedtime, or as indicated.

Overdosage: In addition to symptomatic treatment, gastric lavage, if timely, is recommended in cases of large overdosage.

How Supplied: Peri-Colace® Capsules
NDC 0087-0715-01 Bottles of 30
NDC 0087-0715-02 Bottles of 60
NDC 0087-0715-03 Bottles of 250
NDC 0087-0715-05 Bottles of 1000
NDC 0087-0715-07 Cartons of 100 single unit packs
Note: Peri-Colace capsules should be stored at controlled room temperatures (59°–86°F or 15°–30°C).
Peri-Colace® Syrup
NDC 0087-0721-01 Bottles of 8 fl oz
NDC 0087-0721-02 Bottles of 16 fl oz

Shown in Product Identification Section, page 403

THERAGRAN MULTIVITAMIN FORMULA

Theragran vitamin supplements, formerly Apothecon products, are now marketed by Bristol-Myers Products. For descriptions of Theragran products, please see page 517.

Products are indexed by generic and chemical names in the
YELLOW SECTION.

B.F. Ascher & Company, Inc.
15501 WEST 109th STREET
LENEXA, KS 66219
Mailing address:
P.O. BOX 717
SHAWNEE MISSION, KS
66201-0717

AYR® Saline Nasal Mist and Drops
[ār]

AYR Mist or Drops restores vital moisture to provide prompt relief for dry, crusted and inflamed nasal membranes due to chronic sinusitis, colds, low humidity, overuse of nasal decongestant drops and sprays, allergies, minor nose bleeds and other minor nasal irritations. AYR provides a soothing way to thin thick secretions and aid their removal from the nose and sinuses. AYR can be used as often as needed without the side effects associated with overuse of decongestant nose drops and sprays.

SAFE AND GENTLE ENOUGH FOR CHILDREN AND INFANTS

AYR Drops are particularly convenient for easy application with infants and children. AYR is formulated to prevent stinging, burning and irritation of delicate nasal tissue, even that of babies.

Directions For Use: SPRAY—Squeeze twice in each nostril as often as needed. Hold bottle upright. To spray, give the bottle short, firm squeezes. Take care not to aspirate nasal contents back into bottle. DROPS—Two to four drops in each nostril every two hours as needed, or as directed by your physician.

AYR is a specially formulated, buffered, isotonic saline solution containing sodium chloride 0.65% adjusted to the proper tonicity and pH with monobasic potassium phosphate/sodium hydroxide buffer to prevent nasal irritation. AYR also contains the non-irritating antibacterial and antifungal preservatives thimerosal and benzalkonium chloride and is formulated with deionized water.

How Supplied: AYR Mist in 50 ml spray bottles, AYR Drops in 50 ml dropper bottles.

Shown in Product Identification Section, page 403

ITCH-X GEL®
Dual-acting, itch-relieving gel with aloe vera

Active Ingredients: Benzyl alcohol 10% and pramoxine HCl 1%.

Also contains: Aloe vera gel, carbomer 934, diazolidinyl urea, FD&C blue #1, methylparaben, propylene glycol, propylparaben, SD alcohol 40, styrene/acrylate copolymer, triethanolamine, and water.

Indications: For the temporary relief of pain and itching associated with minor skin irritations, allergic itches, rashes, hives, minor burns, insect bites, sunburns, poison ivy, poison oak, and poison sumac.

Warnings: For external use only. Avoid contact with the eyes. If condition worsens, or if symptoms persist for more than 7 days or clear up and occur again within a few days, discontinue use of this product and consult a physician. KEEP THIS AND ALL DRUGS OUT OF THE REACH OF CHILDREN. In case of accidental ingestion, seek professional assistance or contact a Poison Control Center immediately.

Directions: Adults and children 2 years of age and older: Apply to affected area not more than 3 to 4 times daily. Children under 2 years of age: consult a physician.

How Supplied: 35.4g (1.25 oz) tube

Shown in Product Identification Section, page 403

MOBIGESIC® Analgesic Tablets
[mō ′bĭ-jē ′zĭk]

Breaks the cycle of pain. MOBIGESIC provides pain relief with a mild muscle relaxant effect.

Active Ingredients: Each tablet contains 325 mg of magnesium salicylate with 30 mg of phenyltoloxamine citrate.

Also Contains: Microcrystalline cellulose, magnesium stearate and colloidal silicon dioxide which aid in the formulation of the tablet and its dissolution in the gastrointestinal tract.

Indications: **MOBIGESIC** acts fast to provide relief from stress headache and other painful conditions by breaking the cycle of tension-stress pain. This formula relieves pain while relaxing tense, stiff muscles. Also effective in pain relief after dental procedures and minor surgery.

Caution: When used for the temporary symptomatic relief of colds, if relief does not occur within 7 days (3 days for fever), discontinue use and consult physician. This preparation may cause drowsiness. Do not drive or operate machinery while taking this medication. Do not administer to children under 6 years of age or exceed recommended dosage unless directed by physician.

Warnings: Keep this and all drugs out of the reach of children. In case of accidental overdose, call your doctor or poison control center immediately. As with any drug, if you are pregnant or nursing a baby, seek the advice of a health professional before using this product.

Usual Dosage: Adults—1 or 2 tablets every four hours, up to 10 tablets daily. Children (6 to 12 years)—1 tablet every 4 hours, up to 5 tablets daily. Do not use more than 10 days unless directed by physician.

Store at room temperature (59°–86°F).

How Supplied: Packages of 18's, 50's and 100's.

Shown in Product Identification Section, page 403

MOBISYL® Analgesic Creme
[mō ′bĭ-sĭl]

Penetrates to the site of pain to bring relief.

Active Ingredient: Trolamine salicylate 10%. Also Contains: Glycerin, methylparaben, mineral oil, polysorbate 60, propylparaben, sorbitan stearate, sorbitol, stearic acid, and water.

Description: MOBISYL is a greaseless, odorless, penetrating, non-burning, non-irritating analgesic creme.

Indications: For adults and children, 12 years of age and older, MOBISYL is indicated for the temporary relief of minor aches and pains of muscles and joints, such as simple backache, lumbago, arthritis, neuralgia, strains, bruises and sprains.

Actions: MOBISYL penetrates fast into sore, tender joints and muscles where pain originates. It works to reduce inflammation. Helps soothe stiff joints and muscles and gets you going again.

Warnings: For external use only. Avoid contact with the eyes. Discontinue use if condition worsens or if symptoms persist for more than 7 days, and consult a physician. Do not use on children under 12 years of age except under the advice and supervision of a physician. In case of accidental ingestion, seek professional assistance or contact a Poison Control Center immediately. Close cap tightly. Keep this and all drugs out of the reach of children. Store at room temperature.

Dosage and Administration: Place a liberal amount of MOBISYL Creme in your palm and massage into the area of pain and soreness three or four times a day, especially before retiring. MOBISYL may be worn under clothing or bandages.

How Supplied: MOBISYL is available in 35.4g (1.25 oz) tubes, 100g (3.5 oz) tubes, 226.8g (8 oz) jars.

Shown in Product Identification Section, page 403

PEN•KERA® Creme with Keratin Binding Factor
A Therapeutic Moisturizing Creme for Chronic Dry Skin

Ingredients: Water, octyl palmitate, glycerin, mineral oil, polysorbate 60, sorbitan stearate, polyamino sugar condensate, urea, wheat germ glycerides, carbomer 940, triethanolamine, DMDMH, iodo propynyl butyl carbamate, diazolidinyl urea, and dehydroacetic acid.

Indications: PEN•KERA Therapeutic Creme for Chronic Dry Skin contains Keratin Binding Factor, a polyamino sugar condensate and urea, which is synthesized to match the same biological components as those found in skin. The Keratin Binding Factor in PEN•KERA Creme replaces the missing elements of dehydrated skin which absorb and retain

moisture. The Keratin Binding Factor actually simulates the natural moisturizing mechanism of the skin, relieving itching, flaking, sensitive, dry skin symptoms.
PEN•KERA is fragrance-free, dye-free, paraben-free, lanolin-free, non-comedogenic and non-greasy for smooth, fast absorption.

Dosage and Administration: Apply in a thin layer. Because it penetrates quickly and is non-greasy, PEN•KERA may be used under make-up or sun screens. Regular use will reduce the frequency of application and quantity required to achieve moisturized skin.

Precautions: FOR EXTERNAL USE ONLY

How Supplied: PEN•KERA Therapeutic Creme is available in 8 oz. bottles.

Shown in Product Identification Section, page 403

Astra Pharmaceutical Products, Inc.

50 OTIS ST.
WESTBORO, MA 01581-4500

XYLOCAINE® (lidocaine) 2.5%
[*zī'lo-caine*]
OINTMENT

For temporary relief of pain and itching due to minor burns, sunburn, minor cuts, abrasions, insect bites and minor skin irritations.

Composition: Diethylaminoacet-2,6-xylidide 2.5% in a water miscible ointment vehicle consisting of polyethylene glycols and propylene glycol.

Action and Uses: A topical anesthetic ointment for fast, temporary relief of pain and itching due to minor burns, sunburn, minor cuts, abrasions, insect bites and minor skin irritations. The ointment can be easily removed with water. It is ineffective when applied to intact skin.

Administration and Dosage: Apply topically in liberal amounts for adequate control of symptoms. When the anesthetic effect wears off additional ointment may be applied as needed.

Important Warning: *In persistent, severe or extensive skin disorders, advise patient to use only as directed. In case of accidental ingestion advise patient to seek professional assistance or to contact a poison control center immediately. Keep out of the reach of children.*

Caution: *Do not use in the eyes. Not for prolonged use. If the condition for which this preparation is used persists or if a rash or irritation develops, advise patient to discontinue use and consult a physician.*

How Supplied: Available in tube of 35 grams (approximately 1.25 ounces).

Shown in Product Identification Section, page 403

Au Pharmaceuticals, Inc.

P. O. BOX 131835
TYLER, TX 75713-1835

AURUM–Analgesic Lotion
Topical Analgesic
THERAGOLD–Analgesic Lotion
Topical Analgesic
THERAPEUTIC GOLD–Analgesic Lotion
Topical Analgesic

Active Ingredients: The active ingredients are methyl salicylate 10%; menthol 3%; camphor 2.5%. These are combined in a rich, nonpetroleum base for easy and effective topical application.

Other Selected Ingredients: Special inactive ingredients include Deionized Water, C12–15 Alcohols, Propylene Glycol, Eucalyptus Oil, Stearic Acid, DEA Cetyl Phosphate, PEG 8-Distearate, Carboxy Polymethylene, Methyl Hydroxybenzoate, Ginseng, Imidazolidinyl Urea, Triethanolamine, Disodium EDTA, Urea, Jojoba Oil, Vitamins A & D_3, Vitamin E, FD&C Yellow No. 5, 24 Karat Gold, Aloe.

Indications: These lotions give fast, deep-penetrating, effective temporary relief from stiff, sore, aching muscles and joints associated with arthritis, bursitis, tendinitis and muscle disorders.

Actions: Methyl salicylate, menthol and camphor are classified as counterirritants which combine to provide both heat and cold stimulation to the pain receptors over and around the affected area. The lotions replace the perception of pain with the feeling of heat and/or cold to provide temporary relief of minor aches and pains.

Directions: Apply a liberal amount of lotion to painful area and allow to remain on skin for 30 seconds before rubbing lotion into the affected area. Apply product 3 or 4 times a day or as needed until pain is relieved, then reduce the frequency as needed.

Warnings: Use only as directed. For external use only. Avoid contact with eyes, mucous membranes, broken or irritated skin. Should contact occur, flush area with water. Do not use a heating pad with this lotion until one hour after application. Do not use on children under 12 years of age without advice of a physician. If condition worsens or persists for more than 7 days without relief, discontinue use of this product and consult a physician. Some individuals may experience sensitivity to some ingredients. If so, discontinue use immediately. Do not swallow. If swallowed, induce vomiting and call a physician.

Caution: contains 10% Methyl Salicylate and 24K GOLD. Persons who are allergic or hypersensitive to these ingredients should consult their physician before using this product.

How Supplied: These products are available in 128 ounce, 8 ounce and 2 ounce bottles.
National Drug Code Registration #058796

FEMININE GOLD—Analgesic Lotion
Topical Analgesic

Active Ingredients: The active ingredients are menthol 3%, camphor 2.5%. These are combined in a rich, nonpetroleum base for easy and effective topical application.

Other Selected Ingredients: Special inactive ingredients include Deionized Water, C12–15 Alcohols, Propylene Glycol, Eucalyptus Oil, Stearic Acid, DEA Cetyl Phosphate, PEG 8-Distearate, Carboxy Polymethylene, Methyl Hydroxybenzoate, Ginseng, Imidazolidinyl Urea, Triethanolamine, Disodium EDTA, Urea, Jojoba Oil, Vitamin A & D_3, Vitamin E, FD&C Yellow No. 5, 24 Karat Gold, Aloe.

Indications: This lotion gives fast, deep-penetrating, effective temporary relief from pain and discomfort of cramps and backache suffered during the menstrual cycle.

Actions: Menthol and camphor are classified as counterirritants which combine to provide both heat and cold stimulation to the pain receptors over and around the affected area. The lotion replaces the perception of pain with the feeling of heat and/or cold to provide temporary relief of minor aches and pains.

Directions: Apply a liberal amount of lotion to painful area and allow to remain on skin for 30 seconds before rubbing lotion into the affected area. Apply product 3 or 4 times a day or as needed until pain is relieved, then reduce the frequency to as needed.

Warnings: Use only as directed. For external use only. Avoid contact with eyes, mucous membranes, broken or irritated skin. Should contact occur, flush area with water. Do not use a heating pad with this lotion untl one hour after application. Do not use on children under 12 years of age without advice of a physician. If condition worsens or persists for more than 7 days without relief, discontinue use of this product and consult a physician. Some individuals may experience sensitivity to some ingredients. If so discontinue use immediately. Do not swallow. If swallowed, induce vomiting and call a physician.

Caution: contains 24K GOLD. Persons who are allergic or hypersensitive to these ingredients should consult their physician before using this product.

Continued on next page

Au—Cont.

How Supplied: These products are available in 8 ounce and 2 ounce bottles.
National Drug Code Registration #058796

Ayerst Laboratories
Division of American Home Products Corporation
685 THIRD AVE.
NEW YORK, NY 10017-4071

For information for Ayerst's consumer products, see product listings under Whitehall Laboratories.
Please turn to Whitehall Laboratories, page 774.

Baker Cummins Dermatologicals, Inc.
1950 SWARTHMORE AVENUE
LAKEWOOD, NJ 08701

AQUA-A® Cream

Description: Contains the vitamin A derivative, retinyl palmitate. Moisture-enriched smoothing concentrate.

Ingredients: Water, Caprylic/Capric Triglyceride, Methyl Gluceth-10, Glyceryl Stearate, Squalane, Mineral Oil, PPG-20 Methyl Glucose Ether Distearate, Dimethicone, Stearic Acid, PEG-50 Stearate, Retinyl Palmitate, Sodium Hyaluronate, Lecithin, Sodium Polyglutamate, Ascorbyl Palmitate, Carbomer 934, Dichlorobenzyl Alcohol, Cetyl Alcohol, BHT, Diazolidinyl Urea, Xanthan Gum, Menthol, Sodium Hydroxide, Tetrasodium EDTA.

Directions for Use: Use morning or night or both.

How Supplied: 2 oz. jars

AQUADERM® Sunscreen Moisturizer SPF 15

Description: Aquaderm® Sunscreen Moisturizer SPF 15 developed by leading dermatologists to deliver maximum moisturization. Regular daily use of Aquaderm's dual action moisturizer and sunscreen protects and preserves your youthful appearance. This specially developed formula contains sunscreens (SPF 15) that shield your skin from UVA and UVB rays, to protect it from wrinkles and reduce skin damage and possible skin cancer. Aquaderm® Sunscreen Moisturizer SPF 15 is safe and effective, hypo-allergenic, non-comedogenic, Paraben-free, and will not leave an artificial-feeling film. Aquaderm® Sunscreen Moisturizer SPF 15 is especially suited for patients undergoing Retin-A® therapy, who require maximum moisturization and sun protection. Retin-A® is a registered trademark of Johnson & Johnson.

Active Ingredients: Octyl Methoxycinnamate, 7.5%, Oxybenzone, 6%, in a moisturizing cream base.

Indications: Protects against harmful skin-aging rays of the sun.

Warnings: FOR EXTERNAL USE ONLY. Avoid contact with eyes. If irritation develops, discontinue use. Keep this and all drugs out of the reach of children. In case of accidental ingestion, seek professional assistance or contact a Poison Control Center immediately.

Directions for Use: Apply to face and neck as needed. Effective and compatible for daily use under make-up.

How Supplied: 3.5 oz. tube

AQUADERM® Cream

Description: Ultrarich moisturizing cream concentrate. Softens, smooths, protects, absorbs quickly. Fragrance free—Ideal for use as a compounding base.

Ingredients: Water, Caprylic/Capric Triglyceride, Methyl Gluceth-10, Glyceryl Stearate, Mineral Oil, Squalane, Dimethicone, Stearic Acid, PEG-50 Stearate, Sodium Hyaluronate, Lecithin, Sodium Polyglutamate, Magnesium Aluminum Silicate, Carbomer 934, Dichlorobenzyl Alcohol, Cetyl Alcohol, BHT, Diazolidinyl Urea, Xanthan Gum, Menthol, Sodium Hydroxide, Tetrasodium EDTA.

Directions for Use: Apply to face or other dry areas morning or night or both.

How Supplied: 4 oz. jar (0575-2002-04)
Shown in Product Identification Section, page 403

AQUADERM® Lotion

Description: Ultrarich moisturizing lotion concentrate. Smooths, softens, protects, absorbs quickly. Fragrance Free—Ideal for use as a compounding base.

Ingredients: Water, Caprylic/Capric Triglyceride, Methyl Gluceth-10, Glyceryl Stearate, Dimethicone, Petrolatum, Mineral Oil, Squalane, PEG-50 Stearate, Stearic Acid, Sodium Hyaluronate, Lecithin, Sodium Polyglutamate, Magnesium Aluminum Silicate, Carbomer 934, Dichlorobenzyl Alcohol, Cetyl Alcohol, BHT, Diazolidinyl Urea, Xanthan Gum, Menthol, Tetrasodium EDTA, Sodium Hydroxide.

Directions for Use: Apply to hands and body morning or night or both.

How Supplied: 7.5 fl. oz. bottle (0575-2001-75)
Shown in Product Identification Section, page 403

P&S® Liquid

Ingredients: Mineral Oil, Water, Fragrance, Glycerin, Phenol, Sodium Chloride, D&C Yellow #11, D&C Red #17, D&C Green #6.

Indications: P&S® Liquid, used regularly, helps loosen and remove crusts and scales on the scalp.

Caution: FOR EXTERNAL USE ONLY. Do not apply to large portions of body surfaces. Discontinue use if excessive skin irritation develops. Avoid contact with eyes or mucous membranes. Keep out of the reach of children. In case of accidental ingestion, seek professional assistance or contact a Poison Control Center immediately.

Directions for Use: Apply liberally to scalp lesions each night before retiring. Massage gently to loosen scales and crusts. Leave on overnight and shampoo the next morning. Use daily as needed.

How Supplied: 8 fl. oz. bottle (0575-4001-04); 4 fl. oz. bottle (0575-4001-08)
Shown in Product Identification Section, page 403

P&S® PLUS Tar Gel

Active Ingredient: 8% Coal Tar Solution (equivalent to 1.6% Crude Coal Tar).

Indications: For psoriasis and other scaling conditions. P&S® PLUS relieves the itching, irritation and skin flaking associated with seborrheic dermatitis, psoriasis and dandruff.

Warnings: FOR EXTERNAL USE ONLY. Avoid contact with the eyes; flush with water if product gets into eyes. If irritation develops, discontinue use. If condition worsens or does not improve after regular use of this product as directed, consult a physician. Do not use on children under 2 years of age except as directed by a physician. Use caution in exposing skin to sunlight after applying this product; it may increase your tendency to sunburn for up to 24 hours after application. Do not use this product with other forms of psoriasis therapy such as ultraviolet radiation or prescription drugs unless directed to do so by a doctor. If condition covers a large area of the body, consult your doctor before using this product.

Caution: Keep this and all drugs out of reach of children. In case of accidental ingestion, seek professional assistance or contact a Poison Control Center immediately.

Directions for Use: Apply to affected areas of skin and scalp daily or as directed by physician.

How Supplied: 3.5 oz. tube (NDC 0575-4009-35)

P&S® Shampoo

Active Ingredient: 2% Salicylic Acid.

Indications: P&S® Shampoo relieves the itching, irritation and skin flaking associated with seborrheic dermatitis of the scalp. It also relieves the itching, redness, and scaling associated with psoriasis of the scalp. P&S® Shampoo may be used alone as well as following treatment with P&S® Liquid. Its rich conditioning formula improves hair's manageability and helps prevent tangles.

Warnings: FOR EXTERNAL USE ONLY. Avoid contact with eyes or mucous membranes. If this occurs, rinse thoroughly with water. If condition worsens or does not improve after regular use of this product as directed, consult a physician. Do not use on children under 2 years of age except as directed by a physician. If condition covers a large area of the body, consult your doctor before using this product.

Caution: Keep this and all drugs out of reach of children. In case of accidental ingestion, seek professional assistance or contact a Poison Control Center immediately.

Directions for Use: For best results use twice weekly or as directed by a physician. Wet hair, apply to scalp and massage vigorously. Rinse and repeat.

How Supplied: 4 fl. oz. bottle (NDC 0575-4007-04); 8 fl. oz. bottle (NDC 0575-4007-08)

Shown in Product Identification Section, page 403

ULTRA MIDE 25® Extra Strength Moisturizer

Ingredients: Water, Urea, Mineral Oil, Glycerin, Propylene Glycol, PEG-50 Stearate, Butyrolactone, Hydrogenated Lanolin, Sorbitan Laurate, Glyceryl Stearate, Magnesium Aluminum Silicate, Propylene Glycol Stearate SE, Cetyl Alcohol, Fragrance, Diazolidinyl Urea, Tetrasodium EDTA.

Indications: Intensive moisturizer for extra dry, scaly or calloused skin. Contains ingredients to soften and moisturize areas of very dry, rough, cracked or calloused skin. This unique keratolytic patented formula contains a stabilized form of urea (25%) to help prevent the stinging and irritation often associated with moisturizers containing urea. ULTRA MIDE 25® Lotion contains no parabens.

Warnings: FOR EXTERNAL USE ONLY. Keep out of reach of children. Discontinue use if irritation occurs. Caution should be taken when used near the eyes. In case of accidental ingestion, seek professional assistance or contact a Poison Control Center immediately.

Directions for Use: Apply four times daily, or as directed by a physician. Each application should be rubbed in completely.

How Supplied: 8 fl. oz. bottle (0575-4200-08)

Shown in Product Identification Section, page 403

X–SEB® Shampoo

Active Ingredient: 1% Zinc Pyrithione.

Inactive Ingredients: Purified Water, Ammonium Lauryl Sulfate, Ammonium Laureth Sulfate, Ethylene Glycol Distearate, Lauramide DEA, Salicylic Acid, PEG 75 Lanolin, Ammonium Xylene Sulfate, Triethanolamine, Menthol, Methylchloroisothiazolinone and Methylisothiazolinone, Fragrance, FD&C Blue #1.

Indications: X-SEB® Shampoo provides effective relief of the itching and scalp flaking associated with dandruff. This unique formulation is gentle enough for daily use leaving hair healthy looking and manageable.

Warnings: FOR EXTERNAL USE ONLY. Avoid contact with the eyes. If this happens, rinse thoroughly with water. If condition worsens or does not improve after regular use of this product as directed, consult a physician. Do not use on children under 2 years of age except as directed by a physician.

Caution: Keep this and all drugs out of the reach of children. In case of accidental ingestion, seek professional assistance or contact a Poison Control Center immediately.

Directions for Use: For best results, use X-SEB® Shampoo twice a week or as directed by a physician. Wet hair, apply to scalp and massage vigorously. Rinse and repeat.

How Supplied: 4 fl. oz. bottle (NDC 0575-1006-04); 8 fl. oz. bottle (NDC 0575-1006-08)

Shown in Product Identification Section, page 403

X–SEB® PLUS Conditioning Shampoo

Active Ingredient: 1% Zinc Pyrithione.

Inactive Ingredients: Purified Water, Ammonium Lauryl Sulfate, Ammonium Laureth Sulfate, Ethylene Glycol Distearate, Lauramide DEA, Salicylic Acid, PEG 75 Lanolin, Polyquaternium-7, Ammonium Xylene Sulfate, Triethanolamine, Menthol, Methylchloroisothiazolinone and Methylisothiazolinone, Fragrance, FD&C Blue #1.

Indications: X-SEB® PLUS conditioning shampoo provides effective relief of the itching and scalp flaking associated with dandruff. Ideal for dry, brittle hair. This unique formulation is gentle enough for daily use giving hair extra body, a healthy look and ease of manageability.

Warnings: FOR EXTERNAL USE ONLY. Avoid contact with the eyes; if this happens, rinse thoroughly with water. If condition worsens or does not improve after regular use of this product as directed, consult a physician. Do not use on children under 2 years of age except as directed by a physician.

Caution: Keep this and all drugs out of the reach of children. In case of accidental ingestion, seek professional assistance or contact a Poison Control Center immediately.

Directions for Use: For best results, use X-SEB® PLUS conditioning shampoo twice a week or as directed by a physician. Wet hair, apply to scalp and massage vigorously. Rinse and repeat.

How Supplied: 4 fl. oz. bottle (NDC 0575-1016-04); 8 fl. oz. bottle (NDC 0575-1016-08)

Shown in Product Identification Section, page 403

X–SEB T® Shampoo

Active Ingredient: 10% Coal Tar Solution (2% Crude Coal Tar).

Inactive Ingredients: Purified water, TEA Lauryl Sulfate, Lauramide DEA, Ethylene Glycol Distearate, PEG-75 Lanolin, Salicylic Acid, Polyquaternium-7, Menthol, Hydroxypropyl Methylcellulose, Chloroxylenol, Disodium EDTA, Fragrance, FD&C Blue #1.

Indications: X-SEB T® shampoo relieves the itching, irritation and skin flaking associated with dandruff, seborrheic dermatitis, and psoriasis. This formulation is designed to effectively treat scaly conditions in a mild, gentle cleansing base leaving hair healthy looking and manageable. X-SEB T® will not discolor or damage hair that has been color treated or permed. Ideal for normal to oily hair type.

Warnings: FOR EXTERNAL USE ONLY. Avoid contact with the eyes; if this happens, rinse thoroughly with water. If irritation develops, discontinue use. If condition worsens or does not improve after regular use of this product as directed, consult a physician. Do not use on children under 2 years of age except as directed by a physician. Use caution in exposing skin to sunlight after applying this product; it may increase your tendency to sunburn for up to 24 hours after application. Do not use for prolonged periods without consulting a physician. Do not use this product with other forms of psoriasis therapy such as ultraviolet radiation or prescription drugs unless directed to do so by a physician. If condition covers a large area of the body, consult your physician before using this product.

Continued on next page

Baker Cummins Derm.—Cont.

Caution: Keep this and all drugs out of the reach of children. In case of accidental ingestion, seek professional assistance or contact a Poison Control Center immediately.

Directions for Use: For best results, use X-SEB T® shampoo at least twice a week or as directed by physician. Wet hair, apply to scalp and massage vigorously. Rinse and repeat or as directed by a physician.

How Supplied: 4 fl. oz. bottle (NDC 0575-1005-04); 8 fl. oz. bottle (NDC 0575-1005-08)

Shown in Product Identification Section, page 403

X-SEB T® PLUS Conditioning Shampoo

Active Ingredient: 10% Coal Tar Solution (equivalent to 2% Crude Coal Tar).

Inactive Ingredients: Purified water, TEA Lauryl Sulfate, Lauramide DEA, Ethylene Glycol Distearate, PEG-75 Lanolin, Salicylic Acid, Polyquaternium-7, Menthol, Hydroxypropyl Methylcellulose, Chloroxylenol, Disodium EDTA, Fragrance, FD&C Blue #1.

Indications: X-SEB T® PLUS conditioning shampoo relieves the itching, irritation and skin flaking associated with dandruff, seborrheic dermatitis, and psoriasis. This formulation is designed to effectively treat scaly conditions in a mild, gentle cleansing base leaving hair healthy looking and manageable. X-SEB T® PLUS will not discolor or damage hair that has been color treated or permed. Ideal for normal to dry, brittle hair.

Warnings: FOR EXTERNAL USE ONLY. Avoid contact with the eyes; if this happens, rinse thoroughly with water. If irritation develops, discontinue use. If condition worsens or does not improve after regular use of this product as directed, consult a physician. Do not use on children under 2 years of age except as directed by a physician. Use caution in exposing skin to sunlight after applying this product; it may increase your tendency to sunburn for up to 24 hours after application. Do not use for prolonged periods without consulting a physician. Do not use this product with other forms of psoriasis therapy such as ultraviolet radiation or prescription drugs unless directed to do so by a physician. If condition covers a large area of the body, consult your physician before using this product.

Caution: Keep this and all drugs out of the reach of children. In case of accidental ingestion, seek professional assistance or contact a Poison Control Center immediately.

Directions for Use: For best results, use X-SEB T® PLUS at least twice a week or as directed by physician. Wet hair, apply to scalp and massage vigorously. Rinse and repeat or as directed by physician.

How Supplied: 4 fl. oz. bottle (NDC 0575-1015-04); 8 fl. oz. bottle (NDC 0575-1015-08)

Shown in Product Identification Section, page 403

Beach Pharmaceuticals

Division of Beach Products, Inc.
5220 SOUTH MANHATTAN AVE.
TAMPA, FL 33611

BEELITH Tablets
MAGNESIUM SUPPLEMENT
With PYRIDOXINE HCl
Each tablet supplies 362 mg of magnesium (31.83 mEq).

Directions: As a dietary supplement, take one tablet daily or as directed by a physician. Each tablet yields 362 mg of magnesium and supplies 90% of the Adult U.S. Recommended Daily Allowance (RDA) for magnesium and 1000% of the Adult RDA for vitamin B_6.
Each tablet contains magnesium oxide 600 mg and pyridoxine hydrochloride (Vitamin B_6) 25 mg equivalent to B_6 20 mg. *Also, castor oil, hydroxypropyl methylcellulose, magnesium stearate, microcrystalline cellulose, pharmaceutical glaze, povidone, sodium starch glycolate, D&C Yellow #10, FD&C Yellow #6 (Sunset Yellow), and titanium dioxide.*

Drug Interaction Precautions: Do not take this product if you are presently taking a prescription antibiotic drug containing any form of tetracycline.

Warnings: If you have kidney disease, take only under the supervision of a physician. Excessive dosage may cause laxation. **KEEP OUT OF THE REACH OF CHILDREN.** Do not use if protective printed band around cap is broken or missing.

How Supplied: Golden yellow, film coated tablet with the name **BEACH** and the number **1132** printed on each tablet. Packaged in bottles of 100 (NDC 0486-1132-01) tablets.

Storage: Keep tightly closed. Store at 15°–30°C (59°–86°F). Protect from light.
R4/90

Shown on page 405 in the 1993 PHYSICIANS' DESK REFERENCE

Products are indexed by generic and chemical names in the **YELLOW SECTION.**

Beiersdorf Inc.

P.O. BOX 5529
NORWALK, CT 06856-5529

AQUAPHOR®—Original Formula Ointment
NDC Numbers–10356-020-01
10356-020-02

Composition: Petrolatum, mineral oil, mineral wax and wool wax alcohol.

Actions and Uses: Aquaphor is a stable, neutral, odorless, anhydrous ointment base. Miscible with water or aqueous solutions, Aquaphor will absorb several times its own weight, forming smooth, creamy water-in-oil emulsions. In its pure form, Aquaphor is recommended for use as a topical preparation to help heal severely dry skin. Aquaphor contains no preservatives, fragrances or known irritants.

Administration and Dosages: Use Aquaphor alone or in compounding virtually any ointment using aqueous solutions or in combination with other oil-based substances and all common topical medications. Apply Aquaphor liberally to affected area.

Precautions: For external use only. Avoid contact with eyes. Not to be applied over third degree burns, deep or puncture wounds, infections or lacerations. If condition worsens or does not improve within 7 days, patient should consult a doctor.

How Supplied: 16 oz. jar—List No. 45585; 5 lb. jar—List. No. 45586

Shown in Product Identification Section, page 403

AQUAPHOR® Antibiotic Ointment
NDC Number–10356-022-01

Composition: Polymyxin-B Sulfate/ Bacitracin Zinc, Petrolatum, Mineral Wax, Mineral Oil, Wool Wax Alcohol.

Actions and Uses: Aquaphor Antibiotic Formula is formulated to help reduce wound healing time and the risk of infection.[1] Recommended for prevention of infection in minor first-aid wounds and for use as a post-operative dressing. Aquaphor Antibiotic Formula is preservative-free, fragrance-free and hypoallergenic. It is recommended for patients with sensitive skin.

Administration and Dosage: Use Aquaphor Antibiotic Formula whenever a topical antibiotic ointment is needed to help prevent infection in minor cuts, scrapes and burns. Apply Aquaphor Antibiotic Formula liberally to affected area two to three times a day as needed.

Precautions: For external use only. Avoid contact with eyes, Not to be applied over third degree burns, deep or puncture wounds, infections or lacerations. If condition worsens or does not improve within seven days, patient should consult a physician.

How Supplied: .5 oz. tube.

1. Data on file, BDF Inc

Shown in Product Identification Section, page 403

AQUAPHOR® Natural Healing Ointment
NDC Number–10356-021-01

Composition: Petrolatum, Mineral Oil, Mineral Wax, Wool Wax Alcohol, Panthenol, Bisabolol, Glycerin.

Actions and Uses: Aquaphor Natural Healing Formula is specially formulated for faster healing of severely dry skin, cracked skin and minor burns. It is recommended for patients suffering from severe skin chapping and from skin disorders that result in severely dry, damaged skin. This formula is also indicated as a follow-up skin treatment for patients undergoing radiation therapy or other drying/burning medical therapies. It is preservative-free, fragrance-free and hypoallergenic, and is clinically proven to reduce wound healing time.[1]

Administration and Dosage: Use Aquaphor Natural Healing Formula whenever a mild healing agent is needed. Apply liberally to affected areas two to three times a day. In the case of minor wounds, clean area prior to application.

Precautions: For external use only. Avoid contact with the eyes. Not to be applied over third degree burns, deep or puncture wounds, infections or lacerations. If condition worsens or does not improve within seven days, patient should consult a physician.

How Supplied: 1.75 oz. tube

1. Data on file, BDF Inc

Shown in Product Identification Section, page 403

EUCERIN®
[*ū 'sir-in*]
Dry Skin Care Cleansing Bar

Actions and Uses: Eucerin® Cleansing Bar has been specially formulated for use on sensitive skin. The formulation contains Eucerite®, a special blend of ingredients that closely resemble the natural oils of the skin, thus providing excellent moisturizing properties. This formulation is fragrance-free and noncomedogenic. Additionally, the pH value of Eucerin Cleansing Bar is neutral so as not to affect the skin's normal acid mantle.

Directions: Use during shower, bath, or regular cleansing, or as directed by physician.

How Supplied:
3 ounce bar
List Number 3852

Shown in Product Identification Section, page 404

EUCERIN® Cleansing Lotion
Dry Skin Care

Composition: Water, Sodium Laureth Sulfate, Cocoamphodiacetate, Cocamidopropyl Betaine, PEG-7 Glyceryl Cocoate, Glycol Distearate, PEG-5 Lanolate, Citric Acid, Imidazolidinyl Urea, Cocamide MEA, Lanolin Alcohol.

Actions and Uses: Eucerin Cleansing Lotion is formulated for the care of dry, sensitive or irritated skin. Its soap-free formula combines gentle cleansing with unique moisturizing ingredients to both clean skin and protect it against dryness. It contains no fragrances, is non-comedogenic, and leaves no soapy residue. It is ideal for atopic dermatitis and psoriasis and can also be used as a mild baby bath.

Administration and Dosage: Wash with water; rinse thoroughly.

Precautions: For external use only.

How Supplied:
8 Fluid oz.—List Number 3962
1 Fluid oz.—List Number 3960

Shown in Product Identification Section, page 404

EUCERIN® Creme
[*ū 'sir-in*]
Dry Skin Care
NDC Numbers—10356-090-01
10356-090-05
10356-090-04
10356-090-07

Composition: Water, petrolatum, mineral oil, wool wax alcohol, methylchloroisothiazolinone, methylisothiazolinone.

Actions and Uses: A gentle, noncomedogenic, fragrance-free water-in-oil emulsion. Eucerin can be used as a treatment for dry skin associated with eczema, psoriasis, chapped or chafed skin, sunburn, windburn and itching associated with dryness.

Administration and Dosages: Apply freely to affected areas of the skin as often as necessary or as directed by physician.

Precautions: For external use only.

How Supplied:
16 oz. jar—List Number 0090
8 oz. jar—List Number 3774
4 oz. jar—List Number 3797
2 oz. tube—List Number 3868

Shown in Product Identification Section, page 404

EUCERIN® DAILY FACIAL LOTION
NDC Number–10356-972-01

Composition: Ethylhexyl p-methoxycinnamate, Titanium Dioxide, 2-Phenylbenzamidazole-5-Sulfonic Acid, 2-Ethylhexyl Salicylate. **Other Ingredients:** Triple Purified Water, Caprylic/Capric Triglyceride, Mineral Oil, Octyl Stearate, Cetearyl Alcohol, Glyceryl Stearate, Sodium Hydroxide, PEG-40 Castor Oil, Acrylamide/Sodium Acrylate Copolymer, Sodium Cetearyl Sulfate, Lanolin Alcohol, EDTA, Methylchloroisothiazolinone, Methylisothiazolinone.

Actions and Uses: Eucerin Daily Facial Lotion is fragrance-free, non-comedogenic and non-acnegenic, with an SPF 20 non-sensitive sunscreen to protect skin from UVA and UVB rays. It is specially formulated for dry, sensitive skin or for those undergoing therapies which irritate delicate facial skin such as Retin-A® therapy, chemical peels and treatment with drying medications. This light, oil-in-water formula is non-greasy and is easily absorbed into the skin.

Administration and Dosage: Apply Eucerin Daily Facial Lotion twice a day (especially in the morning), or as directed by a physician, to nourish and moisture skin and protect it from harmful UVA and UVB rays.

Precautions: For external use only, not to be swallowed. Avoid contact with eyes. Discontinue use if signs of irritation or rash appear. Use on children under 6 months of age only with the advice of a physician.

How Supplied:
4-oz. bottle.

Shown in Product Identification Section, page 404

EUCERIN® Lotion
[*ū 'sir-in*]
Dry Skin Care Lotion
NDC Numbers—10356-793-01
10356-793-04
10356-793-06

Composition: Water, Mineral Oil, Isopropyl Myristate, PEG-40 Sorbitan Peroleate, Lanolin Acid Glycerin Ester, Sorbitol, Propylene Glycol, Cetyl Palmitate, Magnesium Sulfate, Aluminum Stearate, Wool Wax Alcohol, BHT, Methylchloroisothiazolinone, Methylisothiazolinone.

Actions and Uses: Eucerin Lotion is a unique non-comedogenic, fragrance-free, water-in-oil formulation that will help to alleviate and soothe excessively dry skin, and provide long-lasting moisturization.

Administration and Dosage: Use daily as preventative care for skin exposed to sun, water, wind, cold or other drying elements.

Precautions: For external use only.

How Supplied:
4 fluid oz. plastic bottle—
List Number 3771
8 fluid oz. plastic bottle—
List Number 3793
16 fluid oz. plastic bottle—
List number 3794

Shown in Product Identification Section, page 404

Continued on next page

Beiersdorf—Cont.

EUCERIN PLUS®
Moisturizing Lotion
NDC #10356-967-01

Composition: Water, Mineral Oil, PEG-7, Hydrogenated Castor Oil, Isohexadecane, Sodium Lactate 5%, Urea 5%, Glycerin, Isopropyl Palmitate, Panthenol, Ozokerite, Magnesium Sulfate, Lanolin Alcohol, Bisabolol, Methylchloroisothiazolinone, Methylisothiazolinone.

Actions and Uses: Eucerin Plus® Moisturizing Lotion is a unique sodium lactate, urea formulation that is clinically proven to relieve chronic dry, scaly skin conditions. Hypo-allergenic and pH balanced, it is not likely to cause transient burning or stinging upon application.[1] Fragrance free and non-comedogenic, it is ideal for xerosis, psoriasis and other hyper keratolitic skin conditions.

Administration and Dosage: Use daily on severely dry, scaly skin or as directed by a physician.

Precautions: Avoid contact with eyes. For external use only. Keep out of the reach of children.

Supplied: 6-oz bottle.

1. Data on File

Shown in Product Identification Section, page 404

BioLink Intl. Inc.
1502 BRITTAIN RD.
AKRON, OHIO 44310

PRODUCT LISTING

BioBars, diet and fitness bar
BioClenz, herbal bowel activator
BioEner-G-Thin, fat-reducing energizer
BioTrim, high-fiber, nonfat drink
CalLink, calcium, magnesium plus
ChildLink, VitaLink II for children
LifeLink, arthritic pain reliever plus
VitaLink II

VITALINK II
Potent Multivitamin and Mineral Supplement

Description: Its advanced antioxidant nutrient formula helps neutralize free radicals that have been indicated to damage healthy cells. It contains all the protector nutrients in high amounts and proper ratios.

Ingredients: Vitamin A (β-carotene), all B complexes, and vitamins C, D, E, and K, plus all essential minerals in chelated form and all 17 L-amino acids.

How Supplied: 60 tablets per bottle

Products are indexed by generic and chemical names in the **YELLOW SECTION.**

The Biopractic Group II, Inc.
99 BROAD STREET
PO BOX 5300
PHILLIPSBURG, NJ 08865

SURGEON'S CHOICE® Powder
(Psyllium Hydrophilic Mucilloid)

Description: A bulk-forming, non-irritant laxative containing ducosate sodium to potentiate water penetration of the psyllium seed husk. Each 7.5 g. adult dose contains 3.4 g. psyllium hydrophilic mucilloid and .01 g. ducosate sodium. Ducosate content per dose is approximately 25% of the amount in an adult dose of Colace.

Inactive Ingredients: Anhydrous dextrose, fructose, gelatin, cherry and orange flavors, citric acid, ducosate sodium, FD&C Red #40.

Actions and Uses: SURGEON'S CHOICE formula is indicated for management of temporary or chronic constipation, especially when easy, comfortable evacuation is desired, as in the case of hemorrhoid patients. An easily dispersed powder with a gel-delaying formula to allow maximized water absorption by the psyllium husk.

Indications: SURGEON'S CHOICE is indicated for management of temporary or chronic constipation. The addition of ducosate sodium as a wetting agent for the psyllium husk provides maximized bulking action and comfortable evacuation.

Contraindications: Fecal impaction, gross intestinal pathology, known sensitivity to formula ingredients.

Dosage and Administration: Stir one heaping teaspoonful (7.5 g.) briskly into at least 8 oz. of liquid and drink entire amount. Drinking a second glass of liquid is helpful.

Adult Dosage: One heaping teaspoon (7.5 g.) 2 to 3 times daily until regularity is established. If recommended by your physician, SURGEON'S CHOICE may be continued once or twice daily. **Children 6 to 12:** One-half the usual adult dose or as recommended by a physician. **Children under 6:** Consult a physician.

Warnings: May cause allergic reaction in people allergic to inhaled or ingested psyllium powder. Do not use laxative products when abdominal pain, nausea or vomiting are present unless directed by a physician. Mix any bulk laxative product with at least 8 oz. of fluid. Using a bulk product without adequate fluid may cause it to swell and block the throat or esophagus and may cause choking. Do not use if you have ever had difficulty swallowing or throat problems.

How Supplied: Powder, 13-oz. jar.

Blaine Company, Inc.
1465 JAMIKE LANE
ERLANGER, KY 41018

MAG–OX 400

Description: Each tablet contains Magnesium Oxide 400 mg. U.S.P. (Heavy), or 241.3 mg. Elemental Magnesium (19.86 mEq.)

Indications and Usage: Hypomagnesemia, magnesium deficiencies and/or magnesium depletion resulting from malnutrition, restricted diet, alcoholism or magnesium depleting drugs. An antacid. For increasing urinary magnesium excretion. For magnesium supplementation during pregnancy.

Warnings: Do not use this product except under the advice and supervision of a physician if you have a kidney disease. May have laxative effect.

Dosage: Adult dose 1 or 2 tablets daily or as directed by a physician.

Professional Labeling: Mag-Ox 400 Tablets for recurring calcium oxalate urinary calculi; for maintenance of tocolysis; for PMS therapy.

How Supplied: Bottles of 100 and 1000.

URO–MAG

Description: Each capsule contains Magnesium Oxide 140 mg. U.S.P. (Heavy), or 84.5 mg. Elemental Magnesium (6.93 mEq.)

Indications and Usage: Hypomagnesemia, magnesium deficiencies and/or magnesium depletion resulting from malnutrition, restricted diet, alcoholism or magnesium depleting drugs. An antacid. For increasing urinary magnesium excretion. For magnesium supplementation during pregnancy.

Warnings: Do not use this product except under the advice and supervision of a physician if you have a kidney disease. May have laxative effect.

Dosage: Adult dose 3–4 capsules daily or as directed by a physician.

Professional Labeling: URO-MAG Capsules for recurring calcium oxalate urinary calculi; for maintenance of tocolysis; for PMS therapy.

How Supplied: Bottles of 100 and 1000.

EDUCATIONAL MATERIAL

Female reproductive system and kidney stone charts, samples and literature available to physicians upon request.

Blairex Laboratories, Inc.
4810 TECUMSEH LANE
P.O BOX 15190
EVANSVILLE, IN 47716-0190

BRONCHO SALINE®
0.9% Sodium Chloride Aerosol for the dilution of bronchodilator inhalation solutions. Sterile normal saline for diluting bronchodilator solutions for oral inhalation.

Description: Broncho Saline® is for patients using bronchodilator solutions for oral inhalation that require dilution with sterile normal saline solution. Broncho Saline is a sterile liquid solution consisting of 0.9% sodium chloride for oral inhalation with a pH of 4.5 to 7.5. Not to be used for injection.

Indications and Usage: Patients who use bronchodilator solutions for inhalation are instructed to dilute the medication with sterile normal saline solution. Bronchodilators that call for dilution with saline for administration by nebulization include:

Alupent Inhalation Solution (Metaproterenol Sulfate, USP, 5%)
Bronkosol (Isoetharine Hydrochloride, USP, 1%)
Isuprel Hydrochloride (Isoproterenol Hydrochloride)
Proventil Solution for Inhalation (Albuterol Sulfate, 0.5%)
Ventolin Solution for Inhalation (Albuterol Sulfate, 0.5%)

Warnings: Use this product only with the approval of your physician, respiratory therapist or pharmacist. Contents under pressure. Do not puncture or incinerate. Keep out of reach of children. If you experience any complications, contact your physician immediately.

Directions for Use:
1. Add the prescribed dosage of bronchodilator medication to the nebulizer cup.
2. Pick up Broncho Saline® and look at the top parts. Line up parts so the half-circle under the valve cap fits over nozzle. This is necessary to press the valve cap down.
3. To dispense Broncho Saline®, aim nozzle, press, and release. Each time you press and release the valve, 1cc (mL) of saline is dispensed. If you need 2cc (mL), depress and release the valve twice. For 3cc (mL), depress and release the valve three times, and so on.
4. Dispense the recommended amount of saline into the nebulizer cup.
5. Proceed with the normal operation of your breathing apparatus.
6. When finished with your treatment, the reservoir should be rinsed clean with warm water. Please follow the cleaning instructions with your breathing apparatus.

How Supplied: Broncho Saline® comes in 90cc (mL) and 240cc (mL) Pressurized Containers.

Store between 15–25°C (59–77°F). Keep out of reach of children. See WARNINGS.

NASAL MOIST®
Sodium Chloride 0.65%

Description: Isotonic saline solution buffered with sodium bicarbonate. Preserved with Benzyl alcohol.

Actions and Uses: Use for dry nasal membranes caused by chronic sinusitis, allergy, asthma, dry air, oxygen therapy. May be used as often as needed.

Directions: Squeeze twice into each nostril as needed.

How Supplied: 45 mL (1.5 oz.) plastic squeeze bottle.

Block Drug Company, Inc.
257 CORNELISON AVENUE
JERSEY CITY, NJ 07302

ARTHRITIS STRENGTH BC® POWDER

Active Ingredients: Aspirin 742 mg in combination with 222 mg Salicylamide and 36 mg Caffeine per powder.

Indications: Arthritis Strength BC Powder is specially formulated to fight occasional minor pain and inflammation of arthritis. Like original formula BC, Arthritis Strength BC provides fast temporary relief of minor arthritis pain and inflammation, neuralgia, neuritis and sciatica; relief of muscular aches, discomfort and fever of colds; and pain of tooth extraction.

Warning: Children and teenagers should not use this medicine for chicken pox or flu symptoms before a doctor is consulted about Reye Syndrome, a rare but serious illness reported to be associated with aspirin. Do not exceed recommended dosage or administer to children, including teenagers, with chicken pox or flu, unless directed by a physician. Do not take this product if you are allergic to aspirin, have asthma, gastric ulcer, or are taking a medication that affects the clotting of blood, except under the advice and supervision of a physician. If pain persists for more than 10 days or redness is present, discontinue use of this product and consult a physician immediately. Keep this and all medication out of children's reach. As with any drug, if you are pregnant or nursing a baby, consult your physician before using this product. IT IS ESPECIALLY IMPORTANT NOT TO USE ASPIRIN DURING THE LAST 3 MONTHS OF PREGNANCY UNLESS SPECIFICALLY DIRECTED TO DO SO BY A DOCTOR BECAUSE IT MAY CAUSE PROBLEMS IN THE UNBORN CHILD OR COMPLICATIONS DURING DELIVERY. Discontinue use if ringing in the ears occurs. In case of accidental overdosage, contact a physician or poison control center immediately.

Dosage and Administration: Place one powder on tongue and follow with liquid. If you prefer, stir powder into glass of water or other liquid. May be used every three to four hours, up to 4 powders each 24 hours. For children under 12, consult a physician.

How Supplied: Available in tamper resistant cellophane wrapped envelopes of 6 powders, and tamper resistant cellophane wrapped boxes of 24 and 50 powders.

BC® COLD POWDER
BC® Cold Powder Multi-Symptom Formula (Cold-Sinus-Allergy)
BC® Cold Powder Non-Drowsy Formula (Cold-Sinus)

Active Ingredients: *BC Cold Powder Multi-Symptom Formula (Cold-Sinus-Allergy)*—Aspirin 650 mg, Phenylpropanolamine Hydrochloride 25 mg, and Chlorpheniramine Maleate 4 mg per powder. *BC Cold Powder Non-Drowsy Formula* (Cold·Sinus) Aspirin 650 mg and Phenylpropanolamine Hydrochloride 25 mg per powder.

Indications: *BC Cold Powder Multi-Symptom* (Cold·Sinus·Allergy) is for relief of cold symptoms such as body aches, fever, nasal congestion, sneezing, running nose, and watery itchy eyes. *BC Cold Powder Non-Drowsy Formula (Cold-Sinus)* is for relief of such symptoms as body aches, fever, and nasal congestions.

Warnings: Children and teenagers should not use this medicine for chicken pox or flu symptoms before a doctor is consulted about Reye syndrome, a rare but serious illness reported to be associated with aspirin. Keep this and all medicines out of children's reach. In case of accidental overdose, contact a physician immediately. As with any drug, if you are pregnant or nursing a baby, seek the advice of a health professional before using this product. IT IS ESPECIALLY IMPORTANT NOT TO USE ASPIRIN DURING THE LAST 3 MONTHS OF PREGNANCY UNLESS SPECIFICALLY DIRECTED TO DO SO BY A DOCTOR BECAUSE IT MAY CAUSE PROBLEMS IN THE UNBORN CHILD OR COMPLICATIONS DURING DELIVERY. Do not exceed recommended dosage. If symptoms do not improve within 7 days, or are accompanied by high fever, consult a physician before continuing use. Do not take this product if you have high blood pressure, heart disease, diabetes, or thyroid disease except under the advice and supervision of a physician. Do not take this product if you are presently taking a prescription antihypertensive or antidepressant drug containing a monoamine oxidase inhibitor except under the advice and supervi-

Continued on next page

Block Drug—Cont.

sion of a physician. This product contains aspirin and should not be taken by individuals who are sensitive to aspirin. BC Cold Powder Multi-Symptom with antihistamine may cause drowsiness. Avoid alcoholic beverages while taking this product. Use caution when driving a motor vehicle or operating machinery.

Dosage and Administration: *Adults*—Stir one powder into a glass of water or other liquid, or place powder on tongue and follow with liquid. May be used every 4 hours up to 4 times a day. *For children under 12*—consult a physician.

How Supplied: Available in tamper-resistant cellophane-wrapped envelopes of 6 powders, as well as tamper-resistant boxes of 24 powders.

BC® POWDER
[*bee-see*]

Active Ingredients: Aspirin 650 mg per powder, Salicylamide 195 mg per powder and Caffeine 32 mg per powder.

Indications: BC Powder is for relief of simple headache; for temporary relief of minor arthritic pain, neuralgia, neuritis and sciatica; for relief of muscular aches, discomfort and fever of colds; and for relief of normal menstrual pain and pain of tooth extraction.

Warning: Children and teenagers should not use this medicine for chicken pox or flu symptoms before a doctor is consulted about Reye Syndrome, a rare but serious illness reported to be associated with aspirin. Do not exceed recommended dosage or administer to children, including teenagers, with chicken pox or flu, unless directed by a physician. Do not take this product if you are allergic to aspirin, have asthma, gastric ulcer, or are taking a medication that affects the clotting of blood, except under the advice and supervision of a physician. If pain persists for more than 10 days or redness is present, discontinue use of this product and consult a physician immediately. Keep this and all medication out of children's reach. As with any drug, if you are pregnant or nursing a baby, consult your physician before using this product. IT IS ESPECIALLY IMPORTANT NOT TO USE ASPIRIN DURING THE LAST 3 MONTHS OF PREGNANCY UNLESS SPECIFICALLY DIRECTED TO DO SO BY A DOCTOR BECAUSE IT MAY CAUSE PROBLEMS IN THE UNBORN CHILD OR COMPLICATIONS DURING DELIVERY. Discontinue use if ringing in the ears occurs.
In case of accidental overdosage, contact a physician or poison control center immediately.

Dosage and Administration: Stir one powder into a glass of water or other liquid, or, place powder on tongue and follow with liquid. May be used every 3 or 4 hours up to 4 times a day. For children under 12 consult a physician.

How Supplied: Available in tamper resistant cellophane wrapped envelopes of 2 or 6 powders, as well as tamper resistant boxes of 24 and 50 powders.

NYTOL® TABLETS

Active Ingredient: Diphenhydramine Hydrochloride, 25 mg per tablet (NYTOL with DPH) and 50 mg per tablet (Maximum Strength NYTOL).

Indications: Diphenhydramine Hydrochloride is an antihistamine with anticholinergic and sedative effects which induces drowsiness and helps in falling asleep.

Warnings: Do not give children under 12 years of age. If sleeplessness persists continuously for more than 2 weeks, consult your doctor. Insomnia may be a symptom of serious underlying medical illness. Do not take this product if you have asthma, glaucoma, emphysema, chronic pulmonary disorders, shortness of breath, difficulty in breathing or difficulty in urination due to enlargement of the prostate gland unless directed by a doctor. Avoid alcoholic beverages while taking this product. Do not take this product if you are taking tranquilizers or sedatives, without first consulting your doctor. In case of accidental overdose seek professional assistance or contact a poison control center immediately. As with any drug, if your are pregnant or nursing a baby, seek the advice of a health professional before using this product. Keep this and all drugs out of the reach of children.

Drug Interaction: Alcohol and other drugs which cause CNS depression will heighten the depressant effect of this product. Monoamine oxidase (MAO) inhibitors will prolong and intensify the anticholinergic effects of antihistamines.

Symptoms and Treatment of Oral Overdosage: In adults overdose may cause CNS depression resulting in hypnosis and coma. In children CNS hyperexcitability may follow sedation; the stimulant phase may bring tremor, delirium and convulsions. Gastrointestinal reactions may include dry mouth, appetite loss, nausea and vomiting. Respiratory distress and cardiovascular complications (hypotension) may be evident. Treatment includes inducing emesis, and controlling symptoms.

Dosage and Administration: Adults and children 12 years of age and over, take 2 NYTOL with DPH or 1 Maximum Strength NYTOL tablet 20 minutes at bedtime if needed, or as directed by a physician.

How Supplied: Available in tamper resistant packages of 16, 32, and 72 tablets NYTOL with DPH; of 8 and 16 tablets Maximum Strength NYTOL.

PROMISE® SENSITIVE TEETH TOOTHPASTE
Desensitizing Dentifrice

Active Ingredients: Potassium Nitrate and Sodium Monofluorophosphate in a pleasantly mint-flavored dentifrice.

Promise contains Potassium Nitrate for relief of dentinal hypersensitivity resulting from the exposure of tooth dentin due to periodontal surgery, cervical (gumline) erosion, abrasion or recession which causes pain on contact with hot, cold, or tactile stimuli. Promise also contains Sodium Monofluorophosphate for cavity prevention.

Indications: Helps reduce painful sensitivity of the teeth to cold, heat, acids, sweets or contact and aids in the prevention of dental cavities.

Actions: Promise significantly reduces tooth hypersensitivity, with response to therapy evident after two weeks of use. Controlled double-blind clinical studies provide substantial evidence of the safety and effectiveness of Promise. The current theory on mechanism of action is that the potassium nitrate in Promise has an effect on neural transmission, interrupting the signal which would result in the sensation of pain. Sodium Monofluorophosphate protects the tooth surfaces to prevent cavities.

Warning: Sensitive teeth may indicate a serious problem that may need prompt care by a dentist. See your dentist if the problem persists or worsens. Do not use this product longer than 4 weeks unless recommended by a dentist or doctor.
Keep this and all drugs out of the reach of children.

Directions: Adults and children 12 years of age and older:
Apply at least a 1-inch strip of the product onto a soft bristle toothbrush. Brush teeth thoroughly for at least 1 minute twice a day (morning and evening) or as recommended by a dentist or doctor.

How Supplied: Promise Toothpaste is supplied in 1.6 oz. and 3.0 oz. tubes.

ORIGINAL FORMULA SENSODYNE® -SC
Toothpaste for Sensitive Teeth

Description: Each tube contains strontium chloride hexahydrate (10%) in a pleasantly flavored cleansing/polishing desensitizing dentifrice.

Actions/Indications: Tooth hypersensitivity is a condition in which individuals experience pain from exposure to hot, cold stimuli, from chewing fibrous foods, or from tactile stimuli (e.g. toothbrushing.) Hypersensitivity usually occurs when the protective enamel covering on teeth wears away (which happens most often at the gum line) or if gum tissue recedes and exposes the dentin underneath.
Running through the dentin are microscopic small "tubules" which, according

to many authorities, carry the pain impulses to the nerve of the tooth.

Sensodyne-SC provides a unique ingredient—strontium chloride—which is believed to be deposited in the tubules where it blocks the pain. The longer Sensodyne-SC is used, the more of a barrier it helps build against pain.

The effect of Sensodyne-SC may not be manifested immediately and may require a few weeks or longer of use for relief to be obtained. A number of clinical studies in the U.S. and other countries have provided substantial evidence of Sensodyne-SC's performance attributes. Complete relief of hypersensitivity has been reported in approximately 65% of users and measurable relief or reduction in hypersensitivity in approximately 90%. The Original Formula has been commercially available for over 30 years. The ADA Council on Dental Therapeutics has given Sensodyne-SC the Seal of Acceptance as an effective desensitizing dentifrice in otherwise normal teeth.

Contraindications: Subjects with severe dental erosion should brush properly and lightly with any dentifrice to avoid further removal of tooth structure.

Dosage and Administration: Apply at least a 1-inch strip of the product onto a soft bristle toothbrush. Brush teeth thoroughly for at least 1 minute twice a day (morning and evening) or as recommended by a dentist or doctor. Make sure to brush all sensitive areas of the teeth. Children under 12 years of age: consult a dentist or doctor.

Warnings: Sensitive teeth may indicate a serious problem that may need prompt care by a dentist. See your dentist if the problem persists or worsens. Do not use this product longer than 4 weeks unless recommended by a dentist or doctor.

How Supplied: SENSODYNE-SC Toothpaste is supplied in 2.1 oz., 4.0 oz., and 6.0 oz. tubes and in 4.0 oz. pumps.
(U.S. Patent No. 3,122,483)

FRESH MINT SENSODYNE®
COOL GEL SENSODYNE®
Toothpaste for Sensitive Teeth and Cavity Prevention
Desensitizing Dentrifice

Active Ingredients: 5% Potassium Nitrate and Sodium Monofluorophosphate (Fresh Mint) or Sodium Fluoride (Cool Gel) in a pleasantly mint-flavored dentifrice.

Fresh Mint Sensodyne and Cool Gel Sensodyne contain Potassium Nitrate for relief of dentinal hypersensitivity resulting from the exposure of tooth dentin due to periodontal surgery, cervical (gum line) erosion, abrasion or recession which causes pain on contact with hot, cold, or tactile stimuli and fluoride for cavity prevention. Fresh Mint Sensodyne has been given the Seal of Acceptance by the ADA Council on Dental Therapeutics as an effective desensitizing dentifrice for otherwise normal teeth.

Actions: Fresh Mint Sensodyne and Cool Gel Sensodyne significantly reduce tooth hypersensitivity, with response to therapy evident after two weeks of use. Controlled double-blind clinical studies provide substantial evidence of the safety and effectiveness of potassium nitrate. The current theory on mechanism of action is that potassium nitrate has an effect on neural transmission, interrupting the signal which would result in the sensation of pain. Fluorides are anticariogenic, forming fluoroapatite in the outer surface of the dental enamel which is resistant to acids and caries.

Warnings: Sensitive teeth may indicate a serious problem that may need prompt care by a dentist. See your dentist if the problem persists or worsens. Do not use this product longer than 4 weeks unless recommended by a dentist or doctor.

Dosage and Administration: Apply at least a 1-inch strip of the product onto a soft bristle toothbrush. Brush teeth thoroughly for at least 1 minute twice a day (morning and evening) or as recommended by a dentist or doctor. Make sure to brush all sensitive areas of the teeth. Children under 12 years of age: consult a dentist or doctor.

How Supplied: Fresh Mint Sensodyne and Cool Gel Sensodyne Toothpastes are supplied in 2.1 and 4.0 oz. tubes and in 4 oz. pumps.
(U.S. Patent No. 3,863,006)

TEGRIN® DANDRUFF SHAMPOO
[tĕg 'rĭn]

Description: Tegrin® Dandruff Shampoo contains 7% coal tar solution equivalent to 1.4% coal tar, in a pleasantly scented, high-foaming, cleansing shampoo base with emollients, conditioners and other formula components.

Actions/Indications: Coal Tar is obtained in the destructive distillation of bituminous coal and is a highly effective agent for controlling the flaking and itching of the scalp associated with dandruff, seborrheic dermatitis and psoriasis. The action of coal tar is believed to be keratolytic, antiseptic, antipruritic and astringent. The coal tar solution used in Tegrin Dandruff Shampoo is prepared in such a way as to reduce the pitch and other irritant components found in crude coal tar without reduction in therapeutic potency.

Coal tar solution has been used clinically for many years as a remedy for dandruff and for scaling associated with scalp disorders such as seborrhea and psoriasis. Its mechanism of action has not been fully established, but it is believed to retard the rate of turnover of epidermal cells with regular use. A number of clinical studies have demonstrated the performance attributes of Tegrin Dandruff Shampoo against dandruff and seborrheic dermatitis. In addition to relieving the above symptoms, Tegrin shampoo, used regularly, maintains scalp and hair cleanliness and leaves the hair lustrous and manageable.

Warnings: For external use only. Avoid contact with eyes. If contact occurs, rinse eyes thoroughly with water. If condition worsens or does not improve after regular use of this product as directed, consult a doctor. Use caution in exposing skin to sunlight after applying this product. It may increase tendency to sunburn for up to 24 hours after application. Do not use for prolonged periods without consulting a doctor. Do not use this product with other forms of psoriasis therapy, such as ultraviolet radiation or prescription drugs, unless directed by a doctor. Keep out of reach of children. In case of accidental ingestion, seek professional assistance or contact a Poison Control Center immediately.

Directions: Shake well. Wet hair thoroughly. Rub Tegrin liberally into hair and scalp. Rinse thoroughly. Briskly massage a second application of the shampoo into a rich lather. Rinse thoroughly. For best results use at least twice a week or as directed by a doctor.

How Supplied: Tegrin Dandruff Shampoo is supplied in 7 fl. oz. (207 ml) plastic bottles.

TEGRIN® for Psoriasis Lotion, Skin Cream and Medicated Soap
[tĕg 'rĭn]

Active Ingredients: Tegrin Lotion, Skin Cream and Medicated Soap each contain 5% coal tar solution, equivalent to 0.8% coal tar. Both the Lotion and Cream also contain alcohol (4.9% and 4.7%, respectively).

Actions/Indications: Coal tar is obtained in the destructive distillation of bituminous coal and is a highly effective agent that helps to relieve the itching, flaking and irritation of the skin associated with psoriasis and seborrheic dermatitis. The action of coal tar is believed to be keratolytic, antiseptic, antipruritic and astringent. The coal tar solution used in the Tegrin products is prepared in such a way as to reduce the pitch and other irritant components found in crude coal tar.

Warnings: For external use only. Avoid contact with eyes. If contact occurs, rinse eyes thoroughly with water. If condition worsens or does not improve after regular use of this product as directed consult a doctor. Do not use this product in or around the rectum or in the genital area or groin except on the advice of a doctor. Use caution in exposing skin to sunlight after applying this product; it may increase tendency to sunburn for up to 24 hours after application. Do not use for prolonged periods without consulting

Continued on next page

Block Drug—Cont.

a doctor. Do not use this product with other forms of psoriasis therapy, such as ultraviolet radiation or prescription drugs, unless directed by a doctor. If the condition covers a large area of the body, consult your doctor before using this product. Keep out of reach of children. In case of accidental ingestion, seek professional assistance or contact a Poison Control Center immediately.

Directions: Apply lotion or cream to affected areas one to four times daily or as directed by a doctor. Use Tegrin Soap on affected areas in place of your regular soap.

How Supplied: Tegrin Lotion 7 fl. oz. (207 ml) bottle, Tegrin Cream 2 oz. (57 g) and 4.4 oz. (124 g) tubes, Tegrin Soap 4.5 oz. (127 g) bars.

TEGRIN®-HC WITH HYDROCORTISONE ANTI-ITCH OINTMENT

Description: Tegrin-HC is a special fragrance-free ointment which contains 1.0% hydrocortisone, an effective anti-itch ingredient in the maximum strength available without a prescription.

Indications: Tegrin-HC is for the temporary relief of itching associated with minor skin irritations, inflammation, rashes due to psoriasis, eczema and seborrheic dermatitis; other uses of this product should be only under the advice and supervision of a doctor.

Warning: For external use only. Avoid contact with the eyes. If condition worsens, or if symptoms persist for more than 7 days, or clear up again within a few days, stop use of this product and do not use any other hydrocortisone products unless you have consulted a doctor. Do not use for the treatment of diaper rash; consult a doctor. In case of accidental ingestion, get professional assistance or contact a poison control center immediately. **KEEP OUT OF THE REACH OF CHILDREN.**

Directions: Adults and children 2 years of age and older: apply to affected area not more than 3 to 4 times daily. Children under 2 years of age: Do not use, consult a doctor.

Products are indexed alphabetically in the **PINK SECTION.**

Bock Pharmacal Company

P.O. BOX 8519
ST. LOUIS, MO 63126-0519

EMETROL®
(Phosphorated Carbohydrate Solution)
For the relief of nausea associated with upset stomach

Description: EMETROL is an oral solution containing balanced amounts of dextrose (glucose) and levulose (fructose) and phosphoric acid with controlled hydrogen ion concentration. Available in original lemon-mint or cherry flavor.

Ingredients: Each 5 mL teaspoonful contains dextrose (glucose), 1.87 g; levulose (fructose), 1.87 g; phosphoric acid, 21.5 mg; and the following inactive ingredients: glycerin, methylparaben, purified water; D&C yellow No. 10 and natural lemon-mint flavor in lemon-mint Emetrol; FD&C red No. 40 and artificial cherry flavor in cherry Emetrol.

Action: EMETROL quickly relieves nausea by local action on the wall of the hyperactive G.I. tract. No delay in therapeutic action such as that associated with systemic drugs.

Indications: For the relief of nausea due to upset stomach from intestinal flu and food or drink indiscretions. For other conditions, take only as directed by your physician.

Advantages:
1. **Fast Action**—works quickly through local action on contact with the hyperactive G.I. tract.
2. **Effectiveness**—clinically proven to stop nausea.
3. **Safety**—all natural active ingredients won't mask symptoms of organic pathology. No known drug interactions.
4. **Convenience**—no ℞ required.
5. **Patient Acceptance**—pleasant tasting lemon-mint or cherry flavor

Usual Adult Dose: One or two tablespoonfuls. Repeat every 15 minutes until distress subsides.

Usual Children's Dose: One or two teaspoonfuls. Repeat dose every 15 minutes until distress subsides.

Important: Never dilute EMETROL or drink fluids of any kind immediately before or after taking a dose.

Caution: Not to be taken for more than one hour (5 doses) without consulting a physician. If upset stomach continues or recurs frequently, consult a physician promptly as it may be a sign of a serious condition.
WARNING: KEEP THIS AND ALL MEDICATIONS OUT OF THE REACH OF CHILDREN. As with any drug, if you are pregnant or nursing a baby, seek the advice of a health professional before using this product.

This product contains fructose and should not be taken by persons with hereditary fructose intolerance (HFI).

> **This product contains sugar and should not be taken by diabetics except under the advice and supervision of a physician.**

In case of accidental overdose, contact a poison control center, emergency medical facility, or physician immediately for advice.

How Supplied: Each 5 mL teaspoonful of EMETROL contains dextrose (glucose), 1.87 g; levulose (fructose), 1.87 g; and phosphoric acid, 21.5 mg in a yellow, lemon-mint or red, cherry-flavored syrup.

Yellow, Lemon-Mint
NDC 0013-2113-45—Bottle of 4 fluid ounces (118 mL)
NDC 0013-2113-65—Bottle of 8 fluid ounces (236 mL)
NDC 0013-2113-51—Bottle of 1 pint (473 mL)

Red, Cherry
NDC 0013-2114-45—Bottle of 4 fluid ounces (118 mL)
NDC 0013-2114-65—Bottle of 8 fluid ounces (236 mL)
NDC 0013-2114-51—Bottle of 1 pint (473 mL)

Store at room temperature.

NOTICE: Each bottle is protected by a printed band around the cap. Do not use if band is damaged or missing.

Shown in Product Identification Section, page 404

Boiron USA

1208 AMOSLAND ROAD
NORWOOD, PA 19074

OSCILLOCOCCINUM®
[ah-sill 'o-cox-see 'num ']

Active Ingredient: Anas Barbariae Hepatis et Cordis Extractum HPUS 200C

Indications: For the relief of flu-like symptoms such as fever, chills, body aches and pains.

Actions: Like most Homeopathic remedies, Oscillococcinum® acts gently by stimulating the patient's natural defense mechanisms.

Warnings: If symptoms persist for more than three days or worsen, consult your physician. Keep all medication out of reach of children. As with any drug if you are pregnant or nursing a baby, seek professional advice before using this product.

Dosage and Administration: (Adults and Children over 2 years)
At the onset of symptoms, place the entire contents of one tube in your mouth and allow to dissolve under your tongue. Repeat every 6 hours as necessary. For maximum results, Oscillococcinum®

should be taken early, at the onset of symptoms, and at least 15 minutes before or 1 hour after meals.

How Supplied: boxes of 3 unit doses or 6 unit doses of 0.04 oz. (1 gram) each (NDC #0220-9280-32 and NDC #0220-9288-33) Tamper resistant package.
Manufactured by Boiron, France.
Distributor: Boiron, Norwood, PA

Shown in Product Identification Section, page 404

EDUCATIONAL MATERIAL

Boiron Product Catalogue
General description of the most popular Boiron remedies and lines.
Oscillococcinum **® Brochure**
Brochure on Oscillococcinum® describing clinical research on the product and its general use.
"What 's Homeopathy?"
Booklet free to physicians and pharmacists.
"An Introduction to Homeopathy for the Practicing Pharmacist"
A free continuing education booklet for pharmacists.

Bristol-Myers Products

(A Bristol-Myers Squibb Company)
345 PARK AVENUE
NEW YORK, NY 10154

ALPHA KERI®
Moisture Rich Body Oil

Composition: Contains mineral oil, Hydroloc™ brand of Westwood's PEG-4 dilaurate, lanolin oil, fragrance, benzophenone-3, D&C green 6.

Indications: ALPHA KERI is a water-dispersible oil for the care of dry skin. ALPHA KERI effectively deposits a thin, uniform, emulsified film of oil over the skin. This film lubricates and softens the skin. ALPHA KERI Moisture Rich Body Oil is an all-over skin moisturizer. Only Alpha Keri contains Hydroloc™—the unique emulsifier that provides a more uniform distribution of the therapeutic oils to moisturize dry skin. ALPHA KERI is valuable as an aid for dry skin and mild skin irritations.

Directions for Use: ALPHA KERI *should always be used with water, either added to water or rubbed on to wet skin.* Because of its inherent cleansing properties it is not necessary to use soap when ALPHA KERI is being used.
For external use only.
Label directions should be followed for use in shower, bath and cleansing.

Precaution: The patient should be warned to guard against slipping in tub or shower.

How Supplied: 4 fl. oz., 8 fl. oz., 12 fl. oz., and 16 fl. oz., plastic bottles. Also available in non-aerosol pump spray, 3.5 oz.

Shown in Product Identification Section, page 405

ALPHA KERI®
Moisture Rich Cleansing Bar
Non-detergent Soap

Composition: Sodium tallowate, sodium cocoate, water, mineral oil, fragrance, PEG-75, glycerin, titanium dioxide, lanolin oil, sodium chloride. May contain: BHT, and/or Trisodium HEDTA, D&C Green 5, D&C Yellow 10.

Indications: ALPHA KERI Moisture Rich Cleansing Bar, rich in emollient oils, thoroughly cleanses as it soothes and softens the skin.

Indications: Adjunctive use in dry skin care.

Directions for Use: To be used as any other soap.

How Supplied: 4 oz. bar.

BUFFERIN®
[*bŭf'fĕr-ĭn*]
Analgesic

Composition:
Active Ingredient: Each coated tablet or caplet contains Aspirin 325 mg in a formulation buffered with Calcium Carbonate, Magnesium Oxide and Magnesium Carbonate.
Other Ingredients: Benzoic Acid, Citric Acid, Corn Starch, FD&C Blue No. 1, Hydroxypropyl Methylcellulose, Magnesium Stearate, Mineral Oil, Polysorbate 20, Povidone, Propylene Glycol, Simethicone Emulsion, Sodium Phosphate, Sorbitan Monolaurate, Titanium Dioxide. May also contain: Carnauba Wax, Zinc Stearate.

Indications: For temporary relief of headaches, pain and fever of colds, muscle aches, minor arthritis pain and inflammation, menstrual pain and toothaches.

Directions: Adults: 2 tablets or caplets with water every 4 hours while symptoms persist, not to exceed 12 tablets or caplets in 24 hours, or as directed by a doctor. Children 6 to under 12 years of age: One tablet or caplet with water every 4 hours, not to exceed 5 tablets or caplets in 24 hours or as directed by a doctor. Children under 6: Consult a doctor.

Warnings: Children and teenagers should not use this medicine for chicken pox or flu symptoms before a doctor is consulted about Reye syndrome, a rare but serious illness reported to be associated with aspirin. KEEP THIS AND ALL OTHER MEDICATIONS OUT OF THE REACH OF CHILDREN. IN CASE OF ACCIDENTAL OVERDOSE, SEEK PROFESSIONAL ASSISTANCE OR CONTACT A POISON CONTROL CENTER IMMEDIATELY. As with any drug, if you are pregnant or nursing a baby, seek the advice of a health professional before using this product. **IT IS ESPECIALLY IMPORTANT NOT TO USE ASPIRIN DURING THE LAST 3 MONTHS OF PREGNANCY UNLESS SPECIFICALLY DIRECTED TO DO SO BY A DOCTOR BECAUSE IT MAY CAUSE PROBLEMS IN THE UNBORN CHILD OR COMPLICATIONS DURING DELIVERY.** Do not take this product for pain for more than 10 days (for adults) or 5 days (for children) or for fever for more than 3 days unless directed by a doctor. If pain or fever persists or gets worse, if new symptoms occur, or if redness or swelling is present, consult a doctor because these could be signs of a serious condition. Consult a dentist promptly for toothache. Do not give this product to children for the pain of arthritis unless directed by a doctor. Do not take this product if you are allergic to aspirin, have asthma, have stomach problems (such as heartburn, upset stomach or stomach pain) that persist or recur, or if you have ulcers or bleeding problems, unless directed by a doctor. If ringing in the ears or loss of hearing occurs, consult a doctor before taking or giving any more of this product.

Drug Interaction Precaution: This product should not be taken by any adult or child who is taking a prescription drug for anticoagulation (thinning of blood), diabetes, gout or arthritis unless directed by a doctor.

How Supplied: BUFFERIN is supplied as:
Coated circular white tablet with letter "B" debossed on one surface.
NDC 19810-0073-2 Bottle of 12's
NDC 19810-0093-3 Bottle of 30's
NDC 19810-0093-4 Bottle of 50's
NDC 19810-0073-5 Bottle of 100's
NDC 19810-0073-6 Bottle of 200's
NDC 19810-0073-7 Bottle of 1000's for hospital and clinical use.
NDC 19810-0073-9 Boxed 150 × 2 tablet foil pack for hospital and clinical use.
NDC 19810-0073-0 Vials of 10
Coated scored white caplet with letter "B" debossed on each side of scoring.
NDC 19810-0072-7 Bottle of 30's
NDC 19810-0072-8 Bottle of 50's
NDC 19810-0072-3 Bottle of 100's
All consumer sizes have child resistant closures except 100's for tablets and 50's for caplets which are sizes recommended for households without young children.
Store at room temperature.
Also described in *PDR* for prescription drugs.

Professional Labeling

1. BUFFERIN® FOR RECURRENT TRANSIENT ISCHEMIC ATTACKS

Indication: For reducing the risk of recurrent transient ischemic attacks (TIA's) or stroke in men who have had transient ischemia of the brain due to fibrin platelet emboli. There is inadequate evidence that aspirin or buffered

Continued on next page

Bristol-Myers—Cont.

aspirin is effective in reducing TIA's in women at the recommended dosage. There is no evidence that aspirin or buffered aspirin is of benefit in the treatment of completed strokes in men or women.

Clinical Trials: The indication is supported by the results of a Canadian study (1) in which 585 patients with threatened stroke were followed in a randomized clinical trial for an average of 26 months to determine whether aspirin or sulfinpyrazone, singly or in combination, was superior to placebo in preventing transient ischemic attacks, stroke, or death. The study showed that, although sulfinpyrazone had no statistically significant effect, aspirin reduced the risk of continuing transient ischemic attacks, stroke, or death by 19 percent and reduced the risk of stroke or death by 31 percent. Another aspirin study carried out in the United States with 178 patients, showed a statistically significant number of "favorable outcomes," including reduced transient ischemic attacks, stroke, and death (2).

Precautions: Patients presenting with signs and symptoms of TIA's should have a complete medical and neurologic evaluation. Consideration should be given to other disorders that resemble TIA's. Attention should be given to risk factors: it is important to evaluate and treat, if appropriate, other diseases associated with TIA's and stroke, such as hypertension and diabetes.
Concurrent administration of absorbable antacids at therapeutic doses may increase the clearance of salicylates in some individuals. The concurrent administration of nonabsorbable antacids may alter the rate of absorption of aspirin, thereby resulting in a decreased acetylsalicylic acid/salicylate ratio in plasma. The clinical significance of these decreases in available aspirin is unknown.
Aspirin at dosages of 1,000 milligrams per day has been associated with small increases in blood pressure, blood urea nitrogen, and serum uric acid levels. It is recommended that patients placed on long-term aspirin treatment be seen at regular intervals to assess changes in these measurements.

Adverse Reactions: At dosages of 1,000 milligrams or higher of aspirin per day, gastrointestinal side effects include stomach pain, heartburn, nausea and/or vomiting, as well as increased rates of gross gastrointestinal bleeding.

Dosage and Administration: Adult oral dosage for men is 1,300 milligrams a day, in divided doses of 650 milligrams twice a day or 325 milligrams four times a day.

References:

(1) The Canadian Cooperative Study Group. "A Randomized Trial of Aspirin and Sulfinpyrazone in Threatened Stroke," *New England Journal of Medicine,* 299:53–59, 1978.

(2) Fields, W.S., et al., "Controlled Trial of Aspirin in Cerebral Ischemia," *Stroke* 8:301–316, 1977.

2. BUFFERIN® FOR MYOCARDIAL INFARCTION

Indication: Aspirin is indicated to reduce the risk of death and/or nonfatal myocardial infarction in patients with a previous infarction or unstable angina pectoris.

Clinical Trials: The indication is supported by the results of six, large, randomized multicenter, placebo-controlled studies[1–7] involving 10,816, predominantly male, post-myocardial infarction (MI) patients and one randomized placebo-controlled study of 1,266 men with unstable angina. Therapy with aspirin was begun at intervals after the onset of acute MI varying from less than 3 days to more than 5 years and continued for periods of from less than one year to four years. In the unstable angina study, treatment was started within 1 month after the onset of unstable angina and continued for 12 weeks and complicating conditions such as congestive heart failure were not included in the study.
Aspirin therapy in MI patients was associated with about a 20 percent reduction in the risk of subsequent death and/or nonfatal reinfarction, a median absolute decrease of 3 percent from the 12 to 22 percent event rates in the placebo groups. In the aspirin-treated unstable angina patients the reduction in risk was about 50 percent, a reduction in the event rate of 5% from the 10% rate in the placebo group over the 12 weeks of the study.
Daily dosage of aspirin in the post-myocardial infarction studies was 300 mg. in one study and 900 and 1500 mg. in five studies. A dose of 325 mg. was used in the study of unstable angina.

Adverse Reactions: Gastrointestinal Reactions: Doses of 1000 mg. per day of aspirin caused gastrointestinal symptoms and bleeding that in some cases were clinically significant. In the largest post-infarction study (The Aspirin Myocardial Infaraction Study (AMIS) with 4,500 people), the percentage incidences of gastrointestinal symptoms for the aspirin (1000 mg. of a standard, solid-tablet formulation) and placebo-treated subjects, respectively, were: stomach pain (14.5%; 4.4%); heartburn (11.9%; 4.8%); nausea and/or vomiting (7.6%; 2.1%); hospitalization for gastrointestinal disorder (4.8%; 3.5%). In the AMIS and other trials, aspirin treated patients had increased rates of gross gastrointestinal bleeding. Symptoms and signs of gastrointestinal irritation were not significantly increased in subjects treated for unstable angina with buffered aspirin in solution.
Cardiovascular and Biochemical: In the AMIS trial, the dosage of 1000 mg. per day of aspirin was associated with small increases in systolic blood pressure (BP) (average 1.5 to 2.1 mm) and diastolic BP (0.5 to 0.6 mm), depending upon whether maximal or last available readings were used. Blood urea nitrogen and uric acid levels were also increased, but by less than 1.0 mg%.
Subjects with marked hypertension or renal insufficiency had been excluded from the trial so that the clinical importance of these observations for such subjects or for any subjects treated over more prolonged periods is not known. It is recommended that patients placed on long-term aspirin treatment, even at doses of 300 mg. per day, be seen at regular intervals to assess changes in these measurements.

Administration and Dosage: Although most of the studies used dosages exceeding 300 mg., two trials used only 300 mg. and pharmacologic data indicate that this dose inhibits platelet function fully. Therefore, 300 mg. or a conventional 325 mg. aspirin dose is a reasonable, routine dose that would minimize gastrointestinal adverse reactions.

References: 1. Elwood P.C., et al., "A Randomized Controlled Trial of Acetylsalicylic Acid in the Secondary Prevention of Mortality from Myocardial Infarction," *British Medical Journal,* 1:436–440, 1974. 2. The Coronary Drug Project Research Group, "Aspirin in Coronary Heart Disease," *Journal of Chronic Disease,* 29:625–642, 1976. 3. Breddin K, et al., "Secondary Prevention of Myocardial Infarction; Comparison of Acetylsalicylic Acid Phenprocoumon and Placebo," *Thromb. Haemost.,* 41:225–236, 1979. 4. Aspirin Myocardial Infarction Study Research Group, "A Randomized, Controlled Trial of Aspirin in Persons Recovered from Myocardial Infarction," *Journal American Medical Association,* 243:661–669, 1980. 5. Elwood P.C., and Sweetnam, P.M., "Aspirin and Secondary Mortality after Myocardial Infarction," *Lancet,* pp. 1313–1315, December 22–29, 1979. 6. The Persantine-Aspirin Reinfarction Study Research Group. "Persantine and Aspirin in Coronary Heart Disease," *Circulation* 62;449–460, 1980. 7. Lewis H.D., et al., "Protective Effects of Aspirin Against Acute Myocardial Infarction and Death in Men with Unstable Angina, Results of a Veterans Administration Cooperative Study," *New England Journal of Medicine,* 309;396–403, 1983.

Shown in Product Identification Section, page 404

BUFFERIN® AF Nite Time

Composition:
Active Ingredients: Each caplet contains Acetaminophen 500 mg. and Diphenhydramine Citrate 38 mg.
Other Ingredients: Benzoic Acid, Carnauba Wax, Corn Starch, D&C Yellow No. 10, D&C Yellow No. 10 Aluminum Lake, FD&C Blue No. 1, FD&C Blue No. 1 Aluminum Lake, Hydroxypropyl Methylcellulose, Methylparaben, Magnesium Stearate, Propylene Glycol, Propylparaben, Simethicone Emulsion,

Stearic Acid, Titanium Dioxide. Remove cotton and recap bottle.

Indications: For temporary relief of occasional minor aches and pains accompanied by sleeplessness.

Warnings: KEEP THIS AND ALL OTHER MEDICATIONS OUT OF THE REACH OF CHILDREN. IN CASE OF ACCIDENTAL OVERDOSE, SEEK PROFESSIONAL ASSISTANCE OR CONTACT A POISON CONTROL CENTER IMMEDIATELY. PROMPT MEDICAL ATTENTION IS CRITICAL FOR ADULTS AS WELL AS FOR CHILDREN EVEN IF YOU DO NOT NOTICE ANY SIGNS OR SYMPTOMS. As with any drug, if you are pregnant or nursing a baby, seek the advice of a health professional before using this product. Do not give this product to children under 12 years of age or use for more than 10 days unless directed by a doctor. Consult a doctor if symptoms persist or get worse or if new ones occur, or if sleeplessness persists continuously for more than 2 weeks because these may be symptoms of serious underlying medical illnesses. Do not take this product if you have asthma, glaucoma, emphysema, chronic pulmonary disease, shortness of breath, difficulty in breathing, or difficulty in urination due to enlargement of the prostate gland unless directed by a doctor. Avoid alcoholic beverages while taking this product. Do not take this product if you are taking sedatives or tranquilizers, without first consulting your doctor.

Directions: Adults: 2 caplets at bedtime if needed or as directed by a doctor.

Overdose: MUCOMYST (acetylcysteine) As An Antidote For Acetaminophen Overdose)
Acetaminophen is rapidly absorbed from the upper gastrointestinal tract with peak plasma levels occurring between 30 and 60 minutes after therapeutic doses and usually within 4 hours following an overdose. The parent compound, which is nontoxic, is extensively metabolized in the liver to form principally the sulfate and glucuronide conjugates which are also nontoxic and are rapidly excreted in the urine. A small fraction of an ingested dose is metabolized in the liver by the cytochrome P-450 mixed function oxidase enzyme system to form a reactive, potentially toxic, intermediate metabolite which preferentially conjugates with hepatic glutathione to form the nontoxic cysteine and mercapturic acid derivatives which are then excreted by the kidney. Therapeutic doses of acetaminophen do not saturate the glucuronide and sulfate conjugation pathways and do not result in the formation of sufficient reactive metabolite to deplete glutathione stores. However, following ingestion of a large overdose (150 mg/kg or greater) the glucuronide and sulfate conjugation pathways are saturated resulting in a larger fraction of the drug being metabolized via the P-450 pathway. The increased formation of reactive metabolite may deplete the hepatic stores of glutathione with subsequent binding of the metabolite to protein molecules within the hepatocyte resulting in cellular necrosis. Acetylcysteine has been shown to reduce the extent of liver injury following acetaminophen overdose. Early symptoms following a potentially hepatotoxic overdose may include: nausea, vomiting, diaphoresis and general malaise. Clinical and laboratory evidence of hepatic toxicity may not be apparent until 48 to 72 hours postingestion. In adults and adolescents, regardless of the quantity of acetaminophen reported to have been ingested, administer MUCOMYST® acetylcysteine immediately. MUCOMYST acetylcysteine therapy should be initiated and continued for a full course of therapy. Its effectiveness depends on early administration, with benefit seen principally in patients treated within 16 hours of the overdose.
If acetaminophen plasma assay capability is not available, and the estimated acetaminophen ingestion exceeds 150 mg/kg, MUCOMYST acetylcysteine therapy should be initiated and continued for a full course of therapy.
For full prescribing information, refer to the MUCOMYST package insert. Do not await the results of assays for acetaminophen level before initiating treatment with MUCOMYST acetylcysteine. The following additional procedures are recommended: The stomach should be emptied promptly by lavage or by induction of emesis with syrup of ipecac. A serum acetaminophen assay should be obtained as early as possible, but no sooner than four hours following ingestion. Liver function studies should be obtained initially and repeated at 24-hour intervals.
For additional emergency information call your regional poison center or toll-free (1-800-525-6115) to the Rocky Mountain Poison Center for assistance in diagnosis and for directions in the use of MUCOMYST acetylcysteine as an antidote.

How Supplied: BUFFERIN® A/F Nite Time is supplied as: Light blue coated caplets with "BUFFERIN® Nite Time" imprinted in dark blue on one side.
NDC 19810-0084-1 Bottles of 24's
NDC 19810-0084-2 Bottles of 50's
The 50 caplet size does not have a child resistant closure and is recommended for households without young children.
Store at room temperature.

Shown in Product Identification Section, page 404

Arthritis Strength BUFFERIN®
[*bŭf′fĕr-ĭn*]
Analgesic

Composition:
Active Ingredient: Aspirin (500 mg) in a formulation buffered with Calcium Carbonate, Magnesium Oxide and Magnesium Carbonate.

Other Ingredients: Benzoic Acid, Citric Acid, Corn Starch, FD&C Blue No. 1, Hydroxypropyl Methylcellulose, Magnesium Stearate, Mineral Oil, Polysorbate 20, Povidone, Propylene Glycol, Simethicone Emulsion, Sodium Phosphate, Sorbitan Monolaurate, Titanium Dioxide. May also contain: Carnauba Wax, Zinc Stearate.

Indications: For temporary relief of the minor aches and pains, stiffness, swelling and inflammation of arthritis.

Directions: Adults: 2 caplets with water every 6 hours while symptoms persist, not to exceed 8 caplets in 24 hours, or as directed by a doctor. Children under 12 years of age: Consult a doctor.

Warnings: Children and teenagers should not use this medicine for chicken pox or flu symptoms before a doctor is consulted about Reye syndrome, a rare but serious illness reported to be associated with aspirin. KEEP THIS AND ALL OTHER MEDICATIONS OUT OF THE REACH OF CHILDREN. IN CASE OF ACCIDENTAL OVERDOSE, SEEK PROFESSIONAL ASSISTANCE OR CONTACT A POISON CONTROL CENTER IMMEDIATELY. As with any drug, if you are pregnant or nursing a baby, seek the advice of a health professional before using this product.
IT IS ESPECIALLY IMPORTANT NOT TO USE ASPIRIN DURING THE LAST 3 MONTHS OF PREGNANCY UNLESS SPECIFICALLY DIRECTED TO DO SO BY A DOCTOR BECAUSE IT MAY CAUSE PROBLEMS IN THE UNBORN CHILD OR COMPLICATIONS DURING DELIVERY. Do not take this product for pain for more than 10 days or for fever for more than 3 days unless directed by a doctor. If pain or fever persists or gets worse, if new symptoms occur, or if redness or swelling is present, consult a doctor because these could be signs of a serious condition. Do not take this product if you are allergic to aspirin, have asthma, have stomach problems (such as heartburn, upset stomach or stomach pain) that persist or recur, or if you have ulcers or bleeding problems, unless directed by a doctor. If ringing in the ears or loss of hearing occurs, consult a doctor before taking any more of this product.

Drug Interaction Precaution: Do not take this product if you are taking a prescription drug for anticoagulation (thinning of blood), diabetes, gout or arthritis unless directed by a doctor.

How Supplied: Arthritis Strength BUFFERIN® is supplied as:
Plain white coated caplet "ASB" debossed on one side.
NDC 19810-0051-1 Bottle of 40's
NDC 19810-0051-2 Bottle of 100's

Continued on next page

Bristol-Myers—Cont.

The 40 caplet size does not have a child resistant closure and is recommended for households without young children.
Store at room temperature.

Shown in Product Identification Section, page 404

Extra Strength BUFFERIN®
[*bŭf'fĕr-ĭn*]
Analgesic

Composition:
Active Ingredient: Aspirin (500 mg) in a formulation buffered with Calcium Carbonate, Magnesium Oxide and Magnesium Carbonate.
Other Ingredients: Benzoic Acid, Citric Acid, Corn Starch, FD&C Blue No. 1, Hydroxypropyl Methylcellulose, Magnesium Stearate, Mineral Oil, Polysorbate 20, Povidone, Propylene Glycol, Simethicone Emulsion, Sodium Phosphate, Sorbitan Monolaurate, Titanium Dioxide. May also contain: Carnauba Wax, Zinc Stearate.

Indications: For temporary relief of headaches, pain and fever of colds, muscle aches, arthritis pain and inflammation, menstrual pain and toothaches.

Directions: Adults: 2 tablets with water every 6 hours while symptoms persist, not to exceed 8 tablets in 24 hours, or as directed by a doctor. Children under 12 years of age: Consult a doctor.

Warnings: Children and teenagers should not use this medicine for chicken pox or flu symptoms before a doctor is consulted about Reye syndrome, a rare but serious illness reported to be associated with aspirin. KEEP THIS AND ALL OTHER MEDICATIONS OUT OF THE REACH OF CHILDREN. IN CASE OF ACCIDENTAL OVERDOSE, SEEK PROFESSIONAL ASSISTANCE OR CONTACT A POISON CONTROL CENTER IMMEDIATELY. As with any drug, if your are pregnant or nursing a baby, seek the advice of a health professional before using this product. **IT IS ESPECIALLY IMPORTANT NOT TO USE ASPIRIN DURING THE LAST 3 MONTHS OF PREGNANCY UNLESS SPECIFICALLY DIRECTED TO DO SO BY A DOCTOR BECAUSE IT MAY CAUSE PROBLEMS IN THE UNBORN CHILD OR COMPLICATIONS DURING DELIVERY.** Do not take this product for more than 10 days or for fever for more than 3 days unless directed by a doctor. If pain or fever persists or gets worse, if new symptoms occur, or if redness or swelling is present, consult a doctor because these could be signs of a serious condition. Consult a dentist promptly for toothache. Do not take this product if you are allergic to aspirin, have asthma, have stomach problems (such as heartburn, upset stomach or stomach pain) that persist or recur, or if you have ulcers or bleeding problems, unless directed by a doctor. If ringing in the ears or loss of hearing occurs, consult a doctor before taking any more of this product.

Drug Interaction Precaution: Do not take this product if you are taking a prescription drug for anticoagulation (thinning of blood), diabetes, gout or arthritis unless directed by a doctor.

How Supplied: Extra Strength BUFFERIN® is supplied as:
White elongated coated tablet with "ESB" debossed on one side.
NDC 19810-0074-1 Bottle of 30's
NDC 19810-0074-4 Bottle of 50's
NDC 19810-0074-3 Bottle of 100's
All sizes have child resistant closures except 50's which is recommended for households without young children.
Store at room temperature.

Shown in Product Identification Section, page 404

COMTREX®
[*cŏm'trĕx*]
Multi-Symptom Cold Reliever

Composition: Each tablet, caplet, liquigel and fluidounce (30 ml.) contains:
[See table below.]

Indications: COMTREX® provides temporary relief of these major cold and flu symptoms: nasal and sinus congestion, runny nose, sneezing, coughing, minor sore throat pain, headache, fever, body aches and pain.

Directions:
Tablets or Caplets: Adults: 2 tablets or caplets every 4 hours while symptoms persist, not to exceed 8 tablets or caplets in 24 hours, or as directed by a doctor. Children 6 to under 12 years of age: One tablet or caplet every 4 hours while symptoms persist, not to exceed 4 tablets or caplets in 24 hours, or as directed by a doctor. Children under 6: Consult a doctor.
Liqui-Gel: Adults: 2 liqui-gels every 4 hours while symptoms persist, not to exceed 12 liqui-gels in 24 hours, or as directed by a doctor. Children 6 to under 12 years of age: 1 liqui-gel every 4 hours while symptoms persist, not to exceed 5 liqui-gels in 24 hours, or as directed by a doctor. Children under 6: Consult a doctor.
Liquid: Adults: One fluidounce (30 ml) in medicine cup provided or 2 tablespoons every 4 hours while symptoms persist, not to exceed 4 doses in 24 hours, or as directed by a doctor. Children 6 to under 12 years of age: ½ fluidounce (15 ml) or one tablespoon every 4 hours while symptoms persist, not to exceed 4 doses in 24 hours, or as directed by a doctor. Children under 6: Consult a doctor.

Warnings: KEEP THIS AND ALL OTHER MEDICATIONS OUT OF THE REACH OF CHILDREN. IN CASE OF ACCIDENTAL OVERDOSE, SEEK

	COMTREX Per Tablet or Caplet	COMTREX Liquid-Gel per Liqui-Gel	COMTREX Liquid Per Fl. Ounce
Acetaminophen:	325 mg.	325 mg.	650 mg.
Pseudoephedrine HCl:	30 mg.	—	60 mg.
Phenylpropanolamine HCl:	—	12.5 mg.	—
Chlorpheniramine Maleate:	2 mg.	2 mg.	4 mg.
Dextromethorphan HBr:	10 mg.	10 mg.	20 mg.

Other Ingredients:

Tablet	Caplet	Liqui-Gels	Liquid
Corn Starch	Benzoic Acid	D&C Yellow No. 10	Alcohol (20% by volume)
D&C Yellow No. 10 Lake	Carnauba Wax	FD&C Red No. 40	Citric Acid
FD&C Red No. 40 Lake	Corn Starch	Gelatin	D&C Yellow No. 10
Magnesium Stearate	D&C Yellow No. 10 Lake	Glycerin	FD&C Blue No. 1
Methylparaben	FD&C Red No. 40 Lake	Polyethylene Glycol	FD&C Red No. 40
Propylparaben	Hydroxypropyl Methylcellulose	Povidone	Flavors
Stearic Acid	Magnesium Stearate	Propylene Glycol	Polyethylene Glycol
May also contain:	Methylparaben	Silicon Dioxide	Povidone
Povidone	Mineral Oil	Sorbitol	Sodium Citrate
	Polysorbate 20	Titanium Dioxide	Sucrose
	Povidone	Water	Water
	Propylene Glycol		
	Propylparaben		
	Simethicone Emulsion		
	Sorbitan Monolaurate		
	Stearic Acid		
	Titanium Dioxide		

PROFESSIONAL ASSISTANCE OR CONTACT A POISON CONTROL CENTER IMMEDIATELY. PROMPT MEDICAL ATTENTION IS CRITICAL FOR ADULTS AS WELL AS FOR CHILDREN EVEN IF YOU DO NOT NOTICE ANY SIGNS OR SYMPTOMS. As with any drug, if you are pregnant or nursing a baby, seek the advice of a health professional before using this product. Do not take this product for more than 7 days (for adults) or 5 days (for children), unless directed by a doctor. If symptoms do not improve or are accompanied by a fever that lasts for more than 3 days, or if new symptoms occur, consult a doctor. Do not exceed recommended dosage because at higher doses nervousness, dizziness or sleeplessness may occur. May cause excitability especially in children. A persistent cough may be a sign of a serious condition. If cough persists for more than 7 days, tends to recur, or is accompanied by rash, persistent headache, fever that lasts for more than 3 days, or if new symptoms occur, consult a doctor. Do not take this product for persistent or chronic cough such as occurs with smoking, asthma or emphysema, or if cough is accompanied by excessive phlegm (mucus/sputum) unless directed by a doctor. If sore throat is severe, persists for more than 2 days, is accompanied or followed by a fever, headache, rash, nausea or vomiting, consult a doctor promptly. This product should not be taken by persons who have asthma, glaucoma, emphysema, chronic pulmonary disease, high blood pressure, heart disease, thyroid disease, diabetes, shortness of breath, difficulty in breathing or difficulty in urination due to enlargement of the prostate gland unless directed by a doctor. May cause marked drowsiness; alcohol may increase the drowsiness effect. Avoid alcoholic beverages, and do not take this product if you are taking sedatives or tranquilizers without first consulting your doctor. Use caution when driving a motor vehicle or operating machinery.

Drug Interaction Precaution: This product should not be taken by any adult or child who is taking a prescription medication for high blood pressure or depression without first consulting a doctor.

Overdose:

MUCOMYST (acetylcysteine) As An Antidote For Acetaminophen Overdose)

Acetaminophen is rapidly absorbed from the upper gastrointestinal tract with peak plasma levels occurring between 30 and 60 minutes after therapeutic doses and usually within 4 hours following an overdose. The parent compound, which is nontoxic, is extensively metabolized in the liver to form principally the sulfate and glucuronide conjugates which are also nontoxic and are rapidly excreted in the urine. A small fraction of an ingested dose is metabolized in the liver by the cytochrome P-450 mixed function oxidase enzyme system to form a reactive, potentially toxic, intermediate metabolite which preferentially conjugates with hepatic glutathione to form the nontoxic cysteine and mercapturic acid derivatives which are then excreted by the kidney. Therapeutic doses of acetaminophen do not saturate the glucuronide and sulfate conjugation pathways and do not result in the formation of sufficient reactive metabolite to deplete glutathione stores. However, following ingestion of a large overdose (150 mg/kg or greater) the glucuronide and sulfate conjugation pathways are saturated resulting in a larger fraction of the drug being metabolized via the P-450 pathway. The increased formation of reactive metabolite may deplete the hepatic stores of glutathione with subsequent binding of the metabolite to protein molecules within the hepatocyte resulting in cellular necrosis. Acetylcysteine has been shown to reduce the extent of liver injury following acetaminophen overdose. Early symptoms following a potentially hepatotoxic overdose may include: nausea, vomiting, diaphoresis and general malaise. Clinical and laboratory evidence of hepatic toxicity may not be apparent until 48 to 72 hours postingestion. In adults and adolescents, regardless of the quantity of acetaminophen reported to have been ingested, administer MUCOMYST® acetylcysteine immediately. MUCOMYST acetylcysteine therapy should be initiated and continued for a full course of therapy. Its effectiveness depends on early administration, with benefit seen principally in patients treated within 16 hours of the overdose.

If acetaminophen plasma assay capability is not available, and the estimated acetaminophen ingestion exceeds 150 mg/kg, MUCOMYST acetylcysteine therapy should be initiated and continued for a full course of therapy.

For full prescribing information, refer to the MUCOMYST package insert. Do not await the results of assays for acetaminophen level before initiating treatment with MUCOMYST acetylcysteine. The following additional procedures are recommended: The stomach should be emptied promptly by lavage or by induction of emesis with syrup of ipecac. A serum acetaminophen assay should be obtained as early as possible, but no sooner than four hours following ingestion. Liver function studies should be obtained initially and repeated at 24-hour intervals.

For additional emergency information call your regional poison center or toll-free (1-800-525-6115) to the Rocky Mountain Poison Center for assistance in diagnosis and for directions in the use of MUCOMYST acetylcysteine as an antidote.

How Supplied:

COMTREX® is supplied as:

Yellow tablet with letter "C" debossed on one surface.

NDC 19810-0790-1 Blister packages of 24's

NDC 19810-0790-2 Bottles of 50's

NDC 19810-0790-3 Vials of 10's

Coated yellow caplet with "Comtrex" printed in red on one side.

NDC 19810-0792-3 Blister packages of 24's

NDC 19810-0792-4 Bottles of 50's

Yellow Liqui-Gel with "Comtrex" printed in red on one side.

NDC 19810-0561-1 Blister packages of 24's

NDC 19810-0561-2 Blister packages of 50's

Clear Red Cherry Flavored liquid:

NDC 19810-0791-1 6 oz. plastic bottles.

All sizes packaged in child resistant closures except for 24's for tablets, caplets and liqui-gels which are sizes recommended for households without young children. Store caplets, tablets and liquid at room temperature.

Store liqui-gels below 86° F. (30° C.). Keep from freezing.

Shown in Product Identification Section, page 404

ALLERGY–SINUS COMTREX

[*cŏm 'trĕx*]

Multi-Symptom Allergy/Sinus Formula

Composition:

Active Ingredients: Each coated tablet or caplet contains 500 mg acetaminophen, 30 mg pseudoephedrine HCl, 2 mg chlorpheniramine maleate.

Other Ingredients: Benzoic acid, carnauba wax, corn starch, D&C yellow No. 10 lake, FD&C blue No. 1 lake, FD&C Red No. 40 lake, hydroxypropyl methylcellulose, mineral oil, polysorbate 20, povidone, propylene glycol, simethicone emulsion, sodium citrate, sorbitan monolaurate, stearic acid, titanium dioxide. May also contain: crospovidone, D&C yellow No. 10, erythorbic acid, FD&C blue No. 1, magnesium stearate, methylparaben, microcrystalline cellulose, polysorbate 80, propylparaben, silicon dioxide, wood cellulose.

Indications:

ALLERGY-SINUS COMTREX provides temporary relief of these upper respiratory allergy, hay fever, and sinusitis symptoms: sneezing, itchy watery eyes, runny nose, headache, nasal and sinus pressure and congestion.

Directions: Adults: 2 tablets or caplets every 6 hours while symptoms persist, not to exceed 8 tablets or caplets in 24 hours, or as directed by a doctor. Children under 12 years of age: Consult a doctor.

Warnings: KEEP THIS AND ALL OTHER MEDICATIONS OUT OF THE REACH OF CHILDREN. IN CASE OF ACCIDENTAL OVERDOSE, SEEK PROFESSIONAL ASSISTANCE OR CONTACT A POISON CONTROL CENTER IMMEDIATELY. PROMPT MEDICAL ATTENTION IS CRITICAL FOR ADULTS AS WELL AS FOR CHIL-

Continued on next page

Bristol-Myers—Cont.

DREN EVEN IF YOU DO NOT NOTICE ANY SIGNS OR SYMPTOMS. As with any drug, if you are pregnant or nursing a baby, seek the advice of a health professional before using this product. Do not take this product for more than 7 days unless directed by a doctor. If symptoms do not improve or are accompanied by a fever that lasts for more than 3 days, or if new symptoms occur, consult a doctor. Do not exceed recommended dosage because at higher doses nervousness, dizziness or sleeplessness may occur. May cause excitability especially in children. This product should not be taken by persons who have asthma, glaucoma, emphysema, chronic pulmonary disease, high blood pressure, heart disease, thyroid disease, diabetes, shortness of breath, difficulty in breathing or difficulty in urination due to enlargement of the prostate gland unless directed by a doctor. May cause drowsiness; alcohol may increase the drowsiness effect. Avoid alcoholic beverages, and do not take this product if you are taking sedatives or tranquilizers without first consulting your doctor. Use caution when driving a motor vehicle or operating machinery.

Drug Interaction Precaution: Do not take this product if you are presently taking a prescription drug for high blood pressure or depression, without first consulting your doctor.

Overdose:

MUCOMYST (acetylcysteine) As An Antidote For Acetaminophen Overdose)

Acetaminophen is rapidly absorbed from the upper gastrointestinal tract with peak plasma levels occurring between 30 and 60 minutes after therapeutic doses and usually within 4 hours following an overdose. The parent compound, which is nontoxic, is extensively metabolized in the liver to form principally the sulfate and glucuronide conjugates which are also nontoxic and are rapidly excreted in the urine. A small fraction of an ingested dose is metabolized in the liver by the cytochrome P-450 mixed function oxidase enzyme system to form a reactive, potentially toxic, intermediate metabolite which preferentially conjugates with hepatic glutathione to form the nontoxic cysteine and mercapturic acid derivatives which are then excreted by the kidney. Therapeutic doses of acetaminophen do not saturate the glucuronide and sulfate conjugation pathways and do not result in the formation of sufficient reactive metabolite to deplete glutathione stores. However, following ingestion of a large overdose (150 mg/kg or greater) the glucuronide and sulfate conjugation pathways are saturated resulting in a larger fraction of the drug being metabolized via the P-450 pathway. The increased formation of reactive metabolite may deplete the hepatic stores of glutathione with subsequent binding of the metabolite to protein molecules within the hepatocyte resulting in cellular necrosis. Acetylcysteine has been shown to reduce the extent of liver injury following acetaminophen overdose. Early symptoms following a potentially hepatotoxic overdose may include: nausea, vomiting, diaphoresis and general malaise. Clinical and laboratory evidence of hepatic toxicity may not be apparent until 48 to 72 hours postingestion. In adults and adolescents, regardless of the quantity of acetaminophen reported to have been ingested, administer MUCOMYST® acetylcysteine immediately. MUCOMYST acetylcysteine therapy should be initiated and continued for a full course of therapy. Its effectiveness depends on early administration, with benefit seen principally in patients treated within 16 hours of the overdose.

If acetaminophen plasma assay capability is not available, and the estimated acetaminophen ingestion exceeds 150 mg/kg, MUCOMYST acetylcysteine therapy should be initiated and continued for a full course of therapy.

For full prescribing information, refer to the MUCOMYST package insert. Do not await the results of assays for acetaminophen level before initiating treatment with MUCOMYST acetylcysteine. The following additional procedures are recommended: The stomach should be emptied promptly by lavage or by induction of emesis with syrup of ipecac. A serum acetaminophen assay should be obtained as early as possible, but no sooner than four hours following ingestion. Liver function studies should be obtained initially and repeated at 24-hour intervals.

For additional emergency information call your regional poison center or toll-free (1-800-525-6115) to the Rocky Mountain Poison Center for assistance in diagnosis and for directions in the use of MUCOMYST acetylcysteine as an antidote.

How Supplied: Allergy-Sinus COMTREX® is supplied as:

Coated green tablets with "Comtrex A/S" printed in black on one side.

NDC 19810-0774-1 Blister packages of 24's

NDC 19810-0774-2 Bottles of 50's

Coated green caplets with "A/S" debossed on one surface.

NDC 19810-0081-4 Blister packages of 24's

NDC 19810-0081-5 Bottles of 50's

All sizes packaged in child resistant closures except 24's for tablets and caplets which are sizes recommended for households without young children.

Store at room temperature.

Shown in Product Identification Section, page 404

Cough Formula COMTREX®

[*cŏm 'trĕx*]

Multi-Symptom Cough Formula

Composition:

Active Ingredients: Each 4 teaspoonfuls (⅔ fl. oz.) contains:

—EXPECTORANT—200 mg Guaifenesin

—COUGH SUPPRESSANT—20 mg Dextromethorphan HBr

—ANALGESIC—500 mg Acetaminophen

—DECONGESTANT—60 mg Pseudoephedrine HCl

Other Ingredients: Alcohol (20% by volume), Citric Acid, FD&C Red No. 40, Flavor, Menthol, Povidone, Saccharin Sodium, Sodium Citrate, Sucrose, Water.

Indications: For temporary relief of cough, nasal and upper chest congestion, minor sore throat pain, and fever and pain due to a chest cold.

Directions: Adults: ⅔ fluidounce (20 ml) in medicine cup provided or four teaspoons every 4 hours while symptoms persist, not to exceed 4 doses in 24 hours, or as directed by a doctor. Children 6 to under 12 years of age: ⅓ fluidounce (10 ml) in medicine cup provided or 2 teaspoons every 4 hours while symptoms persist, not to exceed 4 doses in 24 hours, or as directed by a doctor. Children under 6: Consult a doctor.

Warnings: KEEP THIS AND ALL OTHER MEDICATIONS OUT OF THE REACH OF CHILDREN. IN CASE OF ACCIDENTAL OVERDOSE, SEEK PROFESSIONAL ASSISTANCE OR CONTACT A POISON CONTROL CENTER IMMEDIATELY. PROMPT MEDICAL ATTENTION IS CRITICAL FOR ADULTS AS WELL AS FOR CHILDREN EVEN IF YOU DO NOT NOTICE ANY SIGNS OR SYMPTOMS. As with any drug, if you are pregnant or nursing a baby, seek the advice of a health professional before using this product. Do not take this product for more than 7 days (for adults) or 5 days (for children) unless directed by a doctor. If symptoms do not improve or are accompanied by a fever that lasts for more than 3 days, or if new symptoms occur, consult a doctor. Do not exceed recommended dosage because at higher doses nervousness, dizziness or sleeplessness may occur. A persistent cough may be a sign of a serious condition. If cough persists for more than 7 days, tends to recur or is accompanied by rash, persistent headache, fever that lasts for more than 3 days, or if new symptoms occur, consult a doctor. Do not take this product for persistent or chronic cough such as occurs with smoking, asthma, chronic bronchitis or emphysema or if cough is accompanied by excessive phlegm (mucus/sputum) unless directed by a doctor. If sore throat is severe, persists for more than two days, is accompanied or followed by a fever, headache, rash, nausea or vomiting, consult a doctor promptly. This product should not be taken by persons who have heart disease, high blood pressure, thyroid disease, diabetes or difficulty in urination due to enlargement of the prostate gland unless directed by a doctor.

Overdose:
MUCOMYST (acetylcysteine) As An Antidote For Acetaminophen Overdose)
Acetaminophen is rapidly absorbed from the upper gastrointestinal tract with peak plasma levels occurring between 30 and 60 minutes after therapeutic doses and usually within 4 hours following an overdose. The parent compound, which is nontoxic, is extensively metabolized in the liver to form principally the sulfate and glucuronide conjugates which are also nontoxic and are rapidly excreted in the urine. A small fraction of an ingested dose is metabolized in the liver by the cytochrome P-450 mixed function oxidase enzyme system to form a reactive, potentially toxic, intermediate metabolite which preferentially conjugates with hepatic glutathione to form the nontoxic cysteine and mercapturic acid derivatives which are then excreted by the kidney. Therapeutic doses of acetaminophen do not saturate the glucuronide and sulfate conjugation pathways and do not result in the formation of sufficient reactive metabolite to deplete glutathione stores. However, following ingestion of a large overdose (150 mg/kg or greater) the glucuronide and sulfate conjugation pathways are saturated resulting in a larger fraction of the drug being metabolized via the P-450 pathway. The increased formation of reactive metabolite may deplete the hepatic stores of glutathione with subsequent binding of the metabolite to protein molecules within the hepatocyte resulting in cellular necrosis. Acetylcysteine has been shown to reduce the extent of liver injury following acetaminophen overdose. Early symptoms following a potentially hepatotoxic overdose may include nausea, vomiting, diaphoresis and general malaise. Clinical and laboratory evidence of hepatic toxicity may not be apparent until 48 to 72 hours postingestion. In adults and adolescents, regardless of the quantity of acetaminophen reported to have been ingested, administer MUCOMYST® acetylcysteine immediately. MUCOMYST acetylcysteine therapy should be initiated and continued for a full course of therapy. Its effectiveness depends on early administration, with benefit seen principally in patients treated within 16 hours of the overdose.
If acetaminophen plasma assay capability is not available, and the estimated acetaminophen ingestion exceeds 150 mg/kg, MUCOMYST acetylcysteine therapy should be initiated and continued for a full course of therapy.
For full prescribing information, refer to the MUCOMYST package insert. Do not await the results of assays for acetaminophen level before initiating treatment with MUCOMYST acetylcysteine. The following additional procedures are recommended: The stomach should be emptied promptly by lavage or by induction of emesis with syrup of ipecac. A serum acetaminophen assay should be obtained as early as possible, but no sooner than four hours following ingestion. Liver function studies should be obtained initially and repeated at 24-hour intervals.
For additional emergency information call your regional poison center or toll-free (1-800-525-6115) to the Rocky Mountain Poison Center for assistance in diagnosis and for directions in the use of MUCOMYST acetylcysteine as an antidote.

How Supplied: Cough Formula COMTREX® is supplied as a clear red raspberry flavored liquid:
NDC 19810-0783-1 4 oz. plastic bottle
NDC 19810-0783-2 8 oz. plastic bottle
The 4 oz. size is not child resistant and is recommended for households without young children.
Store at room temperature.

Shown in Product Identification Section, page 404

DAY-NIGHT COMTREX®

Composition:
Active Ingredients: EACH DAYTIME CAPLET CONTAINS 325mg Acetaminophen, 30mg Pseudoephedrine HCl, 10mg Dextromethorphan HBr. EACH NIGHTTIME TABLET CONTAINS 325mg Acetaminophen, 30mg Pseudoephedrine HCl, 10mg Dextromethorphan HBr, 2mg Chlorpheniramine Maleate.
Other Ingredients: DAYTIME CAPLETS AND NIGHTTIME TABLETS BOTH CONTAIN: Corn Starch, D&C Yellow No. 10 Lake, FD&C Red No. 40 Lake, Magnesium Stearate, Methylparaben, Propylparaben, Stearic Acid. DAYTIME CAPLETS ALSO CONTAIN: Benzoic Acid, Carnauba Wax, Hydroxypropyl Methylcellulose, Mineral Oil, Polysorbate 20, Povidone, Propylene Glycol, Simethicone Emulsion, Sorbitan Monolaurate, Titanium Dioxide. NIGHTTIME TABLETS MAY ALSO CONTAIN: Povidone.

Indications: Day/Night COMTREX provides you with two different formulas. COMTREX Daytime Caplets (orange) and COMTREX Nighttime Tablets (yellow), for effective relief. COMTREX Daytime Caplets contain three ingredients for the temporary relief of these major cold and flu symptoms without causing drowsiness: a decongestant—to relieve stuffy nose and sinus congestion; a cough suppressant—to quiet cough; a non-aspirin analgesic—to relieve headache, fever, minor sore throat pain and body aches and pain. COMTREX Nighttime Tablets relieve all these symptoms plus they contain an antihistamine to temporarily relieve runny nose and sneezing.

Warnings for Daytime Caplets and Nighttime Tablets KEEP THESE AND ALL OTHER MEDICATIONS OUT OF THE REACH OF CHILDREN. IN CASE OF ACCIDENTAL OVERDOSE, SEEK PROFESSIONAL ASSISTANCE OR CONTACT A POISON CONTROL CENTER IMMEDIATELY. PROMPT MEDICAL ATTENTION IS CRITICAL FOR ADULTS AS WELL AS FOR CHILDREN EVEN IF YOU DO NOT NOTICE ANY SIGNS OR SYMPTOMS. As with any drug, if you are pregnant or nursing a baby, seek the advice of a health professional before using these products. Do not take these products for more than 7 days or for fever for more than 3 days unless directed by a doctor. If symptoms do not improve or are accompanied by a fever that lasts for more than 3 days, or if new symptoms occur, consult a doctor. Do not exceed recommended dosage because at higher doses nervousness, dizziness or sleeplessness may occur. A persistent cough may be a sign of a serious condition. If cough persists for more than 7 days, tends to recur or is accompanied by rash, persistent headache, fever that lasts for more than 3 days, or if new symptoms occur, consult a doctor. Do not take these products for persistent or chronic cough such as occurs with smoking, asthma or emphysema, or if cough is accompanied by excessive phlegm (mucus/sputum) unless directed by a doctor. If sore throat is severe, persists for more than 2 days, is accompanied or followed by a fever, headache, rash, nausea or vomiting, consult a doctor promptly. These products should not be taken by persons who have asthma, glaucoma, emphysema, chronic pulmonary disease, high blood pressure, heart disease, thyroid disease, diabetes, shortness of breath, difficulty in breathing, or difficulty in urination due to an enlargement of the prostate gland unless directed by a doctor.
Additional Warnings for Nighttime Tablets May cause marked drowsiness; alcohol may increase the drowsiness effect. Avoid alcoholic beverages, and do not take this product if you are taking sedatives or tranquilizers without first consulting your doctor. Use caution when driving a motor vehicle or operating machinery. May cause excitability especially in children.
DRUG INTERACTION PRECAUTION: Do not take these products if you are presently taking a prescription for high blood pressure or depression without first consulting your doctor.

Directions: Adults: 2 Daytime Caplets every 4 hours while symptoms persist, not to exceed 6 Daytime Caplets in 24 hours, or as directed by a doctor. 2 Nighttime Tablets at bedtime, if needed, to be taken no sooner than 4 hours after the last Daytime Caplet dose, or as directed by a doctor. **Children under 12:** Consult a doctor.

Overdose: MUCOMYST (acetylcysteine) As An Antidote For Acetaminophen Overdose)
Acetaminophen is rapidly absorbed from the upper gastrointestinal tract with

Continued on next page

Bristol-Myers—Cont.

peak plasma levels occurring between 30 and 60 minutes after therapeutic doses and usually within 4 hours following an overdose. The parent compound, which is nontoxic, is extensively metabolized in the liver to form principally the sulfate and glucuronide conjugates which are also nontoxic and are rapidly excreted in the urine. A small fraction of an ingested dose is metabolized in the liver by the cytochrome P-450 mixed function oxidase enzyme system to form a reactive, potentially toxic, intermediate metabolite which preferentially conjugates with hepatic glutathione to form the nontoxic cysteine and mercapturic acid derivatives which are then excreted by the kidney. Therapeutic doses of acetaminophen do not saturate the glucuronide and sulfate conjugation pathways and do not result in the formation of sufficient reactive metabolite to deplete glutathione stores. However, following ingestion of a large overdose (150 mg/kg or greater) the glucuronide and sulfate conjugation pathways are saturated resulting in a larger fraction of the drug being metabolized via the P-450 pathway. The increased formation of reactive metabolite may deplete the hepatic stores of glutathione with subsequent binding of the metabolite to protein molecules within the hepatocyte resulting in cellular necrosis. Acetylcysteine has been shown to reduce the extent of liver injury following acetaminophen overdose. Early symptoms following a potentially hepatotoxic overdose may include: nausea, vomiting, diaphoresis and general malaise. Clinical and laboratory evidence of hepatic toxicity may not be apparent until 48 to 72 hours postingestion. In adults and adolescents, regardless of the quantity of acetaminophen reported to have been ingested, administer MUCOMYST® acetylcysteine immediately. MUCOMYST acetylcysteine therapy should be initiated and continued for a full course of therapy. Its effectiveness depends on early administration, with benefit seen principally in patients treated within 16 hours of the overdose.

If acetaminophen plasma assay capability is not available, and the estimated acetaminophen ingestion exceeds 150 mg/kg, MUCOMYST acetylcysteine therapy should be initiated and continued for a full course of therapy.

For full prescribing information, refer to the MUCOMYST package insert. Do not await the results of assays for acetaminophen level before initiating treatment with MUCOMYST acetylcysteine. The following additional procedures are recommended: The stomach should be emptied promptly by lavage or by induction of emesis with syrup of ipecac. A serum acetaminophen assay should be obtained as early as possible, but no sooner than four hours following ingestion. Liver function studies should be obtained initially and repeated at 24-hour intervals.

For additional emergency information call your regional poison center or toll-free (1-800-525-6115) to the Rocky Mountain Poison Center for assistance in diagnosis and for directions in the use of MUCOMYST acetylcysteine as an antidote.

How Supplied: DAY-NIGHT COMTREX® is supplied as:

Day-Coated orange caplet with letter "C" debossed on one surface.

Night-Coated yellow tablet with letter "C" debossed on one surface.

NDC 19810-0078-1 Blister packages of 24's (18 caplets/6 tablets)

Store at room temperature.

Shown in Product Identification Section, page 404

Non-Drowsy COMTREX®

Composition:

Active Ingredients: Each caplet contains 325mg Acetaminophen, 30 mg Pseudoephedrine HCl, 10mg Dextromethorphan HBr. Other Ingredients: Benzoic Acid, Carnauba Wax, Corn Starch, D&C Yellow No. 10 Lake, FD&C Red No. 40 Lake, Hydroxypropyl Methylcellulose, Magnesium Stearate, Methylparaben, Mineral Oil, Polysorbate 20, Povidone, Propylene Glycol, Propylparaben, Simethicone Emulsion, Sorbitan Monolaurate, Stearic Acid, Titanium Dioxide.

Indications: For temporary relief of nasal and sinus congestion, coughing, minor sore throat pain, headache, fever, body aches and pain.

Warnings: KEEP THIS AND ALL OTHER MEDICATIONS OUT OF THE REACH OF CHILDREN. IN CASE OF ACCIDENTAL OVERDOSE, SEEK PROFESSIONAL ASSISTANCE OR CONTACT A POISON CONTROL CENTER IMMEDIATELY. PROMPT MEDICAL ATTENTION IS CRITICAL FOR ADULTS AS WELL AS FOR CHILDREN EVEN IF YOU DO NOT NOTICE ANY SIGNS OR SYMPTOMS. As with any drug, if you are pregnant or nursing a baby, seek the advice of a health professional before using this product. Do not take this product for more than 7 days (for adults) or 5 days (for children) or for fever for more than 3 days unless directed by a doctor. Do not exceed recommended dosage because at higher doses nervousness, dizziness or sleeplessness may occur. A persistent cough may be a sign of a serious condition. If cough persists for more than 7 days, tends to recur or is accompanied by rash, persistent headache, fever that lasts for more than 3 days, or if new symptoms occur, consult a doctor. Do not take this product for persistent or chronic cough such as occurs with smoking, asthma or emphysema, or if cough is accompanied by excessive phlegm (mucus/sputum) unless directed by a doctor. If sore throat is severe, persists for more than 2 days, is accompanied or followed by a fever, headache, rash, nausea or vomiting, consult a doctor promptly. This product should not be taken by persons who have high blood pressure, heart disease, thyroid disease, diabetes or difficulty in urination due to enlargement of the prostate gland unless directed by a doctor.

DRUG INTERACTION PRECAUTION: This product should not be taken by any adult or child who is taking a prescription medication for high blood pressure or depression without first consulting a doctor.

Directions: Adults: 2 caplets every 4 hours while symptoms persist, not to exceed 8 caplets in 24 hours, or as directed by doctor. **Children 6 to under 12 years of age:** One caplet every 4 hours while symptoms persist, not to exceed 4 caplets in 24 hours, or as directed by a doctor. **Children under 6:** Consult a doctor.

Overdose: MUCOMYST (acetylcysteine) As An Antidote For Acetaminophen Overdose)

Acetaminophen is rapidly absorbed from the upper gastrointestinal tract with peak plasma levels occurring between 30 and 60 minutes after therapeutic doses and usually within 4 hours following an overdose. The parent compound, which is nontoxic, is extensively metabolized in the liver to form principally the sulfate and glucuronide conjugates which are also nontoxic and are rapidly excreted in the urine. A small fraction of an ingested dose is metabolized in the liver by the cytochrome P-450 mixed function oxidase enzyme system to form a reactive, potentially toxic, intermediate metabolite which preferentially conjugates with hepatic glutathione to form the nontoxic cysteine and mercapturic acid derivatives which are then excreted by the kidney. Therapeutic doses of acetaminophen do not saturate the glucuronide and sulfate conjugation pathways and do not result in the formation of sufficient reactive metabolite to deplete glutathione stores. However, following ingestion of a large overdose (150 mg/kg or greater) the glucuronide and sulfate conjugation pathways are saturated resulting in a larger fraction of the drug being metabolized via the P-450 pathway. The increased formation of reactive metabolite may deplete the hepatic stores of glutathione with subsequent binding of the metabolite to protein molecules within the hepatocyte resulting in cellular necrosis. Acetylcysteine has been shown to reduce the extent of liver injury following acetaminophen overdose. Early symptoms following a potentially hepatotoxic overdose may include: nausea, vomiting, diaphoresis and general malaise. Clinical and laboratory evidence of hepatic toxicity may not be apparent until 48 to 72 hours postingestion. In adults and adolescents, regardless of the quantity of acetaminophen reported to have been ingested, administer MUCOMYST® acetylcysteine immediately. MUCOMYST acetylcysteine therapy should be initiated and continued for a

full course of therapy. Its effectiveness depends on early administration, with benefit seen principally in patients treated within 16 hours of the overdose.
If acetaminophen plasma assay capability is not available, and the estimated acetaminophen ingestion exceeds 150 mg/kg, MUCOMYST acetylcysteine therapy should be initiated and continued for a full course of therapy.
For full prescribing information, refer to the MUCOMYST package insert. Do not await the results of assays for acetaminophen level before initiating treatment with MUCOMYST acetylcysteine. The following additional procedures are recommended: The stomach should be emptied promptly by lavage or by induction of emesis with syrup of ipecac. A serum acetaminophen assay should be obtained as early as possible, but no sooner than four hours following ingestion. Liver function studies should be obtained initially and repeated at 24-hour intervals.
For additional emergency information call your regional poison center or toll-free (1-800-525-6115) to the Rocky Mountain Poison Center for assistance in diagnosis and for directions in the use of MUCOMYST acetylcysteine as an antidote.

How Supplied: Non-Drowsy Comtrex® is supplied as:
Coated orange caplet with letter "C" debossed on one surface.
NDC 19810-0041-1 Blister packages of 24's
NDC 19810-0041-2 Bottles of 50's
The 24 size does not have a child resistant closure and is recommended for households without young children.
Store at room temperature.

Shown in Product Identification Section, page 404

CONGESPIRIN® for Children Aspirin Free Chewable Cold Tablets

[cŏn "gĕs 'pir-in]

Composition: Each tablet contains acetaminophen 81 mg. (1¼ grains), phenylephrine hydrochloride 1¼ mg. Also Contains: Calcium Stearate, D&C Red No. 30 Aluminum Lake, D&C Yellow No. 10 Aluminum Lake, Ethyl Cellulose, Flavor, Mannitol, Microcrystalline Cellulose, Polyethylene, Saccharin Calcium, Sucrose.

Indications: A non-aspirin analgesic/nasal decongestant that temporarily reduces fever and relieves aches, pains and nasal congestion associated with colds and "flu."

Warnings: KEEP THIS AND ALL MEDICINES OUT OF CHILDREN'S REACH. IN CASE OF ACCIDENTAL OVERDOSE, CONTACT A PHYSICIAN IMMEDIATELY.

Caution: If child is under medical care, do not administer without consulting physician. Do not exceed recommended dosage. Consult your physician if symptoms persist or if high blood pressure, heart disease, diabetes or thyroid disease is present. Do not administer for more than 10 days unless directed by physician.

Directions:
Under 2, consult your physician.

2–3 years	2 tablets
4–5 years	3 tablets
6–8 years	4 tablets
9–10 years	5 tablets
11–12 years	6 tablets
over 12 years	8 tablets

Repeat dose in four hours if necessary. Do not give more than four doses per day unless prescribed by your physician.

Overdose:
MUCOMYST (acetylcysteine) As An Antidote For Acetaminophen Overdose)
Acetaminophen is rapidly absorbed from the upper gastrointestinal tract with peak plasma levels occurring between 30 and 60 minutes after therapeutic doses and usually within 4 hours following an overdose. The parent compound, which is nontoxic, is extensively metabolized in the liver to form principally the sulfate and glucuronide conjugates which are also nontoxic and are rapidly excreted in the urine. A small fraction of an ingested dose is metabolized in the liver by the cytochrome P-450 mixed function oxidase enzyme system to form a reactive, potentially toxic, intermediate metabolite which preferentially conjugates with hepatic glutathione to form the nontoxic cysteine and mercapturic acid derivatives which are then excreted by the kidney. Therapeutic doses of acetaminophen do not saturate the glucuronide and sulfate conjugation pathways and do not result in the formation of sufficient reactive metabolite to deplete glutathione stores. However, following ingestion of a large overdose (150 mg/kg or greater) the glucuronide and sulfate conjugation pathways are saturated resulting in a larger fraction of the drug being metabolized via the P-450 pathway. The increased formation of reactive metabolite may deplete the hepatic stores of glutathione with subsequent binding of the metabolite to protein molecules within the hepatocyte resulting in cellular necrosis. Acetylcysteine has been shown to reduce the extent of liver injury following acetaminophen overdose. Early symptoms following a potentially hepatotoxic overdose may include nausea, vomiting, diaphoresis and general malaise. Clinical and laboratory evidence of hepatic toxicity may not be apparent until 48 to 72 hours postingestion. In adults and adolescents, regardless of the quantity of acetaminophen reported to have been ingested, administer MUCOMYST® acetylcysteine immediately. MUCOMYST acetylcysteine therapy should be initiated and continued for a full course of therapy. Its effectiveness depends on early administration, with benefit seen principally in patients treated within 16 hours of the overdose.
If acetaminophen plasma assay capability is not available, and the estimated acetaminophen ingestion exceeds 150 mg/kg, MUCOMYST acetylcysteine therapy should be initiated and continued for a full course of therapy.
For full prescribing information, refer to the MUCOMYST package insert. Do not await the result of assays for acetaminophen level before initiating treatment with MUCOMYST acetylcysteine. The following additional procedures are recommended: The stomach should be emptied promptly by lavage or by induction of emesis with syrup of ipecac. A serum acetaminophen assay should be obtained as early as possible, but no sooner than four hours following ingestion. Liver function studies should be obtained initially and repeated at 24-hour intervals.
For additional emergency information call your regional poison center or toll-free (1-800-525-6115) to the Rocky Mountain Poison Center for assistance in diagnosis and for directions in the use of MUCOMYST acetylcysteine as an antidote.

How Supplied: CONGESPIRIN Aspirin Free Chewable Cold Tablets are supplied as scored orange tablets with "C" on one side.
NDC 19810-0748-1 Bottles of 24's.
Bottles are child resistant.
Store at room temperature.

Shown in Product Identification Section, page 405

Aspirin Free EXCEDRIN®

Composition: Each caplet contains Acetaminophen 500 mg. and Caffeine 65 mg. Other Ingredients: Benzoic Acid, Carnauba Wax, Corn Starch, Croscarmellose Sodium, D&C Red No. 27 Lake, D&C Yellow No. 10 Lake, FD&C Blue No. 1 Lake, Hydroxypropyl Methylcellulose, Magnesium Stearate, Methylparaben, Microcrystalline Cellulose, Propylparaben, Saccharin Sodium, Simethicone Emulsion, Stearic Acid, Titanium Dioxide. May also contain: Erythorbic Acid, Mineral Oil, Polyethylene Glycol, Polysorbate 20, Polysorbate 80, Povidone, Propylene Glycol, Sorbitan Monolaurate.

Indications: For temporary relief of the pain of headache, sinusitis, colds, muscular aches, menstrual discomfort, toothaches and minor arthritis pain.

Directions: Adults: 2 caplets every 6 hours while symptoms persist, not to exceed 8 caplets in 24 hours, or as directed by a doctor. Children under 12 years of age: Consult a doctor.

Warnings: KEEP THIS AND ALL OTHER MEDICATIONS OUT OF THE REACH OF CHILDREN. IN CASE OF ACCIDENTAL OVERDOSE, SEEK PROFESSIONAL ASSISTANCE OR CONTACT A POISON CONTROL CEN-

Continued on next page

Bristol-Myers—Cont.

TER IMMEDIATELY. PROMPT MEDICAL ATTENTION IS CRITICAL FOR ADULTS AS WELL AS FOR CHILDREN EVEN IF YOU DO NOT NOTICE ANY SIGNS OR SYMPTOMS. As with any drug, if you are pregnant or nursing a baby, seek the advice of a health professional before using this product. Do not take this product for pain for more than 10 days or for fever for more than 3 days unless directed by a doctor. If pain or fever persists or gets worse, if new symptoms occur, or if redness or swelling is present, consult a doctor because these could be signs of a serious condition. Consult a dentist promptly for toothache.

Overdose:
MUCOMYST (acetylcysteine) As An Antidote For Acetaminophen Overdose)
Acetaminophen is rapidly absorbed from the upper gastrointestinal tract with peak plasma levels occurring between 30 and 60 minutes after therapeutic doses and usually within 4 hours following an overdose. The parent compound, which is nontoxic, is extensively metabolized in the liver to form principally the sulfate and glucuronide conjugates which are also nontoxic and are rapidly excreted in the urine. A small fraction of an ingested dose is metabolized in the liver by the cytochrome P-450 mixed function oxidase enzyme system to form a reactive, potentially toxic, intermediate metabolite which preferentially conjugates with hepatic glutathione to form the nontoxic cysteine and mercapturic acid derivatives which are then excreted by the kidney. Therapeutic doses of acetaminophen do not saturate the glucuronide and sulfate conjugation pathways and do not result in the formation of sufficient reactive metabolite to deplete glutathione stores. However, following ingestion of a large overdose (150 mg/kg or greater) the glucuronide and sulfate conjugation pathways are saturated resulting in a larger fraction of the drug being metabolized via the P-450 pathway. The increased formation of reactive metabolite may deplete the hepatic stores of glutathione with subsequent binding of the metabolite to protein molecules within the hepatocyte resulting in cellular necrosis. Acetylcysteine has been shown to reduce the extent of liver injury following acetaminophen overdose. Early symptoms following a potentially hepatotoxic overdose may include: nausea, vomiting, diaphoresis and general malaise. Clinical and laboratory evidence of hepatic toxicity may not be apparent until 48 to 72 hours postingestion. In adults and adolescents, regardless of the quantity of acetaminophen reported to have been ingested, administer MUCOMYST® acetylcysteine immediately. MUCOMYST acetylcysteine therapy should be initiated and continued for a full course of therapy. Its effectiveness depends on early administration, with benefit seen principally in patients treated within 16 hours of the overdose. If acetaminophen plasma assay capability is not available, and the estimated acetaminophen ingestion exceeds 150 mg/kg, MUCOMYST acetylcysteine therapy should be initiated and continued for a full course of therapy.
For full prescribing information, refer to the MUCOMYST package insert. Do not await the results of assays for acetaminophen level before initiating treatment with MUCOMYST acetylcysteine. The following additional procedures are recommended: The stomach should be emptied promptly by lavage or by induction of emesis with syrup of ipecac. A serum acetaminophen assay should be obtained as early as possible, but no sooner than four hours following ingestion. Liver function studies should be obtained initially and repeated at 24-hour intervals.
For additional emergency information call your regional poison center or toll-free (1-800-525-6115) to the Rocky Mountain Poison Center for assistance in diagnosis and for directions in the use of MUCOMYST acetylcysteine as an antidote.

How Supplied: Aspirin Free EXCEDRIN® is supplied as: Coated red caplets with "AF Excedrin" printed in white on one side.
NDC 19810-0089-1 Bottles of 24's
NDC 19810-0089-2 Bottles of 50's
NDC 19810-0089-3 Bottles of 100's
All sizes packaged in child resistant closures except 100's which is recommended for households without young children.
Store at room temperature.

Shown in Product Identification Section, page 405

EXCEDRIN® Extra-Strength Analgesic
[*ĕx ″cĕd ′rĭn*]

Composition:
Each tablet or caplet contains Acetaminophen 250 mg.: Aspirin 250 mg.; and Caffeine 65 mg.
Other Ingredients: (Tablets or Caplets) Benzoic Acid, FD&C Blue No. 1, Hydroxypropyl Methylcellulose, Microcrystalline Cellulose, Mineral Oil, Polysorbate 20, Povidone, Propylene Glycol, Saccharin Sodium, Simethicone Emulsion, Sorbitan Monolaurate, Stearic Acid, Titanium Dioxide. May Also Contain: Carnauba Wax, Hydroxypropylcellulose.

Indications: For temporary relief of the pain of headache, sinusitis, colds, muscular aches, menstrual discomfort, toothaches and minor arthritis pain.

Directions: Adults: 2 tablets or caplets with water every 6 hours while symptoms persist, not to exceed 8 tablets or caplets in 24 hours, or as directed by a doctor. Children under 12 years of age: Consult a doctor.

Warnings: Children and teenagers should not use this medicine for chickenpox or flu symptoms before a doctor is consulted about Reye syndrome, a rare but serious illness reported to be associated with aspirin. KEEP THIS AND ALL OTHER MEDICATIONS OUT OF THE REACH OF CHILDREN. IN CASE OF ACCIDENTAL OVERDOSE, SEEK PROFESSIONAL ASSISTANCE OR CONTACT A POISON CONTROL CENTER IMMEDIATELY. PROMPT MEDICAL ATTENTION IS CRITICAL FOR ADULTS AS WELL AS FOR CHILDREN EVEN IF YOU DO NOT NOTICE ANY SIGNS OR SYMPTOMS. As with any drug, if you are pregnant or nursing a baby, seek the advice of a health professional before using this product. **IT IS ESPECIALLY IMPORTANT NOT TO USE ASPIRIN DURING THE LAST 3 MONTHS OF PREGNANCY UNLESS SPECIFICALLY DIRECTED TO DO SO BY A DOCTOR BECAUSE IT MAY CAUSE PROBLEMS IN THE UNBORN CHILD OR COMPLICATIONS DURING DELIVERY.** Do not take this product for pain for more than 10 days or for fever for more than 3 days unless directed by a doctor. If pain or fever persists or gets worse, if new symptoms occur, or if redness or swelling is present, consult a doctor because these could be signs of a serious condition. Consult a dentist promptly for toothache. Do not take this product if you are allergic to aspirin, have asthma, have stomach problems (such as heartburn, upset stomach or stomach pain) that persist or recur, or if you have ulcers or bleeding problems, unless directed by a doctor. If ringing in the ears or loss of hearing occurs, consult a doctor before taking any more of this product.

Drug Interaction Precaution: Do not take this product if you are taking a prescription drug for anticoagulation (thinning of blood), diabetes, gout or arthritis unless directed by a doctor.

Overdose:
MUCOMYST (acetylcysteine As An Antidote For Acetaminophen Overdose)
Acetaminophen is rapidly absorbed from the upper gastrointestinal tract with peak plasma levels occurring between 30 and 60 minutes after therapeutic doses and usually within 4 hours following an overdose. The parent compound, which is nontoxic, is extensively metabolized in the liver to form principally the sulfate and glucuronide conjugates which are also nontoxic and are rapidly excreted in the urine. A small fraction of an ingested dose is metabolized in the liver by the cytochrome P-450 mixed function oxidase enzyme system to form a reactive, potentially toxic, intermediate metabolite which preferentially conjugates with hepatic glutathione to form the nontoxic cysteine and mercapturic acid derivatives which are then excreted by the kidney. Therapeutic doses of acetaminophen do not saturate the glucuronide and sulfate conjugation pathways and do not result in the formation of sufficient reactive metabolite to deplete glutathione

stores. However, following ingestion of a larger overdose (150 mg/kg or greater) the glucuronide and sulfate conjugation pathways are saturated resulting in larger fraction of the drug being metabolized via the P-450 pathway. The increased formation of reactive metabolite may deplete the hepatic stores of glutathione with subsequent binding of the metabolite to protein molecules within the hepatocyte resulting in cellular necrosis. Acetylcysteine has been shown to reduce the extent of liver injury following acetaminophen overdose. Early symptoms following a potentially hepatotoxic overdose may include nausea, vomiting, diaphoresis and general malaise. Clinical and laboratory evidence of hepatic toxicity may not be apparent until 48 to 72 hours postingestion. In adults and adolescents, regardless of the quantity of acetaminophen reported to have been ingested, administer MUCOMYST® acetylcysteine immediately. MUCOMYST acetylcysteine therapy should be initiated and continued for a full course of therapy. Its effectiveness depends on early administration, with benefit seen principally in patients treated within 16 hours of the overdose.
If acetaminophen plasma assay capability is not available, and the estimated acetaminophen ingestion exceeds 150 mg/kg, MUCOMYST acetylcysteine therapy should be initiated and continued for a full course of therapy.
For full prescribing information, refer to the MUCOMYST package insert. Do not await the results of assays for acetaminophen level before initiating treatment with MUCOMYST acetylcysteine. The following additional procedures are recommended. The stomach should be emptied promptly by lavage or by induction of emesis with syrup of ipecac. A serum acetaminophen assay should be obtained as early as possible, but no sooner than four hours following ingestion. Liver function studies should be obtained initially and repeated at 24-hour intervals.
For additional emergency information call your regional poison center or toll-free (1-800-525-6115) to the Rocky Mountain Poison Center for assistance in diagnosis and for directions in the use of MUCOMYST acetylcysteine as an antidote.

How Supplied: Extra Strength EXCEDRIN® is supplied as:
White circular tablet with letter "E" debossed on one side.
NDC 19810-0700-2 Bottles of 12's
NDC 19810-0782-3 Bottles of 24's
NDC 19810-0782-4 Bottles of 50's
NDC 19810-0700-5 Bottles of 100's
NDC 19810-0782-5 Bottles of 150's
NDC 19810-0782-6 Bottles of 200's
NDC 19810-0700-1 A metal tin of 12's
NDC 19810-0772-1 Vials of 10's
Coated white caplets with "Excedrin" printed in red on one side.
NDC 19810-0002-1 Bottles of 24's
NDC 19810-0002-2 Bottles of 50's
NDC 19810-0002-8 Bottles of 100's
All sizes packaged in child resistant closures except 100's for tablets, 50's for caplets which are sizes recommended for households without young children.
Store at room temperature.

Shown in Product Identification Section, page 405

EXCEDRIN P.M.®
[ĕx ″cĕd ′rĭn]
Analgesic Sleeping Aid

Composition: Each tablet, caplet and fluidounce (30 ml.) contains:
[See table on next page.]

Indications: For temporary relief of occasional headaches and minor aches and pains with accompanying sleeplessness.

Directions:
Tablets or Caplets:
Adults, 2 tablets or caplets at bedtime if needed or as directed by a doctor.
Liquid:
Adults, 1 fluidounce (2 tablespoons) at bedtime if needed, or as directed by a doctor, using the dosage cup provided.

Warnings: KEEP THIS AND ALL OTHER MEDICATIONS OUT OF THE REACH OF CHILDREN. IN CASE OF ACCIDENTAL OVERDOSE, SEEK PROFESSIONAL ASSISTANCE OR CONTACT A POISON CONTROL CENTER IMMEDIATELY. PROMPT MEDICAL ATTENTION IS CRITICAL FOR ADULTS AS WELL AS FOR CHILDREN EVEN IF YOU DO NOT NOTICE ANY SIGNS OR SYMPTOMS. As with any drug, if you are pregnant or nursing a baby, seek the advice of a health professional before using this product. Do not give this product to children under 12 years of age or use for more than 10 days unless directed by a doctor. Consult a doctor if symptoms persist or get worse or if new ones occur, or if sleeplessness persists continuously for more than 2 weeks because these may be symptoms of serious underlying medical illnesses. Do not take this product if you have asthma, glaucoma, emphysema, chronic pulmonary disease, shortness of breath, difficulty in breathing, or difficulty in urination due to enlargement of the prostate gland unless directed by a doctor. Avoid alcoholic beverages while taking this product. Do not take this product if you are taking sedatives or tranquilizers, without first consulting your doctor.

Overdose:
MUCOMYST (acetylcysteine) As An Antidote For Acetaminophen Overdose)
Acetaminophen is rapidly absorbed from the upper gastrointestinal tract with peak plasma levels occurring between 30 and 60 minutes after therapeutic doses and usually within 4 hours following an overdose. The parent compound, which is nontoxic, is extensively metabolized in the liver to form principally the sulfate and glucuronide conjugates which are also nontoxic and are rapidly excreted in the urine. A small fraction of an ingested dose is metabolized in the liver by the cytochrome P-450 mixed function oxidase enzyme system to form a reactive, potentially toxic, intermediate metabolite which preferentially conjugates with hepatic glutathione to form the nontoxic cysteine and mercapturic acid derivatives which are then excreted by the kidney. Therapeutic doses of acetaminophen do not saturate the glucuronide and sulfate conjugation pathways and do not result in the formation of sufficient reactive metabolite to deplete glutathione stores. However, following ingestion of a large overdose (150 mg/kg or greater) the glucuronide and sulfate conjugation pathways are saturated resulting in a larger fraction of the drug being metabolized via the P-450 pathway. The increased formation of reactive metabolite may deplete the hepatic stores of glutathione with subsequent binding of the metabolite to protein molecules within the hepatocyte resulting in cellular necrosis. Acetylcysteine has been shown to reduce the extent of liver injury following acetaminophen overdose. Early symptoms following a potentially hepatotoxic overdose may include: nausea, vomiting, diaphoresis and general malaise. Clinical and laboratory evidence of hepatic toxicity may not be apparent until 48 to 72 hours postingestion. In adults and adolescents, regardless of the quantity of acetaminophen reported to have been ingested, administer MUCOMYST® acetylcysteine immediately. MUCOMYST acetylcysteine therapy should be initiated and continued for a full course of therapy. Its effectiveness depends on early administration, with benefit seen principally in patients treated within 16 hours of the overdose.
If acetaminophen plasma assay capability is not available, and the estimated acetaminophen ingestion exceeds 150 mg/kg, MUCOMYST acetylcysteine therapy should be initiated and continued for a full course of therapy.
For full prescribing information, refer to the MUCOMYST package insert. Do not await the results of assays for acetaminophen level before initiating treatment with MUCOMYST acetylcysteine. The following additional procedures are recommended: The stomach should be emptied promptly by lavage or by induction of emesis with syrup of ipecac. A serum acetaminophen assay should be obtained as early as possible, but no sooner than four hours following ingestion. Liver function studies should be obtained initially and repeated at 24-hour intervals.
For additional emergency information call your regional poison center or toll-free (1-800-525-6115) to the Rocky Moun-

Continued on next page

Bristol-Myers—Cont.

	EXCEDRIN® PM Per Tablet or Caplet	EXCEDRIN® PM Per Fl. Ounce (30 ml.)
Acetaminophen	500 mg.	1000 mg.
Diphenhydramine Citrate:	38 mg.	—
Diphenhydramine HCl:	—	50 mg
Other Ingredients:	Tablet or Caplet	Liquid
	Benzoic Acid	Alcohol (10% by volume)
	Carnauba Wax	Benzoic Acid
	Corn Starch	FD&C Blue No. 1
	D&C Yellow No. 10	Flavor
	D&C Yellow No. 10 Aluminum Lake	Polyethylene Glycol
	FD&C Blue No. 1	Povidone
	FD&C Blue No. 1 Aluminum Lake	Sodium Citrate
	Hydroxypropyl Methylcellulose	Sucrose
	Methylparaben	Water
	Magnesium Stearate	
	Propylene Glycol	
	Propylparaben	
	Simethicone Emulsion	
	Stearic Acid	
	Titanium Dioxide	

tain Poison Center for assistance in diagnosis and for directions in the use of MUCOMYST acetylcysteine as an antidote.

How Supplied: EXCREDRIN P.M.® is supplied as:
Light blue circular coated tablets with "PM" debossed on one side.
NDC 19810-0763-6 Bottles of 10's
NDC 19810-0764-3 Bottles of 24's
NDC 19810-0763-4 Bottles of 50's
NDC 19810-0764-4 Bottles of 100's
NDC 19810-0763-9 Vials of 10's
Light blue coated caplet with "Excedrin P.M." imprinted on one side.
NDC 19810-0032-5 Bottles of 24's
NDC 19810-0032-3 Bottles of 50's
NDC 19810-0032-6 Bottles of 100's
Light blue wild berry flavored liquid.
NDC 19810-0060-1 6 oz. (177 ml) Plastic Bottle
All sizes packaged in child resistant closures except 50's tablets and caplets which are recommended for households without young children.
Store at room temperature

Shown in Product Identification Section, page 405

Sinus EXCEDRIN®
[*ex"cĕd'rĭn*]
Analgesic, Decongestant

Composition: Each coated tablet or caplet contains 500 mg Acetaminophen and 30 mg Pseudoephedrine HCl.

Other Ingredients: Corn Starch, D&C Yellow No. 10 Lake, FD&C Red No. 40 Lake, Hydroxypropyl Methylcellulose, Mineral Oil, Polysorbate 20, Povidone, Propylene Glycol, Simethicone Emulsion, Sorbitan Monolaurate, Stearic Acid, Titanium Dioxide. May also contain: Benzoic Acid, Carnauba Wax.

Indications: For temporary relief of headache, sinus pain and sinus pressure and congestion due to sinusitis or the common cold.

Directions: Adults: 2 tablets or caplets every 6 hours while symptoms persist, not to exceed 8 tablets or caplets in 24 hours, or as directed by a doctor. Children under 12 years of age: Consult a doctor.

Warnings: KEEP THIS AND ALL MEDICATIONS OUT OF THE REACH OF CHILDREN. IN CASE OF ACCIDENTAL OVERDOSE, SEEK PROFESSIONAL ASSISTANCE OR CONTACT A POISON CONTROL CENTER IMMEDIATELY. PROMPT MEDICAL ATTENTION IS CRITICAL FOR ADULTS AS WELL AS FOR CHILDREN EVEN IF YOU DO NOT NOTICE ANY SIGNS OR SYMPTOMS. As with any drug, if you are pregnant or nursing a baby, seek the advice of a health professional before using this product. Do not take this product for more than 10 days unless directed by a doctor. If symptoms do not improve or are accompanied by a fever that lasts for more than 3 days, or if new symptoms occur, consult a doctor. Do not exceed recommended dosage because at higher doses nervousness, dizziness or sleeplessness may occur. Do not take this product if you have heart disease, high blood pressure, thyroid disease, diabetes, or difficulty in urination due to enlargement of the prostate gland unless directed by a doctor.

Drug Interaction Precaution: Do not take this product if you are taking a prescription medication for high blood pressure or depression without first consulting a doctor.

Overdose:
MUCOMYST (acetylcysteine) As An Antidote for Acetaminophen Overdose)
Acetaminophen is rapidly absorbed from the upper gastrointestinal tract with peak plasma levels occurring between 30 and 60 minutes after therapeutic doses and usually within 4 hours following an overdose. The parent compound, which is nontoxic, is extensively metabolized in the liver to form principally the sulfate and glucuronide conjugates which are also nontoxic and are rapidly excreted in the urine. A small fraction of an ingested dose is metabolized in the liver by the cytochrome P-450 mixed function oxidase enzyme system to form a reactive, potentially toxic, intermediate metabolite which preferentially conjugates with hepatic glutathione to form the nontoxic cysteine and mercapturic acid derivatives which are then excreted by the kidney. Therapeutic doses of acetaminophen do not saturate the glucuronide and sulfate conjugation pathways and do not result in the formation of sufficient reactive metabolite to deplete glutathione stores. However, following ingestion of a large overdose (150 mg/kg or greater) the glucuronide and sulfate conjugation pathways are saturated resulting in a larger fraction of the drug being metabolized via the P-450 pathway. The increased formation of reactive metabolite may deplete the hepatic stores of glutathione with subsequent binding of the metabolite to protein molecules within the hepatocyte resulting in cellular necrosis. Acetylcysteine has been shown to reduce the extent of liver injury following acetaminophen overdose. Early symptoms following a potentially hepatotoxic overdose may include: nausea, vomiting, diaphoresis and general malaise. Clinical and laboratory evidence of hepatic toxicity may not be apparent until 48 to 72 hours postingestion. In adults and adolescents, regardless of the quantity of acetaminophen reported to have been ingested, administer MUCOMYST® acetylcysteine immediately. MUCOMYST acetylcysteine therapy should be initiated and continued for a full course of therapy. Its effectiveness depends on early administration, with benefit seen principally in patients treated within 16 hours of the overdose. If acetaminophen plasma assay capability is not available, and the estimated acetaminophen ingestion exceeds 150 mg/kg, MUCOMYST acetylcysteine

therapy should be initiated and continued for a full course of therapy.
For full prescribing information, refer to the MUCOMYST package insert. Do not await the results of assays for acetaminophen level before initiating treatment with MUCOMYST acetylcysteine. The following additional procedures are recommended: The stomach should be emptied promptly by lavage or by induction of emesis with syrup of ipecac. A serum acetaminophen assay should be obtained as early as possible, but no sooner than four hours following ingestion. Liver function studies should be obtained initially and repeated at 24-hour intervals.
For additional emergency information call your regional poison center or toll-free (1-800-525-6115) to the Rocky Mountain Poison Center for assistance in diagnosis and for directions in the use of MUCOMYST acetylcysteine as an antidote.

How Supplied: Sinus EXCEDRIN® is supplied as:
Coated circular orange tablets with "Sinus Excedrin" imprinted in green on one side.
NDC 19810-0080-1 Blister packages of 24's
NDC 19810-0080-2 Bottles of 50's
Coated orange caplets with "Sinus Excedrin" imprinted in green on one side.
NDC 19810-0077-1 Blister packages of 24's
NDC 19810-0077-2 Bottles of 50's
All sizes have child resistant closures except 24's for tablets and caplets which are recommended for households without young children.
Store at room temperature.

Shown in Product Identification Section, page 405

4-WAY® Cold Tablets

Composition: Each tablet contains acetaminophen 325 mg., phenylpropanolamine HCl 12.5 mg., and chlorpheniramine maleate 2 mg. Other Ingredients: Corn Starch, Corn Starch Pregelatinized, Microcrystalline Cellulose, Sodium Starch Glycolate, Stearic Acid, Sucrose.

Indications: For temporary relief of nasal and sinus congestion, runny nose, sneezing, fever, minor sore throat pain, body aches and pain.

Directions:
Adults: 2 tablets every 4 hours while symptoms persist, not to exceed 12 tablets in 24 hours, or as directed by a doctor. Children 6 to under 12 years of age: One tablet every 4 hours while symptoms persist, not to exceed 5 tablets in 24 hours, or as directed by a doctor. Children under 6: Consult a doctor.

Warnings: KEEP THIS AND ALL OTHER MEDICATIONS OUT OF THE REACH OF CHILDREN. IN CASE OF ACCIDENTAL OVERDOSE, SEEK PROFESSIONAL ASSISTANCE OR CONTACT A POISON CONTROL CENTER IMMEDIATELY. PROMPT MEDICAL ATTENTION IS CRITICAL FOR ADULTS AS WELL AS FOR CHILDREN EVEN IF YOU DO NOT NOTICE ANY SIGNS OR SYMPTOMS. As with any drug, if you are pregnant or nursing a baby, seek the advice of a health professional before using this product. Do not take this product for more than 10 days (for adults) or 5 days (for children) unless directed by a doctor. If symptoms do not improve or are accompanied by a fever that lasts for more than 3 days, or if new symptoms occur, consult a doctor. Do not exceed recommended dosage because at higher doses nervousness, dizziness or sleeplessness may occur. May cause excitability especially in children. If sore throat is severe, persists for more than 2 days, is accompanied or followed by a fever, headache, rash, nausea or vomiting, consult a doctor promptly. This product should not be taken by persons who have asthma, glaucoma, emphysema, chronic pulmonary disease, high blood pressure, heart disease, thyroid disease, diabetes, shortness of breath, difficulty in breathing or difficulty in urination due to enlargement of the prostate gland unless directed by a doctor. May cause drowsiness; alcohol may increase the drowsiness effect. Avoid alcoholic beverages, and do not take this product if you are taking sedatives or tranquilizers without first consulting your doctor. Use caution when driving a motor vehicle or operating machinery.

Drug Interaction Precaution: This product should not be taken by any adult or child who is taking a prescription medication for high blood pressure or depression without first consulting a doctor.

Overdose:
MUCOMYST (acetylcysteine) As An Antidote For Acetaminophen Overdose)
Acetaminophen is rapidly absorbed from the upper gastrointestinal tract with peak plasma levels occurring between 30 and 60 minutes after therapeutic doses and usually within 4 hours following an overdose. The parent compound, which is nontoxic, is extensively metabolized in the liver to form principally the sulfate and glucuronide conjugates which are also nontoxic and are rapidly excreted in the urine. A small fraction of an ingested dose is metabolized in the liver by the cytochrome P-450 mixed function oxidase enzyme system to form a reactive, potentially toxic, intermediate metabolite which preferentially conjugates with hepatic glutathione to form the nontoxic cysteine and mercapturic acid derivatives which are then excreted by the kidney. Therapeutic doses of acetaminophen do not saturate the glucuronide and sulfate conjugation pathways and do not result in the formation of sufficient reactive metabolite to deplete glutathione stores. However, following ingestion of a large overdose (150 mg/kg or greater) the glucuronide and sulfate conjugation pathways are saturated resulting in a larger fraction of the drug being metabolized via the P-450 pathway. The increased formation of reactive metabolite may deplete the hepatic stores of glutathione with subsequent binding of the metabolite to protein molecules within the hepatocyte resulting in cellular necrosis. Acetylcysteine has been shown to reduce the extent of liver injury following acetaminophen overdose. Early symptoms following a potentially hepatotoxic overdose may include: nausea, vomiting, diaphoresis and general malaise. Clinical and laboratory evidence of hepatic toxicity may not be apparent until 48 to 72 hours postingestion. In adults and adolescents, regardless of the quantity of acetaminophen reported to have been ingested, administer MUCOMYST® acetylcysteine immediately. MUCOMYST acetylcysteine therapy should be initiated and continued for a full course of therapy. Its effectiveness depends on early administration, with benefit seen principally in patients treated within 16 hours of the overdose.
If acetaminophen plasma assay capability is not available, and the estimated acetaminophen ingestion exceeds 150 mg/kg, MUCOMYST acetylcysteine therapy should be initiated and continued for a full course of therapy.
For full prescribing information, refer to the MUCOMYST package insert. Do not await the results of assays for acetaminophen level before initiating treatment with MUCOMYST acetylcysteine. The following additional procedures are recommended: The stomach should be emptied promptly by lavage or by induction of emesis with syrup of ipecac. A serum acetaminophen assay should be obtained as early as possible, but no sooner than four hours following ingestion. Liver function studies should be obtained initially and repeated at 24-hour intervals.
For additional emergency information call your regional poison center or toll-free (1-800-525-6115) to the Rocky Mountain Poison Center for assistance in diagnosis and for directions in the use of MUCOMYST acetylcysteine as an antidote.

How Supplied: 4-WAY Cold Tablets are supplied as a white tablet with the number "4" debossed on one surface.
NDC 19810-0040-1 Bottle of 36's
All sizes packaged in child resistant bottle closures.
Store at room temperature.

4-WAY® Fast Acting Nasal Spray

Composition:
Phenylephrine hydrochloride 0.5%, naphazoline hydrochloride 0.05%, pyrilamine maleate 0.2%, in a buffered solution. Also Contains: Benzalkonium Chloride, Boric Acid, Sodium Borate, Water. Also available in a mentholated formula containing Phenylephrine hydrochloride 0.5%, naphazoline hydrochloride 0.05%,

Continued on next page

Bristol-Myers—Cont.

pyrilamine maleate 0.2%, in a buffered solution. Also Contains: Benzalkonium Chloride, Boric Acid, Camphor, Eucalyptol, Menthol, Poloxamer 188, Polysorbate 80, Sodium Borate, Water.

Indications: For prompt, temporary relief of nasal congestion due to the common cold, sinusitis, hay fever or other upper respiratory allergies.

Directions and Use Instructions:
Directions: Adults: Spray twice into each nostril not more often than every 4 hours. Do not give to children under 12 years of age unless directed by a doctor.
Use Instructions: For Metered Pump—
Remove protective cap. Hold bottle with thumb at base and nozzle between first and second fingers. With head upright, insert metered pump spray nozzle into nostril. Depress pump all the way down, with a firm even stroke and sniff deeply. Repeat in other nostril. Do not tilt head backward while spraying. Wipe tip clean after each use. Note: This bottle is filled to correct level for proper pump action. Before using the first time, remove the protective cap from the tip and prime the metered pump by depressing pump firmly several times.
Use Instructions: For Atomizer—
With head in a normal upright position, put atomizer tip into nostril. Squeeze bottle with firm, quick pressure while inhaling.

Warnings: KEEP THIS AND ALL OTHER MEDICATIONS OUT OF THE REACH OF CHILDREN. IN CASE OF ACCIDENTAL OVERDOSE OR INGESTION, SEEK PROFESSIONAL ASSISTANCE OR CONTACT A POISON CONTROL CENTER IMMEDIATELY. Do not exceed recommended dosage because burning, stinging, sneezing, or increase of nasal discharge may occur. The use of this container by more than one person may spread infection. Do not use this product for more than 3 days. If symptoms persist, consult a doctor. Adults and children who have heart disease, high blood pressure, thyroid disease, diabetes, or difficulty in urination due to enlargement of the prostate gland should not use this product unless directed by a doctor.

How Supplied:
Regular formula:
NDC 19810-0047-1 Atomizer of ½ fluid ounce.
NDC 19810-0047-2 Atomizer of 1 fluid ounce.
NDC 19810-0047-3 Metered pump of ½ fluid ounce.
New Mentholated formula:
NDC 19810-0049-1 Atomizer of ½ fluid ounce.
NDC 19810-0049-2 Atomizer of 1 fluid ounce.
Store at room temperature.

Shown in Product Identification Section, page 405

4-WAY® Long Lasting Nasal Spray

Composition: Oxymetazoline Hydrochloride 0.05% in an isotonic aqueous solution. Phenylmercuric Acetate 0.002% added as a preservative. **Also Contains:** Benzalkonium Chloride, Glycine, Sorbitol, Water.

Indications: For prompt, temporary relief of nasal congestion due to the common cold, sinusitis, hay fever or other upper respiratory allergies.

Directions and Use Instructions:
Directions: Adults and children 6 to under 12 years of age (with adult supervision): 2 or 3 sprays in each nostril not more often than every 10 to 12 hours. Do not exceed 2 applications in any 24-hour period. Children under 6 years of age: Consult a doctor.
Use Instructions: For Metered Pump—
Remove protective cap. Hold bottle with thumb at base and nozzle between first and second fingers. With head upright, insert metered pump spray nozzle into nostril. Depress pump all the way down, with a firm even stroke and sniff deeply. Repeat in other nostril. Do not tilt head backward while spraying. Wipe tip clean after each use. Note: This bottle is filled to correct level for proper pump action. Before using the first time, remove the protective cap from the tip and prime the metered pump by depressing pump firmly several times.
Use Instructions: For Atomizer—
With head in a normal, upright position, put atomizer tip into nostril. Squeeze bottle with firm, quick pressure while inhaling.

Warnings: KEEP THIS AND ALL OTHER MEDICATIONS OUT OF THE REACH OF CHILDREN. IN CASE OF ACCIDENTAL OVERDOSE OR INGESTION, SEEK PROFESSIONAL ASSISTANCE OR CONTACT A POISON CONTROL CENTER IMMEDIATELY. Do not exceed recommended dosage because burning, stinging, sneezing, or increase of nasal discharge may occur. The use of this container by more than one person may spread infection. Do not use this product for more than 3 days. If symptoms persist, consult a doctor. Adults and children who have heart disease, high blood pressure, thyroid disease, diabetes, or difficulty in urination due to enlargement of the prostate gland should not use this product unless directed by a doctor.

How Supplied: 4-WAY Long Lasting Nasal Spray is supplied as:
NDC 19810-0048-1 Atomizer of ½ fluid ounce.
Store at room temperature.

Shown in Product Identification Section, page 405

KERI LOTION
Skin Lubricant—Moisturizer

Available in three formulations:
KERI Original—recommended for dry skin.

Composition: Mineral oil in water, propylene glycol, glyceryl stearate/PEG-100 stearate, PEG-40 stearate, PEG-4 dilaurate, laureth-4, lanolin oil, methylparaben, propylparaben, fragrance, carbomer-934, triethanolamine, dioctyl sodium sulfosuccinate, quaternium-15.

KERI Silky Smooth with Vitamin E—recommended for daily use on dry skin.

Composition: Water, petrolatum, glycerin, dimethicone, steareth-2, cetyl alcohol, benzyl alcohol, laureth-23, magnesium aluminum silicate, tocopheryl linoleate, carbomer, BHT, fragrance, sodium hydroxide, disodium EDTA, quaternium-15.

KERI Silky Smooth Fragrance Free with Vitamin E—recommended for daily use on dry skin.

Composition: Water, petrolatum, glycerin, dimethicone, steareth-2, cetyl alcohol, benzyl alcohol, laureth-23, magnesium aluminum silicate, tocopheryl linoleate, carbomer, BHT, sodium hydroxide, disodium EDTA, quaternium-15.

Indications: KERI Lotion lubricates and helps hydrate the skin, making it soft and smooth. It relieves itching, helps maintain a normal moisture balance and supplements the protective action of skin lipids. Indicated for generalized dryness; detergent hands; chapped or chafed skin; "winter-itch," diaper rash; heat rash.

Directions for Use: Apply as often as needed. Use particularly after bathing and exposure to sun, water, soaps and detergents. For external use only.

How Supplied: KERI Lotion Original 6½ oz., 11 oz., 15 oz. and 20 oz. plastic bottles. KERI Silky Smooth 6½ oz., 11 oz. and 15 oz. plastic bottles. KERI Silky Smooth Fragrance Free 6½ oz., 11 oz. and 15 oz. plastic bottles.

Shown in Product Identification Section, page 405

NO DOZ® Tablets
[nō ′dōz]

Composition: Each tablet contains 100 mg. Caffeine. Other Ingredients: Cornstarch, Flavors, Mannitol, Microcrystalline Cellulose, Stearic Acid, Sucrose.

Indications: Helps restore mental alertness or wakefulness when experiencing fatigue or drowsiness.

Directions: Adults 1 or 2 tablets not more often than every 3 to 4 hours.

Warnings: KEEP THIS AND ALL OTHER MEDICATIONS OUT OF THE REACH OF CHILDREN. IN CASE OF ACCIDENTAL OVERDOSE, SEEK PROFESSIONAL ASSISTANCE OR CONTACT A POISON CONTROL CENTER IMMEDIATELY. As with any drug, if you are pregnant or nursing a baby, seek the advice of a health professional before using this product. Do not give to children under 12 years of age. For occasional use only. Not intended for use as a substitute for sleep. If fatigue or drowsiness persists or continues to occur, consult a doctor. The recommended dose of this product contains about as much caffeine as a cup of coffee. Limit the use of caffeine-containing medications, foods, or beverages while taking this product because too much caffeine may cause nervousness, irritability, sleeplessness and, occasionally, rapid heart beat.

How Supplied: NO DOZ® is supplied as:
A circular white tablet with "NoDoz" debossed on one side.
NDC 19810-0063-2 Blister pack of 16's
NDC 19810-0063-3 Blister pack of 36's
NDC 19810-0063-5 Bottle of 60's
NDC 19810-0063-1 Vials of 15's
Store at room temperature.

Shown in Product Identification Section, page 405

NO DOZ® Maximum Strength Caplets

Composition: Each caplet contains 200 mg. Caffeine. Other ingredients: Benzoic Acid, Corn Starch, FD&C Blue No. 1, Flavors, Hydroxypropyl Methylcellulose, Microcrystalline Cellulose, Propylene Glycol, Simethicone Emulsion, Stearic Acid, Sucrose, Titanium Dioxide. May also contain: Carnauba Wax, Mineral Oil, Polysorbate 20, Povidone, Sorbitan Monolaurate.

Indications: Helps restore mental alertness or wakefulness when experiencing fatigue or drowsiness.

Directions: Adults: one-half to one caplet not more often than every 3 to 4 hours.

Warnings: KEEP THIS AND ALL OTHER MEDICATIONS OUT OF THE REACH OF CHILDREN. IN CASE OF ACCIDENTAL OVERDOSE, SEEK PROFESSIONAL ASSISTANCE OR CONTACT A POISON CONTROL CENTER IMMEDIATELY. As with any drug, if you are pregnant or nursing a baby, seek the advice of a health professional before using this product. Do not give to children under 12 years of age. For occasional use only. Not intended for use as a substitute for sleep. If fatigue or drowsiness persists or continues to occur, consult a doctor. The recommended dose of this product contains about as much caffeine as a cup of coffee. Limit the use of caffeine-containing medications, foods, or beverages while taking this product because too much caffeine may cause nervousness, irritability, sleeplessness and, occasionally, rapid heart beat.

How Supplied: NO DOZ® Maximum Strength is supplied as: White coated caplets with "NO DOZ" debossed on one side. The opposite side is scored.
NDC 19810-0064-1 Blister Packs of 12's
NDC 19810-0064-3 Bottles of 30
Store at room temperature.

Shown in Product Identification Section, page 405

NUPRIN® (ibuprofen) Analgesic

Warning: ASPIRIN SENSITIVE PATIENTS. Do not take this product if you have had a severe allergic reaction to aspirin, e.g.—asthma, swelling, shock or hives, because even though this product contains no aspirin or salicylates, cross-reactions may occur in patients allergic to aspirin. (See ADDITIONAL WARNINGS BELOW)

Composition: Each tablet or caplet contains ibuprofen USP, 200 mg. **Other Ingredients:** Carnauba wax, cornstarch, D&C Yellow No. 10, FD&C Yellow No. 6, hydroxypropyl methylcellulose, propylene glycol, silicon dioxide, stearic acid, titanium dioxide.

Indications: For the temporary relief of minor aches and pains associated with the common cold, headache, toothache, muscular aches, backache, for the minor pain of arthritis, for the pain of menstrual cramps and for reduction of fever.

Additional Warnings: The following warnings are stated on the Nuprin label: Do not take for pain for more than 10 days or for fever for more than 3 days unless directed by a doctor. If pain or fever persists or gets worse, if new symptoms occur, or if the painful area is red or swollen, consult a doctor. These could be signs of serious illness. If you are under a doctor's care for any serious condition, consult a doctor before taking this product. As with aspirin and acetaminophen, if you have any condition which requires you to take prescription drugs or if you have had any problems or serious side effects from taking any non-prescription pain reliever, do not take NUPRIN without first discussing it with your doctor. If you experience any symptoms which are unusual or seem unrelated to the condition for which you took ibuprofen, consult a doctor before taking any more of it. Although ibuprofen is indicated for the same conditions as aspirin and acetaminophen, it should not be taken with them except under a doctor's direction. Do not combine this product with any other ibuprofen-containing product. As with any drug, if you are pregnant or nursing a baby, seek the advice of a health professional before using this product. IT IS ESPECIALLY IMPORTANT NOT TO USE IBUPROFEN DURING THE LAST 3 MONTHS OF PREGNANCY UNLESS SPECIFICALLY DIRECTED TO DO SO BY A DOCTOR BECAUSE IT MAY CAUSE PROBLEMS IN THE UNBORN CHILD OR COMPLICATIONS DURING DELIVERY. Keep this and all drugs out of the reach of children. In case of accidental overdose, seek professional assistance or contact a poison control center immediately.

Caution: Store at room temperature. Avoid excessive heat 40°C (104°F).

Directions: Adults: Take 1 tablet or caplet every 4 to 6 hours while symptoms persist. If pain or fever does not respond to 1 tablet or caplet, 2 tablets or caplets may be used but do not exceed 6 tablets or caplets in 24 hours, unless directed by a doctor. The smallest effective dose should be used. Take with food or milk if occasional and mild heartburn, upset stomach, or stomach pain occurs with use. Consult a doctor if these symptoms are more than mild or if they persist. Children: Do not give this product to children under 12 except under the advice and supervision of a doctor.

How Supplied:
NUPRIN® is supplied as:
Golden yellow round tablets with "NUPRIN" printed in black on one side.
NDC 19810-0767-2 Bottles of 24's
NDC 19810-0767-3 Bottles of 50's
NDC 19810-0767-4 Bottles of 100's
NDC 19810-0767-7 Bottles of 150's
NDC 19810-0767-8 Bottles of 225's
NDC 19810-0767-9 Vials of 10's
Golden yellow caplets with "NUPRIN" printed in black on one side.
NDC 19810-0796-1 Bottles of 24's
NDC 19810-0796-2 Bottles of 50's
NDC 19810-0796-3 Bottles of 100's
All sizes packaged in child resistant closures except 24's for tablets and 24's for caplets, which are sizes recommended for households without young children.
Store at room temperature. Avoid excessive heat 40°C. (104°F.).
Distributed by Bristol-Myers Company

Shown in Product Identification Section, page 405

PAZO® Hemorrhoid Ointment/Suppositories

Composition:
Ointment: Active Ingredients: Camphor, 2%; Ephedrine Sulfate, 0.2%; Zinc Oxide, 5%. Other Ingredients: Lanolin, Petrolatum.
Suppositories (per suppository): Active Ingredients: Ephedrine Sulfate, 3.86 mg; Zinc Oxide, 96.5 mg. Other Ingredients: Hydrogenated Vegetable Oil.

Indications:
Ointment: For the temporary relief of local pain, itching, and discomfort associated with inflamed hemorrhoidal tissues. Temporarily shrinks hemorrhoidal tissue.
Suppositories: For the temporary relief of local itching and discomfort associated with inflamed hemorrhoidal tissues. Temporarily shrinks hemorrhoidal tissue.

Directions:
Ointment—Adults: When practical, cleanse the affected area with soap and warm water and rinse thoroughly. Gently dry by patting or blotting with toilet tissue or a soft cloth before application of this product. Apply to the affected area up to 4 times daily. Do not put this product into the rectum by using fingers

Continued on next page

Bristol-Myers—Cont.

or any mechanical device or applicator. Children under 12 years of age: consult a doctor.

Suppositories—Adults: When practical, cleanse the affected area with mild soap and warm water and rinse thoroughly. Gently dry by patting or blotting with toilet tissue or a soft cloth before application of this product. Remove foil wrapper and insert suppository into the rectum. Use rectally up to 4 times daily. Children under 12 years of age: consult a doctor.

Warnings: KEEP THIS AND ALL OTHER MEDICATIONS OUT OF THE REACH OF CHILDREN. IN CASE OF ACCIDENTAL INGESTION OR OVERDOSE, SEEK PROFESSIONAL ASSISTANCE OR CONTACT A POISON CONTROL CENTER IMMEDIATELY. As with any drug, if you are pregnant or nursing a baby, seek the advice of a health professional before using this product. If condition worsens or does not improve within 7 days, consult a doctor. Do not exceed the recommended daily dosage unless directed by a doctor. In case of bleeding consult a doctor promptly. Do not use this product if you have heart disease, high blood pressure, thyroid disease, diabetes, or difficulty in urination due to enlargement of the prostate gland unless directed by a doctor. Some users of this product may experience nervousness, tremor, sleeplessness, nausea, and loss of appetite. If these symptoms persist or become worse consult your doctor.

DRUG INTERACTION PRECAUTION: Do not use this product if you are taking a prescription drug for high blood pressure or depression without first consulting your doctor. Store at room temperature.

How Supplied: PAZO® ointment is supplied as:
NDC 19810-0768-1 One ounce tubes
PAZO® suppositories are silver foil wrapped and supplied as:
NDC 19810-0703-1 Box of 12's

Shown in Product Identification Section, page 405

PRESUN® ACTIVE 15 AND 30
Clear Gel Sunscreens

Active Ingredients: Oxybenzone. Octyl Methoxycinnamate. Octyl Salicylate.
PRESUN® 15 Also contains: S.D. Alcohol 40, 71.5% PPG-15 Stearyl Ether, Acrylates/t-Ocylpropenamide Copolymer, Hydroxypropylcellulose.
PRESUN® 30 Also contains: S.D. Alcohol 40, 69% PPG-15 Stearyl Ether, Acrylates/t-Ocylpropenamide Copolymer, Hydroxypropylcellulose.

Indications: 15 OR 30 TIMES NATURAL UVB PROTECTION: Used liberally and regularly PreSun® 15 or 30 Active Clear Gel Sunscreens provide 15 or 30 times your natural UVB sunburn protection and may help reduce the chance of premature wrinkling of the skin caused by repeated and prolonged overexposure to the sun.
UVA/UVB PROTECTION: PreSun® 15 or 30 Active Clear Gel Sunscreens are formulated to provide protection from sunburn caused by both UVA and UVB rays.
CLEAR GEL FORMULA: PreSun® Active Sunscreens are cool refreshing Clear Gels that feel non-greasy. They are fragrance and PABA free, which fits your Active lifestyle.
WATERPROOF: PreSun® 15 or 30 Active Clear Gel Sunscreens maintain their degree of protection even after 80 minutes in the water.

Directions: Smooth evenly and liberally onto dry skin before sun exposure. Massage in gently. Reapply to dry skin after swimming, excessive perspiration or towel drying.

Warnings: For external use only. As with all sunscreens, avoid contact with eyes. Discontinue use if irritation or rash appears. Consult a physician before using on children under six months of age.

How Supplied: 4 oz. plastic bottles

PRESUN® FOR KIDS
Children's Sunscreen

Active Ingredients: Octyl methoxycinnamate, oxybenzone, octyl salicylate.
Also contains: Water, isopropyl myristate, PG dioctanoate, isodecyl neopentanoate, DEA cetyl phosphate, PVP/Eicosene copolymer, stearic acid, cetyl alcohol, dimethicone, diazolidinyl urea, Carbomer-940, triethanolamine, methylchloroisothiazolinone, and methylisothiazolinone.

Indications: 29 TIMES NATURAL PROTECTION: Used as directed, PRESUN For Kids provides 29 times your child's natural sunburn protection and may help reduce the chance of premature aging and wrinkling of the skin.
NONSTINGING: A non-PABA, fragrance-free formula that is designed not to sting sensitive skin. (Avoid contact with eyes since all sunscreens can cause irritation and stinging of the eye.)
HYPOALLERGENIC: PRESUN For Kids is hypoallergenic and, because the known sensitizers common to most sunscreens have been removed, is suitable for your child's sensitive skin.
WATERPROOF 29: PRESUN For Kids maintains its degree of protection (SPF 29) even after 80 minutes in the water.

Warnings: For external use only. Protect from freezing. *As with all sunscreens:* Apply to a small area; check after 24 hours. Discontinue use if irritation or rash appears. Avoid contact with eyes. In case of contact, flush eyes with water. Keep out of the reach of children. Use on children under six months of age only with the advice of a physician.

Directions for Use: For maximum protection, smooth evenly and liberally onto dry skin before sun exposure. Massage in gently. Reapplication to dry skin after prolonged swimming, excessive perspiration or towel drying is recommended for all-day protection.

How Supplied: 4 oz. plastic bottle.

Shown in Product Identification Section, page 406

PRESUN® 8, 15 AND 25 MOISTURIZING SUNSCREENS WITH KERI

PreSun® 8 and 15 Moisturizing Sunscreens

Active Ingredient: Oxybenzone, octyl dimethyl PABA. Also contains: Water, petrolatum, isopropyl myristate, PG dioctanoate, isodecyl neopentanoate, DEA cetyl phosphate, PVP/Eicosene copolymer, stearic acid, cetyl alcohol, dimethicone, diazolidinyl urea, Carbomer-940, triethanolamine, methylchloroisothiazolinone and methylisothiazolinone. May also contain fragrance.

PreSun® 25 Moisturizing Sunscreen

Active Ingredient: Octyl methoxycinnamate, oxybenzone, octyl salicylate. Also contains: Water, isopropyl myristate, isodecyl neopentanoate, propylene glycol dioctanoate, petrolatum, DEA-cetyl phosphate, PVP-Eicosene copolymer, stearic acid, cetyl alcohol, dimethicone, diazolidinyl urea, Carbomer-940, triethanolamince, methylchloroisothiazolinone and methylisothiazolinone.

Indications: 8, 15 or 25 TIMES NATURAL UVB PROTECTION: Used liberally and regularly, PreSun® Moisturizing Sunscreens provide 8, 15 or 25 times your natural UVB sunburn protection and may help reduce the chance of premature wrinkling of the skin caused by repeated and prolonged exposure to the sun. **UVA/UVB Protection:** PreSun® Moisturizing Sunscreens are formulated to provide protection from sunburn caused by both UVA and UVB rays.
Moisturizing: PreSun® Moisturizing Sunscreen with Keri moisturizing is a moisture-rich formula that is absorbed in quickly to provide a high degree of UVB sunburn protection while helping to relieve the drying effects of the sun.
Waterproof: PreSun® Moisturizing Sunscreen maintains its degree of protection even after 80 minutes in the water.

Directions: Smooth evenly and liberally onto dry skin before sun exposure. Massage in gently. Reapply to dry skin after swimming, excessive perspiration or towel drying.

Warning: For external use only. As with all sunscreens, avoid contact with eyes. Discontinue use if irritation or rash appears. Consult a physician before using on children under six months of age.

How Supplied: 4 oz. plastic bottles

PRESUN® 23 and
PRESUN® FOR KIDS
Spray Mist Sunscreens

Active Ingredients: Octyl dimethyl PABA, octyl methoxycinnamate, oxybenzone, octyl salicylate. Also contains: C_{12-15} alcohols benzoate, cyclomethicone, PG dioctanoate, PVP hexadecene, copolymer, and 19% (w/w) SD alcohol 40.

Indications: 23 TIMES NATURAL PROTECTION: Used as directed, PRESUN 23 and PRESUN For Kids Spray Mist Sunscreens provide 23 times your natural sunburn protection and may help reduce the chance of premature aging and wrinkling of the skin.
WATERPROOF 23: PRESUN 23 and PRESUN For Kids Spray Mist Sunscreens maintain their degree of protection (SPF 23) even after 80 minutes in the water.

Convenience Spray: This revolutionary new spray bottle design is non-aerosol.

Directions for Use: For best results, hold bottle about ten inches away from body while spraying. Massage in gently. Reapplication to dry skin after prolonged swimming, excessive perspiration or towel drying is recommended for all-day protection.

Warnings: For external use only. Do not use if sensitive to *p*-aminobenzoic acid (PABA) or related compounds. Avoid flame. Do not expose to heat or store above 86°F. As with all sunscreens: Apply to a small area; check after 24 hours. Discontinue use if irritation or rash appears. Avoid spraying in the eyes. In case of contact, flush eyes with water. Keep out of reach of children. Use on children under six months of age only with the advice of a physician.

How Supplied: 23 Spray Mist Sunscreen: 3.5 oz. plastic bottle with non-aerosol spray. For Kids Spray Mist Sunscreen: 3.5 oz. plastic bottle with non-aerosol spray.

Shown in Product Identification Section, page 406

PRESUN® 15 and 29 SENSITIVE SKIN SUNSCREENS
PABA-FREE Sunscreen Protection

Active Ingredients: Octyl methoxycinnamate, oxybenzone, octyl salicylate. Also contains: Water, isopropyl myristate, PG dioctanoate, isodecyl neopentanoate, DEA cetyl phosphate, PVP/Eicosene copolymer, stearic acid, cetyl alcohol, dimethicone, diazolidinyl urea, Carbomer-940, triethanolamine, methylchloroisothiazolinone, and methylisothiazolinone.

Indications:
15 or 29 TIMES NATURAL PROTECTION: Used as directed, PRESUN 15 or 29 Sensitive Skin Sunscreen provides 15 or 29 times your natural *sunburn* protection and may help reduce the chance of premature aging and wrinkling of the skin as well as skin cancer caused by overexposure to the sun.
PABA-FREE FORMULAS: PABA- and fragrance-free formulas that provide a very high degree of sunburn protection and, because the known sensitizers common to most sunscreens have been removed, is suitable for sensitive skin.
WATERPROOF: PRESUN Sensitive Skin Sunscreen maintains its degree of protection even after 80 minutes in the water.

Directions for Use: For maximum protection, smooth evenly and liberally onto dry skin before sun exposure. Massage in gently. Reapplication to dry skin after prolonged swimming, excessive perspiration or towel drying is recommended for all-day protection.

Warnings: For external use only. Protect from freezing. *As with all sunscreens:* Apply to a small area; check after 24 hours. Discontinue use if irritation or rash appears. Avoid contact with eyes. In case of contact, flush eyes with water. Keep out of the reach of children. Use on children under six months of age only with the advice of a physician.

How Supplied: 29 Sensitive Skin: 4 oz. (NSN 6505-01-267-1483) plastic bottle. 15 Sensitive Skin: 4 oz. plastic bottle.

Shown in Product Identification Section, page 406

PRESUN® 46 MOISTURIZING SUNSCREEN

Active Ingredient: Octyl dimethyl PABA, oxybenzone. Also contains: water, isopropyl myristate, PG dioctanoate, isodecyl neopentanoate, DEA cetyl phosphate, PVP/Eicosene copolymer, stearic acid, cetyl alcohol, dimethicone, diazolidinyl urea, carbomer-940, triethanolamine, methylchloroisothiazolinone and methylisothiazolinone. May also contain fragrance.

Indications: 46 TIMES NATURAL UVB PROTECTION: Used liberally and regularly, PreSun® 46 Moisturizing Sunscreen provides 46 times your natural UVB sunburn protection and may help reduce the chance of premature wrinkling of the skin caused by repeated and prolonged exposure to the sun. UVA/UVB: PreSun 46 Moisturizing Sunscreen is formulated to provide protection from sunburn caused by both UVA nd UVB rays.
Moisturizing: A moisture-rich formula that is absorbed in quickly to provide a high degree of UVB sunburn protection while helping to relieve the drying effects of the sun.
Waterproof: PreSun® 46 Moisturizing Sunscreen maintains its degree of protection even after 80 minutes in the water.

Directions: Smooth evenly and liberally onto dry skin before sun exposure. Massage in gently. Reapply to dry skin after swimming, excessive perspiration or towel drying.

Warnings: For external use only. As with all sunscreens, avoid contact with eyes. Discontinue use if irritation or rash appears. Consult a physician before using on children under six months of age.

How Supplied: 4 oz. plastic bottle

THERAGRAN® LIQUID with Niacin & Vitamin C
High Potency Vitamin Supplement

Each 5 ml. teaspoonful contains:

		Percent US RDA*
Vitamin A	5,000 IU	100
Vitamin D	400 IU	100
Vitamin C	200 mg	333
Thiamine	10 mg	667
Riboflavin	10 mg	588
Niacin	100 mg	500
Vitamin B_6	4.1 mg	205
Vitamin B_{12}	5 mcg	83
Pantothenic Acid	21.4 mg	214

*US Recommended Daily Allowance

Ingredients: purified water, sucrose, glycerine, propylene glycol, sodium ascorbate, niacinamide, polysorbate 80, ascorbic acid, thiamine hydrochloride, d-panthenol, carboxymethylcellulose sodium, riboflavin-5-phosphate sodium, artificial and natural flavors, (sodium benzoate and methylparaben as preservatives), pyridoxine hydrochloride, vitamin A palmitate, cholecalciferol, ferric ammonium citrate, cyanocobalamin
Take 1 teaspoonful daily or as directed by physician.

How Supplied: In bottles of 4 fl. oz. NO REFRIGERATION REQUIRED

Storage: Store at room temperature; avoid excessive heat.
(P9163-00)

Shown in Product Identification Section, page 406

ADVANCED FORMULA THERAGRAN® TABLETS
(High Potency Multivitamin Formula)

FOR ADULTS—PERCENTAGE OF U.S. RECOMMENDED DAILY ALLOWANCE

Vitamins	Quantity	US RDA
Vitamin A	5000 IU	100%
(as Acetate and Beta Carotene)		
Vitamin B_1	3 mg	200%
Vitamin B_2	3.4 mg	200%
Vitamin B_6	3 mg	150%
Vitamin B_{12}	9 mcg	150%
Vitamin C	90 mg	150%
Vitamin D	400 I.U.	100%
Vitamin E	30 I.U.	100%
Niacin	20 mg	100%
Folic Acid	400 mcg	100%
Pantothenic Acid	10.0 mg	100%
Biotin	30 mcg	10%

Continued on next page

Bristol-Myers—Cont.

Ingredients: Lactose, ascorbic acid, microcrystalline cellulose, gelatin, dl-alpha-tocopheryl acetate, niacinamide, starch, calcium pantothenate, sodium caseinate, hydroxypropyl methylcellulose, sucrose, povidone, pyridoxine hydrochloride, riboflavin, silicon dioxide, magnesium stearate, thiamine mononitrate, vitamin A acetate, polyethylene glycol, triacetin, stearic acid, titanium dioxide, annatto, beta carotene, FD&C Red 40, folic acid, biotin, ergocalciferol, cyanocobalamin.

Warning: KEEP OUT OF REACH OF CHILDREN.

Recommended Adult Intake—1 tablet daily or as directed by physician.

How Supplied: Packs of 130; and Unimatic® cartons of 100.

Storage: Store at room temperature; avoid excessive heat; keep tightly closed. UNIMATIC® is a trademark of E.R. Squibb & Sons, Inc.

Shown in Product Identification Section, page 406

COMPLETE FORMULA with Beta Carotene THERAGRAN-M® TABLETS (High Potency Multivitamin Formula with Minerals)

TABLET CONTENTS: FOR ADULTS—PERCENTAGE OF U.S. RECOMMENDED DAILY ALLOWANCE

Vitamins	Quantity	US RDA
Vitamin A	5000 IU	100%
(as Acetate and Beta Carotene)		
Vitamin B_1	3 mg	200%
Vitamin B_2	3.4 mg	200%
Vitamin B_6	3 mg	150%
Vitamin B_{12}	9 mcg	150%
Vitamin C	90 mg	150%
Vitamin D	400 IU	100%
Vitamin E	30 IU	100%
Niacin	20 mg	100%
Folic Acid	400 mcg	100%
Pantothenic Acid	10.0 mg	100%
Biotin	30 mcg	10%
Minerals		
Iron	27 mg	150%
Copper	2 mg	100%
Iodine	150 mcg	100%
Zinc	15 mg	100%
Magnesium	100 mg	25%
Calcium	40 mg	4%
Phosphorus	31 mg	3%
Chromium	15 mcg	*
Molybdenum	15 mcg	*
Selenium	10 mcg	*
Manganese	5 mg	*
ELECTROLYTES		
Chloride	7.5 mg	*
Potassium	7.5 mg	*

*US RDA not established.

Ingredients: Magnesium oxide, dibasic calcium phosphate, lactose, ascorbic acid, ferrous fumarate, gelatin, dl-alpha tocopheryl, acetate, crospovidone, niacinamide, hydroxypropyl methylcellulose, zinc oxide, povidone, manganese sulfate, potassium chloride, starch, calcium pantothenate, sodium caseinate, pyridoxine hydrochloride, cupric sulfate, magnesium stearate, sucrose, silicon dioxide, riboflavin, thiamine mononitrate, stearic acid, polyethylene glycol, triacetin, Vitamin A acetate, FD&C Red 40, potassium citrate, beta carotene, titanium dioxide, folic acid, potassium iodide, FD&C Blue No. 2, chromic chloride, sodium molybdate, biotin, sodium selenate, ergocalciferol, cyanocobalamin

Warning: KEEP OUT OF REACH OF CHILDREN.

Usage: For adults—1 tablet daily

How Supplied: Packs of 90, 130 and 240; and Unimatic® cartons of 100.

Storage: Store at room temperature; avoid excessive heat; keep tightly closed. UNIMATIC® is a trademark of E.R. Squibb & Sons, Inc.

Shown in Product Identification Section, page 406

THERAGRAN® STRESS FORMULA High Potency Multivitamin Stress Formula with Iron and Vitamin C

TABLET CONTENTS: For Adults—Percentage of US Recommended Daily Allowance

Ingredients	Quantity	US RDA
Vitamin B_1	15 mg	1000%
Vitamin B_2	15 mg	882%
Vitamin B_6	25 mg	1250%
Vitamin B_{12}	12 mcg	200%
Vitamin C	600 mg	1000%
Vitamin E	30 IU	100%
Niacin	100 mg	500%
Pantothenic Acid	20 mg	200%
Iron	27 mg	150%
Folic Acid	400 mcg	100%
Biotin	45 mcg	15%

Ingredients: Ascorbic acid, niacinamide, ferrous fumarate, starch, lactose, pyridoxine hydrochloride, crospovidone, dl-alpha tocopheryl acetate, gelatin, calcium pantothenate, riboflavin, povidone, thiamine mononitrate, hydroxypropyl methylcellulose, sodium caseinate, magnesium stearate, silicon dioxide, stearic acid, polyethylene glycol, triacetin, titanium dioxide, FD&C Red No. 40, FD&C Yellow No. 6, folic acid, biotin, cyanocobalamin

Warning: KEEP OUT OF REACH OF CHILDREN.

Recommended Adult Intake—1 tablet daily or as directed by physician.

How Supplied: Bottles of 75.

Storage: Store at room temperature; avoid excessive heat.
(P893-01)

Shown in Product Identification Section, page 406

THERAPEUTIC MINERAL ICE®

Composition:
Active Ingredient: Menthol 2%
Other Ingredients: Ammonium Hydroxide, Carbomer 934, Cupric Sulfate, FD&C Blue No. 1, Isopropyl Alcohol, Magnesium Sulfate, Sodium Hydroxide, Thymol, Water.

Indications: For the temporary relief of minor aches and pains of muscles and joints associated with arthritis, simple backache, strains, bruises, sprains and sports injuries. **USE ONLY AS DIRECTED. Read all warnings before use.**

Warnings: KEEP OUT OF THE REACH OF CHILDREN. For external use only. Not for internal use. Avoid contact with eyes and mucous membranes. Do not use with other ointments, creams, sprays, or liniments. **Do not use with Heating Pads or Heating Devices.** If condition worsens, or if symptoms persist for more than 7 days, or clear up and occur again within a few days, discontinue use of this product and consult your doctor. Do not apply to wounds or damaged skin. Do not bandage tightly. If you have sensitive skin, consult doctor before use. If skin irritation develops, discontinue use and consult your doctor. As with any drug, if you are pregnant or nursing a baby, seek the advice of a health professional before using this product. Keep cap tightly closed. Do not use, pour, spill or store near heat or open flame. **Note:** You can always use Mineral Ice as directed, but its use is never intended to replace your doctor's advice.

Directions: Adults and children 2 years of age and older: Clean skin of all other ointments, creams, sprays, or liniments. Apply to affected areas not more than 3 to 4 times daily. May be used with wet or dry bandages or with ice packs. No protective cover needed. Children under 2 years of age: Consult a doctor.

How Supplied:
NDC 19810-0034-4 3.5 oz.
NDC 19810-0034-2 8 oz.
NDC 19810-0034-3 16 oz.
Store at room temperature.

Shown in Product Identification Section, page 405

THERAPEUTIC MINERAL ICE® Exercise Formula, Pain Relieving Gel

Composition:
Active Ingredient: Menthol 4%.
Other Ingredients: Ammonium Hydroxide, Carbomer 934P or Carbomer 934, Cupric Sulfate, FD&C Blue No. 1, Fragrance, Isopropyl Alcohol, Magnesium Sulfate, Sodium Hydroxide, Thymol, Water.

Indications: For the temporary relief of minor aches and pains of muscles and joints associated with strains, sprains, bruises, sports injuries and simple backache. **USE ONLY AS DIRECTED. Read all warnings before use.**

Warnings: KEEP OUT OF REACH OF CHILDREN. For external use only. Not for internal use. Avoid contact with eyes and mucous membranes. Do not use with other ointments, creams, sprays, or liniments. **Do not use with heating pad or heating devices.** If condition worsens, or if symptoms persist for more than 7 days, or clear up and occur again within a few days, discontinue use of this product and consult your doctor. Do not apply to wounds or damaged skin. Do not bandage tightly. If you have sensitive skin, consult doctor BEFORE use. If skin irritation develops, discontinue use and consult your doctor. As with any drug, if you are pregnant or nursing a baby, seek the advice of a health professional before using this product. Do not use, pour, spill, or store near heat or open flame.
NOTE: You can always use MINERAL ICE® EXERCISE FORMULA as directed, but its use is never intended to replace your doctor's advice.

Directions: Adults and children 2 years of age and older: Clean skin of all other ointments, creams, sprays, or liniments. Apply to affected areas not more than 3 to 4 times daily. May be used with wet or dry bandages or with ice packs. Not greasy. No protective cover needed.
Children: Do not use on children under 2 years of age, except under the advice and supervision of a doctor.

How Supplied: Available in 3 oz. tubes.
STORE AT ROOM TEMPERATURE.
KEEP CAP TIGHTLY CLOSED.

Shown in Product Identification Section, page 406

Burroughs Wellcome Co.
3030 CORNWALLIS ROAD
RESEARCH TRIANGLE PARK
NC 27709

ACTIFED® PLUS Caplets
[*ăk 'tuh-fĕd*]

Product Benefits: Each ACTIFED PLUS Coated Caplet contains three important ingredients for maximum strength relief from symptoms of the common cold, seasonal allergies (hay fever) and sinus congestion.
The **ANTIHISTAMINE** (triprolidine) temporarily dries runny nose and relieves sneezing associated with the common cold, hay fever or other upper respiratory allergies. Also relieves itching of the nose or throat, and itchy, watery eyes due to hay fever.
The **DECONGESTANT** (pseudoephedrine) temporarily relieves nasal congestion due to the common cold, hay fever or other upper respiratory allergies, or associated with sinusitis. Temporarily relieves nasal stuffiness. Reduces the swelling of nasal passages; shrinks swollen membranes; and temporarily restores freer breathing through the nose. Also, helps to decongest sinus openings and passages; relieves sinus pressure.
The non-aspirin **ANALGESIC** (acetaminophen) temporarily relieves occasional minor aches, pains and headache, and reduces fever due to the common cold.

Each ACTIFED PLUS Coated Caplet Contains: acetaminophen 500 mg, pseudoephedrine hydrochloride 30 mg and triprolidine hydrochloride 1.25 mg. Also contains: carnauba wax, crospovidone, FD&C Blue No. 1 Lake, D&C Yellow No. 10 Lake, hydroxypropyl methylcellulose, magnesium stearate, microcrystalline cellulose, polyethylene glycol, polysorbate 80, povidone, pregelatinized corn starch, stearic acid, and titanium dioxide.

Directions: Adults and children 12 years and over, 2 caplets every 6 hours, not to exceed 8 caplets in a 24-hour period. Not recommended for children under 12 years of age.

Warnings: May cause excitability especially in children. May cause drowsiness. Do not exceed recommended dosage because at higher doses nervousness, dizziness, or sleeplessness may occur. Do not take this product for more than 10 days. If symptoms do not improve or are accompanied by fever that lasts for more than 3 days, or if new symptoms occur, consult a physician. Do not take this product if you have high blood pressure, heart disease, diabetes, thyroid disease, asthma, glaucoma, or difficulty in urination due to enlargement of the prostate gland except under the advice and supervision of a physician. As with any drug, if you are pregnant or nursing a baby, seek the advice of a health professional before using this product.
Drug Interaction Precaution: Do not take this product if you are presently taking a prescription antihypertensive or antidepressant drug containing a monoamine oxidase inhibitor except under the advice and supervision of a physician.

Caution: Avoid driving a motor vehicle, operating heavy machinery, or drinking alcoholic beverages while taking this product.
KEEP THIS AND ALL DRUGS OUT OF THE REACH OF CHILDREN. In case of accidental overdose, seek professional assistance or contact a Poison Control Center immediately. Prompt medical attention is critical for adults as well as for children even if you do not notice any signs or symptoms.

Store at 15° to 25°C (59° to 77°F) in a dry place and protect from light. 402894

How Supplied: Boxes of 20, 40.

Shown in Product Identification Section, page 406

ACTIFED® SINUS DAYTIME/ NIGHTTIME Caplets
[*ak 'tuh-fĕd*]

> This package contains 2 separate products. Actifed Sinus DAYTIME (white caplets) is a no-drowsiness product to be used during waking hours. Actifed Sinus NIGHTTIME (blue caplets) may cause marked drowsiness and is for bedtime use or when resting at home. DO NOT TAKE BOTH PRODUCTS AT THE SAME TIME.

ACTIFED® SINUS DAYTIME (white caplets)
CONTAINS NO INGREDIENTS THAT MAY CAUSE DROWSINESS.

Product Benefits: The **DAYTIME** no-drowsiness product (white caplets) contains a non-aspirin pain reliever (acetaminophen) and nasal decongestant (pseudoephedrine) that provide temporary relief of sinus headache pain, sinus pressure and nasal congestion due to the common cold, hay fever, or other allergies.

Directions: Adults and children 12 years and over, 2 caplets every 4 to 6 hours during waking hours. Do not exceed a total of 8 caplets in a 24 hour period. Do not take Actifed Sinus Daytime within 4 hours of Actifed Sinus Nighttime. Not recommended for children under 12.

Each Actifed Sinus Daytime Caplet Contains: acetaminophen 325 mg and pseudoephedrine hydrochloride 30 mg. Also contains: carnauba wax, crospovidone, hydroxypropyl methylcellulose, magnesium stearate, microcrystalline cellulose, polyethylene glycol, povidone, pregelatinized corn starch, sodium starch glycolate, stearic acid, and titanium dioxide.

ACTIFED® SINUS NIGHTTIME (blue caplets)
MAY CAUSE MARKED DROWSINESS.

Product Benefits: The **NIGHTTIME** product (blue caplets) contains a non-aspirin pain reliever (acetaminophen), a nasal decongestant (pseudoephedrine), and an antihistamine (diphenhydramine) that provide temporary relief of sinus headache pain, sinus pressure, nasal congestion, runny nose, and sneezing due to the common cold, hay fever, or other allergies. Also relieves itching of the nose or throat and itchy, watery eyes due to hay fever.

Directions: Adults and children 12 years and over, 2 caplets at bedtime. Do not take during waking hours unless confined to a bed or resting at home; 2 caplets then may be taken every 6 hours. Do

Continued on next page

Burroughs Wellcome—Cont.

not exceed a total of 8 caplets in a 24 hour period. Not recommended for children under 12.

Caution: Alcohol, sedatives, and tranquilizers may increase the drowsiness effect. Avoid driving a motor vehicle, operating heavy machinery, or drinking alcoholic beverages while taking Actifed Sinus Nighttime.

Each Actifed Sinus Nighttime Caplet Contains: acetaminophen 500 mg, diphenhydramine hydrochloride 25 mg and pseudoephedrine hydrochloride 30 mg. Also contains: carnauba wax, crospovidone, FD&C Blue No. 1 Lake, hydroxypropyl methylcellulose, magnesium stearate, microcrystalline cellulose, polyethylene glycol, polysorbate 80, povidone, pregelatinized corn starch, sodium starch glycolate, stearic acid, and titanium dioxide.

ACTIFED SINUS DAYTIME and ACTIFED SINUS NIGHTTIME do not contain triprolidine hydrochloride, the antihistamine found in other ACTIFED products.

Warnings: Do not exceed a combined total of 8 caplets (Actifed Sinus Daytime *plus* Actifed Sinus Nighttime) in a 24 hour period. These products may cause excitability in children. Do not exceed recommended dosage for these products because at higher doses nervousness, dizziness, or sleeplessness may occur. Do not take these products for more than 10 days. If symptoms do not improve or are accompanied by fever that lasts for more than 3 days, or if new symptoms occur, consult a physician. Do not take these products if you have high blood pressure, heart disease, diabetes, thyroid disease, glaucoma, asthma, emphysema, chronic pulmonary disease, shortness of breath, difficulty in breathing, or difficulty in urination due to enlargement of the prostate gland except under the advice and supervision of a physician. As with any drug, if you are pregnant or nursing a baby, seek the advice of a health professional before using these products.

Drug Interaction: Do not take these products if you are presently taking a prescription antihypertensive or antidepressant drug containing a monoamine oxidase inhibitor except under the advice and supervision of a physician.

KEEP THESE AND ALL DRUGS OUT OF THE REACH OF CHILDREN. In case of accidental overdose, seek professional assistance or contact a Poison Control Center immediately. Prompt medical attention is critical for adults as well as for children even if you do not notice any signs or symptoms.

Store at 15° to 25°C (59° to 77°F) in a dry place and protect from light.

How Supplied: Package contains 18 Daytime Caplets and 6 Nighttime Caplets. 402078

Shown in Product Identification Section, page 406

ACTIFED® SINUS DAYTIME/ NIGHTTIME Tablets

[*ak'tuh-fĕd*]

> This package contains 2 separate products. Actifed Sinus DAYTIME (white tablets) is a no-drowsiness product to be used during waking hours. Actifed Sinus NIGHTTIME (blue tablets) may cause marked drowsiness and is for bedtime use or when resting at home. DO NOT TAKE BOTH PRODUCTS AT THE SAME TIME.

ACTIFED® SINUS DAYTIME (white tablets)

CONTAINS NO INGREDIENTS THAT MAY CAUSE DROWSINESS.

Product Benefits: The **DAYTIME** no-drowsiness product (white tablets) contains a non-aspirin pain reliever (acetaminophen) and nasal decongestant (pseudoephedrine) that provide temporary relief of sinus headache pain, sinus pressure and nasal congestion due to the common cold, hay fever, or other allergies.

Directions: Adults and children 12 years and over, 2 tablets every 4 to 6 hours during waking hours. Do not exceed a total of 8 tablets in a 24 hour period. Do not take Actifed Sinus Daytime within 4 hours of Actifed Sinus Nighttime. Not recommended for children under 12.

Each Actifed Sinus Daytime Tablet Contains: acetaminophen 325 mg and pseudoephedrine hydrochloride 30 mg. Also contains: carnauba wax, crospovidone, hydroxypropyl methylcellulose, magnesium stearate, microcrystalline cellulose, polyethylene glycol, povidone, pregelatinized corn starch, sodium starch glycolate, stearic acid, and titanium dioxide.

ACTIFED® SINUS NIGHTTIME (blue tablets)

MAY CAUSE MARKED DROWSINESS.

Product Benefits: The **NIGHTTIME** product (blue tablets) contains a non-aspirin pain reliever (acetaminophen), a nasal decongestant (pseudoephedrine), and an antihistamine (diphenhydramine) that provide temporary relief of sinus headache pain, sinus pressure, nasal congestion, runny nose, and sneezing due to the common cold, hay fever, or other allergies. Also relieves itching of the nose or throat and itchy, watery eyes due to hay fever.

Directions: Adults and children 12 years and over, 2 tablets at bedtime. Do not take during waking hours unless confined to a bed or resting at home; 2 tablets then may be taken every 6 hours. Do not exceed a total of 8 tablets in a 24 hour period. Not recommended for children under 12.

Caution: Alcohol, sedatives, and tranquilizers may increase the drowsiness effect. Avoid driving a motor vehicle, operating heavy machinery, or drinking alcoholic beverages while taking Actifed Sinus Nighttime.

Each Actifed Sinus Nighttime Tablet Contains: acetaminophen 500 mg, diphenhydramine hydrochloride 25 mg and pseudoephedrine hydrochloride 30 mg. Also contains: carnauba wax, crospovidone, FD&C Blue No. 1 Lake, hydroxypropyl methylcellulose, magnesium stearate, microcrystalline cellulose, polyethylene glycol, polysorbate 80, povidone, pregelatinized corn starch, sodium starch glycolate, stearic acid, and titanium dioxide.

ACTIFED SINUS DAYTIME and ACTIFED SINUS NIGHTTIME do not contain triprolidine hydrochloride, the antihistamine found in other ACTIFED products.

Warnings: Do not exceed a combined total of 8 tablets (Actifed Sinus Daytime *plus* Actifed Sinus Nighttime) in a 24 hour period. These products may cause excitability in children. Do not exceed recommended dosage for these products because at higher doses nervousness, dizziness, or sleeplessness may occur. Do not take these products for more than 10 days. If symptoms do not improve or are accompanied by fever that lasts for more than 3 days, or if new symptoms occur, consult a physician. Do not take these products if you have high blood pressure, heart disease, diabetes, thyroid disease, glaucoma, asthma, emphysema, chronic pulmonary disease, shortness of breath, difficulty in breathing, or difficulty in urination due to enlargement of the prostate gland except under the advice and supervision of a physician. As with any drug, if you are pregnant or nursing a baby, seek the advice of a health professional before using these products.

Drug Interaction: Do not take these products if you are presently taking a prescription antihypertensive or antidepressant drug containing a monoamine oxidase inhibitor except under the advice and supervision of a physician.

KEEP THESE AND ALL DRUGS OUT OF THE REACH OF CHILDREN. In case of accidental overdose, seek professional assistance or contact a Poison Control Center immediately. Prompt medical attention is critical for adults as well as for children even if you do not notice any signs or symptoms.

Store at 15° to 25°C (59° to 77°F) in a dry place and protect from light.

How Supplied: Package contains 18 Daytime Tablets and 6 Nighttime Tablets. 402079

Shown in Product Identification Section, page 406

ACTIFED® Syrup
[ăk 'tuh-fĕd]

Product Benefits: ACTIFED Syrup contains two important ingredients for relief from symptoms of the common cold, seasonal allergies (hay fever) and sinus congestion.
The **ANTIHISTAMINE** (triprolidine) temporarily dries runny nose and relieves sneezing associated with the common cold, hay fever, or other upper respiratory allergies. Also relieves itching of the nose or throat, and itchy, watery eyes due to hay fever.
The **DECONGESTANT** (pseudoephedrine) temporarily relieves nasal congestion due to the common cold, hay fever or other upper respiratory allergies, or associated with sinusitis. Temporarily relieves nasal stuffiness. Reduces the swelling of nasal passages; shrinks swollen membranes; and temporarily restores freer breathing through the nose. Also, helps to decongest sinus openings and passages; relieves sinus pressure.

Each 5 mL (1 teaspoonful) Actifed Syrup Contains: pseudoephedrine hydrochloride 30 mg and triprolidine hydrochloride 1.25 mg. Also contains: methylparaben 0.1% and sodium benzoate 0.1% (added as preservatives), D&C Yellow No. 10, glycerin, purified water, and sorbitol.

Directions: Adults and children 12 years of age and over, 2 teaspoonfuls every 4 to 6 hours. Children 6 to under 12 years of age, 1 teaspoonful every 4 to 6 hours. Children under 6 years of age, consult a physician. Do not exceed 4 doses in 24 hours.

Warnings: May cause excitability especially in children. Do not give this product to children under 6 years except under the advice and supervision of a physician. May cause drowsiness. Do not exceed recommended dosage because at higher doses nervousness, dizziness or sleeplessness may occur. If symptoms do not improve within 7 days or are accompanied by high fever, consult a physician before continuing use. Do not take this product if you have high blood pressure, heart disease, diabetes, thyroid disease, asthma, glaucoma or difficulty in urination due to enlargement of the prostate gland except under the advice and supervision of a physician. As with any drug, if you are pregnant or nursing a baby, seek the advice of a health professional before using this product.

Drug Interaction Precaution: Do not take this product if you are presently taking a prescription antihypertensive or antidepressant drug containing a monoamine oxidase inhibitor except under the advice and supervision of a physician.

Caution: Avoid driving a motor vehicle, operating heavy machinery, or drinking alcoholic beverages while taking this product.

KEEP THIS AND ALL DRUGS OUT OF THE REACH OF CHILDREN. In case of accidental overdose, seek professional assistance or contact a Poison Control Center immediately.
Store at 15° to 25°C (59° to 77°F) and protect from light.

How Supplied: Bottles of 4 fl oz and 1 pint. 402359

Shown in Product Identification Section, page 406

ACTIFED® Tablets
[ăk 'tuh-fĕd]

Product Benefits: Each ACTIFED Tablet contains two important ingredients for relief from symptoms of the common cold, seasonal allergies (hay fever) and sinus congestion.
The **ANTIHISTAMINE** (triprolidine) temporarily dries runny nose and relieves sneezing associated with the common cold, hay fever or other upper respiratory allergies. Also relieves itching of the nose or throat, and itchy, watery eyes due to hay fever.
The **DECONGESTANT** (pseudoephedrine) temporarily relieves nasal congestion due to the common cold, hay fever or other upper respiratory allergies, or associated with sinusitis. Temporarily relieves nasal stuffiness. Reduces the swelling of nasal passages; shrinks swollen membranes; and temporarily restores freer breathing through the nose. Also, helps to decongest sinus openings and passages; relieves sinus pressure.

Each Actifed Tablet Contains: pseudoephedrine hydrochloride 60 mg and triprolidine hydrochloride 2.5 mg. Also contains: flavor, hydroxypropyl methylcellulose, lactose, magnesium stearate, polyethylene glycol, potato starch, povidone, sucrose, and titanium dioxide.

Directions: Adults and children 12 years of age and over, 1 tablet every 4 to 6 hours. Children 6 to under 12 years of age, ½ tablet every 4 to 6 hours. Children under 6 years of age, consult a physician. Do not exceed 4 doses in 24 hours.

Warnings: May cause excitability especially in children. Do not give this product to children under 6 years except under the advice and supervision of a physician. May cause drowsiness. Do not exceed recommended dosage because at higher doses nervousness, dizziness or sleeplessness may occur. If symptoms do not improve within 7 days or are accompanied by high fever, consult a physician before continuing use. Do not take this product if you have high blood pressure, heart disease, diabetes, thyroid disease, asthma, glaucoma or difficulty in urination due to enlargement of the prostate gland except under the advice and supervision of a physician. As with any drug, if you are pregnant or nursing a baby, seek the advice of a health professional before using this product.

Drug Interaction Precaution: Do not take this product if you are presently taking a prescription antihypertensive or antidepressant drug containing a monoamine oxidase inhibitor except under the advice and supervision of a physician.

Caution: Avoid driving a motor vehicle, operating heavy machinery, or drinking alcoholic beverages while taking this product.

KEEP THIS AND ALL DRUGS OUT OF THE REACH OF CHILDREN. In case of accidental overdose, seek professional assistance or contact a Poison Control Center immediately.
Store at 15° to 25°C (59° to 77°F) in a dry place and protect from light.

How Supplied: Boxes of 12, 24, 48 and bottles of 100 and 1000; unit dose pack box of 100. 402305

Shown in Product Identification Section, page 406

ACTIFED® PLUS Tablets
[ăk 'tuh-fĕd]

Product Benefits: Each ACTIFED PLUS Coated Tablet contains three important ingredients for maximum strength relief from symptoms of the common cold, seasonal allergies (hay fever) and sinus congestion.
The **ANTIHISTAMINE** (triprolidine) temporarily dries runny nose and relieves sneezing associated with the common cold, hay fever or other upper respiratory allergies. Also relieves itching of the nose or throat, and itchy, watery eyes due to hay fever.
The **DECONGESTANT** (pseudoephedrine) temporarily relieves nasal congestion due to the common cold, hay fever or other upper respiratory allergies, or associated with sinusitis. Temporarily relieves nasal stuffiness. Reduces the swelling of nasal passages; shrinks swollen membranes; and temporarily restores freer breathing through the nose. Also, helps to decongest sinus openings and passages; relieves sinus pressure.
The non-aspirin **ANALGESIC** (acetaminophen) temporarily relieves occasional minor aches, pains and headache, and reduces fever due to the common cold.

Each ACTIFED PLUS Coated Tablet Contains: acetaminophen 500 mg, pseudoephedrine hydrochloride 30 mg and triprolidine hydrochloride 1.25 mg. Also contains: carnauba wax, crospovidone, FD&C Blue No. 1 Lake, D&C Yellow No. 10 Lake, hydroxypropyl methylcellulose, magnesium stearate, microcrystalline cellulose, polyethylene glycol, polysorbate 80, povidone, pregelatinized corn starch, stearic acid, and titanium dioxide.

Directions: Adults and children 12 years and over, 2 tablets every 6 hours, not to exceed 8 tablets in a 24-hour period. Not recommended for children under 12 years of age.

Continued on next page

Burroughs Wellcome—Cont.

Warnings: May cause excitability, especially in children. May cause drowsiness. Do not exceed recommended dosage because at higher doses nervousness, dizziness, or sleeplessness may occur. Do not take this product for more than 10 days. If symptoms do not improve or are accompanied by fever that lasts for more than 3 days, or if new symptoms occur, consult a physician. Do not take this product if you have high blood pressure, heart disease, diabetes, thyroid disease, asthma, glaucoma, or difficulty in urination due to enlargement of the prostate gland except under the advice and supervision of a physician. As with any drug, if you are pregnant or nursing a baby, seek the advice of a health professional before using this product.

Drug Interaction Precaution: Do not take this product if you are presently taking a prescription antihypertensive or antidepressant drug containing a monoamine oxidase inhibitor except under the advice and supervision of a physician.

Caution: Avoid driving a motor vehicle, operating heavy machinery, or drinking alcoholic beverages while taking this product.

KEEP THIS AND ALL DRUGS OUT OF THE REACH OF CHILDREN. In case of accidental overdose, seek professional assistance or contact a Poison Control Center immediately. Prompt medical attention is critical for adults as well as for children even if you do not notice any signs or symptoms.

Store at 15° to 25°C (59° to 77°F) in a dry place and protect from light.

How Supplied: Boxes of 20, 40.

402896

Shown in Product Identification Section, page 406

BOROFAX® Ointment

[*bôr 'uh-făks*]

Description: Contains boric acid 5% and lanolin.

Inactive Ingredients: fragrances, glycerin, mineral oil, purified water and sodium borate.

Indications: A soothing application for burns, abrasions, chafing, and for infants' tender skin.

Directions: Apply topically as required.

Keep this and all medicines out of children's reach.

Store at 15° to 25°C (59° to 77°F).

How Supplied: Tube, 1¾ oz.

433194

EMPIRIN® ASPIRIN

[*ĕm 'puh-rĭn*]

For relief of headache, minor muscular aches and pains, toothache, discomfort and fever of colds and flu, pain of the premenstrual and menstrual periods, and temporary relief of minor arthritis pain (see CAUTION below).

Directions: Adults: 1 or 2 tablets with a full glass of water. Repeat every 4 hours as needed, up to 12 tablets a day. **Children:** Consult a physician (see WARNINGS).

Caution: In arthritic conditions, if pain persists for more than 10 days or redness is present, consult a physician immediately.

Warnings: Children and teenagers should not use this medicine for chicken pox or flu symptoms before a doctor is consulted about Reye syndrome, a rare but serious illness reported to be associated with aspirin. Keep this and all medicines out of children's reach. In case of accidental overdose, contact a physician immediately.

High or continued fever, severe or persistent sore throat especially when accompanied by high fever, headache, nausea or vomiting, may be serious. Consult your physician. Do not exceed dose unless directed by a physician. Do not take this product if you are allergic to aspirin, have asthma, a gastric ulcer or its symptoms, or are taking a medication that affects the clotting of blood, except under the advice of a physician. As with any drug, if you are pregnant or nursing a baby, seek the advice of a health professional before using this product.

IT IS ESPECIALLY IMPORTANT NOT TO USE ASPIRIN DURING THE LAST 3 MONTHS OF PREGNANCY UNLESS SPECIFICALLY DIRECTED TO DO SO BY A DOCTOR BECAUSE IT MAY CAUSE PROBLEMS IN THE UNBORN CHILD OR COMPLICATIONS DURING DELIVERY.

Active Ingredients: Each tablet contains aspirin 325 mg (5 gr).

Inactive Ingredients: microcrystalline cellulose and potato starch.

Store at 15° to 25°C (59° to 77°F) in a dry place.

How Supplied: Bottles of 50, 100.

488216

Shown in Product Identification Section, page 406

MAREZINE® Tablets

[*mâr 'uh-zēn*]

FDA APPROVED USES

Indications: For the prevention and treatment of the nausea, vomiting or dizziness associated with motion sickness.

Directions: Adults and children 12 years of age and over: 1 tablet every 4 to 6 hours, not to exceed 4 tablets in 24 hours or as directed by a doctor. Children 6 to under 12 years of age: ½ tablet every 6 to 8 hours, not to exceed 1½ tablets in 24 hours or as directed by a doctor. For prevention, take the first dose one half-hour before departure.

Warnings: Do not take this product if you have asthma, glaucoma, emphysema, chronic pulmonary disease, shortness of breath, difficulty in breathing or difficulty in urination due to enlargement of the prostate gland unless directed by a doctor. Do not give to children under 6 years of age unless directed by a doctor. May cause drowsiness; alcohol, sedatives and tranquilizers may increase the drowsiness effect. Avoid alcoholic beverages while taking this product. Do not take this product if you are taking sedatives or tranquilizers without first consulting your doctor. Use caution when driving a motor vehicle or operating machinery. As with any drug, if you are pregnant or nursing a baby, seek the advice of a health professional before using this product. Keep this and all drugs out of the reach of children. Overdosage may cause severe agitation or psychosis; seek professional assistance or contact a Poison Control Center immediately.

Active Ingredients: Each scored tablet contains cyclizine hydrochloride 50 mg.

Inactive Ingredients: Corn and potato starch, dextrin, lactose, and magnesium stearate.

Store at 15° to 25°C (59° to 77°F) in a dry place and protect from light.

How Supplied: Box of 12, bottle of 100.

548078

Shown in Product Identification Section, page 406

NEOSPORIN® Ointment

[*nē 'uh-spō 'rĭn*]

Indications: First aid to help prevent infection in minor cuts, scrapes, and burns.

Directions: Clean the affected area. Apply a small amount of this product (an amount equal to the surface area of the tip of a finger) on the area 1 to 3 times daily. May be covered with a sterile bandage.

Warnings: For external use only. Stop use and consult a physician if the condition persists or gets worse, or if a rash or other allergic reaction develops. Do not use this product if you are allergic to any of the listed ingredients. Do not use in the eyes or apply over large areas of the body. In case of deep or puncture wounds, animal bites, or serious burns, consult a physician. Do not use longer than 1 week unless directed by a physician. Keep this and all drugs out of the reach of children. In case of accidental ingestion, seek professional assistance or contact a Poison Control Center immediately.

Each Gram Contains: polymyxin B sulfate 5,000 units, bacitracin zinc 400 units and neomycin 3.5 mg in a special white petrolatum base.

Store at 15° to 25°C (59° to 77°F).

How Supplied: Tubes, ½ oz (with applicator tip), 1 oz; 1/32 oz (approx.) foil packets packed 144 per carton.

Professional Labeling: Consult *1993 Physicians' Desk Reference®*. 561595

Shown in Product Identification Section, page 406

NEOSPORIN® PLUS MAXIMUM STRENGTH Cream

[nē″uh-spō′rŭn]

Indications: First aid to help prevent infection and provide temporary relief of pain or discomfort in minor cuts, scrapes, and burns.

Directions: Adults and children 2 years of age and older: Clean the affected area. Apply a small amount of this product (an amount equal to the surface area of the tip of a finger) on the area 1 to 3 times daily. May be covered with a sterile bandage. Children under 2 years of age: Consult a physician.

Warnings: For external use only. If condition worsens, or if symptoms persist for more than 1 week or clear up and occur again within a few days, or if a rash or other allergic reaction develops, discontinue use of this product and consult a physician. Do not use this product if you are allergic to any of the listed ingredients. Do not use in the eyes or apply over large areas of the body. Do not use in large quantities, particularly over raw surfaces or blistered areas. In case of deep or puncture wounds, animal bites, or serious burns, consult a physician. Do not use longer than 1 week unless directed by a physician. Keep this and all drugs out of the reach of children. In case of accidental ingestion, seek professional assistance or contact a Poison Control Center immediately.

Each Gram Contains: polymyxin B sulfate 10,000 units, neomycin 3.5 mg, and lidocaine 40 mg. Also contains: methylparaben 0.25% (added as a preservative), emulsifying wax, mineral oil, poloxamer 188, propylene glycol, purified water, and white petrolatum.
Store at 15° to 25°C (59° to 77°F).

How Supplied: ½ oz tubes. 561208

Shown in Product Identification Section, page 406

NEOSPORIN® PLUS MAXIMUM STRENGTH Ointment

[nē″uh-spō′rŭn]

Indications: First aid to help prevent infection and provide temporary relief of pain or discomfort in minor cuts, scrapes, and burns.

Directions: Adults and children 2 years of age and older: Clean the affected area. Apply a small amount of this product (an amount equal to the surface area of the tip of a finger) on the area 1 to 3 times daily. May be covered with a sterile bandage. Children under 2 years of age: Consult a physician.

Warnings: For external use only. If condition worsens, or if symptoms persist for more than 1 week or clear up and occur again within a few days, or if a rash or other allergic reaction develops, discontinue use of this product and consult a physician. Do not use this product if you are allergic to any of the listed ingredients. Do not use in the eyes or apply over large areas of the body. Do not use in large quantities, particularly over raw surfaces or blistered areas. In case of deep or puncture wounds, animal bites, or serious burns, consult a physician. Do not use longer than 1 week unless directed by a physician. Keep this and all drugs out of the reach of children. In case of accidental ingestion, seek professional assistance or contact a Poison Control Center immediately.

Each Gram Contains: polymyxin B sulfate 10,000 units, bacitracin zinc 500 units, neomycin 3.5 mg, and lidocaine 40 mg in a special white petrolatum base.
Store at 15° to 25°C (59° to 77°F).

How Supplied: ½ oz and 1 oz tubes. 561204

Shown in Product Identification Section, page 407

NIX®
Permethrin
Lice Treatment

Product Benefits: Nix Creme Rinse kills lice and their unhatched eggs with only one application. Nix protects against head lice reinfestation for a full 14 days. The unique creme rinse formula leaves hair manageable and easy to comb.

Indications: For the treatment of head lice.

Directions for Use: Nix Creme Rinse should be used after hair has been washed with your regular shampoo, rinsed with water and towel dried. A sufficient amount should be applied to saturate hair and scalp (especially behind the ears and on nape of the neck). Leave on hair for 10 minutes but no longer. Rinse with water. A single application is sufficient. Retreatment is required in less than 1% of patients. If live lice are observed seven days or more after the first application of this product, a second treatment should be given. For proper head lice management, remove nits with the nit comb provided.
Head lice live on the scalp and lay small white eggs (nits) on the hair shaft close to the scalp. The nits are most easily found on the nape of the neck or behind the ears. All personal headgear, scarfs, coats, and bed linen should be disinfected by machine washing in hot water and drying, using the hot cycle of a dryer for at least 20 minutes. Personal articles of clothing or bedding that cannot be washed may be dry-cleaned, sealed in a plastic bag for a period of about 2 weeks, or sprayed with a product specifically designed for this purpose. Personal combs and brushes may be disinfected by soaking in hot water (above 130°F) for 5 to 10 minutes. Thorough vacuuming of rooms inhabited by infected patients is recommended.

Warnings: For external use only. Itching, redness, or swelling of the scalp may occur. If skin irritation persists or infection is present or develops, discontinue use and consult a doctor. Do not use near the eyes or permit contact with mucous membranes. If product gets into the eyes, immediately flush with water. Consult a doctor if infestation of eyebrows or eyelashes occurs. This product may cause breathing difficulty or an asthmatic episode in susceptible persons. This product should not be used on children less than 2 months of age. As with any drug, if you are pregnant or nursing a baby, seek the advice of a health professional before using this product. Keep this and all drugs out of the reach of children. In case of accidental ingestion, seek professional assistance or contact a Poison Control Center immediately.

Each Fluid Ounce Contains: permethrin 280 mg (1%). Inactive ingredients are: balsam canada, cetyl alcohol, citric acid, FD&C Yellow No. 6, fragrance, hydrolyzed animal protein, hydroxyethylcellulose, polyoxyethylene 10 cetyl ether, propylene glycol, and stearalkonium chloride. Also contains: isopropyl alcohol 5.6 g (20%) and added as preservatives, methylparaben 56 mg (0.2%) and propylparaben 22 mg (0.08%).
Store at 15° to 25°C (59° to 77°F).

How Supplied: Bottles of 2 fl oz with special comb and Family Pack of 2 bottles, 2 fl oz each, with special comb. 585066

Shown in Product Identification Section, page 407

POLYSPORIN® Ointment

[pŏl′ē-spō′rŭn]

Indications: First aid to help prevent infection in minor cuts, scrapes, and burns.

Directions: Clean the affected area. Apply a small amount of this product (an amount equal to the surface area of the tip of a finger) on the area 1 to 3 times daily. May be covered with a sterile bandage.

Warnings: For external use only. Stop use and consult a physician if the condition persists or gets worse, or if a rash or

Continued on next page

Burroughs Wellcome—Cont.

other allergic reaction develops. Do not use this product if you are allergic to any of the listed ingredients. Do not use in the eyes or apply over large areas of the body. In case of deep or puncture wounds, animal bites, or serious burns, consult a physician. Do not use longer than 1 week unless directed by a physician. Keep this and all drugs out of the reach of children. In case of accidental ingestion, seek professional assistance or contact a Poison Control Center immediately.

Each Gram Contains: polymyxin B sulfate 10,000 units and bacitracin zinc 500 units in a special white petrolatum base.

Store at 15° to 25°C (59° to 77°F).

How Supplied: Tubes, ½ oz with applicator tip, 1 oz; 1/32 oz (approx.) foil packets packed in cartons of 144.

576087

Shown in Product Identification Section, page 407

POLYSPORIN® Powder

[*pŏl 'ē-spō 'rŭn*]

Indications: First aid to help prevent infection in minor cuts, scrapes, and burns.

Directions: Clean the affected area. Apply a light dusting of the powder on the area 1 to 3 times daily. May be covered with a sterile bandage.

Warnings: For external use only. Stop use and consult a physician if the condition persists or get worse, or if a rash or other allergic reaction develops. Do not use this product if you are allergic to any of the listed ingredients. Do not use in the eyes or apply over large areas of the body. In case of deep or puncture wounds, animal bites, or serious burns, consult a physician. Do not use longer than 1 week unless directed by a physician. Keep this and all drugs out of the reach of children. In case of accidental ingestion, seek professional assistance or contact a Poison Control Center immediately.

Each Gram Contains: polymyxin B sulfate 10,000 units and bacitracin zinc 500 units in a lactose base.
Store at 15° to 25°C (59° to 77°F). Do not store under refrigeration.

How Supplied: 0.35 oz (10 g) shaker-vial.

575975

Shown in Product Identification Section, page 407

Children's SUDAFED® Liquid

[*sū 'duh-fĕd*]

Each 5 mL (1 teaspoonful) contains pseudoephedrine hydrochloride 30 mg. Also contains: methylparaben 0.1% and sodium benzoate 0.1% (added as preservatives), citric acid, FD&C Red No. 40, flavor, glycerin, purified water, sorbitol and sucrose.

Indications: For temporary relief of nasal congestion due to the common cold, hay fever or other upper respiratory allergies and nasal congestion associated with sinusitis; promotes nasal and/or sinus drainage.

Directions: To be given every 4 to 6 hours. Do not exceed 4 doses in 24 hours. Children 6 to under 12 years of age, 1 teaspoonful. Children 2 to under 6 years of age, ½ teaspoonful. For children under 2 years of age, consult a physician.

Warnings: Do not exceed recommended dosage because at higher doses nervousness, dizziness or sleeplessness may occur. Do not give this product to children for more than 7 days. If symptoms do not improve or are accompanied by high fever, consult a physician. Do not give this product to children who have heart disease, high blood pressure, thyroid disease, or diabetes unless directed by a physician.

Drug Interaction Precaution: Do not give this product to a child who is taking a prescription drug for high blood pressure or depression, without first consulting the child's physician.

KEEP THIS AND ALL MEDICINES OUT OF CHILDREN'S REACH. In case of accidental overdose, seek professional assistance or contact a Poison Control Center immediately.

Store at 15° to 25°C (59° to 77°F) and protect from light.

How Supplied: Bottles of 4 fl oz.

605225

Shown in Product Identification Section, page 407

SUDAFED® Cough Syrup

[*sū 'duh-fĕd*]

Each 5 mL (1 teaspoonful) contains pseudoephedrine hydrochloride 15 mg, dextromethorphan hydrobromide 5 mg and guaifenesin 100 mg. Also contains: alcohol 2.4%, methylparaben 0.1% and sodium benzoate 0.1% (added as preservatives), citric acid, D&C Yellow No. 10, FD&C Blue No. 1, flavor, glycerin, purified water, saccharin sodium, sodium chloride and sucrose.

Indications: For temporary relief of cough due to minor throat and bronchial irritation as may occur with the common cold or inhaled irritants. For temporary relief of nasal congestion due to the common cold. Helps loosen phlegm (sputum) and thin bronchial secretions to rid the bronchial passageways of bothersome mucus.

Directions: To be given every 4 hours. Do not exceed 4 doses in 24 hours. Adults and children 12 years of age and over, 4 teaspoonfuls. Children 6 to under 12 years of age, 2 teaspoonfuls. Children 2 to under 6 years of age, 1 teaspoonful. For children under 2 years of age, consult a physician.

Warnings: Do not give this product to children under 2 years of age unless directed by a physician. Do not exceed recommended dosage because at higher doses nervousness, dizziness or sleeplessness may occur. Do not take this product for persistent or chronic cough such as occurs with smoking, asthma, chronic bronchitis, or emphysema, or where cough is accompanied by excessive phlegm (sputum) unless directed by a physician. A persistent cough may be a sign of a serious condition. If cough persists for more than 1 week, tends to recur, or is accompanied by fever, rash, or persistent headache, consult a physician. Do not take this preparation if you have high blood pressure, heart disease, diabetes, thyroid disease, or difficulty in urination due to enlargement of the prostate gland, except under the advice and supervision of a physician. As with any drug, if you are pregnant or nursing a baby, seek the advice of a health professional before using this product.

Drug Interaction Precaution: Do not take this product if you are presently taking a prescription antihypertensive or antidepressant drug containing a monoamine oxidase inhibitor except under the advice and supervision of a physician.

KEEP THIS AND ALL DRUGS OUT OF THE REACH OF CHILDREN. In case of accidental overdose, seek professional assistance or contact a Poison Control Center immediately.

Store at 15° to 25°C (59° to 77°F).
DO NOT REFRIGERATE.

How Supplied: Bottles of 4 fl oz and 8 fl oz.

604128

Shown in Product Identification Section, page 407

SUDAFED® Tablets 30 mg

[*sū 'duh-fĕd*]

Each tablet contains pseudoephedrine hydrochloride 30 mg. Also contains: acacia, carnauba wax, dibasic calcium phosphate, FD&C Red No. 40 Lake and Yellow No. 6 Lake, magnesium stearate, pharmaceutical glaze, polysorbate 60, potato starch, povidone, sodium benzoate, stearic acid, talc, and titanium dioxide. Printed with edible black ink.

Indications: For temporary relief of nasal congestion due to the common cold, hay fever or other upper respiratory allergies, and nasal congestion associated with sinusitis; promotes nasal and/or sinus drainage.

Directions: To be given every 4 to 6 hours. Do not exceed 4 doses in 24 hours. Adults and children 12 years of age and over, 2 tablets. Children 6 to under 12 years of age, 1 tablet. Children 2 to under 6 years of age, use Children's Sudafed

Liquid. For children under 2 years of age, consult a physician.

Warnings: Do not exceed recommended dosage because at higher doses nervousness, dizziness or sleeplessness may occur. If symptoms do not improve within 7 days, or are accompanied by a high fever, consult a physician before continuing use. Do not take this preparation if you have high blood pressure, heart disease, diabetes, thyroid disease, or difficulty in urination due to enlargement of the prostate gland, except under the advice and supervision of a physician. As with any drug, if you are pregnant or nursing a baby, seek the advice of a health professional before using this product.

Drug Interaction Precaution: Do not take this product if you are presently taking a prescription antihypertensive or antidepressant drug containing a monoamine oxidase inhibitor except under the advice and supervision of a physician.

KEEP THIS AND ALL MEDICINES OUT OF CHILDREN'S REACH. In case of accidental overdose, seek professional assistance or contact a Poison Control Center immediately.

Store at 15° to 25°C (59° to 77°F) in a dry place and protect from light.

How Supplied: Boxes of 24, 48. Bottles of 100. Institutional Pack, Carton of 500 x 2. 604253

Shown in Product Identification Section, page 407

SUDAFED® Tablets 60 mg (Adult Strength)
[*sū 'duh-fĕd*]

Each tablet contains pseudoephedrine hydrochloride 60 mg. Also contains: acacia, carnauba wax, corn starch, dibasic calcium phosphate, hydroxypropyl methylcellulose, magnesium stearate, pharmaceutical glaze, polysorbate 60, sodium starch glycolate, stearic acid, sucrose, talc, and titanium dioxide. Printed with edible red ink.

Indications: For temporary relief of nasal congestion due to the common cold, hay fever or other upper respiratory allergies, and nasal congestion associated with sinusitis; promotes nasal and/or sinus drainage.

Directions: To be given every 4 to 6 hours. Do not exceed 4 doses in 24 hours. Adults and children 12 years of age and over, 1 tablet. Children 6 to under 12 years of age, use Sudafed 30 mg Tablets. Children 2 to under 6 years of age, use Children's Sudafed Liquid. For children under 2 years of age, consult a physician.

Warnings: Do not exceed recommended dosage because at higher doses nervousness, dizziness or sleeplessness may occur. If symptoms do not improve within 7 days, or are accompanied by a high fever, consult a physician before continuing use. Do not take this preparation if you have high blood pressure, heart disease, diabetes, thyroid disease, or difficulty in urination due to enlargement of the prostate gland, except under the advice and supervision of a physician. As with any drug, if you are pregnant or nursing a baby, seek the advice of a health professional before using this product.

Drug Interaction Precaution: Do not take this product if you are presently taking a prescription antihypertensive or antidepressant drug containing a monoamine oxidase inhibitor, except under the advice and supervision of a physician.

KEEP THIS AND ALL MEDICINES OUT OF CHILDREN'S REACH. In case of accidental overdose, seek professional assistance or contact a Poison Control Center immediately.

Store at 15° to 25°C (59° to 77°F) in a dry place and protect from light.

How Supplied: Bottles of 100. 605656

Shown in Product Identification Section, page 407

SUDAFED PLUS® Liquid
[*sū 'duh-fĕd*]

Each 5 mL (1 teaspoonful) contains pseudoephedrine hydrochloride 30 mg and chlorpheniramine maleate 2 mg. Also contains: methylparaben 0.1% and sodium benzoate 0.1% (added as preservatives), citric acid, D&C Yellow No. 10, FD&C Yellow No. 6, flavor, glycerin, purified water and sucrose.

Indications: For the temporary relief of nasal/sinus congestion associated with the common cold; also sneezing; watery, itchy eyes; runny nose and other hay fever/upper respiratory allergy symptoms.

Directions: To be given every 4 to 6 hours. Do not exceed 4 doses in 24 hours. Adults and children 12 years of age and over, 2 teaspoonfuls. Children 6 to under 12 years of age, 1 teaspoonful. Children under 6 years of age, consult a physician.

Warnings: May cause excitability, especially in children. Do not give to children under 6 years except as directed by a physician. May cause drowsiness. Do not exceed recommended dosage because at higher doses nervousness, dizziness or sleeplessness may occur. If symptoms do not improve within 7 days, or are accompanied by a high fever, consult a physician before continuing use. Do not take this product if you have high blood pressure, heart disease, diabetes, thyroid disease, asthma, glaucoma or difficulty in urination due to enlargement of the prostate gland except under the advice and supervision of a physician. As with any drug, if you are pregnant or nursing a baby, seek the advice of a health professional before using this product.

Drug Interaction Precaution: Do not take this product if you are presently taking a prescription antihypertensive or antidepressant drug containing a monoamine oxidase inhibitor except under the advice and supervision of a physician.

Caution: Avoid driving a motor vehicle or operating heavy machinery. Avoid alcoholic beverages while taking this product.

KEEP THIS AND ALL MEDICINES OUT OF CHILDREN'S REACH. In case of accidental overdose, seek professional assistance or contact a Poison Control Center immediately.

Store at 15° to 25°C (59° to 77°F) and protect from light.

How Supplied: Bottles of 4 fl oz. 605281

Shown in Product Identification Section, page 407

SUDAFED PLUS® Tablets
[*sū 'duh-fĕd*]

Each scored tablet contains pseudoephedrine hydrochloride 60 mg and chlorpheniramine maleate 4 mg. Also contains: lactose, magnesium stearate, potato starch and povidone.

Indications: For the temporary relief of nasal/sinus congestion associated with the common cold; also sneezing; watery, itchy eyes; runny nose and other hay fever/upper respiratory allergy symptoms.

Directions: To be given every 4 to 6 hours. Do not exceed 4 doses in 24 hours. Adults and children 12 years of age and over, 1 tablet. Children 6 to under 12 years of age, ½ tablet. Children under 6 years of age, consult a physician.

Warnings: May cause excitability, especially in children. Do not give to children under 6 years except as directed by a physician. May cause drowsiness. Do not exceed recommended dosage because at higher doses nervousness, dizziness or sleeplessness may occur. If symptoms do not improve within 7 days, or are accompanied by a high fever, consult a physician before continuing use. Do not take this product if you have high blood pressure, heart disease, diabetes, thyroid disease, asthma, glaucoma or difficulty in urination due to enlargement of the prostate gland except under the advice and supervision of a physician. As with any drug, if you are pregnant or nursing a baby, seek the advice of a health professional before using this product.

Drug Interaction Precaution: Do not take this product if you are presently taking a prescription antihypertensive or antidepressant drug containing a monoamine oxidase inhibitor except under the advice and supervision of a physician.

Caution: Avoid driving a motor vehicle or operating heavy machinery. Avoid alcoholic beverages while taking this product.

Continued on next page

Burroughs Wellcome—Cont.

KEEP THIS AND ALL MEDICINES OUT OF CHILDREN'S REACH. In case of accidental overdose, seek professional assistance or contact a Poison Control Center immediately.

Store at 15° to 25°C (59° to 77°F) in a dry place and protect from light.

How Supplied: Boxes of 24, 48.
605385

Shown in Product Identification Section, page 407

SUDAFED® Severe Cold Formula Caplets
[*sū' duh-fĕd*]

Product Benefits: Maximum allowable levels of nasal decongestant, cough suppressant, and non-aspirin pain reliever/fever reducer provide temporary relief from symptoms of the common cold and flu. This product contains no ingredients that may cause drowsiness. The **DECONGESTANT** (pseudoephedrine) temporarily relieves nasal and sinus congestion due to the common cold. It temporarily relieves nasal stuffiness; reduces the swelling of nasal passages; shrinks swollen membranes; and temporarily restores freer breathing through the nose. The **COUGH SUPPRESSANT** (dextromethorphan) temporarily relieves cough due to the common cold. The non-aspirin **PAIN RELIEVER/FEVER REDUCER** (acetaminophen) temporarily relieves headache, body aches and pains, minor sore throat pain, and reduces fever due to the common cold.

Directions: Adults and children 12 years of age and over, 2 caplets every 6 hours, not to exceed 8 caplets in 24 hours. Not recommended for children under 12 years of age.

Each Coated Caplet Contains: acetaminophen 500 mg, dextromethorphan hydrobromide 15 mg, and pseudoephedrine hydrochloride 30 mg. Also contains: carnauba wax, crospovidone, hydroxypropyl methylcellulose, magnesium stearate, microcrystalline cellulose, polyethylene glycol, povidone, pregelatinized corn starch, stearic acid, and titanium dioxide.

Warnings: Do not exceed recommended dosage because at higher doses nervousness, dizziness or sleeplessness may occur. Do not take this product for more than 10 days. A persistent cough may be a sign of a serious condition. If cough persists for more than 7 days, tends to recur, or is accompanied by rash, persistent headache, fever that lasts for more than 3 days, or if new symptoms occur, consult a physician. Do not take this product for persistent or chronic cough such as occurs with smoking, asthma, emphysema, or if cough is accompanied by excessive phlegm (mucus) unless directed by a physician. If sore throat is severe, persists for more than 2 days, is accompanied or followed by fever, headache, rash, nausea, or vomiting, consult a physician promptly. Do not take this product if you have high blood pressure, heart disease, diabetes, thyroid disease, or difficulty in urination due to enlargement of the prostate gland except under the advice and supervision of a physician. As with any drug, if you are pregnant or nursing a baby, seek the advice of a health professional before using this product.

Drug Interaction Precaution: Do not take this product if you are presently taking a prescription antihypertensive or antidepressant drug containing a monoamine oxidase inhibitor except under the advice and supervision of a physician.

KEEP THIS AND ALL DRUGS OUT OF THE REACH OF CHILDREN. In case of accidental overdose, seek professional assistance or contact a Poison Control Center immediately. Prompt medical attention is critical for adults as well as for children even if you do not notice any signs or symptoms.

Store at 15° to 25°C (59° to 77°F) in a dry place.

How Supplied: Boxes of 10, 20.
604210

Shown in Product Identification Section, page 407

SUDAFED® Severe Cold Formula Tablets
[*sū' duh-fĕd*]

Product Benefits: Maximum allowable levels of nasal decongestant, cough suppressant, and non-aspirin pain reliever/fever reducer provide temporary relief from symptoms of the common cold and flu. This product contains no ingredients that may cause drowsiness. The **DECONGESTANT** (pseudoephedrine) temporarily relieves nasal and sinus congestion due to the common cold. It temporarily relieves nasal stuffiness; reduces the swelling of nasal passages; shrinks swollen membranes; and temporarily restores freer breathing through the nose. The **COUGH SUPPRESSANT** (dextromethorphan) temporarily relieves cough due to the common cold. The non-aspirin **PAIN RELIEVER/FEVER REDUCER** (acetaminophen) temporarily relieves headache, body aches and pains, minor sore throat pain, and reduces fever due to the common cold.

Directions: Adults and children 12 years of age and over, 2 tablets every 6 hours, not to exceed 8 tablets in 24 hours. Not recommended for children under 12 years of age.

Each Coated Tablet Contains: acetaminophen 500 mg, dextromethorphan hydrobromide 15 mg, and pseudoephedrine hydrochloride 30 mg. Also contains: carnauba wax, crospovidone, hydroxypropyl methylcellulose, magnesium stearate, microcrystalline cellulose, polyethylene glycol, povidone, pregelatinized corn starch, stearic acid, and titanium dioxide.

Warnings: Do not exceed recommended dosage because at higher doses nervousness, dizziness or sleeplessness may occur. Do not take this product for more than 10 days. A persistent cough may be a sign of a serious condition. If cough persists for more than 7 days, tends to recur, or is accompanied by rash, persistent headache, fever that lasts for more than 3 days, or if new symptoms occur, consult a physician. Do not take this product for persistent or chronic cough such as occurs with smoking, asthma, emphysema, or if cough is accompanied by excessive phlegm (mucus) unless directed by a physician. If sore throat is severe, persists for more than 2 days, is accompanied or followed by fever, headache, rash, nausea, or vomiting, consult a physician promptly. Do not take this product if you have high blood pressure, heart disease, diabetes, thyroid disease, or difficulty in urination due to enlargement of the prostate gland except under the advice and supervision of a physician. As with any drug, if you are pregnant or nursing a baby, seek the advice of a health professional before using this product.

Drug Interaction Precaution: Do not take this product if you are presently taking a prescription antihypertensive or antidepressant drug containing a monoamine oxidase inhibitor except under the advice and supervision of a physician.

KEEP THIS AND ALL DRUGS OUT OF THE REACH OF CHILDREN. In case of accidental overdose, seek professional assistance or contact a Poison Control Center immediately. Prompt medical attention is critical for adults as well as for chilren even if you do not notice any signs or symptoms.

Store at 15° to 25°C (59° to 77°F) in a dry place.

How Supplied: Boxes of 10, 20.
604214

Shown in Product Identification Section, page 407

SUDAFED® SINUS Caplets
[*sū' duh-fĕd sī' nəs*]

Product Benefits:

- Maximum allowable levels of non-aspirin pain reliever and nasal decongestant provide temporary relief of sinus headache pain, pressure and nasal congestion due to colds and flu or hay fever and other allergies.
- Contains no ingredients which may cause drowsiness.

Directions: Adults and children 12 years and over, 2 caplets every 6 hours, not to exceed 8 caplets in a 24-hour period. Not recommended for children under 12 years of age.

Each Coated Caplet Contains: acetaminophen 500 mg and pseudoephedrine hydrochloride 30 mg. Also contains: carnauba wax, crospovidone, FD&C Yellow

No. 6 Lake, hydroxypropyl methylcellulose, magnesium stearate, microcrystalline cellulose, polyethylene glycol, polysorbate 80, povidone, pregelatinized corn starch, stearic acid, and titanium dioxide.

Warnings: Do not exceed recommended dosage because at higher doses nervousness, dizziness, or sleeplessness may occur. Do not take this product for more than 10 days. If symptoms do not improve or are accompanied by fever that lasts for more than 3 days, or if new symptoms occur, consult a physician. Do not take this product if you have high blood pressure, heart disease, diabetes, thyroid disease, or difficulty in urination due to enlargement of the prostate gland except under the advice and supervision of a physician. As with any drug, if you are pregnant or nursing a baby, seek the advice of a health professional before using this product.

Drug Interaction Precaution: Do not take this product if you are presently taking a prescription antihypertensive or antidepressant drug containing a monoamine oxidase inhibitor except under the advice and supervision of a physician.

KEEP THIS AND ALL DRUGS OUT OF THE REACH OF CHILDREN. In case of accidental overdose, seek professional assistance or contact a Poison Control Center immediately. Prompt medical attention is critical for adults as well as children even if you do not notice any signs or symptoms.

Store at 15° to 25°C (59° to 77°F) in a dry place and protect from light.

How Supplied: Boxes of 24 and 48.
605813

Shown in Product Identification Section, page 407

SUDAFED® SINUS Tablets

[*sū' duh-fĕd sī' nəs*]

Product Benefits:

- Maximum allowable levels of non-aspirin pain reliever and nasal decongestant provide temporary relief of sinus headache pain, pressure and nasal congestion due to colds and flu or hay fever and other allergies.
- Contains no ingredients which may cause drowsiness.

Directions: Adults and children 12 years and over, 2 tablets every 6 hours, not to exceed 8 tablets in a 24-hour period. Not recommended for children under 12 years of age.

Each Coated Tablet Contains: Acetaminophen 500 mg and pseudoephedrine hydrochloride 30 mg. Also contains: carnauba wax, crospovidone, FD&C Yellow No. 6 Lake, hydroxypropyl methylcellulose, magnesium stearate, microcrystalline cellulose, polyethylene glycol, polysorbate 80, povidone, pregelatinized corn starch, stearic acid, and titanium dioxide.

Warnings: Do not exceed recommended dosage because at higher doses nervousness, dizziness, or sleeplessness may occur. Do not take this product for more than 10 days. If symptoms do not improve or are accompanied by fever that lasts for more than 3 days, or if new symptoms occur, consult a physician. Do not take this product if you have high blood pressure, heart disease, diabetes, thyroid disease, or difficulty in urination due to enlargement of the prostate gland except under the advice and supervision of a physician. As with any drug, if you are pregnant or nursing a baby, seek the advice of a health professional before using this product.

Drug Interaction Precaution: Do not take this product if you are presently taking a prescription antihypertensive or antidepressant drug containing a monoamine oxidase inhibitor except under the advice and supervision of a physician.

KEEP THIS AND ALL DRUGS OUT OF THE REACH OF CHILDREN. In case of accidental overdose, seek professional assistance or contact a Poison Control Center immediately. Prompt medical attention is critical for adults as well as children even if you do not notice any signs or symptoms.

Store at 15° to 25°C (59° to 77°F) in a dry place and protect from light.

How Supplied: Boxes of 24 and 48.
605807

Shown in Product Identification Section, page 407

SUDAFED® 12 Hour Caplets

[*sū 'duh-fĕd*]

Each coated extended-release caplet contains pseudoephedrine hydrochloride 120 mg in a capsule-shaped tablet. Also contains: hydroxypropyl methylcellulose, magnesium stearate, microcrystalline cellulose, polyethylene glycol, povidone, and titanium dioxide. Printed with edible blue ink.

Indications: For temporary relief of nasal congestion due to the common cold, hay fever, or other upper respiratory allergies, and nasal congestion associated with sinusitis; promotes nasal and/or sinus drainage.

Directions: Adults and children 12 years and over—One caplet every 12 hours, not to exceed two caplets in 24 hours. Sudafed 12 Hour is not recommended for children under 12 years of age.

Warnings: Do not exceed recommended dosage because at higher doses, nervousness, dizziness, or sleeplessness may occur. Do not take this product if you have heart disease, high blood pressure, thyroid disease, diabetes, or difficulty in urination due to enlargement of the prostate gland unless directed by a doctor. If symptoms do not improve within 7 days or are accompanied by fever, consult your doctor before continuing use. As with any drug, if you are pregnant or nursing a baby, seek the advice of a health professional before using this product.

Drug Interaction Precaution: Do not take this product if you are presently taking a prescription drug for high blood pressure or depression, without first consulting your doctor.

KEEP THIS AND ALL DRUGS OUT OF THE REACH OF CHILDREN. In case of accidental overdose, seek professional assistance or contact a Poison Control Center immediately.

Store at 15° to 25°C (59° to 77°F) in a dry place and protect from light.

How Supplied: Boxes of 10 and 20.
605571

Shown in Product Indentification Section, page 407

Campbell Laboratories Inc.

300 EAST 51st STREET
P.O. BOX 812, FDR STATION
NEW YORK, NY 10150

HERPECIN-L® Cold Sore Lip Balm

[*her "puh-sin-el"*]

PRODUCT OVERVIEW

Key Facts: HERPECIN-L Lip Balm is a convenient, easy-to-use treatment for perioral herpes simplex infections. Sunscreens provide an SPF of 15.

Major Uses: HERPECIN-L not only treats cold sores, sun and fever blisters, but with prophylactic use, its sunscreens also protect to help prevent them. Users report early use at the prodromal stages of an attack will often abort the lesions and prevent scabbing. Prescribe: Apply "early, often and liberally."

Safety Information: For topical use only. A rare sensitivity may occur.

PRESCRIBING INFORMATION

HERPECIN-L® Cold Sore Lip Balm

Composition: A soothing, emollient, lip balm incorporating allantoin, the sunscreen, Padimate O, in a balanced, slightly acidic lipid base that includes petrolatum and titanium dioxide at a cosmetically acceptable level. (Does not contain any caines, antibiotics, phenol or camphor.) (NDC 38083-777-31)

Actions and Uses: HERPECIN-L® relieves dryness and chapping by providing a lipid barrier to help restore normal moisture balance to the lips. Skin protectants help to soften the crusts and scabs of "cold sores." The sunscreen is effective in 2900-3200 AU range while titanium dioxide, though at low levels, helps to block, scatter and reflect the sun's rays. Applied as a lip balm, SPF is 15. Regular reapplication during sun exposure, is advised.

Continued on next page

Campbell—Cont.

Administration: (1) *Recurrent "cold sores, sun and fever blisters":* Simply put, use **soon** and **often.** Frequent sufferers report that with *prophylactic* use (BID/PRN), attacks are fewer and less severe. Most recurrent herpes labialis patients are aware of the prodromal symptoms: tingling, itching, burning. At this stage, or if the lesion has already developed, HERPECIN-L should be applied liberally as often as convenient —at least *every hour.* (2) *Outdoor protection:* Apply before and during sun exposure, after swimming and again at bedtime (h.s.). (3) *Dry, chapped lips:* Apply as needed.

Adverse Reactions: If sensitive to any of the ingredients, discontinue use.

Contraindications: None.

How Supplied: 2.8 gm. swivel tubes.

Samples Available: Yes. (Request on professional letterhead or Rx pad.)

Care-Tech Laboratories

Div. of Consolidated Chemical, Inc.
3224 SOUTH KINGSHIGHWAY BOULEVARD
ST. LOUIS, MO 63139

BARRI-CARE®

Composition: Active Ingredient: Chloroxylenol
Inactive Ingredients: Petrolatum, Water, Paraffin, Propylene Glycol, Milk Protein, Cod Liver Oil, Aloe Vera Gel, Fragrance, Potassium Hydroxide, Methyl Paraben, Propyl Paraben, Vitamin A & D_3, (E) dl Alpha-Tocopheryl Acetate, (E) dl-Alpha-Tocopherol, D&C Yellow #11 and D&C Red #17.

Actions and Uses: Barri-Care is an antimicrobial ointment formulated to provide a moisture proof barrier against urine, detergent irritants, feces and drainage from wounds or skin lesions. Proven antimicrobial action against E. coli, MRSA, S. aureus and Pseudomonas aeruginosa. Protects perineal area of the incontinent patient from painful skin rashes and relieves irritation around stoma sites. Utilize on Grades I–IV pressure ulcers to halt skin breakdown. Can be used also on minor burns. Will not melt under feverish conditions.

Precautions: External Use Only. Non-Toxic. Avoid eye contact.

Directions: Cleanse affected area with Satin thoroughly. Apply ointment topically to affected area. Reapply 2–3 times daily or as directed by physician.

How Supplied: 2 oz. jar, 4 oz. tubes, 8 oz. jar. NDC #46706-206

CARE CREME®

Composition: Active Ingredient: Chloroxylenol
Inactive Ingredients: Water, Cetyl Alcohol, Lanolin Oil, Cod Liver Oil, Sodium Laureth Sulfate, Triethanolamine, Propylene Glycol, Petrolatum, Lanolin Alcohol, Methyl Gluceth 20 Distearate, Beeswax, Citric Acid, Methyl Paraben, Fragrance, Propyl Paraben, Vitamins A, D_3 and E-dl Alpha-Tocopherol.

Actions and Uses: Care Creme is an antimicrobial skin care creme specially formulated for use on severely dry skin such as Sjogren's Syndrome, atopic dermatitis, psoriasis, minor burns, urine or fecal exposure, scaling and inter-tissue ammonia related rash. Extremely effective on oncology radiation burns. Use at first sign of reddened skin or initial breakdown. Vitamin and oil enriched to promote skin integrity. Contains no metallic ions.

Precautions: Non-toxic, External Use Only. Avoid use around eye area.

Directions: Cleanse affected area with Satin and gently massage Care Creme into skin until completely absorbed or as directed by physician.

How Supplied: 2 oz., 4 oz. tubes, 9 oz. jar. NDC #46706-205

CLINICAL CARE® WOUND CLEANSER

Composition: Active Ingredient: Benzethonium Chloride
Inactive Ingredients: Water, Amphoteric 2, Aloe Vera Gel, DMDM Hydantoin, Citric Acid.

Actions and Uses: Clinical Care is an antimicrobial, emulsifying solution which aids in removing debris and particulate matter from open, dermal wounds. Clinical Care inhibits the growth of pathogenic organisms. Proven effective at eliminating S. aureus, P. aeruginosa, S. typhimurium, Aspergillus, E. coli, MRSA, S. pyogenes and K. pneumonia. Will not produce dermal irritation.

Precautions: External Use Only. Non-Toxic. No contra-indicators.

Directions: Spray affected area as necessary to debride. Use sterile gauze to gently remove debris and necrotic tissue at dermal surface.

How Supplied: 4 oz. spray, 8 oz. spray

CONCEPT®

Composition: Active Ingredient: Chloroxylenol
Inactive Ingredients: Water, Amphoteric 9, Polysorbate 20, PEG-150 Distearate, Cocamide DEA, Cocoyl Sarcosine, Fragrance, D&C Green #5.

Actions and Uses: Concept is a geriatric shampoo and body wash for patients whose skin is irritated by soaps and harsh detergents. Concept is non-eye irritating and reduces bacteria on the skin. Excellent for replenishing moisture in dry, flaky dermal tissues and eliminating body odors. Utilize on children over 6 months of age to address rashing or atopic dermatitis.

Precautions: External Use Only. Non-Toxic.

Directions: Use in normal manner of bathing and shampooing. Rinse thoroughly.

How Supplied: 8 oz., Gallons

FORMULA MAGIC®

Composition: Active Ingredient: Benzethonium Chloride
Inactive Ingredients: Talc, Mineral Oil, Magnesium Carbonate, Fragrance, DMDM Hydantoin.

Actions and Uses: Formula Magic is primarily a geriatric care powder and nursing lubricant. Aids in preventing excoriation, friction chafing and eliminating odor. Antibacterial action proven effective at 99.9% inhibition where Formula Magic is applied. Excellent for use on diabetic patients, feet and under breasts to relieve redness and skin irritation.

Precautions: Non-irritating to skin, non-toxic, slightly irritating to eyes.

Directions: Apply liberally to body and rub gently into skin.

How Supplied: 4 oz. and 12 oz. NDC #46706-202

ORCHID FRESH II®
Perineal/Ostomy Cleanser

Composition: Active Ingredient: Benzethonium Chloride
Inactive Ingredients: Water, Amphoteric 2, DMDM Hydantoin, Fragrance, Citric Acid.

Actions and Uses: Orchid Fresh II is an amphoteric, topical antimicrobial cleansing solution which gently cleans and emulsifies feces and urine on the incontinent patient. Use also on stoma sites and ostomy bags to deodorize and eliminate odor. Outstanding antimicrobial action on Pseudomonas, E. coli, Staphylococcus aureus, MRSA, etc. Orchid Fresh II will aid in reducing skin breakdown.

Precautions: External Use Only, Non-Toxic—Non-Dermal Irritating

Directions: Spray topically and remove feces and urine with warm, moist washcloth. Spray directly on peristomal skin areas, clean gently and pat dry. Utilize Care Creme on reddened skin areas.

How Supplied: 4 oz., 8 oz. and Gallons NDC #46706-115

SATIN® ANTIMICROBIAL SKIN CLEANSER

Composition: Active Ingredient: Chloroxylenol
Inactive Ingredients: Water, Sodium Laureth Sulfate, Cocamidopropyl Betaine, PEG-8, Cocamide DEA, Glycol Stearate, Lanolin Oil, Tetrasodium EDTA, D&C Yellow #10.

Actions and Uses: Satin has been specially formulated for use on sensitive or aging dermal tissue, atopic dermatitis and psoriasis. Effective in eliminating gram-positive and gram-negative pathogens such as E. coli, S. aureus, Pseudomonas, etc. Contains emollients to replenish natural oils and proteins. Satin also eliminates skin odor and dry, itchy skin.

Precautions: No contra-indicators. External use only. Non-Toxic.

Directions: Use during shower, bath or regular cleansing or as directed by physician.

How Supplied: 4 oz., 8 oz., 12 oz. 16 oz., 1 Gallon NDC #46706-101

TECHNI-CARE® SURGICAL SCRUB

Composition: Active Ingredient: Chloroxylenol 3%
Inactive Ingredients: Water, Sodium Lauryl Sulfate, Cocamide DEA, Propylene Glycol, Cocamidopropyl Betaine, Cocamidopropyl PG-Dimonium Chloride Phosphate, Citric Acid, Tetrasodium EDTA, Aloe Vera Gel, Hydrolyzed Animal Protein, D&C Yellow #10.

Actions and Uses: Techni-Care represents entirerly new technology in a broad-spectrum, topical, antiseptic microbicide for skin degerming. 99.99% Bacterial reduction in 30 second contact usage. Techni-Care may be used for disinfection of wounds, for pre-op and post-op along with surgical scrub applications. Non-staining and non-irritating to dermal tissue. Techni-Care conditions dermal tissue and promotes more rapid rate of healing.

Precautions: Non-Toxic, Non-Irritating, External Use Only. Can be used safely around ears and eyes or as directed by a physician.

Directions: Apply, lather and rinse well. For pre-op, apply and let dry, no rinsing required.

How Supplied: 20 mL packets, 8 oz., 16 oz., 32 oz., Gallons and peel paks

---

Products are indexed
by product category
in the
BLUE SECTION.

Chattem Consumer Products

Division of Chattem, Inc.
1715 WEST 38TH STREET
CHATTANOOGA, TN 37409

FLEX-ALL 454® PAIN RELIEVING GEL

Active Ingredient: Menthol 7%.

Inactive Ingredients: Alcohol, Allantoin, Aloe Vera Gel, Boric Acid Carbomer 940, Diazolidinyl Urea, Eucalyptus Oil, Glycerin, Iodine, Methylparaben, Methyl Salicylate, Peppermint Oil, Polysorbate 60, Potassium Iodide, Propylene Glycol, Propylparaben, Thyme Oil, Triethanolamine, Water.

Indications: To relieve the pain of minor arthritis, simple backache, strains, sprains, bruises, and cramps.

Actions: Flex-all is classified as a counterirritant which provides relief of deep-seated pain through cutaneous stimulation rather than through a direct analgesic effect.

Warnings: For external use only. Keep out of reach of children. If swallowed, call a physician or contact a poison control center. Keep away from eyes and mucous membranes, broken or irritated skin. Do not bandage tightly or use heating pad. If skin redness or irritation develops, or pain lasts more than 10 days, discontinue use and call a physician.

Dosage and Administration: Apply generously to painful muscles and joints and gently massage until Flex-all 454 disappears. Use before and after exercise. Repeat as needed for temporary relief of minor arthritis pain, simple backache, strains, sprains, bruises, and cramps.

How Supplied: Available in 2 oz., 4 oz. and 8 oz. bottles.

ICY HOT® Balm
[*ī'see hot*]
(topical analgesic balm)
ICY HOT® Cream
(topical analgesic cream)
ICY HOT® Stick
(topical analgesic stick)

Active Ingredients: Icy Hot Balm contains methyl salicylate 29%, menthol 7.6%. Icy Hot Cream contains methyl salicylate 30%, menthol 10%. Icy Hot Stick contains methyl salicylate 30%, menthol 10%.
Inactive ingredients of Icy Hot Balm include paraffin and white petrolatum. Inactive ingredients of Icy Hot Cream include carbomer, cetyl esters wax, emulsifying wax, oleth-3 phosphate, stearic acid, trolamine, and water. Inactive ingredients of Icy Hot Stick include ceresin, cyclomethicone, hydrogenated castor oil, microcrystalline wax, paraffin, PEG-150 distearate, propylene glycol, stearic acid, and stearyl alcohol.

Description: Icy Hot Balm, Icy Hot Cream, and Icy Hot Stick are topically applied analgesics containing two active ingredients, methyl salicylate and menthol. It is the particular concentration of these ingredients, in combination with inert ingredients, that results in the distinct, combined heating/cooling sensation of Icy Hot.

Actions: Icy Hot is classified as a counterirritant which, when rubbed into the intact skin, provides relief of deep-seated pain through a counterirritant action rather than through a direct analgesic effect. In acting as a counterirritant, Icy Hot replaces the perception of pain with another sensation that blocks deep pain temporarily by its action on or near the skin surface.

Indications: For the temporary relief of minor aches and pains of muscles and joints associated with arthritis, simple backache, strains, bruises, and sprains.

Directions: Adults and children 2 years of age and older: Apply to affected area not more than 3 to 4 times daily. Children under 2 years of age: Do not use, consult a doctor.
Stick: Twist base to raise Icy Hot approximately one quarter inch above container.
Adults and children 2 years of age and older: Apply to affected area not more than 3 to 4 times daily. Children under 2 years of age: Do not use, consult a doctor.

Warnings: For external use only. Do not use otherwise than as directed. Keep this and all drugs out of the reach of children. In case of accidental ingestion, seek professional assistance or contact a poison control center immediately. Avoid contact with eyes. Avoid contact with mouth, genitalia, and mucous membranes, irritated, or very sensitive skin. If you have diabetes or impaired circulation, use Icy Hot only upon the advice of a physician. Do not apply to wounds or damaged skin. Do not bandage tightly. Do not apply external heat or hot water. If condition worsens, or if symptoms persist for more than 7 days or clear up and occur again within a few days, discontinue use of this product and consult a doctor.
CAUTION: Discontinue use if excessive irritation of the skin develops.

Adverse Reactions: The most common adverse reactions that may occur with Icy Hot use are skin irritation and blistering. The most serious adverse reaction is severe toxicity that occurs if the product is ingested.

How Supplied: Icy Hot Balm is available in a 3½ oz jar. Icy Hot Cream is available in tubes in two sizes, 1¼ oz and 3 oz. Icy Hot Stick is available as a 1¾ oz stick.

Continued on next page

Chattem Consumer—Cont.

NORWICH® ASPIRIN
Aspirin (acetylsalicylic acid) Tablets

Active Ingredient: Each tablet contains:
Regular: 325 mg. (5 grains) of pure aspirin.
Maximum: 500 mg. (7.7 grains) of pure aspirin.

Inactive Ingredients: Hydroxypropyl Methylcellulose, Polyethylene Glycol, Starch.

Actions: Analgesic and antipyretic.

Indications: For fast, effective relief of headache, minor aches and pains, and for reduction of fever, as well as temporary relief of minor aches and pains of arthritis, muscular aches, colds and flu, and menstrual discomfort.

Warnings: Children and teenagers should not use this medicine for chicken pox or flu symptoms before a doctor is consulted about Reye syndrome, a rare but serious illness reported to be associated with aspirin. As with any drug, if you are pregnant or nursing a baby, seek the advice of a health professional before using this product. IT IS ESPECIALLY IMPORTANT NOT TO USE ASPIRIN DURING THE LAST 3 MONTHS OF PREGNANCY UNLESS SPECIFICALLY DIRECTED TO DO SO BY A DOCTOR BECAUSE IT MAY CAUSE PROBLEMS IN THE UNBORN CHILD OR COMPLICATIONS DURING DELIVERY. Keep this and all medicines out of reach of children. In case of accidental overdose, seek professional assistance or contact a poison control center immediately.

Caution: If pain persists for more than 10 days or if redness is present, or in conditions affecting children under 12, consult physician immediately. Do not take if you have ulcers, ulcer symptoms or bleeding problems. If asthmatic or taking medicines for anticoagulation (thinning the blood), diabetes, gout, or arthritis, consult physician before use. Discontinue if ringing in the ears occurs.

Treatment of Oral Overdosage: IN CASE OF ACCIDENTAL OVERDOSE, SEEK PROFESSIONAL ASSISTANCE OR CONTACT A POISON CONTROL CENTER IMMEDIATELY.

Dosage and Administration: 325 mg: Adults: 1 or 2 tablets every 3–4 hours up to 6 times a day. Children: under 3 years, consult physician; 3–6 years, ½ to 1 tablet; over 6 years, 1 tablet. May be taken every 3–4 hours up to 3 times a day.
500 mg: Adults: Initial dose 2 caplets followed by 1 caplet every 3 hours or 2 caplets every 6 hours, not to exceed 8 caplets in any 24-hour period, or as directed by a physician. NOT RECOMMENDED FOR CHILDREN UNDER 12.

Professional Labeling: Same as outlined under indications. Aspirin is also indicated to reduce the risk of death and/or nonfatal myocardial infarction in patients with a previous infarction or unstable angina pectoris.

How Supplied: 325 mg: In child-resistant bottles of 500 tablets and 100 tablets and easy to open screw cap, 250 tablets.
500 mg: In child-resistant bottles of 150 caplets.
Tablet identification:
325 mg. Imprinted **(N)** in a shield.
500 mg. "NORWICH"

NORWICH ENTERIC SAFETY COATED ASPIRIN
Aspirin (acetylsalicylic acid) Tablets

Active Ingredients: Norwich® Enteric Safety Coated Aspirin tablets are available in 325 mg and 500 mg dosage units.
The enteric coating covers a core of aspirin and is designed to resist disintegration in the stomach, dissolving in the more neutral-to-alkaline environment of the duodenum. Such action helps to protect the stomach from injury that may result from ingestion of plain or buffered aspirin.

Inactive Ingredients: Dioctyl Sodium Sulfosuccinate, Hydroxypropyl Cellulose, Hydroxypropyl Methylcellulose, Iron Oxide, Microcrystalline Cellulose, Pharmaceutical Glaze, Polyethylene Glycol, Polyvinyl Acetate Phthalate, Pregelatinized Starch, Silicon Dioxide, Stearic Acid, Talc, Titanium Dioxide, Triethyl Citrate, Yellow # 6 (Sunset Yellow), Yellow # 10.

Indications: Norwich® Enteric Safety Coated Aspirin is for temporary relief of minor aches and pains and inflammation due to arthritis and rheumatism. The enteric safety coating is designed so the aspirin is safer for the stomach than plain or buffered aspirin and is safe for daily aspirin users.

Dosage: For analgesic or anti-inflammatory indications, the maximum OTC dosage for aspirin is 4000 mg per day in divided dosages, i.e., two 325 mg tablets every 4 hours or two 500 mg tablets every 6 hours.

Caution: If pain persists for more than 10 days, or if redness is present, or in conditions affecting children under 12, consult physician immediately. Consult a physician before use if you have ulcers, ulcer symptoms or bleeding problems or if you are asthmatic or taking medicines for anticoagulation (thinning the blood), diabetes, gout or arthritis. Discontinue use if ringing in the ears occurs.

Consumer Warning: Children and teenagers should not use this medicine for chicken pox or flu symptoms before a doctor is consulted about Reye syndrome, a rare but serious illness reported to be associated with aspirin. As with any drug, if you are pregnant or nursing a baby, seek the advise of a health professional before using this product. **IT IS ESPECIALLY IMPORTANT NOT TO USE ASPIRIN DURING THE LAST 3 MONTHS OF PREGNANCY UNLESS SPECIFICALLY DIRECTED TO DO SO BY A DOCTOR BECAUSE IT MAY CAUSE PROBLEMS IN THE UNBORN CHILD OR COMPLICATIONS DURING DELIVERY. Keep this and all medicines out of the reach of children.** In case of accidental overdose, seek professional assistance or contact a poison control center immediately.

Avoid excessive heat (over 104°F or 40°C).

Professional Warning: There have been occasional reports in the literature concerning individuals with impaired gastric emptying in whom there may be retention of one or more aspirin tablets over time. This unusual phenomenon may occur as a result of outlet obstruction from ulcer disease alone or combined with hypotonic gastric peristalsis. Because of the integrity of the enteric coating in an acidic environment, these tablets may accumulate and form a bezoar in the stomach. Individuals with this condition may present with complaints of early satiety or of vague upper abdominal distress. Diagnosis may be made by endoscopy or by abdominal films which show opacities suggestive of a mass of small tablets (Ref.: Bogacz, K. and Caldron, P.: Enteric-coated Aspirin Bezoar: Elevation of Serum Salicylate Level by Barium Study. *Amer. J. Med.* 1987:83, 783–6). Management may vary according to the condition of the patient. Options include: gastrotomy and alternating slightly basic and neutral lavage (Ref.: Baum, J.: Enteric-Coated Aspirin and the Problem of Gastric Retention. *J. Rheum,* 1984:11, 250–1). While there have been no clinical reports, it has been suggested that such individuals may also be treated with parenteral cimetidine (to reduce acid secretion) and then given sips of slightly basic liquids to effect gradual dissolution of the enteric coating. Progress may be followed with plasma salicylate levels or via recognition of tinnitus by the patient.
It should be kept in mind that individuals with a history of partial or complete gastrectomy may produce reduced amounts of acid and therefore have less acidic gastric pH. Under these circumstances, the benefits offered by the acid-resistant enteric coating may not exist.

Safety: The safety of enteric-coated aspirin has been demonstrated in a number of endoscopic studies comparing enteric-coated aspirin and plain aspirin, as well as plain buffered and "arthritis strength" preparations. In these studies, endoscopies were performed in healthy volunteers before and after either two-day or 14-day administration of aspirin doses of 3,900 or 4,000 mg/day. Compared to all the other preparations, the enteric-coated aspirin produced significantly less damage to the gastric mucosa.

There was also statistically less duodenal damage when compared with the plain, i.e., non-enteric-coated, aspirin.

Antiplatelet Effect: FDA approved professional labeling permits the use of aspirin to reduce the risk of death and/or nonfatal myocardial infarction (MI) in patients with a previous infarction or unstable angina pectoris and its use in reducing the risk of transient ischemic attacks in men.
Labeling for both indications follows:

ASPIRIN FOR MYOCARDIAL INFARCTION

Indication: Aspirin is indicated to reduce the risk of death and/or nonfatal myocardial infarction in patients with a previous infarction or unstable angina pectoris.

Clinical Trials: The indication is supported by the results of six, large, randomized multicenter, placebo-controlled studies involving 10,816 predominantly male, post-myocardial infarction (MI) patients and one randomized placebo-controlled study of 1,266 men with unstable angina. (1–7) Therapy with aspirin was begun at intervals after the onset of acute MI varying from less than three days to more than five years and continued for periods of from less than one year to four years. In the unstable angina study, treatment was started within one month after the onset of unstable angina and continued for 12 weeks, and patients with complicating conditions such as congestive heart failure were not included in the study.

Aspirin therapy in MI patients was associated with about a 20 percent reduction in the risk of subsequent death and/or nonfatal reinfarction, a median absolute decrease of 3 percent from the 12 to 22 percent event rates in the placebo groups. In aspirin-treated unstable angina patients, the reduction in risk was about 50 percent, a reduction in event rate to 5% from the 10% in the placebo group over the 12 weeks of the study.

Daily dosage of aspirin in the post-myocardial infarction studies was 300 mg in one study and 900 to 1500 mg in five studies. A dose of 325 mg was used in the study of unstable angina.

Adverse Reactions: Gastrointestinal Reactions: Doses of 1000 mg per day of plain aspirin caused gastrointestinal symptoms and bleeding that in some cases were clinically significant. In the largest postinfarction study (the Aspirin Myocardial Infarction Study [AMIS] with 4,500 people), the percentage incidences of gastrointestinal symptoms of a standard, solid-tablet formulation and placebo-treated subjects, respectively, were: stomach pain (14.5%; 4.4%); heartburn (11.9%; 4.8%); nausea and/or vomiting (7.6%; 2.1%); hospitalization for gastrointestinal disorder (4.9%; 3.5%). In the AMIS and other trials plain aspirin treated patients had increased rates of gross gastrointestinal bleeding. Symptoms and signs of gastrointestinal irritation were not significantly increased in subjects treated for unstable angina with buffered aspirin in solution.

Cardiovascular and Biochemical: In the AMIS trial, the dosage of 1000 mg per day of plain aspirin was associated with small increases in systolic blood pressure (BP) (average 1.5 to 2.1 mmHg), depending upon whether maximal or last available readings were used. Blood urea nitrogen and uric acid levels were also increased, but by less than 1.0 mg%. Subjects with marked hypertension or renal insufficiency had been excluded from the trial so that the clinical importance of these observations for such subjects or for any subjects treated over more prolonged periods is not known. It is recommended that patients placed on long-term aspirin treatment, even at doses of 300 mg per day, be seen at regular intervals to assess changes in these measurements.

Dosage and Administration: Although most of the studies used dosages exceeding 300 mg daily, two trials used only 300 mg and pharmacologic data indicate that this dose inhibits platelet function fully. Therefore, 300 mg or a conventional 325 mg aspirin dose daily is a reasonable, routine dose that would minimize gastrointestinal adverse reactions for both solid oral dosage forms (buffered and plain aspirin) and buffered aspirin in solution.

References: 1. Elwood, P.C., et al.: A Randomized Controlled Trial of Acetylsalicylic Acid in the Secondary Prevention of Mortality from Myocardial Infarction, *Br. Med. J.* 1:436–440, 1974. 2. The Coronary Drug Project Research Group: Aspirin in Coronary Heart Disease, *J. Chronic Dis.* 29:625–642, 1976. 3. Breddin, K., et al.: Secondary Prevention of Myocardial Infarction: A Comparison of Acetylsalicylic Acid, Phenprocoumon or Placebo, *Homeostasis* 470:263–268, 1979. 4. Aspirin Myocardial Infarction Study Research Group: A Randomized Controlled Trial of Aspirin in Persons Recovered from Myocardial Infarction, *J.A.M.A.*, 243:661–669, 1980. 5. Elwood, P.C., and Sweetnam, P.M.: Aspirin and Secondary Mortality After Myocardial Infarction, *Lancet* pp. 1313–1315, Dec. 22–29, 1979. 6. The Persantine-Aspirin Reinfarction Study Research Group, Persantine and Aspirin in Coronary Heart Disease, *Circulation* 62:449–469, 1980. 7. Lewis, H.D., et al.: Protective Effects of Aspirin Against Acute Myocardial Infarction and Death in Men with Unstable Angina, Results of a Veterans Administration Cooperative Study, *N. Engl. J. Med.* 309:396–403, 1983.

Aspirin for Transient Ischemic Attacks

Indication: For reducing the risk of recurrent transient attacks (TIA's) or stroke in men who have had transient ischemia of the brain due to fibrin platelet emboli. There is inadequate evidence that aspirin or buffered aspirin is effective in reducing TIA's in women at the recommended dosage. There is no evidence that aspirin or buffered aspirin is of benefit in the treatment of completed strokes in men or women.

Clinical Trials: The indication is supported by the results of a Canadian study (1) in which 585 patients with threatened stroke were followed in a randomized clinical trial for an average of 26 months to determine whether aspirin or sulfinpyrazone, singly or in combination, was superior to placebo in preventing transient ischemic attacks, stroke or death. The study showed that, although sulfinpyrazone had no statistically significant effect, aspirin reduced the risk of continuing transient ischemic attacks or stroke or death by 19 percent and reduced the risk of stroke or death by 31 percent. Another aspirin study carried out in the United States with 178 patients showed a statistically significant number of "favorable outcomes", including reduced transient ischemic attacks, stroke and death (2).

Precautions: Patients presenting with signs and/or symptoms of TIA's should have a complete medical and neurologic evaluation. Consideration should be given to other disorders that resemble TIA's. Attention should be given to risk factors: it is important to evaluate and treat, if appropriate, other diseases associated with TIA's and stroke, such as hypertension and diabetes.
Concurrent administration of absorbable antacids at therapeutic doses may increase the clearance of salicylates in some individuals. The concurrent administration of nonabsorbable antacids may alter the rate of absorption of aspirin, thereby resulting in a decreased acetylsalicylic acid/salicylate ratio in plasma. The clinical significance of these decreases in available aspirin is unknown.
Aspirin at dosages of 1,000 mg per day has been associated with small increases in blood pressure, blood urea nitrogen, and serum uric acid levels. It is recommended that patients placed on long-term aspirin treatment be seen at regular intervals to assess changes in these measurements.

Adverse Reactions: At dosages of 1,000 mg or higher of aspirin per day, gastrointestinal side effects include stomach pain, heartburn, nausea and/or vomiting, as well as increased rates of gross gastrointestinal bleeding.

Dosage and Administration: Adult dosage for men is 1,300 mg per day, in divided doses of 650 mg twice a day or 325 mg four times a day.

References: 1. The Canadian Cooperative Study Group: Randomized Trial of Aspirin and Sulfinpyrazone in Threatened Stroke, N. *Engl. J. Med.* 299:53, 1978. 2. Fields, W.S., et al.: Controlled Trial of Aspirin in Cerebral Ischemia, *Stroke* 8:301–316, 1980.

Continued on next page

Chattem Consumer—Cont.

How Supplied: Norwich® Enteric Safety Coated 325 mg Tablets in child-resistant bottles of 150. 500 mg Tablets in child-resistant bottles of 100.

Maximum Strength Multi-Symptom PAMPRIN Menstrual Relief Tablets/Caplets

Active Ingredients: Each tablet/caplet contains acetaminophen 500 mg, pamabrom 25 mg, and pyrilamine maleate 15 mg.

Inactive Ingredients: Crospovidone; Magnesium Stearate; Povidone; Pregelatinized Starch; Sodium Starch Glycolate; Stearic Acid.

Indications: Clinically tested and found to be safe and effective in the relief of menstrual pain of cramps, backache, headache, water weight gain, premenstrual tension, and irritability.

Warning: Keep this and all drugs out of the reach of children. In case of accidental overdose, seek professional assistance or contact a poison control center immediately.

Precautions: IF DROWSINESS OCCURS, DO NOT DRIVE OR OPERATE MACHINERY. As with any drug, if you are pregnant or nursing a baby, seek the advice of a health professional before using this product.

Dosage and Administration: Two tablets (or caplets) and repeat every three to four hours as needed, not to exceed 8 tablets (or caplets) in a 24 hour period.

How Supplied: Non-child resistant packages of foil pouches containing 24 tablets or caplets and child resistant bottles containing 12 or 48 tablets or 48 caplets.

Product Identification: White, round tablets with PAMPRIN debossed in the center of the tablet surrounded by three rosette shaped designs on the top and bottom of the word PAMPRIN **OR** white capsule shaped caplets with PAMPRIN debossed in the center of the caplet and faced on either end by a single rosette.

Maximum Pain Relief PAMPRIN Menstrual Relief Caplets

Active Ingredients: Each caplet contains acetaminophen 250 mg, magnesium salicylate 250 mg, and pamabrom 25 mg.

Inactive Ingredients: Blue #1; Cellulose; Hydroxypropyl Methylcellulose; Magnesium Stearate; Microcrystalline Cellulose; Propylene Glycol; Silicon Dioxide; Starch; Stearic Acid; Titanium Dioxide.

Indications: Clinically tested and found to provide safe and effective relief of menstrual pain of cramps, backache, headache, and legaches that occur before and during the menstrual period. It also contains a mild diuretic to relieve the water gain experienced by many women.

CAUTION: Do not take for more than 10 days or for fever for more than 3 days unless directed by a doctor. If ringing in the ears or a loss of hearing occurs, consult a doctor before taking any more of this product. If pain or fever persists or gets worse, if new symptoms occur, or if redness or swelling is present, consult a doctor because these could be signs of a serious condition. Do not take if you are taking a prescription for anticoagulation (thinning the blood), diabetes, gout or arthritis unless directed by a doctor. Do not take if you are allergic to salicylates (including aspirin) unless directed by a doctor. As with any drug, if you are pregnant or nursing a baby, seek the advice of a health professional before using this product. **IT IS ESPECIALLY IMPORTANT NOT TO USE SALICYLATES DURING THE LAST 3 MONTHS OF PREGNANCY UNLESS SPECIFICALLY DIRECTED TO DO SO BY A DOCTOR BECAUSE IT MAY CAUSE PROBLEMS IN THE UNBORN CHILD OR COMPLICATIONS DURING DELIVERY.**

WARNINGS: Children and teenagers should not use this medicine for chicken pox or flu symptoms before a doctor is consulted about Reye syndrome, a rare but serious illness reported to be associated with salicylates. Keep this and all drugs out of the reach of children. In case of accidental overdose, seek professional assistance or contact a poison control center immediately.

Dosage and Administration: Two caplets and repeat every three to four hours as needed, not to exceed 8 caplets in a 24 hour period. Drink a full glass of water with each dose.

How Supplied: Non-child resistant foil pouches containing 16 caplets and child resistant bottles containing 32 caplets.

Product Identification: Coated white capsule shaped caplets with PAMPRIN printed in blue on the center of the caplet.

PRĒMSYN PMS®
[*preem 'sin pms*]
Premenstrual Syndrome Caplets

Active Ingredients: Each caplet contains Acetaminophen 500 mg., Pamabrom 25 mg., and Pyrilamine Maleate 15 mg.

Indications: PRĒMSYN PMS® has been clinically proven to safely and effectively relieve premenstrual tension, irritability, nervousness, edema, backaches, legaches, and headaches that often accompany premenstrual syndrome.

Warning: KEEP THIS AND ALL DRUGS OUT OF THE REACH OF CHILDREN. In case of accidental overdose, seek professional assistance or contact a poison control center immediately.

Precautions: If drowsiness occurs, do not drive or operate machinery. As with any drug, if pregnant or nursing a baby, seek the advice of a health professional before using this product.

Dosage and Administration: Two caplets at first sign of premenstrual discomfort and repeat every three or four hours as needed, not to exceed 8 caplets in a 24-hour period.

How Supplied: Tamper-resistant bottles of 20 and 40 caplets.

Product Identification Marks: White caplet with PRĒMSYN PMS debossed on one surface.

EDUCATIONAL MATERIAL

PRĒMSYN PMS®
PMS—Practical Advice for the Period Before Your Period
This booklet is written to the woman who suffers from PMS. It describes PMS, the various symptoms associated with the syndrome, a three-month symptom dairy and treatments including dietary tips, stress reduction and exercise. Free to physicians, pharmacists and other health professionals for distribution to patients. This can be obtained by writing Chattem, Inc.

Chesebrough-Pond's Inc.
33 BENEDICT PLACE
GREENWICH, CT 06830

VASELINE® Pure Petroleum Jelly Skin Protectant

Composition: White Petrolatum U.S.P.

Indication: A soothing protectant for minor skin irritations such as burns, scrapes, abrasions, chafing, detergent hands, dry or chapped skin, and sunburn. Provides temporary relief of external hemorrhoids and scaling due to psoriasis. Helps prevent diaper rash, soothes chapped skin and temporarily soothes minor sunburn due to its emollient and lubricant properties. Helps prevent and heal dry, chapped sun- and wind-burned skin. Vaseline products are non-comedogenic.

Directions: Cleanse affected areas with soap and water prior to application, then apply generously to provide a continuous protective film. Apply as needed, before, during and following exposure to sun, wind, water, and cold weather.

Drug Interaction: No known drug interactions. Product is innocuous, physiologically inert with no known sensitization potential.

Warning: Not meant for puncture wounds, serious burns, or cuts.

How Supplied: 1 oz. and 2.5 oz. plastic tubes. (NDC 0521-8120-01, -31). 1.75 oz., 3.75 oz., 7.5 oz., and 13 oz. plastic jars (NDC 0521-8120-24, -28, -29, -32).

VASELINE® INTENSIVE CARE® MOISTURIZING SUNBLOCK LOTION

Active Ingredients: Ethylhexyl *p*-methoxycinnamate, oxybenzone, 2-ethylhexyl salicylate.*

Inactive Ingredients: Water, glycerin, stearic acid, aloe vera gel, PVP/Eicosene copolymer, dimethicone, TEA, DEA-cetylphosphate, cetyl alcohol, petrolatum, tocopheryl acetate, magnesium aluminum silicate, carbomer, fragrance, methylparaben, propylparaben, disodium EDTA, DMDM hydantoin.

Indications/Actions: Vaseline Intensive Care Moisturizing Sunblock Lotion is a non-greasy, fragrance-free formula which provides broad-spectrum protection from the sun's harmful UVA and UVB rays. These effective moisturizers are hypo-allergenic and will penetrate into the skin quickly to replenish moisture loss due to sun and wind exposure. Vaseline Intensive Care Moisturizing Sunblock Lotion is also PABA-free; gentle and non-stinging, and waterproof for 80 minutes.

Directions: Apply generously and evenly to exposed areas. Apply product liberally prior to exposure to sun. Reapply after prolonged swimming or excessive perspiration or every two hours.

Warnings: Avoid contact with eyes. For external use only.

How Supplied: 4 oz., 6 oz., and 10 oz. SPF 15 and SPF 25.

*SPF 25, only.

VASELINE® INTENSIVE CARE® ULTRA VIOLET (UV) DAILY DEFENSE LOTION FOR HAND AND BODY—SPF 15

Active Ingredients: Ethylhexyl *p*-methoxycinnamate, oxybenzone.

Inactive Ingredients: Water, glycerin, stearic acid, C11–13 isoparaffin, glycol stearate, TEA, tocopheryl acetate (Vitamin E acetate), cetyl acetate, glyceryl stearate, cetyl alcohol, dimethicone, DEA-cetyl phosphate, magnesium aluminum silicate, acetylated lanolin alcohol, stearamide AMP, methylparaben, propylparaben, fragrance, carbomer, disodium EDTA, DMDM hydantoin.

Indications/Actions: Vaseline Intensive Care Ultra Violet Daily Defense Lotion is a light, non-greasy hand and body lotion that contains a UVA and UVB sunscreen to provide daily protection from the harmful burning rays which can cause premature aging and other long-term skin damage. It provides 15 times the natural sunburn protection. In addition, Vaseline Intensive Care UV Daily Defense Lotion has been formulated with a special blend of moisturizers to soften and smooth the skin without a greasy after-feel. It is also dermatologist tested and PABA free.

Directions: Use every day. Apply liberally to all areas of the body, especially on the back of hands, arms, legs, and neck to guard against sun damage and to soften skin.

Warnings: For external use only. Avoid contact with eyes. Keep out of the reach of children.

How Supplied: SPF #15 4 oz. and 10 oz.

VASELINE® INTENSIVE CARE® Extra Strength LOTION

Active Ingredient: Dimethicone

Other Ingredients: Water, glycerin, stearic acid, C11–13 isoparaffin, glycol stearate, petrolatum, glyceryl stearate, TEA, zinc oxide, cetyl alcohol, potassium cetyl phosphate, carbomer, cetyl acetate, acetylated lanolin alcohol, stearamide AMP, fragrance, magnesium aluminum silicate, methylparaben, propylparaben, disodium EDTA, DMDM hydantoin

Indications: Vaseline® Intensive Care® Extra Strength Lotion is specially formulated to help treat and prevent severe dry skin. Its clinically tested formula contains a proven healing ingredient—Dimethicone—to treat extremely dry, red, sore skin. The Vaseline Intensive Care Extra Strength Lotion is hypo-allergenic and non-comedogenic.

Directions: Apply liberally to severely dry skin, particularly hands, elbows and feet. Use to moisturize and treat skin after bathing/showering; under shaving cream; after shaving; overnight.

Warnings: Keep out of reach of children. For external use only. Avoid contact with eyes. If condition worsens or does not improve within 7 days, consult a doctor. Not to be applied over deep or puncture wounds, infections or lacerations.

How Supplied: 6 oz., 10 oz. and 15 oz.

Products are indexed by generic and chemical names in the **YELLOW SECTION.**

Church & Dwight Co., Inc.

469 N. HARRISON STREET
PRINCETON, NJ 08540

ARM & HAMMER® Pure Baking Soda

Active Ingredient: Sodium Bicarbonate U.S.P.

Indications: For alleviation of acid indigestion, also known as heartburn or sour stomach. Not a remedy for other types of stomach complaints such as nausea, stomachache, abdominal cramps, gas pains, or stomach distention caused by overeating and/or overdrinking. In the latter case, one should not ingest solids, liquids or antacid but rather refrain from all physical activity and—if uncomfortable—call a physician.

Actions: ARM & HAMMER® Pure Baking Soda provides fast-acting, effective neutralization of stomach acids. Each level ½ teaspoon dose will neutralize 20.9 mEq of acid.

Warnings: Except under the advice and supervision of a physician: (1) do not administer to children under five years of age, (2) do not take more than eight level ½ teaspoons per person up to 60 years old or four level ½ teaspoons per person 60 years or older in a 24-hour period, (3) do not use this product if you are on a sodium restricted diet, (4) do not use the maximum dose for more than two weeks, (5) do not ingest food, liquid or any antacid when stomach is overly full to avoid possible injury to the stomach.

Dosage and Administration: Level ½ teaspoon in ½ glass (4 fl. oz.) of water every two hours up to maximum dosage or as directed by a physician. Accurately measure level ½ teaspoon. Each level ½ teaspoon contains 20.9 mEq (.476 gm) sodium.

How Supplied: Available in 8 oz., 16 oz., 32 oz., and 64 oz. boxes.

IDENTIFICATION PROBLEM?
Consult the
Product Identification Section
where you'll find
products pictured
in full color.

CIBA Consumer Pharmaceuticals
Division of CIBA-GEIGY Corporation
MACK WOODBRIDGE II
WOODBRIDGE, NJ 07095

ACUTRIM® 16 HOUR* STEADY CONTROL APPETITE SUPPRESSANT TABLETS
Caffeine Free

ACUTRIM® II—MAXIMUM STRENGTH APPETITE SUPPRESSANT TABLETS
Caffeine Free

ACUTRIM LATE DAY® STRENGTH* APPETITE SUPPRESSANT TABLETS
Caffeine Free

*Peak strength and duration claims relate solely to blood levels.

Description:
ACUTRIM® tablets deliver their maximum strength dosage of appetite suppressant at a precisely controlled, even rate.
This steady release is scientifically targeted to effectively distribute the appetite suppressant all day.
ACUTRIM makes it easier to follow the kind of reduced calorie diet needed for best weight control results.
A diet plan developed by an expert dietician is included in the package for your personal use as a further aid.

Formula: Each ACUTRIM® tablet contains: Active Ingredient—phenylpropanolamine HCl 75 mg (appetite suppressant).
Inactive Ingredients—ACUTRIM® 16 HOUR Steady Control: Cellulose Acetate, Hydroxypropyl Methylcellulose, Stearic Acid—ACUTRIM® II MAXIMUM STRENGTH: Cellulose Acetate, D&C Yellow #10, FD&C Blue #1, FD&C Yellow #6, Hydroxypropyl Methylcellulose, Povidone, Propylene Glycol, Stearic Acid, Titanium Dioxide—ACUTRIM LATE DAY® Strength: Cellulose Acetate, FD&C Yellow #6, Hydroxypropyl Methylcellulose, Isopropyl Alcohol, Propylene Glycol, Riboflavin, Stearic Acid, Titanium Dioxide.

Directions: Adult oral dosage is **one tablet** at mid-morning with a full glass of water. Exceeding the recommended dose has not been shown to result in greater weight loss. This product's effectiveness is directly related to the degree to which you reduce your usual daily food intake. Attempts at weight reduction which involve the use of this product should be limited to periods not exceeding 3 months, because this should be enough time to establish new eating habits. Read and follow important Diet Plan enclosed.
WARNINGS: FOR ADULT USE ONLY. Do not take more than one tablet per day (24 hours). Exceeding the recommended dose may cause serious health problems. Do not give this product to children under 12 years of age. Persons between 12 and 18 are advised to consult their physician before using this product. If nervousness, dizziness, sleeplessness, palpitations or headache occurs, stop taking this medication and consult your physician. If you are being treated for high blood pressure, depression, or an eating disorder or have heart disease, diabetes, or thyroid disease, do not take this product except under the supervision of a physician. As with any drug, if you are pregnant or nursing a baby, seek the advice of a health professional before using this product.

Drug Interaction Precaution: If you are taking a cough/cold or allergy medication containing any form of phenylpropanolamine, or any type of nasal decongestant, do not take this product. Do not take this product if you are taking any prescription drug, except under the advice and supervision of a physician. Do not use this product if you are presently taking a prescription monoamine oxidase inhibitor (MAOI) for depression or for two weeks after stopping use of a MAOI without first consulting a physician.
KEEP THIS AND ALL MEDICATION OUT OF THE REACH OF CHILDREN.
In case of accidental overdose, seek professional assistance or contact a poison control center immediately.

How Supplied: Tamper-evident blister packages of 20 and 40 tablets. Do not use if individual seals are broken.
DO NOT STORE ABOVE 86°F
PROTECT FROM MOISTURE

Shown in Product Identification Section, page 407

EXTRA STRENGTH DOAN'S®
Analgesic Caplets

Indications: For temporary relief of occasional minor backache.

Directions: Adults—Two caplets 3 or 4 times daily, not to exceed 8 caplets during a 24-hour period or as directed by a physician. Not intended for use by children or teenagers except under the advice of a physician. If pain persists for more than 10 days, discontinue use and consult your physician.

Warning: Children and teenagers should not use this medicine for chicken pox or flu symptoms before a doctor is consulted about Reye's syndrome, a rare but serious illness. As with any drug, if you are pregnant or nursing a baby, seek the advice of a health professional before using this product. Do not use this product if you are under medical care or are allergic to aspirin or salicylates, except under the advice and supervision of your physician. **Keep this and all medicines out of the reach of children.** In case of accidental overdose, seek professional assistance or consult a Poison Control Center immediately.

Active Ingredient: Each caplet contains Magnesium Salicylate 500 mg.

Also Contains: Hydroxypropyl methylcellulose, magnesium stearate, microcrystalline cellulose, polyethylene glycol, polysorbate 80, propylene glycol, stearic acid and titanium dioxide.

How Supplied: Tamper-evident blister packages of 24 and 48 caplets. Do not use if individual seals are broken.
Store at 15°–30°C (59°–86°F). Protect from moisture.

Shown in Product Identification Section, page 407

Extra Strength
DOAN'S® P.M.
Magnesium Salicylate/ Diphenhydramine
Analgesic/Sleep Aid Caplets

Active Ingredients: Magnesium salicylate USP 500 mg, and Diphenhydramine HCl 25 mg. Also contains: Colloidal silicon dioxide, dibasic calcium phosphate, croscarmellose sodium, lactose, microcrystalline cellulose, magnesium stearate, stearic acid, Opadry blue color, Opadry clear.

Indications: For temporary relief of occasional minor back pain accompanied by sleeplessness.

Directions: Adults: Take 2 caplets at bedtime if needed, or as directed by a doctor.

Warnings: KEEP THIS AND ALL OTHER MEDICATIONS OUT OF THE REACH OF CHILDREN. IN CASE OF ACCIDENTAL OVERDOSE, SEEK PROFESSIONAL ASSISTANCE OR CONTACT A POISON CONTROL CENTER IMMEDIATELY. DO NOT GIVE THIS PRODUCT TO CHILDREN UNDER 12 YEARS OF AGE. As with any drug, if you are pregnant or nursing a baby, seek the advice of a health professional before using this product. If pain or sleeplessness persist continuously for more than 2 weeks, consult your doctor. Insomnia may be a symptom of a serious underlying medical illness. Do not take this product if you have asthma, glaucoma, emphysema, chronic pulmonary disease, shortness of breath, difficulty in breathing, or difficulty in urination due to enlargement of the prostate gland, or if you are allergic to aspirin or salicylates unless directed by a doctor. Avoid alcoholic beverages while taking this product. Do not take this product if you are taking sedatives or tranquilizers without first consulting your doctor. Children and teenagers should not use this medicine if chicken pox or flu symptoms exist before a doctor is consulted about Reye syndrome, a rare but serious disease.

How Supplied: Extra Strength Doan's P.M. is available in tamper resistant foil blister packages of 20 caplets. See back of blister pack and carton flap for lot number and expiration date. Store at room temperature. Protect from moisture.
NDC 0083-0245

Shown in Product Identification Section, page 407

REGULAR STRENGTH DOAN'S®
Analgesic Caplets

Indications: For temporary relief of occasional minor backache.

Directions: Adults—Two caplets every 4 hours as needed, not to exceed 12 caplets during a 24-hour period or as directed by a physician. Not intended for use by children or teenagers except under the advice of a physician. If pain persists for more than 10 days, discontinue use and consult your physician.

Warning: Children and teenagers should not use this medicine for chicken pox or flu symptoms before a doctor is consulted about Reye's syndrome, a rare but serious illness. As with any drug, if you are pregnant or nursing a baby, seek the advice of a health professional before using this product. Do not use this product if you are under medical care or are allergic to aspirin or salicylates, except under the advice and supervision of your physician. **Keep this and all medicines out of the reach of children.** In case of accidental overdose, seek professional assistance or consult a Poison Control Center immediately.

Active Ingredient: Each caplet contains Magnesium Salicylate 325 mg. **Also Contains:** Magnesium Stearate, Microcrystalline Cellulose, Opadry Olive Green, Polyethylene Glycol, Purified Water, Stearic Acid.

How Supplied: Tamper-evident blister packages of 24 and 48 caplets. Do not use if individual seals are broken.
Store at 15°–30°C (59°–86°F). Protect from moisture.

Shown in Product Identification Section, page 407

DULCOLAX®
[dul'co-lax]
brand of bisacodyl USP
Tablets of 5 mg
Suppositories of 10 mg
Laxative

Ingredients: Each enteric coated tablet contains: Active: Bisacodyl USP 5 mg. Also contains: Acacia, acetylated monoglyceride, carnauba wax, cellulose acetate phthalate, corn starch, D&C Red No. 30 aluminum lake, D&C Yellow No. 10 aluminum lake, dibutyl phthalate, docusate sodium, gelatin, glycerin, iron oxides, kaolin, lactose, magnesium stearate, methylparaben, pharmaceutical glaze, polyethylene glycol, povidone, propylparaben, sodium benzoate, sorbitan monooleate, sucrose, talc, titanium dioxide, white wax.
Each suppository contains: Active: Bisacodyl USP 10 mg. Also contains: Hydrogenated vegetable oil.
SODIUM CONTENT: Tablets and suppositories contain less than 0.2 mg per dosage unit and are thus dietetically sodium free.

Indications: For the relief of occasional constipation and irregularity. Physicians should refer to the "Professional Labeling" section for additional indications and information.

Directions:
Tablets
Adults and children 12 years of age and over: Take 2 or 3 tablets (usually 2) in a single dose once daily.
Children 6 to under 12 years of age: Take 1 tablet once daily.
Children under 6 years of age: Consult a physician.
Expect results in 8–12 hours if taken at bedtime or within 6 hours if taken before breakfast.
Suppositories
Adults and children 12 years of age and over: 1 suppository once daily. Remove foil wrapper. Lie on your side and, with pointed end first, push suppository high into the rectum so it will not slip out. Retain it for 15 to 20 minutes. If you feel the suppository must come out immediately, it was not inserted high enough and should be pushed higher.
Children 6 to under 12 years of age: ½ suppository once daily.
Children under 6 years of age: Consult a physician.
If the suppository seems soft, hold in foil wrapper under cold water for one or two minutes. In the presence of anal fissures or hemorrhoids, suppository may be coated at the tip with petroleum jelly before insertion.

Warnings: Do not use laxative products when abdominal pain, nausea, or vomiting are present unless directed by a physician. The process of restoring normal bowel function by use of a laxative may result in some abdominal discomfort. Laxative products should not be used for a period longer than 1 week unless directed by a physician. Rectal bleeding or failure to have a bowel movement after use of a laxative may indicate a serious condition. If this occurs, discontinue use and consult your physician. As with any drug, if you are pregnant or nursing a baby, seek the advice of a health care professional before using this product. KEEP THIS AND ALL MEDICATION OUT OF THE REACH OF CHILDREN. In case of accidental overdose or ingestion, seek professional assistance or contact a poison control center immediately. For tablets: Do not chew or crush. Do not give to children under 6 years of age unless directed by a physician. Do not take this product within 1 hour after taking an antacid or milk.

How Supplied: Dulcolax, brand of bisacodyl: Yellow, enteric-coated tablets of 5 mg in boxes of 10, 25, 50 and 100; suppositories of 10 mg in boxes of 4, 8, 16 and 50.
NDC 0083-6200 (tablets)
NDC 0083-6100 (suppositories)

Note: Store Dulcolax suppositories and tablets at temperatures below 77°F (25°C). Avoid excessive humidity.

Also Available: Dulcolax® Bowel Prep Kit. Each kit contains:
1 Dulcolax suppository of 10 mg bisacodyl;
4 Dulcolax tablets of 5 mg bisacodyl;
Complete patient instructions.

PROFESSIONAL LABELING:

Description and Clinical Pharmacology: Dulcolax is a contact stimulant laxative, administered either orally or rectally, which acts directly on the colonic mucosa to produce normal peristalsis throughout the large intestine. The active ingredient in Dulcolax, bisacodyl, is a colorless, tasteless compound that is practically insoluble in water or alkaline solution. Its chemical name is: bis(p-acetoxyphenyl)-2-pyridylmethane. Bisacodyl is very poorly absorbed, if at all, in the small intestine following oral administration, nor in the large intestine following rectal administration. On contact with the mucosa or submucosal plexi of the large intestine, bisacodyl stimulates sensory nerve endings to produce parasympathetic reflexes resulting in increased peristaltic contractions of the colon. It has also been shown to promote fluid and ion accumulation in the colon, which increases the laxative effect. A bowel movement is usually produced approximately 6 hours after oral administration (8–12 hours if taken at bedtime), and approximately 15 minutes to 1 hour after rectal administration, providing satisfactory cleansing of the bowel which may, under certain circumstances, obviate the need for colonic irrigation.

Indications and Usage: For use as part of a bowel cleansing regimen in preparing the patient for surgery or for preparing the colon for x-ray endoscopic examination. Dulcolax will not replace the colonic irrigations usually given patients before intracolonic surgery, but is useful in the preliminary emptying of the colon prior to these procedures.
Also for use as a laxative in postoperative care (i.e., restoration of normal bowel hygiene), antepartum care, postpartum care, and in preparation for delivery.

Contraindications: Stimulant laxatives, such as Dulcolax, are contraindicated for patients with acute surgical abdomen, appendicitis, rectal bleeding, or intestinal obstruction.

Continued on next page

The full prescribing information for each CIBA Consumer Pharmaceuticals product is contained herein and is that in effect as of December 15, 1992

CIBA Consumer—Cont.

Precautions: Long-term administration of Dulcolax is not recommended in the treatment of chronic constipation.

Dosage and Administration:
Preparation for x-ray endoscopy: For barium enemas, no food should be given following oral administration to prevent reaccumulation of material in the cecum, and a suppository should be administered one to two hours prior to examination.
Children under 6 years of age: Oral administration is not recommended due to the requirement to swallow tablets whole. For rectal administration, the suppository dosage is 5 mg (½ of 10 mg suppository) in a single daily dose.

Shown in Product Identification Section, page 407

EUCALYPTAMINT®
Arthritis Pain Reliever
100% All Natural Ointment
External Analgesic

Description: An all-natural, deep-penetrating topical analgesic that provides hours of soothing relief.

Active Ingredient: Natural Menthol (15%)

Inactive Ingredients: Lanolin and Eucalyptus Oil

Indications: For the temporary relief of minor aches and pains of muscles and joints associated with arthritis, backache, strains, bruises, and sprains.

Directions: Adults and children 2 years of age and older: Gently massage a conservative amount into affected area not more than 3 to 4 times daily.
Children under 2 years of age: Consult a physician.

Warning: FOR EXTERNAL USE ONLY. Avoid contact with eyes. Do not apply to wounds or damaged skin. Do not bandage tightly. Do not use with heating pads or heating devices. If condition worsens, or if symptoms persist for more than 7 days, discontinue use of this product and consult a physician. Keep this and all drugs out of the reach of children. In case of accidental ingestion, seek professional assistance or contact a Poison Control Center immediately.

How Supplied: Eucalyptamint Ointment is supplied in 2 oz. and 4 oz. bottles.

Shown in Product Identification Section, page 407

EUCALYPTAMINT®
Muscle Pain Relief Formula
External Analgesic

Description: A uniquely scented gel creme formulation providing hours of effective pain relief for overworked muscles.

Active Ingredient: Menthol 8%

Other Ingredients: Carbomer 980, Eucalyptus Oil, Fragrance, Propylene Glycol, SD 3A Alcohol, Triethanolamine, TWEEN 80, Water.

Indications: For the temporary relief of minor aches and pains of muscles associated with simple backache, strains, sprains and sports injuries.

Directions: Adults and children 2 years of age and older: Gently massage a conservative amount into affected area not more than 3 to 4 times daily. Children under 2 years of age: Consult a physician.

Warning: FOR EXTERNAL USE ONLY. Avoid contact with eyes. Do not apply to wounds or damaged skin. Do not bandage tightly. Do not use with heating pads or heating devices. If condition worsens, or if symptoms persist for more than 7 days, discontinue use of this product and consult a physician. Keep this and all drugs out of the reach of children. In case of accidental ingestion, seek professional assistance or contact a Poison Control Center immediately. Store at room temperature 15°–30°C (59°–86°F). DO NOT FREEZE.

How Supplied: Eucalyptamint Muscle Pain Relief Formula is supplied in 2.25 oz. bottles and is available in two scents: Alpine Breeze and Powder Fresh.

Shown in Product Identification Section, page 407

FIBERALL® Chewable Tablets
[fi 'ber-all]
Lemon Creme Flavor

Description: Fiberall Chewable Tablets are a bulk-forming, nonirritant laxative which contain less than 1.5 grams of sugar per tablet. The active ingredient is calcium polycarbophil, a bulk-forming man-made fiber. The smooth gelatinous bulk formed by Fiberall Chewable Tablets encourages peristaltic activity and a more normal elimination of the bowel contents.
The recommended dose of one tablet contains the equivalent to 1 gram of polycarbophil.
Inactive Ingredients: Crospovidone, dextrose, flavors, magnesium stearate and yellow No. 10 aluminum lake. Each dose contains less than 1 mg of sodium, 225 mg of calcium and less than 6 calories.

Indications: Fiberall Chewable Tablets are indicated for the management of chronic constipation, temporary constipation caused by illness or pregnancy, irritable bowel syndrome, and for constipation related to duodenal ulcer or diverticulosis. Fiberall Chewable Tablets are also indicated for stool softening in patients with hemorrhoids or after anorectal surgery.

Actions: After the tablet is chewed it readily disperses and acts without irritants or stimulants. Polycarbophil absorbs water in the gastrointestinal tract to form a gelatinous bulk which encourages a more normal bowel movement.

Dosage and Administration: *Adults and children 12 years and older:* chew and swallow 1 tablet, 1–4 times a day. *Children 6 to under 12 years:* one-half the usual adult dose or as recommended by a physician. *Children under 6:* consult a physician. **Drink a full glass (8 fl oz) of liquid with each dose.** Drinking additional liquid helps Fiberall work even more effectively. Continued use for 2 to 3 days may be desired for maximum laxative benefits.

Contraindications: Fecal impaction or intestinal obstruction. Any disease state in which consumption of extra calcium is contraindicated.

Drug Interactions: This product contains calcium, which may interact with some forms of TETRACYCLINE if taken concomitantly. The tetracycline product should be taken 1 hour before or 2–3 hours after taking a Fiberall Chewable Tablet.

How Supplied: Boxes containing 18 tablets.

FIBERALL® Fiber Wafers
[fi 'ber-all]
Fruit & Nut, Oatmeal Raisin

Description: Fiberall Fiber Wafers are a bulk-forming, nonirritant laxative. The active ingredient is psyllium hydrophilic mucilloid, a dietary fiber extracted from the seed husk of blond psyllium seed *(Plantago ovata)*. The smooth gelatinous bulk formed by Fiberall Wafers encourages peristaltic activity and a more normal elimination of the bowel contents.
One (1) Fiberall Fiber Wafer contains 3.4 g of psyllium hydrophilic mucilloid in a good-tasting wafer form, of which approximately 2.2 g is soluble fiber. One wafer is equivalent to one teaspoonful of Fiberall Powder.
Inactive Ingredients: Fruit & Nut Flavor: Baking powder, brown sugar, butter flavor, cinnamon, corn syrup, crisp rice, dried ground apricots, flour, glycerin, granulated sugar, granulated walnuts, lecithin, margarine, molasses, oats, salt, vegetable oil shortening (soybean and cottonseed oil), water and wheat bran. Fiberall Fruit & Nut Fiber Wafers contain approximately 79 calories and 110 mg of sodium per wafer.
Oatmeal Raisin Flavor: Baking powder, cinnamon, cinnamon flavor, cloves, corn syrup, flour, glycerin, granulated sugar, lecithin, molasses, oats, raisins, vegetable oil shortening (soybean and cottonseed oil), water and wheat bran. Fiberall Oatmeal Raisin Fiber Wafers contain approximately 78 calories and 30 mg of sodium per wafer.

Indications: Fiberall Fiber Wafers are indicated for the management of chronic constipation, temporary constipation caused by illness or pregnancy, irritable bowel syndrome, and for constipation related to duodenal ulcer or diverticulosis. Fiberall Wafers are also indicated for stool softening in patients with hemorrhoids or after anorectal surgery.

Actions: The homogenous high-fiber formula of Fiberall Fiber Wafers, eaten with 8 oz of a beverage of the patient's choice, acts without irritants or stimulants in the gastrointestinal tract.

Dosage and Administration: The recommended dosage for adults is one to two Fiberall Fiber Wafers 1 to 3 times daily, with a full 8 oz glass of water or other liquid with each wafer. The recommended daily dose for children 6 to under 12 years old is one-half the usual adult dose (with liquid), or as recommended by a physician. For children under 6, consult a physician. Drinking additional liquid is recommended and helps Fiberall work even more effectively. Two to three days' usage may be required for optimal laxative benefits.

Contraindications: Fecal impaction or intestinal obstruction.

Precaution: As with any grain product, inhaled or ingested psyllium powder may cause an allergic reaction in individuals sensitive to it.

How Supplied: Boxes containing 14 wafers.

Shown in Product Identification Section, page 407

FIBERALL® Powder, Orange or Natural Flavor
[fi 'ber-all]

Description: Fiberall is a bulk-forming, nonirritant laxative which contains no sugar. The active ingredient is psyllium hydrophilic mucilloid, a dietary fiber extracted from the seed husk of blond psyllium seed *(Plantago ovata)*. The smooth gelatinous bulk formed by Fiberall encourages peristaltic activity and a more normal elimination of the bowel contents.
The recommended dose contains 3.4 g psyllium hydrophilic mucilloid, of which approximately 2.2 g is soluble fiber.

Inactive Ingredients: Natural Flavor: Citric acid, flavor, polysorbate 60 and wheat bran. Orange Flavor: Beta-carotene, citric acid, flavor, polysorbate 60, saccharin, wheat bran and yellow No. 6 lake. Each dose contains less than 10 mg of sodium, less than 60 mg of potassium, and provides less than 6 calories (10 calories for Orange).

Indications: Fiberall is indicated for the management of chronic constipation, temporary constipation caused by illness or pregnancy, irritable bowel syndrome, and for constipation related to duodenal ulcer or diverticulosis. Fiberall is also indicated for stool softening in patients with hemorrhoids or after anorectal surgery.

Actions: The homogenous, high-fiber formula of Fiberall is readily dispersed in liquids and acts without irritants or stimulants in the gastro-intestinal tract.

Dosage and Administration:
Adults: Natural: Place one scoopful filled to the line (5 g) or one slightly rounded teaspoonful in a glass and add 8 oz. of cool water or other liquid. Stir to mix. Orange: Place one level scoopful (5.9 g) or one rounded teaspoonful in glass and add liquid as above. Take orally one to three times daily according to individual response.
Children 6 to under 12 years old: One-half the usual adult dose (with liquid) or as recommended by a physician. Drinking additional liquid is recommended and helps Fiberall work even more effectively. Two to three days' usage may be required for maximum laxative benefits.
New Users: Start by taking 1 dose each day. Gradually increase to 3 doses per day if needed or recommended by doctor. If minor gas or bloating occurs, reduce the amount taken until system adjusts.

Contraindications: Fecal impaction or intestinal obstruction.

Precaution: As with any grain product, inhaled or ingested psyllium powder may cause an allergic reaction in individuals sensitive to it.

How Supplied: Powder, in 10 or 15 oz containers.

Shown in Product Identification Section, page 407

NŌSTRIL® Nasal Decongestant
[nō 'stril]
phenylephrine HCl, USP

Active Ingredient: phenylephrine HCl 0.25% (¼% Mild strength) or phenylephrine HCl 0.5% (½% Regular strength). Also contains benzalkonium chloride 0.004% as a preservative, boric acid, sodium borate, water.

Indications: For temporary relief of nasal congestion due to the common cold, hay fever, other upper respiratory allergies, or associated with sinusitis.

Actions: NŌSTRIL metered pump spray for nasal decongestion delivers measured, uniform doses. The medication constricts the smaller arterioles of the nasal passages, producing a gentle, predictable, decongestant effect. Nōstril penetrates and shrinks swollen membranes, restoring freer breathing and unclogs sinus passages, bringing the effective medication in contact with inflamed, swollen tissues. It will not hurt tender membranes since it is formulated to match the pH of normal nasal secretions. The one-way pump helps prevent draw-back contamination of the medication.

Warnings: Do not exceed recommended dosage because burning, stinging, sneezing, or increased nasal discharge may occur. Do not use for more than 3 days. If symptoms persist, consult a physician. Use of the dispenser by more than one person may spread infection. Do not use this product if you have heart disease, high blood pressure, thyroid disease, diabetes or difficulty in urination due to enlargement of the prostate gland, unless directed by a physician. Keep this and all drugs out of reach of children.

Symptoms and Treatment of Oral Overdosage: In case of accidental ingestion, seek professional assistance or consult a poison control center immediately.

Dosage and Administration:
¼% Mild—Adults and children 6 to under 12 years of age (with adult supervision): 2 or 3 sprays in each nostril not more often than every 4 hours. Children under 6 years of age: consult a doctor.
½% Regular—Adults: 2 or 3 sprays in each nostril not more often than every 4 hours. Do not give to children under 12 years of age unless directed by a doctor.
Remove protective cap. Hold bottle with thumb at base and nozzle between first and second fingers. With head upright, insert nozzle into nostril. Depress pump 2 or 3 times, all the way down, and sniff deeply. Repeat in other nostril. Before using the first time, prime pump by depressing it firmly several times.

How Supplied: Metered nasal pump spray in white plastic bottles of ½ fl. oz. (15 ml) packaged in tamper-resistant outer cartons.
0.25% (¼% Mild strength) for children 6 years and over and adults who prefer a milder decongestant (NDC 0083-7200-52).
0.5% (½% Regular strength) for adults and children 12 years or older (NDC 0083-7100-52).

Shown in Product Identification Section, page 408

NŌSTRILLA® Long Acting
[nō-stril 'a]
Nasal Decongestant
oxymetazoline HCl, USP

Active Ingredient: oxymetazoline HCl 0.05%. Also contains benzalkonium chloride 0.02% as a preservative, glycine, sorbitol solution, water. (Mercury preservatives are not used in this product.)

Indications: For temporary relief of nasal congestion due to the common cold, hay fever, other upper respiratory allergies, or associated with sinusitis.

Actions: NŌSTRILLA metered pump spray for nasal decongestion delivers measured, uniform doses. The medica-

Continued on next page

The full prescribing information for each CIBA Consumer Pharmaceuticals product is contained herein and is that in effect as of December 15, 1992

CIBA Consumer—Cont.

tion constricts the smaller arterioles of the nasal passages, producing a prolonged (up to 12 hours), gentle, predictable, decongestant effect. Nōstrilla penetrates and shrinks swollen membranes, restoring freer breathing and unclogs sinus passages, bringing the effective medication in contact with inflamed, swollen tissues. It will not hurt tender membranes since it is formulated to match the pH of normal nasal secretions. Use at bedtime restores freer nasal breathing through the night. The one-way pump helps prevent draw-back contamination of the medication.

Warnings: Do not exceed recommended dosage because burning, stinging, sneezing or increased nasal discharge may occur. Do not use for more than 3 days. If symptoms persist, consult a physician. Use of the dispenser by more than one person may spread infection. Do not use this product if you have heart disease, high blood pressure, thyroid disease, diabetes or difficulty in urination due to enlargement of the prostate gland unless directed by a doctor. Keep this and all drugs out of reach of children.

Symptoms and Treatment of Oral Overdosage: In case of accidental ingestion, seek professional assistance or contact a poison control center immediately.

Dosage and Administration: Adults and children 6 to under 12 years of age (with adult supervision): 2 or 3 sprays in each nostril not more often than every 10 to 12 hours. Do not exceed 2 applications in any 24-hour period. Children under 6 years of age: consult a doctor.
Remove protective cap. Hold bottle with thumb at base and nozzle between first and second fingers. With head upright, insert nozzle into nostril. Depress pump 2 or 3 times, all the way down, and sniff deeply. Repeat in other nostril. Before using the first time, prime pump by depressing it firmly several times.

How Supplied: Metered nasal pump spray in white plastic bottles of ½ fl. oz. (15 ml) packaged in tamper-resistant outer cartons (NDC 0083-7300-52).

Shown in Product Identification Section, page 408

NUPERCAINAL®
Dibucaine Hemorrhoidal and Anesthetic Ointment

Active Ingredient: 1% dibucaine USP.
Also contains: acetone sodium bisulfite, lanolin, light mineral oil, purified water, and white petrolatum.

Indications: For prompt, temporary relief of pain, itching and burning due to hemorrhoids or other anorectal disorders. May also be used topically for temporary relief of pain and itching associated with sunburn, minor burns, cuts, scrapes, insect bites, or minor skin irritation.

Directions: Adults: When practical, cleanse the affected area with mild soap and water and rinse thoroughly. Gently dry by patting or blotting with toilet tissue or a soft cloth before application of this product. Puncture tube seal with cap or sharp object. Apply externally to the affected area up to 3 or 4 times daily. Children 2–12: Do not use except under the advice and supervision of a physician. DO NOT USE IN INFANTS UNDER 2 YEARS OF AGE OR LESS THAN 35 LBS. WEIGHT.

Warnings: IF SWALLOWED, CONSULT A PHYSICIAN OR POISON CONTROL CENTER IMMEDIATELY. **Do not use in or near the eyes.** If condition worsens or does not improve within 7 days, consult a physician. Do not put this product into the rectum by using fingers or any mechanical device. Do not exceed recommended daily dosage unless directed by a physician. Certain persons can develop allergic reactions to ingredients in this product. If the symptom being treated does not subside or if redness, irritation, swelling, pain, bleeding or other symptoms develop or increase, discontinue use and consult a physician promptly. As with any drug, if you are pregnant or nursing a baby, seek the advice of a health care professional before using this product. KEEP THIS AND ALL MEDICATION OUT OF REACH OF CHILDREN.

How Supplied: Nupercainal Hemorrhoidal and Anesthetic Ointment is available in tamper-evident packaged tubes of 1 and 2 ounces. See crimp of tube for lot number and expiration date. Store between 59–86°.
NDC 0083-5812.

Shown in Product Identification Section, page 408

NUPERCAINAL®
Pain Relief Cream

Active Ingredient: 0.5% dibucaine USP.
Also contains: acetone sodium bisulfite, fragrance, glycerin, potassium hydroxide, purified water, stearic acid, and trolamine.

Indications: For prompt, temporary relief of pain and itching due to sunburn, minor burns, cuts, scrapes, scratches, and nonpoisonous insect bites.

Directions: Puncture tube seal with cap or sharp object. Apply to affected area, rub in gently. **Do not use in or near eyes.**

Caution: IF SWALLOWED, CONSULT A PHYSICIAN OR POISON CONTROL CENTER IMMEDIATELY. Not for prolonged use. Not more than ⅔ tube should be applied in 24 hours for adults or ⅙ tube to a child. If the symptom being treated does not subside or rash, irritation, swelling, pain, or other symptoms develop or increase, discontinue use and consult a physician.

How Supplied: Nupercainal Pain-Relief Cream is available in tamper-evident packaged tubes of 1½ ounces. See crimp of tube for lot number and expiration date. NDC 0083-5830-91.

Shown in Product Identification Section, page 408

NUPERCAINAL®
Suppositories

Indications: Nupercainal Rectal Suppositories give temporary relief of itching, burning, and discomfort associated with hemorrhoids or other anorectal disorders.
Each suppository contains 2.1 grams cocoa butter, NF and .25 gram zinc oxide. Also contains acetone sodium bisulfite and bismuth subgallate.

Directions: ADULTS—When practical, cleanse the affected area. Tear one suppository at the "V" cut, peel foil downward and remove foil wrapper before inserting into the rectum. Gently insert the suppository rectally, rounded end first. Use one suppository up to 6 times daily or after each bowel movement. CHILDREN UNDER 12 YEARS OF AGE—Consult a physician.

WARNING: IF ACCIDENTALLY SWALLOWED, CONSULT A PHYSICIAN OR POISON CONTROL CENTER IMMEDIATELY.
If condition worsens or does not improve within 7 days, consult a physician. Do not exceed the recommended daily dosage unless directed by a physician. In case of bleeding consult a physician promptly. As with any drug, if you are pregnant or nursing a baby, seek the advice of a health professional before using this product.
Keep this and all medications out of reach of children.
Nupercainal Suppositories are available in tamper-evident packages of 12 and 24. Do not store above 86 °F.

C86-42 (Rev. 9/86)

Shown in Product Identification Section, page 408

OTRIVIN®
xylometazoline hydrochloride USP Nasal Spray and Nasal Drops 0.1% Pediatric Nasal Drops 0.05% Nasal Decongestant

One application provides rapid and long-lasting relief of nasal congestion for up to 10 hours.
Quickly clears stuffy noses due to common cold, sinusitis, hay fever.
Nasal congestion can make life miserable—you can't breathe, smell, taste, or sleep comfortably. That is why Otrivin is so helpful. It clears away that stuffy feeling.
Otrivin has been prescribed by doctors for many years. Here is how you use it:

Nasal Spray 0.1%—for adults and children 12 years and older. Spray 2 or 3 times into each nostril every 8–10 hours. With head upright, squeeze sharply and firmly while inhaling (sniffing) through the nose. For adult use only.

Nasal Drops 0.1%—for adults and children 12 years and older. Put 2 or 3 drops into each nostril every 8 to 10 hours. Tilt head as far back as possible. Immediately bend head forward toward knees, hold for a few seconds, then return to upright position.

Do not give Nasal Spray 0.1% or Nasal Drops 0.1% to children under 12 years except under the advice and supervision of a physician.

Pediatric Nasal Drops 0.05%—for children 2 to 12 years of age. Put 2 or 3 drops into each nostril every 8 to 10 hours. Tilt head as far back as possible. Immediately bend head forward toward knees, hold a few seconds, then return to upright position.

Do not give this product to children under 2 years except under the advice and supervision of a physician.

Otrivin Nasal Spray/Nasal Drops contain 0.1% xylometazoline hydrochloride, USP. Also contains benzalkonium chloride, dibasic sodium phosphate, disodium edetate, monobasic sodium phosphate, purified water and sodium chloride. They are available in an unbreakable plastic spray package of 0.66 fl oz (20 ml) and in a plastic dropper bottle of 0.83 fl oz (25 ml).

Otrivin Pediatric Nasal Drops contain 0.05% xylometazoline hydrochloride, USP. Also contains benzalkonium chloride, dibasic sodium phosphate, disodium edetate, monobasic sodium phosphate, purified water and sodium chloride. It is available in a plastic dropper bottle of 0.83 fl oz (25 ml).

Warnings: Do not exceed recommended dosage, because symptoms such as burning, stinging, sneezing, or increase of nasal discharge may occur. Do not use this product for more than 3 days. If symptoms persist, consult a physician. The use of this dispenser by more than one person may cause infection.

Keep this and all medicines out of the reach of children. Overdosage in young children may cause marked sedation. In case of accidental ingestion, seek professional assistance or contact a Poison Control Center immediately.

Caution: Do not use if the clear overwrap with the name Otrivin® or the printed band on the bottle is missing or damaged.
Store between 59°–86°F.

Shown in Product Identification Section, page 408

PRIVINE®
naphazoline hydrochloride, USP 0.05% Nasal Solution 0.05% Nasal Spray Nasal Decongestant

Privine is a nasal decongestant that comes in three forms: Nasal Drops (in a bottle with a dropper), Nasal Spray (in a plastic squeeze bottle) and Nasal Solution (in a 16 fl oz bottle). All are for prompt, and prolonged relief of nasal congestion due to common colds, sinusitis, hay fever, etc.
Privine is an effective nasal decongestant **when you use it in the recommended dosage.** If you use too much, too long, or too often, Privine may be harmful to your nasal mucous membranes and cause burning, stinging, sneezing or an increased runny nose.
Do not use Privine by mouth.

IF NASAL STUFFINESS PERSISTS AFTER 3 DAYS OF TREATMENT, DISCONTINUE USE AND CONSULT A DOCTOR.
Keep this and all medications out of the reach of children. Do not use Privine in children under 12 years of age, except with the advice and supervision of a doctor.

Caution: Do not use Privine if you have glaucoma.

OVERDOSAGE IN YOUNG CHILDREN MAY CAUSE MARKED SEDATION AND IF SEVERE, EMERGENCY TREATMENT MAY BE NECESSARY. IN CASE OF ACCIDENTAL INGESTION, SEEK PROFESSIONAL ASSISTANCE OR CONTACT A POISON CONTROL CENTER IMMEDIATELY.

How to use Nasal Drops.
Use only 1 to 2 drops in each nostril. Do not repeat this dosage more than every 6 hours. Squeeze rubber bulb to fill dropper with proper amount of medication. For best results, tilt head as far back as possible and put 1 to 2 drops of solution into your right nostril. Then lean head forward, inhaling and turning your head to the left. Refill dropper by squeezing bulb. Now tilt head as far back as possible and put 1 to 2 drops of solution into your left nostril. Then lean head forward, inhaling, and turning your head to the right.
The Privine dropper bottle is designed to make administration of the proper dosage easy. Privine will not cause sleeplessness, so you may use it before going to bed.

Important: After use, be sure to rinse the dropper with very hot water. This helps prevent contamination of the bottle with bacteria from nasal secretions. Use of the dispenser by more than one person may spread infection.

Note: Privine Nasal Solution may be used on contact with glass, plastic, stainless steel and specially treated metals used in atomizers. Do not let the solution come in contact with reactive metals, especially aluminum. If solution becomes discolored, it should be discarded.

How to use Nasal Spray.
Spray 1 or 2 times in each nostril, not more often than every 6 hours. Avoid overdosage. Follow directions for use carefully. For best results do **not** shake the plastic squeeze bottle.
Remove cap. With head held upright, spray twice into each nostril. Squeeze the bottle sharply and firmly while sniffing through the nose.
Privine Nasal Drops contain 0.05% naphazoline HCl, USP. It also contains benzalkonium chloride, dibasic sodium phosphate, disodium edetate, monobasic sodium phosphate, purified water and sodium chloride.
Privine Nasal Solution contains 0.05% naphazoline hydrochloride, USP. It also contains benzalkonium chloride, disodium edetate dihydrate, hydrochloric acid, purified water, sodium chloride, and trolamine. It is available in bottles of 16 fl. oz. (473 ml).
Privine Nasal Spray contains 0.05% naphazoline hydrochloride USP. It also contains benzalkonium chloride, dibasic sodium phosphate, disodium edetate, monobasic sodium phosphate, purified water, and sodium chloride. It is available in plastic squeeze bottles of 0.66 fl oz (20 ml).

Caution: Do not use if the clear overwrap on the box with the name Privine® or the printed band on the bottle is missing or damaged.
Store the nasal drops, nasal solution and nasal spray between 59°–86°F.

Shown in Product Identification Section, page 408

Q-VEL®
Muscle Relaxant/Pain Reliever

Active Ingredient: Quinine Sulfate 1 gr. (64.8 mg).

Contains: Vitamin E (400 I.U. *dl*-alpha tocopheryl acetate) in a lecithin base.

Indications: For prevention and temporary relief of night leg cramps.

Warnings: Do not take if pregnant or nursing a baby. Q-Vel is also not indicated for those sensitive to quinine or under 12 years of age. Discontinue use and consult your physician if ringing in the ears, deafness, diarrhea, nausea, skin rash, bruising or visual disturbances occur. In case of accidental overdose, seek medical assistance or contact Poison Control Center at once. Keep this and all medicine out of reach of children.

Dosage: To prevent night leg cramps take 2 soft caplets after the evening meal plus 2 at bedtime. For relief in case of

Continued on next page

The full prescribing information for each CIBA Consumer Pharmaceuticals product is contained herein and is that in effect as of December 15, 1992

CIBA Consumer—Cont.

sudden attack, take 2 soft caplets at once plus 2 after ½ hour if needed. Do not exceed 4 soft caplets daily.

How Supplied: Bottles of 16, 30, 50 and 100 softgels.
Store at 15°–30°C (59°–86°F) and protect from moisture.

Shown in Product Identification Section, page 408

SLOW FE®
Slow Release Iron Tablets

Description: SLOW FE supplies ferrous sulfate for the treatment of iron deficiency and iron deficiency anemia with a significant reduction in the incidence of the common side effects of oral iron preparations. The wax matrix delivery system of SLOW FE is designed to maximize the release of ferrous sulfate in the duodenum and the jejunum where it is best tolerated and absorbed. SLOW FE has been clinically shown to be associated with a lower incidence of constipation, diarrhea and abdominal discomfort when compared to regular iron tablets and the leading capsule.

Formula: Each tablet contains 160 mg. dried ferrous sulfate USP, equivalent to 50 mg. elemental iron. Also contains cetostearyl alcohol, colloidal silicon dioxide, hydroxypropyl methylcellulose, shellac, lactose, magnesium stearate, polyethylene glycol.

Dosage: ADULTS—one or two tablets daily or as recommended by a physician. A maximum of four tablets daily may be taken. CHILDREN—one tablet daily. Tablets must be swallowed whole.

Warning: The treatment of any anemic condition should be on the advice and under the supervision of a physician. As oral iron products interfere with absorption of oral tetracycline antibiotics, these products should not be taken within two hours of each other. As with any drug, if you are pregnant or nursing a baby, seek the advice of a health professional before using this product.

Keep this and all medicines out of reach of children. In case of accidental overdose, contact your physician or poison control center immediately.
Tamper-Evident Packaging.

How Supplied: Blister packages of 30, 60 and bottles of 100. Do Not Store Above 86°F. Protect From Moisture.

Shown in Product Identification Section, page 408

SUNKIST CHILDREN'S CHEWABLE MULTIVITAMINS—REGULAR

Vitamin Ingredients: Each tablet contains:
[See table above.]

VITAMINS	QUANTITY PER TABLET	PERCENT U.S. RDA FOR CHILD. 2 TO 4 YRS OF AGE (1 TABLET)	PERCENT U.S. RDA FOR ADULTS & CHILD. OVER 4 YRS OF AGE (1 TABLET)
Vitamin A (as Palmitate + Beta Carotene)	2500 IU	100	50
Vitamin D-3	400 IU	100	100
Vitamin E	15 IU	150	50
Vitamin C	60 mg	150	100
Folic Acid	0.3 mg	150	75
Niacinamide	13.5 mg	150	68
Vitamin B-6	1.05 mg	150	53
Vitamin B-12	4.5 mcg	150	75
Vitamin B-1	1.05 mg	150	70
Vitamin B-2	1.20 mg	150	71
Vitamin K-1	5 mcg	*	*

*Recognized as essential in human nutrition, but no U.S. RDA established.

Indication: Dietary supplementation.

Dosage and Administration: One chewable tablet daily for children two years and older.

Warning: Phenylketonurics: Contains Phenylalanine

How Supplied: SUNKIST Children's Multivitamins-Regular are supplied in bottles of 60 chewable tablets with child resistant caps.
SUNKIST® is a registered trademark of SUNKIST Growers, Inc., Sherman Oaks, CA 91423. ©

Shown in Product Identification Section, page 408

SUNKIST CHILDREN'S CHEWABLE MULTIVITAMINS—PLUS EXTRA C

Vitamin Ingredients: Each tablet contains the ingredients of the Regular vitamin product plus extra Vitamin C (a total of 250 mg).

Indication: Dietary supplementation.

Dosage and Administration: One chewable tablet daily for adults and children two years and older.

Warning: Phenylketonurics: Contains Phenylalanine.

How Supplied: SUNKIST Children's Multivitamins Plus Extra C are supplied in bottles of 60 chewable tablets with child resistant caps.
Sunkist® is a registered trademark of Sunkist Growers, Inc., Sherman Oaks, CA 91423.©

Shown in Product Identification Section, page 408

SUNKIST CHILDREN'S CHEWABLE MULTIVITAMINS—PLUS IRON

Vitamin Ingredients: Each tablet contains the vitamins of the Regular product plus 15 mg of Iron.

Indication: Dietary supplementation.

Dosage and Administration: One chewable tablet daily for children two years and older.

Warning: Phenylketonurics: Contains Phenylalanine.

Precaution: Contains iron, which can be harmful in large doses. Close tightly and keep out of reach of children. In case of overdose, contact a physician or poison control center immediately.

How Supplied: SUNKIST Children's Multivitamins Plus Iron are supplied in bottles of 60 chewable tablets with child resistant caps.
Sunkist® is a registered trademark of Sunkist Growers, Inc., Sherman Oaks, CA 91423.©

Shown in Product Identification Section, page 408

SUNKIST CHILDREN'S CHEWABLE MULTIVITAMINS—COMPLETE

Vitamin Ingredients: Each tablet contains the following ingredients:
[See table bottom of next page.]

Indication: Dietary supplementation.

Dosage and Administration: Children ages 2 to 4 one-half chewable tablet daily; One chewable tablet daily for children four years and older.

Warning: Phenylketonurics: Contains Phenylalanine.

Precautions: Contains iron, which can be harmful in large doses. Close tightly and keep out of reach of children. In case of overdose, contact a physician or poison control center immediately.

How Supplied: SUNKIST Children's Multivitamins Complete are supplied in bottles of 60 chewable tablets with child resistant caps.
Sunkist® is a registered trademark of Sunkist Growers, Inc., Sherman Oaks, CA 91423.©

Shown in Product Identification Section, page 408

SUNKIST® VITAMIN C
Citrus Complex
Chewable Tablets
Easy to Swallow Caplets

Description: All Sunkist Vitamin C chewable tablets have a delicious orange flavor unlike any other Vitamin C tablet. Each 60 mg chewable tablet contains 100% of the U.S. RDA* of Vitamin C. Each 250 mg chewable tablet contains 417% of the U.S. RDA* of Vitamin C. Each 500 mg chewable tablet contains 833% of the U.S. RDA* of Vitamin C.

Each 500 mg easy to swallow caplet contains 833% of the U.S. RDA* of Vitamin C.

Sunkist Vitamin C chewable tablets and easy to swallow caplets do not contain artificial flavors, colors or preservatives.

Indication: Dietary supplement.

How Supplied: 60 mg Chewable Tablets—Rolls of 11.
250 mg and 500 mg Chewable Tablets—Bottles of 60.
500 mg Easy to Swallow Caplets—Bottles of 60.

Sunkist® is a registered trademark of Sunkist Growers, Inc., Sherman Oaks, CA 91423.©

*U.S. Recommended Daily Allowance for adults and children over 4 years of age.

Shown in Product Identification Section, page 408

Age	Initial Dose	Maximum Dose per 24 hours
Adults and children over 12 years	4 tsp or 4 Tablets	12 tsp or 12 Tablets
Children 6–12 years	2 tsp or 2 Tablets	6 tsp or 6 Tablets
Children 3–6 years	1 tsp or 1 Tablet	3 tsp or 3 Tablets
Infants and children under 3 years	Only as directed by a physician	

Columbia Laboratories, Inc.
4000 HOLLYWOOD BLVD.
HOLLYWOOD, FL 33021

DIASORB®
[*dī 'ă-zorb*]
Activated Nonfibrous Attapulgite
Liquid and Tablets

Description: Diasorb relieves cramps and pain associated with diarrhea. It is available as a pleasant-tasting cola-flavored liquid and as easy-to-swallow tablets. Diasorb is safe for children.

Active Ingredient: Each liquid teaspoonful and tablet contains 750 mg activated nonfibrous attapulgite.

Inactive Ingredients: *Liquid*—Benzoic acid, citric acid, flavor, glycerin, magnesium aluminum silicate, methylparaben, polysorbate, propylene glycol, propylparaben, saccharin, sodium hypochlorite solution, sorbitol, xanthan gum, and water. *Tablet*—D&C Red No. 30 Al Lake, Gelatin, Hydroxypropyl Cellulose, Hydroxypropyl Methylcellulose, Magnesium Stearate, Pharmaceutical Shellac, Polyethylene Glycol, Povidone, Propylene Glycol, Sorbitol, Titanium Dioxide, and Water.

Directions for Use: Take the full recommended starting dose at the first sign of diarrhea, and repeat after each subsequent bowel movement. Do not exceed maximum recommended dose per day. Shake liquid well before using.
Swallow tablets with water. Do not chew.

Caution: Do not use if foil seal around tablet is broken.

Warning: Do not use for more than 2 days or in the presence of fever or in infants or children under 3, unless directed by a physician. In case of accidental overdose, seek professional assistance or contact a poison control center immediately.
Store at room temperature (59° to 86° F) in a dry place.
KEEP THIS AND ALL MEDICATIONS OUT OF THE REACH OF CHILDREN.

Dosage: See Table for recommended dosage for acute diarrhea.
[See table above.]

How Supplied: *Liquid*—In plastic bottles of 4 fl oz (120 mL).
Tablets—Packaged in blister packs of 24.

Shown in Product Identification Section, page 408

VITAMINS	QUANTITY PER TABLET	PERCENT U.S. RDA FOR CHILD. 2 TO 4 YRS OF AGE (½ TABLET)	PERCENT U.S. RDA FOR ADULTS & CHILD. OVER 4 YRS OF AGE (1 TABLET)
Vitamin A (as Palmitate + Beta Carotene)	5000 IU	100	100
Vitamin D-3	400 IU	50	100
Vitamin E	30 IU	150	100
Vitamin C	60 mg	75	100
Folic Acid	0.4 mg	100	100
Biotin	40 mcg	13	13
Pantothenic Acid	10 mg	100	100
Niacinamide	20 mg	111	100
Vitamin B-6	2 mg	143	100
Vitamin B-12	6 mcg	100	100
Vitamin B-1	1.5 mg	107	100
Vitamin B-2	1.7 mg	106	100
Vitamin K-1	10 mcg	*	*
MINERALS			
Iron	18 mg	90	100
Magnesium	20 mg	5	5
Iodine	150 mcg	107	100
Zinc	10 mg	63	67
Manganese	1 mg	*	*
Calcium	100 mg	6	10
Phosphorus	78 mg	5	8
Copper	2 mg	100	100

*Recognized as essential in human nutrition, but no U.S. RDA established.

LEGATRIN®
[*leg'a-trin*]

Active Ingredient: Quinine Sulfate, 162.5 mg per tablet.

Other Ingredients: Calcium phosphate dibasic, cellulose, croscarmellose sodium, FD&C blue No. 2 aluminum lake, FD&C red No. 40 aluminum lake, gelatin, hydroxypropyl cellulose, hydroxypropyl methylcellulose, magnesium stearate, polyethylene glycol 400, silica, starch, stearic acid, titanium dioxide.

Indications: For relief of night leg cramps, muscle spasms, restless legs.

Warnings: Discontinue use and consult a physician immediately if swelling,

Continued on next page

Columbia—Cont.

bruising, skin rash, skin discoloration or bleeding occurs. These symptoms may indicate a serious condition. Discontinue use if ringing in the ears, deafness, diarrhea, nausea or visual disturbances occur. In case of accidental overdose, seek medical assistance or contact Poison Control Center immediately. Do not take if pregnant, nursing a baby, allergic or sensitive to quinine or under 12 years of age. Keep this and all medication out of reach of children.

Caution: Do not use if Legatrin printed foil seal is damaged or missing.

Dosage: When a leg cramp occurs, take two tablets at once. To help prevent future night leg cramp attacks, take two tablets two hours before bedtime. Do not exceed two tablets daily. Consult a physician if symptoms persist longer than ten days.

How Supplied: Blister packages of 30 and 50 tablets.

Shown in Product Identification Section, page 408

Copley Pharmaceutical Inc.

25 JOHN RD
CANTON, MA 02021

LICE·ENZ® FOAM
Shampoo Aerosol
Lice Killing Shampoo Kit

Description: Lice·Enz® Foam shampoo is supplied as a metered aerosol delivery system for ease of application to the patient for the treatment of lice infestation.

Active Ingredients: Pyrethrins 0.3%, Piperonyl Butoxide, 3.0%; inert ingredients, 96.7%.

Indications: Lice·Enz® is indicated for the treatment of human pediculosis—head lice, body lice, pubic lice and their eggs. Lice·Enz® is specially formulated for head lice in children. The mousse application allows complete control of the amount of pesticide the child is exposed to; no messy shampoo to drip onto the child. Lice·Enz® is user friendly and easy to apply.

Actions: Lice·Enz® is a pediculicide for control of head lice, pubic lice and body lice and their nits.
SHOULD NOT BE USED BY RAGWEED-SENSITIZED PERSONS.
KEEP THIS AND ALL DRUGS OUT OF THE REACH OF CHILDREN.
CAUTIONS: For external use only. Harmful if swallowed. Do not inhale. Keep out of eyes and avoid contact with mucous membranes.

First Aid: In case this product should get in eyes, flush immediately with water. In case of infection or skin irritation, discontinue use and consult a physician. Consult a physician if infestation of eyebrows and eyelashes occur. Avoid contamination of food or foodstuffs. Use only as directed. Intentional misuse by deliberately concentrating and inhaling the contents can be harmful or fatal.

Physical or Chemical Hazard: Contents under pressure. Do not use or store near heat or open flame. Do not puncture or incinerate container. Exposure to temperatures above 120°F may cause bursting.

Storage: Store away from heat, sparks and open flame in original container and in an area inaccessible to children.

Disposal: Do not reuse empty container. Replace cap and discard container in trash. Do not incinerate or puncture.

Directions for Use: It is a violation of Federal Law to use this product in a manner inconsistent with its labeling. 1. Shake well. Apply as much LICE·ENZ® FOAM as needed to the hair and scalp or any other infested areas until entirely wet. Do not use on eyelashes or eyebrows. 2. Massage LICE·ENZ® FOAM into scalp and allow it to remain for no more than 10 minutes. 3. Wash hair thoroughly with warm water and shampoo or soap. 4. If desired, apply creme rinse to ease the nit removal process. 5. Comb hair with special no-nit comb to remove dead lice and eggs. 6. After combing, rinse hair thoroughly. 7. Repeat treatment in 7–10 days if reinfestation has occurred. 8. Do not exceed two consecutive applications within 24 hours. To help eliminate infestation, it is important to sterilize all clothing and bedding of infested person at time of treatment.
Note: The manufacturer of this product endorses the National Pediculosis Association's "No Nit Policy."

How Supplied: LICE·ENZ® FOAM aerosol is supplied in a 2-ounce aerosol container (ozone-friendly propellant).

Literature Available: Additional patient literature available upon request.

Shown in Product Identification Section, page 408

Del Pharmaceuticals, Inc.

A Subsidiary of Del Laboratories, Inc.
163 E. BETHPAGE ROAD
PLAINVIEW, NY 11803

DERMAREST® DriCort™
Anti-Itch Creme
(Hydrocortisone 1.0%)

Description: Dermarest DriCort contains the maximum strength of hydrocortisone available without a prescription. However, through a unique patented base, DriCort goes on feeling powder dry immediately. As a result, it gives dry, scaly skin a soft, silky feeling.

Active Ingredients: Hydrocortisone Acetate (equivalent to Hydrocortisone, 1.0%)

Other Ingredients: Caprylic/Capric Triglyceride, Colloidal Silicon Dioxide, Polyethylene, White Petrolatum.

Indications: For the temporary relief of itching associated with minor skin irritations, inflammation, and rashes due to eczema, insect bites, psoriasis, seborrheic dermatitis, poison ivy, poison oak, or poison sumac, soaps, detergents, cosmetics, jewelry, and for external genital, feminine, and anal itching. Other uses of this product should be only under the advice and supervision of a physician.

Warnings: For external use only. Avoid contact with the eyes. If condition worsens, or if symptoms persist for more than 7 days or clear up and occur again within a few days, stop use of this product and do not begin use of any other hydrocortisone product unless you have consulted a physician. Do not use for the treatment of diaper rash. Consult a physician. Do not use if you have a vaginal discharge. Consult a physician. For external anal itching use: Do not exceed the recommended daily dosage unless directed by a physician. In case of bleeding, consult a physician promptly. Do not put this product into the rectum by using fingers or any mechanical device or applicator. Keep this and all drugs out of the reach of children. In case of accidental ingestion, seek professional assistance or contact a Poison Control Center immediately.

Dosage and Administration: Adults and children 2 years of age and older: Apply to affected area not more than 3 to 4 times daily. Children under 2 years of age: Do not use, consult a physician. For external anal itching use: Adults: When practical, cleanse the affected area with mild soap and warm water and rinse thoroughly. Gently dry by patting or blotting with toilet tissue or a soft cloth before application of this product. Children under 12 years of age: Consult a physician.

How supplied: 0.5 oz (14 g) and 1 oz (28 g) tubes

Shown in Product Identification Section, page 408

BABY ORAJEL®

Active Ingredients: *Baby Orajel:* Benzocaine 7.5%.

Inactive Ingredients: *Baby Orajel:* FD&C Red No. 40, flavor, glycerin, polyethylene glycols, sodium saccharin, sorbic acid, sorbitol.

Indications: Baby Orajel is a soothing, cherry-flavored product which quickly relieves teething pain.

Actions: Benzocaine is a topical, local anesthetic commonly used for pain, discomfort, or pruritis associated with wounds, mucous membranes and skin irritations.

Warnings: Do not use if tube tip is out prior to opening. As with all products containing benzocaine, localized allergic reactions may occur after prolonged or repeated use. Keep this and all medications out of reach of children.

Precaution: For persistent or excessive teething pain, consult your physician.

Dosage and Administration: Wash hands. Cut open tip of tube on score mark. For infants 4 months of age and older, apply a *small* amount with fingertip or cotton applicator on affected area no more than four times daily.

How Supplied: Baby Orajel: Gel in ⅓ oz (9.45 g) tube.

Shown in Product Identification Section, page 408

BABY ORAJEL® TOOTH & GUM CLEANSER

Active Ingredients: Microdent™ (Poloxamer 407 2.0%, Simethicone 0.12%).

Inactive Ingredients: Carboxymethylcellulose Sodium, Citric Acid, Flavor, Glycerin, Methylparaben, Potassium Sorbate, Propylene Glycol, Propylparaben, Purified Water, Sodium Saccharin, Sorbitol.

Indications and Actions: Baby Orajel Tooth & Gum Cleanser is the first and only oral cleanser specially formulated to remove the plaque-like film on babies' teeth and gums. It's fluoride-Free, nonabrasive and does not foam so it's safe to use every day. It's sugar-free and has a flavor babies love. Only Baby Orajel Tooth & Gum Cleanser contains patented Microdent™—shown in clinical testing to help remove plaque and fight its buildup.

Warnings: Keep out of the reach of children. Do not use if tube tip is cut prior to opening.

Dosage and Administration: Wash hands. Cut open tip of tube on score mark. Apply a small amount to baby's gums and teeth with your finger or a gauze pad or a toothbrush. Gently rub the gums and teeth to remove food and plaque-like film. For best results, use in the morning and at bedtime.

How Supplied: Gel in ½ oz. (14.2g) tube and 1 oz. (28.3g) tube. Available in Vanilla or Fruit flavor.

Maximum Strength ORAJEL®

[*ōr 'ah-jel*]

Active Ingredient: Benzocaine 20% in a special base.

Inactive Ingredients: Clove oil, flavors, polyethylene glycols, sodium saccharin, sorbic acid.

Indications: Maximum Strength Orajel is formulated to provide faster relief from toothache pain for hours.

Actions: Benzocaine is a topical, local anesthetic commonly used for pain, discomfort, or pruritis associated with wounds, mucous membranes and skin irritation.

Warnings: Keep this and all drugs out of the reach of children. Do not use if tube tip is cut prior to opening.

Precaution: This preparation is intended for use in cases of toothache only as a temporary expedient until a dentist can be consulted. Do not use continuously.

Directions: Cut open tip of tube on score mark. Squeeze a small quantity of Maximum Strength Orajel directly into cavity and around gum surrounding the teeth.

How Supplied: Gel in two sizes—³⁄₁₆ oz (5.3 g) and ⅓ oz (9.45 g) tubes.

Shown in Product Identification Section, page 408

ORAJEL® Mouth-Aid®

[*ōr 'ah-jel*]

Active Ingredients: Benzocaine 20%, benzalkonium chloride 0.12%, zinc chloride 0.1% in a special emollient base.

Inactive Ingredients: Allantoin, flavor, polyethylene glycols, propyl gallate, propylene glycol, purified water, sodium saccharin, sorbic acid, trisodium EDTA.

Indications: Orajel Mouth-Aid combines a fast-acting maximum strength pain reliever, soothing ingredients which aid healing, a germicide and an astringent to help provide relief of minor mouth and lip irritations.

Actions: Benzocaine is a topical, local anesthetic commonly used for pain, discomfort, or pruritis associated with wounds, mucous membranes and skin irritations. Benzalkonium chloride is a rapidly acting surface disinfectant and detergent. Zinc chloride provides an astringent effect.

Warnings: Keep this and all medications out of reach of children. Do not use if tube tip is cut prior to opening.

Precaution: If condition persists, discontinue use and consult your physician or dentist. Not for prolonged use.

Directions: Cut open tip of tube on score mark. Apply directly to affected area as needed.

How Supplied: Gel in a ⅓ oz (9.45 g) tube.

Shown in Product Identification Section, page 408

PRONTO® Lice Killing Shampoo Kit

Description: Pronto Concentrate Lice Killing Shampoo contains the maximum strength of pyrethrins and piperonyl butoxide. In addition, a conditioner is included in the formulation to reduce tangles, for easy, effective comb-out of lice and eggs.

Active Ingredients: Pyrethrins 0.33%, piperonyl butoxide technical 4.00% [equivalent to 3.2% butylcarbityl (6-propylpiperonyl) ether and 0.80% related compounds].

Indications: One treatment pediculicide shampoo kills head, body and pubic lice on contact.

Actions: Pronto Lice Killing Shampoo contains the maximum strength of pyrethrins and piperonyl butoxide. Pyrethrins act directly on the nervous system of insects and piperonyl butoxide enhances the neurotoxic effect of pyrethrins by inhibiting the oxidative breakdown of the pyrethrins by the insect's detoxification system. This results in a longer amount of time which the pyrethrins may exert their toxic effect on the insect.

Warnings: May cause eye injury. Do not use near eyes or permit contact with eyes or nose. May cause skin irritation. Wash thoroughly with soap and water after handling. If product should get into eyes, immediately flush with water. Follow directions carefully.

Not to be used by persons allergic to ragweed. Harmful if swallowed. In case of infection or skin irritation, discontinue use and consult a physician. In order to prevent reinfestation with lice, all clothing and bedding must be sterilized or treated concurrent with the application of this preparation. Do not exceed two consecutive applications within 24 hours.

Precaution: If in eyes, flush with plenty of water and get medical attention.

Directions for Use: It is a violation of Federal Law to use this product in a manner inconsistent with its labeling.

Instruct child to close eyes and cover eyes with clean wet towel. Apply Pronto Shampoo Concentrate cautiously to dry hair, scalp or any affected areas. Add a generous amount of water to work Pronto Shampoo Concentrate into a rich lather. Allow the shampoo to remain on area for 10 minutes, but no longer. Rinse treated areas thoroughly with warm water. Rinse eyes out with water following use. A fine-toothed comb (included) may be used to help remove dead lice and their eggs (nits) from hair. Handy applicator gloves are provided for convenience in applying the shampoo to avoid contact with lice.

Storage and Disposal: Do not reuse empty container. Rinse thoroughly. Securely wrap original container in several layers of newspaper and discard in waste container.

How Supplied: 2 fl oz (59 ml) and 4 fl oz (118 ml) plastic bottles.

Shown in Product Identification Section, page 408

Continued on next page

Del—Cont.

EDUCATIONAL MATERIAL

Teething Booklet From Baby Orajel®
Facts parents should know about tooth development and the teething process.
Free to physicians, pharmacists and patients

Fact and Fallacy Booklet From Pronto®
Answers questions about head lice control.
Free to physicians, pharmacists and patients.

Effcon Laboratories, Inc.

P.O. BOX 71206
MARIETTA, GA 30007-1206

PIN-X®
Pinworm Treatment

Description: Each 1 mL of liquid for oral administration contains:
Pyrantel base .... 50 mg
(as Pyrantel Pamoate)

Indication: For the treatment of pinworms.

Warnings: Keep this and all drugs out of the reach of children. In case of accidental overdose, seek professional assistance or contact a poison control center immediately.
If you are pregnant or have liver disease, do not take this product unless directed by a doctor.

Directions for Use: Adults and children 2 years to under 12 years of age: oral dosage is a single dose of 5 milligrams of pyrantel base per pound, or 11 milligrams per kilogram, of body weight not to exceed 1 gram. Dosage information is summarized on the following dosing schedule:

Weight		Dosage (taken as a single dose)
25 to 37 lbs.	=	½ tsp.
38 to 62 lbs.	=	1 tsp.
63 to 87 lbs.	=	1½ tsp.
88 to 112 lbs.	=	2 tsp.
113 to 137 lbs.	=	2½ tsp.
138 to 162 lbs.	=	3 tsp. (1 tbsp.)
163 to 187 lbs.	=	3½ tsp.
188 lbs. & over	=	4 tsp.

SHAKE WELL BEFORE USING

How Supplied: Pin-X is supplied as a tan to yellowish, caramel-flavored suspension which contains 50 mg of pyrantel base (as pyrantel pamoate) per mL, in bottles of 30 mL (1 fl oz). NDC 55806-024-10.
Store at controlled room temperature 15°–30°C (59°–86°F).
Manufactured for:
Effcon Laboratories Inc.
Marietta, GA 30007-1206

Manufactured by:
MIKART, INC.
Atlanta, GA 30318
Rev. 1/89
Code 587A00
Shown in Product Identification Section, page 409

Emutech International, Inc

4790 IRVINE BLVD.
SUITE 105-418
IRVINE, CA 92720

ALOE UP
Aloe Vera Juice Drink
with Vitamin C
Natural Peach Flavor

Description: *ALOE UP* is a delicious, naturally peach flavored aloe vera juice drink with vitamin C, beta-carotene and vitamin E as antioxidants. The aloe used in *ALOE UP* is aloin-free and cold processed to protect all the naturally occurring nutritional factors in the juice. It is flavored with natural peach to provide an excellent taste. Each 8-oz serving provides 120 mg (200% U.S. RDA) of vitamin C, 150 mg of potassium and contains 90 calories.

Uses: *ALOE UP* can be used as a refreshing, great tasting beverage with meals or anytime in between. It can also be used as a liquid base to mix with other nutritional products such as EMUTECH'S *CHEATER'S DELIGHT* or *ULTRA MEAL. ALOE UP* is an excellent alternative to soft drinks and can be enjoyed equally by children, adults and senior citizens.

Directions: Simply pour an 8-oz glass of *ALOE UP* and enjoy it. It is ready to drink. After opening, it is best to refrigerate to preserve flavor and integrity.

How Supplied: *ALOE UP* is packaged in a sealed, quart-size, food-grade PET bottle.

CHEATER'S DELIGHT
Chromium Supplement
with Potassium, Fiber and Herbs

Description: *CHEATER'S DELIGHT* is a chromium supplement with potassium, fiber and herbs in a delicious, easy-to-blend powder form. Each 7-gram serving (1 scoop—approximately 1 level tablespoon), contains 25 mcg of elemental chromium (as polynicotinate), 150 mg of potassium and 5 grams of dietary fiber, along with lecithin and gymnema sylvestre. Sweetened with aspartame, one serving has only 8 calories.

Uses: *CHEATER'S DELIGHT* is designed to be used as part of an overall weight management program which includes meal substitution, calorie reduction and exercise. When taken ½ hour before meals, it provides a sense of fullness, which helps reduce the craving for additional calories, particularly from sweets and fatty foods.

Directions: Stir one scoop (7 grams), of *CHEATER'S DELIGHT* in 8 oz. of cold water to make a great-tasting fruit-flavored drink. It can also be mixed with fruit juices or *ALOE UP*, EMUTECH'S peach flavored aloe drink.

How Supplied: *CHEATER'S DELIGHT* is packaged in a sealed can containing 10.6 oz (210 grams—30 servings), along with a 7-gram scoop.

Warning: Phenylketonurics: contains phenylalanine.

KICK START
B Vitamin Supplement
with Other Nutritional Factors

Description: *KICK START* is a unique B vitamin supplement that acts as an energy source by providing both complex and simple carbohydrates in a great-tasting powder. *KICK START*, in addition to the B vitamins, contains maltodextrin, a special co-crystallized honey-apple-cinnamon blend and a concentrated guarana bean extract. Each 10-gram serving (1 scoop—approximately 1 level tablespoon), contains 35 calories, all from energy-producing carbohydrates.

Uses: *KICK START* can be taken in the morning to start your day or anytime when you feel a need for an energy lift. It can be used before physical activity or exercise, as well as part of a reduced calorie weight management program.

Directions: Stir one scoop (10 grams) of *KICK START* in 4 oz of cold water to make a great tasting apple-flavored cold beverage or in 4 oz of hot water to make a delicious honey-apple-flavored hot tea. It can also be mixed into other juices or hot drinks.

How Supplied: *KICK START* is packaged in a sealed can containing 10.6 oz (300 grams—30 servings), along with a 10-gram scoop. It also is available in single-serving foil packets.

RENEW
Omega-3 Fatty Acid Supplement
with Vitamins A & E

Description: *RENEW* is an Omega-3 fatty supplement with vitamins A and E in a soft gelatin capsule. It is micellized using the EMUSOL®-patented technology to ensure complete solubility in water. Water solubility greatly enhances the absorption of the fat-soluble nutrients.

Nutritional Information: Two capsules supply:

Omega-3 Fatty Acids	250 mg
Vitamin A	1500 I.U.
Vitamin E	10 I.U.

Uses: As a dietary supplement, *RENEW* supplies nutritional factors directly involved with maintenance of normal circulatory processes.

®EMUSOL is a registered trademark of Bioglan, Inc.

Directions: Take two capsules per day with food.

How Supplied: *RENEW* is packaged in a white plastic sealed bottle containing 60 soft gelatin capsules.

ULTRA MEAL
Meal Replacement Nutritional Drink

Description: *ULTRA MEAL* is a nutritionally balanced powdered drink mix that provides proper levels of protein, carbohydrate, fat, fiber and other nutrients for use as a filling and delicious meal replacement that mixes easily in water. It was developed to be part of an overall weight management program that includes behavior modification, reduced calories, increased physical activity and energy level maintenance. *ULTRA MEAL* provides a nutritious and satisfying alternative to high-fat, high-calorie meals. It contains 8 grams of protein, 3 grams of dietary fiber and less than 1 gram of fat derived from lecithin and medium chain triglycerides (MCT's). Partially sweetened with aspartame, *ULTRA MEAL* contains only 75 calories per serving, (25 grams—1 scoop). It comes in 3 delicious flavors—French Vanilla, Chocolate Fudge and Tropical Banana.

Nutritional Information: Serving size: 25 grams (1 scoop). Servings per container: 26

Each Serving Provides:

Calories	75
Protein	8 grams
Carbohydrate	10 grams
Fat	less than 1 gram
Sodium	90 mg
Potassium	200 mg
Fiber	3 grams

Percentage of Adult U.S. Recommended Daily Allowance (U.S. RDA):

Protein	15%
Vitamin A	35%
Vitamin C	35%
Thiamine	35%
Riboflavin	35%
Niacin	35%
Calcium	10%
Iron	0%
Vitamin D	35%
Vitamin E	35%
Vitamin B_6	35%
Folic Acid	35%
Vitamin B_{12}	35%
Phosphorus	10%
Iodine	35%
Magnesium	10%
Zinc	35%
Copper	35%
Biotin	35%
Pantothenic Acid	35%
Selenium	25 mcg*
Chromium	25 mcg*
Manganese	1.0 mg*

* No U.S. RDA established.

Uses: *ULTRA MEAL* can be used as a low-calorie, filling, occasional meal replacement or as a routine part of an overall weight management program.

Directions: Add 1 scoop (25 grams) of *ULTRA MEAL* to 8 oz of cold water. Mix thoroughly. For best results, use a shaker or a blender. For best taste, add ice. As part of a fast weight loss program, have one delicious *UTLRA MEAL* for breakfast and another for lunch. Then have a sensible low-calorie meal for dinner.

How Supplied: *ULTRA MEAL* is packaged in a sealed can containing 1.3 lb (600 grams—24 servings), along with a 25-gram scoop.

Warning: Phenylketonurics: contains phenylalanine.

VITA FUEL
Liquid Vitamin & Mineral Supplement

Description: *VITA FUEL* is a delicious, tropical fruit-flavored liquid vitamin and mineral supplement with aloe juice. It supplies all the nutrients in a water-soluble form to insure rapid absorption. This includes the fat-soluble nutrients, vitamins A, D, E and beta-carotene which are micellized using the patented EMUSOL® process. This insures the maximum absorption of these nutrients. *VITA FUEL* provides 100% of the U.S. RDA of most vitamins, including 100% of vitamin A from micellized beta-carotene, 200% of vitamin C and 150 mg of potassium in 1 tablespoon (15 ml) serving. Sweetened with aspartame and flavored with natural tropical fruit flavors, 1 serving contains only 5 calories.

Nutritional Information: Per 1 tablespoon serving (15ml)
[See table below.]

Uses: *VITA FUEL* can be used whenever vitamin and mineral supplementation is desired. Because of its liquid nature, it can easily be added to drinks or to food. It is easily taken by children and the elderly who have difficulty in taking tablets. *VITA FUEL* can be taken with *ULTRA MEAL, ALOE UP* or any other EMUTECH nutritional product.

Directions: Place 1 tablespoon (15 ml) in 4 oz of cold water or any other liquid drink. It is particularly good in *ALOE UP.*

How Supplied: *VITA FUEL* is packaged in a 16 oz (450 ml—30 servings) food-grade sealed PET bottle.

Warning: Phenylketonurics: contains phenylalanine.

®EMUSOL is a registered trademark of Bioglan, Inc.

INGREDIENT	AMT	% U.S. RDA
Vitamin A (Beta-Carotene)	5000 I.U.	100
Vitamin E	30 I.U.	100
Vitamin D	200 I.U.	50
Vitamin B_1	1.5 mg	100
Vitamin B_2	1.7 mg	100
Vitamin B_3 (Niacinamide)	20.0 mg	100
Vitamin B_6	2.0 mg	100
Vitamin B_{12}	6.0 mcg	100
Biotin	150.0 mcg	50
Panothenic Acid	10.0 mg	100
Vitamin C	120.0 mg	200
Calcium	50.0 mg	5
Magnesium	20.0 mg	5
Zinc	15.0 mg	100
Copper	0.5 mg	25
Manganese	0.5 mg	*
Selenium	50.0 mcg	*
Chromium	5.0 mcg	*
Postassium	150.0 mg	*

*No U.S. RDA established.

Fisons Consumer Health

Fisons Corporation
P.O. BOX 1212
ROCHESTER, NY 14603

ALLEREST® MAXIMUM STRENGTH TABLETS, NO DROWSINESS TABLETS, HEADACHE STRENGTH TABLETS, SINUS PAIN FORMULA TABLETS, CHILDREN'S CHEWABLE TABLETS AND 12 HOUR CAPLETS

Active Ingredients:
Maximum Strength Tablets—Chlorpheniramine maleate 2 mg, pseudoephedrine HCl 30 mg.
No Drowsiness Tablets—Acetaminophen 325 mg, pseudoephedrine HCl 30 mg.
Headache Strength Tablets—Acetaminophen 325 mg, chlorpheniramine maleate 2 mg, pseudoephedrine HCl 30 mg.
Sinus Pain Formula Tablets—Acetaminophen 500 mg, chlorpheniramine maleate 2 mg, pseudoephedrine HCl 30 mg.

Continued on next page

Fisons Consumer—Cont.

Children's Chewable Tablets—Chlorpheniramine maleate 1 mg, phenylpropanolamine HCl 9.4 mg.
12 Hour Caplets—Chlorpheniramine maleate 12 mg, phenylpropanolamine HCl 75 mg.

Other Ingredients:
Maximum Strength Tablets—Blue 1 lake, dibasic calcium phosphate, magnesium stearate, microcrystalline cellulose, povidone, pregelatinized starch, sodium starch glycolate. *No Drowsiness and Headache Strength Tablets*—Magnesium stearate, microcrystalline cellulose, povidone, pregelatinized starch.
Sinus Pain Formula Tablets—Magnesium stearate, microcrystalline cellulose, povidone, pregelatinized starch, sodium starch glycolate.
Children's Chewable Tablets—Calcium stearate, citric acid, flavor, magnesium trisilicate, mannitol, saccharin sodium, sorbitol.
12 Hour Caplets—Carnauba wax, colloidal silicon dioxide, lactose, methylcellulose, polyethylene glycol, povidone, Red 30, stearic acid, titanium dioxide, Yellow 6.

Indications: *Maximum Strength, Headache Strength, Sinus Pain Formula, Children's Chewable Tablets and 12 Hour Caplets*—Temporarily relieves nasal congestion, runny nose, sneezing, itching of the nose or throat, and itchy, watery eyes due to hay fever or other upper respiratory allergies; also *Headache Strength and Sinus Pain Formula Tablets*—For the temporary relief of minor aches, pains, and headache; also *12 Hour Caplets*—For temporary relief of nasal congestion due to the common cold and associated with sinusitis.
No Drowsiness Tablets—Temporarily relieves nasal congestion due to hay fever or other upper respiratory allergies. For the temporary relief of minor aches, pains, and headache.

Warnings: *All Products*—Do not exceed recommended dosage because at higher doses, nervousness, dizziness, or sleeplessness may occur. Do not take this product if you have heart disease, high blood pressure, thyroid disease, diabetes, or difficulty in urination due to enlargement of the prostate gland, unless directed by a physician. As with any drug, if you are pregnant or nursing a baby, seek the advice of a health professional before using this product. **Keep this and all drugs out of the reach of children.** In case of accidental overdose, seek professional assistance or contact a Poison Control Center immediately. Prompt medical attention (for products containing acetaminophen) is critical for adults as well as children even if you do not notice any signs or symptoms. And, *All Products Except No Drowsiness Tablets*—Do not take this product if you have asthma, glaucoma, emphysema, chronic pulmonary disease, shortness of breath, or difficulty in breathing unless directed by a physician. May cause excitability, especially in children. May cause drowsiness; alcohol, sedatives, and tranquilizers may increase the drowsiness effect. Avoid alcoholic beverages while taking this product. Do not take this product if you are taking sedatives or tranquilizers, without first consulting your physician. Use caution when driving a motor vehicle or operating machinery.
Maximum Strength Tablets, Children's Chewable Tablets and 12 Hour Caplets—Do not take this product for more than 7 days. If symptoms do not improve or are accompanied by fever, consult a physician.
Headache Strength, Sinus Pain Formula, and No Drowsiness Tablets—Do not take this product for more than 10 days (for adults) or 5 days (for children). If symptoms do not improve or are accompanied by fever that lasts more than 3 days, or if new symptoms occur, consult a physician.

Drug Interaction Precaution: *All Products*—Do not take this product if you are presently taking a prescription drug for high blood pressure or depression, without first consulting your physician; and *Children's Chewable Tablets and 12 Hour Caplets*—Do not take this product if you are presently taking another medication containing phenylpropanolamine.

Directions: Dose as follows while symptoms persist, or as directed by a physician.
Maximum Strength, No Drowsiness and Headache Strength Tablets—Adults and children 12 years of age and older: 2 tablets every 4 hours, not to exceed 8 tablets in 24 hours. Children 6 to under 12 years of age: 1 tablet every 4 hours, not to exceed 4 tablets in 24 hours. Children under 6 years of age: Consult a physician.
Sinus Pain Formula Tablets—Adults and children 12 years of age and older: 2 tablets every 6 hours, not to exceed 8 tablets in 24 hours. Children under 12 years of age: Consult a physician.
Children's Chewable Tablets—Children 6 to under 12 years of age: 2 tablets every 4 hours, not to exceed 8 tablets in 24 hours. Children under 6 years of age: Consult a physician.
12 Hour Caplets—Adults and children over 12 years of age: 1 caplet swallowed whole every 12 hours, not to exceed 2 caplets in 24 hours.

How Supplied:
Maximum Strength Tablets—Boxes of 24, 48, and 72.
No Drowsiness Tablets—Boxes of 20.
Headache Strength Tablets—Boxes of 24.
Sinus Pain Formula Tablets—Boxes of 20.
Children's Chewable Tablets—Boxes of 24.
12 Hour Caplets—Boxes of 10.
ALLEREST is a registered trademark of Fisons BV.

Shown in Product Identification Section, page 409

AMERICAINE® HEMORRHOIDAL OINTMENT
[*a-mer ′i-kān*]

Active Ingredient: Benzocaine 20%.

Other Ingredients: Benzethonium chloride, polyethylene glycol 300, polyethylene glycol 3350.

Indications: For the temporary relief of local pain, itching and soreness associated with hemorrhoids and anorectal inflammation.

Warnings: If condition worsens, or does not improve within 7 days, consult a physician. Do not exceed the recommended daily dosage unless directed by a physician. In case of bleeding, consult a physician promptly. Do not put this product into the rectum by using fingers or any mechanical device or applicator. Certain persons can develop allergic reactions to ingredients in this product. If the symptom being treated does not subside or if redness, irritation, swelling, pain, or other symptoms develop or increase, discontinue use and consult a physician. **Keep this and all drugs out of the reach of children.** In case of accidental ingestion, seek professional assistance or contact a Poison Control Center immediately.

Directions: *Adults:* When practical, cleanse the affected area with mild soap and warm water and rinse thoroughly. Gently dry by patting or blotting with toilet tissue or a soft cloth before application of this product. Apply externally to the affected area up to 6 times daily. *Children under 12 years of age:* Consult a physician.

How Supplied: *Hemorrhoidal Ointment*—1 oz. tube.
AMERICAINE is a registered trademark of Fisons BV.

Shown in Product Identification Section, page 409

AMERICAINE® TOPICAL ANESTHETIC SPRAY AND FIRST AID OINTMENT
[*a-mer ′i-kān*]

Active Ingredient: Benzocaine 20%.

Other Ingredients: *Spray*—Butane (propellant), isobutane (propellant), polyethylene glycol 200, propane (propellant). *Ointment*—Benzethonium chloride, polyethylene glycol 300, polyethylene glycol 3350.

Indications: For the temporary relief of pain and itching associated with minor cuts, scrapes, burns, sunburn, insect bites, or minor skin irritations.

Warnings: For external use only. Avoid contact with the eyes. If condition worsens, or if symptoms persist for more than 7 days or clear up and occur again within a few days, discontinue use of this product and consult a physician. **Keep this and all drugs out of the reach of children.** In case of accidental ingestion, seek professional assistance or contact a Poison Control Center immediately. *For Spray only*—Contents under pressure. Do not puncture or incinerate. Flammable mixture; do not use near fire or flame. Do not store at temperature above 120°F. Use only as directed. Intentional misuse by deliberately concentrating and inhaling the contents can be harmful or fatal.

Directions: Adults and children 2 years of age and older: Apply liberally to affected area not more than 3 to 4 times daily. Children under 2 years of age: Consult a physician.

How Supplied: *Topical Anesthetic Spray*—2/3 oz., 2 oz. and 4 oz. aerosol containers. *First Aid Ointment*—3/4 oz. tube, which is a clear, fragrance-free gel formula that is nonstaining, easy to apply, and is easily removed with soap and water.

AMERICAINE is a registered trademark of Fisons BV.

Shown in Product Identification Section, page 409

CALDECORT® ANTI-ITCH CREAM AND SPRAY; CALDECORT LIGHT® CREAM

[*kal 'de-kort*]

Active Ingredient: *Cream*—Hydrocortisone acetate (equivalent to hydrocortisone 1%). *Light Cream*—Hydrocortisone acetate (equivalent to hydrocortisone 1/2%). *Spray*—Hydrocortisone 1%.

Other Ingredients: *Cream*—Isopropyl myristate, methylparaben, polysorbate 60, propylparaben, purified water, sorbitan monostearate, sorbitol solution, stearic acid. *Light Cream*—Aloe vera gel, isopropyl myristate, methylparaben, polysorbate 60, propylparaben, purified water, sorbitan monostearate, sorbitol solution, stearic acid. *Spray*—Isobutane (propellant), isopropyl myristate, SD alcohol 40-B 62.7% (w/w).

Indications: For the temporary relief of itching associated with minor skin irritations, inflammation, and rashes due to eczema, insect bites, poison ivy, poison oak, poison sumac, soaps, detergents, cosmetics, jewelry, seborrheic dermatitis, psoriasis, and for external feminine itching. Other uses of this product should be only under the advice and supervision of a doctor.

Warnings: For external use only. Avoid contact with the eyes. If condition worsens, or if symptoms persist for more than 7 days or clear up and occur again within a few days, stop use of this product and do not begin use of any other hydrocortisone product unless you have consulted a doctor. Do not use for the treatment of diaper rash. Consult a doctor. Do not use if you have a vaginal discharge. Consult a doctor. **Keep this and all drugs out of the reach of children.** In case of accidental ingestion, seek professional assistance or contact a Poison Control Center immediately. *For Spray only*—Avoid contact with the eyes or on other mucous membranes. Contents under pressure. Do not puncture or incinerate. Flammable mixture, do not use near fire or flame. Do not store at temperature above 120°F. Use only as directed. Intentional misuse by deliberately concentrating and inhaling the contents can be harmful or fatal.

Directions: Adults and children 2 years of age and older: Apply to affected area not more than 3 or 4 times daily. Children under 2 years of age: Do not use, consult a doctor.

How Supplied: *Cream*—1/2 oz. and 1 oz. tubes. *Light Cream*—1/2 oz. tubes. *Spray*—1.5 oz. aerosol container.

CALDECORT and CALDECORT LIGHT are registered trademarks of Fisons BV.

Shown in Product Identification Section, page 409

CALDESENE® MEDICATED POWDER AND OINTMENT

[*kal 'de-sēn*]

Active Ingredients: *Powder*—Calcium undecylenate 10%. *Ointment*—Petrolatum 53.9%; zinc oxide 15%.

Other Ingredients: *Powder* — Fragrance, talc. *Ointment*—Cod liver oil, fragrance, lanolin oil, methylparaben, propylparaben, talc.

Indications: Caldesene Medicated Powder is indicated to help heal, relieve and prevent diaper rash, prickly heat and chafing. Caldesene Ointment helps treat and prevent diaper rash, protects against urine and other irritants, soothes chafed skin, and promotes healing.

Actions: Only Caldesene Medicated Powder contains calcium undecylenate, an antibacterial that inhibits growth of the organisms frequently associated with diaper rash (including *S aureus, S epidermidis, E coli, and P aeruginosa*). Also forms a protective coating to repel moisture, soothe and comfort minor skin irritations, help heal and prevent chafing and prickly heat. Caldesene Ointment forms a protective skin coating to repel moisture and promote healing of diaper rash, while its natural ingredients protect irritated skin against wetness and other irritants. Unlike other ointments containing zinc oxide, Caldesene Ointment has a mild fragrance and is easily removed from the diaper area with soap and water.

Warnings: For external use only. Avoid contact with eyes. If condition worsens or does not improve within 7 days, consult a doctor. **Keep this and all drugs out of the reach of children.** In case of accidental ingestion, seek professional assistance or contact a Poison Control Center immediately.

Powder only: Keep powder away from child's face to avoid inhalation, which can cause breathing problems. Do not use on broken skin.

Ointment only: Do not apply over deep puncture wounds, infections and lacerations.

Directions: Use on baby after every bath or diaper change as directed by a pediatrician. Cleanse and thoroughly dry baby's skin, then smooth on Caldesene. Powder only: Apply powder close to the body away from child's face.

How Supplied: *Medicated Powder*—2 oz. and 4 oz. shaker containers. *Medicated Ointment*—1.25 oz.

CALDESENE is a registered trademark of Fisons BV.

Shown in Product Identification Section, page 409

CRUEX® ANTIFUNGAL POWDER, SPRAY POWDER AND CREAM

[*kru 'ex*]

Active Ingredients: *Powder*—Calcium undecylenate 10%. *Spray Powder* — Total undecylenate 19%, as undecylenic acid and zinc undecylenate. *Cream*—Total undecylenate 20%, as undecylenic acid and zinc undecylenate.

Other Ingredients: *Powder*—Colloidal silicon dioxide, fragrance, isopropyl myristate, talc. *Spray Powder*—Fragrance, isobutane (propellant), isopropyl myristate, menthol, talc, trolamine. *Cream*—Fragrance, glycol stearate SE, lanolin, methylparaben, PEG-8 laurate, PEG-6 stearate, propylparaben, purified water, sorbitol solution, stearic acid, trolamine, white petrolatum.

Indications: For the treatment of jock itch (tinea cruris) and relief of itching, chafing, burning rash and irritation in the groin area. Cruex powders also absorb perspiration.

Warnings: Do not use on children under 2 years of age except under the advice and supervision of a doctor. For external use only. If irritation occurs, or if there is no improvement within 2 weeks, discontinue use and consult a doctor or pharmacist. **Keep this and all drugs out of the reach of children.** In case of accidental ingestion, seek professional assistance or contact a Poison Control Center immediately. *For Spray Powder only*—Avoid spraying in eyes or on other mucous membranes. Contents under pressure. Do not puncture or incinerate. Flammable mixture, do not use near a fire or flame. Do not store at temperature above 120° F. Use only as directed. Intentional misuse by deliberately concentrating and inhaling the contents can be harmful or fatal.

Directions: Cleanse skin with soap and water and dry thoroughly. Apply Cruex to affected area morning and night, before and after athletic activity, or as directed by a doctor. Best results are usually obtained with 2 weeks' use of this product. If satisfactory results have not occurred within this time, consult a

Continued on next page

Fisons Consumer—Cont.

doctor or pharmacist. Children under 12 years of age should be supervised in the use of this product. This product is not effective on the scalp or nails.

How Supplied: *Powder*—1.5 oz. plastic squeeze bottle. *Spray Powder*—1.8 oz., 3.5 oz. and 5.5 oz. aerosol containers. *Cream*—½ oz. tube.
CRUEX is a registered trademark of Fisons BV.

Shown in Product Identification Section, page 409

DESENEX® ANTIFUNGAL POWDER, SPRAY POWDER, CREAM, OINTMENT, SPRAY LIQUID AND PENETRATING FOAM

[*dess 'i-nex*]

Active Ingredients: *Cream, Ointment, Powder, and Spray Powder,*—Total undecylenate 25%, as undecylenic acid and zinc undecylenate. *Spray Liquid*—Tolnaftate 1%. *Penetrating Foam*—Undecylenic acid 10%.

Other Ingredients: *Cream, Ointment*—Fragrance, glycol stearate SE, lanolin, methylparaben, PEG-8 laurate, PEG-6 stearate, propylparaben, purified water, sorbitol solution, stearic acid, trolamine, white petrolatum. *Powder*—Fragrance, talc. *Spray Powder*—Fragrance, isobutane (propellant), isopropyl myristate, menthol, talc, trolamine. *Spray Liquid*—BHT, fragrance, isobutane (propellant), polyethylene glycol 400, SD alcohol 40-B (41% w/w). *Penetrating Foam*—Emulsifying wax, fragrance, isobutane (propellant), isopropyl alcohol (29.2% w/w), purified water, sodium benzoate, trolamine.

Indications: Desenex Antifungal Products cure athlete's foot (tinea pedis) exclusive of the nails and scalp. Relieves itching, burning, and cracking. Desenex Spray Liquid prevents the recurrence of athlete's foot with daily use.

Warnings: Do not use on children under 2 years of age except under the advice and supervision of a doctor. For external use only. Avoid contact with the eyes. If irritation occurs, or if there is no improvement within 4 weeks, discontinue use and consult a doctor. **Keep this and all drugs out of the reach of children.** In case of accidental ingestion, seek professional assistance or contact a Poison Control Center immediately. *For Spray Powder, Spray Liquid, and Penetrating Foam*—Avoid spraying in the eyes or on other mucous membranes. Contents under pressure. Do not puncture or incinerate. Flammable mixture, do not use near fire or flame. Do not store at temperature above 120° F. Use only as directed. Intentional misuse by deliberately concentrating and inhaling the contents can be harmful or fatal.

Directions: Cleanse skin with soap and water and dry thoroughly. Apply over affected area morning and night or as directed by a doctor, paying special attention to the spaces between the toes. It is also helpful to wear well-fitting, ventilated shoes and to change shoes and socks at least once daily. Best results are usually obtained with 4 weeks' use of this product. If satisfactory results have not occurred within this time, consult a doctor. Children under 12 years of age should be supervised in the use of this product. This product is not effective on the scalp or nails. For persistent cases of athlete's foot, use Desenex Ointment or Cream at night and Desenex Powder or Spray Powder during the day. To prevent recurrence of athlete's foot, apply Desenex Spray Liquid to feet once or twice daily.

How Supplied: *Cream*—½ oz. tube. *Ointment*—½ oz. and 1 oz. tubes. *Powder*—1.5 oz. and 3 oz. shaker containers. *Spray Powder*—2.7 oz. and 5.5 oz. aerosol containers. *Spray Liquid*—3 oz. aerosol container. *Penetrating Foam*—1.5 oz. aerosol container.
DESENEX is a registered trademark of Fisons BV.

Shown in Product Identification Section, page 409

DESENEX® FOOT & SNEAKER DEODORANT SPRAY

[*dess 'i-nex*]

Ingredients: Isobutane (propellant), SD alcohol 40-B, talc, aluminum chlorohydrex, silica, diisopropyl adipate, fragrance, menthol, tartaric acid.

Description: Foot & Sneaker Deodorant Spray cools and comforts feet, helping them feel clean and refreshed, Helps foster good foot hygiene with regular use. Specially formulated to absorb wetness, deodorize and relieve the discomfort of hot, perspiring, active feet. Sprays on like a liquid—dries quickly to a fine powder.

Directions: **Shake well,** hold 6 inches from area and spray onto soles of your feet and between your toes daily. Also, spray liberally over entire area of shoes or sneakers before wearing.

Warnings: Avoid spraying in eyes. Contents under pressure. Do not puncture or incinerate. Flammable mixture, do not use near fire or flame. Do not store at temperature above 120° F. Use only as directed. Intentional misuse by deliberately concentrating and inhaling the contents can be harmful or fatal. **Keep out of reach of children.**

How Supplied: *Desenex Foot & Sneaker Deodorant Spray Powder*—3 oz. aerosol container. Also available, Desenex Foot & Sneaker Deodorant Powder Plus with an antifungal—2 oz. shaker container.
DESENEX is a registered trademark of Fisons BV.

Shown in Product Identification Section, page 409

ISOCLOR® TIMESULE® Capsules

[*īs 'ō-klŏr*]

Active Ingredients: Chlorpheniramine maleate 8 mg and pseudoephedrine HCl 120 mg.

Other Ingredients: Castor wax, ethylcellulose, gelatin, mineral oil, silicone oil, sugar spheres, white petrolatum.

Indications: For temporary relief of nasal congestion due to the common cold, hay fever, or other upper respiratory allergies, or associated with sinusitis. Helps decongest sinus openings, sinus passages. Reduces swelling of nasal passages, shrinks swollen membranes, and temporarily restores freer breathing through the nose. Alleviates runny nose, sneezing, itching of the nose or throat, and itchy and watery eyes as may occur in allergic rhinitis (such as hay fever).

Warnings: Do not exceed recommended dosage because, at higher doses, nervousness, dizziness, or sleeplessness may occur. Do not give this product to children under 12 years except under the advice and supervision of a physician. Do not take this product if you have asthma, glaucoma, emphysema, chronic pulmonary disease, shortness of breath, difficulty in breathing, difficulty in urination due to enlargement of the prostate gland, high blood pressure, heart disease, diabetes, or thyroid disease except under the advice and supervision of a physician. If symptoms do not improve within seven days or are accompanied by a high fever, consult a physician before continuing use. May cause drowsiness; alcohol may increase the drowsiness effect. May cause excitability especially in children. As with any drug, if you are pregnant or nursing a baby, seek the advice of a health professional before using this product.
Avoid driving a motor vehicle or operating heavy machinery. Avoid alcoholic beverages while taking this product.
Keep this and all drugs out of the reach of children. In case of accidental overdose, seek professional assistance or contact a Poison Control Center immediately.

Drug Interaction Precaution: Do not take this product if you are currently taking a prescription drug for high blood pressure or depression without first consulting your physician.

Directions: Adults and children 12 years and older—one capsule every 12 hours. Do not exceed two capsules in 24 hours.

How Supplied: Packaged on blister cards in cartons of 10's and 20's, and bottles of 100.
ISOCLOR® and TIMESULE® are registered trademarks of Fisons Corporation.
Distributed by:
FISONS
Consumer Health
Rochester, NY 14623 USA

Shown in Product Identification Section, page 409

MYOFLEX® ANALGESIC CREME

[*mī'ō-flex*]

Active Ingredient: Trolamine salicylate 10%.

Other Ingredients: Cetyl alcohol, disodium EDTA, fragrance, propylene glycol, purified water, sodium lauryl sulfate, stearyl alcohol, white wax.

Indications: For the temporary pain relief of minor backache, sore muscles, and aching joints caused by arthritis, overexertion, muscle strain and rheumatism.

Warning: For external use only. Use only as directed. Do not apply to irritated skin or if excessive irritation develops. Avoid contact with eyes or mucous membranes. If pain persists for more than 10 days or redness is present, consult a physician. For children under 12, consult a physician. **Keep this and all other medication out of the reach of children.** In case of accidental ingestion, seek professional assistance or contact a Poison Control Center immediately. As with any drug, if you are pregnant or nursing a baby, seek the advice of a health professional before using this product.

Directions: Adults—Rub into areas of soreness three or four times daily. Affected areas may be wrapped loosely with two- or three-inch elastic bandage after liberal application.

How Supplied: As an odorless, stainless, non-burning creme in 2 oz. and 4 oz. tubes, and 8 oz. and 16 oz. jars.
MYOFLEX is a registered trademark of Fisons Corporation.

Shown in Product Identification Section, page 409

SINAREST® TABLETS, EXTRA STRENGTH TABLETS AND NO DROWSINESS TABLETS

[*sīn 'a-rest*]

Active Ingredients:
Tablets—Acetaminophen 325 mg, chlorpheniramine maleate 2 mg, pseudoephedrine HCl 30 mg.
Extra Strength Tablets—Acetaminophen 500 mg, chlorpheniramine maleate 2 mg, pseudoephedrine HCl 30 mg.
No Drowsiness Tablets—Acetaminophen 500 mg, pseudoephedrine HCl 30 mg.

Other Ingredients:
All Products—Magnesium stearate, microcrystalline cellulose, povidone, pregelatinized starch.
Extra Strength and No Drowsiness Tablets also contain—Sodium starch glycolate. *Tablets and Extra Strength Tablets* also contain—Yellow 6 lake, Yellow 10 lake.

Indications:
Tablets and Extra Strength Tablets—Temporarily relieves nasal congestion, runny nose, sneezing, itching of the nose and throat, and itchy, watery eyes due to hay fever or other upper respiratory allergies, or associated with sinusitis. For temporary relief of minor aches, pains, and headache.
No Drowsiness Tablets—Temporarily relieves nasal congestion due to hay fever or other upper respiratory allergies, or associated with sinusitis. For temporary relief of minor aches, pains, and headache.

Warnings: *Tablets*—Do not take this product for more than 10 days (for adults) or 5 days (for children). *Extra Strength and No Drowsiness Tablets*—Do not take this product for more than 10 days. *All Products*—Do not exceed recommended dosage because at higher doses, nervousness, dizziness, or sleeplessness may occur. If symptoms do not improve or are accompanied by fever that lasts more than 3 days, or if new symptoms occur, consult a physician. Do not take this product if you have heart disease, high blood pressure, thyroid disease, diabetes, or difficulty in urination due to enlargement of the prostate gland, unless directed by a physician. As with any drug, if you are pregnant or nursing a baby, seek the advice of a health professional before using this product. **Keep this and all drugs out of the reach of children.** In case of accidental overdose, seek professional assistance or contact a Poison Control Center immediately. Prompt medical attention is critical for adults as well as children even if you do not notice any signs or symptoms. Also, *Tablets and Extra Strength Tablets*—Do not take this product if you have asthma, glaucoma, emphysema, chronic pulmonary disease, shortness of breath, or difficulty in breathing unless directed by a physician. May cause excitability, especially in children. May cause drowsiness; alcohol, sedatives, and tranquilizers may increase the drowsiness effect. Avoid alcoholic beverages while taking this product. Do not take this product if you are taking sedatives or tranquilizers, without first consulting your physician. Use caution when driving a motor vehicle or operating machinery.

Drug Interaction Precautions: *All Products*—Do not take this product if you are presently taking a prescription drug for high blood pressure or depression, without first consulting your physician.

Directions: Dose as follows while symptoms persist, or as directed by a physician.
Tablets—Adults and children 12 years of age and older: 2 tablets every 4 hours, not to exceed 8 tablets in 24 hours. Children 6 to under 12 years of age: 1 tablet every 4 hours, not to exceed 4 tablets in 24 hours. Children under 6 years of age: Consult a physician.
Extra Strength and No Drowsiness Tablets—Adults and children 12 years of age and older: 2 tablets every 6 hours, not to exceed 8 tablets in 24 hours. Children under 12 years of age: Consult a physician.

How Supplied:
Tablets—Boxes of 20, 40, and 80.
Extra Strength Tablets—Boxes of 24.
No Drowsiness Tablets—Boxes of 20.
SINAREST is a registered trademark of Fisons BV.

TING® ANTIFUNGAL CREAM, POWDER, SPRAY LIQUID, and SPRAY POWDER

Active Ingredient: Tolnaftate, 1%.

Other Ingredients: *Cream*—BHT, fragrance, polyethylene glycol 400, polyethylene glycol 3350, titanium dioxide. *Powder*—Corn starch, fragrance, talc. *Spray Liquid*—BHT, fragrance, isobutane (propellant), polyethylene glycol 400, SD alcohol 40-B (41% w/w). *Spray Powder*—BHT, fragrance, isobutane (propellant), PPG-12-buteth-16, SD alcohol 40-B (14% w/w), talc.

Indications: Cures athlete's foot and jock itch with a clinically proven ingredient. Relieves itching and burning. Prevents recurrence of athlete's foot with daily use.

Warnings: Do not use on children under 2 years of age except under the advice and supervision of a doctor. For external use only. Avoid contact with the eyes. If irritation occurs, or if there is no improvement within 4 weeks for athlete's foot, or within 2 weeks for jock itch, discontinue use and consult a doctor or pharmacist. **Keep this and all drugs out of the reach of children.** In case of accidental ingestion, seek professional assistance or contact a Poison Control Center immediately. *For Spray Liquid and Spray Powder only*—Avoid spraying in eyes or on other mucous membranes. Contents under pressure; do not puncture or incinerate. Flammable mixture, do not use near fire or flame. Do not store at temperature above 120°F. Use only as directed. Intentional misuse by deliberately concentrating and inhaling contents can be harmful or fatal.

Directions: Cleanse skin with soap and water and dry thoroughly. Apply over affected area morning and night or as directed by a doctor. For athlete's foot pay special attention to the spaces between the toes. It is also helpful to wear well-fitting, ventilated shoes and to change shoes and socks at least once daily. Best results in athlete's foot are usually obtained within 4 weeks' use of this product, and in jock itch, with two weeks' use. If satisfactory results have not occurred within these times, consult a doctor or pharmacist. Children under 12 years of age should be supervised in the use of this product. This product is not effective on the scalp or nails. To prevent recurrence of athlete's foot, apply Ting to feet once or twice daily following the above directions.

Continued on next page

Fisons Consumer—Cont.

How Supplied: *Cream*—½ oz. tube, *Powder*—1.5 oz. shaker container, *Spray Liquid and Spray Powder*—3 oz. aerosol containers.
TING is a registered trademark of Fisons BV.

Shown in Product Identification Section, page 409

VITRON-C® TABLETS
[*vī 'tron c*]

Active Ingredients: Each tablet contains
Ferrous fumarate, USP .... 200 mg
66 mg elemental iron (365% U.S. RDA)
Ascorbic acid ..125 mg (200% U.S. RDA)
Present in part as sodium ascorbate, USP

Other Ingredients: Colloidal silicon dioxide, flavor, glycine, hydroxypropyl methylcellulose, iron oxides, magnesium stearate, microcrystalline cellulose, polyethylene glycol, polysorbate 80, povidone, saccharin sodium, talc, titanium dioxide.

Indications: For iron deficiency anemia.

Actions: Vitron-C contains ferrous fumarate with ascorbic acid to enhance iron absorption. Vitron-C, a well-tolerated formula, is especially useful when pregnancy, menstruation, or chronic blood loss increases iron needs. The chewable, fruit-flavored, sugar-free tablets are easy to take and help improve patient compliance.

Warnings: The treatment of any anemic condition should be under the advice and supervision of a physician. As with any drug, if you are pregnant or nursing a baby, seek the advice of a health professional before using this product. **Keep this and all drugs out of the reach of children.** In case of accidental overdose, seek professional assistance or contact a Poison Control Center immediately.

Directions: Adults—one or two tablets daily or as directed by a physician. Tablet is palatable, and may be swallowed whole, chewed or sucked like a lozenge.

How Supplied: Bottles of 100 and 1000 tablets.
VITRON-C is a registered trademark of Fisons Corporation.

EDUCATIONAL MATERIAL

Americaine® Hemorrhoidal Ointment
Comforting Facts On a Painful Subject
Booklet with cents-off coupon describing hemorrhoidal conditions, with instructions on self-treatment, and when to consult a doctor.
Samples
To order FREE booklets and Americaine® Hemorrhoidal patient samples, write to Fisons Consumer Health.

Americaine® Topical Anesthetic
Make It All Better
Booklet with cents-off coupon featuring basic information on child safety/accident prevention, with instructions on self-treatment of minor pain and itching, and when to consult a doctor. To order FREE booklet, write to Fisons Consumer Health.

Caldesene®
Health and Safety Tips
Booklets with cents-off coupon and basic information on prevention of diaper rash, with instructions on home treatment, and when to consult a doctor (English and Spanish).
Samples
To order FREE booklets and Caldesene® Medicated Powder and Caldesene® Ointment patient samples, write to Fisons Consumer Health.

Fisons Corporation
P.O. BOX 1766
ROCHESTER, NY 14603

DELSYM®
(dextromethorphan polistirex)
12-Hour Cough Relief
[*del 'sĭm*]

Active Ingredient: Each teaspoonful (5 mL) contains dextromethorphan polistirex equivalent to 30 mg dextromethorphan hydrobromide.

Other Ingredients: Citric acid, ethylcellulose, FD&C Yellow No. 6, flavor, high fructose corn syrup, methylparaben, polyethylene glycol 3350, polysorbate 80, propylene glycol, propylparaben, purified water, sucrose, tragacanth, vegetable oil, xanthan gum.

Indications: Temporarily relieves cough due to minor throat and bronchial irritation as may occur with the common cold or inhaled irritants.

Warnings: Do not take this product for persistent or chronic cough such as occurs with smoking, asthma, emphysema, or if cough is accompanied by excessive phlegm (mucus) unless directed by a physician. A persistent cough may be a sign of a serious condition. If cough persists for more than 1 week, tends to recur, or is accompanied by fever, rash, or persistent headache, consult a physician. As with any drug, if you are pregnant or nursing a baby, seek the advice of a health professional before using this product. **Keep this and all drugs out of the reach of children.** In case of accidental overdose, seek professional assistance or contact a Poison Control Center immediately.

Directions: Shake Bottle Well Before Using. Dose as follows or as directed by a physician.

Adults and Children 12 years of age and over: 2 teaspoonfuls every 12 hours, not to exceed 4 teaspoonfuls in 24 hours.
Children 6 to under 12 years of age: 1 teaspoonful every 12 hours, not to exceed 2 teaspoonfuls in 24 hours.
Children 2 to under 6 years of age: ½ teaspoonful every 12 hours, not to exceed 1 teaspoonful in 24 hours.
Children under 2 years of age: Consult a physician.

How Supplied: 3 fl. oz. bottles
NDC 0585-0842-61
***FISONS* Pharmaceuticals**
Fisons Corporation
Rochester, NY 14623 USA
DELSYM is a registered trademark of Fisons Corporation.

Fleming & Company
1600 FENPARK DR.
FENTON, MO 63026

CHLOR-3
Medicinal Condiment

Active Ingredients: A troika of sodium chloride (50% 24.3 mEq/half tsp. iodized); potassium chloride (30% 11.5 mEq/half tsp.); magnesium chloride (20% 5.6 mEq/half tsp.).

Indications: The first medicinal condiment to restore needed K^+ & Mg^{++} lost during diuresis, at the expense of Na^+. To restore electrolytes lost by overcooking foods, or to add to diets that lack green vegetables, bananas, etc. And to replace conventional salting of foods in culinary and gourmet arts.

Symptoms and Treatment of Oral Overdosage: Hyperkalemia and hypermagnesemia are not end-stage results of usage.

How Supplied: In 8-oz plastic shaker, tamper-evident bottles.

IMPREGON Concentrate

Active Ingredient: Tetrachlorosalicylanilide 2%

Indications: Diaper Rash Relief, 'Staph' control, Mold inhibitor.

Actions: This is a bacteriostatic/fungistatic agent for home usage and hospital usage.

Warnings: Impregon should not be exposed to direct sunlight for long periods after applications.

Precaution: Addition of bleach prior to diaper treatment negates application effects.

Dosage and Administration: One capful (5ml) per gallon of water to impregnate diapers in the diaper pail. Dilutions for many home areas accompany the full package.

Note: For disposable-type diapers, add one teaspoonful to 8 oz of water to a 'Windex-type' sprayer. Spray middle half area of diapers until damp, and allow to dry before using, to prevent rashes.

How Supplied: Four ounce amber plastic bottles.

MAGONATE TABLETS
MAGONATE LIQUID
Magnesium Gluconate (Dihydrate)

Active Ingredients: Each tablet contains magnesium gluconate (dihydrate) 500mg (27mg of Mg^{++}). Each 5cc of Magonate Liquid contains magnesium gluconate (dihydrate) 1000mg (54mg of Mg^{++}).

Indications: For all patients in negative magnesium balance.

Precaution: Excessive dosage may cause loose stools.

Dosage and Administration: Magonate is recommended during and for three weeks after a course in chemotherapy, then monitored regularly.
Adults and children over 12 yrs.—one or two tablets or ½ to 1 teaspoon of liquid t.i.d. Under 12 yrs.—one tablet or ½ teaspoon of liquid t.i.d. Dosage may be increased in severe cases.

How Supplied: Magonate Tablets are supplied in bottles of 100 and 1000 tablets. Magonate Liquid is supplied in pints and gallons.

MARBLEN Suspensions and Tablet

Composition: A modified 'Sippy Powder' antacid containing magnesium and calcium carbonates.

Action and Uses: The peach/apricot (pink) or unflavored (green) antacid suspensions are sugar-free and neutralize 18 mEq acid per teaspoonful with a low sodium content of 18mg per fl. oz. Each pink tablet consumes 18.0 mEq acid.

Administration and Dosage: One teaspoonful rather than a tablespoonful or one tablet to reduce patient cost by ⅔.

How Supplied: Plastic pints and bottles of 100 and 1000.

NEPHROX SUSPENSION
(aluminum hydroxide)
Antacid Suspension

Composition: A watermelon flavored aluminum hydroxide (320mg as gel)/ mineral oil (10% by volume) antacid per teaspoonful.

Action and Uses: A sugar-free/saccharin-free pink suspension containing no magnesium and low sodium (19mg/oz). Extremely palatable and especially indicated in renal patients. Each teaspoon consumes 9 mEq acid.

Administration and Dosage: Two teaspoonfuls or as directed by a physician.

Caution: To be taken only at bedtime. Do not use at any other time or administer to infants, expectant women, and nursing mothers except upon the advice of a physician as this product contains mineral oil.

How Supplied: Plastic pints and gallons.

NICOTINEX Elixir
nicotinic acid

Composition: Contains niacin 50 mg./tsp. in a sherry wine base (amber color).

Action and Uses: Produces flushing when tablets fail. To increase micro-circulation of inner-ear in Meniere's, tinnitus and labyrinthine syndromes. For 'cold hands & feet', and as a vehicle for additives.

Administration and Dosage: One or two teaspoonsful on fasting stomach.

Side Effects: Patients should be warned of dermal flush. Ulcer and gout patients may be affected by 14% alcoholic content.

Contraindications: Severe hypotension and hemorrhage.

How Supplied: Plastic pints and gallons.

OCEAN MIST
(buffered saline)

Composition: Special isotonic saline, buffered with sodium bicarbonate to proper pH so as not to irritate the nose.

Action and Uses: Rhinitis medicamentosa, rhinitis sicca and atrophic rhinitis. For patients 'hooked on nose drops' and glaucoma patients on diuretics having dry nasal capillaries. OCEAN may be used as a mist or drop.

Administration and Dosage: One or two squeezes in each nostril.

Supplied: Plastic 45cc spray bottles and pints.

PURGE
(flavored castor oil)

Composition: Contains 95% castor oil (USP) in a sweetened lemon flavored base that completely masks the odor and taste of the oil.

Indications: Preparation of the bowel for x-ray, surgery and proctological procedures, IVPs, and constipation.

Dosage: Infants—1–2 teaspoonfuls. Children—adjust between infant and adult dose. Adult—2–4 tablespoonfuls.

Precaution: Not indicated when nausea, vomiting, abdominal pain or symptoms of appendicitis occur. Pregnancy, use only on advice of physician.

Supplied: Plastic 1 oz. & 2 oz. bottles.

Gebauer Company
9410 ST. CATHERINE AVENUE
CLEVELAND, OH 44104

SALIVART®
[*sal 'ĭ-vart*]
Saliva Substitute

Description: Prompt, lasting relief of dryness of the mouth or throat (hyposalivation, xerostomia).

Active Ingredients:

	%W/W
Sodium carboxymethylcellulose	1.000
Sorbitol	3.000
Sodium chloride	0.084
Potassium chloride	0.120
Calcium chloride, dihydrate	0.015
Magnesium chloride, hexahydrate	0.005
Potassium phosphate, dibasic	0.034
Inactive Ingredients:	
Purified water	95.742
	100.000

No preservatives
Propellant: Nitrogen

Indications: For reduced salivary flow, caused by medications, radiation therapy near the mouth or throat, salivary gland infection, mouth or throat inflammation, dental or oral surgery, fever, emotional factors. Also for relieving nasal crusting and bad taste.

Actions: Moistens and lubricates the oral cavity like natural saliva to allow normal eating, swallowing, and talking. Improves adherence of dentures.

Warnings: Avoid spraying in eyes. Keep out of reach of children. Contents under pressure. Do not puncture or incinerate. Protect from direct sunlight and from heat above 50°C (120°F).

Dosage and Administration: Spray Salivart directly into the mouth or throat, for 1 or 2 seconds, using it as often as needed to maintain moistness, or as instructed by physician. Nasal crusting can be relieved by applying Salivart with a cotton swab.

How Supplied:

75 Gram	NDC 0386-0009-75
25 Gram	NDC 0386-0009-25

Products are indexed by generic and chemical names in the **YELLOW SECTION.**

Herald Pharmacal, Inc.
6503 WARWICK ROAD
RICHMOND, VA 23225

AQUA GLYCOLIC LOTION

Description: Aqua Glycolic lotion is a high-potency moisturizer containing 10 per cent partially neutralized Glycolic Acid in an unscented lanolin-free lotion base.

How Supplied: 4 oz. bottles and 8 oz. bottles

AQUA GLYCOLIC SHAMPOO®

Description: Cosmetically elegant shampoo, non-irritating, containing Glycolic Acid, leaves hair soft, manageable, helps eliminate itching, leaves scalp free from scale.

How Supplied: 8 oz. bottles and 16 oz. bottles

AQUA GLYDE CLEANSER®

Description: A cleanser for acne and other oily skin conditions. Contains special denatured alcohol #40, purified water, and Glycolic Acid.

How Supplied: 8 oz. plastic bottles.

AQUARAY® 20 SUNSCREEN

Description: AQUARAY Sunscreen is free of the sensitizing ingredients PABA, Padimate O, fragrance, lanolin, alcohol and parabens. It offers a wide range of protection from both UVA and UVB sun rays.

How Supplied: 4 fl. oz. bottles.

CAM LOTION®

Description: Lipid-free, soap-free skin cleanser for atopic dermatitis and other diseases aggravated by oily, greasy substances of animal and vegetable origin.

How Supplied: 8 and 16 oz. bottles.

IDENTIFICATION PROBLEM?
Consult the
Product Identification Section
where you'll find
products pictured
in full color.

Inter-Cal Corporation
427 MILLER VALLEY RD.
PRESCOTT, AZ 86301

ESTER–C®
(Calcium Ascorbate)

Description: Each Ester-C tablets & caplets contains 500 mg Vitamin C in the form of Calcium Ascorbate 550 mg, vegetable-derived cellulose, stearic acid, and magnesium stearate. Ester-C contains no preservatives, sugars, artificial colorings, or flavorings.
As the calcium salt of L-ascorbic acid, Ester-C has an empirical formula of $CaC_{12}H_{14}O_{12}$ and a formula weight of 390.3.

Actions: Vitamin C has been found to be essential for the prevention of scurvy. In humans, an exogenous source of the vitamin is required for collagen formation and tissue repair. Ascorbate ion is reversibly oxidized to dehydroascorbate ion in the body. Both of these are active forms of the vitamin and are considered to play important roles in biochemical oxidation-reduction reactions. The vitamin is involved in tyrosine metabolism, carbohydrate metabolism, iron metabolism, folic acid-folinic acid conversion, synthesis of lipids and proteins, resistance to infections, and cellular respiration.

Indications and Usage: Vitamin C and its salts, such as Calcium Ascorbate, are recommended as nutritional supplements in the prevention of scurvy. In scurvy, collagenous structures are primarily affected, and lesions develop in blood vessels and bones. Symptoms of mild deficiency may include faulty development of teeth and bones, bleeding gums, gingivitis, and loose teeth. An increased need for the vitamin exists in febrile states, chronic illness and infection, e.g., rheumatic fever, pneumonia, tuberculosis, whooping cough, diphtheria, sinusitis, etc. Additional increases in the daily intake of ascorbate are indicated in burns, delayed healing of bone fractures and wounds, and hemovascular disorders. Immature and premature infants require relatively larger amounts of Vitamin C.

Contraindications: Because of its calcium content, Ester-C is contraindicated in hypercalcemic states, e.g., from dosing with parathyroid hormone or overdosage of Vitamin D.

Adverse Reactions: There are no known adverse reactions following ingestion of Ester-C tablets, caplets & powder. The gastric disturbances characteristic of large doses of ascorbic acid are absent or greatly diminished when the pH-neutral form of calcium ascorbate present in Ester-C tablets, caplets & powder are utilized as the source of Vitamin C supplementation.

Dosage and Administration: The minimum U.S. Recommended Daily Allowance for Vitamin C for the prevention of diseases such as scurvy is 60 mg per day. Optimum daily allowances, e.g., for the maintenance of increased plasma and cellular reserves, are significantly greater. For adults, the recommended average preventative dose of the vitamin is 70 to 150 mg daily. The recommended average optimum dose of Ester-C is 550 to 1650 mg (1 to 3 tablets or caplets) daily.
For frank scurvy, doses of 300 mg to one gram of Vitamin C daily have been recommended. Normal adults, however, have received as much as six grams of the vitamin without evidence of toxicity.
For enhancement of wound healing, doses of the vitamin approximating two Ester-C tablets, caplets and powder daily for a week or ten days both preoperatively and postoperatively are generally considered adequate, although considerably larger amounts may be recommended. In the treatment of burns, the daily number of Ester-C tablets, caplets and powder recommended is governed by the extent of tissue injury. For severe burns, daily doses of 2 to 4 tablets or caplets (approximately one to two grams of Vitamin C) are recommended.
In other conditions in which the need for increased Vitamin C is recognized, three to five times the optimum allowance appears to be adequate.

How Supplied: 550 mg tablets and caplets of Ester-C in plastic bottles of 100, 250, 90, and 225's. 4 oz. and 8 oz. powders, 275 mg tablet also available.
Store at room temperature.
U.S. Patent granted April 18, 1989; No. 4,822,816.

Literature revised: December, 1989.
Mfd. by Inter-Cal Corp.
Prescott, AZ 86301

Johnson & Johnson Consumer Products, Inc.
GRANDVIEW RD
SKILLMAN, NJ 08558

K-Y® BRAND JELLY PERSONAL LUBRICANT

Description: **K-Y® Brand Jelly Personal Lubricant** is a greaseless, water-soluble jelly which is clear, spreads easily, is non-irritating, and is safe to use with latex products.

Indications: **K-Y® Jelly** provides vaginal moisture, lubricates condoms and helps ease insertion of tampons, rectal thermometers, enemas, douches and other devices inserted into body cavities. **K-Y® Jelly** will not harm rubber, plastic, diaphragms or glass surfaces.

Actions: Helps lubricate body cavities for easier insertion. When used as a sexual lubricant, **K-Y® Jelly** helps overcome vaginal dryness from sexual intercourse, menopause, childbirth, lactation or stressful periods.

Directions: Squeeze tube to obtain desired amount of lubricant (a 1–2 inch strip should be sufficient). Reapply as needed.

Ingredients: Chlorhexidine Gluconate, Glucono Delta Lactone, Glycerin, Hydroxyethyl Cellulose, Methylparaben, Purified Water, Sodium Hydroxide

THIS PRODUCT IS NOT A CONTRACEPTIVE AND DOES NOT CONTAIN A SPERMICIDE. Store at room temperature.

How Supplied: K-Y® Jelly is available in 2 and 4 oz. tubes and a convenient 3-pack (containing 0.4 oz. tubes).

Shown in Product Identification Section, page 409

Johnson & Johnson • MERCK

Consumer Pharmaceuticals Co.
CAMP HILL ROAD
FORT WASHINGTON, PA 19034

ALternaGEL™
[al-tern 'a-jel]
Liquid
High-Potency Aluminum Hydroxide Antacid

Description: ALternaGEL is available as a white, pleasant-tasting, high-potency aluminum hydroxide liquid antacid.

Ingredients: Each 5 mL teaspoonful contains: Active: 600 mg aluminum hydroxide (equivalent to dried gel, USP) providing 16 milliequivalents (mEq) of acid-neutralizing capacity (ANC), and less than 2.5 mg (0.109 mEq) of sodium and no sugar. Inactive: butylparaben, flavors, propylparaben, purified water, simethicone, and other ingredients.

Indications: ALternaGEL is indicated for the symptomatic relief of hyperacidity associated with peptic ulcer, gastritis, peptic esophagitis, gastric hyperacidity, hiatal hernia, and heartburn.
ALternaGEL will be of special value to those patients for whom magnesium-containing antacids are undesirable, such as patients with renal insufficiency, patients requiring control of attendant G.I. complications resulting from steroid or other drug therapy, and patients experiencing the laxation which may result from magnesium or combination antacid regimens.

Directions: One to two teaspoonfuls, as needed, between meals and at bedtime, or as directed by a physician: May be followed by a sip of water if desired. Concentrated product. Shake well before using. Keep tightly closed.

Warnings: Keep this and all drugs out of the reach of children.
Except under the advice and supervision of a physician: do not take more than 18 teaspoonfuls in a 24-hour period, or use the maximum dose of ALternaGEL for more than two weeks. ALternaGEL may cause constipation.
Prolonged use of aluminum-containing antacids in patients with renal failure may result in or worsen dialysis osteomalacia. Elevated tissue aluminum levels contribute to the development of the dialysis encephalopathy and osteomalacia syndromes. Small amounts of aluminum are absorbed from the gastrointestinal tract and renal excretion of aluminum is impaired in renal failure. Aluminum is not well removed by dialysis because it is bound to albumin and transferrin, which do not cross dialysis membranes. As a result, aluminum is deposited in bone, and dialysis osteomalacia may develop when large amounts of aluminum are ingested orally by patients with impaired renal function.
Aluminum forms insoluble complexes with phosphate in the gastrointestinal tract, thus decreasing phosphate absorption. Prolonged use of aluminum-containing antacids by normophosphatemic patients may result in hypophosphatemia if phosphate intake is not adequate. In its more severe forms, hypophosphatemia can lead to anorexia, malaise, muscle weakness, and osteomalacia.

Drug Interaction Precaution:
Do not use this product for any patient receiving a prescription antibiotic containing any form of tetracycline.

How Supplied: ALternaGEL is available in bottles of 12 fluid ounces and 5 fluid ounces, and 1 fluid ounce hospital unit doses. NDC 16837-860

Shown in Product Identification Section, page 409

DIALOSE® Tablets
[di 'a-lose]
Stool Softener Laxative

Description: DIALOSE is a very low sodium, nonhabit forming, stool softener containing 100 mg docusate sodium per tablet.
The docusate in DIALOSE is a highly efficient surfactant which facilitates absorption of water by the stool to form a soft, easily evacuated mass. Unlike stimulant laxatives, DIALOSE does not interfere with normal peristalsis, neither does it cause griping nor sensations of urgency.

Ingredients: Active: docusate sodium, 100 mg per tablet
Inactive: Colloidal silicon dioxide, D & C Red No. 28, D & C Red No. 27, Dextrates, FD & C Blue No. 1, FD & C Red No. 40, Flavors, Hydroxypropyl Methylcellulose, Magnesium Stearate, Microcrystalline Cellulose, Polyethylene Glycol, Polysorbate 80, Pregelatinized Starch, Propylene Glycol, Sodium Starch Glycolate, Titanium Dioxide.

Indications: DIALOSE is indicated for the relief of occasional constipation (irregularity).
DIALOSE is an effective aid to soften or prevent formation of hard stools in a wide range of conditions that may lead to constipation. DIALOSE helps to eliminate straining associated with obstetric, geriatric, cardiac, surgical, anorectal, or proctologic conditions. In cases of mild constipation, the fecal softening action of DIALOSE can prevent constipation from progressing and relieve painful defecation.

Directions: *Adults:* One tablet, one to three times daily: adjust dosage as needed.
Children 6 to under 12 years: One tablet daily or as directed by physician.
Children under 6 years: As directed by physician.
It is helpful to increase the daily intake of fluids by taking a glass of water with each dose.

Warnings: Unless directed by a physician: Do not use when abdominal pain, nausea, or vomiting are present. Do not use for a period longer than one week. Do not take this product if you are presently taking a prescription drug or mineral oil. As with any drug, if you are pregnant or nursing a baby, seek the advice of a health professional before using this product.
Keep out of the reach of children.

How Supplied: Bottles of 36 and 100 pink tablets. Also available in 100 tablet unit dose boxes (10 strips of 10 tablets each). NDC 16837-870.

Shown in Product Identification Section, page 409

DIALOSE® PLUS Tablets
[di 'a-lose Plus]
Stool Softener/Stimulant Laxative

Description: DIALOSE PLUS provides a very low sodium tablet formulation of 100 mg docusate sodium and 65 mg yellow phenolphthalein.

Ingredients: Each tablet contains: Actives: docusate sodium, 100 mg., yellow phenolphthalein, 65 mg.
Inactives: D & C Yellow No. 10, Dextrates, Dibasic Calcium Phosphate Dihydrate, FD & C Red No. 40, Flavors, Hydroxypropyl Methylcellulose, Magnesium Stearate, Microcrystalline Cellulose, Polydextrose, Polyethylene Glycol, Polysorbate 80, Sodium Starch Glycolate, Titanium Dioxide, Triacetin.

Indications: DIALOSE PLUS is indicated for the treatment of constipation characterized by lack of moisture in the intestinal contents, resulting in hardness of stool and decreased intestinal motility. DIALOSE PLUS combines the advantages of the stool softener, docusate sodium, with the peristaltic activating effect of yellow phenolphthalein.

Directions: *Adults:* One or two tablets daily as needed, at bedtime or on arising.
Children 6 to under 12 years: One tablet daily as needed
Children under 6 years: As directed by physician.

Continued on next page

J&J • Merck —Cont.

It is helpful to increase the daily intake of fluids by taking a glass of water with each dose.

Warnings: Unless directed by a physician: Do not use when abdominal pain, nausea, or vomiting are present. Do not use for a period longer than one week. If skin rash appears do not use this product or any other preparation containing phenolphthalein. Frequent or prolonged use may result in dependence on laxatives. Do not take this product if you are presently taking a prescription drug or mineral oil.
As with any drug, if you are pregnant or nursing a baby, seek the advice of a health professional before using this. Keep out of the reach of children.

How Supplied: Bottles of 36 and 100 yellow tablets. Also available in 100 capsule unit dose boxes (10 strips of 10 capsules each). NDC 16837-871.

Shown in Product Identification Section, page 409

EFFER-SYLLIUM®

[*ef'fer-sil'lium*]

Natural Fiber Bulking Agent

Description: EFFER-SYLLIUM is a tan, granular powder. Each rounded teaspoonful, or individual packet (7 g) contains psyllium hydrocolloid, 3 g.

Ingredients: Active: psyllium hydrocolloid. Inactive: citric acid, ethyl vanillin, lemon and lime flavors, potassium bicarbonate, potassium citrate, saccharin calcium, starch, sucrose.
EFFER-SYLLIUM contains less than 5 mg sodium per rounded teaspoonful and is considered dietetically sodium free.

Indications: EFFER-SYLLIUM is indicated to restore normal bowel habits in chronic constipation, to promote normal elimination in irritable bowel syndrome, and to ease passage of stools in presence of anorectal disorders. EFFER-SYLLIUM produces a soft, lubricating bulk which promotes natural elimination.
EFFER-SYLLIUM is not a one-dose, fast-acting bowel regulator. Administration for several days may be needed to establish regularity.

Directions:
Adults: One rounded teaspoonful, or one packet, in a glass of water one to three times a day, or as directed by physician. *Children, 6 years and over:* One level teaspoonful, or one-half packet (3.5 g) in one-half glass of water at bedtime, or as directed by physician. *Children, under 6 years:* As directed by physician.

Instructions: Pour EFFER-SYLLIUM into a *dry* glass, add water and stir briskly. Drink immediately. To avoid caking, always use a *dry* spoon to remove EFFER-SYLLIUM from its container. Replace cap tightly. Keep in a dry place.

Warning: Avoid inhalation. May cause a potentially severe reaction when inhaled by persons sensitive to psyllium powder or suffering from respiratory disorders. As with all medications, keep out of the reach of children.

How Supplied: Bottles of 9 oz and 16 oz, and individual convenience packets (7 g each) packaged in boxes of 24. NDC 16837-440.

Shown in Product Identification Section, page 409

FERANCEE®

[*fer'an-see*]

Chewable Hematinic

Two Tablets Daily Provide:

	US RDA*	
Iron	744%	134 mg
Vitamin C	500%	300 mg

*Percentage of US Recommended Daily Allowances for adults and children 4 or more years of age.

Ingredients: Active: ferrous fumarate, sodium ascorbate, ascorbic acid. Inactive: confectioner's sugar, flavors, magnesium stearate, mannitol, povidone, saccharin calcium, starch, Yellow 5 (tartrazine), Yellow 6.

Indications: A pleasant-tasting hematinic for iron deficiency anemias, well-tolerated FERANCEE is particularly useful when chronic blood loss, onset of menses, or pregnancy create additional demands for iron supplementation. Available information indicates a low incidence of staining of the teeth by ferrous fumarate, alone or in combination with ascorbic acid. The peach-cherry flavored chewable tablets dissolve quickly in the mouth and may be either chewed or swallowed.

Directions:
Adults: Two tablets daily, or as directed by physician.
Chidren over 6 years of age: One tablet daily, or as directed by physician.
Children under 6 years of age: As directed by physician.

Warnings: As with any drug, if you are pregnant or nursing a baby, seek the advice of a health professional before using this product. Keep out of the reach of children. In case of accidental overdose, seek professional assistance or contact a Poison Control Center immediately.

How Supplied: FERANCEE is supplied in bottles of 100 brown and yellow, two-layer tablets. A child-resistant cap is standard on each bottle as a safeguard against accidental ingestion by children. Keep in a dry place. Replace cap tightly. NDC 16837-650.

Shown in Product Identification Section, page 409

FERANCEE®-HP Tablets

[*fer-an-see hp*]

High Potency Hematinic

One Tablet Daily Provides:

	US RDA*	
Iron	611%	110 mg
Vitamin C	1000%	600 mg

*Percentage of US Recommended Daily Allowances for adults and children 4 or more years of age.

Ingredients: Active: ferrous fumarate, sodium ascorbate, ascorbic acid. Inactive: flavor, hydrogenated vegetable oil, microcrystalline cellulose, povidone, Red 40, and other ingredients.

Indications: FERANCEE-HP is a high potency formulation of iron and vitamin C and is intended for use as either:
(1) a maintenance hematinic for those patients needing a daily iron supplement to maintain normal hemoglobin levels, or
(2) intensive therapy for the acute and/or severe iron deficiency anemia where a high intake of elemental iron is required.

The use of well-tolerated ferrous fumarate provides high levels of elemental iron with a low incidence of gastric distress. The inclusion of 600 mg of vitamin C per tablet serves to maintain more of the iron in the absorbable ferrous state.

Precautions: Because FERANCEE-HP contains 110 mg of elemental iron per tablet, it is recommended that its use be limited to adults, ie over 12 years of age.

Directions: One tablet per day after a meal or as directed by a physician should be sufficient to maintain normal hemoglobin levels in most patients with a history of recurring iron deficiency anemia. Not recommended for children under 12 years of age.
For acute and/or severe iron deficiency anemia, two or three tablets per day taken one tablet per dose after meals. (Each tablet provides 110 mg elemental iron.)

Warnings: As with all medications, keep out of the reach of children. In case of accidental overdose, seek professional assistance or contact a Poison Control Center immediately.

How Supplied: FERANCEE-HP is supplied in bottles of 60 red, film coated, oval shaped tablets.
NDC 16837-863.
Note: A child-resistant safety cap is standard on each bottle of 60 tablets as a safeguard against accidental ingestion by children.

Shown in Product Identification Section, page 410

MYLANTA®

[*my-lan'ta*]

Alumina, Magnesia and Simethicone Liquid and Tablets Antacid/Anti-Gas

Description: MYLANTA is a well-balanced, pleasant-tasting antacid/anti-gas medication that provides consistent, effective relief of symptoms associated with gastric hyperacidity and excess gas. Non-constipating and dietetically sodium-free, MYLANTA contains two proven antacids, magnesium hydroxide and aluminum hydroxide, plus simethicone for gas relief.

Ingredients: Each 5mL (one teaspoonful) of liquid suspension or each chewable tablet contains: **Active:** Magnesium hydroxide 200 mg, Aluminum hydroxide (Dried Gel, USP in tablet and equiv. to Dried Gel USP in liquid) 200 mg and Simethicone 20 mg. **Inactive:** Tablets: Colloidal silicon dioxide, dextrates, flavors, magnesium stearate, mannitol, sodium saccharin, sorbitol, FD & C Blue 1 or FD & C Red 27 or D & C Yellow 10. Liquid: Butylparaben, carboxymethylcellulose sodium, flavors, hydroxypropyl methylcellulose, microcrystalline cellulose, propylparaben, purified water, saccharin sodium and sorbitol.
Sodium Content: MYLANTA contains an insignificant amount of sodium per daily dose and is considered dietetically sodium-free. Typical values are 0.68 mg (0.03 mEq) sodium per 5 mL teaspoonful of liquid and 0.77 mg (0.03 mEq) per tablet.
Acid Neutralizing Capacity: Two teaspoonfuls of MYLANTA liquid has an acid neutralizing capacity, as measured in laboratory testing, of 25.4 mEq. Two MYLANTA tablets have an acid neutralizing capacity of 23.0 mEq.

Indications: As an antacid for symptomatic relief of hyperacidity associated with the diagnosis of peptic ulcer, gastritis, peptic esophagitis, heartburn and hiatal hernia. As an antiflatulent to alleviate the symptoms of mucus-entrapped gas, including postoperative gas pain.

Advantages: MYLANTA is homogenized for a smooth, creamy taste. The choice of two pleasant-tasting liquid flavors and the non-constipating formula encourage patient acceptance, thereby minimizing the skipping of prescribed doses. MYLANTA is also available in tablets, and both the liquid and tablet forms are sodium-free. MYLANTA provides consistent relief in patients suffering from distress associated with hyperacidity, mucus-entrapped gas, or swallowed air.

Directions:
Liquid: Shake well. 2–4 teaspoonfuls between meals and at bedtime or as directed by a physician.
Tablets: 2–4 tablets, well chewed, between meals and at bedtime or as directed by a physician.

Warnings: Keep this and all other drugs out of the reach of children. Do not take more than 24 tsps/tablets in a 24 hour period or use the maximum dose of this product for more than two weeks, except under the advice and supervision of a physician. Do not use this product if you have kidney disease.

Prolonged use of aluminum-containing antacids in patients with renal failure may result in or worsen dialysis osteomalacia. Elevated tissue aluminum levels contribute to the development of the dialysis encephalopathy and osteomalacia syndromes. Small amounts of aluminum are absorbed from the gastrointestinal tract and renal excretion of aluminum is impaired in renal failure. Aluminum is not well removed by dialysis because it is bound to albumin and transferrin, which do not cross dialysis membranes. As a result, aluminum is deposited in bone, and dialysis osteomalacia may develop when large amounts of aluminum are ingested orally by patients with impaired renal function.
Aluminum forms insoluble complexes with phosphate in the gastrointestinal tract, thus decreasing phosphate absorption. Prolonged use of aluminum-containing antacids by normophosphatemic patients may result in hypophosphatemia if phosphate intake is not adequate. In its more severe forms, hypophosphatemia can lead to anorexia, malaise, muscle weakness, and osteomalacia.

Drug Interaction Precaution: Do not use this product for any patient receiving a prescription antibiotic containing any form of tetracycline.

How Supplied: MYLANTA is available as a white liquid suspension in pleasant-tasting flavors, Original Cherry Creme, and Cool Mint Creme, and as a two-layer green and white chewable Cool Mint Creme flavored tablet, as well as a two-layer pink and white Cherry Creme flavored tablet identified as "MYLANTA." Liquid supplied in bottles of 5 oz, 12 oz, and 24 oz. Tablets supplied in bottles of 48 and 100 count sizes and in 12 tablet rollpacks. Also available for hospital use in liquid unit dose bottles of 1 oz, and bottles of 5 oz.
NDC 16837-610 (original liquid). NDC 16837-620 (cool mint creme tablets).
NDC 16837-621 (cherry creme liquid).
NDC 16837-628 (cherry creme tablets).
NDC 16837-629 (cool mint creme liquid).

Shown in Product Identification Section, page 410

MYLANTA® DOUBLE STRENGTH
[*my-lan 'ta*]
Alumina, Magnesia and Simethicone Liquid and Tablets
Double-Strength Antacid/Anti-Gas

Description: MYLANTA DOUBLE STRENGTH is a well-balanced, high-potency antacid/anti-gas medication that provides rapid, effective, and long-lasting relief of symptoms associated with gastric hyperacidity and excess gas. Pleasant-tasting, non-constipating and dietetically sodium-free, MYLANTA DOUBLE STRENGTH contains two proven antacids, magnesium hydroxide and aluminum hydroxide, plus simethicone for gas relief.

Ingredients: Each 5 mL (one teaspoonful) of liquid suspension or each chewable tablet contains: Active: Magnesium hydroxide 400 mg, Aluminum hydroxide (Dried Gel, USP in tablet and equiv. to Dried Gel USP in liquid) 400 mg and Simethicone 40 mg. Inactive: Tablets: Colloidal silicon dioxide, dextrates, flavors, magnesium stearate, mannitol, sodium saccharin, sorbitol, FD & C Blue 1 or FD & C Red 27 or D & C Yellow 10. Liquid: Butylparaben, carboxymethylcellulose sodium, flavors, hydroxypropyl methylcellulose, microcrystalline cellulose, potassium citrate, propylparaben, purified water, saccharin sodium and sorbitol.
Sodium Content: MYLANTA DOUBLE STRENGTH contains an insignficant amount of sodium per daily dose. Typical values are 1.14 mg (0.05 mEq) sodium per 5 mL teaspoonful of liquid and 1.3 mg (0.06 mEq) per tablet.
Acid Neutralizing Capacity: Two teaspoonfuls of MYLANTA DOUBLE STRENGTH liquid has an acid neutralizing capacity of 50.8 mEq, as measured in laboratory testing. Two MYLANTA DOUBLE STRENGTH tablets have an acid neutralizing capacity of 46.0 mEq.

Indications: As an antacid for symptomatic relief of hyperacidity associated with the diagnosis of peptic ulcer, gastritis, peptic esophagitis, heartburn and hiatal hernia. As an antiflatulent to alleviate the symptoms of mucus-entrapped gas, including postoperative gas pain.

Advantages: MYLANTA DOUBLE STRENGTH is homogenized for a smooth, creamy taste. The choice of three pleasant-tasting liquid flavors and the non-constipating formula encourage patient acceptance, thereby minimizing the skipping of prescribed doses. MYLANTA DOUBLE STRENGTH is also available in tablets, and both the liquid and tablet forms are sodium-free. The high potency of MYLANTA DOUBLE STRENGTH is achieved through greater concentration of two proven antacid ingredients, plus simethicone. MYLANTA DOUBLE STRENGTH provides rapid, consistent and long-lasting relief in patients suffering from distress associated with hyperacidity, mucus-entrapped gas, or swallowed air.

Directions:
Liquid: Shake well. 2–4 teaspoonfuls between meals and at bedtime, or as directed by a physician.
Tablets: 2–4 tablets, well chewed, between meals and at bedtime, or as directed by a physician.
Because patients with peptic ulcer vary greatly in both acid output and gastric emptying time, the amount and schedule of dosages should be varied accordingly.

Warnings: Keep this and all drugs out of the reach of children. Do not take more than 12 tsps/tablets in a 24-hour period or use the maximum dose of this product for more than two weeks, except under

Continued on next page

J&J • Merck —Cont.

advice and supervision of a physician. Do not use this product if you have kidney disease.

Prolonged use of aluminum-containing antacids in patients with renal failure may result in or worsen dialysis osteomalacia. Elevated tissue aluminum levels contribute to the development of the dialysis encephalopathy and osteomalacia syndromes. Small amounts of aluminum are absorbed from the gastrointestinal tract and renal excretion of aluminum is impaired in renal failure. Aluminum is not well removed by dialysis because it is bound to albumin and transferrin, which do not cross dialysis membranes. As a result, aluminum is deposited in bone, and dialysis osteomalacia may develop when large amounts of aluminum are ingested orally by patients with impaired renal function.

Aluminum forms insoluble complexes with phosphate in the gastrointestinal tract, thus decreasing phosphate absorption. Prolonged use of aluminum-containing antacids by normophosphatemic patients may result in hypophosphatemia if phosphate intake is not adequate. In its more severe forms, hypophosphatemia can lead to anorexia, malaise, muscle weakness, and osteomalacia.

Drug Interaction Precaution: Do not use this product for any patient receiving a prescription antibiotic containing any form of tetracycline.

How Supplied: MYLANTA DOUBLE STRENGTH is available as a white liquid suspension in three pleasant-tasting flavors, Original, Cherry Creme, and Cool Mint Creme, and in a two-layer, green and white chewable Cool Mint Creme flavored tablet, as well as a two-layer pink and white Cherry Creme flavored tablet identified as "Mylanta DS". Liquid supplied in 5 oz, 12 oz and 24 oz bottles. Tablets supplied in bottles of 30 and 60 count sizes, and 8 tablet roll packs. Also available for hospital use in liquid unit dose bottles of 1 oz, and bottles of 5 oz.

NDC 16837-652 (original liquid). NDC 16837-651 (cool mint creme tablets).
NDC 16837-624 (cool mint creme liquid).
NDC 16837-622 (cherry creme liquid).
NDC 16837-627 (cherry creme tablets).

Professional Labeling

Indications: Stress-induced upper gastrointestinal hemorrhage: MYLANTA DOUBLE STRENGTH is indicated for the prevention of stress-induced upper gatrointestinal hemorrhage.

Hyperacidic conditions: As an antacid, for the symptomatic relief of hyperacidity associated with the diagnosis of peptic ulcer and other gastrointestinal conditions where a high degree of acid neutralization is desired.

Directions: Prevention of stress-induced upper gastrointestinal hemorrhage: 1) Aspirate stomach via nasogastric tube* and record pH. 2) Instill 10 mL of MYLANTA DOUBLE STRENGTH followed by 30 mL of water via nasogastric tube. Clamp tube. 3) Wait one hour. Aspirate stomach and record pH. 4a) If pH equals or exceeds 4.0, apply drainage or intermittent suction for one hour, then repeat the cycle. 4b) If pH is less than 4.0, instill double (20 mL) MYLANTA DOUBLE STRENGTH followed by 30 mL of water. Clamp tube. 5) Wait one hour. If pH equals or exceeds 4.0, see number 7, if pH is still less than 4.0, instill double (40 mL) MYLANTA DOUBLE STRENGTH followed by 30 mL of water. Clamp tube. 6) Wait one hour. If pH equals or exceeds 4.0, see number 7. If pH is still less than 4.0, instill double (80 mL)† MYLANTA DOUBLE STRENGTH followed by 30 mL of water. 7) Drain for one hour and repeat cycle with the effective dosage of MYLANTA DOUBLE STRENGTH.

In hyperacid states for symptomatic relief: One or two teaspoonfuls as needed between meals and at bedtime or as directed by a physician. Higher dosage regimens may be employed under the direct supervision of a physician in the treatment of active peptic ulcer disease.

Precaution: Aluminum-magnesium hydroxide containing antacids should be used with caution in patients with renal impairment.

Adverse Effects: Occasional regurgitation and mild diarrhea have been reported with the dosage recommended for the prevention of stress-induced upper gastrointestinal hemorrhage.

References: 1. Zinner MJ, Zuidema GD, Smigh PL, Mignosa M: The prevention of upper gastrointestinal tract bleeding in patients in an intensive care unit. *Surg Gynecol Obster* 153:214–220, 1981. 2. Lucas CE, Sugawa C, Riddle J, et al.: Natural history and surgical dilemma of "stress" gastric bleeding. *Arch Surg* 102:266–273, 1971. 3. Hastings PR, Skillman JJ, Bushnell LS, Silen W: Antacid titration in the prevention of acute gastrointestinal bleeding: a controlled, randomized trial in 100 critically ill patients. *N Engl J Med* 298:1042–1045, 1978. 4. Day SB, MacMillan BG, Altemeier WA: *Curling's Ulcer, An Experience of Nature.* Springfield, IL, Charles C Thomas Co., 1972, p. 205. 5. Skillman JJ, Bushnell LS, Goldman H, Silen W: Respiratory failure, hypotension, sepsis, and jaundice. A clinical syndrome associated with lethal hemorrhage from acute stress ulceration of the stomach. *Am J Surg* 117:523–530, 1969. 6. Priebe HJ, Skillman J, Bushnell LS, et al. Antacid versus cimetidine in preventing acute gastrointestinal bleeding. *N Engl J Med* 302:426–430, 1980. 7. Silen W: The prevention and management of stress ulcers. *Hosp Pract* 15:93–97, 1980. 8. Herrmann V, Kaminski DL: Evaluation of intragastric pH in acutely ill patients. *Arch Surg* 114:511–514, 1979. 9. Martin LF, Staloch DK, Simonowitz DA, et al.: Failure of cimetidine prophylaxis in the critically ill. *Arch Surg* 114:492–496, 1979. 10. Zinner MJ, Turtinen L, Gurll NJ, Reynolds DG: The effect of metiamide on gastric mucosal injury in rat restraint. *Clin Res* 23:484A, 1975. 11. Zinner M, Turtinen BA, Gurll NJ: The role of acid and ischemia in production of stress ulcers during canine hemorrhagic shock. *Surgery* 77:807–816, 1975. 12. Winans CS: Prevention and treatment of stress ulcer bleeding: Antacids or cimetidine? *Drug Ther Bull* (hospital) 12:37–45, 1981.

*If nasogastric tube is not in place, administer 20 mL of MYLANTA DOUBLE STRENGTH orally q2h.

†In a recent clinical study[1] 20 mL of MYLANTA DOUBLE STRENGTH, q2h, was sufficient in more than 85 percent of the patients. No patient studied required more than 80 mL of MYLANTA DOUBLE STRENGTH q2h.

Shown in Product Identification Section, page 410

MYLANTA® GAS—40 mg Tablets
MYLICON® Drops

[my'li-con]

Antiflatulent

Ingredients: Each tablet or 0.6 mL of drops contains: Active: simethicone, 40 mg. Inactive: Tablets: calcium silicate, lactose, povidone, saccharin calcium. Drops: carbomer 934P, citric acid, flavors, hydroxypropyl methylcellulose, purified water, Red 3, saccharin calcium, sodium benzoate, sodium citrate.

Indications: Adults and children: For relief of the painful symptoms of excess gas in the digestive tract. Such gas is frequently caused by excessive swallowing of air or by eating foods that disagree. MYLANTA Gas-40 mg is a valuable adjunct in the treatment of many conditions in which the retention of gas may be a problem, such as: postoperative gaseous distention, air swallowing, peptic ulcer, spastic or irritable colon, diverticulosis. If condition persists, consult your physician.

Infants: MYLICON drops are also useful for relief of the painful symptoms of excess gas associated with excessive swallowing of air or food intolerance.

The defoaming action of MYLICON relieves flatulence by dispersing and preventing the formation of mucus-surrounded gas pockets in the gastrointestinal tract. MYLICON acts in the stomach and intestines to change the surface tension of gas bubbles enabling them to coalesce; thus the gas is freed and is eliminated more easily by belching or passing flatus.

Directions:

Tablets—One or two tablets four times daily after meals and at bedtime. May also be taken as needed up to 12 tablets daily or as directed by a physician. TABLETS SHOULD BE CHEWED THOROUGHLY.

Drops—Adults and Children: 0.6 mL four times daily after meals and at bedtime or

as directed by a physician. Shake well before using.
Infants (under 2 years): Initially, 0.3 mL four times daily, after meals and at bedtime, or as directed by a physician.
The dosage can also be mixed with 1 oz of cool water, infant formula, or other suitable liquids to ease administration.

Warnings: Do not exceed 12 doses per day except under the advice and supervision of a physician. Keep this and all drugs out of the reach of children.

How Supplied: Bottles of 100 white, scored, chewable tablets, identified MYL GAS 40, and dropper bottles of 15 mL (0.5 fl. oz) and 30 mL (1 fl oz) pink, pleasant tasting liquid. Also available in 100 tablet unit dose boxes (10 strips of 10 tablets each).
NDC 16837-450 (tablets).
NDC 16837-630 (drops).

Shown in Product Identification Section, page 410

MYLANTA® GAS Tablets
High-Capacity Antiflatulent

Ingredients: Each tablet contains:
Active: simethicone, 80 mg.
Inactive: dextrates, flavor, sorbitol, stearic acid, tricalcium phosphate.

Indications: For relief of the painful symptoms of excess gas in the digestive tract. Such gas is frequently caused by excessive swallowing of air or by eating foods that disagree. MYLANTA® GAS is a high capacity antiflatulent for adjunctive treatment of many conditions in which the retention of gas may be a problem, such as the following: air swallowing, postoperative gaseous distention, peptic ulcer, spastic or irritable colon, diverticulosis. If condition persists, consult your physician.
MYLANTA® GAS has a defoaming action that relieves flatulence by dispersing and preventing the formation of mucus-surrounded gas pockets in the gastrointestinal tract. MYLANTA® GAS acts in the stomach and intestines to change the surface tension of gas bubbles enabling them to coalesce; thus, the gas is freed and is eliminated more easily by belching or passing flatus.

Directions: One tablet four times daily after meals and at bedtime. May also be taken as needed up to 6 tablets daily or as directed by a physician. TABLETS SHOULD BE CHEWED THOROUGHLY.

Warnings: Keep this and all drugs out of the reach of children.

How Supplied: Economical bottles of 100 and convenience packages of individually wrapped 12 and 48 pink, scored, chewable tablets identified MYL GAS 80. Also available in 100 tablet unit dose boxes (10 strips of 10 tablets each).
NDC 16837-858.

Shown in Product Identification Section, page 410

MYLANTA® GELCAPS ANTACID
[mīlăntă]
Antacid

Description: MYLANTA® GELCAPS are a tasteless, non-chalky, easy to swallow antacid. The better way to get potent antacid relief.

Ingredients: Each MYLANTA® GELCAP contains:
Active: Calcium carbonate 311 mg, magnesium carbonate 232 mg.
Inactives: Benzyl alcohol, butylparaben, castor oil, D&C yellow 10, disodium calcium edetate, FD&C blue 1, gelatin, hydroxypropyl cellulose, magnesium stearate, methylparaben, microcrystalline cellulose, propylparaben, sodium croscarmellose, sodium lauryl sulfate, sodium propionate, titanium dioxide.
Acid Neutralizing Capacity: Two Mylanta® GELCAPS have an acid neutralizing capacity of 23.0 Meq.

Indications: For the relief of acid indigestion, heartburn, sour stomach and upset stomach associated with these symptoms.

Directions: Take 2-4 gelcaps as needed or as directed by a physician.

Warnings: Keep this and all other drugs out of the reach of children. Do not take more than 24 gelcaps in a 24 hour period or use the maximum dosage for more than two weeks or use if you have kidney disease, except under the advice and supervision of a physician.

How Supplied: MYLANTA® GELCAPS are available as a swallowable blue and white gelcap identified "MYLANTA GELCAP." Supplied in bottles of 50 and boxes of 24 individual blisterpacks.
NDC 16837-850

Shown in Product Identification Section, page 410

Maximum Strength MYLANTA® GAS Tablets
Maximum Strength Antiflatulent

Ingredients: Each tablet contains:
Active: simethicone, 125 mg.
Inactive: dextrates, flavor, sorbitol, stearic acid, tricalcium phosphate.

Indications: Maximum Strength MYLANTA® GAS is useful for relief of the painful symptoms of excess gas in the digestive tract. Such gas is frequently caused by excessive swallowing of air or by eating foods that disagree. Maximum Strength MYLANTA® GAS is the strongest possible antiflatulent for adjunctive treatment of many conditions in which the retention of gas may be a problem, such as the following: air swallowing, postoperative gaseous distention, peptic ulcer, spastic or irritable colon, diverticulosis. If condition persists, consult your physician.
Maximum Strength MYLANTA® GAS has a defoaming action that relieves flatulence by dispersing and preventing the formation of mucus-surrounded gas pockets in the gastrointestinal tract. Maximum Strength MYLANTA® GAS acts in the stomach and intestines to change the surface tension of gas bubbles enabling them to coalesce; thus, the gas is freed and is eliminated more easily by belching or passing flatus.

Directions: One tablet four times daily after meals and at bedtime or as directed by physician. TABLETS SHOULD BE CHEWED THOROUGHLY.

Warnings: Keep this and all drugs out of the reach of children.

How Supplied: Convenience packages of individually wrapped 12 and 60 white, scored chewable tablets identified MYL GAS 125. NDC 16837-455.

Shown in Product Identification Section, page 410

THE STUART FORMULA® Tablets
Multivitamin/Multimineral Supplement

One Tablet Daily Provides:

VITAMINS:	US RDA*	
A	100%	5,000 IU
D	100%	400 IU
E	50%	15 IU
C	100%	60 mg
Folic Acid	100%	0.4 mg
B_1 (thiamin)	80%	1.2 mg
B_2 (riboflavin)	100%	1.7 mg
Niacin	100%	20 mg
B_6 (pyridoxine hydrochloride)	100%	2 mg
B_{12} (cyanocobalamin)	100%	6 mcg
MINERALS:	**US RDA**	
Calcium	16%	160 mg
Phosphorus	12%	125 mg
Iodine	100%	150 mcg
Iron	100%	18 mg
Magnesium	25%	100 mg

*Percentage of US Recommended Daily Allowances for adults and children 4 or more years of age.

Ingredients: Each tablet contains:
Active: dibasic calcium phosphate, magnesium oxide, ascorbic acid, ferrous fumarate, dl-alpha tocopheryl acetate, folic acid, niacinamide, vitamin A palmitate, cyanocobalamin, pyridoxine hydrochloride, riboflavin, thiamin mononitrate, ergocalciferol, potassium iodide. Inactive: calcium sulfate, carnauba wax, pharmaceutical glaze, povidone, sodium starch glycolate, starch, sucrose, titanium dioxide, white wax.

Indications: The STUART FORMULA tablet provides a well-balanced multivitamin/multimineral formula intended for use as a daily dietary supplement for adults and children over age four.

Directions: One tablet daily or as directed by physician.

Warnings: Keep this and all drugs out of the reach of children. In case of acci-

Continued on next page

J&J • Merck —Cont.

dental overdose, seek professional assistance or contact a Poison Control Center immediately.

How Supplied: Bottles of 100 and 250 white round tablets. Child-resistant safety caps are standard on both bottles as a safeguard against accidental ingestion by children.
NDC 16837-866.

Shown in Product Identification Section, page 410

STUARTINIC® Tablets
[*stu "are-tin 'ic*]
Hematinic

One Tablet Daily Provides:

	US RDA*	
Iron	556%	100 mg
VITAMINS:		
C	833%	500 mg
B_1 (thiamin)	327%	4.9 mg
B_2 (riboflavin)	353%	6 mg
Niacin	100%	20 mg
B_6 (pyridoxine hydrochloride)	40%	0.8 mg
B_{12} (cyanocobalamin)	417%	25 mcg
Pantothenic Acid	92%	9.2 mg

*Percentage of US Recommended Daily Allowances for adults and children 4 or more years of age.

Ingredients: Active: ferrous fumarate, ascorbic acid, sodium ascorbate, niacinamide, calcium pantothenate, thiamin mononitrate, riboflavin, pyridoxine hydrochloride, cyanocobalamin. Inactive: flavor, hydrogenated vegetable oil, microcrystalline cellulose, povidone, Yellow 6, Yellow 10, and other ingredients.

Indications: STUARTINIC is a complete hematinic for patients with history of iron deficiency anemia who also lack proper amounts of vitamin C and B-complex vitamins due to inadequate diet.
The use of well-tolerated ferrous fumarate in STUARTINIC provides a high level of elemental iron with a low incidence of gastric distress. The inclusion of 500 mg of Vitamin C per tablet serves to maintain more of the iron in the absorbable ferrous state. The B-complex vitamins improve nutrition where B-complex deficient diets contribute to the anemia.

Warnings: As with any drug, if you are pregnant or nursing a baby, seek the advice of a health professional before using this product. Keep out of the reach of children. In case of accidental overdose, seek professional assistance or contact a Poison Control Center immediately.

Dosage: One tablet daily taken after a meal or as directed by physician. Because of the high amount of iron per tablet, STUARTINIC is not recommended for children under 12 years of age.

How Supplied: STUARTINIC is supplied in bottles of 60 yellow, film coated, oval shaped tablets. NDC 16837-862.
Note: A child-resistant safety cap is standard on each 60 tablet bottle as a safeguard against accidental ingestion by children.

Shown in Product Identification Section, page 410

Konsyl Pharmaceuticals, Inc.
4200 S. HULEN
FORT WORTH, TX 76109

KONSYL® POWDER
(psyllium hydrophilic mucilloid)
Sugar Free, Sugar Substitute Free.
6.0 grams of psyllium per TEASPOON

Description: Konsyl is a bulk-forming natural therapeutic fiber for restoring and maintaining regularity. Konsyl contains 100% hydrophilic mucilloid, a highly efficient dietary fiber derived from the husk of the psyllium seed. Konsyl contains no chemical stimulants and is non-addictive. Each dose contains 6.0 grams of psyllium compared to 3.4 grams of psyllium in most other products.

Inactive Ingredients: None. Each 6 gram dose provides 3 calories. Konsyl is sodium free. Since Konsyl is sugar free, it is excellent for diabetics who require a bowel normalizer.

Actions: Konsyl provides bulk that promotes normal elimination. The product is uniform, instantly miscible, palatable, and non-irritative in the gastrointestinal tract.

Indications: Konsyl is indicated in the management of chronic constipation, irritable bowel syndrome, as adjunctive therapy in the constipation of diverticular disease, bowel management of patients with hemorrhoids, and for constipation during pregnancy, convalescence, and senility. Konsyl is also indicated for other indications as prescribed by physician.

Contraindications: May cause allergic reaction in people sensitive to inhaled or ingested psyllium powder.

Dosage and Administration:
ADULTS: Place one rounded teaspoon (6.0 grams) into a dry shaker cup or container that can be closed. Add 8 oz. of juice or other beverage rather than water. Shake, don't stir, for 3–5 seconds. Drink immediately. Follow with an 8 oz. glass of juice or water to aid product action. Konsyl can be taken one to three times daily, depending on need and response. It may require continued use for 2–3 days to provide optimal benefit. When taking Konsyl, one should drink several 8 oz. glasses of water a day to aid product action.
CHILDREN: (6–12 years old) Use ½ adult dose in 8 oz. of liquid, 1–3 times daily.

New Users: Easy Does It. Medical research shows that higher fiber intake is important for good digestive health. To help the body adjust and avoid minor gas and bloating sometimes associated with high fiber intake, it may be necessary to take one half dose over several days and then slowly increase the dosage over several days. Always follow with 8 oz. of liquid.

How Supplied: Powder, containers of 10.6 oz. (300 g), 15.9 oz. (450 g) and 30 single dose (6.0 g) packets.

Is this product OTC? Yes.

KONSYL-D® POWDER
(Psyllium hydrophilic mucilloid)
3.4 grams of psyllium per TEASPOON with dextrose added

Description: Konsyl-D is a bulk-forming natural therapeutic fiber for restoring and maintaining regularity. Konsyl-D contains 3.4 grams of psyllium hydrophilic mucilloid, a highly efficient dietary fiber derived from the husk of the psyllium seed. Konsyl-D contains no chemical stimulants and is non-addictive. Each teaspoon dose contains 3.4 grams of psyllium which is unflavored and can be mixed with a variety of juices.

Inactive Ingredients: Dextrose. Each 6.5 gram dose provides 14 calories. Konsyl-D is sodium free.

Actions: See Konsyl description of Actions.

Indications: See Konsyl description of Indications.

Contraindications: Intestinal obstruction, fecal impaction.

Precaution: May cause allergic reaction in people sensitive to inhaled or ingested psyllium powder.

Dosage and Administration:
ADULTS: Place one rounded teaspoon (6.5 grams) into a dry glass. Add 8 oz. of juice or other beverage. Stir for 3–5 seconds. Drink immediately. Follow with an 8 oz. glass of juice or water to aid product action. Konsyl-D can be taken one to three times daily, depending on need and response. It may require 2 to 3 days continued use to provide optimal benefit. When taking Konsyl-D, one should drink several 8 oz. glasses of water a day to aid product action.
CHILDREN: (6–12 years old) ½ adult dose in 8 oz. of liquid, 1–3 times daily.

New Users: See Konsyl instructions for New Users.

How Supplied: Powder, containers of 11.5 oz (325 g), 17.6 oz (500 g) and 30 single dose (6.5 g) packets.

Is the Product OTC? Yes.

KONSYL®-ORANGE POWDER
(psyllium hydrophilic mucilloid)
Ultra Fine Texture . . . Easy to Mix Formula
3.4 grams of psyllium per TABLESPOON

Description: Konsyl-Orange is a bulk-forming natural therapeutic fiber for restoring and maintaining regularity. Konsyl-Orange contains 3.4 grams of psyllium hydrophilic mucilloid, a highly efficient dietary fiber derived from the husk of the psyllium seed. Konsyl-Orange contains no chemical stimulants and is non-addictive. Each TABLESPOON dose contains 3.4 grams of psyllium which is ultrafine texture for easy mixing.

Inactive Ingredients: Sucrose, citric acid, FD&C Yellow #6 and D&C Yellow #10 and flavoring. Each 12 gram dose provides 35 calories. Konsyl-Orange is sodium free.

Actions: See Konsyl description of Actions.

Indications: See Konsly description of Indication.

Contraindications: Intestinal obstruction, fecal impaction.

Precaution: May cause allergic reaction in people sensitive to inhaled or ingested psyllium powder.

Dosage and Administration:
ADULTS: Place one rounded tablespoon (12.0 grams) into a dry glass. Add 8 oz. of water or other beverage. Stir 3–5 seconds. Drink immediately. Follow with an 8 oz. glass of water to aid product action. Konsyl-Orange can be taken one to three times daily, depending on need and response. It may require 2–3 days continued use to provide optimal benefit. When taking Konsyl-Orange, one should drink several 8 oz. glasses of water daily to aid product action.
CHILDREN: (6–12 years old) ½ adult dose in 8 oz. of liquid, 1–3 times daily.

New Users: See Konsyl instructions for New Users.

How Supplied: Ultra fine powder container of 19 oz (538 g) and 30 single dose (12.0 g) packets.

Is the product OTC? Yes.

IDENTIFICATION PROBLEM?
Consult the
Product Identification Section
where you'll find
products pictured
in full color.

Lactaid, Inc.
PLEASANTVILLE, NJ 08232

LACTAID® Caplets
(lactase enzyme)

PRODUCT OVERVIEW

KEY FACTS
Lactaid® lactase enzyme hydrolyzes lactose into two digestible simple sugars: glucose and galactose. Lactaid Caplets are taken orally for *in vivo* hydrolysis of lactose.

MAJOR USES
Lactase insufficiency, suspected from gastrointestinal discomfort (ie, gas, bloating, flatulence, cramps, and diarrhea) after the ingestion of milk or lactose-containing products.

PRESCRIBING INFORMATION

Description: Each Caplet contains 3000 FCC (Food Chemical Codex) units of lactase enzyme (derived from *Aspergillus oryzae*).

Action: Lactase enzyme hydrolyzes the lactose sugar (a double sugar) into its simple sugar components, glucose and galactose.

Indications: Lactase insufficiency, suspected from gastrointestinal discomfort (ie, gas, bloating, flatulence, cramps, and diarrhea) after the ingestion of milk or lactose-containing products.

Usual Dosage: These convenient, portable caplets are easy to swallow or chew and can be used with milk or any dairy food. We recommend taking 2 or 3 caplets with the first bite of any meal containing dairy. Take no more than 6 caplets at a time. Don't be discouraged if at first Lactaid does not work to your satisfaction. Because the degree of enzyme deficiency naturally varies from person to person and from food to food, you may have to adjust the number of caplets up or down to find your own level of comfort. Lactaid Caplets are nonhabit-forming, and because they work only on the food as you eat it, use them every time you enjoy dairy foods.

Warning: If you experience any discomfort which is unusual or seems unrelated to the condition for which you took this product, consult a doctor before taking any more of it. Do not use if carton is opened or if printed plastic neckwrap is broken.

Inactive Indgredients: Dextrates, Dibasic Calcium Phosphate, Microcrystalline Cellulose, Croscarmellose Sodium, Hydrogenated Vegetable Oil and Cornstarch.

Nutritional Information: Serving size: 2 Caplets; Calories: 2; Protein: 0 g; Carbohydrate: 0 g; Fat: 0 g; Sodium: 0 mg. Percentage of U.S. Recommended Daily Allowances (U.S.RDA): Contains less than 2% of the U.S. RDA of Protein, Vitamin A, Vitamin C and Thiamine.

How Supplied: Lactaid Caplets are available in bottles of 12, 50, and 100 counts. Store at or below room temperature (below 77°F) but do not refrigerate. Keep away from heat.

Shown in Product Identification Section, page 413

Lavoptik Company, Inc.
661 WESTERN AVENUE N.
ST. PAUL, MN 55103

LAVOPTIK® Eye Wash

Description: Isotonic LAVOPTIK Eye Wash is a buffered solution designed to help physically remove contaminants from the surface of the eye and lids. Formulated to buffer contaminants toward the safe range and help restore normal salts and water ratios in the tears.

Contents: Each 100 ml

Sodium Chloride	0.49 gram
Sodium Biphosphate	0.40 gram
Sodium Phosphate	0.45 gram
Preservative Agent	
Benzalkonium Chloride	0.005 gram

Precautions: If you experience severe eye pain, headache, rapid change in vision (side or straight ahead); sudden appearance of floating objects, acute redness of the eyes, pain on exposure to light or double vision consult a physician at once. If symptoms persist or worsen after use of this product, consult a physician. If solution changes color or becomes cloudy do not use. Keep this and all medicines out of reach of children. Keep container tightly closed. Do not use if safety seal is broken at time of purchase.

Administration: 6 ounce size with Eye Cup.
Rinse cup with clean water immediately before and after each use, avoid contamination of rim and inside surfaces of cup. Apply cup, half-filled with LAVOPTIK Eye Wash tightly to the eye. Tilt head backward. Open eyelids wide, rotate eyeball and blink several times to insure thorough washing. Discard washings. Repeat other eye. Tightly cap bottle.
32 ounce size.
Break seal as you remove cap and pour directly on contaminated area.

How Supplied: 6 ounce bottle with eyecup, NDC 10651-01040.
32 ounce bottle, NDC 10651-01019.

Products are
indexed alphabetically
in the
PINK SECTION.

Lederle Laboratories
A Division of American Cyanamid Co.
ONE CYANAMID PLAZA
WAYNE, NJ 07470

LEDERMARK®
Product Identification Code

Many Lederle tablets and capsules bear an identification code. A current listing appears in the Product Information Section of the 1993 *PDR* for prescription drugs.

CALTRATE® 600
[*căl-trāte*]
High Potency Calcium Supplement
Nature's Most Concentrated Form of Calcium™
No Sugar, No Salt, No Lactose, No Cholesterol, No Preservatives, Film-Coated for Easy Swallowing

Inactive Ingredients: Croscarmellose Sodium, Hydroxypropyl Methylcellulose, Magnesium Stearate, Microcrystalline Cellulose, PVPP, Sodium Lauryl Sulfate, and Titanium Dioxide.

TWO TABLETS DAILY PROVIDE:

	For Adults—Percentage of US Recommended Daily Allowance (US RDA)
3000 mg Calcium Carbonate which provides 1200 mg elemental calcium	120%

Recommended Intake: One or two tablets daily or as directed by the physician.

Warning: Keep out of the reach of children.

How Supplied: Bottle of 60—NDC 0005-5510-19
Store at Room Temperature.
 11643-91
D15

Shown in Product Identification Section, page 410

CALTRATE® 600+Iron & Vitamin D
[*căl-trāte*]
High Potency Calcium Supplement
Nature's Most Concentrated Form of Calcium™
No Sugar, No Salt, No Lactose, No Cholesterol, Film-Coated for Easy Swallowing

Inactive Ingredients: Blue 2, Croscarmellose Sodium, Hydroxypropyl Cellulose, Magnesium Stearate, Microcrystalline Cellulose, Polysorbate 80, Povidone, PVPP, Red 40, Sodium Lauryl Sulfate, Titanium Dioxide, and Triethyl Citrate.

- CALTRATE + Iron contains pure calcium and time-release iron for diets deficient in both minerals.
- Plus Vitamin D to help absorb calcium.

ONE TABLET DAILY CONTAINS:

	For Adults—Percentage of US Recommended Daily Allowance (RDA)
1500 mg Calcium Carbonate which provides 600 mg elemental calcium	60%
18 mg elemental Iron in the Optisorb® Time-Release System (as ferrous fumarate)	100%
125 IU Vitamin D	31%

Recommended Intake: One or two tablets daily or as directed by the physician.

Warning: Keep out of the reach of children.

How Supplied: Bottle of 60—NDC 0005-5523-19
Store at Room Temperature.
 11602-91
D9

Shown in Product Identification Section, page 410

CALTRATE® 600 + Vitamin D
[*căl-trāte*]
High Potency Calcium Supplement
Nature's Most Concentrated Form of Calcium™
No Sugar, No Salt, No Lactose, No Cholesterol, Film-Coated for Easy Swallowing

Inactive Ingredients: Blue 2, Croscarmellose Sodium, FD&C Yellow No. 6, Hydroxypropyl Methylcellulose, Magnesium Stearate, Microcrystalline Cellulose, Povidone, PVPP, Red 40, Sodium Lauryl Sulfate, and Titanium Dioxide.

TWO TABLETS DAILY PROVIDE:

	For Adults—Percentage of US Recommended Daily Allowance (RDA)
3000 mg Calcium Carbonate which provides 1200 mg elemental calcium	120%
250 IU Vitamin D	62%

Recommended Intake: One or two tablets daily or as directed by the physician.

Warning: Keep out of the reach of children.

How Supplied: Bottle of 60—NDC-0005-5509-19
Store at Room Temperature.
 11642-91
D12

Shown in Product Identification Section, page 410

CENTRUM®
[*sĕn-trŭm*]
High Potency Multivitamin-Multimineral Formula, Advanced Formula
From A to Zinc®

Each tablet contains:

		For Adults—Percentage of US Recommended Daily Allowance (US RDA)
VITAMINS		
Vitamin A (as Acetate and Beta Carotene)	5000 IU	(100%)
Vitamin D	400 IU	(100%)
Vitamin E (as *dl*-Alpha Tocopheryl Acetate)	30 IU	(100%)
Vitamin K_1	25 mcg*	
Vitamin C	60 mg	(100%)
Folic Acid	400 mcg	(100%)
Vitamin B_1	1.5 mg	(100%)
Vitamin B_2	1.7 mg	(100%)
Niacinamide	20 mg	(100%)
Vitamin B_6	2 mg	(100%)
Vitamin B_{12}	6 mcg	(100%)
Pantothenic Acid	10 mg	(100%)
Biotin	30 mcg	(10%)
MINERALS		
Calcium	162 mg	(16%)
Phosphorus	109 mg	(11%)
Iodine	150 mcg	(100%)
Iron	18 mg	(100%)
Magnesium	100 mg	(25%)
Copper	2 mg	(100%)
Zinc	15 mg	(100%)
Manganese	2.5 mg*	
Potassium	40 mg*	
Chloride	36.3 mg*	
Chromium	25 mcg*	
Molybdenum	25 mcg*	
Selenium	20 mcg*	
Nickel	5 mcg*	
Tin (as Stannous Chloride)	10 mcg*	
Silicon	2 mg*	
Vanadium	10 mcg*	
Boron	150 mcg*	

*No US RDA established

Inactive Ingredients: FD&C Yellow No. 6, Hydroxypropyl Methylcellulose, Lactose, Magnesium Stearate, Microcrystalline Cellulose, Polysorbate 80, Polyvinylpyrrolidone, Stearic Acid, Titanium Dioxide, and Triethyl Citrate.

Recommended Intake: Adults, 1 tablet daily.

How Supplied:
Light peach, engraved CENTRUM C1.
Bottle of 60—NDC 0005-4239-19
Combopack*—NDC 0005-4239-30
*Bottles of 100 plus 30
Store at Room Temperature.
 20112-92
D36

Shown in Product Identification Section, page 410

CENTRUM® Liquid
High Potency
Multivitamin-Multimineral Formula
Advanced Formula

Each 15 mL (1 tablespoon) contains:

		For Adults—Percentage of US Recommended Daily Allowance (US RDA)
Vitamin A (as Palmitate)	2500 IU	(50%)
Vitamin E (as *dl*-Alpha Tocopheryl Acetate)	30 IU	(100%)
Vitamin C (as Ascorbic Acid)	60 mg	(100%)
Vitamin B_1 (as Thiamine Hydrochloride)	1.5 mg	(100%)
Vitamin B_2 (as Riboflavin)	1.7 mg	(100%)
Niacinamide	20 mg	(100%)
Vitamin B_6 (as Pyridoxine Hydrochloride)	2 mg	(100%)
Vitamin B_{12} (as Cyanocobalamin)	6 mcg	(100%)
Vitamin D_2	400 IU	(100%)
Biotin	300 mcg	(100%)
Pantothenic Acid (as Panthenol)	10 mg	(100%)
Iodine (as Potassium Iodide)	150 mcg	(100%)
Iron (as Ferrous Gluconate)	9 mg	(50%)
Zinc (as Zinc Gluconate)	3 mg	(20%)
Manganese (as Manganese Chloride)	2.5 mg	*
Chromium (as Chromium Chloride)	25 mcg	*
Molybdenum (as Sodium Molybdate)	25 mcg	*

*No US RDA established

Inactive Ingredients: Alcohol 6.6%, Artificial and Natural Flavors, Citric Acid, Glycerin, Polysorbate 80, Sodium Benzoate, and Sucrose.

Recommended Intake: Adults, 1 tablespoonful (15 mL) daily.

Warning: Keep this and all medication out of the reach of children.

How Supplied: 8 oz Bottle—
NDC 0005-4343-61
Store at Controlled Room Temperature 15°–30°C (59°–86°F).
PROTECT FROM FREEZING.

23317
D3

Shown in Product Identification Section, page 411

Products are indexed by generic and chemical names in the **YELLOW SECTION.**

CENTRUM, JR.®
Children's Chewable
Vitamin/Mineral Formula + Extra C

	Quantity per tablet	Percentage of US Recommended Daily Allowance (US RDA) For Children 2 to 4 (½ tablet)	For Children Over 4 (1 tablet)
EACH TABLET CONTAINS:			
VITAMINS			
Vitamin A (as Acetate)	5,000 IU	(100%)	(100%)
Vitamin D	400 IU	(50%)	(100%)
Vitamin E (as Acetate)	30 IU	(150%)	(100%)
Vitamin C (as Ascorbic Acid and Sodium Ascorbate)	300 mg	(375%)	(500%)
Folic Acid	400 mcg	(100%)	(100%)
Biotin	45 mcg	(15%)	(15%)
Thiamine (as Thiamine Mononitrate)	1.5 mg	(107%)	(100%)
Pantothenic Acid (as Calcium Pantothenate)	10 mg	(100%)	(100%)
Riboflavin	1.7 mg	(107%)	(100%)
Niacinamide	20 mg	(111%)	(100%)
Vitamin B_6	2 mg	(143%)	(100%)
Vitamin B_{12} (as Cyanocobalamin)	6 mcg	(100%)	(100%)
Vitamin K_1 (as Phytonadione)	10 mcg*		
MINERALS			
Iron (as Ferrous Fumarate)	18 mg	(90%)	(100%)
Magnesium (as Magnesium Oxide)	40 mg	(10%)	(10%)
Iodine (as Potassium Iodide)	150 mcg	(107%)	(100%)
Copper (as Cupric Oxide)	2 mg	(100%)	(100%)
Phosphorus (as Tribasic Calcium Phosphate)	50 mg	(3.12%)	(5.0%)
Calcium (as Tribasic Calcium Phosphate)	108 mg	(6.75%)	(10.8%)
Zinc (as Zinc Oxide)	15 mg	(93%)	(100%)
Manganese (as Manganese Sulfate)	1 mg*		
Molybdenum (as Sodium Molybdate)	20 mcg*		
Chromium (as Chromium Chloride)	20 mcg*		

*Recognized as essential in human nutrition but no US RDA established

CENTRUM, JR.®
[*sĕn-trŭm*]
Children's Chewable
Vitamin/Mineral Formula + Extra C Tablets
Nutritional Support From Head to Toe®

[See table above.]

Inactive Ingredients: Acacia, Artificial Flavorings, Blue 1, Blue 2, Colloidal Silicon Dioxide, Dextrins, Dextrose, Gelatin, Hydrogenated Vegetable Oil, Hydrolyzed Protein, Lactose, Magnesium Stearate, Methylparaben, Microcrystalline Cellulose, Modified Food Starch, Mono- and Di-glycerides, Potassium Sorbate, Povidone, Propylparaben, Red 40, Sodium Benzoate, Sorbic Acid, Stearic Acid, Sucrose, Yellow 6.

Warnings: CONTAINS IRON, WHICH CAN BE HARMFUL IN LARGE DOSES. CLOSE TIGHTLY AND KEEP OUT OF THE REACH OF CHILDREN. IN CASE OF ACCIDENTAL OVERDOSE, CONTACT A PHYSICIAN OR POISON CONTROL CENTER IMMEDIATELY.

How Supplied: Bottle of 60—
NDC 0005-4249-19
Store at Room Temperature.

20416-92
D9

Shown in Product Identification Section, page 411

CENTRUM, JR.®
[*sĕn-trŭm*]
Children's Chewable
Vitamin/Mineral Formula + Extra Calcium
Nutritional Support From Head to Toe®

[See table top of next page.]

Inactive Ingredients:
Artificial Flavorings, Citric Acid, Lactose, Magnesium Stearate, Microcrystalline Cellulose, Modified Food Starch, Red 40, Silica Gel, Sodium Starch Glycolate, Stearic Acid, Sucrose.

Warnings: CONTAINS IRON, WHICH CAN BE HARMFUL IN LARGE DOSES. CLOSE TIGHTLY AND KEEP OUT OF THE REACH OF CHILDREN. IN CASE OF ACCIDENTAL OVERDOSE, CONTACT A PHYSICIAN OR POISON CONTROL CENTER IMMEDIATELY.

Recommended Intake: 2 to 4 years of age: chew one-half tablet daily. Over 4 years of age: chew one tablet daily.

How Supplied: Bottle of 60—
NDC 0005-4222-19
Store at Room Temperature.

20415-92
D7

Shown in Product Identification Section, page 411

Continued on next page

Lederle—Cont.

CENTRUM, JR.®
Children's Chewable
Vitamin/Mineral Formula + Extra Calcium

EACH TABLET CONTAINS:	Quantity per tablet	Percentage of US Recommended Daily Allowance (US RDA) For Children 2 to 4 (½ tablet)	For Children Over 4 (1 tablet)
VITAMINS			
Vitamin A (as Acetate)	5,000 IU	(100%)	(100%)
Vitamin D	400 IU	(50%)	(100%)
Vitamin E (as Acetate)	30 IU	(150%)	(100%)
Vitamin C (as Ascorbic Acid)	60 mg	(75%)	(100%)
Folic Acid	400 mcg	(100%)	(100%)
Biotin	45 mcg	(15%)	(15%)
Thiamine (as Thiamine Mononitrate)	1.5 mg	(107%)	(100%)
Pantothenic Acid (as Calcium Pantothenate)	10 mg	(100%)	(100%)
Riboflavin	1.7 mg	(107%)	(100%)
Niacinamide	20 mg	(111%)	(100%)
Vitamin B_6	2 mg	(143%)	(100%)
Vitamin B_{12} (as Cyanocobalamin)	6 mcg	(100%)	(100%)
Vitamin K_1 (as Phytonadione)	10 mcg*		
MINERALS			
Iron (as Ferrous Fumarate)	18 mg	(90%)	(100%)
Magnesium (as Magnesium Oxide)	40 mg	(10%)	(10%)
Iodine (as Potassium Iodide)	150 mcg	(107%)	(100%)
Copper (as Cupric Oxide)	2 mg	(100%)	(100%)
Phosphorus (as Dibasic Calcium Phosphate)	50 mg	(3.12%)	(5.0%)
Calcium (as Dibasic Calcium Phosphate and Calcium Carbonate)	160 mg	(10%)	(16%)
Zinc (as Zinc Oxide)	15 mg	(93%)	(100%)
Manganese (as Manganese Sulfate)	1 mg*		
Molybdenum (as Sodium Molybdate)	20 mcg*		
Chromium (as Chromium Chloride)	20 mcg*		

*Recognized as essential in human nutrition but no US RDA established

CENTRUM, JR.®
Children's Chewable
Vitamin/Mineral Formula + Iron

EACH TABLET CONTAINS:	Quantity per tablet	Percentage of US Recommended Daily Allowance (US RDA) For Children 2 to 4 (½ tablet)	For Children Over 4 (1 tablet)
VITAMINS			
Vitamin A (as Acetate)	5,000 IU	(100%)	(100%)
Vitamin D	400 IU	(50%)	(100%)
Vitamin E (as Acetate)	30 IU	(150%)	(100%)
Vitamin C (as Ascorbic Acid)	60 mg	(75%)	(100%)
Folic Acid	400 mcg	(100%)	(100%)
Biotin	45 mcg	(15%)	(15%)
Thiamine (as Thiamine Mononitrate)	1.5 mg	(107%)	(100%)
Pantothenic Acid (as Calcium Pantothenate)	10 mg	(100%)	(100%)
Riboflavin	1.7 mg	(107%)	(100%)
Niacinamide	20 mg	(111%)	(100%)
Vitamin B_6	2 mg	(143%)	(100%)
Vitamin B_{12} (as Cyanocobalamin)	6 mcg	(100%)	(100%)
Vitamin K_1 (as Phytonadione)	10 mcg*		
MINERALS			
Iron (as Ferrous Fumarate)	18 mg	(90%)	(100%)
Magnesium (as Magnesium Oxide)	40 mg	(10%)	(10%)
Iodine (as Potassium Iodide)	150 mcg	(107%)	(100%)
Copper (as Cupric Oxide)	2 mg	(100%)	(100%)
Phosphorus (as Dibasic Calcium Phosphate)	50 mg	(3.12%)	(5.0%)
Calcium (as Dibasic Calcium Phosphate and Calcium Carbonate)	108 mg	(6.75%)	(10.8%)
Zinc (as Zinc Oxide)	15 mg	(93%)	(100%)
Manganese (as Manganese Sulfate)	1 mg*		
Molybdenum (as Sodium Molybdate)	20 mcg*		
Chromium (as Chromium Chloride)	20 mcg*		

*Recognized as essential in human nutrition but no US RDA established

CENTRUM, JR.®
[sĕn-trŭm]
Children's Chewable Vitamin/Mineral Formula + Iron Tablets
Nutritional Support From Head to Toe®

[See table on preceding page.]

Inactive Ingredients: Acacia, Artificial Flavorings, Blue 1, Blue 2, Colloidal Silicon Dioxide, Dextrins, Dextrose, Gelatin, Hydrogenated Vegetable Oil, Hydrolyzed Protein, Lactose, Magnesium Stearate, Methylparaben, Microcrystalline Cellulose, Modified Food Starch, Mono- and Di-glycerides, Potassium Sorbate, Propylparaben, Red 40, Sodium Benzoate, Sodium Starch Glycolate, Sorbic Acid, Stearic Acid, Sucrose, Yellow 6.

Recommended Intake: 2 to 4 years of age: Chew one-half tablet daily. Over 4 years of age: Chew one tablet daily.

Warnings: CONTAINS IRON, WHICH CAN BE HARMFUL IN LARGE DOSES. CLOSE TIGHTLY AND KEEP OUT OF THE REACH OF CHILDREN. IN CASE OF ACCIDENTAL OVERDOSE, CONTACT A PHYSICIAN OR POISON CONTROL CENTER IMMEDIATELY.

How Supplied: Assorted Flavors—Uncoated Tablet—Partially Scored—Engraved Lederle C2 and CENTRUM, JR.
Bottle of 60—NDC 0005-4234-19
Store at Room Temperature.
© 1989 20413-92
D10

Shown in Product Identification Section, page 410

CENTRUM SILVER®
Specially Formulated Multivitamin-Multimineral for Adults 50+
Complete From A to Zinc®

Each tablet contains:
[See table top of next column]

Inactive Ingredients: Blue 2, Crospovidone, FD&C Yellow No. 6, Gelatin, Hydroxypropyl Methylcellulose, Lactose, Magnesium Stearate, Microcrystalline Cellulose, Polyethylene Glycol, Polysorbate 80, Red 40, Silica Gel, Stearic Acid, and Titanium Dioxide.

Gel-Tabs™ —Specially coated supplement to assure ease of swallowing.

Recommended Intake:
Adults, 1 tablet daily.

How Supplied: Bottle of 60—
NDC 0005-4177-19
Bottle of 100—NDC 0005-4177-23
Store at Room Temperature.
© 1991 11630-91
D3

Shown in Product Identification Section, page 411

CENTRUM SILVER®

		For Adults—Percentage of US Recommended Daily Allowance (US RDA)
Vitamin A (as Acetate and Beta Carotene)	6000 IU	(120%)
Vitamin B_1	1.5 mg	(100%)
Vitamin B_2	1.7 mg	(100%)
Vitamin B_6	3 mg	(150%)
Vitamin B_{12}	25 mcg	(416%)
Biotin	30 mcg	(10%)
Folic Acid	200 mcg	(50%)
Niacinamide	20 mg	(100%)
Pantothenic Acid	10 mg	(100%)
Vitamin C	60 mg	(100%)
Vitamin D	400 IU	(100%)
Vitamin E	45 IU	(150%)
Vitamin K_1	10 mcg*	
Calcium	200 mg	(20%)
Copper	2 mg	(100%)
Iodine	150 mcg	(100%)
Iron	9 mg	(50%)
Magnesium	100 mg	(25%)
Phosphorus	48 mg	(5%)
Zinc	15 mg	(100%)
Chloride	72 mg*	
Chromium	100 mcg*	
Manganese	2.5 mg*	
Molybdenum	25 mcg*	
Nickel	5 mcg*	
Potassium	80 mg*	
Selenium	25 mcg*	
Silicon	10 mcg*	
Vanadium	10 mcg*	

*No US RDA established

Dual Action
FERRO-SEQUELS®
[fĕrrō-sēquals]
High Potency Iron Supplement
Time-Release Iron Plus
Clinically Proven Anticonstipant
Easy-to-Swallow Tablets
Low Sodium, No Sugar

Active Ingredients: Each tablet contains 150 mg of ferrous fumarate equivalent to 50 mg of elemental iron and 100 mg of docusate sodium (DSS).

Inactive Ingredients: Blue 1, Corn Starch, Crospovidone, Hydroxypropyl Methylcellulose, Lactose, Magnesium Stearate, Microcrystalline Cellulose, Modified Food Starch, Povidone, Silica Gel, Sodium Lauryl Sulfate, Titanium Dioxide, and Yellow 10.

Warnings: As with any drug, if you are pregnant or nursing a baby, seek the advice of a health professional before using this product. Keep this and all medications out of the reach of children. In case of accidental overdose, seek professional assistance or contact a Poison Control Center immediately.

Recommended Intake: One tablet, once or twice daily or as prescribed by a physician.

How Supplied: Boxes of 30—
NDC 0005-5267-68
Bottle of 30—NDC 0005-5267-13
Bottle of 60—NDC 0005-5267-19
Bottle of 100—NDC 0005-5267-23
Unit Dose Pack 10×10—
NDC 0005-5267-60
Green, capsule-shaped, film-coated tablets engraved LL and F2.
Store at Room Temperature. 27533
D3

Shown in Product Identification Section, page 411

FIBERCON®
[fī-bĕr-cŏn]
Calcium Polycarbophil
Bulk-Forming Fiber Laxative

Less than one calorie per tablet, Sodium- and Preservative-free, Film-coated for easy swallowing, Calcium rich, No chemical stimulants, Non-habit forming.

Active Ingredient: Each tablet contains 625 mg calcium polycarbophil equivalent to 500 mg polycarbophil.

Inactive Ingredients: Calcium Carbonate, Caramel, Crospovidone, Hydroxypropyl Methylcellulose, Magnesium Stearate, Microcrystalline Cellulose, Povidone, and Silica Gel.

Indications: Relief of constipation. FIBERCON restores and maintains regularity and promotes normal function of the bowel.

Actions: FIBERCON works naturally so continued use for 1 to 3 days is normally required to provide full benefit.

Warnings: Any sudden change in bowel habits may indicate a more serious condition than constipation. Consult your physician if symptoms such as nausea, vomiting, abdominal pain, or rectal bleeding occur or if this product has no effect within 1 week.
For chronic or continued constipation consult your physician.

Interaction Precaution: If you are taking any form of tetracycline antibiotic, FIBERCON should be taken at least 1 hour before or 2 hours after you have taken the antibiotic.

KEEP THIS AND ALL MEDICINES OUT OF THE REACH OF CHILDREN. STORE AT CONTROLLED ROOM TEMPERATURE 15°–30°C (59°–86°F). PROTECT CONTENTS FROM MOISTURE.

Recommended Intake: FIBERCON dosage will vary according to diet, exercise, previous laxative use or severity of constipation. Recommended adult starting dose: 2 or 4 tablets daily. May be increased up to eight tablets daily. Children 6 to 12 years: swallow one tablet one to three times a day. Children under 6 years: consult a physician.
A FULL GLASS (8 fl oz) OF LIQUID SHOULD BE TAKEN WITH EACH

Continued on next page

Lederle—Cont.

DOSE. See package insert for additional information.

How Supplied:
Film coated tablets, scored, engraved LL and F66.
Package of 36 tablets, NDC 0005-2500-02
Package of 60 tablets, NDC 0005-2500-86
Package of 90 tablets, NDC 0005-2500-33
Bottle of 500 tablets, NDC 0005-2500-31
Unit Dose Pkg, NDC 0005-2500-28

10995-91
D8

Shown in Product Identification Section, page 411

FILIBON®

[fĭ-lĭ-bōn]

Multivitamin-Multimineral Supplement for Pregnant or Lactating Women Prenatal Tablets

Each tablet contains:

	For Pregnant or Lactating Women–Percentage of US Recommended Daily Allowance (US RDA)
Vitamin A (as Acetate)	5000 I.U. (63%)
Vitamin D_2	400 I.U. (100%)
Vitamin E (as *dl*-Alpha Tocopheryl Acetate)	30 I.U. (100%)
Vitamin C (as Ascorbic Acid)	60 mg (100%)
Folic Acid	0.4 mg (50%)
Vitamin B_1 (as Thiamine Mononitrate)	1.5 mg (88%)
Vitamin B_2 (as Riboflavin)	1.7 mg (85%)
Niacinamide	20 mg (100%)
Vitamin B_6	2 mg (80%)
Vitamin B_{12} (as Cyanocobalamin)	6 mcg (75%)
Calcium (as Calcium Carbonate)	125 mg (10%)
Iodine (as Potassium Iodide)	150 mcg (100%)
Iron (as Ferrous Fumarate)	18 mg (100%)
Magnesium (as Magnesium Oxide)	100 mg (22%)

Inactive Ingredients: Ethylcellulose, Hydroxypropyl Methylcellulose, Lactose, Magnesium Stearate, Microcrystalline Cellulose, Povidone, Pregelatinized Starch, Red 40, Silicon Dioxide, Sodium Lauryl Sulfate, Sodium Starch Glycolate, Titanium Dioxide, and Stearic Acid.

Recommended Intake: 1 daily, or as prescribed by the physician.

How Supplied: Capsule-shaped tablets (film-coated, pink) engraved LL and F4.
Bottle of 100—NDC-0005-4294-23
Store at Room Temperature.

10999-91
D12

GEVRABON®

[jĕv-ra băn]

Vitamin-Mineral Supplement

Composition: Each fluid ounce (30 mL) contains:

	For Adults—Percentage of US Recommended Daily Allowance (US RDA)
Vitamin B_1 (as Thiamine Hydrochloride)	5 mg (333%)
Vitamin B_2 (as Riboflavin-5-Phosphate Sodium)	2.5 mg (147%)
Niacinamide	50 mg (250%)
Vitamin B_6 (Pyridoxine Hydrochloride)	1 mg (50%)
Vitamin B_{12} (as Cyanocobalamin)	1 mcg (17%)
Pantothenic Acid (as D-Pantothenyl Alcohol)	10 mg (100%)
Iodine (as Potassium Iodide)	100 mcg (67%)
Iron (as Ferrous Gluconate)	15 mg (83%)
Magnesium (as Magnesium Chloride)	2 mg (0.5%)
Zinc (as Zinc Chloride)	2 mg (13%)
Choline (as Tricholine Citrate)	100 mg*
Manganese (as Manganese Chloride)	2 mg*

*Recognized as essential in human nutrition but no U.S. RDA established.

Alcohol 18%

Inactive Ingredients: Alcohol, Citric Acid, Glycerin, Sherry Wine, Sucrose.

Indications: For use as a nutritional supplement. Shake well.

Warnings: As with any drug, if you are pregnant or nursing a baby, seek the advice of a health professional before using this product. Keep this preparation out of the reach of children.

Administration and Dosage: Adult: One ounce (30 mL) daily or as prescribed by the physician as a nutritional supplement.

Important Note: In time a slight natural deposit, characteristic of the sherry wine base, may occur. This does not indicate in any way a loss of quality.

How Supplied: Syrup (sherry flavor) decanters of 16 fl oz—NDC 0005-5250-35
Keep Out of Direct Sunlight.
Store at Room Temperature, 15°-30°C (59°-86°F).
DO NOT FREEZE.

16520
D4

GEVRAL® T

[jĕv-ral t]

High Potency Multivitamin and Multimineral Supplement Tablets

Each tablet contains:
[See table next column]

Inactive Ingredients: BHA, BHT, Blue 2, Gelatin, Hydrolyzed Protein, Hydroxypropyl Methylcellulose, Lactose,

	For Adults—Percentage of US Recommended Daily Allowance (US RDA)
Vitamin A (as Acetate)	5000 IU (100%)
Vitamin E (as *dl*-Alpha Tocopheryl Acetate)	45 IU (150%)
Vitamin C (as Ascorbic Acid)	90 mg (150%)
Folic Acid	0.4 mg (100%)
Vitamin B_1 (as Thiamine Mononitrate)	2.25 mg (150%)
Vitamin B_2 (as Riboflavin)	2.6 mg (153%)
Niacinamide	30 mg (150%)
Vitamin B_6 (as Pyridoxine Hydrochloride)	3 mg (150%)
Vitamin B_{12} (as Cyanocobalamin)	9 mcg (150%)
Vitamin D_2	400 IU (100%)
Calcium (as Dibasic Calcium Phosphate)	162 mg (16%)
Phosphorus (as Dibasic Calcium Phosphate)	125 mg (13%)
Iodine (as Potassium Iodide)	225 mcg (150%)
Iron (as Ferrous Fumarate)	27 mg (150%)
Magnesium (as Magnesium Oxide)	100 mg (25%)
Copper (as Cupric Oxide)	1.5 mg (75%)
Zinc (as Zinc Oxide)	22.5 mg (150%)

Magnesium Stearate, Methylparaben, Microcrystalline Cellulose, Modified Food Starch, Mono- and Di-glycerides, Polacrilin, Polysorbate 60, Potassium Sorbate, Propylparaben, PVPP, Red 40, Silica Gel, Sodium Benzoate, Sodium Lauryl Sulfate, Sorbic Acid, Stearic Acid, Sucrose, Titanium Dioxide, and other ingredients.

Indications: For the treatment of vitamin and mineral deficiencies.

Recommended Intake: 1 tablet daily or as prescribed by physician.

Warnings: Keep this and all medications out of the reach of children.

How Supplied: Tablets (film-coated, maroon). Engraved LL and G2.
Bottle of 100—NDC 0005-4286-23
Store at Room Temperature.
A SPECTRUM® Product

D7
14170

INCREMIN®

[ĭn-cre-mĭn]

WITH IRON SYRUP
Vitamins + Iron
DIETARY SUPPLEMENT
(Cherry Flavored)

Composition: Each teaspoonful (5 mL) contains:
[See table on next page.]

Inactive Ingredients: Alcohol 0.75%, Cherry Flavor, Red 33, Sodium Benzoate, Sodium Hydroxide, Sorbic Acid and Sorbitol.

Indications: For the prevention of iron deficiency anemia in children and adults.

		Percentage of US Recommended Daily Allowance (US RDA)	
		Children Under 4	Children Over 4 and Adults
Vitamin B_1 (as Thiamine Hydrochloride)	5 mg	714%	333%
Vitamin B_6	5 mg	714%	250%
Vitamin B_{12} (as Cyanocobalamin)	25 mcg	833%	417%
Iron (as Ferric Pyrophosphate)	30 mg	300%	167%
*L-Lysine Hydrochloride	300 mg		

*No US RDA established

Warnings: As with any drug, if you are pregnant or nursing a baby, seek the advice of a health professional before using this product.
Keep this and all medications out of the reach of children.

Recommended Dosages (or as prescribed by a physician):
Children: One teaspoonful (5 mL) daily for the prevention of iron deficiency anemia.
Adults: One teaspoonful (5 mL) daily for the prevention of iron deficiency anemia.

Notice: To protect from light always dispense in this container or in an amber bottle.
Store at Room Temperature.

How Supplied: Syrup (cherry flavor)—Bottles of 4 fl oz—NDC 0005-5604-58

20421-92
DS15

PROTEGRA™
[*prō-tĕg-ră*]
Antioxidant Vitamin & Mineral Supplement

Each softgel contains:

		For Adults–Percentage of US Recommended Daily Allowance (US RDA)
Vitamin E	200 IU	667%
Vitamin C	250 mg	417%
Beta Carotene	3 mg	100%*
Zinc	7.5 mg	50%
Copper	1 mg	50%
Selenium	15 mcg	**
Manganese	1.5 mg	**

*US RDA for Vitamin A
**No US RDA established

Inactive Ingredients: Gelatin, cottonseed oil, glycerin, dibasic calcium phosphate, lecithin, partially hydrogenated cottonseed and soybean oils, beeswax, titanium dioxide, FD&C Yellow #6, and FD&C Red #40.

Recommended Intake: Adults: One softgel daily or as directed by a physician. PROTEGRA™ can be taken by itself or with a multiple vitamin.

How Supplied: Bottle of 50—NDC-0005-4377-18
Store at room temperature.

Warning: Keep out of the reach of children.

20156-92

Shown in Product Identification Section, page 411

STRESSTABS® Advanced Formula
[*strĕss-tăbs*]
High Potency Stress Formula Vitamins

Each tablet contains:

	For Adults–Percentage of US Recommended Daily Allowance (US RDA)
Vitamin E (as *dl*-Alpha Tocopheryl Acetate)	30 IU (100%)
Vitamin C (as Ascorbic Acid)	500 mg (833%)
B VITAMINS	
Folic Acid	400 mcg (100%)
Vitamin B_1 (as Thiamine Mononitrate)	10 mg (667%)
Vitamin B_2 (as Riboflavin)	10 mg (588%)
Niacinamide	100 mg (500%)
Vitamin B_6 (as Pyridoxine Hydrochloride)	5 mg (250%)
Vitamin B_{12} (as Cyanocobalamin)	12 mcg (200%)
Biotin	45 mcg (15%)
Pantothenic Acid (as Calcium Pantothenate, USP)	20 mg (200%)

Inactive Ingredients: Calcium Carbonate, FD&C Yellow No. 6, Magnesium Stearate, Microcrystalline Cellulose, Modified Food Starch, Silica Gel, and Stearic Acid.

Recommended Intake: Adults, 1 tablet daily or as directed by the physician.

How Supplied:
Bottle of 30—NDC 0005-4124-13
Bottle of 60—NDC 0005-4124-19
Store at Room Temperature.

20457-92
D19

Shown in Product Identification Section, page 411

STRESSTABS® + IRON Advanced Formula
[*strĕss-tăbs*]
High Potency Stress Formula Vitamins

Each tablet contains:
[See table next column]

Inactive Ingredients: Calcium Carbonate, FD&C Yellow No. 6, Magnesium Stearate, Microcrystalline Cellulose, Modified Food Starch, Red 40, Silica Gel, and Stearic Acid.

Recommended Intake: Adults, 1 tablet daily or as directed by the physician.

	For Adults–Percentage of US Recommended Daily Allowance (US RDA)
Vitamin E (as *dl*-Alpha Tocopheryl Acetate)	30 IU (100%)
Vitamin C (as Ascorbic Acid)	500 mg (833%)
B VITAMINS	
Folic Acid	400 mcg (100%)
Vitamin B_1 (as Thiamine Mononitrate)	10 mg (667%)
Vitamin B_2 (as Riboflavin)	10 mg (588%)
Niacinamide	100 mg (500%)
Vitamin B_6	5 mg (250%)
Vitamin B_{12} (as Cyanocobalamin)	12 mcg (200%)
Biotin	45 mcg (15%)
Pantothenic Acid (as Calcium Pantothenate, USP)	20 mg (200%)
Iron (as Ferrous Fumarate)	27 mg (150%)

How Supplied: Capsule-shaped tablets (film-coated, orange-red, scored). Engraved LL and S2.
Bottle of 60—NDC 0005-4126-19
Store at Room Temperature.

20459-92
D17

Shown in Product Identification Section, page 411

STRESSTABS® + ZINC Advanced Formula
[*strĕss-tăbs*]
High Potency Stress Formula Vitamins

Each tablet contains:

	For Adults—Percentage of US Recommended Daily Allowance (US RDA)
Vitamin E (as *dl*-Alpha Tocopheryl Acetate)	30 IU (100%)
Vitamin C (as Ascorbic Acid)	500 mg (833%)
B VITAMINS	
Folic Acid	400 mcg (100%)
Vitamin B_1 (as Thiamine Mononitrate)	10 mg (667%)
Vitamin B_2 (as Riboflavin)	10 mg (588%)
Niacinamide	100 mg (500%)
Vitamin B_6	5 mg (250%)
Vitamin B_{12} (as Cyanocobalamin)	12 mcg (200%)
Biotin	45 mcg (15%)
Pantothenic Acid (as Calcium Pantothenate, USP)	20 mg (200%)
Copper (as Cupric Oxide)	3 mg (150%)
Zinc (as Zinc Sulfate)	23.9 mg (159%)

Inactive Ingredients: Calcium Carbonate, FD&C Yellow No. 6, Magnesium Stearate, Microcrystalline Cellulose, Modified Food Starch, Silica Gel, and Stearic Acid.

Recommended Intake: Adults, 1 tablet daily or as directed by the physician.

Continued on next page

Lederle—Cont.

How Supplied: Capsule-shaped tablet (film-coated, peach color). Engraved LL and S3.
Bottle of 60—NDC 0005-4125-19
Store at Room Temperature.

20458-92
D19

Shown in Product Identification Section, page 411

ZINCON®
[zinc-ŏn]
Dandruff Shampoo

Contains: Pyrithione Zinc (1%), Water, Sodium Methyl Cocoyl Taurate, Cocamide MEA, Sodium Chloride, Magnesium Aluminum Silicate, Sodium Cocoyl Isethionate, Fragrance, Glutaraldehyde, D&C Green #5, Citric Acid or Sodium Hydroxide to adjust pH if necessary.

Indications: Relieves the itching and scalp flaking associated with dandruff. Relieves the itching, irritation, and skin flaking associated with seborrheic dermatitis of the scalp.

Directions: For best results use twice a week. Wet hair, apply to scalp and massage vigorously. Rinse and repeat. SHAKE WELL BEFORE USING.

Warnings: Keep this and all drugs out of the reach of children. For external use only. Avoid contact with the eyes—if this happens, rinse thoroughly with water. If condition worsens or does not improve after regular use of this product as directed, consult a doctor. Do not use on children under 2 years of age except as directed by a doctor.

How Supplied:
4 oz Bottle—NDC 0005-5455-58
8 oz Bottle—NDC 0005-5455-61

13918
D4

Shown in Product Identification Section, page 411

If desired, additional information on any Lederle product will be provided by contacting Lederle Professional Services Dept.

EDUCATIONAL MATERIAL

Calcium Supplements: The Differences Are Real
8-page pamphlet describing why today's women need to supplement their diet with calcium.
Write to: Lederle Promotional Center
2200 Bradley Hill Road
Blauvelt, NY 10913

Lever Brothers Company
390 PARK AVENUE
NEW YORK, NY 10022

DOVE® BAR AND LIQUID DOVE® BEAUTY WASH

Active Ingredients: Sodium Cocoyl Isethionate, Stearic Acid, Sodium Tallowate, Water, Sodium Isethionate, Coconut Acid, Sodium Stearate, Sodium Dodecylbenzenesulfonate, Sodium Cocoate, Fragrance, Sodium Chloride, Titanium Dioxide.

Actions and Uses: Dove is specially formulated to be predictably gentle to all kinds of skin—dry, oily, normal skin, as well as sensitive pediatric or senescent skin. Dove is not a soap but a neutral cleanser with a pH of 7 that leaves skin soft, moist, and healthy looking.

Directions: Instruct patients to use Dove as they would any other cleanser.

How Supplied: Original Dove 3.5 oz. and 4.75 bars; Unscented Dove 4.75 oz.; 6 oz. pump dispenser—Liquid Dove Beauty Wash.

Shown in Product Identification Section, page 411

LEVER 2000®

Active Ingredients: Sodium tallowate, sodium cocoyl, isethionate, water, sodium cocoate, stearic acid, sodium isethionate, coconut fatty acid, fragrance, titanium dioxide, sodium chloride, triclosan tetrasodium EDTA, disodium phosphate, trisodium etidronate, BHT.

Actions and Uses: Lever 2000® is the mildest antibacterial bar soap available. Lever 2000® offers the broadest spectrum of gram-negative and gram-positive antibacterial efficacy. It is a useful adjunct to any therapeutic regimen that fights topical bacterial infection. It is also milder to the skin than any other antibacterial or deodorant bar soap. Lever 2000® has been proven mild enough for children's tender skin as young as 18 months and can also be used by adolescents and adults.

Directions: Instruct patients to use Lever 2000® as they would any other mild antibacterial or deodorant soap.

How Supplied: 3.5 oz., 5 oz., and 6.5 oz. bars.

Shown in Product Identification Section, page 411

Products are indexed by generic and chemical names in the **YELLOW SECTION.**

Macsil, Inc.
1326 FRANKFORD AVENUE
PHILADELPHIA, PA 19125

BALMEX® BABY POWDER

Composition: Contains: Active Ingredient—zinc oxide; Inactive Ingredients—corn starch, calcium carbonate, BALSAN® (especially purified balsam Peru).

Action and Uses: Absorbent, emollient, soothing—for diaper irritation, intertrigo, and other common dermatological conditions. In acute, simple miliaria, itching ceases in minutes and lesions dry promptly. For routine use after bathing and each diaper change.

How Supplied: 8 oz. shaker-top plastic containers.

BALMEX® EMOLLIENT LOTION

Gentle and effective scientifically compounded infant's skin conditioner.

Composition: Contains a special lanolin oil (non-sensitizing, dewaxed, moisturizing fraction of lanolin), BALSAN® (specially purified balsam Peru) and silicone.

Action and Uses: The special Lanolin Oil aids nature lubricate baby's skin to keep it smooth and supple. Balmex Emollient Lotion is also highly effective as a physiologic conditioner on adult's skin.

How Supplied: Available in 6 oz. dispenser-top plastic bottles.

BALMEX® OINTMENT

Composition: Contains: Active Ingredients—Bismuth Subnitrate, Zinc Oxide; Inactive Ingredients—Balsan (Specially Purified Balsam Peru), Benzoic Acid, Beeswax, Mineral Oil, Silicone, Synthetic White Wax, Purified Water, and other ingredients.

Action and Uses: Emollient, protective, anti-inflammatory, promotes healing—for diaper rash, minor burns, sunburn, and other simple skin conditions; also decubitus ulcers, skin irritations associated with ileostomy and colostomy drainage. Nonstaining, readily washes out of diapers and clothing.

How Supplied: 1, 2, 4 oz. tubes; 1 lb. plastic jars (½ oz. tubes for Hospitals only). Balmex Ointment-All Commercial Sizes-Safety Sealed.

Products are indexed by product category in the **BLUE SECTION.**

Marion Merrell Dow Inc.
See SmithKline Beecham Consumer Brands.

Marlyn Health Care
14851 N. SCOTTSDALE RD
SCOTTSDALE, AZ 85254

MARLYN FORMULA 50®

PRODUCT OVERVIEW

Key Facts: MARLYN FORMULA 50 is a combination of amino acids and B6 in a gelatin capsule which provides protein "building blocks" important to growth and development of all protein containing tissue including nails, hair and skin.

Major Uses: Dermatologists recommend Formula 50 not only for splitting, peeling nails but also prescribe it in conjunction with their favorite topical cream for control of nail fungus. OB-Gyn's recommend it for help in controlling excessive hair fallout after child birth.
The recommended daily dose is six capsules daily.

Safety Information: There are no known contraindications or adverse reactions.

PRESCRIBING INFORMATION

MARLYN FORMULA 50®

Composition: Each capsule contains:
Amino Acids .... 0.3 Gm*
Vitamin B6 (pyridoxine HCl) ...... 1.0 mg.
*Approximate analysis of the amino acids: indispensable amino acids (lysine, tryptophan, phenylalanine, methionine, threonine, leucine, isoleucine, valine), 35.30%; semi-dispensable amino acids (arginine, histidine, tyrosine, cystine, glycine), 19.18%; dispensable amino acids (glutamic acid, alanine, aspartic acid, serine, proline), 45.56%.
Amino acids: Protein "building blocks" important to growth and development of all protein containing tissue including nails, hair, and skin.

Dosage and Administration: The recommended daily dose is 6 capsules daily.

Supply: Bottles of 100, 250 and 1000 capsules.

MARLYN FORMULA 50 MEGA FORTE

PRODUCT OVERVIEW

Key Facts: MARLYN FORMULA 50 MEGA FORTE is a combination of amino acids and B6 in a gelatin capsule which provides protein "building blocks" important to growth and development of all protein containing tissues including nails, hair, and skin. In addition FORMULA 50 MEGA FORTE has the added advantages of Silicon, L-Cysteine and natural Mucopolysaccharides (from bovine cartilage.)

Major Uses: Dermatologists recommend FORMULA 50 MEGA FORTE not only for splitting, peeling nails but also prescribe it in conjunction with their favorite topical cream for control of nail fungus. OB-Gyn's recommend it for help in controlling excessive hair fallout after childbirth.
The recommended daily dose is six capsules daily.

Safety Information: There are no known contraindications or adverse reactions.

PRESCRIBING INFORMATION

MARLYN FORMULA 50 MEGA FORTE

Each 6 capsules contain:
Amino Acids .... 1980 mg
Vitamin B_6 .... 6 mg
Silicon
(from Amino Acid Chelate) .... 90 mg
L-Cysteine HCl .... 120 mg
(Natural Extract)
Mucopolysaccharides .... 60 mg
(from Bovine cartilage extract)
Approximate analysis of amino acids: indispensable amino acids (lysine, tryptophan, phenylalanine, methionine, threonine, leucine, isoleucine, valine), 35.30%; semi-dispensable amino acids (arginine, histidine, tyrosine, cystine, glycine), 19.18%; dispensable amino acids (glutamic acids, alanine, aspartic acid, serine, proline), 45.56%.
Amino Acids; Protein "building blocks" important to growth and development of all protein containing tissue including nails, hair, and skin.

Dosage and Administration: The recommended daily dose is 6 capsules daily.

Supply: Bottles of 90, 180, 500.

WOBENZYM N™
[wō-bĕn-zy-m]

Manufactured by Mucos Pharma GMbH in Germany. Exclusively distributed by Maryln Co., Scottsdale, AZ USA.

Description: Each enteric coated Wobenzym N tablet contains:
Pancreatin 8 NF .... 100 mg
Trypsin 720 FIP-U .... 24 mg
Chymotrypsin 300 FIP-U .... 1 mg
Bromelain 225 FIP-U .... 45 mg
Papain 164 FIP-U .... 60 mg
Rutosid 3 H_2O .... 50 mg

Dosage and Administration: Take 2 (two) tablets 3 (three) times daily after each meal.

How Supplied: Tamper-resistant blister packs of either 40 enteric coated tablets or 200 enteric coated tablets. Available without a prescription.

McNeil Consumer Products Company
Division of McNeil-PPC, Inc.
FORT WASHINGTON, PA 19034

IMODIUM® A–D
(loperamide hydrochloride)

Description: Each 5 ml (teaspoon) of Imodium A-D liquid contains loperamide hydrochloride 1 mg. Imodium A-D liquid is stable, cherry flavored, and clear in color.
Each caplet of Imodium AD contains 2 mg of loperamide and is scored and colored green.

Actions: Imodium A-D contains a clinically proven antidiarrheal medication. Loperamide HCl acts by slowing intestinal motility and by affecting water and electrolyte movement through the bowel.

Indication: Imodium A-D is indicated for the control and symptomatic relief of acute nonspecific diarrhea.

Usual Dosage: Adults: Take four teaspoonfuls or two caplets after first loose bowel movement. If needed, take two teaspoonfuls or one caplet after each subsequent loose bowel movement. Do not exceed eight teaspoonfuls or four caplets in any 24 hour period, unless directed by a physician.
9–11 years old (60–95 lbs.): Two teaspoonfuls or one caplet after first loose bowel movement, followed by one teaspoonful or one-half caplet after each subsequent loose bowel movement. Do not exceed six teaspoonfuls or three caplets a day.
6–8 years old (48–59 lbs.): Two teaspoonfuls or one caplet after first loose bowel movement, followed by one teaspoonful or one-half caplet after each subsequent loose bowel movement. Do not exceed four teaspoonfuls or two caplets a day.
Professional Dosage Schedule for children two-five years old (24–47 lbs): one teaspoon after first loose bowel movement, followed by one after each subsequent loose bowel movement. Do not exceed three teaspoonfuls a day.

Warnings: DO NOT USE FOR MORE THAN TWO DAYS UNLESS DIRECTED BY A PHYSICIAN. Do not use if diarrhea is accompanied by high fever (greater than 101°F), or if blood is present in the stool, or if you have had a rash or other allergic reaction to loperamide HCl. If you are taking antibiotics or have a history of liver disease, consult a physician before using this product. As with any drug, if you are pregnant or nursing a baby, seek the advice of a physician before using this product. Keep this and all drugs out of the reach of children. In case of accidental overdose, seek professional assistance or contact a poison control center immediately. Store at room temperature.

Overdosage: Overdosage of loperamide HCl in man may result in constipation, CNS depression and nausea. A

Continued on next page

McNeil Consumer—Cont.

slurry of activated charcoal administered promptly after ingestion of loperamide hydrochloride can reduce the amount of drug which is absorbed. If vomiting occurs spontaneously upon ingestion, a slurry of 100 grams of activated charcoal should be administered orally as soon as fluids can be retained. If vomiting has not occurred, and CNS depression is evident, gastric lavage should be performed followed by administration of 100 gms of the activated charcoal slurry through the gastric tube. In the event of overdosage, patients should be monitored for signs of CNS depression for at least 24 hours. Children may be more sensitive to central nervous system effects than adults. If CNS depression is observed, naloxone may be administered. If responsive to naloxone, vital signs must be monitored carefully for recurrence of symptoms of drug overdose for at least 24 hours after the last dose of naloxone.

Inactive Ingredients: Liquid: Alcohol (5.25%), citric acid, flavors, glycerin, methylparaben, propylparaben and purified water.

Caplets: Corn starch, lactose, magnesium stearate, microcrystalline cellulose, FD&C Blue #1 and D&C yellow #10.

How Supplied: Cherry flavored liquid (clear) 2 fl. oz., 3 fl. oz., and 4 fl. oz. tamper resistant bottles with child resistant safety caps and special dosage cups. Green Scored caplets in 6's and 12's and 18's blister packaging which is tamper resistant and child resistant.

Shown in Product Identification Section, page 413

PEDIACARE® Cold-Allergy Chewable Tablets
PEDIACARE® Cough-Cold Liquid and Chewable Tablets
PEDIACARE® NightRest Cough-Cold Liquid
PEDIACARE® Infants' Oral Decongestant Drops

Description: Each PEDIACARE Cold-Allergy Chewable Tablet contains chlorpheniramine maleate 1 mg and pseudoephedrine hydrochloride 15 mg. Each 5 ml of PEDIACARE Cough-Cold Liquid contains pseudoephedrine hydrochloride 15 mg, chlorpheniramine maleate 1 mg and dextromethorphan hydrobromide 5 mg. Each Pediacare Cough-Cold Formula Chewable Tablet contains pseudoephedrine hydrochloride 15 mg, chlorpheniramine maleate 1 mg and dextromethorphan hydrobromide 5 mg. Each 0.8 ml oral dropper of PEDIACARE Infants' Oral Decongestant Drops contains pseudoephedrine hydrochloride 7.5 mg. PEDIACARE NightRest Cough-Cold liquid contains pseudoephedrine hydrochloride 15 mg, chlorpheniramine maleate 1 mg and dextromethorphan hydrobromide 7.5 mg per 5 ml. PEDIACARE Cough-Cold Liquid and Infants' Drops are stable, cherry flavored and red in color. PEDIACARE Cold-Allergy Chewable Tablets are fruit flavored and pink in color. PEDIACARE Cough-Allergy Chewable Tablets are fruit flavored and pink in color.

Actions: PEDIACARE Products are available in four different formulas, allowing you to select the ideal product to temporarily relieve the patient's symptoms. PEDIACARE Cold-Allergy Chewable Tablets contain an antihistamine and a nasal decongestant to relieve children's cold and allergy symptoms. PEDIACARE Cough-Cold liquid and 6–12 Chewable Tablets contain both of the above ingredients plus a cough suppressant, dextromethorphan hydrobromide, to provide temporary relief of nasal congestion, runny nose, sneezing and coughing due to the common cold, hay fever or other upper respiratory allergies. PEDIACARE NightRest Cough-Cold Liquid contains a decongestant, pseudoephedrine hydrochloride, an antihistamine, chlorpheniramine maleate, and a cough suppressant, dextromethorphan hydrobromide, to provide temporary relief of coughs, nasal congestion, runny nose and sneezing due to the common cold. PEDIACARE NightRest may be used day or night to relieve cough and cold symptoms. PEDIACARE Infants' Oral Decongestant Drops contain a decongestant, pseudoephedrine hydrochloride, to provide temporary relief of nasal congestion due to the common cold, hay fever or other upper respiratory allergies.

Professional Dosage: A calibrated dosage cup is provided for accurate dosing of the PEDIACARE Liquid formulas. A calibrated oral dropper is provided for accurate dosing of PEDIACARE Infants' Drops. All doses of PEDIACARE Cold-Allergy Chewable Tablets, PEDIACARE Cough-Cold Liquid and Chewable Tablets, as well as PEDIACARE Infants' Drops may be repeated every 4–6 hours, not to exceed 4 doses in 24 hours. PEDIACARE NightRest Liquid may be repeated every 6–8 hrs, not to exceed 4 doses in 24 hours.

[See table below.]

"**WARNINGS:** Do not use if carton is opened, or if printed plastic bottle wrap or foil inner seal is broken. Keep this and all medication out of the reach of children. In case of accidental overdosage, contact a physician or poison control center immediately."

The following information appears on the appropriate package labels:

PEDIACARE Cold-Allergy Chewable Tablets: Do not exceed the recommended dosage because nervousness, dizziness or sleeplessness may occur. Do not give this product to children for more than 7 days. If symptoms do not improve, or are accompanied by fever, consult a physician. May cause excitability especially in children. May cause drowsiness. Do not give this product to children who have heart disease, high blood pressure, thyroid disease, diabetes, asthma or glaucoma unless directed by a physician.

PEDIACARE Cough-Cold Liquid, NightRest Cough-Cold Liquid and Chewable Tablets: Do not exceed the recommended dosage because nervousness, dizziness or sleeplessness may occur. Do not give this product to children for more than 7 days. If symptoms do not improve, or are accompanied by fever, consult a doctor. A persistent cough may be a sign of a serious condition. If cough persists for more than one week, tends to recur or is accompanied by fever, rash, or persistent headache, consult a doctor. Do not give this product for persistent or chronic cough such as occurs with asthma or if cough is accompanied by excessive phlegm (mucus) unless directed by a doctor. This preparation may cause drowsiness or, in some cases, excitability. Do not give this product to children who have heart disease, high blood pressure, thyroid disease, glaucoma or asthma unless directed by a doctor.

DRUG INTERACTION PRECAUTION: Do not give this product to a child who is taking a prescription drug for high blood pressure or depression,

Age Group	0–3 mos	4–11 mos	12–23 mos	2–3 yrs	4–5 yrs	6–8 yrs	9–10 yrs	11 yrs	Dosage
Weight (lbs)	6–11 lb	12–17 lb	18–23 lb	24–35 lb	36–47 lb	48–59 lb	60–71 lb	72–95 lb	
PEDIACARE Infants' Drops*	½ dropper (0.4 ml)	1 dropper (0.8 ml)	1½ droppers (1.2 ml)	2 droppers (1.6 ml)					q4–6h
PEDIACARE Cold-Allergy Chewable Tablets**				1 tab	1½ tabs	2 tabs	2½ tabs	3 tabs	q4–6h
PEDIACARE Cough-Cold Liquid**				1 tsp	1½ tsp	2 tsp	2½ tsp	3 tsp	q4–6h
and Chewable Tablets**				1 tab	1½ tabs	2 tabs	2½ tabs	3 tabs	q4–6h
PEDIACARE NightRest Liquid**				1 tsp	1½ tsp	2 tsp	2½ tsp	3 tsp	q6–8h

*Administer to children under 2 years only on the advice of a physician.
**Administer to children under 6 years only on the advice of a physician.

without first consulting the child's doctor.

PEDIACARE Infants' Oral Decongestant Drops: "Do not exceed the recommended dosage because at higher doses nervousness, dizziness or sleeplessness may occur. Do not give this product to children who have heart disease, high blood pressure, thyroid disease or diabetes unless directed by a physician. Do not give this product to children for more than seven days. If symptoms do not improve or are accompanied by fever, consult a physician. Do not give this product to children who are taking a prescription drug for high blood pressure or depression without first consulting a physician. Take by mouth only. Not for nasal use."
PEDIACARE Cold-Allergy Chewable Tablets also contain the warning, "Phenylketonurics: Contains phenylalanine 3 mg per tablet", and the inactive ingredient listing, "Inactive Ingredients: Aspartame, Cellulose, Citric Acid, Corn Starch, Flavors, Mannitol, Colloidal Silicon Dioxide, Stearic Acid, and Red #7."
PEDIACARE Cough-Cold Liquid: Inactive Ingredients: Benzoic acid, citric acid, flavors, glycerin, polyethylene glycol, propylene glycol, sodium benzoate, sorbitol, sucrose, purified water, Red #33, Blue #1 and Red #40.
PEDIACARE NightRest Cough-Cold Liquid: Inactive ingredients: Benzoic acid, citric acid, flavors, glycerin, polyethylene glycol. proplene glycol, sodium benzoate, sorbitol, sucrose, purified water. Red #33, blue #1 and Red #40.
PEDIACARE Cough-Cold Chewable Tablets also contain the warning, "Phenylketonurics: contains phenylalanine 3 mg per tablet", and the inactive ingredient listing, "Inactive Ingredients: Aspartame, cellulose, citric acid, flavors, magnesium stearate, magnesium trisilicate, mannitol, starch and Red #7."
PEDIACARE Infants' Oral Decongestant Drops: "Inactive Ingredients: Benzoic acid, citric acid, flavors, glycerin, polyethylene glycol, propylene glycol, purified water, sodium benzoate, sorbitol, sucrose and Red #40."

Overdosage: Acute dextromethorphan overdose usually does not result in serious signs and symptoms unless massive amounts have been ingested. Signs and symptoms of a substantial overdose may include nausea and vomiting, visual disturbances, CNS disturbances, and urinary retention. Symptoms from pseudoephedrine overdose consist most often of mild anxiety, tachycardia and/or mild hypertension. Symptoms usually appear within 4 to 8 hours of ingestion and are transient, usually requiring no treatment. Chlorpheniramine toxicity should be treated as you would an antihistamine/anticholinergic overdose and is likely to be present within a few hours after acute ingestion.

How Supplied: PEDIACARE Cough-Cold Liquid and NightRest Cough-Cold Liquid (colored red)—bottles of 4 fl. oz. with child-resistant safety cap and calibrated dosage cup. PEDIACARE Cold-Allergy Chewable Tablets (pink, scored)—blister packs of 16. PEDIACARE Cough-Cold Chewable Tablets (pink, scored)—blister packs of 16. PEDIACARE Infants' Drops (colored red)—bottles of ½ fl. oz with calibrated dropper.

Shown in Product Identification Section, page 413

MAXIMUM STRENGTH SINE-AID® Sinus Headache Gelcaps, Caplets and Tablets

Description: Each MAXIMUM STRENGTH SINE-AID® Gelcap, Caplet or Tablet contains acetaminophen 500 mg and pseudoephedrine hydrochloride 30 mg.

Actions: MAXIMUM STRENGTH SINE-AID® Gelcaps, Caplets and Tablets contain a clinically proven analgesic-antipyretic and a decongestant. Maximum allowable non-prescription levels of acetaminophen and pseudophedrine provide temporary relief of sinus congestion and pain. Acetaminophen is equal to aspirin in analgesic and antipyretic effectiveness and it is unlikely to produce many of the side effects associated with aspirin and aspirin-containing products. Acetaminophen produces analgesia by elevation of the pain threshold and antipyresis through action on the hypothalamic heat-regulating center. Pseudoephedrine hydrochloride is a sympathomimetic amine that promotes sinus cavity drainage by reducing nasopharyngeal mucosal congestion.

Indications: MAXIMUM STRENGTH SINE-AID® Gelcaps, Caplets and Tablets provide effective symptomatic relief from sinus headache pain and congestion. SINE-AID® is particularly well-suited in patients with aspirin allergy, hemostatic disturbances (including anticoagulant therapy), and bleeding diatheses (e.g. hemophilia) and upper gastrointestinal disease (e.g. ulcer, gastritis, hiatus hernia).

Precautions: If a rare sensitivity occurs, the drug should be discontinued. Although pseudoephedrine is virtually without pressor effect in normotensive patients, it should be used with caution in hypertensives.

Usual Dosage: Adult dosage: Two gelcaps, caplets or tablets every four to six hours. Do not exceed eight gelcaps, caplets or tablets in any 24 hour period.
Warning: Do not administer to children under 12 or exceed the recommended dosage because at higher doses nervousness, dizziness or sleeplessness may occur. Do not take this product for more than 7 days. If symptoms do not improve or are accompanied by a fever, consult a physician. Do not take this product if you have heart disease, high blood pressure, thyroid disease, diabetes or difficulty in urination due to enlargement of the prostate gland unless directed by a doctor.
Drug Interaction Precaution: Do not take this product if you are presently taking a prescription drug for high blood pressure or depression without first consulting your doctor.
Do not use if carton is open or if blister unit is broken, or if printed neck wrap or printed foil inner seal is broken. Keep this and all medication out of the reach of children. As with any drug, if you are pregnant or nursing a baby, seek the advice of a health professional before using this product. In case of accidental overdosage, contact a physician or poison control center immediately.

Overdosage: Acetaminophen in massive overdosage may cause hepatic toxicity in some patients. In adults and adolescents, hepatic toxicity has rarely been reported following ingestion of acute overdoses of less than 10 grams. Fatalities are infrequent (less than 3–4% of untreated cases) and have rarely been reported with overdoses of less than 15 grams. In children, an acute overdosage of less than 150 mg/kg has not been associated with hepatic toxicity.
Early symptoms following a potentially hepatotoxic overdose may include: nausea, vomiting, diaphoresis and general malaise. Clinical and laboratory evidence of hepatic toxicity may not be apparent until 48 to 72 hours postingestion. In adults and adolescents, regardless of the quantity of acetaminophen reported to have been ingested, administer MUCOMYST® acetylcysteine immediately if 24 hours or less have elapsed from the reported time of ingestion. For full prescribing information, refer to the MUCOMYST package insert. Do not await results of assays for acetaminophen level before initiating treatment with MUCOMYST acetylcysteine. The following additional procedures are recommended: The stomach should be emptied promptly by lavage or by induction of emesis with syrup of ipecac. A serum acetaminophen assay should be obtained as early as possible, but no sooner than four hours following ingestion. Liver function studies should be obtained initially and repeated at 24-hour intervals.
Serious toxicity or fatalities are extremely infrequent in children, possibly due to differences in the way they metabolize acetaminophen. In children, the maximum potential amount ingested can be more easily estimated. If more than 150 mg/kg or an unknown amount was ingested, obtain an acetaminophen plasma level. The acetaminophen plasma level should be obtained as soon as possible, but no sooner than 4 hours following the ingestion. Induce emesis using syrup of ipecac. If the plasma level is obtained and falls above the broken line on the acetaminophen overdose nomogram, the MUCOMYST acetylcysteine therapy should be initiated and continued for a full course of therapy. If acetaminophen plasma assay capability is not available, and the estimated acetami-

Continued on next page

McNeil Consumer—Cont.

nophen ingestion exceeds 150 mg/kg, MUCOMYST acetylcysteine therapy should be initiated and continued for a full course of therapy.

For additional emergency information, call your regional poison center or call the Rocky Mountain Poison Center toll-free, (1-800-525-6115).

Symptoms from pseudoephedrine overdose consist most often of mild anxiety, tachycardia and/or mild hypertension. Symptoms usually appear within 4 to 8 hours of ingestion and are transient, usually requiring no treatment.

Inactive Ingredients: Gelcaps: Benzyl Alcohol, Butylparaben, Castor Oil, Cellulose, Corn Starch, Edetate Calcium Disodium, Gelatin, Hydroxypropyl Methylcellulose, Iron Oxide Black, Magnesium Stearate, Methylparaben, Propylparaben, Sodium Lauryl Sulfate, Sodium Propionate, Sodium Starch Glycolate, Titanium Dioxide, FD&C Red #40.

Caplets: Cellulose, Corn Starch, Hydroxypropyl Methylcellulose, Magnesium Stearate, Polyethylene Glycol, Sodium Starch Glycolate, Titanium Dioxide, Blue #1 and Red #40.

Tablets: Cellulose, Corn Starch, Magnesium Stearate and Sodium Starch Glycolate.

How Supplied:

Gelcaps (colored red and white imprinted "SINE-AID")—blister package of 20 and tamper resistant bottle of 40.

Caplets (colored white imprinted "Maximum SINE-AID")—blister package of 24 and tamper resistant bottle of 50.

Tablets (colored white embossed "Sine-Aid")—blister package of 24 and tamper resistant bottle of 50.

Shown in Product Identification Section, page 414

CHILDREN'S TYLENOL®
acetaminophen
Chewable Tablets, Elixir, Drops Suspension Liquid, Drops

Description: Infants' TYLENOL acetaminophen Drops are stable, alcohol-free, fruit-flavored and orange in color. Infants' TYLENOL Suspension Drops are alcohol-free, grape-flavored and purple in color. Each 0.8 ml (one calibrated dropperful) contains 80 mg acetaminophen. Children's TYLENOL Elixir is stable and alcohol-free, cherry-flavored, and red in color or grape-flavored, and purple in color. Children's TYLENOL Suspension Liquid is alcohol-free, cherry-flavored and red in color. Each 5 ml contains 160 mg acetaminophen. Each Children's TYLENOL Chewable Tablet contains 80 mg acetaminophen in a grape- or fruit-flavored tablet.

Actions: Acetaminophen is a clinically proven analgesic/antipyretic. Acetaminophen produces analgesia by elevation of the pain threshold and antipyresis through action on the hypothalamic heat regulating center. Acetaminophen is equal to aspirin in analgesic and antipyretic effectiveness and it is unlikely to produce many of the side effects associated with aspirin and aspirin containing products.

Indications: Children's TYLENOL Chewable Tablets, Elixir, Drops, Suspension Liquid and Suspension Drops are designed for treatment of infants and children with conditions requiring temporary relief of fever and discomfort due to colds and "flu," and of simple pain and discomfort due to teething, immunizations and tonsillectomy.

Precautions: If a rare sensitivity reaction occurs, the drug should be stopped.

Usual Dosage: All dosages may be repeated every 4 hours, but not more than 5 times daily. Administer to children under 2 years only on the advice of a physician. Children's TYLENOL Chewable Tablets: 2–3 years: two tablets. 4–5 years: three tablets, 6–8 years: four tablets. 9–10 years: five tablets. 11–12 years: six tablets.

Children's TYLENOL Elixir and Suspension Liquid: (special cup for measuring dosage is provided) 4–11 months: one-half teaspoon. 12–23 months: three-quarters teaspoon, 2–3 years: one teaspoon. 4–5 years: one and one-half teaspoons. 6–8 years: 2 teaspoons. 9–10 years: two and one-half teaspoons. 11–12 years: three teaspoons.

Infants' TYLENOL Drops and Suspension Drops: 0–3 months: 0.4 ml. 4–11 months: 0.8 ml. 12–23 months: 1.2 ml. 2–3 years: 1.6 ml. 4–5 years: 2.4 ml.

Warning: Keep this and all medication out of reach of children. In case of accidental overdose, contact a physician or poison control center immediately. Consult your physician if fever persists for more than 3 days or if pain continues for more than 5 days. Store at room temperature.

NOTE: In addition to the above:

Children's TYLENOL® Drops and Suspension Drops—Do not use if printed carton overwrap or printed plastic bottle wrap is broken or missing or if carton is opened.

Children's TYLENOL Elixir and Suspension Liquid—Do not use if printed carton overwrap is broken or missing or if carton is opened. Do not use if printed plastic bottle wrap or printed foil inner seal is broken. Not a USP elixir.

Children's TYLENOL Chewables—Do not use if carton is opened or if printed plastic bottle wrap or printed foil inner seal is broken. Phenylketonurics: contains phenylalanine 3mg per tablet.

Overdosage: Acetaminophen in massive overdosage may cause hepatic toxicity in some patients. In adults and adolescents, hepatic toxicity has rarely been reported following ingestion of acute overdoses of less than 10 grams. Fatalities are infrequent (less than 3–4% of untreated cases) and have rarely been reported with overdoses of less than 15 grams. In children, an acute overdosage of less than 150 mg/kg has not been associated with hepatic toxicity.

Early symptoms following a potentially hepatotoxic overdose may include: nausea, vomiting, diaphoresis and general malaise. Clinical and laboratory evidence of hepatic toxicity may not be apparent until 48 to 72 hours postingestion.

In adults and adolescents, regardless of the quantity of acetaminophen reported to have been ingested, administer MUCOMYST® acetylcysteine immediately if 24 hours or less have elapsed from the reported time of ingestion. For full prescribing information, refer to the MUCOMYST package insert. Do not await results of assays for acetaminophen level before initiating treatment with MUCOMYST acetylcysteine. The following additional procedures are recommended: The stomach should be emptied promptly by lavage or by induction of emesis with syrup of ipecac. A serum acetaminophen assay should be obtained as early as possible, but no sooner than four hours following ingestion. Liver function studies should be obtained initially and repeated at 24-hour intervals.

Serious toxicity or fatalities are extremely infrequent in children, possibly due to differences in the way they metabolize acetaminophen. In children, the maximum potential amount ingested can be more easily estimated. If more than 150 mg/kg or an unknown amount was ingested, obtain an acetaminophen plasma level. The acetaminophen plasma level should be obtained as soon as possible, but no sooner than 4 hours following the ingestion. Induce emesis using syrup of ipecac. If the plasma level is obtained and falls above the broken line on the acetaminophen overdose nomogram, the MUCOMYST acetylcysteine therapy should be initiated and continued for a full course of therapy. If acetaminophen plasma assay capability is not available, and the estimated acetaminophen ingestion exceeds 150 mg/kg, MUCOMYST acetylcysteine therapy should be initiated and continued for a full course of therapy.

For additional emergency information, call your regional poison center or call the Rocky Mountain Poison Center toll free, (1-800-525-6115).

Inactive Ingredients: Children's Tylenol Chewable Tablets—Aspartame, Cellulose, Citric Acid, Ethylcellulose, Flavors, Hydroxypropyl Methylcellulose, Mannitol, Starch, Magnesium Stearate, Red #7 and Blue #1 (Grape only).

Children's Tylenol Elixir—Benzoic Acid, Citric Acid, Flavors, Glycerin, Polyethylene Glycol, Propylene Glycol, Sodium Benzoate, Sorbitol, Sucrose, Purified Water, Red #40. In addition to the above ingredients cherry flavored elixir contains Red #33 and grape flavored elixir contains malic acid and Blue #1.

Children's TYLENOL Suspension Liquid—Butylparaben, Cellulose, Citric Acid, Corn Syrup, Flavors, Glycerin, Pu-

rified Water, Sodium Benzoate, Sorbitol, Xanthan Gum, FD&C Red #40.
Infant's Tylenol Drops—Butylparaben, Citric Acid, Glycerin, Polyethylene Glycol, Propylene Glycol, Saccharin, Sodium Citrate, purified water and yellow #6.
Infant's TYLENOL Suspension Drops—Butylparaben, Cellulose, Citric Acid, Corn Syrup, Flavors, Glycerin, Purified Water, Sodium Benzoate, Sorbitol, Xanthan Gum, FD&C Red #33 and FD&C Blue #1.

How Supplied: Chewable Tablets (pink colored fruit, purple colored grape, scored, imprinted "TYLENOL")—Bottles of 30 and child resistant blister packs of 48 (fruit only). Elixir (cherry colored red and grape colored purple) Suspension liquid (cherry flavored colored red)—bottles of 2 and 4 fl. oz. Drops (colored orange)—bottles of ½ oz. (15 ml.) and 1 oz. (30 ml.) with calibrated plastic dropper. Suspension drops (grape flavored colored purple)—bottles of ½ oz (15 ml) with calibrated plastic dropper.
All packages listed above have child-resistant safety caps.

Shown in Product Identification Section, pages 412 and 413

Junior Strength TYLENOL® acetaminophen Coated Caplets and Chewable Tablets

Description: Each Junior Strength Caplet or Chewable tablet contains 160 mg acetaminophen in a small, coated, capsule shaped tablet or grape or fruit chewable tablet.

Actions: Acetaminophen is a clinically proven analgesic/antipyretic. Acetaminophen produces analgesia by elevation of the pain threshold and antipyresis through action on the hypothalamic heat-regulating center. Acetaminophen is equal to aspirin in analgesic and antipyretic effectiveness and it is unlikely to produce many of the side effects associated with aspirin and aspirin-containing products.

Indications: Junior Strength TYLENOL Caplets are designed for easy swallowability in older children and young adults. Both Junior Strength TYLENOL Caplets and Junior Strength Chewable Tablets provide fast, effective temporary relief of fever and discomfort due to colds and "flu," and pain and discomfort due to simple headaches, minor muscle aches, sprains and overexertion.

Precautions: If a rare sensitivity reaction occurs, the drug should be stopped.

Usual Dosage: Caplets should be taken with liquid. Chewable tablets should be well chewed. All dosages may be repeated every 4 hours, but not more than 5 times daily. For ages: 6–8 years: two Caplets or tablets, 9–10 years: two and one-half Caplets or tablets, 11 years: three Caplets or tablets, 12 years: four Caplets or tablets.

Warning: Do not use if carton is opened or if a blister unit is broken. Keep this and all medications out of the reach of children. In case of accidental overdosage, contact a physician or poison control center immediately. Consult your physician if fever persists for more than three days or if pain continues for more than five days. As with any drug, if you are pregnant or nursing a baby, seek the advice of a health professional before using this product. In addition the caplet package states: Not for children who have difficulty swallowing tablets. In addition the chewable tablet package states: Phenylketonurics: contains phenylalanine 5 mg per tablet.

Overdosage: Acetaminophen in massive overdosage may cause hepatic toxicity in some patients. In adults and adolescents, hepatic toxicity has rarely been reported following ingestion of acute overdosage of less than 10 grams. Fatalities are infrequent (less than 3–4% of untreated cases) and have rarely been reported with overdoses of less than 15 grams. In children, an acute overdosage of less than 150 mg/kg has not been associated with hepatic toxicity.
Early symptoms following a potentially hepatotoxic overdose may include: nausea, vomiting, diaphoresis and general malaise. Clinical and laboratory evidence of hepatic toxicity may not be apparent until 48 to 72 hours postingestion.
In adults and adolescents, regardless of the quantity of acetaminophen reported to have been ingested, administer MUCOMYST® acetylcysteine immediately if 24 hours or less have elapsed from the reported time of ingestion. For full prescribing information, refer to the MUCOMYST package insert. Do not await the results of assays for acetaminophen level before initiating treatment with MUCOMYST acetylcysteine. The following additional procedures are recommended: The stomach should be emptied promptly by lavage or by induction of emesis with syrup of ipecac. A serum acetaminophen assay should be obtained as early as possible, but no sooner than four hours following ingestion. Liver function studies should be obtained initially and repeated at 24-hour intervals.
Serious toxicity or fatalities are extremely infrequent in children, possibly due to differences in the way they metabolize acetaminophen. In children, the maximum potential amount ingested can be more easily estimated. If more than 150 mg/kg or an unknown amount was ingested, obtain an acetaminophen plasma level. The acetaminophen plasma level should be obtained as soon as possible, but no sooner than 4 hours following the ingestion. Induce emesis using syrup of ipecac. If the plasma level is obtained and falls above the broken line on the acetaminophen overdose nomogram, the MUCOMYST acetylcysteine therapy should be initiated and continued for a full course of therapy. If acetaminophen plasma assay capability is not available, and the estimated acetaminophen ingestion exceeds 150 mg/kg, MUCOMYST acetylcysteine therapy should be initiated and continued for a full course of therapy.
For additional emergency information, call your regional poison center or call the Rocky Mountain Poison Center toll-free (1-800-525-6115).

Inactive Ingredients: Caplets: Cellulose, Ethylcellulose, Magnesium Stearate, Sodium Lauryl Sulfate, Sodium Starch Glycolate, Starch.
Tablets: Aspartame, Cellulose, Citric Acid, Ethylcellulose, Flavors, Magnesium Stearate, Mannitol, Starch, Blue #1 and Red #7.

How Supplied: Coated Caplets, (colored white, coated, scored, imprinted "TYLENOL 160") Package of 30.
Chewable tablets (colored purple or pink, imprinted "TYLENOL 160") Package of 24.
All packages are safety sealed and use child resistant blister packaging.

Shown in Product Identification Section, page 413

Regular Strength TYLENOL® acetaminophen Tablets and Caplets

Description: Each Regular Strength TYLENOL Tablet or Caplet contains acetaminophen 325 mg.

Actions: Acetaminophen is a clinically proven analgesic and antipyretic. Acetaminophen produces analgesia by elevation of the pain threshold and antipyresis through action on the hypothalamic heat-regulating center. Acetaminophen is equal to aspirin in analgesic and antipyretic effectiveness and it is unlikely to produce many of the side effects associated with aspirin and aspirin-containing products.

Indications: Acetaminophen acts safely and quickly to provide temporary relief from: simple headache; minor muscular aches; the minor aches and pains associated with bursitis, neuralgia, sprains, overexertion, menstrual cramps; and from the discomfort of fever due to colds and "flu". Also for temporary relief of minor aches and pains of arthritis and rheumatism.

Precautions: If a rare sensitivity reaction occurs, the drug should be discontinued.

Usual Dosage: Adults and Children 12 years of Age and Older: 1 to 2 tablets 3 or 4 times daily. Children (6-12): ½ to 1 tablet 3 or 4 times daily. Consult a physician for use by children under 6.
WARNING: DO NOT USE IF PRINTED RED NECK WRAP IS BROKEN OR MISSING. DO NOT TAKE FOR PAIN FOR MORE THAN 10 DAYS OR FOR FEVER FOR MORE THAN 3 DAYS UNLESS DIRECTED BY A PHYSICIAN. SEVERE OR RECURRENT

Continued on next page

McNeil Consumer—Cont.

PAIN OR HIGH OR CONTINUED FEVER MAY BE INDICATIVE OF SERIOUS ILLNESS. UNDER THESE CONDITIONS, CONSULT A PHYSICIAN. KEEP THIS AND ALL MEDICATION OUT OF THE REACH OF CHILDREN. AS WITH ANY DRUG, IF YOU ARE PREGNANT OR NURSING A BABY, SEEK THE ADVICE OF A HEALTH PROFESSIONAL BEFORE USING THIS PRODUCT. IN THE CASE OF ACCIDENTAL OVERDOSAGE, CONTACT A PHYSICIAN OR POISON CONTROL CENTER IMMEDIATELY.

Overdosage: Acetaminophen in massive overdosage may cause hepatic toxicity in some patients. In adults and adolescents, hepatic toxicity has rarely been reported following ingestion of acute overdoses of less than 10 grams. Fatalities are infrequent (less than 3–4% of untreated cases) and have rarely been reported with overdoses of less than 15 grams. In children, an acute overdosage of less than 150 mg/kg has not been associated with hepatic toxicity.
Early symptoms following a potentially hepatotoxic overdose may include: nausea, vomiting, diaphoresis and general malaise. Clinical and laboratory evidence of hepatic toxicity may not be apparent until 48 to 72 hours postingestion. In adults and adolescents, regardless of the quantity of acetaminophen reported to have been ingested, administer MUCOMYST® acetylcysteine immediately if 24 hours or less have elapsed from the reported time of ingestion. For full prescribing information, refer to the MUCOMYST package insert. Do not await results of assays for acetaminophen level before initiating treatment with MUCOMYST acetylcysteine. The following additional procedures are recommended: The stomach should be emptied promptly by lavage or by induction of emesis with syrup of ipecac. A serum acetaminophen assay should be obtained as early as possible, but no sooner than four hours following ingestion. Liver function studies should be obtained initially and repeated at 24-hour intervals.
Serious toxicity or fatalities are extremely infrequent in children, possibly due to differences in the way they metabolize acetaminophen. In children, the maximum potential amount ingested can be more easily estimated. If more than 150 mg/kg or an unknown amount was ingested, obtain an acetaminophen plasma level. The acetaminophen plasma level should be obtained as soon as possible, but no sooner than 4 hours following the ingestion. Induce emesis using syrup of ipecac. If the plasma level is obtained and falls above the broken line on the acetaminophen overdose nomogram, the MUCOMYST acetylcysteine therapy should be initiated and continued for a full course of therapy. If acetaminophen plasma assay capability is not available, and the estimated acetaminophen ingestion exceeds 150 mg/kg, MUCOMYST acetylcysteine therapy should be initiated and continued for a full course of therapy.
For additional emergency information, call your regional poison center or call the Rocky Mountain Poison Center toll-free (1-800-525-6115).

Inactive Ingredients: Tablets—Magnesium Stearate, Cellulose, Sodium Starch Glycolate, and Starch. Caplets—Cellulose, Hydroxpropyl Methylcellulose, Magnesium Stearate, Polyethylene Glycol, Sodium Starch Glycolate, Starch and Red #40.

How Supplied: Tablets (colored white, scored, imprinted "TYLENOL")—tins of 12, and tamper-resistant bottles of 24, 50, 100 and 200. Caplets (colored white, "TYLENOL")—tamper-resistant bottles of 24, 50, 100. For additional pain relief, Extra-Strength TYLENOL® Gelcaps, Caplets and Tablets, 500 mg, and Extra-Strength TYLENOL® Adult Liquid Pain Reliever are available (colored green; 1 fl. oz. = 1000 mg.)

Shown in Product Identification Section, page 411

Extra Strength TYLENOL® acetaminophen Gelcaps, Caplets, Tablets

Description: Each Extra-Strength TYLENOL Gelcap, Caplet or Tablet contains acetaminophen 500 mg.

Actions: Acetaminophen is a clinically proven analgesic and antipyretic. Acetaminophen produces analgesia by elevation of the pain threshold and antipyresis through action on the hypothalamic heat-regulating center. Acetaminophen is equal to aspirin in analgesic and antipyretic effectiveness and it is unlikely to produce many of the side effects associated with aspirin and aspirin-containing products.

Indications: For the temporary relief of minor aches, pains, headaches and fever.

Precautions: If a rare sensitivity reaction occurs, the drug should be discontinued.

Usual Dosage: Adults and children 12 years of Age and Older: Two Gelcaps, Caplets or Tablets 3 or 4 times daily. No more than a total of 8 Gelcaps, Caplets or Tablets in any 24-hour period.
Warning: Do not take for pain for more than 10 days or for fever for more than 3 days unless directed by a doctor. Severe or recurrent pain or high or continued fever may be indicative of serious illness. Under these conditions, consult a doctor. **Do not use if printed red neck wrap or printed foil inner seal is broken. Keep this and all medication out of the reach of children. As with any drug, if you are pregnant or nursing a baby, seek the advice of a health professional before using this product. In case of accidental overdosage, contact a doctor or poison control center immediately.**

Overdosage: Acetaminophen in massive overdosage may cause hepatic toxicity in some patients. In adults and adolescents, hepatic toxicity has rarely been reported following ingestion of acute overdosage of less than 10 grams. Fatalities are infrequent (less than 3–4% of untreated cases) and have rarely been reported with overdoses of less than 15 grams. In children, an acute overdosage of less than 150 mg/kg has not been associated with hepatic toxicity.
Early symptoms following a potentially hepatotoxic overdose may include: nausea, vomiting, diaphoresis and general malaise. Clinical and laboratory evidence of hepatic toxicity may not be apparent until 48 to 72 hours postingestion. In adults and adolescents, regardless of the quantity of acetaminophen reported to have been ingested, administer MUCOMYST® acetylcysteine immediately if 24 hours or less have elapsed from the reported time of ingestion. For full prescribing information, refer to the MUCOMYST package insert. Do not await the results of assays for acetaminophen level before initiating treatment with MUCOMYST acetylcysteine. The following additional procedures are recommended: The stomach should be emptied promptly by lavage or by induction of emesis with syrup of ipecac. A serum acetaminophen assay should be obtained as early as possible, but no sooner than four hours following ingestion. Liver function studies should be obtained initially and repeated at 24-hour intervals.
Serious toxicity or fatalities are extremely infrequent in children, possibly due to differences in the way they metabolize acetaminophen. In children, the maximum potential amount ingested can be more easily estimated. If more than 150 mg/kg or an unknown amount was ingested, obtain an acetaminophen plasma level. The acetaminophen plasma level should be obtained as soon as possible, but no sooner than 4 hours following the ingestion. Induce emesis using syrup of ipecac. If the plasma level is obtained and falls above the broken line on the acetaminophen overdose nomogram, the MUCOMYST acetylcysteine therapy should be initiated and continued for a full course of therapy. If acetaminophen plasma assay capability is not available, and the estimated acetaminophen ingestion exceeds 150 mg/kg, MUCOMYST acetylcysteine therapy should be initiated and continued for a full course of therapy.
For additional emergency information, call your regional poison center or call the Rocky Mountain Poison Center toll-free, (1-800-525-6115).

Inactive Ingredients: Tablets—Magnesium Stearate, Cellulose, Sodium Starch Glycolate and Starch. Caplets—Cellulose, Hydroxypropyl Methylcellulose, Magnesium Stearate, Polyethylene

Glycol, Sodium Starch Glycolate, Starch and Red #40.
Gelcaps—Benzyl Alcohol, Butylparaben, Castor Oil, Cellulose, Edetate Calcium Disodium, Gelatin, Hydroxypropyl Methylcellulose, Magnesium Stearate, Methylparaben, Propylparaben, Sodium Lauryl Sulfate, Sodium Propionate, Sodium Starch Glycolate, Starch, Titanium Dioxide, Blue #1 and #2, Red #40 and Yellow #10.

How Supplied: Tablets (colored white, imprinted "TYLENOL" and "500")—vials of 10 and tamper-resistant bottles of 30, 60, 100, and 200. Caplets (colored white, imprinted "TYLENOL 500 mg")—vials of 10 and tamper-resistant bottles of 24, 50, 100, 175, and 250's.
Gelcaps (colored yellow and red, imprinted "Tylenol 500") tamper-resistant bottles of 24, 50, 100, and 150. For adults who prefer liquids or can't swallow solid medication, Extra-Strength TYLENOL® Adult Liquid Pain Reliever, mint flavored, is also available (colored green; 1 fl. oz. = 1000 mg.).

Shown in Product Identification Section, pages 411 and 412

Extra-Strength TYLENOL® acetaminophen Adult Liquid Pain Reliever

Description: Each 15 ml. (½ fl. oz. or one tablespoonful) contains 500 mg. acetaminophen (alcohol 7%).

Actions: TYLENOL acetaminophen is a clinically proven analgesic and antipyretic. Acetaminophen produces analgesia by elevation of the pain threshold and antipyresis through action on the hypothalamic heat-regulating center. Acetaminophen is equal to aspirin in analgesic and antipyretic effectiveness and it is unlikely to produce many of the side effects associated with aspirin and aspirin-containing products.

Indications: Acetaminophen provides temporary relief of minor aches, pains, headaches and fevers.

Precautions: If a rare sensitivity reaction occurs, the drug should be discontinued.

Usual Dosage: Extra-Strength TYLENOL Adult Liquid Pain Reliever is an adult preparation for those adults who prefer liquids or can't swallow solid medication. Not for use in children under 12. Measuring cup is marked for accurate dosage. Extra-Strength Dose—1 fl. oz. (30 ml or 2 tablespoonsful, 1000 mg), which is equivalent to two 500 mg Extra-Strength TYLENOL Tablets, Caplets or Gelcaps. Take every 4–6 hours, no more than 4 doses in any 24-hour period.
"**Warning:** Do not take for pain for more than 10 days or for fever for more than 3 days unless directed by a doctor. Severe or recurrent pain or high or continued fever may be indicative of serious illness. Under these conditions, consult a physician. **Do not use if printed plastic overwrap or printed foil inner seal is broken. Keep this and all medication out of the reach of children. As with any drug, if you are pregnant or nursing a baby, seek the advice of a health professional before using this product. In case of accidental overdosage, contact a doctor or poison control center immediately.**"

Overdosage: Acetaminophen in massive overdosage may cause hepatic toxicity in some patients. In adults and adolescents, hepatic toxicity has rarely been reported following ingestion of acute overdosage of less than 10 grams. Fatalities are infrequent (less than 3–4% of untreated cases) and have rarely been reported with overdoses of less than 15 grams. In children, an acute overdosage of less than 150 mg/kg has not been associated with hepatic toxicity.
Early symptoms following a potentially hepatotoxic overdose may include: nausea, vomiting, diaphoresis and general malaise. Clinical and laboratory evidence of hepatic toxicity may not be apparent until 48 to 72 hours postingestion.
In adults and adolescents, regardless of the quantity of acetaminophen reported to have been ingested, administer MUCOMYST® acetylcysteine immediately if 24 hours or less have elapsed from the reported time of ingestion. For full prescribing information, refer to the MUCOMYST package insert. Do not await the results of assays for acetaminophen level before initiating treatment with MUCOMYST acetylcysteine. The following additional procedures are recommended: The stomach should be emptied promptly by lavage or by induction of emesis with syrup of ipecac. A serum acetaminophen assay should be obtained as early as possible, but no sooner than four hours following ingestion. Liver function studies should be obtained initially and repeated at 24-hour intervals.
Serious toxicity or fatalities are extremely infrequent in children, possibly due to differences in the way they metabolize acetaminophen. In children, the maximum potential amount ingested can be more easily estimated. If more than 150 mg/kg or an unknown amount was ingested, obtain an acetaminophen plasma level. The acetaminophen plasma level should be obtained as soon as possible, but no sooner than 4 hours following the ingestion. Induce emesis using syrup of ipecac. If the plasma level is obtained and falls above the broken line on the acetaminophen overdose nomogram, the MUCOMYST acetylcysteine therapy should be initiated and continued for a full course of therapy. If acetaminophen plasma assay capability is not available, and the estimated acetaminophen ingestion exceeds 150 mg/kg, MUCOMYST acetylcysteine therapy should be initiated and continued for a full course of therapy.
For additional emergency information, call your regional poison center or call the Rocky Mountain Poison Center toll-free, (1-800-525-6115).

Inactive Ingredients: Alcohol, Citric Acid, Flavors, Glycerin, Polyethylene Glycol, Purified Water, Sodium Benzoate, Sorbitol, Sucrose, Yellow #6 (Sunset Yellow), Yellow #10 and Blue #1.

How Supplied: Mint-flavored liquid (colored green), 8 fl. oz. tamper-resistant bottle with child resistant safety cap and special dosage cup.

EXTRA STRENGTH TYLENOL® Headache Plus Pain Reliever with Antacid Caplets

Description: Each Extra Strength TYLENOL® Headache Plus Pain Reliever with Antacid caplet contains acetaminophen 500 mg. and calcium carbonate 250 mg.

Indications: TYLENOL® Headache Plus provides temporary relief of minor aches and pains with heartburn or acid indigestion and upset stomach associated with these symptoms.

Actions: TYLENOL® Headache Plus contains a clinically proven analgesic and antacid. Acetaminophen produces analgesia by elevation of the pain threshold. Acetaminophen is equal to aspirin in analgesic effectiveness, and it is unlikely to produce many of the side effects associated with aspirin and aspirin-containing products. The antacid, calcium carbonate, provides fast relief of heartburn or acid indigestion and upset stomach associated with these symptoms.

Usual Dosage: Adults and children 12 years of age and older: Two caplets every 6 hours. No more than a total of 8 caplets in any 24 hour period or as directed by a physician.

Precautions: If a rare sensitivity reaction occurs, the drug should be stopped.

Warning: Do not give this product to children under 12 years of age. Do not use the maximum dosage of this product for more than 10 days except under the advice and supervision of a physician. Do not take the product for pain for more than 10 days, or for fever for more than 3 days unless directed by a physician. If pain or fever persists or gets worse, if new symptoms occur, or if redness or swelling is present, consult a physician because these could be signs of a serious condition. **Do not use if carton is opened, or if printed neck wrap or printed foil seal is broken. Keep this and all medication out of the reach of children. As with any drug, if you are pregnant or nursing a baby, seek the advice of a health professional before using this product. In the case of accidental overdose, seek professional assistance or contact a poison control center immediately. Prompt medical**

Continued on next page

McNeil Consumer—Cont.

attention is critical for adults as well as for children even if you do not notice any signs or symptoms.

Overdosage: Acetaminophen in massive overdosage may cause hepatic toxicity in some patients. In adults and adolescents, hepatic toxicity has rarely been reported following ingestion of acute overdosage of less than 10 grams. Fatalities are infrequent (less than 3–4% of untreated cases) and have rarely been reported with overdoses of less than 15 grams. In children, an acute overdosage of less than 150 mg/kg has not been associated with hepatic toxicity.

Early symptoms following a potentially hepatotoxic overdose may include: nausea, vomiting, diaphoresis and general malaise. Clinical and laboratory evidence of hepatic toxicity may not be apparent until 48 to 72 hours postingestion. In adults and adolescents, regardless of the quantity of acetaminophen reported to have been ingested, administer MUCOMYST® acetylcysteine immediately if 24 hours or less have elapsed from the reported time of ingestion. For full prescribing information, refer to the MUCOMYST package insert. Do not await results of assays for acetaminophen level before initiating treatment with MUCOMYST acetylcysteine. The following additional procedures are recommended: The stomach should be emptied promptly by lavage or by induction of emesis with syrup of ipecac. A serum acetaminophen assay should be obtained as early as possible, but no sooner than four hours following ingestion. Liver function studies should be obtained initially and repeated at 24-hour intervals.

Serious toxicity or fatalities are extremely infrequent in children, possibly due to differences in the way they metabolize acetaminophen. In children, the maximum potential amount ingested can be more easily estimated. If more than 150 mg/kg or an unknown amount was ingested, obtain an acetaminophen plasma level. The acetaminophen plasma level should be obtained as soon as possible, but no sooner than 4 hours following the ingestion. Induce emesis using syrup of ipecac. If the plasma level is obtained and falls above the broken line on the acetaminophen overdose nomogram, the MUCOMYST acetylcysteine therapy should be initiated and continued for a full course of therapy. If acetaminophen, plasma assay capability is not available, and the estimated acetaminophen ingestion exceeds 150 mg/kg, MUCOMYST acetylcysteine therapy should be initiated and continued for a full course of therapy.

For additional emergency information, call your regional poison center or call the Rocky Mountain Poison Center toll-free (1-800-525-6115).

Inactive Ingredients: Acacia, Cellulose, Corn Starch, Croscarmellose Sodium, Hydroxypropyl Methylcellulose, Magnesium Stearate, Maltodextrin, Propylene Glycol, Sodium Starch Glycolate, Titanium Dioxide, Triacetin, Blue #1 and Blue #2.

How Supplied: Caplets (white with royal blue imprinted "TYLENOL Headache Plus"). Tamper resistant bottles of 24, 50 and 100.

Shown in Product Identification Section, page 412

EXTRA STRENGTH TYLENOL® PM

Pain Reliever/Sleep Aid Gelcaps, Caplets and Tablets

Description: Each EXTRA STRENGTH TYLENOL® PM Gelcap, Caplet or Tablet contains acetaminophen 500 mg and diphenhydramine HCl 25 mg.

Actions: EXTRA STRENGTH TYLENOL® PM gelcaps, caplets and tablets contain a clinically proven analgesic-antipyretic and an antihistamine. Maximum allowable non-prescription levels of acetaminophen and diphenhydramine provide temporary relief of occasional headaches and minor aches and pains accompanying sleeplessness. Acetaminophen is equal to aspirin in analgesic and antipyretic effectiveness and it is unlikely to produce many of the side effects associated with aspirin containing products. Acetaminophen produces analgesia by elevation of the pain threshold. Diphenhydramine HCl is an antihistamine with sedative properties.

Indications: EXTRA STRENGTH TYLENOL® PM gelcaps, caplets and tablets provide effective symptomatic relief from occasional headaches and minor aches and pains with accompanying sleeplessness.

Precautions: If a rare sensitivity occurs, the drug should be discontinued.

Usual Dosage: Adults and Children 12 years of Age and Older: Two gelcaps, caplets or tablets at bedtime or as directed by physician. Do not exceed recommended dosage.

"**WARNINGS:** Do not give to children under 12 years of age or use for more than 10 days unless directed by a physician. Consult your physician if symptoms persist or new ones occur, or if fever persists for more than 3 days, or if sleeplessness persists continuously for more than 2 weeks. Insomnia may be a symptom of serious underlying medical illness. Do not take this product if you have asthma, glaucoma, emphysema, chronic pulmonary disease, shortness of breath, difficulty in breathing or difficulty in urination due to enlargement of the prostate gland unless directed by a physician. Avoid alcoholic beverages while taking this product. Do not take if you are taking sedatives or tranquilizers without first consulting your physician. **Do not use if carton is open or if printed neck wrap or printed foil inner seal is broken. Keep this and all medications out of the reach of children. In case of accidental overdose, contact a physician or poison control center immediately. As with any drug, if you are pregnant or nursing a baby, seek the advice of a health professional before using this product.**

Caution: This product will cause drowsiness. Do not drive a motor vehicle or operate machinery after use.

Overdosage: Acetaminophen in massive overdosage may cause hepatic toxicity in some patients. In adults and adolescents, hepatic toxicity has rarely been reported following ingestion of acute overdosage of less than 10 grams. Fatalities are infrequent (less than 3–4% of untreated cases) and have rarely been reported with overdoses of less than 15 grams. In children, an acute overdosage of less than 150 mg/kg has not been associated with hepatic toxicity.

Early symptoms following a potentially hepatotoxic overdose may include: nausea, vomiting, diaphoresis and general malaise. Clinical and laboratory evidence of hepatic toxicity may not be apparent until 48 to 72 hours postingestion. In adults and adolescents, regardless of the quantity of acetaminophen reported to have been ingested, administer MUCOMYST® acetylcysteine immediately if 24 hours or less have elapsed from the reported time of ingestion. For full prescribing information, refer to the MUCOMYST package insert. Do not await results of assays for acetaminophen level before initiating treatment with MUCOMYST acetylcysteine. The following additional procedures are recommended: The stomach should be emptied promptly by lavage or by induction of emesis with syrup of ipecac. A serum acetaminophen assay should be obtained as early as possible, but no sooner than four hours following ingestion. Liver function studies should be obtained initially and repeated at 24-hour intervals. Serious toxicity or fatalities are extremely infrequent in children, possibly due to differences in the way they metabolize acetaminophen. In children, the maximum potential amount ingested can be more easily estimated. If more than 150 mg/kg or an unknown amount was ingested, obtain an acetaminophen plasma level. The acetaminophen plasma level should be obtained as soon as possible, but no sooner than 4 hours following the ingestion. Induce emesis using syrup of ipecac. If the plasma level is obtained and falls above the broken line on the acetaminophen overdose nomogram, the MUCOMYST acetylcysteine therapy should be initiated and continued for a full course of therapy. If acetaminophen plasma assay capability is not available, and the estimated acetaminophen ingestion exceeds 150 mg/kg, MUCOMYST acetylcysteine therapy should be initiated and continued for a full course of therapy.

For additional emergency information, call your regional poison center or call

the Rocky Mountain Poison Center toll-free, (1-800-525-6115).
Diphenhydramine toxicity should be treated as you would an antihistamine/anticholinergic overdose and is likely to be present within a few hours after acute ingestion.

Inactive Ingredients: Gelcaps: Benzyl Alcohol, Butylparaben, Castor Oil, Cellulose, Cornstarch, Edetate Calcium Disodium, Gelatin, Hydroxypropyl Methylcellulose, Magnesium Stearate, Propylparaben, Sodium Lauryl Sulfate, Sodium Citrate, Sodium Propionate, Sodium Starch Glycolate, Titanium Dioxide, Blue #1 and Red #28.
Tablets: Cellulose, colloidal silicon dioxide, corn starch, sodium citrate, sodium starch glycolate, stearic acid, and Blue #1. Caplets: Cellulose, colloidal silicon dioxide, corn starch, hydroxypropyl methylcellulose, polyethylene glycol, sodium citrate, sodium starch glycolate, stearic acid, titanium dioxide, Blue #1 and Blue #2.

How Supplied: Gelcaps (colored blue and white imprinted "TYLENOL PM") tamper-resistant bottles of 20 and 40.
Caplets (colored light blue imprinted "Tylenol PM") tamper-resistant bottles of 24 and 50. Tablets (colored light blue embossed with "Tylenol" on one side and "PM" on the other) tamper-resistant bottles of 24 and 50.

Shown in Product Identification Section, page 413

CHILDREN'S TYLENOL COLD®
Multi Symptom Chewable Tablets and Liquid

Description: Each Children's Tylenol Cold Chewable Grape-Flavored Tablet contains acetaminophen 80 mg, chlorpheniramine maleate 0.5 mg and pseudoephedrine hydrochloride 7.5 mg. Children's Tylenol Cold Liquid is grape flavored and contains no alcohol. Each teaspoon (5 ml) contains acetaminophen 160 mg, chlorpheniramine maleate 1 mg, and pseudoephedrine hydrochloride 15 mg.

Actions: Children's Tylenol Cold Chewable Tablets and Liquid combine the analgesic-antipyretic acetaminophen with the decongestant pseudoephedrine hydrochloride and the antihistamine chlorpheniramine maleate to help relieve nasal congestion, dry runny noses and prevent sneezing as well as to relieve the fever, aches, pains and general discomfort associated with colds and upper respiratory infections.
Acetaminophen is equal to aspirin in analgesic and antipyretic effectiveness and it is unlikely to produce the side effects often associated with aspirin or aspirin-containing products.

Indications: Provides fast, effective temporary relief of nasal congestion, runny nose, sneezing, minor aches and pains, headaches and fever due to the common cold, hay fever or other upper respiratory allergies.

Usual Dosage: Administer to children under 6 years only on the advice of a physician. Children's Tylenol Cold Chewable Tablets: 2–5 years—2 tablets, 6–11 years—4 tablets.
Children's Tylenol Cold Liquid Formula: 2–5 years—1 teaspoonful; 6–11 years—2 teaspoonsful. Measuring cup is provided and marked for accurate dosing.
Doses may be repeated every 4-6 hours as needed, not to exceed 4 doses in 24 hours. The Warnings are identical for the two dosage forms except the Liquid Cold Formula does not contain the phenylketonurics statement since the product does not contain aspartame.
Warning: Do not use if carton is opened, or if printed plastic bottle wrap or printed foil inner seal is broken.
Keep this and all medication out of the reach of children. In case of accidental overdosage, contact a physician or poison control center immediately. Phenylketonurics: contains phenylalanine, 4 mg per tablet. Do not exceed the recommended dosage because nervousness, dizziness or sleeplessness may occur. Do not take this product for more than 7 days. If fever persists for more than three days, or if symptoms do not improve or new ones occur within five days or are accompanied by high fever, consult a physician before continuing use. This preparation may cause drowsiness, or in some cases, excitability. Do not give this product to children who have heart disease, high blood pressure, thyroid disease, diabetes, glaucoma or asthma or are taking a prescription drug for high blood pressure or depression, except under the advice and supervision of a physician.

Overdosage: Acetaminophen in massive overdosage may cause hepatic toxicity in some patients. In adults and adolescents, hepatic toxicity has rarely been reported following ingestion of acute overdosage of less than 10 grams. Fatalities are infrequent (less than 3–4% of untreated cases) and have rarely been reported with overdoses of less than 15 grams. In children, an acute overdosage of less than 150 mg/kg has not been associated with hepatic toxicity.
Early symptoms following a potentially hepatotoxic overdose may include: nausea, vomiting, diaphoresis and general malaise. Clinical and laboratory evidence of hepatic toxicity may not be apparent until 48 to 72 hours postingestion.
In adults and adolescents, regardless of the quantity of acetaminophen reported to have been ingested, administer MUCOMYST® acetylcysteine immediately if 24 hours or less have elapsed from the reported time of ingestion. For full prescribing information, refer to the MUCOMYST package insert. Do not await the results of assays for acetaminophen level before initiating treatment with MUCOMYST acetylcysteine. The following additional procedures are recommended: The stomach should be emptied promptly by lavage or by induction of emesis with syrup of ipecac. A serum acetaminophen assay should be obtained as early as possible, but no sooner than four hours following ingestion. Liver function studies should be obtained initially and repeated at 24-hour intervals.
Serious toxicity or fatalities are extremely infrequent in children, possibly due to differences in the way they metabolize acetaminophen. In children, the maximum potential amount ingested can be more easily estimated. If more than 150 mg/kg or an unknown amount was ingested, obtain an acetaminophen plasma level. The acetaminophen plasma level should be obtained as soon as possible, but no sooner than 4 hours following the ingestion. Induce emesis using syrup of ipecac. If the plasma level is obtained and falls above the broken line on the acetaminophen overdose nomogram, the MUCOMYST acetylcysteine therapy should be initiated and continued for a full course of therapy. If acetaminophen plasma assay capability is not available, and the estimated acetaminophen ingestion exceeds 150 mg/kg, MUCOMYST acetylcysteine therapy should be initiated and continued for a full course of therapy.
For additional emergency information, call your regional poison center or call the Rocky Mountain Poison Center toll-free, (1-800-525-6115).
Chlorpheniramine toxicity should be treated as you would an antihistamine/anticholinergic overdose and is likely to be present within a few hours after acute ingestion.
Symptoms from pseudoephedrine overdose consist most often of mild anxiety, tachycardia and/or mild hypertension. Symptoms usually appear within 4 to 8 hours of ingestion and are transient, usually requiring no treatment.

Inactive Ingredients: Chewable Tablets—Aspartame, citric acid, ethylcellulose, flavors, magnesium stearate, mannitol, microcrystalline cellulose, pregelatinized starch, sucrose, Blue #1 and Red #7.
Liquid—Benzoic acid, citric acid, flavors, glycerin, malic acid, polyethylene glycol, propylene glycol, sodium benzoate, sorbitol, sucrose, purified water, Blue #1 and Red #40.

How Supplied: Chewable Tablets (colored purple, scored, imprinted "Tylenol Cold") on one side and "TC" on opposite side—bottles of 24. Cold Formula—bottles (colored purple) of 4 fl. oz.

Shown in Product Identification Section, page 412

CHILDREN'S TYLENOL® COLD PLUS COUGH
Multi Symptom Liquid

Description: Children's Tylenol Cold Plus Cough Liquid is cherry flavored and

Continued on next page

McNeil Consumer—Cont.

contains no alcohol. Each teaspoon (5 ml) contains acetaminophen 160 mg, chlorpheniramine maleate 1 mg, dextromethorphan hydrobromide 5 mg and pseudoephedrine hydrochloride 15 mg.

Actions: Children's Tylenol Cold Plus Cough Liquid combine the analgesic-antipyretic acetaminophen with the decongestant pseudoephedrine hydrochloride, the cough suppressant dextromethorphan hydrobromide, and the antihistamine chlorpheniramine maleate to help relieve nasal congestion, coughs, dry runny noses and prevent sneezing as well as to relieve the fever, aches, pains and general discomfort associated with colds and upper respiratory infections.
Acetaminophen is equal to aspirin in analgesic and antipyretic effectiveness and it is unlikely to produce the side effects often associated with aspirin or aspirin-containing products.

Indications: Provides fast, effective temporary relief of nasal congestion, coughs, runny nose, sneezing, minor aches and pains, headaches and fever due to the common cold, hay fever or other upper respiratory allergies.

Usual Dosage: Administer to children under 6 years only on the advice of a physician.
Children's Tylenol Cold Plus Cough Liquid Formula: 2–5 years—1 teaspoonful; 6–11 years—2 teaspoonsful. Measuring cup is provided and marked for accurate dosing.
Doses may be repeated every 4-6 hours as needed, not to exceed 4 doses in 24 hours.

Warning: Do not use if carton is opened, or if printed plastic bottle wrap or printed foil inner seal is broken. Keep this and all medication out of the reach of children. In case of accidental overdosage, contact a physician or poison control center immediately. Do not exceed recommended dosage because at higher doses nervousness, dizziness or sleeplessness may occur. Do not give this product to children for more than 7 days. If fever persists for more than 3 days, or if symptoms do not improve or new ones occur within 5 days or are accompanied by fever, consult a physician before continuing use. This preparation may cause drowsiness or in some cases, excitability. Do not give this product to children who have heart disease, high blood pressure, thyroid disease, diabetes, asthma or glaucoma unless directed by a doctor. A persistent cough may be a sign of a serious condition. If cough persists for more than 1 week, tends to recur, or is accompanied by fever, rash or persistent headache, consult a physician. Do not give this product for persistent or chronic cough such as occurs with asthma or if cough is accompanied by excessive phlegm (mucus) unless directed by a physician.

Drug Interaction Precaution: Do not give this product to a child who is taking a prescription drug for high blood pressure or depression without first consulting the child's physician.

Overdosage: Acetaminophen in massive overdosage may cause hepatic toxicity in some patients. In adults and adolescents, hepatic toxicity has rarely been reported following ingestion of acute overdosage of less than 10 grams. Fatalities are infrequent (less than 3–4% of untreated cases) and have rarely been reported with overdoses of less than 15 grams. In children, an acute overdosage of less than 150 mg/kg has not been associated with hepatic toxicity.
Early symptoms following a potentially hepatotoxic overdose may include: nausea, vomiting, diaphoresis and general malaise. Clinical and laboratory evidence of hepatic toxicity may not be apparent until 48 to 72 hours postingestion.
In adults and adolescents, regardless of the quantity of acetaminophen reported to have been ingested, administer MUCOMYST® acetylcysteine immediately if 24 hours or less have elapsed from the reported time of ingestion. For full prescribing information, refer to the MUCOMYST package insert. Do not await the results of assays for acetaminophen level before initiating treatment with MUCOMYST acetylcysteine. The following additional procedures are recommended: The stomach should be emptied promptly by lavage or by induction of emesis with syrup of ipecac. A serum acetaminophen assay should be obtained as early as possible, but no sooner than four hours following ingestion. Liver function studies should be obtained initially and repeated at 24-hour intervals.
Serious toxicity or fatalities are extremely infrequent in children, possibly due to differences in the way they metabolize acetaminophen. In children, the maximum potential amount ingested can be more easily estimated. If more than 150 mg/kg or an unknown amount was ingested, obtain an acetaminophen plasma level. The acetaminophen plasma level should be obtained as soon as possible, but no sooner than 4 hours following the ingestion. Induce emesis using syrup of ipecac. If the plasma level is obtained and falls above the broken line on the acetaminophen overdose nomogram, the MUCOMYST acetylcysteine therapy should be initiated and continued for a full course of therapy. If acetaminophen plasma assay capability is not available, and the estimated acetaminophen ingestion exceeds 150 mg/kg, MUCOMYST acetylcysteine therapy should be initiated and continued for a full course of therapy.
For additional emergency information, call your regional poison center or call the Rocky Mountain Poison Center toll-free, (1-800-525-6115).
Chlorpheniramine toxicity should be treated as you would an antihistamine/anticholinergic overdose and is likely to be present within a few hours after acute ingestion.
Symptoms from pseudoephedrine overdose consist most often of mild anxiety, tachycardia and/or mild hypertension. Symptoms usually appear within 4 to 8 hours of ingestion and are transient, usually requiring no treatment.

Inactive Ingredients: Citric Acid, Corn Syrup, Flavors, Polyethylene Glycol, Propylene Glycol, Sodium Benzoate, Sodium Carboxymethylcellulose, Sorbitol, Purified Water, Red #33 and Red #40.

How Supplied: Cold Plus Cough Formula—bottles (red colored) of 4 fl. oz.

Shown in Product Identification Section, page 412

Effervescent Formula TYLENOL® Cold Medication Tablets

Description: Each Effervescent TYLENOL Cold Tablet contains acetaminophen 325 mg., chlorpheniramine maleate 2 mg., and phenylpropanolamine hydrochloride 12.5 mg.

Actions: TYLENOL Cold Medication Tablets contain a clinically proven analgesic-antipyretic, decongestant and antihistamine. Acetaminophen produces analgesia by elevation of the pain threshold and antipyresis through action on the hypothalamic heat-regulating center. Acetaminophen is equal to aspirin in analgesic and antipyretic effectiveness and it is unlikely to produce many of the side effects associated with aspirin and aspirin-containing products. Phenylpropanolamine is a sympathomimetic amine which provides temporary relief of nasal congestion. Chlorpheniramine is an antihistamine which helps provide temporary relief of runny nose, sneezing and watery and itchy eyes.

Indications: TYLENOL Cold Medication provides effective temporary relief of runny nose, sneezing, watery and itchy eyes, nasal congestion, and aches, pains, sore throat and fever due to a cold or "flu."

Precautions: If a rare sensitivity reaction occurs, the drug should be stopped. Although phenylpropanolamine is virtually without pressor effect in normotensive patients, it should be used with caution in hypertensives.

Usual Dosage: Effervescent TYLENOL® Cold must be dissolved in water before taking.
ADULTS (12 years and over): 2 tablets every 4 hours, not to exceed 12 tablets in 24 hours.
CHILDREN (6–11): 1 tablet every 4 hours, not to exceed 6 tablets in 24 hours.
WARNINGS: Do not administer to children under 6. Do not take this product for more than 7 days (Adults) or 5 days (Children) or for fever for more than 3 days unless directed by a doctor. If sore throat is severe, persists for more than 2 days, is accompanied or followed by fever, headache, rash, nausea or vomiting,

consult a physician promptly. Do not exceed recommended dosage because at higher doses nervousness, dizziness or sleeplessness may occur. May cause excitability, especially in children. May cause drowsiness; alcohol may increase the drowsiness effect. Avoid alcoholic beverages while taking this product. Use caution when driving a motor vehicle or operating machinery. Do not take this product if you have asthma, glaucoma, emphysema, chronic pulmonary disease, shortness of breath, difficulty in breathing, heart disease, high blood pressure, thyroid disease, diabetes or difficulty in urination due to enlargement of the prostate gland unless directed by a doctor. **DO NOT USE IF GLUED CARTON FLAP IS OPENED OR IF FOIL PACK IS TORN OR BROKEN. KEEP THIS AND ALL MEDICATION OUT OF THE REACH OF CHILDREN. AS WITH ANY DRUG, IF YOU ARE PREGNANT OR NURSING A BABY, SEEK THE ADVICE OF A HEALTH PROFESSIONAL BEFORE USING THIS PRODUCT. IN CASE OF ACCIDENTAL OVERDOSAGE, CONTACT A PHYSICIAN OR POISON CONTROL CENTER IMMEDIATELY. DO NOT TAKE THIS PRODUCT IF YOU ARE ON A SODIUM RESTRICTED DIET, EXCEPT UNDER THE ADVICE AND SUPERVISION OF A DOCTOR. EACH TABLET CONTAINS 525 MG. OF SODIUM.**

DRUG INTERACTION PRECAUTION: Do not take this product if you are presently taking a prescription drug for high blood pressure or depression without first consulting your doctor.

Overdosage: Acetaminophen in massive overdosage may cause hepatic toxicity in some patients. In adults and adolescents, hepatic toxicity has rarely been reported following ingestion of acute overdosage of less than 10 grams. Fatalities are infrequent (less than 3–4% of untreated cases) and have rarely been reported with overdoses of less than 15 grams. In children, an acute overdosage of less than 150 mg/kg has not been associated with hepatic toxicity.

Early symptoms following a potentially hepatotoxic overdose may include: nausea, vomiting, diaphoresis and general malaise. Clinical and laboratory evidence of hepatic toxicity may not be apparent until 48 to 72 hours postingestion.

In adults and adolescents, regardless of the quantity of acetaminophen reported to have been ingested, administer MUCOMYST® acetylcysteine immediately if 24 hours or less have elapsed from the reported time of ingestion. For full prescribing information, refer to the MUCOMYST package insert. Do not await results of assays for acetaminophen level before initiating treatment with MUCOMYST acetylcysteine. The following additional procedures are recommended: The stomach should be emptied promptly by lavage or by induction of emesis with syrup of ipecac. A serum acetaminophen assay should be obtained as early as possible, but no sooner than four hours following ingestion. Liver function studies should be obtained initially and repeated at 24-hour intervals.

Serious toxicity or fatalities are extremely infrequent in children, possibly due to differences in the way they metabolize acetaminophen. In children, the maximum potential amount ingested can be more easily estimated. If more than 150 mg/kg or an unknown amount was ingested, obtain an acetaminophen plasma level. The acetaminophen plasma level should be obtained as soon as possible, but no sooner than 4 hours following the ingestion. Induce emesis using syrup of ipecac. If the plasma level is obtained and falls above the broken line on the acetaminophen overdose nomogram, the MUCOMYST acetylcysteine therapy should be initiated and continued for a full course of therapy. If acetaminophen plasma assay capability is not available, and the estimated acetaminophen ingestion exceeds 150 mg/kg, MUCOMYST acetylcysteine therapy should be initiated and continued for a full course of therapy.

For additional emergency information, call your regional poison center or call the Rocky Mountain Poison Center toll-free, (1-800-525-6115).

Symptoms from phenylpropanolamine overdose consist most often of mild anxiety, tachycardia and/or mild hypertension. Symptoms usually appear within 4 to 8 hours of ingestion and are transient, usually requiring no treatment.

INACTIVE INGREDIENTS: Citric Acid, Flavor, Potassium Benzoate, Povidone, Saccharin, Sodium Bicarbonate, Sodium Carbonate, Sodium Docusate, Sorbitol.

How Supplied: Tablets: carton of 20 tablets in 10 foil twin packs.

Shown in Product Identification Section, page 412

Hot Medication
TYLENOL® Cold & Flu Medication Packets

Description: Each packet of TYLENOL Cold & Flu contains acetaminophen 650 mg., chlorpheniramine maleate 4 mg., pseudoephedrine hydrochloride 60 mg. and dextromethorphan hydrobromide 30 mg.

Actions: TYLENOL Cold and Flu Medication contains a clinically proven analgesic-antipyretic, decongestant, cough suppressant and antihistamine. Acetaminophen produces analgesia by elevation of the pain threshold and antipyresis through action on the hypothalamic heat-regulating center. Acetaminophen is equal to aspirin in analgesic and antipyretic effectiveness and it is unlikely to produce many of the side effects associated with aspirin and aspirin-containing products. Pseudoephedrine hydrochloride is a sympathomimetic amine which provides temporary relief of nasal congestion. Dextromethorphan is a cough suppressant which provides temporary relief of coughs due to minor throat irritations that may occur with the common cold. Chlorpheniramine is an antihistamine which helps provide temporary relief of runny nose, sneezing and watery and itchy eyes.

Indications: TYLENOL Cold and Flu Medication provides effective temporary relief of runny nose, sneezing, watery and itchy eyes, nasal congestion, coughing, and aches, pains, sore throat and fever due to a cold or "flu."

Precautions: If a rare sensitivity reaction occurs, the drug should be stopped. Although pseudoephedrine is virtually without pressor effect in normotensive patients, it should be used with caution in hypertensives.

Usual Dosage: Adults (12 years and over): Dissolve one packet in 6 oz. cup of hot water. Sip while hot. Sweeten to taste, if desired. May repeat every 6 hours, not to exceed 4 doses in 24 hours.

WARNINGS: Do not administer to children under 12 or exceed the recommended dosage because nervousness, dizziness or sleeplessness may occur. Do not take this product for more than 7 days. If fever persists for more than 3 days, or if symptoms do not improve or are accompanied by high fever, consult a doctor. A persistent cough may be a sign of a serious condition. If cough persists for more than 1 week, tends to recur or is accompanied by fever, rash or persistent headache, consult a doctor. Do not take this product for persistent or chronic cough such as occurs with smoking, asthma, emphysema, or if cough is accompanied by excessive phlegm (mucus) unless directed by a doctor. If sore throat is severe, persists for more than 2 days, is accompanied or followed by fever, headache, rash, nausea or vomiting, consult a doctor promptly. Do not exceed recommended dosage because at higher doses nervousness, dizziness, or sleeplessness may occur. May cause excitability, especially in children. Do not take this product if you have asthma, glaucoma, heart disease, high blood pressure, emphysema, chronic pulmonary disease, shortness of breath, difficulty in breathing, diabetes, thyroid disease or difficulty in urination due to enlargement of the prostate gland unless directed by a doctor. May cause drowsiness, alcohol may increase the drowsiness effect. Avoid alcoholic beverages while taking this product. Use caution when driving a motor vehicle or operating machinery.

DO NOT USE IF GLUED CARTON FLAP IS OPENED OR IF FOIL PACKET IS TORN OR BROKEN. KEEP THIS AND ALL MEDICATION OUT OF THE REACH OF CHILDREN. AS WITH ANY DRUG, IF YOU ARE PREGNANT OR NURSING A BABY, SEEK THE ADVICE OF A HEALTH PROFESSIONAL BEFORE USING

Continued on next page

McNeil Consumer—Cont.

THIS PRODUCT. IN CASE OF ACCIDENTAL OVERDOSAGE, CONTACT A PHYSICIAN OR POISON CONTROL CENTER IMMEDIATELY. PHENYLKETONURICS: CONTAINS PHENYLALANINE 11 MG PER PACKET.
DRUG INTERACTION PRECAUTION: Do not take this product if you are presently taking a prescription drug for high blood pressure or depression without first consulting your doctor.

Overdosage: Acetaminophen in massive overdosage may cause hepatic toxicity in some patients. In adults and adolescents, hepatic toxicity has rarely been reported following ingestion of acute overdosage of less than 10 grams. Fatalities are infrequent (less than 3–4% of untreated cases) and have rarely been reported with overdoses of less than 15 grams. In children, an acute overdosage of less than 150 mg/kg has not been associated with hepatic toxicity.
Early symptoms following a potentially hepatotoxic overdose may include: nausea, vomiting, diaphoresis and general malaise. Clinical and laboratory evidence of hepatic toxicity may not be apparent until 48 to 72 hours postingestion.
In adults and adolescents, regardless of the quantity of acetaminophen reported to have been ingested, administer MUCOMYST® acetylcysteine immediately if 24 hours or less have elapsed from the reported time of ingestion. For full prescribing information, refer to the MUCOMYST package insert. Do not await results of assays for acetaminophen level before initiating treatment with MUCOMYST acetylcysteine. The following additional procedures are recommended: The stomach should be emptied promptly by lavage or by induction of emesis with syrup of ipecac. A serum acetaminophen assay should be obtained as early as possible, but no sooner than four hours following ingestion. Liver function studies should be obtained initially and repeated at 24-hour intervals.
Serious toxicity or fatalities are extremely infrequent in children, possibly due to differences in the way they metabolize acetaminophen. In children, the maximum potential amount ingested can be more easily estimated. If more than 150 mg/kg or an unknown amount was ingested, obtain an acetaminophen plasma level. The acetaminophen plasma level should be obtained as soon as possible, but no sooner than 4 hours following the ingestion. Induce emesis using syrup of ipecac. If the plasma level is obtained and falls above the broken line on the acetaminophen overdose nomogram, the MUCOMYST acetylcysteine therapy should be initiated and continued for a full course of therapy. If acetaminophen plasma assay capability is not available, and the estimated acetaminophen ingestion exceeds 150 mg/kg, MUCOMYST acetylcysteine therapy should be initiated and continued for a full course of therapy.
For additional emergency information, call your regional poison center or call the Rocky Mountain Poison Center toll-free, (1-800-525-6115).
Symptoms from pseudoephedrine overdose consist most often of mild anxiety, tachycardia and/or mild hypertension. Symptoms usually appear within 4 to 8 hours of ingestion and are transient, usually requiring no treatment.
Acute dextromethorphan overdose usually does not result in serious signs and symptoms unless massive amounts have been ingested. Signs and symptoms of a substantial overdose may include nausea and vomiting, visual disturbances, CNS disturbances, and urinary retention.
Chlorpheniramine toxicity should be treated as you would an antihistamine/anticholinergic overdose and is likely to be present within a few hours after acute ingestion.

Inactive Ingredients: Aspartame, Citric Acid, Corn Starch, Flavors, Sodium Citrate, Sucrose, Red #40 and Yellow #10.

How Supplied: Packets of powder (yellow colored) in cartons of 6 foil packets and cartons of 12 tamper-resistant foil cartons.

Shown in Product Identification Section, page 412

TYLENOL® Cold Medication No Drowsiness Formula Caplets and Gelcaps

Description: Each TYLENOL Cold Medication No Drowsiness Formula Caplet or Gelcap contains acetaminophen 325 mg., pseudoephedrine hydrochloride 30 mg. and dextromethorphan hydrobromide 15 mg.

Actions: TYLENOL Cold Medication No Drowsiness Formula Caplets and Gelcaps contain a clinically proven analgesic-antipyretic, decongestant and cough suppressant. Acetaminophen produces analgesia by elevation of the pain threshold and antipyresis through action on the hypothalamic heat-regulating center. Acetaminophen is equal to aspirin in analgesic and antipyretic effectiveness and it is unlikely to produce many of the side effects associated with aspirin and aspirin-containing products. Pseudoephedrine hydrochloride is a sympathomimetic amine which provides temporary relief of nasal congestion. Dextromethorphan is a cough suppressant which provides temporary relief of coughs due to minor throat irritations that may occur with the common cold.

Indications: TYLENOL Cold Medication No Drowsiness Formula provides effective temporary relief of the nasal congestion, sore throat, coughing, and aches, pains and fever due to a cold or "flu."

Precautions: If a rare sensitivity reaction occurs, the drug should be stopped. Although pseudoephedrine is virtually without pressor effect in normotensive patients, it should be used with caution in hypertensives.

Usual Dosage: Adults (12 years and older): Two caplets or gelcaps every 6 hours, not to exceed 8 caplets in 24 hours. Children (6–12 years): One caplet or gelcap every 6 hours, not to exceed 4 caplets or gelcaps in 24 hours for 5 days.

WARNING: Do not administer to children under 6 or exceed the recommended dosage because nervousness, dizziness or sleeplessness may occur. Do not take this product for more than 7 days. If fever persists for more than three days, or if symptoms do not improve or are accompanied by high fever, consult a physician. A persistent cough may be a sign of a serious condition. If cough persists for more than 1 week, tends to recur or is accompanied by fever, rash or persistent headache, consult a physician. Do not take this product for persistent or chronic cough such as occurs with smoking, asthma, emphysema or if cough is accompanied by excessive phlegm (mucus) unless directed by a physician. If sore throat is severe, persists for more than 2 days, is accompanied or followed by fever, headache, rash, nausea or vomiting, consult a physician promptly. Do not take this product if you have heart disease, high blood pressure, thyroid disease, diabetes, or difficulty in urination due to enlargement of the prostate gland unless directed by a physician.
DO NOT USE IF CARTON IS OPENED OR IF A BLISTER UNIT IS BROKEN. KEEP THIS AND ALL MEDICATION OUT OF THE REACH OF CHILDREN. AS WITH ANY DRUG, IF YOU ARE PREGNANT OR NURSING A BABY, SEEK THE ADVICE OF HEALTH PROFESSIONAL BEFORE USING THIS PRODUCT. IN THE CASE OF ACCIDENTAL OVERDOSAGE CONTACT A PHYSICIAN OR POISON CONTROL CENTER IMMEDIATELY.
DRUG INTERACTION PRECAUTION: Do not take this product if you are presently taking a prescription drug for high blood pressure or depression without first consulting your physician.

Overdosage: Acetaminophen in massive overdosage may cause hepatic toxicity in some patients. In adults and adolescents, hepatic toxicity has rarely been reported following ingestion of acute overdosage of less than 10 grams. Fatalities are infrequent (less than 3–4% of untreated cases) and have rarely been reported with overdosage of less than 15 grams. In children, an acute overdosage of less than 150 mg/kg has not been associated with hepatic toxicity.
Early symptoms following a potentially hepatotoxic overdose may include: nausea, vomiting, diaphoresis and general malaise. Clinical and laboratory evidence of hepatic toxicity may not be apparent until 48 to 72 hours postingestion.

In adults and adolescents, regardless of the quantity of acetaminophen reported to have been ingested, administer MUCOMYST® acetylcysteine immediately if 24 hours or less have elapsed from the reported time of ingestion. For full prescribing information, refer to the MUCOMYST package insert. Do not await results of assays for acetaminophen level before initiating treatment with MUCOMYST acetylcysteine. The following additional procedures are recommended: The stomach should be emptied promptly by lavage or by induction of emesis with syrup of ipecac. A serum acetaminophen assay should be obtained as early as possible, but no sooner than four hours following ingestion. Liver function studies should be obtained initially and repeated at 24-hour intervals.

Serious toxicity or fatalities are extremely infrequent in children, possibly due to differences in the way they metabolize acetaminophen. In children, the maximum potential amount ingested can be more easily estimated. If more than 150 mg/kg or an unknown amount was ingested, obtain an acetaminophen plasma level. The acetaminophen plasma level should be obtained as soon as possible, but no sooner than 4 hours following the ingestion. Induce emesis using syrup of ipecac. If the plasma level is obtained and falls above the broken line on the acetaminophen overdose nomogram, the MUCOMYST acetylcysteine therapy should be initiated and continued for a full course of therapy. If acetaminophen plasma assay capability is not available, and the estimated acetaminophen ingestion exceeds 150 mg/kg. MUCOMYST acetylcysteine therapy should be initiated and continued for a full course of therapy.

For additional emergency information, call your regional poison center or call the Rocky Mountain Poison Center toll-free, (1-800-525-6115).

Symptoms from pseudoephedrine overdose consist most often of mild anxiety, tachycardia and/or mild hypertension. Symptoms usually appear within 4 to 8 hours of ingestion and are transient, usually requiring no treatment.

Acute dextromethorphan overdose usually does not result in serious signs and symptoms unless massive amounts have been ingested. Signs and symptoms of a substantial overdose may include nausea and vomiting, visual disturbances, CNS disturbances, and urinary retention.

Inactive Ingredients: Caplet: Cellulose, Glyceryl Triacetate, Hydroxypropyl Methylcellulose, Magnesium Stearate, Sodium Starch Glycolate, Starch, Titanium Dioxide, Blue #1 and Yellow #10. Gelcap: Benzyl Alcohol, Butylparaben, Castor Oil, Cellulose, Corn Starch, Edetate Calcium Disodium, Gelatin, Hydroxpropyl Methylcellose, Magnesium Sterate, Methylparaben, Propylparaben, Sodium Propionate, Sodium Lauryl Sulfate, Sodium Starch Glycolate, Titanium Dioxide, Red #40 and Yellow #10.

How Supplied: Caplets (colored white, imprinted "TYLENOL Cold")—blister packs of 24 and tamper-resistant bottles of 50.

Gelcaps (colored red and tan, imprinted "TYLENOL COLD")—blister packs of 20 and tamper-resistant bottles of 40.

Shown in Product Identification Section, page 412

No Drowsiness Formula TYLENOL®Cold & Flu Hot Medication Packets

Description: Each packet of No Drowsiness TYLENOL Cold & Flu contains acetaminophen 650 mg., pseudoephedrine hydrochloride 60 mg and dextromethorphan hydrobromide 30 mg.

Actions: No Drowsiness TYLENOL Cold and Flu Hot Medication contains a clinically proven analgesic-antipyretic, decongestant, and cough suppressant. Acetaminophen produces analgesia by elevation of the pain threshold and antipyresis through action on the hypothalamic heat-regulating center. Acetaminophen is equal to aspirin in analgesic and antipyretic effectiveness and it is unlikely to produce many of the side effects associated with aspirin and aspirin-containing products. Pseudoephedrine hydrochloride is a sympathomimetic amine which provides temporary relief of nasal congestion. Dextromethorphan is a cough suppressant which provides temporary relief of coughs due to minor throat irritations that may occur with the common cold.

Indications: No Drowsiness TYLENOL Cold and Flu Hot Medication provides effective temporary relief of nasal congestion, coughing, and aches, pains, sore throat and fever due to a cold or "flu."

Precautions: If a rare sensitivity reaction occurs, the drug should be stopped. Although pseudoephedrine is virtually without pressor effect in normotensive patients, it should be used with caution in hypertensives.

Usual Dosage: Adults (12 years and over): Dissolve one packet in 6 oz. cup of hot water. Sip while hot. Sweeten to taste, if desired. May repeat every 6 hours, not to exceed 4 doses in 24 hours.

WARNING: Do not administer to children under 12 or exceed the recommended dosage because nervousness, dizziness or sleeplessness may occur. Do not take this product for more than 7 days. If fever persists for more than 3 days, or if symptoms do not improve or are accompanied by high fever, consult a doctor. A persistent cough may be a sign of a serious condition. If cough persists for more than 1 week, tends to recur or is accompanied by fever, rash or persistent headache, consult a doctor. Do not take this product for persistent or chronic cough such as occurs with smoking, asthma, emphysema, or if cough is accompanied by excessive phlegm (mucus) unless directed by a doctor. If sore throat is severe, persists for more than 2 days, is accompanied or followed by fever, headache, rash, nausea or vomiting, consult a doctor promptly. Do not take this product if you have asthma, glaucoma, heart disease, high blood pressure, emphysema, chronic pulmonary disease, shortness of breath, difficulty in breathing, diabetes, thyroid disease or difficulty in urination due to enlargement of the prostate gland unless directed by a doctor.

DO NOT USE IF GLUED CARTON FLAP IS OPENED OR IF FOIL PACKET IS TORN OR BROKEN. KEEP THIS AND ALL MEDICATION OUT OF THE REACH OF CHILDREN. AS WITH ANY DRUG, IF YOU ARE PREGNANT OR NURSING A BABY, SEEK THE ADVICE OF A HEALTH PROFESSIONAL BEFORE USING THIS PRODUCT. IN CASE OF ACCIDENTAL OVERDOSAGE, CONTACT A PHYSICIAN OR POISON CONTROL CENTER IMMEDIATELY. PHENYLKETONURICS: CONTAINS PHENYLALANINE 11 MG PER PACKET.

DRUG INTERACTION PRECAUTION: Do not take this product if you are presently taking a prescription drug for high blood pressure or depression without first consulting your doctor.

Overdosage: Acetaminophen in massive overdosage may cause hepatic toxicity in some patients. In adults and adolescents, hepatic toxicity has rarely been reported following ingestion of acute overdosage of less than 10 grams. Fatalities are infrequent (less than 3–4% of untreated cases) and have rarely been reported with overdoses of less than 15 grams. In children, an acute overdosage of less than 150 mg/kg has not been associated with hepatic toxicity.

Early symptoms following a potentially hepatotoxic overdose may include: nausea, vomiting, diaphoresis and general malaise. Clinical and laboratory evidence of hepatic toxicity may not be apparent until 48 to 72 hours postingestion.

In adults and adolescents, regardless of the quantity of acetaminophen reported to have been ingested, administer MUCOMYST® acetylcysteine immediately if 24 hours or less have elapsed from the reported time of ingestion. For full prescribing information, refer to the MUCOMYST package insert. Do not await results of assays for acetaminophen level before initiating treatment with MUCOMYST acetylcysteine. The following additional procedures are recommended. The stomach should be emptied promptly by lavage or by induction of emesis with syrup of ipecac. A serum acetaminophen assay should be obtained as early as possible, but no sooner than four hours following ingestion. Liver function studies should be ob-

Continued on next page

McNeil Consumer—Cont.

tained initially and repeated at 24-hour intervals.

Serious toxicity or fatalities are extremely infrequent in children, possibly due to differences in the way they metabolize acetaminophen. In children, the maximum potential amount ingested can be more easily estimated. If more than 150 mg/kg or an unknown amount was ingested, obtain an acetaminophen plasma level. The acetaminophen plasma level should be obtained as soon as possible, but not sooner than 4 hours following the ingestion. Induce emesis using syrup of ipecac. If the plasma level is obtained and falls above the broken line on the acetaminophen overdose nomogram, the MUCOMYST acetylcysteine therapy should be initiated and continued for a full course of therapy. If acetaminophen plasma assay capability is not available, and the estimated acetaminophen ingestion exceeds 150 mg/kg, MUCOMYST acetylcysteine therapy should be initiated and continued for a full course of therapy.

For additional emergency information, call your regional poison center or call the Rocky Mountain Poison Control toll-free, (1-800-525-6115).

Symptoms from pseudoephedrine overdose consist most often of mild anxiety, tachycardia and/or mild hypertension. Symptoms usually appear within 4 to 8 hours of ingestion and are transient, usually requiring no treatment.

Acute dextromethorphan overdose usually does not result in serious signs and symptoms unless massive amounts have been ingested. Signs and symptoms of a substantial overdose may include nausea and vomiting, visual disturbances. CNS disturbances and urinary retention.

Inactive Ingredients: Aspartame, Citric Acid, Corn Starch, Flavors, Sodium Citrate, Sucrose, Red #40 and Yellow #10.

How Supplied: Packets of powder (yellow colored) in cartons of 6 foil packets and cartons of 12 tamper-resistant foil cartons.

Shown in Product Identification Section, page 412

Multisymptom TYLENOL® Cold Medication Tablets and Caplets

Description: Each TYLENOL Cold Tablet or Caplet contains acetaminophen 325 mg., chlorpheniramine maleate 2 mg., pseudoephedrine hydrochloride 30 mg. and dextromethorphan hydrobromide 15 mg.

Actions: TYLENOL Cold Medication Tablets and Caplets contain a clinically proven analgesic-antipyretic, decongestant, cough suppressant and antihistamine. Acetaminophen produces analgesia by elevation of the pain threshold and antipyresis through action on the hypothalamic heat-regulating center. Acetaminophen is equal to aspirin in analgesic and antipyretic effectiveness and it is unlikely to produce many of the side effects associated with aspirin and aspirin-containing products. Pseudoephedrine hydrochloride is a sympathomimetic amine which provides temporary relief of nasal congestion. Dextromethorphan is a cough suppressant which provides temporary relief of coughs due to minor throat irritations that may occur with the common cold. Chlorpheniramine is an antihistamine which helps provide temporary relief of runny nose, sneezing and watery and itchy eyes.

Indications: TYLENOL Cold Medication provides effective temporary relief of runny nose, sneezing, watery and itchy eyes, nasal congestion, coughing, and aches, pains, sore throat and fever due to a cold or "flu."

Precautions: If a rare sensitivity reaction occurs, the drug should be stopped. Although pseudoephedrine is virtually without pressor effect in normotensive patients, it should be used with caution in hypertensives.

Usual Dosage: Adults: Two tablets or caplets every 6 hours, not to exceed 8 tablets or caplets in 24 hours. Children (6–12 years): One caplet or tablet every 6 hours, not to exceed 4 tablets or caplets in 24 hours for 5 days.

WARNING: Do not administer to children under 6 or exceed the recommended dosage because nervousness, dizziness or sleeplessness may occur. May cause excitability especially in children. Do not take this product for more than 7 days. If fever persists for more than three days, or if symptoms do not improve or are accompanied by high fever, consult a physician. A persistent cough may be a sign of a serious condition. If cough persists for more than 1 week, tends to recur or is accompanied by fever, rash or persistent headache, consult a physician. Do not take this product for persistent or chronic cough such as occurs with smoking, asthma, emphysema or if cough is accompanied by excessive phlegm (mucus) unless directed by a physician. This preparation may cause drowsiness, alcohol may increase the drowsiness effect. Avoid alcoholic beverages while taking this product. Use caution when driving a motor vehicle or operating machinery. If sore throat is severe, persists for more than 2 days, is accompanied or followed by fever, headache, rash, nausea or vomiting, consult a physician promptly. Do not take this product if you have heart disease, high blood pressure, thyroid disease, diabetes, asthma, glaucoma, emphysema, chronic pulmonary disease, shortness of breath, difficulty in breathing or difficulty in urination due to enlargement of the prostate gland unless directed by a physician.

DO NOT USE IF CARTON IS OPENED OR IF A BLISTER UNIT IS BROKEN. KEEP THIS AND ALL MEDICATION OUT OF THE REACH OF CHILDREN. AS WITH ANY DRUG, IF YOU ARE PREGNANT OR NURSING A BABY, SEEK THE ADVICE OF A HEALTH PROFESSIONAL BEFORE USING THIS PRODUCT. IN THE CASE OF ACCIDENTAL OVER-DOSAGE CONTACT A PHYSICIAN OR POISON CONTROL CENTER IMMEDIATELY.

DRUG INTERACTION PRECAUTION: Do not take this product if you are presently taking a prescription drug for high blood pressure or depression without first consulting your physician.

Overdosage: Acetaminophen in massive overdosage may cause hepatic toxicity in some patients. In adults and adolescents, hepatic toxicity has rarely been reported following ingestion of acute overdosage of less than 10 grams. Fatalities are infrequent (less than 3–4% of untreated cases) and have rarely been reported with overdoses of less than 15 grams. In children, an acute overdosage of less than 150 mg/kg has not been associated with hepatic toxicity.

Early symptoms following a potentially hepatotoxic overdose may include: nausea, vomiting, diaphoresis and general malaise. Clinical and laboratory evidence of hepatic toxicity may not be apparent until 48 to 72 hours postingestion. In adults and adolescents, regardless of the quantity of acetaminophen reported to have been ingested, administer MUCOMYST® acetylcysteine immediately if 24 hours or less have elapsed from the reported time of ingestion. For full prescribing information, refer to the MUCOMYST package insert. Do not await results of assays for acetaminophen level before initiating treatment with MUCOMYST acetylcysteine. The following additional procedures are recommended: The stomach should be emptied promptly by lavage or by induction of emesis with syrup of ipecac. A serum acetaminophen assay should be obtained as early as possible, but no sooner than four hours following ingestion. Liver function studies should be obtained initially and repeated at 24-hour intervals.

Serious toxicity or fatalities are extremely infrequent in children, possibly due to differences in the way they metabolize acetaminophen. In children, the maximum potential amount ingested can be more easily estimated. If more than 150 mg/kg or an unknown amount was ingested, obtain an acetaminophen plasma level. The acetaminophen plasma level should be obtained as soon as possible, but no sooner than 4 hours following the ingestion. Induce emesis using syrup of ipecac. If the plasma level is obtained and falls above the broken line on the acetaminophen overdose nomogram, the MUCOMYST acetylcysteine therapy should be initiated and continued for a full course of therapy. If acetaminophen plasma assay capability is not available, and the estimated acetaminophen ingestion exceeds 150 mg/kg, MUCOMYST acetylcysteine therapy

should be initiated and continued for a full course of therapy.
For additional emergency information, call your regional poison center or call the Rocky Mountain Poison Center toll-free, (1-800-525-6115).
Chlorpheniramine toxicity should be treated as you would an antihistamine/anticholinergic overdose and is likely to be present within a few hours after acute ingestion.
Symptoms from pseudoephedrine overdose consist most often of mild anxiety, tachycardia and/or mild hypertension. Symptoms usually appear within 4 to 8 hours of ingestion and are transient, usually requiring no treatment.
Acute dextromethorphan overdose usually does not result in serious signs and symptoms unless massive amounts have been ingested. Signs and symptoms of a substantial overdose may include nausea and vomiting, visual disturbances, CNS disturbances, and urinary retention.

Inactive Ingredients: Tablets: Cellulose, Starch, Magnesium Stearate, Yellow #6 and Yellow #10. Caplets: Cellulose, Glyceryl Triacetate, Hydroxypropyl Methylcellulose, Magnesium Stearate, Sodium Starch Glycolate, Starch, Titanium Dioxide, Blue #1 and Yellow #6 & #10.

How Supplied: Tablets (colored yellow, imprinted "TYLENOL Cold")—blister packs of 24 and tamper-resistant bottles of 50. Caplets (light yellow, imprinted "TYLENOL Cold")—blister packs of 24 and tamper-resistant bottles of 50.

Shown in Product Identification Section, page 412

TYLENOL® Cold Night Time Medication Liquid

Description: Each 30 ml (1 fl. oz.) contains acetaminophen 650 mg., diphenhydramine hydrochloride 50 mg., pseudoephedrine hydrochloride 60 mg., (alcohol 10%).

Actions: TYLENOL Cold Night Time Medication Liquid contains a clinically proven analgesic-antipyretic, decongestant, and antihistamine. Acetaminophen produces analgesia by elevation of the pain threshold and antipyresis through action on the hypothalamic heat-regulating center. Acetaminophen is equal to aspirin in analgesic and antipyretic effectiveness and it is unlikely to produce many of the side effects associated with aspirin and aspirin-containing products. Pseudoephedrine hydrochloride is a sympathomimetic amine which provides temporary relief of nasal congestion. Diphenhydramine is an antihistamine which helps provide temporary relief of runny nose, sneezing and watery and itchy eyes.

Indications: TYLENOL Cold Night Time Medication Liquid provides effective temporary relief of runny nose, sneezing, watery and itchy eyes, nasal congestion, and aches, pains, sore throat and fevers due to a cold or "flu."

Precautions: If a rare sensitivity reaction occurs, the drug should be stopped. Although pseudoephedrine is virtually without pressor effect in normotensive patients, it should be used with caution in hypertensives.

Usual Dosage: Measuring cup is provided and marked for accurate dosing. Adults (12 years and over): 1 fluid ounce (2 tbsp.) in measuring cup provided every 6 hours, not to exceed 4 doses in 24 hours. Not recommended for children.
WARNINGS: Do not take this product for more than 7 days or for fever for more than 3 days unless directed by a doctor. If symptoms do not improve or are accompanied by fever, consult a doctor. If sore throat is severe, persists for more than 2 days, is accompanied or followed by fever, headache, rash, nausea or vomiting, consult a physician promptly. Do not exceed recommended dosage because at higher doses nervousness, dizziness or sleeplessness may occur. May cause excitability, especially in children. Do not take this product if you have asthma, glaucoma, heart disease, high blood pressure, emphysema, chronic pulmonary disease, shortness of breath, difficulty in breathing, diabetes, thyroid disease or difficulty in urination due to enlargement of the prostate gland, or if you are taking sedatives or tranquilizers, unless directed by a doctor. May cause marked drowsiness; alcohol, sedatives and tranquilizers may increase the drowsiness effect. Avoid alcoholic beverages while taking this product. Use caution when driving a motor vehicle or operating machinery.
DO NOT USE IF CARTON IS OPENED OR IF PRINTED PLASTIC WRAP OR PRINTED FOIL INNER SEAL IS BROKEN. KEEP THIS AND ALL MEDICATION OUT OF THE REACH OF CHILDREN. AS WITH ANY DRUG, IF YOU ARE PREGNANT OR NURSING A BABY, SEEK THE ADVICE OF A HEALTH PROFESSIONAL BEFORE USING THIS PRODUCT. IN CASE OF ACCIDENTAL OVERDOSAGE, CONTACT A PHYSICIAN OR POISON CONTROL CENTER IMMEDIATELY.
DRUG INTERACTION PRECAUTION: Do not take this product if you are presently taking a prescription drug for high blood pressure or depression without first consulting your doctor.

Overdosage: Acetaminophen in massive overdosage may cause hepatic toxicity in some patients. In adults and adolescents, hepatic toxicity has rarely been reported following ingestion of acute overdosage of less than 10 grams. Fatalities are infrequent (less than 3–4% of untreated cases) and have rarely been reported with overdoses of less than 15 grams. In children, an acute overdosage of less than 150 mg/kg has not been associated with hepatic toxicity.
Early symptoms following a potentially hepatotoxic overdose may include: nausea, vomiting, diaphoresis and general malaise. Clinical and laboratory evidence of hepatic toxicity may not be apparent until 48 to 72 hours postingestion.
In adults and adolescents, regardless of the quantity of acetaminophen reported to have been ingested, administer MUCOMYST® acetylcysteine immediately if 24 hours or less have elapsed from the reported time of ingestion. For full prescribing information, refer to the MUCOMYST package insert. Do not await results of assays for acetaminophen level before initiating treatment with MUCOMYST acetylcysteine. The following additional procedures are recommended: The stomach should be emptied promptly by lavage or by induction of emesis with syrup of ipecac. A serum acetaminophen assay should be obtained as early as possible, but no sooner than four hours following ingestion. Liver function studies should be obtained initially and repeated at 24-hour intervals.
Serious toxicity or fatalities are extremely infrequent in children, possibly due to differences in the way they metabolize acetaminophen. In children, the maximum potential amount ingested can be more easily estimated. If more than 150 mg/kg or an unknown amount was ingested, obtain an acetaminophen plasma level. The acetaminophen plasma level should be obtained as soon as possible, but no sooner than 4 hours following the ingestion. Induce emesis using syrup of ipecac. If the plasma level is obtained and falls above the broken line on the acetaminophen overdose nomogram, the MUCOMYST acetylcysteine therapy should be initiated and continued for a full course of therapy. If acetaminophen plasma assay capability is not available, and the estimated acetaminophen ingestion exceeds 150 mg/kg, MUCOMYST acetylcysteine therapy should be initiated and continued for a full course of therapy.
For additional emergency information, call your regional poison center or call the Rocky Mountain Poison Center toll-free, (1-800-525-6115).
Diphenhydramine toxicity should be treated as you would an antihistamine/anticholinergic overdose and is likely to be present within a few hours after acute ingestion.
Symptoms from pseudoephedrine overdose consist most often of mild anxiety, tachycardia and/or mild hypertension. Symptoms usually appear within 4 to 8 hours of ingestion and are transient, usually requiring no treatment.

Inactive Ingredients: Alcohol (10%), Citric Acid, Flavors, Glycerin, Polyethylene Glycol, Purified Water, Sodium Benzoate, Sucrose, Red #40, Red #33 and Blue #1.

How Supplied: Cherry flavored (colored red) in 5 oz. bottles with child-resistant safety cap, special dosage cup graded in ounces and tablespoons, and tamper-resistant packaging.

Shown in Product Identification Section, page 412

Continued on next page

McNeil Consumer—Cont.

Maximum-Strength TYLENOL® Allergy Sinus Medication Caplets, Gelcaps

Description: Each TYLENOL® Allergy Sinus Caplet or Gelcap contains acetaminophen 500 mg, chlorpheniramine maleate 2 mg, and pseudoephedrine hydrochloride 30 mg.

Actions: TYLENOL® Allergy Sinus Caplets or Gelcaps contain a clinically proven analgesic-antipyretic, decongestant, and antihistamine. Acetaminophen produces analgesia by elevation of the pain threshold and antipyresis through action on the hypothalamic heat-regulating center. Acetaminophen is equal to aspirin in analgesic and antipyretic effectiveness, and it is unlikely to produce many of the side effects associated with aspirin and aspirin-containing products. Pseudoephedrine hydrochloride is a sympathomimetic amine which provides temporary relief of nasal congestion. Chlorpheniramine is an antihistamine which helps provide temporary relief of runny nose, sneezing and watery and itchy eyes.

Indications: TYLENOL® Allergy Sinus provides effective temporary relief of these upper respiratory allergy, hay fever and sinusitis symptoms: sneezing, itchy, watery eyes, runny nose, itching of the nose or throat, nasal and sinus congestion and sinus pain and headaches.

Precautions: If a rare sensitivity reaction occurs, the drug should be stopped. Although pseudoephedrine is virtually without pressor effect in normotensive patients, it should be used with caution in hypertensives.

Usual Dosage: Adults: Two caplets or gelcaps every 6 hours, not to exceed 8 caplets or gelcaps in 24 hours.
"WARNING: Do not administer to children under 12 or exceed the recommended dosage because nervousness, dizziness, or sleeplessness may occur. May cause excitability, especially in children. This preparation may cause drowsiness; alcohol may increase the drowsiness effect. Avoid alcoholic beverages when taking this product. Use caution when driving a motor vehicle or operating machinery. Do not take this product if you have heart disease, high blood pressure, thyroid disease, diabetes, asthma, glaucoma, emphysema, chronic pulmonary disease, shortness of breath, difficulty in breathing or difficulty in urination due to enlargement of prostate gland unless directed by a doctor. Do not take this product for more than 7 days. If symptoms do not improve or are accompanied by a high fever, consult a physician." **DO NOT USE IF CARTON IS OPEN OR IF A BLISTER UNIT IS BROKEN. KEEP THIS AND ALL MEDICATION OUT OF THE REACH OF CHILDREN. AS WITH ANY DRUG, IF YOU ARE PREGNANT OR NURSING A BABY, SEEK THE ADVICE OF A HEALTH PROFESSIONAL BEFORE USING THIS PRODUCT. IN THE CASE OF ACCIDENTAL OVERDOSE, CONTACT A PHYSICIAN OR POISON CONTROL CENTER IMMEDIATELY. DRUG INTERACTION PRECAUTION:** Do not take this product if you are presently taking a prescription drug for high blood pressure or depression without first consulting your doctor.

Overdosage: Acetaminophen in massive overdosage may cause hepatic toxicity in some patients. In adults and adolescents, hepatic toxicity has rarely been reported following ingestion of acute overdosage of less than 10 grams. Fatalities are infrequent (less than 3–4% of untreated cases) and have rarely been reported with overdoses of less than 15 grams. In children, an acute overdosage of less than 150 mg/kg has not been associated with hepatic toxicity.
Early symptoms following a potentially hepatotoxic overdose may include: nausea, vomiting, diaphoresis and general malaise. Clinical and laboratory evidence of hepatic toxicity may not be apparent until 48 to 72 hours postingestion.
In adults and adolescents, regardless of the quantity of acetaminophen reported to have been ingested, administer MUCOMYST® acetylcysteine immediately if 24 hours or less have elapsed from the reported time of ingestion. For full prescribing information, refer to the MUCOMYST package insert. Do not await results of assays for acetaminophen level before initiating treatment with MUCOMYST acetylcysteine. The following additional procedures are recommended: The stomach should be emptied promptly by lavage or by induction of emesis with syrup of ipecac. A serum acetaminophen assay should be obtained as early as possible, but no sooner than four hours following ingestion. Liver function studies should be obtained initially and repeated at 24-hour intervals.
Several toxicity or fatalities are extremely infrequent in children, possibly due to differences in the way they metabolize acetaminophen. In children, the maximum potential amount ingested can be easily estimated. If more than 150 mg/kg or an unknown amount was ingested, obtain an acetaminophen plasma level. The acetaminophen plasma level should be obtained as soon as possible, but no sooner than 4 hours following ingestion. Induce emesis using syrup of ipecac. If the plasma level is obtained and falls above the broken line on the acetaminophen overdose nomogram, the MUCOMYST acetylcysteine therapy should be initiated and continued for a full course of therapy. If acetaminophen plasma assay capability is not available, and the estimated acetaminophen ingestion exceeds 150 mg/kg, MUCOMYST acetylcysteine therapy should be initiated and continued for a full course of therapy.
For additional emergency information, call your regional poison center or call the Rocky Mountain Poison Control Center toll-free, (1-800-525-6115).
Chlorpheniramine toxicity should be treated as you would an antihistamine/anticholinergic overdose and is likely to be present within a few hours after acute ingestion.
Symptoms from pseudophedrine overdose consist most often of mild anxiety, tachycardia and/or hypertension. Symptoms usually appear within 4 to 8 hours of ingestion and are transient, usually requiring no treatment.

Inactive Ingredients: CAPLET: Cellulose, hydroxypropyl cellulose, hydroxypropyl methylcellulose, magnesium stearate, polyethylene glycol, sodium starch glycolate, corn starch, titanium dioxide, blue #1, yellow #6, yellow #10.
GELCAP: Benzyl Alcohol, Butylparaben, Castor oil, Cellulose, Edetate Calcium Disodium, Gelatin, Hydroxypropyl Methylcellulose, Magnesium Stearate, Methylparaben, Propylparaben, Sodium Lauryl Sulfate, Sodium Propionate, Sodium Starch Glycolate, Starch, Titanium Dioxide Blue #1 and #2 and Yellow #10.

How Supplied: Caplets: (dark yellow, imprinted "TYLENOL Allergy Sinus")—Blister packs of 24 and tamper-resistant bottles of 50.
Gelcaps: (dark green and dark yellow, imprinted "TYLENOL A/S")—Blister packs of 20 and tamper-resistant bottles of 40.

Shown in Product Identification Section, page 413

MAXIMUM STRENGTH TYLENOL® COUGH MEDICATION

Description: Each 20 ml (4 tsp.) adult dose contains dextromethorphan HBr 30 mg., and acetaminophen 1,000mg.

Actions: MAXIMUM STRENGTH TYLENOL® COUGH Medication Liquid contains a clinically proven cough suppressant and analgesic-antipyretic. Acetaminophen produces analgesia by elevation of the pain threshold and antipyresis through action on the hypothalamic heat-regulating center. Dextromethorphan is a cough suppressant which provides temporary relief of coughs due to minor throat irritations that may occur with the common cold.

Indications: MAXIMUM STRENGTH TYLENOL® COUGH Medication provides effective, temporary relief of coughing, and the aches, pains and sore throat that may accompany a cough due to a cold.

Usual Dosage: A specially marked dosage cup is provided for accurate dosing. Adults: (12 years and older) 4 teaspoons or 20ml as marked on dosage cup every 6–8 hours, not to exceed 4 doses in 24 hours. Children: (ages 6–11) 1 1/4 teaspoons or 6.25ml as marked on dosage cup every 4 hours, not to exceed 5 doses in 24 hours. Not recommended for children under 6 years.

WARNING: Do not take this product for more than 10 days or for fever for more than 3 days unless directed by a physician. Severe or recurrent pain or high or continued fever may be indicative of serious illness. Under these conditions, consult a physician. A persistent cough may be a sign of a serious condition. If cough persists for more than 1 week, tends to recur or is accompanied by fever, rash or persistent headache, consult a doctor. Do not take this product for persistent or chronic cough such as occurs with smoking, asthma, emphysema, or if cough is accompanied by excessive phlegm (mucus) unless directed by a doctor. If sore throat is severe, persists for more than 2 days, is accompanied or followed by fever, headache, rash, nausea or vomiting, consult a doctor promptly.

Do not use if carton is opened or if printed neck wrap (under dosage cup) or printed foil inner seal is broken. Keep this and all medication out of the reach of children. As with any drug, if you are pregnant or nursing a baby, seek the advice of a health professional before using this product. In case of accidental overdosage, contact a doctor or poison control center immediately.

Drug Interaction Precaution: Do not take this product if you are presently taking a prescription drug (MAOI) without first consulting your doctor.

Overdosage: Acetaminophen in massive dosage may cause hepatic toxicity in some patients. In adults and adolescents, hepatic toxicity has rarely been reported following ingestion of acute overdosage of less than 10 grams. Fatalities are infrequent (less than 3–4% of untreated cases) and have rarely been reported with overdoses of less than 15 grams. In children, an acute overdosage of less than 150mg/kg has not been associated with hepatic toxicity.

Early symptoms following a potentially hepatotoxic overdose may include: nausea, vomiting, diaphoresis and general malaise. Clinical and laboratory evidence of hepatic toxicity may not be apparent until 48 to 72 hours postingestion.

In adults and adolescents, regardless of the quantity of acetaminophen reported to have been ingested, administer MUCOMYST® acetylcysteine immediately if 24 hours or less have elapsed from the reported time of ingestion. For full prescribing information, refer to the MUCOMYST package insert. Do not await results of assays for acetaminophen level before initiating treatment with MUCOMYST acetylcysteine. The following additional procedures are recommended: The stomach should be emptied by lavage or by induction of emesis with syrup of ipecac. A serum acetaminophen assay should be obtained as early as possible, but no sooner than four hours following ingestion. Liver function studies should be obtained initially and repeated at 24-hour intervals.

Serious toxicity or fatalities are extremely infrequent in children, possibly due to differences in the way they metabolize acetaminophen. In children, the maximum potential amount ingested can be more easily estimated. If more than 150mg/kg or an unknown amount was ingested, obtain an acetaminophen plasma level. The acetaminophen plasma level should be obtained as soon as possible, but no sooner than 4 hours following the ingestion. Induce emesis using syrup of ipecac. If the plasma level is obtained and falls above the broken line on the acetaminophen overdose nomogram, the MUCOMYST acetylcysteine therapy should be initiated and continued for a full course of therapy. If acetaminophen plasma assay capability is not available, and the estimated acetaminophen ingestion exceeds 150mg/kg, MUCOMYST acetycysteine therapy should be initiated and continued for a full course of therapy.

For additional emergency information, call your regional poison center or call the Rocky Mountain Poison Center toll free (1-800-526-6115).

Acute dextromethorphan overdose usually does not result in serious signs and symptoms unless massive amounts have been ingested. Signs and symptoms of a substantial overdose may include nausea and vomiting, visual disturbances, CNS disturbances, and urinary retention.

Inactive Ingredients: Alcohol (10%), Citric Acid, Flavors, Glycerin, Polyethylene Glycol, Purified Water, Sodium Benzoate, Sodium Carboxymethylcellulose, Sodium Saccharin, Sorbitol, Sucrose, Red #33, and Red #40.

How Supplied: MAXIMUM STRENGTH TYLENOL® COUGH is available in a 4 oz. bottle with child-resistant safety cap, special dosing cup marked in ml, and tamper resistant packaging.

Shown in Product Identification Section, page 412

MAXIMUM STRENGTH TYLENOL® COUGH MEDICATION WITH DECONGESTANT

Description: Each 20 ml (4 tsp.) adult dose contains dextromethorphan HBr 30 mg., and acetaminophen 1,000mg, and pseudoephedrine HCl 60mg.

Actions: MAXIMUM STRENGTH TYLENOL® COUGH with Decongestant Medication Liquid contains a clinically proven cough suppressant, an analgesic-antipyretic, and decongestant. Acetaminophen produces analgesia by elevation of the pain threshold and antipyresis through action on the hypothalamic heat-regulating center. Dextromethorphan is a cough suppressant which provides temporary relief of coughs due to minor throat irritations that may occur with the common cold. Pseudoephedrine hydrochloride is a sympathomimetic amine which provides temporary relief of nasal congestion.

Indications: MAXIMUM STRENGTH TYLENOL® COUGH with Decongestant Medication provides effective, temporary relief of coughing, nasal congestion and the aches, pains and sore throat that may accompany a cough due to a cold.

Usual Dosage: A specially marked dosage cup is provided for accurate dosing. Adults: (12 years and older) 4 teaspoons or 20ml as marked on dosage cup every 6–8 hours, not to exceed 4 doses in 24 hours. Children: (ages 6–11) 1 1/4 teaspoons or 6.25ml as marked on dosage cup every 4 hours, not to exceed 5 doses in 24 hours. Not recommended for children under 6 years.

WARNING: Do not take this product for more than 7 days or for fever for more than 3 days unless directed by a doctor. If symptoms do not improve or are accompanied by fever, consult a physician. A persistent cough may be a sign of a serious condition. If cough persists for more than 1 week, tends to recur or is accompanied by fever, rash or persistent headache, consult a doctor. Do not take this product for persistent or chronic cough such as occurs with smoking, asthma, emphysema, or if cough is accompanied by excessive phlegm (mucus) unless directed by a doctor. Do not exceed the recommended dosage because at higher doses nervousness, dizziness or sleeplessness may occur. Do not take this product if you have heart disease, high blood pressure, thyroid disease, diabetes or difficulty in urination due to enlargement of the prostate gland unless directed by a doctor. If sore throat is severe, persists for more than 2 days, is accompanied or followed by fever, headache, rash, nausea or vomiting, consult a doctor promptly.

Do not use if carton is opened or if printed neck wrap (under dosage cup) or printed foil inner seal is broken. Keep this and all medication out of the reach of children. As with any drug, if you are pregnant or nursing a baby, seek the advice of a health professional before using this product. In case of accidental overdosage, contact a doctor or poison control center immediately.

Drug Interaction Precaution: Do not take this product if you are presently taking a prescription drug for high blood pressure or depression, without first consulting your doctor.

Overdosage: Acetaminophen in massive dosage may cause hepatic toxicity in some patients. In adults and adolescents, hepatic toxicity has rarely been reported following ingestion of acute overdosage of less than 10 grams. Fatalities are infrequent (less than 3–4% of untreated

Continued on next page

cases) and have rarely been reported with overdoses of less than 15 grams. In children, an acute overdosage of less than 150mg/kg has not been associated with hepatic toxicity.

Early symptoms following a potentially hepatotoxic overdose may include: nausea, vomiting, diaphoresis and general malaise. Clinical and laboratory evidence of hepatic toxicity may not be apparent until 48 to 72 hours postingestion. In adults and adolescents, regardless of the quantity of acetaminophen reported to have been ingested, administer MUCOMYST® acetylcysteine immediately if 24 hours or less have elapsed from the reported time of ingestion. For full prescribing information, refer to the MUCOMYST package insert. Do not await results of assays for acetaminophen level before initiating treatment with MUCOMYST acetylcysteine. The following additional procedures are recommended: The stomach should be emptied by lavage or by induction of emesis with syrup of ipecac. A serum acetaminophen assay should be obtained as early as possible, but no sooner than four hours following ingestion. Liver function studies should be obtained initially and repeated at 24-hour intervals.

Serious toxicity or fatalities are extremely infrequent in children, possibly due to differences in the way they metabolize acetaminophen. In children, the maximum potential amount ingested can be more easily estimated. If more than 150mg/kg or an unknown amount was ingested, obtain an acetaminophen plasma level. The acetaminophen plasma level should be obtained as soon as possible, but no sooner than 4 hours following the ingestion. Induce emesis using syrup of ipecac. If the plasma level is obtained and falls above the broken line on the acetaminophen overdose nomogram, the MUCOMYST acetylcysteine therapy should be initiated and continued for a full course of therapy. If acetaminophen plasma assay capability is not available, and the estimated acetaminophen ingestion exceeds 150mg/kg, MUCOMYST acetycysteine therapy should be initiated and continued for a full course of therapy. For additional emergency information, call your regional poison center or call the Rocky Mountain Poison Center toll free (1-800-526-6115).

Acute dextromethorphan overdose usually does not result in serious signs and symptoms unless massive amounts have been ingested. Signs and symptoms of a substantial overdose may include nausea and vomiting, visual disturbances, CNS disturbances, and urinary retention.

Symptoms from pseudoephedrine overdose consist most often of mild anxiety, tachycardia and/or mild hypertension. Symptoms usually appear witin 4 to 8 hours of ingestion and are transient, usually requiring no treatment.

Inactive Ingredients: Alcohol (10%), Citric Acid, Flavors, Glycerin, Polyethylene Glycol, Purified Water, Sodium Benzoate, Sodium Carboxymethylcellulose, Sodium Saccharin, Sorbitol, Sucrose, Red #33, Red #40 and Blue #1.

How Supplied: MAXIMUM STRENGTH TYLENOL COUGH with Decongestant is available in a 4 oz. and 8 oz. bottles with child-resistant safety cap, special dosing cup marked in ml, and tamper resistant packaging.

Shown in Product Identification Section, page 412

Maximum-Strength TYLENOL® Sinus Medication Gelcaps, Caplets and Tablets

Description: Each Maximum-Strength TYLENOL® Sinus Medication Gelcap, Caplet or Tablet contains acetaminophen 500 mg and pseudoephedrine hydrochloride 30 mg.

Actions: TYLENOL Sinus Medication contains a clinically proven analgesic-antipyretic and a decongestant. Maximum allowable non-prescription levels of acetaminophen and pseudoephedrine provide temporary relief of sinus headache and congestion. Acetaminophen is equal to aspirin in analgesic and antipyretic effectiveness and it is unlikely to produce many of the side effects associated with aspirin and aspirin-containing products.

Acetaminophen produces analgesia by elevation of the pain threshold and antipyresis through action on the hypothalamic heat-regulating center. Pseudoephedrine hydrochloride is a sympathomimetic amine which promotes sinus cavity drainage by reducing nasopharyngeal mucosal congestion.

Indications: Maximum-Strength TYLENOL Sinus Medication provides effective symptomatic relief from sinus headache pain and congestion. Maximum-Strength TYLENOL Sinus Medication is particularly well-suited in patients with aspirin allergy, hemostatic disturbances (including anticoagulant therapy), and bleeding diatheses (e.g., hemophilia) and upper gastrointestinal disease (e.g., ulcer, gastritis, hiatus hernia).

Precautions: If a rare sensitivity occurs, the drug should be discontinued. Although pseudoephedrine is virtually without pressor effect in normotensive patients, it should be used with caution in hypertensives.

Usual Dosage: Adults and Children 12 years of Age and Older: Two Tablets, Caplets or Gelcaps every 4–6 hours. Do not exceed eight Tablets, Caplets or Gelcaps in any 24-hour period.

WARNING: Do not administer to children under 12 or exceed the recommended dosage because at higher doses nervousness, dizziness, or sleeplessness may occur. Do not take this product for more than 7 days. If symptoms do not improve or are accompanied by fever, consult a physician. Do not take this product if you have heart disease, high blood pressure, thyroid disease, diabetes, or difficulty in urination due to enlargement of the prostate gland unless directed by a doctor.

DRUG INTERACTION PRECAUTION: Do not take this product if you are presently taking a prescription drug for high blood pressure or depression without first consulting your doctor. **Do not use if carton is opened or if blister unit is broken or if printed green neck wrap or printed foil inner seal is broken. Keep this and all medication out of the reach of children. As with any drug, if you are pregnant or nursing a baby, seek the advice of a health professional before using this product. In case of accidental overdosage, contact a physician or poison control center immediately.**

Overdosage: Acetaminophen in massive overdosage may cause hepatic toxicity in some patients. In adults and adolescents, hepatic toxicity has rarely been reported following ingestion of acute overdosage of less than 10 grams. Fatalities are infrequent (less than 3–4% of untreated cases) and have rarely been reported with overdoses of less than 15 grams. In children, an acute overdosage of less than 150 mg/kg has not been associated with hepatic toxicity.

Early symptoms following a potentially hepatotoxic overdose may include: nausea, vomiting, diaphoresis and general malaise. Clinical and laboratory evidence of hepatic toxicity may not be apparent until 48 to 72 hours postingestion. In adults and adolescents, regardless of the quantity of acetaminophen reported to have been ingested, administer MUCOMYST® acetylcysteine immediately if 24 hours or less have elapsed from the reported time of ingestion. For full prescribing information, refer to the MUCOMYST package insert. Do not await the results of assays for acetaminophen level before initiating treatment with MUCOMYST acetylcysteine. The following additional procedures are recommended: The stomach should be emptied promptly by lavage or by induction of emesis with syrup of ipecac. A serum acetaminophen assay should be obtained as early as possible, but no sooner than four hours following ingestion. Liver function studies should be obtained initially and repeated at 24-hour intervals.

Serious toxicity or fatalities are extremely infrequent in children, possibly due to differences in the way they metabolize acetaminophen. In children, the maximum potential amount ingested can be more easily estimated. If more than 150 mg/kg or an unknown amount was ingested, obtain an acetaminophen plasma level. The acetaminophen plasma level should be obtained as soon as possible, but no sooner than 4 hours following the ingestion. Induce emesis using syrup of ipecac. If the plasma level

is obtained and falls above the broken line on the acetaminophen overdose nomogram, the MUCOMYST acetylcysteine therapy should be initiated and continued for a full course of therapy. If acetaminophen plasma assay capability is not available, and the estimated acetaminophen ingestion exceeds 150 mg/kg, MUCOMYST acetylcysteine therapy should be initiated and continued for a full course of therapy.
For additional emergency information, call your regional poison center or call the Rocky Mountain Poison Center toll-free, (1-800-525-6115).
Symptoms from pseudoephedrine overdose consist most often of mild anxiety, tachycardia and/or mild hypertension. Symptoms usually appear within 4 to 8 hours of ingestion and are transient, usually requiring no treatment.

Inactive Ingredients: Caplets—Cellulose, Hydroxypropyl Methylcellulose, Magnesium Stearate, Polyethylene Glycol, Polysorbate 80, Sodium Starch Glycolate, Starch, Titanium Dioxide, Blue #1, Red #40 and Yellow #10. Tablets—Cellulose, Magnesium Stearate, Sodium Lauryl Sulfate, Starch, Yellow #6, Yellow #10, and Blue #1.
Gelcaps—Benzyl alcohol, butylparaben, castor oil, cellulose, edetate calcium disodium, gelatin, hydroxypropyl methylcellulose, iron oxide black, magnesium stearate, methylparaben, propylparaben, sodium lauryl sulfate, sodium propionate, sodium starch glycolate, starch, titanium dioxide, Blue #1 and Yellow #10.

How Supplied: Tablets (colored light green, imprinted "Maximum-Strength TYLENOL Sinus")—tamper-resistant bottles of 24 and 50. Caplets (light green coating, printed "TYLENOL Sinus" in dark green) tamper-resistant bottles of 24 and 50.
Gelcaps (colored green and white), imprinted "TYLENOL Sinus" in tamper-resistant packages of 20 and 40.

Shown in Product Identification Section, page 413

Mead Johnson Nutritionals

A Bristol-Myers Squibb Company
2400 W. LLOYD EXPRESSWAY
EVANSVILLE, IN 47721

Enfamil® Infant Formula[1]
Enfamil® With Iron Infant Formula[1]
Enfamil® Infant Formula Nursette®
Enfamil® Premature Formula
Enfamil® Premature Formula With Iron
Enfamil® Human Milk Fortifier
Fer-In-Sol® Iron Supplement Drops, Syrup, Capsules
Nutramigen® Hypoallergenic Protein Hydrolysate Formula[1]

[1]Concentrated liquid, powder, and ready to use

Poly-Vi-Sol® Vitamins, Chewable Tablets and Drops (without Iron)
Poly-Vi-Sol® Vitamins, Peter Rabbit[2] Shaped Chewable Tablets (without Iron)
Poly-Vi-Sol® Vitamins with Iron, Peter Rabbit[2] Shaped Chewable Tablets
Poly-Vi-Sol® Vitamins with Iron, Drops
ProSobee® Soy Formula[1]
ProSobee® Soy Formula Nursette®[1]

[2]Registered trademark of F. Warne & Co., Inc.

Special Metabolic Diets:
Lofenalac® Iron Fortified Low Phenylalanine Diet Powder
Low Methionine Diet Powder (Product 3200K)
Low PHE/TYR Diet Powder (Product 3200AB)
Mono- and Disaccharide-Free Diet Powder (Product 3232A)
MSUD Diet Powder
Phenyl-Free® Phenylalanine-Free Diet Powder
Pregestimil® Iron Fortified Protein Hydrolysate Formula with Medium Chain Triglycerides
Ricelyte® Oral Electrolyte Maintenance Solution Made With Rice Syrup Solids
Special Metabolic Modules:
HIST 1
HIST 2
HOM 1
HOM 2
LYS 1
LYS 2
MSUD 1
MSUD 2
OS 1
OS 2
PKU 1
PKU 2
PKU 3
Protein-Free Diet Powder (Product 80056)
TYR 1
TYR 2
UCD 1
UCD 2
Tempra® 1 Acetaminophen Infant Drops
Tempra® 2 Acetaminophen Toddlers Syrup
Tempra® 3 Chewable Tablets, Regular or Double-Strength
Trind® Liquid, Antihistamine, Nasal Decongestant, Sugar-Free
Trind-DM® Liquid, Cough Suppressant, Antihistamine, Nasal Decongestant, Sugar-Free
Tri-Vi-Sol® Vitamin Drops
Tri-Vi-Sol® Vitamin Drops with Iron
Detailed information may be obtained by contacting Mead Johnson Nutritionals Medical Affairs Department at (812) 429-6437.

Products are indexed by generic and chemical names in the **YELLOW SECTION.**

Menley & James Laboratories, Inc.

COMMONWEALTH CORPORATE CENTER
100 TOURNAMENT DRIVE, SUITE 310
HORSHAM, PA 19044-3697

A.R.M.® Allergy Relief Medicine Maximum Strength Caplets

Product Information: A.R.M. combines two important medicines in one safe, fast-acting caplet:
- The highest level of antihistamine available without prescription—for better relief of sneezing, runny nose and itchy, weepy eyes.
- A clinically proven sinus decongestant to help ease breathing and drain sinus congestion for hours.

Directions: Adults and Children 12 years of age and over: ONE CAPLET every 4 hours, not to exceed 6 caplets in 24 hours. Children (6–11 years of age): ONE-HALF CAPLET every 4 hours, not to exceed 6 half caplets in 24 hours. Children under 6 years of age: Consult a physician.

Active Ingredients: Each caplet contains Chlorpheniramine Maleate, 4 mg, Phenylpropanolamine Hydrochloride, 25 mg. **Inactive Ingredients:** Carnauba Wax, D&C Yellow 10, FD&C Yellow 6, Gelatin, Hydroxypropyl Methylcellulose, Lactose, Magnesium Stearate, Polyethylene Glycol, Sodium Starch Glycolate, Starch and trace amounts of other ingredients.

TAMPER-RESISTANT PACKAGE FEATURES FOR YOUR PROTECTION:
- Each caplet is encased in a clear plastic cell with a foil back.
- The name A.R.M. appears on each caplet (see product illustration on front of carton).
- **DO NOT USE THIS PRODUCT IF EITHER OF THESE TAMPER-RESISTANT FEATURES IS MISSING OR BROKEN. IF YOU HAVE ANY QUESTIONS, PLEASE CALL 1-800-321-1834 TOLL FREE.**

Warning: Do not exceed recommended dosage. If symptoms do not improve within 7 days, or are accompanied by high fever, consult a physician before continuing use. Stop use if dizziness, sleeplessness or nervousness occurs. If you have or are being treated for depression, high blood pressure, glaucoma, diabetes, asthma, heart disease, thyroid disease or difficulty in urination due to enlargement of the prostate gland, use only as directed by a physician. Do not take this product if you are taking another medication containing phenylpropanolamine.
Avoid alcoholic beverages while taking this product. Do not drive or operate heavy machinery. May cause drowsiness. May cause excitability, especially in children. **Keep this and all medication out**

Continued on next page

Menley & James—Cont.

of reach of children. In case of accidental overdose, seek professional assistance or contact a Poison Control Center immediately. As with any drug, if you are pregnant or nursing a baby, seek the advice of a health professional before using this product.
Store at controlled room temperature (59°–86°F) in a dry place.

How Supplied: Consumer packages of 20 and 40 caplets.

Shown in Product Identification Section, page 414

ACNOMEL®
Acne Medication Cream
For External Use Only

Indications: For the management of acne.

Directions: Cleanse the skin thoroughly before applying medication. Cover the entire affected area with a thin layer one to three times daily. Because excessive drying of the skin may occur, start with one application daily, then gradually increase to two or three times daily if needed or as directed by a physician. If bothersome dryness or peeling occurs, reduce application to once a day or every other day.

Active Ingredients: Resorcinol 2%, Sulfur 8%. **Inactive Ingredients:** Alcohol 11% (w/w), Bentonite, Fragrance, Iron Oxides, Potassium Hydroxide, Propylene Glycol, Titanium Dioxide, Purified Water.

Warnings: Apply to affected areas only. Do not use on broken skin or apply to large areas of the body. Do not get into eyes. If excessive skin irritation develops or increases, discontinue use and consult a physician. Using other topical acne medications at the same time or immediately following use of this product may increase dryness or irritation of the skin. If this occurs, only one medication should be used unless directed by a physician. **Keep this and all medication out of the reach of children.** In case of accidental ingestion, seek professional assistance or contact a Poison Control Center immediately.
Store at controlled room temperature (59°–86°F).

How Supplied: Cream—in specially lined 1 oz. tubes.

Shown in Product Identification Section, page 414

AQUA CARE® CREAM
With 10% Urea
Effective Medication for Dry Skin Relief

Product Information: AQUA CARE, with 10% urea, is a topical cream formulated to restore nature's moisture balance to rough, dry skin. The special urea ingredient penetrates the surface of the skin to both restore lost moisture and soften dry, rough skin.

Directions: Apply two or three times daily to areas of need or as directed by a physician.

Active Ingredient: Urea 10%. **Also Contains:** Purified Water, Cetyl Esters, DEA-Oleth-3 Phosphate, Petrolatum, Triethanolamine, Carbomer, Glycerin, Lanolin Oil, Mineral Oil, Lanolin Alcohol, Benzyl Alcohol, Fragrance.

Warning: Discontinue use if irritation occurs.
Store at controlled room temperature (59°–86°F).
FOR EXTERNAL USE ONLY

How Supplied: Available in 2.5 oz. tubes.

Shown in Product Identification Section, page 414

AQUA CARE® LOTION
With 10% Urea
Effective Medication for Dry Skin Relief

Product Information: AQUA CARE, with 10% urea, is a topical lotion formulated to restore nature's moisture balance to rough, dry skin. The special urea ingredient penetrates the surface of the skin to both restore lost moisture and soften dry, rough skin.

Directions: Apply two or three times daily to areas of need or as directed by a physican.

Active Ingredient: Urea 10%. **Also Contains:** Purified Water, Mineral Oil, Petrolatum, Propylene Glycol Stearate, Sorbitan Monostearate, Cetyl Alcohol, Lactic Acid, Magnesium Aluminum Silicate, Sodium Lauryl Sulfate, Methylparaben, Propylparaben, may also contain Sodium Hydroxide.

Warning: Discontinue use if irritation occurs.
Store at controlled room temperature (59°–86°F).
FOR EXTERNAL USE ONLY

How Supplied: Available in 8 oz. bottles.

Shown in Product Identification Section, page 414

ASTHMAHALER®
Epinephrine Bitartrate
Inhalation Aerosol
(300 metered inhalations)
Alcohol Free Formula

Indications: For temporary relief of shortness of breath, tightness of chest, and wheezing due to bronchial asthma.

Dosage and Administration: For oral inhalation only. Each inhalation contains the equivalent of 0.16 milligram of epinephrine base.
Inhalation dosage for adults and children 4 years of age and older: Start with one inhalation, then wait at least 1 minute. If not relieved, use once more. Do not use again for at least 3 hours. Use of this product by children should be supervised by an adult. Children under 4 years of age: consult a physician.

Directions: Shake well before each use.

1. Remove plastic dust cap, take mouthpiece off metal vial and fit other end of mouthpiece onto top of vial, turn vial upside down. Shake well.
2. Breathe out fully and place mouthpiece well into mouth, aimed at the back of the throat.
3. As you begin to breathe in deeply, press the vial firmly down into the adapter with the index finger. This releases one dose.
4. Release pressure on vial and remove unit from mouth. Hold the breath as long as possible, then breathe out slowly.

The plastic mouthpiece should be cleaned daily. Remove metal vial and wash adapter with soap and hot water and rinse thoroughly. Dry and replace with vial.

Active Ingredients: Contains Epinephrine Bitartrate 7 mg per mL in inert propellant. **Inactive Ingredients:** Cetylpyridinium Chloride, Propellants 11, 12, & 114, Sorbitan Trioleate.

Warnings: Do not use this product unless a diagnosis of asthma has been made by a physician. Do not use this product if you have heart disease, high blood pressure, thyroid disease, diabetes, or difficulty in urination due to enlargement of the prostate gland unless directed by a physician. Do not use this product if you have ever been hospitalized for asthma or if you are taking any prescription drug for asthma unless directed by a physician.
DO NOT USE THIS PRODUCT MORE FREQUENTLY OR AT HIGHER DOSES THAN RECOMMENDED UNLESS DIRECTED BY A PHYSICIAN. Excessive use may cause nervousness and rapid heart beat, and possibly, adverse effects on the heart.
DO NOT CONTINUE TO USE THIS PRODUCT, BUT SEEK MEDICAL ASSISTANCE IMMEDIATELY IF SYMPTOMS ARE NOT RELIEVED WITHIN 20 MINUTES OR BECOME WORSE.

Drug Interaction Precaution: Do not use this product if you are presently taking a prescription drug for high blood pressure or depression, without first consulting your physician.
Contents under pressure. Do not puncture or incinerate container. Do not expose to heat. Store at controlled room temperature (59°–86°F).
As with any drug, if you are pregnant or nursing a baby, seek the advice of a health professional before using this product. **Keep this and all medication out of the reach of children.** In case of accidental overdose, consult a physician immediately.

How Supplied: ½ fl. oz. (15 mL). Available as combination package metal vial plus plastic mouthpiece, or as refill metal vial only.

ASTHMANEFRIN®
Solution "A" Bronchodilator

Indications: For temporary relief of shortness of breath, tightness of chest, and wheezing due to bronchial asthma.

Directions: For use in hand-held rubber bulb nebulizer. Pour at least 8 drops of solution into ASTHMANEFRIN NEBULIZER.

Care of Solution: Refrigerate once bottle has been opened.

Active Ingredients: Racepinephrine Hydrochloride Equivalent to 2.25% Epinephrine base (activity 50%). **Inactive Ingredients:** Benzoic Acid, Chlorobutanol, Glycerin, Hydrochloric Acid, Sodium Bisulfite, Sodium Chloride, Water.

Warnings: **Do not use this product unless a diagnosis of asthma has been made by a physician.** Do not use this product if you have heart disease, high blood pressure, thyroid disease, diabetes, or difficulty in urination due to enlargement of the prostate gland unless directed by a physician. Do not use this product if you have ever been hospitalized for asthma or if you are taking any prescription drug for asthma unless directed by a physician.
DO NOT USE THIS PRODUCT MORE FREQUENTLY OR AT HIGHER DOSES THAN RECOMMENDED UNLESS DIRECTED BY A PHYSICIAN. Excessive use may cause nervousness and rapid heart beat, and possibly, adverse effects on the heart. **DO NOT CONTINUE TO USE THIS PRODUCT, BUT SEEK MEDICAL ASSISTANCE IMMEDIATELY IF SYMPTOMS ARE NOT RELIEVED WITHIN 20 MINUTES OR BECOME WORSE.**
Do not use this product if it is pinkish or darker than slightly yellow or if it contains a precipitate.

Drug Interaction Precaution: Do not use this product if you are presently taking a prescription drug for high blood pressure or depression, without first consulting your physician.
As with any drug, if you are pregnant or nursing a baby, seek the advice of a physician before using this product.
Keep this and all medication out of the reach of children.
Store at 59° to 75° F. Avoid excessive heat.

Dosage and Administration: Inhalation dosage for adults and children 4 years of age and older: 1 to 3 inhalations not more often than every 3 hours. The use of this product by children should be supervised by an adult. Children under 4 years of age: consult a physician.

How Supplied: ½ fl. oz. (15 mL) and 1 fl. oz. (30 mL) Solutions. FOR USE WITH ASTHMANEFRIN® NEBULIZER.

BENZEDREX® INHALER
Nasal Decongestant

Indications: For the temporary relief of nasal congestion due to the common cold, hay fever, or associated with sinusitis.

Directions: This product delivers in each 800 milliliters of air 0.04 to 0.50 milligrams of propylhexedrine. Adults and children 6 to 12 years of age (with adult supervision): 2 inhalations in each nostril not more often than every 2 hours. Children under 6 years of age: consult a physician.
This inhaler is effective for a minimum of 3 months after first use. KEEP INHALER TIGHTLY CLOSED.

Active Ingredient: Propylhexedrine 250 mg. **Inactive Ingredients:** Lavender Oil, Menthol.

Warnings: Do not use this product continuously for more than 3 days. If symptoms persist, consult a physician. Do not exceed recommended dosage because burning, stinging, sneezing, or increase of nasal discharge may occur. The use of this container by more than one person may spread infection. **Keep this and all medication out of the reach of children.** Ill effects may result if taken internally. In case of accidental overdose or ingestion of contents, seek professional assistance or contact a Poison Control Center immediately. As with any drug, if you are pregnant or nursing a baby, seek the advice of a health professional before using this product.
Store at controlled room temperature (59°–86°F).
TAMPER-RESISTANT PACKAGE FEATURE FOR YOUR PROTECTION:
- Inhaler sealed with imprinted cellophane. Do not use if missing or broken.

Comments or questions? Call 1-800-321-1834 Toll Free.

How Supplied: In single plastic tubes.
Shown in Product Identification Section, page 414

BENZEDREX® NASAL SPRAY REGULAR
Nasal Decongestant

Indications: For the temporary relief of nasal congestion due to colds, hay fever, sinusitis or other upper respiratory allergies.

Directions: Adults and children 12 years of age and over: With head upright, spray 2 or 3 times into each nostril. Spray quickly and firmly while inhaling. Wipe nozzle clean after use. Repeat every 4 hours as needed. Children under 12 years of age: consult a physician.

Active Ingredient: Phenylephrine Hydrochloride 0.5%. **Inactive Ingredients:** Benzalkonium Chloride, Citric Acid, Methylparaben, Sodium Chloride, Sodium Citrate, Water.

TAMPER-RESISTANT PACKAGE FEATURE FOR YOUR PROTECTION:
- Bottle is sealed with a white neckband printed with "SEALED FOR YOUR PROTECTION." Do not use if missing or broken.

Warnings: Do not exceed recommended dosage because burning, stinging, sneezing or increase of nasal discharge may occur. Do not use this product continuously for more than 3 days. If symptoms persist, consult a physician. Do not use this product if you have heart disease, high blood pressure, thyroid disease, diabetes, or difficulty in urination due to enlargement of the prostate gland unless directed by a physician. The use of this container by more than one person may spread infection. In case of accidental overdose or ingestion of contents, seek professional assistance or contact a Poison Control Center immediately. **Keep this and all medication out of the reach of children.** As with any drug, if you are pregnant or nursing a baby, seek the advice of a health professional before using this product.
Store at controlled room temperature (59°–86°F).
Comments or questions? Call 1-800-321-1834 Toll Free.

How Supplied: In 15mL plastic squeeze bottle.
Shown in Product Identification Section, page 414

BENZEDREX® NASAL SPRAY 12 HOUR
Nasal Decongestant

Indications: For up to 12 hour relief of nasal congestion due to colds, hay fever, sinusitis or other upper respiratory allergies.

Directions: Adults and children 6 to under 12 years of age (with adult supervision): 2 or 3 sprays in each nostril not more often than every 10 to 12 hours. To spray, with head upright, squeeze bottle quickly and firmly while inhaling. Wipe nozzle clean after use. Do not exceed 2 applications in any 24-hour period. Children under 6 years of age: consult a physician.

Active Ingredient: Oxymetazoline Hydrochloride 0.05%. **Inactive Ingredients:** Benzalkonium Chloride, Glycine, Phenylmercuric Acetate, Sorbitol, Water.

TAMPER-RESISTANT PACKAGE FEATURE FOR YOUR PROTECTION:
- Bottle is sealed with a white neckband printed with "SEALED FOR YOUR PROTECTION." Do not use if missing or broken.

Warnings: Do not exceed recommended dosage because burning, stinging, sneezing or increase of nasal discharge may occur. Do not use this product continuously for more than 3 days. If symptoms persist, consult a physician. Do not use this product if you have heart

Continued on next page

Menley & James—Cont.

disease, high blood pressure, thyroid disease, diabetes or difficulty in urination due to enlargement of the prostate gland unless directed by a physician. The use of this container by more than one person may spread infection. In case of accidental overdose or ingestion of contents, seek professional assistance or contact a Poison Control Center immediately. **Keep this and all medication out of the reach of children.** As with any drug, if you are pregnant or nursing a baby, seek the advice of a health professional before using this product.
Store at controlled room temperature (59°–86°F).
Comments or questions? Call 1-800-321-1834 Toll Free.

How Supplied: In 15mL plastic squeeze bottle.

Shown in Product Identification Section, page 414

CONGESTAC®
Congestion Relief Medicine
Nasal Decongestant/Expectorant Caplets

Indications: For the temporary relief of nasal congestion due to the common cold, hay fever, or associated with sinusitis. Helps loosen mucus and thin bronchial secretions to drain bronchial tubes and make coughs more productive.

Directions: ONE CAPLET every 4 hours not to exceed 4 caplets in 24 hours. Children (6 to 12 years): one-half the adult dose (break caplet in half). Children under 6 years use only as directed by physician.

Active Ingredients: Each caplet contains Guaifenesin 400 mg, Pseudoephedrine Hydrochloride 60 mg. **Inactive Ingredients:** Croscarmellose Sodium, Hydroxypropyl Methylcellulose, Magnesium Stearate, Microcrystalline Cellulose, Polyethylene Glycol, Povidone, Silicon Dioxide, Starch and trace amounts of other ingredients.

TAMPER-RESISTANT PACKAGE FEATURES FOR YOUR PROTECTION:

- Each caplet is encased in a clear plastic cell with a foil back.
- The letter "C" appears on each caplet (see product illustration on front of carton).
- **DO NOT USE THIS PRODUCT IF EITHER OF THESE TAMPER-RESISTANT FEATURES IS MISSING OR BROKEN. IF YOU HAVE ANY QUESTIONS, PLEASE CALL 1-800-321-1834 TOLL FREE.**

Warnings: Do not exceed recommended dosage because at higher doses nervousness, dizziness or sleeplessness may occur. Do not take this product for more than 7 days. If symptoms do not improve or are accompanied by a fever, consult a physician. Do not take this product if you have heart disease, high blood pressure, thyroid disease, diabetes, or difficulty in urination due to enlargement of the prostate gland, unless directed by a physician. Do not take this product for persistent or chronic cough such as occurs with smoking, asthma, chronic bronchitis or emphysema, or where cough is accompanied by excessive mucus unless directed by a physician. **Keep this and all medication out of reach of children.** In case of accidental overdose, seek professional assistance or contact a Poison Control Center immediately. As with any drug, if you are pregnant or nursing a baby, seek the advice of a health professional before using this product.

Drug Interaction Precaution: Do not take this product or give to a child if you or the child are presently taking a prescription antihypertensive or antidepressant drug containing a monoamine oxidase inhibitor except under the advice and supervision of a pysician.
Store at controlled room temperature (59°–86°F).
The CONGESTAC horizontal color bar is a trademark.

How Supplied: In consumer packages of 12 and 24 caplets.

Shown in Product Identification Section, page 414

FEMIRON® MultiVitamins and Iron
[fem 'i 'ern]

Indications: For use as an iron and vitamin supplement.

Dosage and Administration: Women: One tablet daily.
Each Tablet Contains:

	Quantity	% of U.S. RDA
Vitamin A	5,000 I.U.	100
Vitamin D	400 I.U.	100
Vitamin E	15 I.U.	50
Vitamin C	60 mg	100
Folic Acid	0.4 mg	100
Vitamin B_1	1.5 mg	100
Vitamin B_2	1.7 mg	100
Niacinamide	20 mg	100
Vitamin B_6	2 mg	100
Vitamin B_{12}	6 mcg	100
Pantothenic Acid	10 mg	100
Iron	**20 mg**	**111**

Ingredients: Calcium Carbonate, Ferrous Fumarate, Ascorbic Acid, Gelatin, Niacinamide, Vitamin E Acetate, Starch, Calcium Pantothenate, Microcrystalline Cellulose, Calcium Silicate, Alginic Acid, Hydroxypropyl Methylcellulose, Crospovidone, Stearic Acid, Sodium Lauryl Sulfate, Vitamin A Acetate, Pyridoxine Hydrochloride, Artificial Colors (FD&C Red 40, Titanium Dioxide, FD&C Blue 2), Riboflavin, Thiamine Mononitrate, Polyethylene Glycol. Magnesium Stearate, Folic Acid, Polysorbate 80, Vitamin D, Cyanocobalamin.

Actions: Helps ensure adequate intake of iron and vitamins.

Warning: Keep this and all medication out of the reach of children.

Precaution: Alcoholics and individuals with chronic liver or pancreatic disease may have enhanced iron absorption with the potential for iron overload. NOTE: Unabsorbed iron may cause some darkening of the stool.

Symptoms and Treatment of Oral Overdosage: Toxicity and symptoms are primarily due to iron overdose. Abdominal pain, nausea, vomiting and diarrhea may occur, with possible subsequent acidosis and cardiovascular collapse with severe poisoning. **Treatment:** Induce vomiting immediately. Administer milk, eggs to reduce gastric irritation. Contact a physician immediately.

TAMPER-RESISTANT PACKAGE FEATURE:

- Bottle has imprinted seal under cap.
- **DO NOT USE IF SEAL IS BROKEN OR MISSING. IF YOU HAVE ANY QUESTIONS, PLEASE CALL 1-800-321-1834 TOLL FREE.**

Store at controlled room temperature (59°–86°F).

How Supplied: Bottles of 35, 60, and 90 tablets. Femiron Iron Supplement (no added vitamins) is also available.

Shown in Product Identification Section, page 414

GARFIELD
Chewable Multivitamins Regular

Indications: Dietary supplementation.

Directions: For adults and children 2 years and older, chew one tablet daily.

EACH TABLET CONTAINS:
[See table top of next page.]

Ingredients: SUCROSE (A NATURAL SWEETENER) ASCORBIC ACID, MONO AND DIGLYCERIDES, TALC, GELATIN, VITAMIN E ACETATE, NIACINAMIDE, NATURAL AND ARTIFICIAL FLAVORS, STARCH, CALCIUM CARBONATE, ARTIFICIAL COLORS (INCLUDING FD&C RED 40, FD&C YELLOW 6, FD&C BLUE 2 AND FD&C BLUE 1), SILICA, STEARIC ACID, MAGNESIUM STEARATE, PYRIDOXINE HYDROCHLORIDE, RIBOFLAVIN, THIAMINE MONONITRATE, BETA CAROTENE, LACTOSE, VITAMIN A ACETATE, FOLIC ACID, VITAMIN D, VITAMIN B-12.

Warnings: CLOSE TIGHTLY AND KEEP THIS AND ALL MEDICATION OUT OF THE REACH OF CHILDREN. IN CASE OF ACCIDENTAL OVERDOSE, SEEK PROFESSIONAL ASSISTANCE OR CONTACT A POISON CONTROL CENTER IMMEDIATELY.
Store at controlled room temperature (59°–86°F).

ONE TABLET DAILY PROVIDES: VITAMINS	QUANTITY PER TABLET	Percent U.S. RDA For Children 2 to 4 Years of Age	Percent U.S. RDA For Adults & Children Over 4 Years of Age
Vitamin A (as Acetate)	1250 IU	100	50
Vitamin A (as Beta Carotene)	1250 IU		
Vitamin D	400 IU	100	100
Vitamin E	15 IU	150	50
Vitamin C	60 mg	150	100
Folic Acid	0.3 mg	150	75
Thiamine (Vitamin B_1)	1.05 mg	150	70
Riboflavin (Vitamin B_2)	1.2 mg	150	70
Niacin	13.5 mg	150	67
Vitamin B_6	1.05 mg	150	52
Vitamin B_{12}	4.5 mcg	150	75

Child-Resistant Cap

TAMPER-RESISTANT PACKAGE FEATURE:

- Bottle has imprinted seal under cap.
- **DO NOT USE IF SEAL IS BROKEN OR MISSING. IF YOU HAVE ANY QUESTIONS, PLEASE CALL 1-800-321-1834 TOLL FREE.**

How Supplied: Bottles of 60 tablets. Garfield Chewable Multivitamin Plus Extra C, Plus Iron and Complete with Minerals also available.

Shown in Product Identification Section, page 414

GARFIELD
Chewable Multivitamins Plus Extra C

Indications: Dietary supplementation.

Directions: For adults and children 2 years and older, chew one tablet daily.

EACH TABLET CONTAINS:

[See table below.]

Ingredients: SUCROSE (A NATURAL SWEETENER), SODIUM ASCORBATE, ASCORBIC ACID, MONO AND DIGLYCERIDES, MICROCRYSTALLINE CELLULOSE, TALC, GELATIN, VITAMIN E ACETATE, STARCH, NATURAL AND ARTIFICIAL FLAVORS, NIACINAMIDE, ARTIFICIAL COLORS INCLUDING FD&C RED 40, FD&C YELLOW 6, FD&C BLUE 2 AND FD&C BLUE 1), SILICA, MAGNESIUM STEARATE, HYDROGENATED COTTONSEED OIL, RIBOFLAVIN, PYRIDOXINE HYDROCHLORIDE, THIAMINE MONONITRATE, BETA CAROTENE, LACTOSE, VITAMIN A ACETATE, FOLIC ACID, VITAMIN D, VITAMIN B-12.

Warnings: CLOSE TIGHTLY AND KEEP THIS AND ALL MEDICATION OUT OF THE REACH OF CHILDREN. IN CASE OF ACCIDENTAL OVERDOSE, SEEK PROFESSIONAL ASSISTANCE OR CONTACT A POISON CONTROL CENTER IMMEDIATELY.

Store at controlled room temperature (59°–86°F).

Child-Resistant Cap

ONE TABLET DAILY PROVIDES: VITAMINS	QUANTITY PER TABLET	Percent U.S. RDA For Children 2 to 4 Years of Age	Percent U.S. RDA For Adults & Children Over 4 Years of Age
Vitamin A (as Acetate)	1250 IU	100	50
Vitamin A (as Beta Carotene)	1250 IU		
Vitamin D	400 IU	100	100
Vitamin E	15 IU	150	50
Vitamin C	**250 mg**	**625**	**417**
Folic Acid	0.3 mg	150	75
Thiamine (Vitamin B_1)	1.05 mg	150	70
Riboflavin (Vitamin B_2)	1.2 mg	150	70
Niacin	13.5 mg	150	67
Vitamin B_6	1.05 mg	150	52
Vitamin B_{12}	4.5 mcg	150	75

TAMPER-RESISTANT PACKAGE FEATURE:

- Bottle has imprinted seal under cap.
- **DO NOT USE IF SEAL IS BROKEN OR MISSING. IF YOU HAVE ANY QUESTIONS, PLEASE CALL 1-800-321-1834 TOLL FREE.**

How Supplied: Bottles of 60 tablets. Garfield Chewable Multivitamins Regular, Plus Iron and Complete with Minerals also available.

Shown in Product Identification Section, page 414

GARFIELD
Chewable Multivitamins Plus Iron

Indications: Dietary supplementation.

Directions: For adults and children 2 years and older, chew one tablet daily.

EACH TABLET CONTAINS:

[See table top of next page.]

Ingredients: SUCROSE (A NATURAL SWEETENER), ASCORBIC ACID, FERROUS FUMARATE, MONO AND DIGLYCERIDES, TALC, GELATIN, VITAMIN E ACETATE, NIACINAMIDE, STARCH, NATURAL AND ARTIFICIAL FLAVORS, CALCIUM CARBONATE, ARTIFICIAL COLORS (INCLUDING FD&C RED 40, FD&C YELLOW 6, FD&C BLUE 2 AND FD&C BLUE 1), SILICA, MAGNESIUM STEARATE, STEARIC ACID, PYRIDOXINE HYDROCHLORIDE, RIBOFLAVIN, THIAMINE MONONITRATE, BETA CAROTENE, LACTOSE, VITAMIN A ACETATE, FOLIC ACID, VITAMIN D, VITAMIN B-12.

Warnings: CONTAINS IRON, WHICH CAN BE HARMFUL IN LARGE DOSES. CLOSE TIGHTLY AND KEEP THIS AND ALL MEDICATION OUT OF THE REACH OF CHILDREN. IN CASE OF ACCIDENTAL OVERDOSE, SEEK PROFESSIONAL ASSISTANCE OR CONTACT A POISON CONTROL CENTER IMMEDIATELY.

Store at controlled room temperature (59°–86°F).

Child-Resistant Cap

TAMPER-RESISTANT PACKAGE FEATURE:

- Bottle has imprinted seal under cap.
- **DO NOT USE IF SEAL IS BROKEN OR MISSING. IF YOU HAVE ANY QUESTIONS, PLEASE CALL 1-800-321-1834 TOLL FREE.**

How Supplied: Bottles of 60 tablets. Garfield Chewable Multivitamins Regular, Plus Extra C, and Complete with Minerals also available.

Shown in Product Identification Section, page 414

Continued on next page

Menley & James—Cont.

ONE TABLET DAILY PROVIDES: VITAMINS	QUANTITY PER TABLET	Percent U.S. RDA For Children 2 to 4 Years of Age	Percent U.S. RDA For Adults & Children Over 4 Years of Age
Vitamin A (as Acetate)	1250 IU	100	50
Vitamin A (as Beta Carotene)	1250 IU		
Vitamin D	400 IU	100	100
Vitamin E	15 IU	150	50
Vitamin C	60 mg	150	100
Folic Acid	0.3 mg	150	75
Thiamine (Vitamin B_1)	1.05 mg	150	70
Riboflavin (Vitamin B_2)	1.2 mg	150	70
Niacin	13.5 mg	150	67
Vitamin B_6	1.05 mg	150	52
Vitamin B_{12}	4.5 mcg	150	75
MINERALS			
IRON (ELEMENTAL)	15 mg	150	83

GARFIELD
Chewable Multivitamins
COMPLETE WITH MINERALS

Indications: Dietary supplementation.

Directions: For children 2 to 4 years of age, chew one-half tablet daily. For adults and children over 4, chew one tablet daily.

EACH TABLET CONTAINS:
[See table below.]

Ingredients: DICALCIUM PHOSPHATE, SORBITOL, SODIUM ASCORBATE, FERROUS FUMARATE, MONO AND DIGLYCERIDES, GELATIN, MAGNESIUM OXIDE, MICROCRYSTALLINE CELLULOSE, VITAMIN E ACETATE, TALC, NATURAL AND ARTIFICIAL FLAVORS, NIACINAMIDE, STEARIC ACID, ZINC OXIDE, ARTIFICIAL COLORS (INCLUDING FD&C RED 40, FD&C BLUE 2 AND FD&C YELLOW 6), CITRIC ACID, CALCIUM PANTOTHENATE, MAGNESIUM STEARATE, SILICA, TARTARIC ACID, STARCH, HYDROGENATED COTTONSEED OIL, ASPARTAME (A SWEETENER), CUPRIC OXIDE, PYRIDOXINE HYDROCHLORIDE, BETA CAROTENE, VITAMIN A ACETATE, RIBOFLAVIN, THIAMINE MONONITRATE, FOLIC ACID, POTASSIUM IODIDE, BIOTIN, VITAMIN D, VITAMIN B-12.

VITAMINS	QUANTITY PER TABLET	Percent U.S. RDA For Children 2 to 4 Years of Age (½ Tablet)	Percent U.S. RDA For Adults & Children Over 4 Years of Age (1 Tablet)
Vitamin A (as Acetate)	2500 IU	100	100
Vitamin A (as Beta Carotene)	2500 IU		
Vitamin D	400 IU	50	100
Vitamin E	30 IU	150	100
Vitamin C	60 mg	75	100
Folic Acid	0.4 mg	100	100
Thiamine (Vitamin B_1)	1.5 mg	107	100
Riboflavin (Vitamin B_2)	1.7 mg	106	100
Niacin	20 mg	111	100
Vitamin B_6	2 mg	143	100
Vitamin B_{12}	6 mcg	100	100
Biotin	40 mcg	13	13
Pantothenic Acid	10 mg	100	100
MINERALS			
IRON (ELEMENTAL)	**18 mg**	**90**	**100**
CALCIUM	**100 mg**	**6**	**10**
Copper	2 mg	100	100
Phosphorus	100 mg	6	10
Iodine	150 mcg	107	100
Magnesium	20 mg	5	5
Zinc	15 mg	94	100

Warnings: CONTAINS IRON, WHICH CAN BE HARMFUL IN LARGE DOSES. CLOSE TIGHTLY AND KEEP THIS AND ALL MEDICATION OUT OF THE REACH OF CHILDREN. IN CASE OF ACCIDENTAL OVERDOSE, SEEK PROFESSIONAL ASSISTANCE OR CONTACT A POISON CONTROL CENTER IMMEDIATELY.
PHENYLKETONURICS: CONTAINS PHENYLALANINE
Store at controlled room temperature (59°–86°F).
Child-Resistant Cap
TAMPER-RESISTANT PACKAGE FEATURE:
- Bottle has imprinted seal under cap.
- **DO NOT USE IF SEAL IS BROKEN OR MISSING. IF YOU HAVE ANY QUESTIONS, PLEASE CALL 1-800-321-1834 TOLL FREE**

How Supplied: Bottles of 60 tablets. Garfield Chewable Multivitamins Regular, Plus Extra C, and Plus Iron also available.

Shown in Product Identification Section, page 414

HOLD® DM
Dextromethorphan Cough Suppressant Lozenge

Indications: Temporarily suppresses coughs due to minor sore throat and bronchial irritation associated with a cold or inhaled irritants.

Directions: Adults: Take two lozenges one after the other every 4 hours as needed. **Children** (6-12 years): Take one lozenge every 4 hours as needed. Let dissolve fully.

Active Ingredient: Each lozenge contains Dextromethorphan Hydrobromide 5 mg. **Inactive Ingredients:** Original Flavor—Corn Syrup, D&C Yellow 10, Flavors, Sucrose, Vegetable Oil and trace amounts of other ingredients.
Cherry Flavor—Corn Syrup, FD&C Blue 1, FD&C Red 40, Imitation Flavor, Sucrose, Vegetable Oil and trace amounts of other ingredients.
Honey Lemon Flavor—Corn Syrup, FD&C Yellow 5, Flavors, Sucrose, Vegetable Oil and trace amounts of other ingredients.

Actions: Dextromethorphan is the most widely used, non-narcotic/non-habit forming antitussive. A 10-20 mg dose has been recognized as being effective in relieving the discomfort of coughs up to 4 hours by reducing cough intensity and frequency.

Warnings: Do not take this product for persistent or chronic cough such as occurs with smoking, asthma, chronic bronchitis, or emphysema, or where cough is accompanied by excessive phlegm (mucus), unless directed by a physician. A persistent cough may be a sign of a serious condition. If cough persists for more than one week, tends to recur, or is accompanied by fever, rash or persistent headache, consult a physician. Do not give this product to children under 6 years of age unless directed by a physician. As with any drug, if you are pregnant or nursing a baby, seek the advice of a health professional before using this product. **Keep this and all medication out of the reach of children.** In case of accidental overdose, seek professional assistance or contact a Poison Control Center immediately.

How Supplied: Available in Original, Cherry and Honey Lemon flavors. 10 individually wrapped lozenges come packaged in a plastic tube container.

Shown in Product Identification Section, page 414

LIQUIPRIN®
Infants' Drops
(acetaminophen)

Description: LIQUIPRIN is a nonsalicylate analgesic and antipyretic particularly suitable for infants and children. LIQUIPRIN Drops is a raspberry-flavored, reddish pink solution. It contains no alcohol and no saccharin.

Indications: LIQUIPRIN is indicated for use in the treatment of infants and children with conditions requiring reduction of fever and/or relief of pain such as mild upper respiratory infections (tonsillitis, common cold, flu), teething, headache, myalgia, postimmunization reactions, posttonsillectomy discomfort and gastroenteritis. As adjunctive therapy with antibiotics or sulfonamides, LIQUIPRIN may be useful as an analgesic and antipyretic in bacterial or viral infections, such as bronchitis, pharyngitis, tracheobronchitis, sinusitis, pneumonia, otitis media and cervical adenitis.

Usual Dosage: LIQUIPRIN may be given alone or mixed with milk, juices, applesauce or other beverages and foods. All dosages may be repeated every 4 hours, if pain and fever persist, but not to exceed 5 times daily or as directed by physician.

LIQUIPRIN should be administered in the following dosages:
0–3 months: 40 mg—½ dropperful
4–11 months: 80 mg—1 dropperful
12–23 months: 120 mg—1½ droppersful
2–3 years, 24–35 lbs.: 160 mg—2 droppersful
4–5 years, 36–47 lbs.: 240 mg—3 droppersful

Active Ingredient: Acetaminophen 80 mg per 1.66 mL (top mark on dropper). **Inactive Ingredients:** Artificial Raspberry and other artificial and natural flavors, Citric Acid, D&C Red 33, Dextrose, FD&C Red 40, Fructose, Glycerin, Methylparaben, Polyethylene Glycol, Propylene Glycol, Propylparaben, Sodium Citrate, Sodium Gluconate, Sucrose, Water.

Actions: LIQUIPRIN safely and effectively reduces fever and pain in infants and children without the hazards of salicylate therapy (e.g., gastric mucosal irritation).

Warnings: If fever persists for more than three days, or if pain continues for five days, or if new symptoms occur, consult a physician.

Precautions and Adverse Reactions: If a sensitivity reaction occurs, the drug should be discontinued. LIQUIPRIN has rarely been found to produce side effects. It is usually well tolerated by patients who are sensitive to products containing aspirin.

Store at controlled room temperature (59°–86°F). Avoid excessive heat.

How Supplied: LIQUIPRIN is available in a 1 fl. oz. (30 mL) plastic bottle with a calibrated dropper and child-resistant cap, and safety-sealed package.

Shown in Product Identification Section, page 414

ORNEX®
Nasal Decongestant/Analgesic
Caplets

Product Information: For temporary relief of nasal congestion, headache, aches, pains and fever due to colds, sinusitis and flu.

Directions: Adults and Children 12 years of age and over: TWO CAPLETS every 4 hours, not to exceed 8 caplets in 24 hours. Children (6 to 11 years): ONE CAPLET every 4 hours, not to exceed 4 caplets in 24 hours. Children under 6 years of age: Consult a physician.

NO ANTIHISTAMINE DROWSINESS

Active Ingredients: Each caplet contains Acetaminophen 325 mg, Pseudoephedrine Hydrochloride 30 mg. **Inactive Ingredients:** Cellulose, Crospovidone, FD&C Blue 1, Hydroxypropyl Methylcellulose, Magnesium Stearate, Microcrystalline Cellulose, Polyethylene Glycol, Polysorbate 80, Povidone, Starch, Titanium Dioxide and trace amounts of other ingredients.

TAMPER-RESISTANT PACKAGE FEATURES FOR YOUR PROTECTION:

- Each caplet is encased in a clear plastic cell with a foil back.
- The name ORNEX appears on each caplet (see product illustration on front of carton).
- **DO NOT USE THIS PRODUCT IF EITHER OF THESE TAMPER-RESISTANT FEATURES IS MISSING OR BROKEN. IF YOU HAVE ANY QUESTIONS, PLEASE CALL 1-800-321-1834 TOLL FREE.**

Warnings: Do not exceed recommended dosage. Do not use for more than 10 days or give to children under 6, unless directed by a physician. If you have, or are being treated for depression, high blood pressure, diabetes, heart disease, thyroid disease, or difficulty in urination due to enlargement of the prostate gland, use only as directed by a physician. Stop use if dizziness, sleeplessness or nervousness occurs. **Keep this and all medication out of reach of children.** In case of accidental overdose, seek professional assistance or contact a Poison Control Center immediately. As with any drug, if you are pregnant or nursing a baby, seek the advice of a health professional before using this product.

Store at controlled room temperature (59°–86°F) in a dry place.

How Supplied: In consumer packages of 24 and 48 caplets. Also, Dispensary Packages of 792 caplets for industrial dispensaries and student health clinics only.

Shown in Product Identification Section, page 414

MAXIMUM STRENGTH
ORNEX®
Decongestant/Analgesic
Caplets

Product Information: For temporary relief of nasal congestion, headache, aches, pains and fever due to colds, sinusitis and flu.

Directions: Adults and Children 12 years of age and over: TWO CAPLETS every 6 hours, not to exceed 8 caplets in any 24-hour period. Children under 12 years of age: Consult a physician.

NO ANTIHISTAMINE DROWSINESS

Active Ingredients: Each caplet contains Acetaminophen 500 mg, Pseudoephedrine Hydrochloride 30 mg. **Inactive Ingredients:** Cellulose, Crospovidone, Hydroxypropyl Methylcellulose, Magnesium Stearate, Polyethylene Glycol, Polysorbate 80, Povidone, Starch, Titanium Dioxide and trace amounts of other ingredients.

TAMPER-RESISTANT PACKAGE FEATURES FOR YOUR PROTECTION:

- Each caplet is encased in a clear plastic cell with a foil back.
- The name ORNEX MAX appears on each caplet (see product illustration on front of carton).
- **DO NOT USE THIS PRODUCT IF EITHER OF THESE TAMPER-RESISTANT FEATURES IS MISSING OR BROKEN. IF YOU HAVE ANY QUESTIONS, PLEASE CALL 1-800-321-1834 TOLL FREE.**

Warnings: Do not exceed recommended dosage. Do not use for more than 10 days or give to children under 12, unless directed by a physician. If you have, or are being treated for depression, high blood pressure, diabetes, heart disease, thyroid disease, or difficulty in urination due to enlargement of the prostate gland,

Continued on next page

Menley & James—Cont.

use only as directed by a physician. Stop use if dizziness, sleeplessness or nervousness occurs. **Keep this and all medication out of reach of children.** In case of accidental overdose, seek professional assistance or contact a Poison Control Center immediately. As with any drug, if you are pregnant or nursing a baby, seek the advice of a health professional before using this product.
Store at controlled room temperature (59°–86°F) in a dry place.

How Supplied: In consumer packages of 24 and 48 caplets.

Shown in Product Identification Section, page 414

ORNEX®
SEVERE COLD FORMULA
Nasal Decongestant/Analgesic/ Cough Suppressant Caplets

Product Information: For temporary relief of nasal and sinus congestion, headache, aches, pains, fever and coughing due to colds, sinusitis, flu and cough.

Directions: Adults and Children 12 years of age and over: TWO CAPLETS every 6 hours, not to exceed 8 caplets in any 24-hour period. Children under 12 years of age: Consult a physician.

NO ANTIHISTAMINE DROWSINESS

Active Ingredients: Each caplet contains Acetaminophen 500 mg, Pseudoephedrine Hydrochloride 30 mg, Dextromethorphan Hydrobromide 15 mg. **Inactive Ingredients:** Cellulose, Crospovidone, D&C Red 30, D&C Yellow 10, FD&C Blue 2, FD&C Yellow 6, Hydroxypropyl Methylcellulose, Magnesium Stearate, Polyethylene Glycol, Povidone, Starch, Titanium Dioxide, and trace amounts of other ingredients.

TAMPER-RESISTANT PACKAGE FEATURES FOR YOUR PROTECTION:
- Each caplet is encased in a clear plastic cell with foil back.
- The name ORNEX SC appears on each caplet (see product illustration on front of carton).
- **DO NOT USE THIS PRODUCT IF EITHER OF THESE TAMPER-RESISTANT FEATURES IS MISSING OR BROKEN. IF YOU HAVE ANY QUESTIONS, PLEASE CALL 1-800-321-1834 TOLL FREE.**

Warnings: Do not exceed recommended dosage because at higher doses nervousness, dizziness, or sleeplessness may occur. Do not take this product for persistent or chronic cough such as occurs with smoking, asthma, or emphysema, or if cough is accompanied by excessive phlegm (mucus) unless directed by a physician. Do not use for more than 10 days, unless directed by a physician. A persistent cough may be a sign of a serious condition. If cough persists for more than 7 days, tends to recur, or is accompanied by rash, persistent headache, fever that lasts for more than 3 days, or if new symptoms occur, consult a physician. If sore throat is severe, persists for more than 2 days, is accompanied or followed by a fever, headache, rash, nausea or vomiting, consult a physician promptly. Do not take this product if you have high blood pressure, heart disease, diabetes, thyroid disease, or difficulty in urination due to enlargement of the prostate gland, unless directed by a physician. **Keep this and all medication out of the reach of children.** In case of accidental overdose, seek professional assistance or contact a Poison Control Center immediately. As with any drug, if you are pregnant or nursing a baby, seek the advice of a health professional before using this product.
Store at controlled room temperature (59°–86°F) in a dry place.

Drug Interaction Precaution: Do not take this product if you are presently taking a prescription drug for high blood pressure or depression, without first consulting your physician.

How Supplied: In consumer packages of 24 and 48 caplets.

Shown in Product Identification Section, page 414

SERUTAN®
Toasted Granules (brand of psyllium hydrophilic mucilloid)

Description: SERUTAN TOASTED GRANULES are an effective, natural way to restore or maintain regularity. They contain psyllium, one of the richest natural sources of soluble dietary fiber available. Unlike other psyllium products that are powdered, SERUTAN GRANULES need no mixing. Crunchy and lightly sweetened, they can be sprinkled on everday foods like cereal or oatmeal, salads, applesauce, casseroles, yogurt and desserts, accompanied by an 8 oz. beverage. SERUTAN GRANULES contain no chemical stimulants, are not habit forming, and can be used daily to maintain regularity by those who may not otherwise get enough fiber in their diets.

Product Information per heaping teaspoon (6.5g)

Calories	14
Cholesterol	0
Fat	0.25g
Sodium	0.03g
Total Dietary Fiber	3g

Indications: For the management of chronic constipation, irritable bowel syndrome and constipation due to pregnancy, convalescence or senility. Also for stool softening in hemorrhoid patients.

Directions: Adults: One to three heaping teaspoons 1 to 3 times daily sprinkled on food (cereals, salads, casseroles, desserts, etc.). Be sure to drink at least 8 oz. of liquid (a full glass) with your food each time you use SERUTAN GRANULES. SERUTAN GRANULES should always be put on food, not taken directly from a spoon. Children 6–12: give half the adult dose with 8 oz. of liquid. Do not exceed 9 teaspoons per day or five teaspoons per day for children 6–12. Note: it may require two to three days' therapy to produce full effectiveness.

Action: SERUTAN GRANULES promotes normal elimination and regularity by increasing bulk volume and water content of the stool.

Contraindications: Fecal impaction or intestinal obstruction.

TAMPER-RESISTANT FEATURE FOR YOUR PROTECTION: Imprinted neck seal under cap. Do not use if seal is missing or broken. If you have any questions, please call 1-800-321-1834 toll free.

Warning: Keep this and all medications out of reach of children. May cause allergic reaction in those individuals sensitive to psyllium.

Active Ingredient: Psyllium Hydrophilic Mucilloid, 2.5 grams per heaping teaspoon. **Inactive Ingredients:** Acacia, BHA, Calcium Propionate, Caprylic/ Capric Triglyceride, Caramel Color, Carboxymethylcellulose Sodium, Corn Starch, Invert Sugar, Magnesium Stearate, Oat Flour, Sodium Benzoate, Sodium Saccharin, Sucrose, Vegetable Oil, Wheat Germ.
Low sodium—0.03 grams per teaspoon.

How Supplied: Available in 6 oz. and 18 oz. plastic jars. SERUTAN is also available in two other formulas: Regular Powder (in 7 oz., 14 oz. and 21 oz. sizes) and Fruit Flavored Powder (in 6 oz., 12 oz. and 18 oz. sizes).
Store at controlled room temperature (59°–86°F).

Shown in Product Identification Section, page 414

TROPH-IRON®
Vitamins B_1, B_{12} and Iron

Indications: For deficiencies of vitamins B_1, B_{12} and iron.

Directions: One teaspoonful daily, or as directed by physician. While its effectiveness is in no way affected, TROPH-IRON Liquid may darken as it ages.

Active Ingredients: Each 5 mL (1 teaspoonful) contains Thiamine Hydrochloride (vitamin B_1), 10 mg; Cyanocobalamin (vitamin B_{12}), 25 mcg; Iron, 20 mg, present as soluble ferric pyrophosphate. **Inactive Ingredients:** Citric Acid, FD&C Red 40, Flavor, Glucose, Glycerin, Methylparaben, Propylparaben, Sodium Citrate, Sodium Saccharin, Purified Water.

TAMPER-RESISTANT PACKAGE FEATURE: Sealed, imprinted bottle cap; do not use if broken.

Warning: The treatment of any anemic condition should be under the advice and supervision of a physician. Since oral

iron products interfere with absorption of oral tetracycline antibiotics, these products should not be taken within two hours of each other.
Iron-containing medications may occasionally cause gastrointestinal discomfort, such as nausea, constipation or diarrhea. **Keep this and all medication out of reach of children.** In case of accidental overdose, seek professional assistance or contact a Poison Control Center immediately. As with any drug, if you are pregnant or nursing a baby, seek the advice of a health professional before using this product.

Store at controlled room temperature (59°–86°F).

How Supplied: 4 fl. oz. (118 mL) bottles.

TROPHITE®
Vitamins B_1 and B_{12}

Indications: For deficiencies of vitamins B_1 and B_{12}.

Directions: One teaspoonful daily, or as directed by physician.

Active Ingredients: Each 5 mL (1 teaspoonful) contains Thiamine Hydrochloride (vitamin B_1), 10 mg; and Cyanocobalamin (vitamin B_{12}), 25 mcg. **Inactive Ingredients:** D&C Red 33, D&C Yellow 10, Dextrose, FD&C Blue 1, Flavor, Glycerin, Methylparaben, Propylparaben, Sodium Tartrate, Tartaric Acid, Purified Water.

Important: Dispense liquid only in original bottle or an amber bottle. This product is light-sensitive. Never dispense in a flint, green, or blue bottle.
TROPHITE Liquid may be mixed with water, milk, or fruit or vegetable juices immediately before taking.
TAMPER-RESISTANT PACKAGE FEATURE: Sealed, imprinted bottle cap; do not use if broken.

Warning: Keep this and all medication out of reach of children. In case of accidental overdose, seek professional assistance or contact a Poison Control Center immediately. As with any drug, if you are pregnant or nursing a baby, seek the advice of a health professional before using this product.
Store at controlled room temperature (59°–86°F).

How Supplied: 4 fl. oz. (118 mL) bottles.

Products are
indexed alphabetically
in the
PINK SECTION.

Miles Inc.
P. O. BOX 340
ELKHART, IN 46515

ALKA-MINTS® Chewable Antacid Rich in Calcium

Active Ingredient: Each ALKA-MINTS Chewable Antacid tablet contains calcium carbonate 850 mg. (340 mg of elemental calcium). Each tablet contains less than .5 mg sodium per tablet, and is dietarily sodium free.

Inactive Ingredients: Dioctyl sodium sulfosuccinate, flavor, hydrolyzed cereal solids, magnesium stearate, polyethylene glycol, sorbitol, sugar (compressible)

Indications: ALKA-MINTS is an antacid for occasional use for relief of acid indigestion, heartburn and sour stomach.

Actions: ALKA-MINTS has a natural, clean, spearmint taste that leaves the mouth feeling refreshed. Measured by the in-vitro standard established by the Food and Drug Administration, one ALKA-MINTS tablet neutralizes 15.9 mEq of acid.

Warnings: Do not take more than 9 tablets in a 24 hour period, or use the maximum dosage of this product for more than 2 weeks, except under the advice and supervision of a physician. May cause constipation. As with any drug, if you are pregnant or nursing a baby, seek the advice of a health professional before using this product. Keep this and all drugs out of the reach of children.

Dosage and Administration: Chew 1 tablet every 2 hours or as directed by a physician.

How Supplied: Cartons of 30's. Each carton contains convenient pocket-sized packs with individually sealed tablets so ALKA-MINTS stay fresh wherever you go.

Product Identification Mark:
ALKA-MINTS embossed on each tablet.
Shown in Product Identification Section, page 415

ALKA-SELTZER® Effervescent Antacid & Pain Reliever With Specially Buffered Aspirin

Active Ingredients: Each tablet contains: aspirin 325 mg., heat treated sodium bicarbonate 1916 mg., citric acid 1000 mg. ALKA-SELTZER® in water contains principally the antacid sodium citrate and the analgesic sodium acetylsalicylate. Buffered pH is between 6 and 7.

Inactive Ingredients: None.

Indications: ALKA-SELTZER® Effervescent Antacid & Pain Reliever is an analgesic and an antacid and is indicated for relief of sour stomach, acid indigestion or heartburn with headache or body aches and pains. Also for fast relief of upset stomach with headache from overindulgence in food and drink—especially recommended for taking before bed and again on arising. Effective for pain relief alone: headache or body and muscular aches and pains.

Actions: When the ALKA-SELTZER® Effervescent Antacid & Pain Reliever tablet is dissolved in water, the acetylsalicylate ion differs from acetylsalicylic acid chemically, physically and pharmacologically. Being fat insoluble, it is not absorbed by the gastric mucosal cells. Studies and observations in animals and man including radiochrome determinations of fecal blood loss, measurement of ion fluxes and direct visualization with gastrocamera, have shown that, as contrasted with acetylsalicylic acid, the acetylsalicylate ion delivered in the solution does not alter gastric mucosal permeability to permit back-diffusion of hydrogen ion, and gastric damage and acute gastric mucosal lesions are therefore not seen after administration of the product. ALKA-SELTZER® Effervescent Antacid & Pain Reliever has the capacity to neutralize gastric hydrochloric acid quickly and effectively. In-vitro, 154 ml. of 0.1 N hydrochloric acid are required to decrease the pH of one tablet of ALKA-SELTZER® Effervescent Antacid & Pain Reliever in solution to 4.0. Measured against the in vitro standard established by the Food and Drug Administration one tablet neutralizes 17.2 mEq of acid. In vivo, the antacid activity of two ALKA-SELTZER® Antacid & Pain Reliever tablets is comparable to that of 10 ml. of milk of magnesia. ALKA-SELTZER® Effervescent Antacid & Pain Reliever is able to resist pH changes caused by the continuing secretion of acid in the normal individual and to maintain an elevated pH until emptying occurs.
ALKA-SELTZER® Effervescent Antacid & Pain Reliever provides highly water soluble acetylsalicylate ions which are fat insoluble. Acetylsalicylate ions are not absorbed from the stomach. They empty from the stomach and thereby become available for absorption from the duodenum. Thus, fast drug absorption and high plasma acetylsalicylate levels are achieved. Plasma levels of salicylate following the administration of ALKA-SELTZER® Effervescent Antacid & Pain Reliever solution (acetylsalicylate ion equivalent to 648 mg. acetylsalicylic acid) can reach 29 mg./liter in 10 minutes and rise to peak levels as high as 55 mg./liter within 30 minutes.

Warnings: Children and teenagers should not use this medicine for chicken pox or flu symptoms before a doctor is consulted about Reye syndrome, a rare but serious illness reported to be associated with aspirin. As with any drug, if you are pregnant or nursing a baby, seek the advice of a health professional before using this product. IT IS ESPECIALLY IMPORTANT NOT TO USE ASPIRIN

Continued on next page

Miles—Cont.

DURING THE LAST 3 MONTHS OF PREGNANCY UNLESS SPECIFICALLY DIRECTED TO DO SO BY A DOCTOR BECAUSE IT MAY CAUSE PROBLEMS IN THE UNBORN CHILD OR COMPLICATIONS DURING DELIVERY. Except under the advice and supervision of a physician, do not take more than, Adults: 8 tablets in a 24 hour period. (60 years of age or older: 4 tablets in a 24 hour period), or use the maximum dosage for more than 10 days. Do not use if you are allergic to aspirin or have asthma, if you have a coagulation (bleeding) disease, or if you are on a sodium restricted diet. Each tablet contains 567 mg. of sodium.
Keep this and all drugs out of the reach of children.

Dosage and Administration:
ALKA-SELTZER® must be dissolved in water before taking.
Adults: 2 tablets every 4 hours.
CAUTION: If symptoms persist or recur frequently, or if you are under treatment for ulcer, consult your physician.

Professional Labeling:

ASPIRIN FOR MYOCARDIAL INFARCTION

Indication: The Aspirin contained in ALKA-SELTZER® is indicated to reduce the risk of death and/or non-fatal myocardial infarction in patients with a previous infarction or unstable angina pectoris.

Clinical Trials: The indication is supported by the results of six, large, randomized multicenter, placebo-controlled studies[1–7] involving 10,816, predominantly male, post-myocardial infarction (MI) patients and one randomized placebo-controlled study of 1,266 men with unstable angina. Therapy with aspirin was begun at intervals after the onset of acute MI varying from less than 3 days to more than 5 years and continued for periods of from less than one year to four years. In the unstable angina study, treatment was started within 1 month after the onset of unstable angina and continued for 12 weeks and complicating conditions such as congestive heart failure were not included in the study.
Aspirin therapy in MI patients was associated with about a 20 percent reduction in the risk of subsequent death and/or non-fatal reinfarction, a median absolute decrease of 3 percent from the 12 to 22 percent event rates in the placebo groups. In aspirin-treated unstable angina patients the reduction in risk was about 50 percent, a reduction in event rate of 5 percent from the 10 percent rate in the placebo group over the 12 weeks of the study.
Daily dosage of aspirin in the post-myocardial infarction studies was 300 mg in one study and 900 to 1500 mg in five studies. A dose of 325 mg was used in the study of unstable angina.

Adverse Reactions: Gastrointestinal Reactions: Symptoms and signs of gastrointestinal irritation were not significantly increased in subjects treated for unstable angina with buffered aspirin in solution (ALKA-SELZER®). Doses of 1000 mg per day of aspirin tablets caused gastrointestinal symptoms and bleeding that in some cases were clinically significant. In the largest post-infarction study (the Aspirin Myocardial Infarction Study (AMIS) with 4,500 people), the percentage incidences of gastrointestinal symptoms for the aspirin (1000 mg of a standard, solid-tablet formulation) and placebo-treated subjects, respectively, were: stomach pain (14.5%; 4.4%); heartburn (11.9%; 4.8%); nausea and/or vomiting (7.6%; 2.1%); hospitalization for gastrointestinal disorder (4.9%; 3.5%). In the AMIS and other trials, aspirin treated patients had increased rates of gross gastrointestinal bleeding. As with all aspirin products ALKA-SELTZER is contraindicated in patients with aspirin sensitivity, with asthma, or with coagulation disease.

Cardiovascular and Biochemical: In the AMIS trial, the dosage of 1000 mg per day of aspirin was associated with small increases in systolic blood pressure (BP) (average 1.5 to 2.1 mm) and diastolic BP (0.5 to 0.6 mm), depending upon whether maximal or last available readings were used. Blood urea nitrogen and uric acid levels were also increased, but by less than 1.0 mg%. Subjects with marked hypertension or renal insufficiency had been excluded from the trial so that the clinical importance of these observations for such subjects or for any subjects treated over more prolonged periods is not known. It is recommended that patients placed on long-term aspirin treatment, even at doses of 300 mg per day, be seen at regular intervals to assess changes in these measurements.

Sodium in Buffered Aspirin for Solution Formulations: One tablet daily of buffered aspirin in solution adds 567 mg of sodium to that in the diet and may not be tolerated by patients with active sodium-retaining states such as congestive heart or renal failure. This amount of sodium adds about 30 percent to the 70 to 90 meq intake suggested as appropriate for dietary treatment of essential hypertension in the 1984 Report of the Joint National Committee on Detection, Evaluation, and Treatment of High Blood Pressure.[8]

Dosage and Administration: Although most of the studies used dosages exceeding 300 mg, daily, two trials used only 300 mg and pharmacologic data indicate that this dose inhibits platelet function fully. Therefore, 300 mg or a conventional 325 mg aspirin dose daily is a reasonable, routine dose that would minimize gastrointestinal adverse reactions. This use of aspirin applies to both solid, oral dosage forms (buffered and plain aspirin) and buffered aspirin in solution.

References:

(1) Elwood, P. C., et al., A Randomized Controlled Trial of Acetysalicylic Acid in the Secondary Prevention of Mortality from Myocardial Infarction," *British Medical Journal* 1:436–440, 1974.
(2) The Coronary Drug Project Research Group, "Aspirin in Coronary Heart Disease," *Journal of Chronic Diseases,* 29:625–642, 1976.
(3) Breddin K., et al., "Secondary Prevention of Myocardial Infarction: A Comparison of Acetylsalicylic Acid, Phenprocoumon or Placebo," *International Congress Series* 470:263–268, 1979.
(4) Aspirin Myocardial Infarction Study Research Group, "A Randomized, Controlled Trial of Aspirin in Persons Recovered from Myocardial Infarction," *Journal American Medical Association* 245:661–669, 1980.
(5) Elwood, P. C., and P. M. Sweetnam, "Aspirin and Secondary Mortality after Myocardial Infarction," *Lancet* pp. 1313–1315, December 22–29, 1979.
(6) The Persantine-Aspirin Reinfarction Study Research Group, "Persantine and Aspirin in Coronary Heart Disease," *Circulation,* 62: 449–460, 1980.
(7) Lewis, H. D., et al., "Protective Effects of Aspirin Against Acute Myocardial Infarction and Death in Men with Unstable Angina, Results of a Veterans Administration Cooperative Study," *New England Journal of Medicine* 309:396–403, 1983.
(8) "1984 Report of the Joint National Committee on Detection, Evaluation, Treatment of High Blood Pressure," U.S. Department of Health and Human Services and United States Public Health Service, National Institutes of Health.

How Supplied: Tablets: foil sealed; box of 12 in 6 foil twin packs; box of 24 in 12 foil twin packs; box of 36 tablets in 18 foil twin packs; 100 tablets in 50 foil twin packs; carton of 72 tablets in 36 foil twin packs. Product Identification Mark: "ALKA-SELTZER" embossed on each tablet.

Shown in Product Identification Section, page 414

Flavored ALKA-SELTZER®
Effervescent Antacid & Pain Reliever

Active Ingredients: Each tablet contains: Aspirin 325 mg, heat treated sodium bicarbonate 1710 mg, citric acid 1220 mg. Alka-Seltzer in water contains principally the antacid sodium citrate and the analgesic sodium acetylsalicylate.

Inactive Ingredients: Flavors, Saccharin Sodium.

Indications: For fast relief of ACID INDIGESTION, SOUR STOMACH or HEARTBURN with HEADACHE, or BODY ACHES AND PAINS. Also for fast relief of UPSET STOMACH with

HEADACHE from overindulgence in food and drink—especially recommended for taking before bed and again on arising. EFFECTIVE FOR PAIN RELIEF ALONE: HEADACHE or BODY and MUSCULAR ACHES and PAINS.

Warnings: Children and teenagers should not use this medicine for chicken pox or flu symptoms before a doctor is consulted about Reye syndrome, a rare but serious illness reported to be associated with aspirin.

As with any drug, if you are pregnant or nursing a baby, seek the advice of a health professional before using this product. IT IS ESPECIALLY IMPORTANT NOT TO USE ASPIRIN DURING THE LAST 3 MONTHS OF PREGNANCY UNLESS SPECIFICALLY DIRECTED TO DO SO BY A DOCTOR BECAUSE IT MAY CAUSE PROBLEMS IN THE UNBORN CHILD OR COMPLICATIONS DURING DELIVERY.

Except under the advice and supervision of a physician: Do not take more than, ADULTS: 6 tablets in a 24-hour period, (60 years of age or older: 4 tablets in a 24-hour period), or use the daily maximum dosage for more than 10 days. Do not use if you are allergic to aspirin or have asthma, if you have a coagulation (bleeding) disease, or if you are on a sodium restricted diet. Each tablet contains 506 mg of sodium.

Keep this and all drugs out of the reach of children.

Directions: Alka-Seltzer must be dissolved in water before taking. ADULTS: 2 tablets every 4 hours. CAUTION: If symptoms persist or recur frequently or if you are under treatment for ulcer, consult your physician.

Professional Labeling:

ASPIRIN FOR MYOCARDIAL INFARCTION

Indication: The Aspirin contained in Alka-Seltzer is indicated to reduce the risk of death and/or non-fatal myocardial infarction in patients with a previous infarction or unstable angina pectoris.

Clinical Trials: The indication is supported by the results of six, large, randomized multicenter, placebo-controlled studies[1–7] involving 10,816, predominantly male, post-myocardial infarction (MI) patients and one randomized placebo-controlled study of 1,266 men with unstable angina. Therapy with aspirin was begun at intervals after the onset of acute MI varying from less than 3 days to more than 5 years and continued for periods of from less than one year to four years. In the unstable angina study, treatment was started within 1 month after the onset of unstable angina and continued for 12 weeks and complicating conditions such as congestive heart failure were not included in the study.

Aspirin therapy in MI patients was associated with about a 20 percent reduction in the risk of subsequent death and/or non-fatal reinfarction, a median absolute decrease of 3 percent from the 12 to 22 percent event rates in the placebo groups. In aspirin-treated unstable angina patients the reduction in risk was about 50 percent, a reduction in event rate of 5 percent from the 10 percent rate in the placebo group over the 12 weeks of the study.

Daily dosage of aspirin in the post-myocardial infarction studies was 300 mg in one study and 900 to 1500 mg in five studies. A dose of 325 mg was used in the study of unstable angina.

Adverse Reactions: Gastrointestinal Reactions: Symptoms and signs of gastrointestinal irritation were not significantly increased in subjects treated for unstable angina with buffered aspirin in solution (ALKA-SELZER®). Doses of 1000 mg per day of aspirin tablets caused gastrointestinal symptoms and bleeding that in some cases were clinically significant. In the largest post-infarction study (the Aspirin Myocardial Infarction Study (AMIS) with 4,500 people), the percentage incidences of gastrointestinal symptoms for the aspirin (1000 mg of a standard, solid-tablet formulation) and placebo-treated subjects, respectively, were: stomach pain (14.5%; 4.4%); heartburn (11.9%; 4.8%); nausea and/or vomiting (7.6%; 2.1%); hospitalization for gastrointestinal disorder (4.9%; 3.5%). In the AMIS and other trials, aspirin treated patients had increased rates of gross gastrointestinal bleeding. As with all aspirin products Alka-Seltzer is contraindicated in patients with aspirin sensitivity, with asthma, or with coagulation disease.

Cardiovascular and Biochemical: In the AMIS trial, the dosage of 1000 mg per day of aspirin was associated with small increases in systolic blood pressure (BP) (average 1.5 to 2.1 mm) and diastolic BP (0.5 to 0.6 mm), depending upon whether maximal or last available readings were used. Blood urea nitrogen and uric acid levels were also increased, but by less than 1.0 mg%. Subjects with marked hypertension or renal insufficiency had been excluded from the trial so that the clinical importance of these observations for such subjects or for any subjects treated over more prolonged periods is not known. It is recommended that patients placed on long-term aspirin treatment, even at doses of 300 mg per day, be seen at regular intervals to assess changes in these measurements.

Sodium in Buffered Aspirin for Solution Formulations: One tablet daily of flavored buffered aspirin in solution adds 506 mg of sodium to that in the diet and may not be tolerated by patients with active sodium-retaining states such as congestive heart or renal failure. This amount of sodium adds about 30 percent to the 70 to 90 meq intake suggested as appropriate for dietary treatment of essential hypertension in the 1984 Report of the Joint National Committee on Detection, Evaluation, and Treatment of High Blood Pressure.[8]

Dosage and Administration: Although most of the studies used dosages exceeding 300 mg, daily, two trials used only 300 mg and pharmacologic data indicate that this dose inhibits platelet function fully. Therefore, 300 mg or a conventional 325 mg aspirin dose daily is a reasonable, routine dose that would minimize gastrointestinal adverse reactions. This use of aspirin applies to both solid, oral dosage forms (buffered and plain aspirin) and buffered aspirin in solution.

References:

(1) Elwood, P. C., et al., A Randomized Controlled Trial of Acetysalicylic Acid in the Secondary Prevention of Mortality from Myocardial Infarction," *British Medical Journal* 1:436–440, 1974.

(2) The Coronary Drug Project Research Group, "Aspirin in Coronary Heart Disease," *Journal of Chronic Diseases,* 29:625–642, 1976.

(3) Breddin K., et al., "Secondary Prevention of Myocardial Infarction: A Comparison of Acetylsalicylic Acid, Phenprocoumon or Placebo," *International Congress Series* 470:263–268, 1979.

(4) Aspirin Myocardial Infarction Study Research Group, "A Randomized, Controlled Trial of Aspirin in Persons Recovered from Myocardial Infarction," *Journal American Medical Association* 245:661–669, 1980.

(5) Elwood, P. C., and P. M. Sweetnam, "Aspirin and Secondary Mortality after Myocardial Infarction," *Lancet* pp. 1313–1315, December 22–29, 1979.

(6) The Persantine-Aspirin Reinfarction Study Research Group, "Persantine and Aspirin in Coronary Heart Disease," *Circulation,* 62: 449–460, 1980.

(7) Lewis, H. D., et al., "Protective Effects of Aspirin Against Acute Myocardial Infarction and Death in Men with Unstable Angina, Results of a Veterans Administration Cooperative Study," *New England Journal of Medicine* 309:396–403, 1983.

(8) "1984 Report of the Joint National Committee on Detection, Evaluation, Treatment of High Blood Pressure," U.S. Department of Health and Human Services and United States Public Health Service, National Institutes of Health.

How Supplied: Foil sealed effervescent tablets in cartons of 12's in 6 foil twin packs; 24's in 12 foil twin packs; 36's in 18 foil twin packs.

Shown in Product Identification Section, page 414

ALKA-SELTZER® Effervescent Antacid

Active Ingredients: Each tablet contains heat treated sodium bicarbonate 958 mg., citric acid 832 mg., potassium bicarbonate 312 mg. ALKA-SELTZER®

Continued on next page

Miles—Cont.

Effervescent Antacid in water contains principally the antacids sodium citrate and potassium citrate.

Inactive Ingredient: A tableting aid.

Indications: ALKA-SELTZER® Effervescent Antacid is indicated for relief of acid indigestion, sour stomach or heartburn.

Actions: The ALKA-SELTZER® Effervescent Antacid solution provides quick and effective neutralization of gastric acid. Measured by the in vitro standard established by the Food and Drug Administration one tablet will neutralize 10.6 mEq of acid.

Warnings: Except under the advice and supervision of a physician, do not take more than: Adults: 8 tablets in a 24 hour period (60 years of age or older: 7 tablets in a 24 hour period), Children: 4 tablets in a 24 hour period; or use the maximum dosage of this product for more than 2 weeks.
Do not use this product if you are on a sodium restricted diet. Each tablet contains 311 mg. of sodium.
Keep this and all drugs out of the reach of children. As with any drug, if you are pregnant or nursing a baby, seek the advice of a health professional before using this product.

Dosage and Administration: Adults: Take 1 or 2 tablets fully dissolved in water every 4 hours. Children: ½ the adult dosage.

How Supplied: Boxes of 20 tablets in 10 foil twin packs; 36 tablets in 18 foil twin packs.

Shown in Product Identification Section, page 415

ALKA-SELTZER® Extra Strength Antacid & Pain Reliever

Active Ingredients: Each tablet contains: Aspirin 500mg, heat treated sodium bicarbonate 1985mg, citric acid 1000mg. Alka-Seltzer in water contains principally the antacid sodium citrate and the analgesic sodium acetylsalicylate.

Inactive Ingredient: Flavors

Indications: For fast relief of acid indigestion, sour stomach or heartburn with headache or body aches and pains. Also, for fast relief of upset stomach with headache from overindulgence in food and drink—especially recommended for taking before bed and again on arising. Effective for pain relief alone: headache or body and muscular aches and pains.

Warnings: Children and teenagers should not use this medicine for chicken pox or flu symptoms before a doctor is consulted about Reye syndrome, a rare but serious illness reported to be associated with aspirin. As with any drug, if you are pregnant or nursing a baby, seek the advice of a health professional before using this product. IT IS ESPECIALLY IMPORTANT NOT TO USE ASPIRIN DURING THE LAST 3 MONTHS OF PREGNANCY UNLESS SPECIFICALLY DIRECTED TO DO SO BY A DOCTOR BECAUSE IT MAY CAUSE PROBLEMS IN THE UNBORN CHILD OR COMPLICATIONS DURING DELIVERY. Except under the advice and supervision of a physician, do not take more than, Adults: 7 tablets in a 24-hour period (60 years of age or older, 4 tablets in a 24-hour period), or use the daily maximum dosage for more than 10 days. Do not use if you are allergic to aspirin or have asthma, if you have a coagulation (bleeding) disease, or if you are on a sodium restricted diet. Each tablet contains 588mg of sodium. Keep this and all drugs out of the reach of children.

Dosage and Administration: Extra Strength Alka-Seltzer must be dissolved in water before taking. Adults: 2 tablets every 4 hours. Caution: If symptoms persist, or recur frequently, or if you are under treatment for ulcer, consult your physician.

How Supplied: Foil sealed effervescent tablets in cartons of 12's in 6 foil twin packs; 24's in 12 foil twin packs.

Shown in Product Identification Section, page 415

ALKA-SELTZER PLUS® Cold Medicine

Active Ingredients:
Each dry ALKA-SELTZER PLUS® Cold Tablet contains the following active ingredients: Phenylpropanolamine bitartrate 24.08 mg., chlorpheniramine maleate 2 mg., aspirin 325 mg. The product is dissolved in water prior to ingestion and the aspirin is converted into its soluble ionic form, sodium acetylsalicylate.

Inactive Ingredients: Citric acid, flavors, sodium bicarbonate.

Indications: For relief of the symptoms of common colds and flu.

Actions: Provides temporary relief of these major cold and flu symptoms: nasal and sinus congestion, runny nose, sneezing, headache, scratchy sore throat, fever, body aches and pains.

Warnings: Children and teenagers should not use this medicine for chicken pox or flu symptoms before a doctor is consulted about Reye syndrome, a rare but serious illness reported to be associated with aspirin. Do not exceed recommended dosage because at higher doses nervousness, dizziness or sleeplessness may occur. May cause excitability, especially in children. Do not take this product if you are allergic to aspirin or have asthma, glaucoma, bleeding problems, emphysema, chronic pulmonary disease, shortness of breath, difficulty in breathing, heart disease, high blood pressure, thyroid disease, diabetes or difficulty in urination due to enlargement of the prostate gland or on a sodium-restricted diet unless directed by a doctor. Each tablet contains 506 mg of sodium. May cause drowsiness; alcohol, sedatives and tranquilizers may increase drowsiness effect. Avoid alcoholic beverages while taking this product. Do not take this product if you are taking sedatives or tranquilizers without first consulting your doctor. Use caution when driving a motor vehicle or operating machinery. If sore throat is severe, persists for more than 2 days, is accompanied by a high fever, headache, nausea or vomiting, consult a physician promptly. Do not take this product for more than 7 days. If symptoms do not improve or are accompanied by fever or if fever persists for more than 3 days, consult a doctor. As with any drug, if you are pregnant or nursing a baby, seek the advice of a health professional before using this product. IT IS ESPECIALLY IMPORTANT NOT TO USE ASPIRIN DURING THE LAST 3 MONTHS OF PREGNANCY UNLESS SPECIFICALLY DIRECTED TO DO SO BY A DOCTOR BECAUSE IT MAY CAUSE PROBLEMS IN THE UNBORN CHILD OR COMPLICATIONS DURING DELIVERY. Keep this and all drugs out of the reach of children.

Drug Interaction Precaution: Do not take this product if you are presently taking a prescription drug for anticoagulation (thinning the blood), diabetes, gout, arthritis, high blood pressure or depression without first consulting your doctor.

Dosage and Administration:
ALKA-SELTZER PLUS® is taken in solution; 2 tablets dissolved in approximately 4 ounces of water. Adults: two tablets every 4 hours up to 8 tablets in 24 hours.

How Supplied: Tablets: carton of 12 tablets in 6 foil twin packs; 20 tablets in 10 foil twin packs; carton of 36 tablets in 18 foil twin packs; carton of 48 tablets in 24 foil twin packs.

Product Identification Mark:
"Alka-Seltzer Plus" embossed on each tablet.

Shown in Product Identification Section, page 415

ALKA-SELTZER PLUS® Night-Time Cold Medicine

Active Ingredients: Each tablet contains aspirin 500 mg, brompheniramine maleate 2 mg, phenylpropanolamine bitartrate 20 mg, dextromethorphan hydrobromide 10 mg. In water the aspirin is converted into its soluble ionic form, sodium acetylsalicylate.

Inactive Ingredients: Aspartame, citric acid, flavor, sodium bicarbonate, tableting aids.

Indications: For fast, effective nighttime relief of the major symptoms of cold and flu without alcohol.

Actions: Provides temporary relief of these major cold and flu symptoms: coughing, nasal and sinus congestion, body aches and pains, runny nose, headache, sneezing, fever, scratchy sore throat so you can get the rest you need.

Warning: Children and teenagers should not use this medicine for chicken pox or flu symptoms before a doctor is consulted about Reye syndrome, a rare but serious illness reported to be associated with aspirin. If sore throat is severe, persists for more than 2 days, is accompanied by high fever, headache, nausea or vomiting, consult a physician promptly. As with any drug, if you are pregnant or nursing a baby, seek the advice of a health professional before using this product. **IT IS ESPECIALLY IMPORTANT NOT TO USE ASPIRIN DURING THE LAST 3 MONTHS OF PREGNANCY UNLESS SPECIFICALLY DIRECTED TO DO SO BY A DOCTOR BECAUSE IT MAY CAUSE PROBLEMS IN THE UNBORN CHILD OR COMPLICATIONS DURING DELIVERY.** Do not exceed recommended dosage because at higher doses nervousness, dizziness or sleeplessness may occur. May cause excitability, especially in children. Do not take this product unless directed by a doctor if you are allergic to aspirin, have chronic pulmonary disease, heart disease, glaucoma, asthma, shortness of breath, bleeding problems, difficulty in breathing, thyroid disease, diabetes, emphysema, high blood pressure or difficulty in urination due to enlargement of the prostate gland or on a sodium restricted diet. Each tablet contains 506 mg of sodium. May cause marked drowsiness; alcohol, sedatives and tranquilizers may increase drowsiness effect. Avoid alcoholic beverages while taking this product. Do not take this product if you are taking sedatives or tranquilizers without first consulting your doctor. Use caution when driving a motor vehicle or operating machinery. Do not take this product for persistent or chronic cough such as occurs with smoking, asthma, emphysema, or if cough is accompanied by excessive phlegm (mucus), unless directed by a doctor. A persistent cough may be a sign of a serious condition. If cough persists for more than 1 week, tends to recur or is accompanied by fever, rash, or persistent headache, consult a doctor. Do not take this product for more than 7 days. If symptoms do not improve or are accompanied by fever or if fever persists for more than 3 days, consult a doctor. Keep this and all drugs out of the reach of children, **PHENYLKETONURICS:** Contains Phenylalanine 9 mg per tablet.

Drug Interaction Precaution: Do not take this product if you are presently taking a prescription drug for anticoagulation (thinning the blood), diabetes, gout, arthritis, high blood pressure or depression without first consulting your doctor.

Dosage and Administration: Adults: Take 2 tablets fully dissolved in 4 ounces of water (use more or less water to taste). Additional fluid intake is encouraged for cold sufferers. Repeat every 4 hours, not to exceed 8 tablets in any 24-hour period.

How Supplied: Tablets: carton of 12 tablets in 6 foil twin packs; carton of 20 tablets in 10 foil twin packs; carton of 36 tablets in 18 foil twin packs.

Product Identification Mark: "A/S PLUS NIGHT-TIME" etched on each tablet

Shown in Product Identification Section, page 415

ALKA-SELTZER PLUS®
Sinus Allergy Medicine

Active Ingredients: Phenylpropanolamine bitartrate 24.08 mg, brompheniramine maleate 2 mg, aspirin 500 mg. In water the aspirin is converted into its soluble ionic form, sodium acetylsalicylate.

Inactive Ingredients: Aspartame, citric acid, flavors, heat-treated sodium bicarbonate, tableting aids

Indications: For the temporary relief of nasal congestion, sinus pain and pressure, headache, runny nose, sneezing and itchy, watery eyes due to sinusitis, allergic rhinitis, hay fever or other upper respiratory allergies.

Warnings: Children and teenagers should not use this medicine for chicken pox or flu symptoms before a doctor is consulted about Reye syndrome, a rare but serious illness reported to be associated with aspirin. Do not exceed recommended dosage because at higher doses nervousness, dizziness or sleeplessness may occur. Adults: Do not take this product for more than 7 days. If symptoms do not improve or are accompanied by fever or if fever persists for more than 3 days, consult a doctor. May cause excitability, especially in children. Do not take this product if you have thyroid or heart disease, diabetes, high blood pressure, asthma, glaucoma, emphysema, chronic pulmonary disease, shortness of breath, difficulty in breathing, difficulty in urination due to enlargement of the prostate gland, bleeding problems, allergy to aspirin or are on a sodium restricted diet, unless directed by a doctor. Each tablet contains 506 mg of sodium. May cause drowsiness. Alcohol, sedatives and tranquilizers may increase the drowsiness effect. Avoid alcoholic beverages while taking this product. Do not take this product if you are taking sedatives or tranquilizers without first consulting your doctor. Use caution when driving a motor vehicle or operating machinery. As with any drug, if you are pregnant or nursing a baby, seek the advice of a health professional before using this product. IT IS ESPECIALLY IMPORTANT NOT TO USE ASPIRIN DURING THE LAST 3 MONTHS OF PREGNANCY UNLESS SPECIFICALLY DIRECTED TO DO SO BY A DOCTOR BECAUSE IT MAY CAUSE PROBLEMS IN THE UNBORN CHILD OR COMPLICATIONS DURING DELIVERY. Keep this and all drugs out of the reach of children.

Drug Interaction: Do not take this product if you are presently taking a prescription drug for anticoagulation (thinning of the blood), diabetes, gout, arthritis, high blood pressure or depression without first consulting your doctor.
PHENYLKETONURICS: Contains 8.98 mg phenylalanine per tablet.

Directions: Adults: Take 2 tablets dissolved in approximately 4 ounces (½ glass) of water every 4 hours. Do not exceed 8 tablets in any 24-hour period.

How Supplied: Boxes of 32 tablets in 16 foil twin packs; 16 tablets in 8 foil twin packs

Product Identification Mark: "AS + Sinus Allergy" embossed on each tablet.

Shown in Product Identification Section, page 415

ALKA-SELTZER PLUS® COLD & COUGH MEDICINE

Active Ingredients: Each ALKA-SELTZER PLUS® COLD AND COUGH tablet contains the following active ingredients: Aspirin 500 mg, Chlorpheniramine Maleate 2 mg, Phenylpropanolamine Bitartrate 24.08 mg, Dextromethorphan Hydrobromide 10 mg. In water the aspirin is converted into its soluble ionic form, sodium acetylsalicylate.

Inactive Ingredients: Aspartame, Citric Acid, Flavor, Sodium Bicarbonate, Tableting Aids.

Indications: Provides temporary relief of the major symptoms of colds and flu with cough.

Actions: Provides temporary relief of these major symptoms of colds and flu with cough: nasal and sinus congestion, body aches and pains, runny nose, coughing, headache, scratchy sore throat, sneezing, fever.

Warnings: Children and teenagers should not use this medicine for chicken pox or flu symptoms before a doctor is consulted about Reye syndrome, a rare but serious illness reported to be associated with aspirin. If sore throat is severe, persists for more than 2 days, is accompanied by high fever, headache, nausea or vomiting, consult a physician promptly. As with any drug, if you are pregnant or nursing a baby, seek the advice of a health professional before using this product. **IT IS ESPECIALLY IMPORTANT NOT TO USE ASPIRIN DURING THE LAST 3 MONTHS OF PREGNANCY UNLESS SPECIFICALLY DIRECTED TO DO SO BY A DOCTOR BECAUSE IT MAY CAUSE PROB-**

Continued on next page

Miles—Cont.

LEMS IN THE UNBORN CHILD OR COMPLICATIONS DURING DELIVERY. Do not exceed recommended dosage because at higher doses nervousness, dizziness or sleeplessness may occur. May cause excitability, especially in children. Do not take this product unless directed by a doctor if you are allergic to aspirin, have chronic pulmonary disease, heart disease, glaucoma, asthma, shortness of breath, bleeding problems, difficulty in breathing, thyroid disease, diabetes, emphysema, high blood pressure or difficulty in urination due to enlargement of the prostate gland or on a sodium restricted diet. Each tablet contains 506 mg of sodium. May cause marked drowsiness; alcohol, sedatives, and tranquilizers may increase drowsiness effect. Avoid alcoholic beverages while taking this product. Do not take this product if you are taking sedatives or tranquilizers without first consulting your doctor. Use caution when driving a motor vehicle or operating machinery. Do not take this product for persistent or chronic cough such as occurs with smoking, asthma, emphysema, or if cough is accompanied by excessive phlegm (mucus) unless directed by a doctor. A persistent cough may be a sign of a serious condition. If cough persists for more than 1 week, tends to recur or is accompanied by fever, rash, or persistent headache, consult a doctor. Do not take this product for more than 7 days. If symptoms do not improve or are accompanied by fever or if fever persists for more than 3 days, consult a doctor. Keep this and all drugs out of the reach of children.

PHENYLKETONURICS: Contains Phenylalanine 7 mg per tablet.

Drug Interaction Precaution: Do not take this product if you are presently taking a prescription drug for anticoagulation (thinning the blood), diabetes, gout, arthritis, high blood pressure or depression without first consulting your doctor.

Dosage and Administration: ALKA-SELTZER PLUS® COLD & COUGH MEDICINE is taken in solution; approximately 4 ounces of water. Additional fluid intake is encouraged for cold sufferers. Adults: 2 tablets every 4 hours up to 8 tablets in 24 hours.

How Supplied: Tablets: carton of 36 tablets in 18 foil twin packs: carton of 20 tablets in 10 foil twin packs: carton of 48 tablets in 24 foil packs, carton of 12 tablets in 6 foil packs.

Product Identification Mark: "AS + Cold Cough" embossed on each tablet.

Shown in Product Identification Section, page 415

BACTINE® Antiseptic·Anesthetic First Aid Liquid

Active Ingredients: Benzalkonium Chloride 0.13% w/w, Lidocaine HCl 2.5% w/w.

Inactive Ingredients: Edetate Disodium, Fragrances, Octoxynol 9, Propylene Glycol, Purified Water.

Indications: Antiseptic/anesthetic for helping prevent infection, cleanse wounds, and for the temporary relief of pain and itching due to insect bites, minor burns, sunburn, minor cuts and minor skin irritations.

Warnings: For external use only. Do not use in large quantities, particularly over raw surfaces or blistered areas. Avoid spraying in eyes, mouth, ears or on sensitive areas of the body. This product is not for use on wild or domestic animal bites. If you have an animal bite or puncture wound, consult your physician immediately. If condition worsens or if symptoms persist for more than 7 days, discontinue use of this product and consult a physician. Do not bandage tightly. Keep this and all drugs out of reach of children. In case of accidental ingestion, seek professional assistance or contact a Poison Control Center immediately.

Dosage and Administration: For adults and children 2 years of age or older. For superficial skin wounds, cuts, scratches, scrapes, cleanse affected area thoroughly.

Directions: To apply, hold bottle 2 to 3 inches from injured area and squeeze repeatedly. To aid in removing foreign particles, dab injured area with clean gauze saturated with product. For sunburn, minor burns, insect bites, and minor skin irritations, apply to affected area of skin for temporary relief. Product can be applied to affected area with clean gauze saturated with product.

How Supplied: 2 oz., 4 oz. and 16 oz. liquid, and 3.5 oz. pump spray.

Shown in Product Identification Section, page 415

BACTINE® First Aid Antibiotic Plus Anesthetic Ointment

Active Ingredients: Each gram contains Polymyxin B Sulfate 5000 units; Bacitracin 400 units; Neomycin Sulfate 5 mg (equivalent to 3.5 mg Neomycin base); Diperodon HCl 10 mg (pain reliever).

Inactive Ingredients: Mineral Oil, White Petrolatum.

Indications: First aid to help prevent infection, guard against bacterial contamination, relieve pain and itching in minor cuts, scrapes and burns.

Warning: For external use only. Do not use in the eyes or apply over large areas of the body. In case of deep or puncture wounds, animal bites or serious burns, consult a physician. Stop use and consult a physician if the condition persists or gets worse. Do not use longer than one (1) week unless directed by a physician. Keep this and all medicines out of children's reach. In case of accidental ingestion, seek professional assistance or contact a Poison Control Center immediately.

Directions: Clean the affected area. Apply a small amount of this product (an amount equal to the surface area of the tip of a finger) one to three times daily. May be covered with a sterile bandage.

How Supplied: ½ oz. tube.

Shown in Product Identification Section, page 415

BACTINE® Brand Hydrocortisone Anti-Itch Cream

Active Ingredient: Hydrocortisone 0.5%.

Inactive Ingredients: Butylated Hydroxyanisole, Butylated Hydroxytoluene, Butylparaben, Carbomer, Cetyl Alcohol, Colloidal Silicon Dioxide, Corn oil (and) Gylceryl Oleate (and) Propylene Glycol (and) (BHA) (and) BHT (and) Propyl Gallate (and) Citric Acid, DEA-Oleth-3 Phosphate, Diisopropyl Sebacate, Edetate Disodium, Glycerin, Hydroxypropyl Methylcellulose 2906, Lanolin Alcohol, Methylparaben, Mineral Oil (and) Lanolin Alcohol, Propylene Glycol Stearate SE, Propylparaben, Purified Water.

Indications: For the temporary relief of minor skin irritations, itching, and rashes due to eczema, insect bites, poison ivy, poison oak, poison sumac, soaps, detergents, cosmetics, and jewelry.

Warnings: For external use only. Avoid contact with the eyes. If condition worsens or if symptoms persist for more than seven days, discontinue use and consult a physician.
Do not use on children under 2 years of age except under the advice and supervision of a physician.
Keep this and all drugs out of the reach of children. In case of accidental ingestion, seek professional assistance or contact a Poison Control Center immediately.

Directions: For adults and children 2 years of age and older. Gently massage into affected skin area not more than 3 or 4 times daily.

How Supplied: ½ oz. plastic tube.

Shown in Product Identification Section, page 415

BUGS BUNNY™ Children's Chewable Vitamins Plus Iron (Sugar Free)
FLINTSTONES™ Children's Chewable Vitamins Plus Iron

One Tablet Provides Vitamins	Quantity	% of U.S. RDA For Children 2 to 4 Years of Age	For Adults and Children over 4 Years of Age
Vitamin A (as Acetate and Beta Carotene)	2500 I.U.	100	50
Vitamin D	400 I.U.	100	100
Vitamin E	15 I.U.	150	50
Vitamin C	60 mg.	150	100
Folic Acid	0.3 mg.	150	75
Thiamine	1.05 mg.	150	70
Riboflavin	1.20 mg.	150	70
Niacin	13.50 mg.	150	67
Vitamin B_6	1.05 mg.	150	52
Vitamin B_{12}	4.5 mcg.	150	75
Mineral:			
Iron (Elemental)	15 mg.	150	83

BUGS BUNNY™ With Extra C Children's Chewable Vitamins (Sugar Free)
FLINTSTONES™ With Extra C Children's Chewable Vitamins

One Tablet Provides Vitamins	Quantity	% of U.S. RDA For Children 2 To 4 Years of Age	For Adults and Children Over 4 Years of Age
Vitamin A (as Acetate and Beta Carotene)	2500 I.U.	100	50
Vitamin D	400 I.U.	100	100
Vitamin E	15 I.U.	150	50
Vitamin C	250 mg.	625	417
Folic Acid	0.3 mg.	150	75
Thiamine	1.05 mg.	150	70
Riboflavin	1.20 mg.	150	70
Niacin	13.50 mg.	150	67
Vitamin B_6	1.05 mg.	150	52
Vitamin B_{12}	4.5 mcg.	150	75

FLINTSTONES™ COMPLETE Children's Chewable Vitamins
BUGS BUNNY™ COMPLETE Children's Chewable Vitamins + Minerals (Sugar Free)

Vitamins	Quantity Per Tablet	Percentage of U.S. Recommended Daily Allowance (U.S. RDA) For Children 2 to 4 Years of Age (½ tablet)	For Adults & Children Over 4 Years of Age (1 tablet)
Vitamin A (as Acetate and Beta Carotene)	5000 I.U.	100	100
Vitamin D	400 I.U.	50	100
Vitamin E	30 I.U.	150	100
Vitamin C	60 mg.	75	100
Folic Acid	0.4 mg.	100	100
Vitamin B-1 (Thiamine)	1.5 mg.	107	100
Vitamin B-2 (Riboflavin)	1.7 mg.	106	100
Niacin	20 mg.	111	100
Vitamin B-6 (Pyridoxine)	2 mg.	143	100
Vitamin B-12 (Cyanocobalamin)	6 mcg.	100	100
Biotin	40 mcg.	13	13
Pantothenic Acid	10 mg.	100	100
Minerals	**Quantity**	**Percent U.S. RDA**	
Iron (elemental)	18 mg.	90	100
Calcium	100 mg.	6	10
Copper	2 mg.	100	100
Phosphorus	100 mg.	6	10
Iodine	150 mcg.	107	100
Magnesium	20 mg.	5	5
Zinc	15 mg.	94	100

BUGS BUNNY™ Children's Chewable Vitamins (Sugar Free)
BUGS BUNNY™ Children's Chewable Vitamins Plus Iron (Sugar Free)
FLINTSTONES™ Children's Chewable Vitamins
FLINTSTONES™ Children's Chewable Vitamins Plus Iron

Vitamin Ingredients: Each multivitamin supplement with iron contains the ingredients listed in the chart. [See chart top left.]
BUGS BUNNY™ Children's Chewable Vitamins and FLINTSTONES™ Children's Chewable Vitamins provide the same quantities of vitamins, but do not provide iron.

Indication: Dietary supplementation.

Dosage and Administration: One chewable tablet daily. For adults and children two years and older; tablet must be chewed.

Warning For Bugs Bunny Only: Phenylketonurics: Contains Phenylalanine.

Precaution:
IRON SUPPLEMENTS ONLY.
Contains iron, which can be harmful in large doses. Close tightly and keep out of reach of children. In case of overdose contact a Poison Control Center immediately.

How Supplied: Flintstones are supplied in bottles of 60 and 100, Bugs Bunny in bottles of 60 with child-resistant caps.

Shown in Product Identification Section, page 415

FLINTSTONES™ With Extra C Children's Chewable Vitamins
BUGS BUNNY™ With Extra C Children's Chewable Vitamins (Sugar Free)

Vitamin Ingredients: Each multivitamin supplement contains the ingredients listed in the chart above: [See second chart.]

Indication: Dietary supplementation.

Dosage and Administration: One tablet daily for adults and children two years and older; tablet must be chewed.

Warning For Bugs Bunny Only: Phenylketonurics: Contains Phenylalanine.

Continued on next page

Miles—Cont.

How Supplied: Flintstones in bottles of 60's & 100's, Bugs Bunny in bottles of 60 with child-resistant caps.

Shown in Product Identification Section, page 415

FLINTSTONES™ COMPLETE
With Iron, Calcium & Minerals
Children's Chewable Vitamins
BUGS BUNNY™ COMPLETE
Children's Chewable
Vitamins + Minerals
With Iron and Calcium
(Sugar Free)

Ingredients: Each supplement provides the ingredients listed in the chart.
[See bottom chart on preceding page.]

Indication: Dietary Supplementation.

Dosage and Administration: 2–4 years of age: Chew one-half tablet daily. Over 4 years of age: Chew one tablet daily.

Warning: Phenylketonurics: Contains Phenylalanine.

Precaution: Contains iron, which can be harmful in large doses. Close tightly and keep out of reach of children. In case of overdose, contact a physician or Poison Control Center immediately.

How Supplied: Bottles of 60's with child-resistant caps.

Shown in Product Identification Section, page 415

DOMEBORO® Astringent Solution Powder Packets

Active Ingredients: Each powder packet contains aluminum sulfate 1191 mg and calcium acetate 938 mg. DOMEBORO in water contains principally, the astringent aluminum acetate buffered to an acid pH.

Inactive Ingredient: Dextrin

Indications: For temporary relief of minor skin irritations due to poison ivy, poison oak, poison sumac, insect bites, athlete's foot or rashes caused by soaps, detergents, cosmetics or jewelry.

Actions: DOMEBORO provides soothing, effective relief of minor skin irritations. For over 50 years, doctors have been recommending DOMEBORO ASTRINGENT SOLUTION to help relieve minor skin irritations.

Warnings: If condition worsens or symptoms persist for more than 7 days, discontinue use of the product and consult a doctor. For external use only. Avoid contact with the eyes. Do not cover compress or wet dressing with plastic to prevent evaporation. Keep this and all drugs out of the reach of children. In case of accidental ingestion, seek professional assistance or contact a Poison Control Center immediately.

Directions: One packet dissolved in 16 ounces of water makes a modified Burow's Solution approximately equivalent to a 1:40 dilution; two packets, a 1:20 dilution; and four packets, a 1:10 dilution. Dissolve one or two packets in water and stir the solution until fully dissolved. Do not strain or filter the solution. Can be used as a compress, wet dressing or as a soak. AS A COMPRESS OR WET DRESSING: Saturate a clean, soft, white cloth or gauze in the solution; gently squeeze and apply loosely to the affected area. Saturate the cloth in the solution every 15 to 30 minutes and apply to the affected area. Repeat as often as necessary. Discard remaining solution after use. AS A SOAK: Soak affected area in the solution for 15 to 30 minutes. Repeat 3 times a day. Discard remaining solution after use.

How Supplied: Boxes of 12 or 100 powder packets.

Shown in Product Identification Section, page 415

DOMEBORO® Astringent Solution Effervescent Tablets

Active Ingredients: Aluminum sulfate 878 mg and calcium acetate 604 mg. DOMEBORO in water contains principally the astringent aluminum acetate buffered to an acid pH.

Inactive Ingredients: Dextrin, polyethylene glycol, sodium bicarbonate

Indications: For temporary relief of minor skin irritations due to poison ivy, poison oak, poison sumac, insect bites, athlete's foot or rashes caused by soaps, detergents, cosmetics or jewelry.

Actions: DOMEBORO provides soothing, effective relief of minor skin irritations. For over 50 years doctors have been recommending DOMEBORO ASTRINGENT SOLUTION to help relieve minor skin irritations.

Warnings: If conditions worsens or symptoms persist for more than 7 days, discontinue use of the product and consult a doctor. For external use only. Avoid contact with the eyes. Do not cover compress or wet dressing with plastic to prevent evaporation. Keep this and all drugs out of the reach of children. In case of accidental ingestion, seek professional assistance or contact a Poison Control Center immediately.

Directions: One tablet dissolved in 12 ounces of water makes a modified Burow's Solution approximately equivalent to a 1:40 dilution; two tablets, a 1:20 dilution; and four tablets, a 1:10 dilution. Dissolve one or two tablets in water and stir the solution until fully dissolved. Do not strain or filter the solution. Can be used as a compress, wet dressing or as a soak. AS A COMPRESS OR WET DRESSING: Saturate a clean, soft, white cloth or gauze in the solution; gently squeeze and apply loosely to the affected area. Saturate the cloth in the solution every 15 to 30 minutes and apply to the affected area. Repeat as often as necessary. Discard remaining solution after use. AS A SOAK: Soak affected area in the solution for 15 to 30 minutes. Repeat 3 times a day. Discard remaining solution after use.

How Supplied: Boxes of 12 or 100 effervescent tablets

Shown in Product Identification Section, page 415

MILES® Nervine Nighttime Sleep-Aid

Active Ingredient: Each capsule-shaped tablet contains diphenhydramine HCl 25 mg.

Inactive Ingredients: Calcium Phosphate Dibasic, Calcium Sulfate, Carboxymethylcellulose Sodium, Corn Starch, Magnesium Stearate, Microcrystalline Cellulose.

Indications: Miles® Nervine helps you fall asleep and relieves occasional sleeplessness.

Actions: Antihistamines act on the central nervous system and produce drowsiness.

Warnings: Do not give to children under 12 years of age. Avoid alcoholic beverages while taking this product. Do not take this product if you are taking sedatives or tranquilizers without first consulting your doctor. If sleeplessness persists continuously for more than 2 weeks, consult your doctor. Insomnia may be a symptom of serious underlying medical illness. Do not take this product if you have asthma, glaucoma, emphysema, chronic pulmonary disease, shortness of breath, difficulty in breathing or difficulty in urination due to enlargement of the prostate gland unless directed by a doctor. As with any drug, if you are pregnant or nursing a baby, seek the advice of a health professional before using this product. Keep this and all drugs out of the reach of children. In case of accidental overdose, seek professional assistance or contact a poison control center immediately.

Dosage and Administration: Two caplets once daily at bedtime or as directed by a physician.

How Supplied: Blister pack 12's, bottle of 30's with a child-resistant cap.

Shown in Product Identification Section, page 416

MYCELEX® OTC
CREAM ANTIFUNGAL

Active Ingredient: Clotrimazole 1%

Inactive Ingredients: Benzyl alcohol (1%) as a preservative, cetostearyl alcohol, cetyl esters wax, octyldodecanol, polysorbate 60, purified water, sorbitan monostearate.
Store between 2°–30°C (36°–86°F).

Indications: Cures athlete's foot (tinea pedis), jock itch (tinea cruris), and ringworm (tinea corporis). For effective relief of the itching, cracking, burning and discomfort which can accompany these conditions.

Warnings: For external use only. Do not use on children under 2 years of age except under the advice and supervision of a doctor. If irritation occurs or if there is no improvement within 4 weeks (for athlete's foot or ringworm) or within 2 weeks (for jock itch) discontinue use and consult a doctor or pharmacist. Keep this and all drugs out of the reach of children. In case of accidental ingestion seek professional assistance or contact a Poison Control Center immediately. Use only as directed.

Directions: Cleanse skin with soap and water and dry thoroughly. Apply a thin layer and gently massage over affected area morning and evening or as directed by a doctor. For athlete's foot, pay special attention to the spaces between the toes. It is also helpful to wear well-fitting, ventilated shoes and to change shoes and socks at least once daily. Best results in athlete's foot and ringworm are usually obtained with 4 weeks' use of this product and in jock itch with 2 weeks' use. If satisfactory results have not occurred within these times, consult a doctor or pharmacist. Children under 12 years of age should be supervised in the use of this product. This product is not effective on the scalp or nails.
FOR BEST RESULTS, FOLLOW DIRECTIONS AND CONTINUE TREATMENT FOR LENGTH OF TIME INDICATED.

How Supplied: Cream Tube 15 g
Shown in Product Identification Section, page 416

MYCELEX® OTC
SOLUTION ANTIFUNGAL

Active Ingredient: Clotrimazole 1%

Inactive Ingredient: Polyethylene glycol 400
Store between 2°–30°C (36°–86°F).

Indications: Cures athlete's foot (tinea pedis), jock itch (tinea cruris), and ringworm (tinea corporis). For effective relief of the itching, cracking, burning and discomfort which can accompany these conditions.

Warnings: For external use only. Do not use on children under 2 years of age except under the advice and supervision of a doctor. If irritation occurs or if there is no improvement within 4 weeks (for athlete's foot or ringworm) or within 2 weeks (for jock itch) discontinue use and consult a doctor or pharmacist. Keep this and all drugs out of the reach of children. In case of accidental ingestion seek professional assistance or contact a Poison Control Center immediately. Use only as directed.

Directions: Cleanse skin with soap and water and dry thoroughly. Apply a thin layer and gently massage over affected area morning and evening as directed by a doctor. For athlete's foot, pay special attention to the spaces between the toes. It is also helpful to wear well-fitting, ventilated shoes and to change shoes and socks at least once daily. Best results in athlete's foot and ringworm are usually obtained with 4 weeks' use of this product and in jock itch with 2 weeks' use. If satisfactory results have not occurred within these times, consult a doctor or pharmacist. Children under 12 years of age should be supervised in the use of this product. This product is not effective on the scalp or nails.
FOR BEST RESULTS, FOLLOW DIRECTIONS AND CONTINUE TREATMENT FOR LENGTH OF TIME INDICATED.

How Supplied: Solution Bottle 10 mL
Shown in Product Identification Section, page 416

MYCELEX-7®
VAGINAL CREAM ANTIFUNGAL

Active Ingredient: Clotrimazole 1%

Inactive Ingredients: Benzyl alcohol, cetostearyl alcohol, cetyl esters wax, octyldodecanol, polysorbate 60, purified water, sorbitan monostearate

Indications: For treatment of vaginal yeast (Candida) infection.

Actions: Cures most vaginal yeast infections. MYCELEX®-7 Antifungal Vaginal Cream can kill the yeast that may cause vaginal infection. It is greaseless and does not stain clothes.

Precautions: IF THIS IS THE FIRST TIME YOU HAVE HAD VAGINAL ITCH AND DISCOMFORT, CONSULT YOUR DOCTOR. IF YOU HAVE HAD A DOCTOR DIAGNOSE A VAGINAL YEAST INFECTION BEFORE AND HAVE THE SAME SYMPTOMS NOW, USE THIS CREAM AS DIRECTED FOR 7 CONSECUTIVE DAYS.

WARNING: **DO NOT USE IF YOU HAVE ABDOMINAL PAIN, FEVER, OR FOUL-SMELLING DISCHARGE. CONTACT YOUR DOCTOR IMMEDIATELY.**
IF YOU DO NOT IMPROVE IN 3 DAYS OR IF YOU DO NOT GET WELL IN 7 DAYS, YOU MAY HAVE A CONDITION OTHER THAN A YEAST INFECTION. CONSULT YOUR DOCTOR. Do not use during pregnancy except under the advice and supervision of a doctor. Do not use tampons while using this medication. If symptoms return within a two-month period, contact your doctor. Keep this and all drugs out of the reach of children. In case of accidental ingestion, seek professional assistance or contact a Poison Control Center immediately. NOT FOR USE IN CHILDREN LESS THAN 12 YEARS OF AGE.

Dosage and Administration: Before using, read the enclosed pamphlet. **Directions:** Fill the applicator and insert one applicatorful of cream into the vagina, preferably at bedtime. Repeat this procedure daily for 7 consecutive days.

How Supplied: 1.5 oz. tube and applicator.
Shown in Product Identification Section, page 415

MYCELEX-7®
VAGINAL INSERTS ANTIFUNGAL

Active Ingredient: Each insert contains 100 mg clotrimazole.

Inactive Ingredients: Corn starch, lactose, magnesium stearate, povidone.

Indications: For treatment of vaginal yeast (Candida) infection.

Actions: Cures most vaginal yeast infections. MYCELEX-7 Antifungal Vaginal Inserts can kill the yeast that may cause vaginal infection. They do not stain clothes.

Precautions: IF THIS IS THE FIRST TIME YOU HAVE HAD VAGINAL ITCH AND DISCOMFORT, CONSULT YOUR DOCTOR. IF YOU HAVE HAD A DOCTOR DIAGNOSE A VAGINAL YEAST INFECTION BEFORE AND HAVE THE SAME SYMPTOMS NOW, USE THESE INSERTS AS DIRECTED FOR 7 CONSECUTIVE DAYS.

WARNING: DO NOT USE IF YOU HAVE ABDOMINAL PAIN, FEVER, OR FOUL-SMELLING DISCHARGE. CONTACT YOUR DOCTOR IMMEDIATELY.
IF YOU DO NOT IMPROVE IN 3 DAYS OR IF YOU DO NOT GET WELL IN 7 DAYS, YOU MAY HAVE A CONDITION OTHER THAN A YEAST INFECTION. CONSULT YOUR DOCTOR. Do not use during pregnancy except under the advice and supervision of a doctor. Do not use tampons while using this medication. If symptoms return within a two-month period, contact your doctor. Keep this and all drugs out of the reach of children. In case of accidental ingestion, seek professional assistance or contact a Poison Control Center immediately. NOT FOR USE IN CHILDREN LESS THAN 12 YEARS OF AGE.

Dosage and Administration: Before using, read the enclosed pamphlet. **Directions:** Unwrap one insert, place it in the applicator, and use the applicator

Continued on next page

Miles—Cont.

to place the insert into the vagina, preferably at bedtime. Repeat this procedure daily for 7 consecutive days.

How Supplied: 7 vaginal inserts and applicator.

ONE–A–DAY® Essential Vitamins 11 Essential Vitamins

Ingredients: One tablet daily of ONE-A-DAY® Essential provides:

Vitamins	Quantity	U.S. RDA
Vitamin A (as Acetate and Beta Carotene)	5000 I. U.	100
Vitamin C	60 mg.	100
Thiamine (B_1)	1.5 mg.	100
Riboflavin (B_2)	1.7 mg.	100
Niacin	20 mg.	100
Vitamin D	400 I.U.	100
Vitamin E	30 I.U.	100
Vitamin B_6	2 mg.	100
Folic Acid	0.4 mg.	100
Vitamin B_{12}	6 mcg.	100
Pantothenic Acid	10 mg.	100

Indication: Dietary supplementation.

Dosage and Administration: One tablet daily for adults and teens.

How Supplied: ONE-A-DAY® Essential, bottles of 60 and 100.

Shown in Product Identification Section, page 416

ONE-A-DAY® Maximum Formula Vitamins and Minerals Supplement for adults and teens The most complete ONE-A-DAY® brand.

Ingredients:
One tablet daily of ONE-A-DAY® Maximum Formula provides:

Vitamins	Quantity	% of U.S. RDA
Vitamin A (as Acetate and Beta Carotene)	5000 I.U.	100
Vitamin C	60 mg.	100
Thiamine (B_1)	1.5 mg.	100
Riboflavin (B_2)	1.7 mg.	100
Niacin	20 mg.	100
Vitamin D	400 I.U.	100
Vitamin E	30 I.U.	100
Vitamin B_6	2 mg.	100
Folic Acid	0.4 mg.	100
Vitamin B_{12}	6 mcg.	100
Biotin	30 mcg.	10
Pantothenic Acid	10 mg.	100

Minerals [See top next column.]

Indication: Dietary supplementation.

Dosage and Administration: One tablet daily for adults and teens.

Precaution: Contains iron, which can be harmful in large doses. Close tightly and keep out of reach of children. In case of overdose, contact a physician or Poison Control Center immediately.

Minerals	Quantity	% of U.S. RDA
Iron (Elemental)	18 mg.	100
Calcium	130 mg.	13
Phosphorus	100 mg.	10
Iodine	150 mcg.	100
Magnesium	100 mg.	25
Copper	2 mg.	100
Zinc	15 mg.	100
Chromium	10 mcg.	*
Selenium	10 mcg.	*
Molybdenum	10 mcg.	*
Manganese	2.5 mg.	*
Potassium	37.5 mg.	*
Chloride	34 mg.	*

*No U.S. RDA established

How Supplied: Bottles of 30, 60, and 130 with child-resistant caps.

Shown in Product Identification Section, page 416

ONE-A-DAY® Plus Extra C Vitamins. For adults and teens.

Vitamin ingredients: One tablet daily of ONE-A-DAY® Plus Extra C provides:

Vitamins	Quantity	% of U.S. RDA
Vitamin A (as Acetate and Beta Carotene)	5000 I.U.	100
Vitamin C	300 mg.	500
Thiamine (B_1)	1.5 mg.	100
Riboflavin (B_2)	1.7 mg.	100
Niacin	20 mg.	100
Vitamin D	400 I.U.	100
Vitamin E	30 I.U.	100
Vitamin B_6	2 mg.	100
Folic Acid	0.4 mg.	100
Vitamin B_{12}	6 mcg.	100
Pantothenic Acid	10 mg.	100

Indication: Dietary supplementation.

Dosage and Administration: One tablet daily.

How Supplied: Bottles of 60's with child resistant caps.

Shown in Product Identification Section, page 416

ONE-A-DAY STRESSGARD® FORMULA High Potency B Complex and C plus A, D, E, Iron and Zinc Multivitamin/Multimineral Supplement For Adults

Ingredients:

Vitamins	Quantity	% of U.S. RDA
Vitamin A (as Acetate and Beta Carotene)	5000 I.U.	100
Vitamin C	600 mg.	1000
Thiamine (B_1)	15 mg.	1000
Riboflavin (B_2)	10 mg.	588
Niacin	100 mg.	500
Vitamin D	400 I.U.	100
Vitamin E	30 I.U.	100
Vitamin B_6	5 mg.	250
Folic Acid	400 mcg.	100
Vitamin B_{12}	12 mcg.	200
Pantothenic Acid	20 mg.	200

Minerals	Quantity	% of U.S. RDA
Iron (Elemental)	18 mg.	100
Zinc	15 mg.	100
Copper	2 mg.	100

Indication: Dietary supplementation.

Dosage and Administration: Adults—one tablet daily with food.

Precaution: Contains iron, which can be harmful in large doses. Close tightly and keep out of reach of children. In case of overdose, contact a physician or Poison Control Center immediately.

How Supplied: Bottles of 60 with child-resistant caps.

Shown in Product Identification Section, page 416

ONE-A-DAY® WOMEN'S FORMULA Advanced Multivitamin Formula with Calcium, Extra Iron, Zinc and Beta Carotene.

Provides calcium and extra iron Plus the daily nutritional support of 11 essential vitamins.

Ingredients: One tablet daily of ONE-A-DAY® WOMEN'S FORMULA provides:

Vitamins	Quantity	% of U.S. RDA
Vitamin A (as Acetate and Beta Carotene)	5000 I.U.	100
Vitamin C	60 mg.	100
Thiamine (B_1)	1.5 mg.	100
Riboflavin (B_2)	1.7 mg.	100
Niacin	20 mg.	100
Vitamin D	400 I.U.	100
Vitamin E	30 I.U.	100
Vitamin B_6	2 mg.	100
Folic Acid	0.4 mg.	100
Vitamin B_{12}	6 mcg.	100
Pantothenic Acid	10 mg.	100

Mineral	Quantity	% of U.S. RDA
Iron (Elemental)	27 mg.	150
Calcium (Elemental)	450 mg.	45
Zinc	15 mg.	100

Indication: Dietary supplementation.

Dosage and Administration: One tablet daily.

Precaution: Contains iron, which can be harmful in large doses. Close tightly and keep out of reach of children. In case of overdose, contact a physician or Poison Control Center immediately.

How Supplied: Bottles of 60 and 130 with child-resistant caps.

Shown in Product Identification Section, page 416

Muro Pharmaceutical, Inc.
890 EAST STREET
TEWKSBURY, MA 01876-1496

BROMFED® SYRUP
Antihistamine-Nasal Decongestant (alcohol free)
ORANGE-LEMON FLAVOR

Each 5 mL (1 teaspoonful) contains: 2 mg brompheniramine maleate and 30 mg pseudoephedrine hydrochloride; also contains citric acid, FD & C Yellow #6, flavor, glycerin, methyl paraben, sodium benzoate, sodium citrate, sodium saccharin, sorbitol, sucrose, purified water.

Indications: For temporary relief of nasal congestion, sneezing, itchy and watery eyes and running nose due to common cold, hay fever or other upper respiratory allergies.

Directions: Adults and children 12 years of age and over: 2 teaspoonfuls every 4–6 hours. Children 6 to 12 years of age: 1 teaspoonful every 4–6 hours. Do not exceed 4 doses in 24 hours. Children under 6 years of age, consult a physician.

Warnings: If symptoms do not improve within 7 days or are accompanied by high fever, consult a physician before continuing use. May cause drowsiness. May cause excitability especially in children. DO NOT exceed recommended daily dosage because at higher doses nervousness, dizziness, or sleeplessness may occur. **Except under the advice and supervision of a physician:** DO NOT give this product to children under 6 years. DO NOT take this product if you have asthma, glaucoma, difficulty in urination due to enlargement of the prostate gland, high blood pressure, heart disease, diabetes, or thyroid disease. As with any drug, if you are pregnant or nursing a baby, seek the advice of a health professional before using this product.

Caution: Avoid operating a motor vehicle or heavy machinery and alcoholic beverages while taking this product. Keep this and all drugs out of the reach of children.

Drug Interaction Precaution: Do not take this product if you are presently taking a prescription antihypertensive or antidepressant drug containing a monoamine oxidase inhibitor except under the advice and supervision of a physician.

Overdosage: In case of accidental overdose, seek professional assistance or contact a Poison Control Center immediately.
Store between 15° and 30°C (59° and 86°F). Dispense in tight, light resistant, child resistant containers as defined in USP.

How Supplied: NDC 0451-4201-16—16 fl. oz. (480 mL), NDC 0451-4201-04—4 fl. oz. (120 mL).

GUAIFED® SYRUP
Expectorant/Nasal Decongestant

A red colored, berry citrus flavored syrup.
Each 5mL (teaspoonful) contains:

Pseudoephedrine HCl, USP	30mg
Guaifenesin, USP	200mg

CONTAINS NO ANTIHISTAMINE which may cause drowsiness or excessive drying.
Guaifed® Syrup also contains inactive ingredients:
Benzoic Acid, Berry Citrus Flavor, Citric Acid, FD&C Red #40, Glycerin, Menthol, Polyethylene Glycol, Povidone, Purified Water, Saccharin Sodium, Sodium Citrate, Sorbitol, Vanillin.

Directions: Guaifed® Syrup—Adults and Children 12 years of age and over: Two teaspoonfuls every 4–6 hours, not to exceed eight teaspoonfuls in 24 hours. Children 6 to under 12 years of age: One teaspoonful every 4–6 hours, not to exceed four teaspoonfuls in 24 hours. Children 2 to under 6 years of age: ½ teaspoonful every 4–6 hours, not to exceed two teaspoonfuls in 24 hours. Children under 2 years of age: consult a physician.

How Supplied: Guaifed® Syrup is a red colored, berry citrus flavored syrup supplied in 473 mL bottles (NDC #0451-2601-16) and 118 mL bottles (NDC #0451-2601-04).
Store at controlled room temperature between 15°C and 30°C (59°F and 86°F).
Dispense in Child Resistant, tight and light resistant containers.
See GUAITAB® product listing for additional information.

GUAITAB® TABLETS
Expectorant/Nasal Decongestant

A purple layered tablet
Each tablet contains:

Pseudoephedrine HCl	60mg
Guaifenesin	400mg

GUAITAB® TABLET also contains inactive ingredients: colloidal silicon dioxide, lactose, magnesium stearate, microcrystalline cellulose, pharmaceutical glaze, sodium starch glycolate, starch, talc, FD&C Blue #2, D&C Red #27.

Indications: For the temporary relief of nasal congestion associated with the common cold, sinusitis, hay fever or other upper respiratory allergies. Also helps loosen phlegm (mucus) and thin bronchial secretions to rid the bronchial passageways of bothersome mucus, drain bronchial tubes, and make coughs more productive.

Warnings: Do not exceed recommended dosage because at higher doses nervousness, dizziness or sleeplessness may occur. Do not use if you have high blood pressure, heart disease, diabetes, thyroid disease or a persistent chronic cough, except under the advice and supervision of a physician. Do not take this product for persistent or chronic cough such as occurs with smoking, asthma, chronic bronchitis, or emphysema, or where cough is accompanied by excessive phlegm (mucus) unless directed by a doctor. A persistent cough may be a sign of a serious condition. If cough persists for more than 1 week, tends to recur, or is accompanied by a fever, rash or persistent headache, consult a doctor.

Contraindications: Hypersensitivity to guaifenesin or sympathomimetic amines; marked hypertension, hyperthyroidism; or in patients receiving monoamine oxidase (MAO) inhibitors.

Adverse Reactions: Possible side effects include nausea, vomiting, nervousness, restlessness, rash (including urticaria), headache, or dry mouth.
Drug Interaction Precautions: Do not take this medication if you are presently taking a prescription antihypertensive or antidepressant drug containing a monoamine oxidase inhibitor except under the advice and supervision of a physician.

Geriatrics: Pseudoephedrine should be used with caution in the elderly because they may be more sensitive to the effect of the sympathomimetics.

Note: As with any drug, if you are pregnant or nursing a baby, seek the advice of a health professional before using this product.
In the case of accidental overdose, seek professional assistance or contact a Poison Control Center immediately.
Guaifenesin has been shown to produce a color interference with certain clinical laboratory determinations of 5-hydroxyindoleacetic acid (5-HIAA) and vanillylmandelic acid (VMA).

Directions: GUAITAB® TABLETS—Adults and Children 12 years of age and over: One Tablet every 4–6 hours, not to exceed four tablets in 24 hours. Children 6 to under 12 years of age: ½ the adult dosage (break tablet in half): ½ tablet every 4–6 hours, not to exceed two tablets in 24 hours.

How Supplied: GUAITAB® TABLET is a purple layered Tablet in bottles of 100's. Each scored Tablet is coded "60/400" on one side and "Muro" on the other side. NDC 0451-4600-50.

SALINEX® NASAL MIST AND DROPS
Buffered Isotonic Saline Solutions

Ingredients: Sodium Chloride 0.4%. Also contains disodium phosphate, edetate disodium, hydroxypropyl methylcellulose, monosodium phosphate, polyethylene glycol, propylene glycol and purified water. Preservative used is benzalkonium chloride 0.01%.

Indications: Rhinitis Medicamentosa and Rhinitis Sicca. For relief of nasal congestion associated with overuse of nasal sprays, drops and inhalers.

Continued on next page

Muro—Cont.

To alleviate crusting due to nose bleeds; to compensate for nasal stuffiness and dryness due to lack of humidity.

Directions: Squeeze twice in each nostril as needed.

How Supplied: SPRAY: 50 ml plastic spray bottle. DROPS: 15 ml plastic dropper bottle.

Natren Inc.
3105 WILLOW LANE
WESTLAKE VILLAGE, CA 91361

BIFIDO FACTOR®
Bifidobacterium bifidum
Powder
Malyoth Strain

Ingredients: Active—Two billion viable *Bifidobacterium bifidum* strain Malyoth per gram with naturally occurring metabolic products retained in the supernatant. Potency guaranteed through expiration date. Inactive—Non-fat milk, whey.

Dosage: Low Frequency—¼ to ½ tsp. once daily. High Frequency—1 tsp. three times daily.

Precautions: Individuals sensitive to milk should not use this product.

How Supplied: Powder—

1.25 oz.	NDC-53983-200-05
2.5 oz.	NDC-53983-200-25
4.5 oz.	NDC-53983-200-45

PRO-BIFIDONATE®
Bifidobacterium bifidum
Powder
Malyoth Strain

Ingredients: Active—Two billion viable *Bifidobacterium bifidum* strain Malyoth per gram with naturally occurring metabolic products retained in the supernatant. Potency guaranteed through expiration date. Inactive—Garbanzo bean (chick-pea) extract; powder also contains cellulose.

Dosage: Low Frequency—¼ to ½ tsp. once daily. High Frequency—1 tsp. three times daily.

How Supplied: Powder—

1.75 oz.	NDC-53983-700-15
3.0 oz.	NDC-53983-700-25

PRO-BIONATE®
Lactobacillus acidophilus
Powder and Capsules
NAS Strain

Ingredients: Active—Two billion viable *Lactobacillus acidophilus* strain NAS per capsule/gram with naturally occurring metabolic products retained in the supernatant. Potency guaranteed through expiration date. Inactive—Garbanzo bean (chick-pea) extract; powder also contains cellulose.

Dosage:
Capsule - Low Frequency—1 capsule per day. High Frequency—1 capsule three times per day.
Powder - Low Frequency—¼ to ½ tsp. once daily. High Frequency—1 tsp. three times daily.

How Supplied:
Powder—

1.75 oz.	NDC-53983-600-25
3.0 oz.	NDC-53983-600-35

Capsules—

30 count	NDC-53983-600-20
60 count	NDC-53983-600-15

SUPERDOPHILUS®
Lactobacillus acidophilus
POWDER
DDS-1 Strain

Ingredients: Active—Two billion viable *Lactobacillus acidophilus* strain DDS-1 per gram with naturally occurring metabolic products retained in the supernatant. Potency guaranteed through expiration date. Inactive—Non-fat milk, whey.

Dosage: Low Frequency—¼ to ½ tsp. once daily. High Frequency—1 tsp. three times daily.

Precautions: Individuals sensitive to milk should not use this product.

How Supplied: Powder—

1.25 oz.	NDC-53983-100-05
2.5 oz.	NDC-53983-100-15
4.5 oz.	NDC-53983-100-35

Nature's Bounty, Inc.
90 ORVILLE DRIVE
BOHEMIA, NY 11716

ENER-B®
Vitamin B-12 Nasal Gel
Dietary Supplement

Description: ENER-B™ is the first intra-nasal application for Vitamin B-12. Each delivery supplies 400 mcg. of Vitamin B-12. This method of delivery provides the highest Vitamin B-12 blood levels that can be obtained without a prescription. Clinical tests show that ENER-B produced 8.4 to 10 times more Vitamin B-12 in the blood than tablets.

[See illustration next column.]

Clinical Tests results are available by writing Nature's Bounty.

Potency and Administration: Each nasal applicator delivers 1⁄10 cc of gel into the nose which adheres to the mucous membranes providing 400 mcg. of Vitamin B-12. Odorless and non-irritating to the nose.

Directions: As a dietary supplement, one unit every two to three days.

Measured Vitamin B-12 Increase in Blood Levels

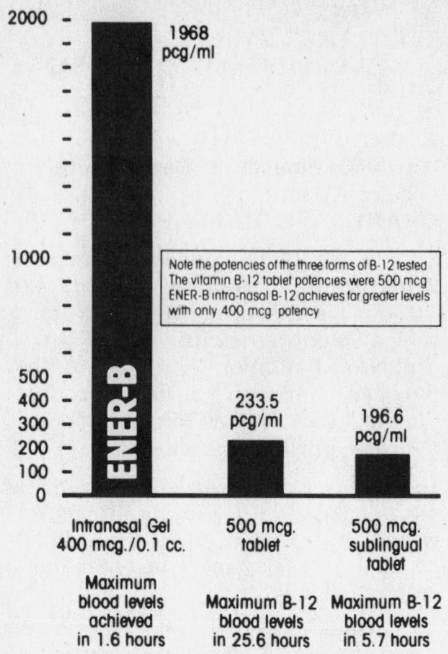

How Supplied: Packages of 12 unit doses. Supplies 400 mcg. of B-12 each.

Shown in Product Identification Section, page 416

Neutrogena Corporation
5760 W. 96TH ST.
LOS ANGELES, CA 90045

NEUTROGENA® CLEANSING WASH

Inactive Ingredients: Purified water, glycerin, sodium oleate, disodium lauroamphodiacetate, sodium trideceth sulfate, sodium cocoate, cocamidopropyl betaine, lauramide DEA, triethanolamine, BHA, BHT, trisodium HEDTA, citric acid.

Indications: A mild-lather cleanser especially formulated for dry, sensitive skin, for skin irritated by drying medications, or for use in conjunction with dermabrasions, chemical peels or facial surgery.

Actions: Neutrogena Cleansing Wash is a gentle, glycerin-enriched formula designed to effectively cleanse skin, extremely sensitive skin or skin made hyperirritable by drying medications or facial procedures. It is residue-free so as not to interfere with skin treatments. It is fragrance-free, contains no color and is noncomedogenic.

Dosage and Administration: Use twice daily, or as directed by physician. Mix with water, work Neutrogena Cleansing Wash into a creamy lather and apply to face. Gently massage in a circular motion. Rinse completely.

How Supplied: Available in 6 fl oz pump dispenser bottle.

Shown in Product Identification Section, page 416

NEUTROGENA MOISTURE®

Active Ingredient: Octyl methoxycinnamate (SPF 5).

Inactive Ingredients: Purified water, petrolatum, glycerin, isopropyl isostearate, octyl palmitate, soya sterol, cetyl alcohol, glyceryl stearate, PEG-100 stearate, sodium hydroxide, PEG-10 soya sterol, methylparaben, diazolidinyl urea, ethylparaben, propylparaben, tetrasodium EDTA, carbomer.

Actions: Neutrogena Moisture is an extremely effective facial moisturizer for even the most fragile complexions. It is noncomedogenic, fragrance-free, and contains no color. Hypoallergenic. Provides an SPF 5 protection for the skin.

Dosage and Administration: Apply Neutrogena Moisture over face and throat morning and night, after thoroughly cleansing the skin.

How Supplied: 2 fl oz and 4 fl oz bottle.
Shown in Product Identification Section, page 416

NEUTROGENA MOISTURE® SPF 15 UNTINTED

Active Ingredients: Octyl methoxycinnamate and benzophenone-3.

Inactive Ingredients: Purified water, propylene glycol, isoceteth-3 acetate, glycerin, emulsifying wax NF, dimethicone, PEG-150 stearate, glyceryl stearate, PEG-100 stearate, diazolidinyl urea, triethanolamine, methylparaben, ethylparaben, propylparaben, carbomer.

Actions: Effective 8 hour moisturization with broad spectrum (UVA/UVB) sunblock protection (SPF 15) in a noncomedogenic facial moisturizer. Fragrance-free, hypoallergenic.

Dosage and Administration: Use daily after thorough cleansing of skin, alone or under makeup.

How Supplied: 4 fl oz bottle.
Shown in Product Identification Section, page 416

NEUTROGENA MOISTURE® SPF 15 WITH SHEER TINT

Active Ingredients: Octyl methoxycinnamate and benzophenone-3.

Inactive Ingredients: Purified water, propylene glycol isoceteth-3 acetate, glycerin, emulsifying wax NF, dimethicone, PEG-150 stearate, glyceryl stearate, PEG-100 stearate, diazolidinyl urea, triethanolamine, methylparaben, ethylparaben, propylparaben, carbomer, iron oxides.

Actions: A PABA-free, non-comedogenic facial moisturizer that provides broad spectrum (UVA/UVB) sunblock protection (SPF 15). Fragrance-free, hypoallergenic. Moisturizes for 8 hours with just a hint of color.

Dosage and Administration: Use during the day with or without makeup.

How Supplied: 4 fl oz bottle.

NEUTROGENA® NORWEGIAN FORMULA® EMULSION

Inactive Ingredients: Purified Water, Glycerin, Caprylic/Capric Triglyceride, Dimethicone, Octyldodecanol, Petrolatum, Cetyl Alcohol, Glyceryl Laurate, Stearic Acid, Stearyl Alcohol, Hydrogenated Lanolin, Triethanolamine, Fragrance (scented only), Dimethicone Copolyol, Methylparaben, Imidazolidinyl Urea, Steapyrium Chloride, Sodium Cetearyl Sulfate, Propylparaben, BHA, BHT, Sodium Sulfate.

Indications: Neutrogena® Norwegian Formula® Emulsion has a glycerin-enriched formula that provides 17 hours of moisturizing relief for dry hands and skin.

Dosage and Administration: Apply liberally to arms, legs, and body as needed or as directed by a physician.

How Supplied: Available in 5.25 fl. oz. and 10.5 fl. oz. pump bottles, scented and fragrance-free.
Shown in Product Identification Section, page 416

NEUTROGENA® NORWEGIAN FORMULA® HAND CREAM

Inactive Ingredients: Purified Water, Glycerin, Cetearyl Alcohol, Sodium Cetearyl Sulfate, Fragrance (scented only), Stearic Acid, Methylparaben, Propylparaben, Sodium Sulfate, Dilauryl Thiodipropionate.

Indications: Neutrogena® Norwegian Formula® Hand Cream is a concentrated, emollient-rich cream for localized topical application. The non-comedogenic, cosmetically acceptable formula is effective for a wide range of dry skin conditions, including chronic hand dermatoses, xeroses and other conditions responsive to adjunctive hydration.

Dosage and Administration: Apply a small amount to affected area as needed or as directed by a physician.

How Supplied: Available in 2 oz. tube, scented and fragrance-free.
Shown in Product Identification Section, page 416

NEUTROGENA® SUNBLOCK SPF 15

Active Ingredients: Octyl methoxycinnamate, Octyl salicylate, and Menthyl anthranilate.

Inactive Ingredients: Mineral oil, aluminum starch octenylsuccinate, silica, PVP/eicosene copolymer, phenyltrimethicone, cyclomethicone, tribehenin, calcium behenate, titanium dioxide, dimethiconol, propylparaben, C_{18}–C_{36} acid triglyceride.

Indications: Neutrogena Sunblock SPF 15 provides broad spectrum protection (UVA/UVB/IR) from the damaging rays of the sun.

Actions: Provides broad spectrum protection with a SPF 15 effective in preventing sun damage. Liberal and regular use of Neutrogena Sunblock SPF 15 may help reduce the chance of premature aging of the skin and protects against the cancer-causing rays of the sun.

Waterproof: Stays on the skin even after 6 hours exposure in the water. Excellent for children above the age of 6 months. Remove with soap and water.

Rubproof/Sweatproof: Abrasion-resistant. Stays on even after rubbing or towel drying. Lower potential to run into eyes and cause stinging.

PABA-Free/Non-comedogenic: Suitable for those sensitive to PABA and its related compounds; won't clog pores. Fragrance-free. Hypoallergenic.

Warnings: For external use only, not to be swallowed. Avoid contact with eyes. Discontinue use if irritation or rash develops.

Dosage and Administration: For best results, apply to face and body 15 minutes before sun exposure. Reapply after rigorous swimming or exercise.

How Supplied: 2¼ oz tube.
Shown in Product Identification Section, page 416

NEUTROGENA® SUNBLOCK SPF 30

Active Ingredients: Octyl methoxycinnamate, Octocrylene, Menthyl anthranilate.

Inactive Ingredients: Mineral oil, Aluminum starch octenylsuccinate, Silica, Phenyl trimethicone, Tricontanyl PVP, Tribehenin (and) Calcium behenate, Cyclomethicone (and) Dimethiconol, Stearyl dimethicone, Zinc oxide, Tocopheryl acetate, BHT, C_{18-36} Acid triglyceride.

Indications: Neutrogena Sunblock SPF 30 provides broad spectrum protection (UVA/UVB/IR) from the damaging rays of the sun.

Actions: Provides broad spectrum protection with a SPF 30 effective in preventing sun damage. Liberal and regular use of Neutrogena Sunblock SPF 30 may help reduce the chance of premature aging of the skin and protects against the cancer-causing rays of the sun.

Waterproof: Stays on the skin even after 6 hours exposure in the water.

Continued on next page

Neutrogena—Cont.

Excellent for children above the age of 6 months. Remove with soap and water.

Rubproof/Sweatproof: Abrasion-resistant. Stays on even after rubbing or towel drying. Lower potential to run into eyes and cause stinging.

PABA-free/Non-comedogenic: Suitable for those sensitive to PABA and its related compounds; won't clog pores. Fragrance-free. Hypoallergenic.

Warnings: For external use only. Not to be swallowed. Avoid contact with eyes. Discontinue use if irritation or rash develops.

Dosage and Administration: For best results, apply to face and body 15 minutes before sun exposure. Reapply after rigorous swimming or exercise.

How Supplied: 2¼ oz. tube.

Shown in Product Identification Section, page 416

NEUTROGENA® T/DERM® TAR EMOLLIENT

Ingredients: 5% Neutar® Solubilized Coal Tar Extract (1.2% Coal Tar) in a soothing, emollient oil base.

Indications: Neutrogena® T/Derm® is the cosmetically acceptable liquid tar preparation for soothing relief of itching and scaling associated with psoriasis and other chronic, crusted, pruritic skin conditions.

Actions: Neutar® Solubilized Coal Tar Extract is biologically equivalent to crude coal tar and proven to reduce hyper-keratotic cell turnover by inhibiting DNA synthesis.

Dosage and Administration: Gently rub into affected areas of the skin once or twice a day (or as directed by a physician). Allow 15–20 minutes to dry. Any excess may be removed by gently patting the area dry with a soft cloth or tissue.

Caution: FOR EXTERNAL USE ONLY. Use caution in exposing skin to sunlight after applying this product. It may increase your tendency to sunburn for up to 24 hours after application. Do not use this product with other forms of psoriasis therapy such as ultraviolet radiation or prescription drugs unless directed to do so by a physician. If condition covers a large area of the body, consult your physician before using this product. Do not use this product in or around the rectum or in the genital area or groin except on the advice of a physician. Do not use on broken or inflamed skin. If irritation occurs, discontinue use and consult physician. If condition worsens or does not improve after regular use of the product as directed, consult a physician. Do not use this product for prolonged periods without consulting a physician. Avoid contact with eyes. If contact occurs, rinse eyes thoroughly with water. Keep this and all drugs out of the reach of children. In case of accidental ingestion, seek professional assistance or contact a Poison Control Center immediately. Slight staining of clothing may occur. Standard laundry procedures will remove most stains. Store away from direct sunlight.

How Supplied: 4 fl. oz. bottle.

NEUTROGENA® T/GEL® THERAPEUTIC SHAMPOO

Ingredients: 2% Neutar® Solubilized Coal Tar Extract (0.5% Coal Tar) in a bland shampoo base.

Indications: The clear amber formula of Neutrogena® T/Gel® Therapeutic Shampoo provides significant relief of symptoms associated with serious scalp conditions such as psoriasis, seborrheic dermatitis and dandruff, leaving hair clean and fresh smelling, with no residual tar odor.

Actions: Neutar® Solubilized Coal Tar Extract is biologically equivalent to crude coal tar and proven to reduce hyper-keratotic cell turnover by inhibiting DNA synthesis.

Dosage and Administration: Use daily or as directed by a physician. Wet hair thoroughly. Massage a liberal amount of T/Gel® into scalp and leave on for several minutes. Rinse thoroughly and repeat.

Caution: FOR EXTERNAL USE ONLY. Use caution in exposing skin to sunlight after applying this product. It may increase your tendency to sunburn for up to 24 hours after application. Do not use this product with other forms of psoriasis therapy such as ultraviolet radiation or prescription drugs unless directed to do so by a physician. If condition covers a large area of the body, consult your physician before using this product. Do not use on broken or inflamed skin. If irritation occurs, discontinue use and consult physician. If condition worsens or does not improve after regular use of the product as directed, consult a physician. Do not use this product for prolonged periods without consulting a physician. Avoid contact with eyes. If contact occurs, rinse eyes thoroughly with water. Keep this and all drugs out of reach of children. In case of accidental ingestion, seek professional assistance or contact a Poison Control Center immediately. In rare instances, temporary discoloration of gray, blonde, or tinted hair may occur. Slight staining of clothing may occur. Standard laundry procedures will remove most stains. Store away from direct sunlight.

How Supplied: 4.4 fl. oz., 8.5 fl. oz and 16 fl. oz. bottles.

Shown in Product Identification Section, page 416

NEUTROGENA® T/SAL® THERAPEUTIC SHAMPOO

Ingredients: Salicylic Acid 2% in a bland shampoo base.

Indications: The clear amber formula of Neutrogena® T/Sal® Therapeutic Shampoo provides significant relief of symptoms associated with serious scalp conditions requiring keratolytic action, such as psoriasis and seborrheic dermatitis, leaving hair clean and fresh smelling, with no residual tar odor.

Actions: The keratolytic activity of salicyclic acid reduces hyperkeratotic lesions.

Dosage and Administration: Use daily or as directed by a physician. Wet hair thoroughly. Massage a liberal amount of T/Sal® into scalp and leave on for several minutes. Rinse thoroughly and repeat.

Caution: FOR EXTERNAL USE ONLY. If condition covers a large area of the body, consult your physician before using this product. Do not use on broken or inflamed skin. If irritation occurs, discontinue use and consult physician. If condition worsens or does not improve after regular use of the product as directed, consult a physician. Avoid contact with eyes. If contact occurs, rinse eyes thoroughly with water. Keep this and all drugs out of reach of children. In case of accidental ingestion, seek professional assistance or contact a Poison Control Center immediately. Store away from direct sunlight.

How Supplied: 4.5 fl. oz. bottle.

Shown in Product Identification Section, page 416

Niché Pharmaceuticals, Inc.

300 TROPHY CLUB DRIVE #400
ROANOKE, TX 76262

MAGTAB® SR

[*măg-tăb*]
(Magnesium Lactate)
Sustained release Magnesium Supplement

Description: MagTab® SR is a sustained release oral magnesium supplement. Each pale yellow caplet contains 7mEq (84 Mg) magnesium as magnesium lactate in a wax matrix.

Ingredients: Each caplet contains 7mEq (84 Mg) elemental magnesium as magnesium L. Lactate dihydrate (835 Mg) in a sustained release wax matrix formulation. Inactive ingredients: polyethylene glycol, microcrystalline cellulose, carnauba wax, stearic acid, calcium stearate, and D & C yellow No. 10.

Indications/Uses: As a dietary supplement, MagTab® SR is indicated for patients with, or at risk for, magnesium deficiency. Hypomagnesemia and/or magnesium deficiency can result from inadequate nutritional intake or absorption, magnesium depleting drugs such as diuretics, or alcoholism.

Warnings: Patients with renal disease should not take magnesium supplements without the advice and direct supervision of a physician.

Side Effects: Excessive dosage of magnesium can cause loose stools or diarrhea.

Dosage: As a dietary supplement, take 1 or 2 caplets b.i.d. or as directed by a physician. Four caplets of MagTab® SR will meet the USRDA range for average adult males and females (300–350 mg) where magnesium depleting drugs are being used, supplementation with higher dosages may be required and should be considered.

How Supplied: MagTab® SR is available for oral administration as uncoated yellow caplets, coded Niche/420. Caplets are supplied as follows:

59016-42016	Bottles of 60
59016-42017	Bottles of 100

Store at 15°–30°C (59°–86°F)
U.S. Patent Number: 5,002,774

Ohm Laboratories, Inc.
P. O. BOX 279
FRANKLIN PARK, NJ 08823

CRAMP END
Ibuprofen Tablets, USP, 200 mg
Menstrual Pain & Cramp Reliever

WARNING: **ASPIRIN-SENSITIVE PATIENTS: Do not take this product if you have had a severe allergic reaction to aspirin, e.g., asthma, swelling, shock or hives, because even though this product contains no aspirin or salicylates, cross-reactions may occur in patients allergic to aspirin.**

Indications: For the temporary relief of painful menstrual cramps (Dysmenorrhea); also headaches, backaches and muscular aches and pains associated with Premenstrual Syndrome.

Directions: Adults: Take 1 tablet every 4 to 6 hours at the onset of menstrual symptoms and while pain persists. If pain does not respond to 1 tablet, 2 tablets may be used but do not exceed 6 tablets in 24 hours, unless directed by a doctor. The smallest effective dose should be used. Take with food or milk if occasional and mild heartburn, upset stomach, or stomach pain occurs with use. Consult a doctor if these symptoms are more than mild or if they persist.
Children: Do not give this product to children under 12 except under the advice and supervision of a doctor.

Warnings: Do not take for pain for more than 10 days unless directed by a doctor. If pain persists or gets worse, or if new symptoms occur, consult a doctor. These could be signs of serious illness. If you are under a doctor's care for any serious condition, consult a doctor before taking this product. As with aspirin and acetaminophen, if you have any condition which requires you to take prescription drugs or if you have had any problems or serious side effects from taking any non-prescription pain reliever, do not take this product without first discussing it with your doctor. If you experience any symptoms which are unusual or seem unrelated to the condition for which you took ibuprofen, consult a doctor before taking any more of it. Although ibuprofen is indicated for the same conditions as aspirin and acetaminophen, it should not be taken with them except under a doctor's direction. Do not combine this product with any other ibuprofen-containing product. As with any drug, if you are pregnant or nursing a baby, seek the advice of a health professional before using this product. **IT IS ESPECIALLY IMPORTANT NOT TO USE IBUPROFEN DURING THE LAST 3 MONTHS OF PREGNANCY UNLESS SPECIFICALLY DIRECTED TO DO SO BY A DOCTOR BECAUSE IT MAY CAUSE PROBLEMS IN THE UNBORN CHILD OR COMPLICATIONS DURING DELIVERY.** Keep this and all drugs out of the reach of children. In case of accidental overdose, seek professional assistance or contact a poison control center immediately.

How Supplied: Coated tablets in blister packs of 12's
Store at room temperature; avoid excessive heat 40°C (104°F).

Active Ingredient: Each tablet contains Ibuprofen 200 mg.
Manufactured by OHM LABORATORIES, INC, Franklin Park, NJ 08823

Shown in Product Identification Section, page 416

IBUPROHM®
Ibuprofen Tablets, USP
Ibuprofen Caplets, USP

Active Ingredient: Each tablet contains Ibuprofen USP, 200 mg.

Warning: ASPIRIN SENSITIVE PATIENTS: Do not take this product if you have had a severe allergic reaction to aspirin, e.g., asthma, swelling, shock or hives, because even though this product contains no aspirin or salicylates, cross-reactions may occur in patients allergic to aspirin.

Indications: For the temporary relief of minor aches and pains associated with the common cold, headache, toothache, muscular aches, backache, for the minor pain of arthritis, for the pain of menstrual cramps, and for reduction of fever.

Directions: *Adults:* Take 1 tablet every 4 to 6 hours while symptoms persist. If pain or fever does not respond to 1 tablet, 2 tablets may be used but do not exceed 6 tablets in 24 hours, unless directed by a doctor. The smallest effective dose should be used. Take with food or milk if occasional and mild heartburn, upset stomach, or stomach pain occurs with use. Consult a doctor if these symptoms are more than mild or if they persist.
Children: Do not give this product to children under 12 except under the advice and supervision of a doctor.

Warnings: Do not take for pain for more than 10 days or for fever for more than 3 days unless directed by a doctor. If pain or fever persists or gets worse, if new symptoms occur, or if the painful area is red or swollen, consult a doctor. These could be signs of serious illness. If you are under a doctor's care for any serious condition, consult a doctor before taking this product. As with aspirin and acetaminophen, if you have any condition which requires you to take prescription drugs or if you have had any problems or serious side effects from taking any nonprescription pain reliever, do not take this product without first discussing it with your doctor. If you experience any symptoms which are unusual or seem unrelated to the condition for which you took ibuprofen, consult a doctor before taking any more of it. Although ibuprofen is indicated for the same conditions as aspirin and acetaminophen, it should not be taken with them except under a doctor's direction. Do not combine the product with any other ibuprofen-containing product. As with any drug, if you are pregnant or nursing a baby, seek the advice of a health professional before using this product. IT IS ESPECIALLY IMPORTANT NOT TO USE IBUPROFEN DURING THE LAST 3 MONTHS OF PREGNANCY UNLESS SPECIFICALLY DIRECTED TO DO SO BY A DOCTOR BECAUSE IT MAY CAUSE PROBLEMS IN THE UNBORN CHILD OR COMPLICATIONS DURING DELIVERY. Keep this and all drugs out of the reach of children. In case of accidental overdose, seek professional assistance or contact a poison control center immediately.

How Supplied: Coated tablets in bottles of 24, 50, 100, 165, 250, 500 and 1000. Coated caplets in bottles of 24, 50, 100 and 250.

Storage: Store at room temperature; avoid excessive heat 40° (104°F).

Shown in Product Identification Section, page 416

LOPERAMIDE HYDROCHLORIDE CAPLETS*
2 mg (Nonprescription Formula)
(Antidiarrheal)

Loperamide Hydrochloride Caplet relieves diarrhea for both adults and children 6 years of age and older, in many cases with just one dose. Each caplet contains loperamide hydro-

*Each Caplet (capsule-shaped tablet) contains 2 mg of Loperamide Hydrochloride.

Continued on next page

Ohm—Cont.

Adults and Children 12 Years of Age and Older	Take 2 caplets after the first loose bowel movement and 1 caplet after each subsequent loose bowel movement but no more than 4 caplets a day for no more than two days.
Children 9–11 Years (60–95 lbs)	Take 1 caplet after the first loose bowel movement and ½ caplet after each subsequent loose bowel movement but no more than 3 caplets a day for no more than two days.
Children 6–8 Years (48–59 lbs)	Take 1 caplet after the first loose bowel movement and ½ caplet after each subsequent loose bowel movement but no more than 2 caplets a day for no more than two days.
Under 6 years old (up to 47 lbs):	**Consult a physician. Not intended for children under 6 years old.**

chloride, previously available only in a prescription product. This ingredient has been prescribed for millions of people, and has proven to be an exceptionally safe and effective antidiarrheal medication. Loperamide HCl caplets are small and easy to swallow.

Indication: Loperamide hydrchloride controls the symptoms of diarrhea.

Directions: Drink plenty of clear fluids to help prevent dehydration, which may accompany diarrhea.

Dosage and Administration:
[See table above.]

Warnings: DO NOT USE FOR MORE THAN TWO DAYS UNLESS DIRECTED BY A PHYSICIAN. Do not use if diarrhea is accompanied by high fever (greater than 101°F), or if blood is present in the stool, or if you have had a rash or other allergic reaction to loperamide HCl. If you are taking antibiotics or have a history of liver disease, consult a physican before using this product. As with any drug, if you are pregnant or nursing a baby, seek the advice of a health professional before using this product. Keep this and all drugs out of the reach of children. In case of accidental overdose, seek professional assistance or contact a poison control center immediately.

Active Ingredient: Loperamide HCl 2 mg per caplet.

Inactive Ingredients: Croscarmellose sodium, Crospovidone, Hydrogenated vegetable oil, lactose, magnesium stearate, powdered cellulose, pregelatinized starch, FD&C Blue #1 and D&C Yellow #10.
See side panel for expiration date. Store at room temperature 15°–25°C (59°–77°F).

How Supplied: Green scored caplet with "122" engraved on the other side. The caplets in 6's, 10's, 12's, and 20's blister packaging which is tamper resistant and child resistant.

Shown in Product Identification Section, page 416

Ortho Pharmaceutical Corporation
Advanced Care Products
RARITAN, NJ 08869

CONCEPTROL®
Contraceptive Gel/Inserts

Description: CONCEPTROL Contraceptive Gel: An unscented, unflavored, colorless, greaseless and non-staining gel in convenient, easy-to-use disposable plastic applicators. Each applicator is filled with a single, pre-measured dose containing the active spermicide Nonoxynol-9—4.0%, (100 mg per application) at pH 4.5.
CONCEPTROL Contraceptive Inserts: A non-foaming, single dose vaginal contraceptive containing the active spermicide Nonoxynol-9-8.34% (150 mg per insert).

Indication: Contraception.

Actions and Uses: Spermicidal products for use whenever control of conception is desirable.

Warning: Occasional burning and/or irritation of the vagina or penis have been reported. If this occurs, discontinue use and consult a physician as necessary. Not effective if taken orally. Keep out of reach of children. When pregnancy is contraindicated, the contraceptive program should be discussed with a health care professional.

Dosage and Administration:
CONCEPTROL Contraceptive Gel: One applicatorful of CONCEPTROL Contraceptive Gel should be inserted deeply into the vagina just before intercourse. An additional applicatorful is required each time intercourse is repeated.
CONCEPTROL Contraceptive Inserts: One insert should be placed into the vagina at least ten minutes prior to male penetration to insure proper dispersion. An additional insert is required each time intercourse is repeated.
CONCEPTROL Contraceptive Gel/Inserts:
If intercourse has not occurred within one hour after the application of CONCEPTROL, repeat application. Add a new application each time intercourse is repeated. Douching after use of CONCEPTROL is not recommended; however should you desire to do so, wait at least six hours to avoid interfering with contraceptive protection.
CONCEPTROL is an effective method of contraception. While no method of birth control can provide an absolute guarantee against becoming pregnant, for maximum protection, CONCEPTROL must be used according to directions.

How Supplied:
CONCEPTROL Contraceptive Gel is available in packages of 6 or 10 easy-to-use single-dose applicators.
CONCEPTROL Contraceptive Inserts are available in packages containing 10 inserts.

Inactive Ingredients:
CONCEPTROL Contraceptive Gel:
Lactic Acid, Methylparaben, Povidone, Propylene Glycol, Purified Water, Sodium Carboxymethylcellulose, Sorbic Acid, Sorbitol Solution.
CONCEPTROL Contraceptive Inserts:
Lauroamphodiacetate Sodium Trideceth Sulfate, Polyethylene Glycol 1000, Polyethylene Glycol 1450, Povidone.

Storage: Avoid excessive heat (over 86°F or 30°C).

Shown in Product Identification Section, page 417

DELFEN®
Contraceptive Foam

Description: A contraceptive foam in an aerosol dosage formulation containing 12.5% Nonoxynol-9 (100 mg. per application) and buffered to normal vaginal pH 4.5.

Indication: Contraception.

Action and Uses: A spermicidal foam for intravaginal contraception.

Warning: Occasional burning and/or irritation of the vagina or penis have been reported. In such cases, the use of the product should be discontinued and a physician consulted as necessary. Not effective if taken orally. Keep out of reach of children.
When pregnancy is contraindicated, the contraceptive program should be discussed with a health care professional.

Dosage and Administration: Insert DELFEN Contraceptive Foam just prior to each act of intercourse. You may have intercourse any time up to one hour after you have inserted the foam. If you repeat intercourse, insert another applicatorful of DELFEN Foam. After shaking the can, remove cap and place can upright on a level surface. Place the measured-dose (5cc) applicator on top of the can, then press applicator down very gently to fill. Fill to the top of the ribbed section of the applicator. Remove applicator from can to stop flow of foam. Insert the filled applicator well into the vagina and depress the plunger. Remove the applicator with the plunger in depressed position. Douching is not recommended after using DELFEN Foam. However, if douching is desired for cleansing purposes, wait at least six hours after intercourse. Refer to direction circular in package for diagrams and detailed instructions. While no method of contraception can provide an absolute guarantee against becoming pregnant, for maximum protection, DELFEN Foam must be used according to directions.

How Supplied: DELFEN Contraceptive Foam 0.60 oz. Starter can with applicator. Also 1.40 oz. refill can without applicator.

Inactive Ingredients: Benzoic Acid, Cetyl Alcohol, Cellulose Gum, Glacial Acetic Acid, Methylparaben, Perfume, Phosphoric Acid, Polyvinyl Alcohol, Propellant A-31, Propylene Glycol, Purified Water, Stearamidoethyl Diethylamine, Sorbic Acid, Stearic Acid.

Storage: Contents under pressure. Do not puncture or incinerate container. Do not expose to heat or store at temperatures above 120°F.

Shown in Product Identification Section, page 417

GYNOL II® Original Formula ORTHO-GYNOL® Contraceptive Jelly

Description:
GYNOL II Original Formula:
A colorless, unscented, unflavored, greaseless and non-staining contraceptive jelly containing the active spermicide Nonoxynol-9 (2%, 100 mg. per application) and having a pH of 4.5.
ORTHO-GYNOL: Is a water-dispersible spermicidal jelly having a pH of 4.5 and contains the active spermicide Octoxynol-9 (1%, 50 mg per application).

Indication: Contraception.

Actions and Uses: An aesthetically pleasing spermicidal vaginal jelly for use with a vaginal diaphragm whenever the control of conception is desired.

Warning: Occasional burning and/or irritation of the vagina or penis have been reported. In such cases, use of the product should be discontinued and a physician consulted as necessary. Not effective if taken orally. Keep out of reach of children. When pregnancy is contraindicated, the contraceptive program should be discussed with a health care professional.

Dosage and Administration: Used in conjunction with a vaginal diaphragm. Prior to insertion, put about a teaspoonful of contraceptive jelly into the cup of the dome of the diaphragm and spread a small amount around the edge with your fingertip. This will aid in insertion and provide protection.
It is also important to remember that if intercourse occurs more than six hours after insertion, or if repeated intercourse takes place, an additional application of contraceptive jelly is necessary. DO NOT REMOVE THE DIAPHRAGM—simply add more contraceptive jelly with an applicator, being careful not to dislodge the diaphragm. Remember, another application of contraceptive jelly is required each time intercourse is repeated, regardless of how little time has transpired since the diaphragm has been in place.
IMPORTANT—An association has been reported between diaphragm use and toxic shock syndrome (TSS), a serious condition which can be fatal. For contraceptive effectiveness, the diaphragm should remain in place for six hours after intercourse and *should be removed as soon as possible thereafter.* Continuous wearing of a contraceptive diaphragm for more than twenty-four hours is not recommended. Retention of the diaphragm for any period of time may encourage the growth of certain bacteria in the vaginal tract. It has been suggested that under certain as yet unestablished conditions overgrowth of these bacteria may lead to symptoms of TSS. For further information, please contact your physician. Women with a known or suspected history of TSS should not use the diaphragm.
If a douche is desired for cleansing purposes, wait at least six hours after intercourse. While no method of contraception can provide an absolute guarantee against becoming pregnant, for maximum protection, the contraceptive jelly must be used according to directions. Refer to direction circular enclosed in the package for diagrams and complete instructions.

Inactive Ingredients:
GYNOL II Original Formula:
Lactic Acid, Methylparaben, Povidone, Propylene Glycol, Purified Water, Sodium Carboxymethylcellulose, Sorbic acid, Sorbitol Solution.
ORTHO-GYNOL:
Benzoic Acid, Castor Oil, Fragrance, Glacial Acetic Acid, Methylparaben, Potassium Hydroxide, Propylene Glycol, Purified Water, Sodium Carboxymethylcellulose, Sorbic Acid.

How Supplied: 2.5 oz and 3.8 oz tube packages for GYNOL II Original Formula, 3.8 oz tube for ORTHO-GYNOL.

Storage: Should be stored at room temperature.

Shown in Product Identification Section, page 417

GYNOL II EXTRA STRENGTH CONTRACEPTIVE JELLY

Description: GYNOL II Extra Strength Contraceptive Jelly is a clear, unscented, water-soluble, greaseless gel. It is mildly lubricating and non-staining. Each applicatorful contains 150 mg of nonoxynol-9 (3%), a potent spermicide which provides effective protection against pregnancy when used with a diaphragm or a condom or alone. A diaphragm alone is not effective protection against pregnancy.

Indication: Contraception.

Actions and Uses: An aesthetically pleasing spermicidal jelly for use alone, with a condom or a diaphragm whenever control of contraception is desired.

Warning: Occasional burning and/or irritation of the vagina or penis have been reported. In such cases, the medication should be discontinued and a physician consulted as necessary. Not effective if taken orally. Keep out of reach of children. When pregnancy is contraindicated, the contraceptive program should be discussed with a health care professional.

Dosage and Administration: When used in conjunction with a vaginal diaphragm. Prior to insertion, put about a teaspoonful of GYNOL II Extra Strength Contraceptive Jelly into the cup of the dome of the diaphragm and spread a small amount around the edge with your fingertip then insert.
It is also important to remember that if intercourse occurs more than six hours after insertion, or if repeated intercourse takes place, an additional application of GYNOL II Extra Strength is necessary. DO NOT REMOVE THE DIAPHRAGM, simply add more GYNOL II Extra Strength with the applicator provided in the applicator package, being careful not to dislodge the diaphragm. Remember, another application of GYNOL II Extra Strength is required each time intercourse is repeated, regardless of how little time has transpired since the diaphragm has been in place.
IMPORTANT—An association has been reported between diaphragm use and toxic shock syndrome (TSS), a serious condition which can be fatal. For contraceptive effectiveness, the diaphragm should remain in place for six hours after intercourse and *should be removed as soon as possible thereafter.* Continuous wearing of a contraceptive diaphragm for more than twenty-four hours is not recommended. Retention of the diaphragm for any period of time may encourage the growth of certain bacteria in the vaginal tract. It has been suggested that under certain as yet unestablished conditions overgrowth of these bacteria may lead to symptoms of TSS. For further information, please contact your physician. Women with a known or suspected history of TSS should not use the diaphragm.

Dosage and Administration: For use with a condom or as a use-alone product. Insert an applicatorful of GYNOL II Extra Strength into the vagina as shown in the illustration. Intercourse should occur within one hour after GYNOL II Extra Strength has been inserted. An additional application must be used prior to each additional act of intercourse. This method of contraception must be used each and every time intercourse takes place, regardless of the time of the month.

Inactive Ingredients: Lactic Acid, Methylparaben, Povidone, Propylene Glycol, Purified Water, Sodium Carboxy-

Continued on next page

Ortho—Cont.

methylcellulose, Sorbic Acid, Sorbitol Solution.

How Supplied: 2.85 oz. tube with applicator.

Storage: Should be stored at room temperature.

Shown in Product Identification Section, page 417

MICATIN®
['mī-kə-tin]
Antifungal For Athlete's Foot and Ringworm

Description: An antifungal containing the active ingredient miconazole nitrate 2%, clinically proven to cure athlete's foot and ringworm.

Indications: Athlete's foot (tinea pedis), jock itch (tinea cruris), and ringworm (tinea corporis).

Actions and Uses: Proven clinically effective in the treatment of athlete's foot (tinea pedis), jock itch (tinea cruris), and ringworm (tinea corporis). For effective relief of the itching, cracking, scaling, burning and discomfort that can accompany these conditions.

Directions: Cleanse skin with soap and water and dry thoroughly. Apply a thin layer of MICATIN over affected area morning and night or as directed by a doctor. For athlete's foot, pay special attention to the spaces between the toes. It is also helpful to wear well-fitting, ventilated shoes and to change shoes and socks at least once daily. Best results in athlete's foot and ringworm are usually obtained with 4 weeks' use of this product. If satisfactory results have not occurred within this time, consult a doctor or pharmacist. Children under 12 years of age should be supervised in the use of this product. This product is not effective on the scalp or nails.
Do not use on children under 2 years of age except under the advice and supervision of a doctor. For external use only. If irritation occurs, or if there is no improvement within 4 weeks, discontinue use and consult a doctor or pharmacist. Keep this and all drugs out of the reach of children. In case of accidental ingestion, seek professional assistance or contact a Poison Control Center immediately.

How Supplied:
MICATIN® Antifungal Cream is available in a 0.5 oz. tube and a 1.0 oz. tube.
MICATIN Antifungal Spray Powder is available in a 3.0 oz. aerosol can.
MICATIN Antifungal Odor Control Spray Powder is available in a 3.0 oz. aerosol can.
MICATIN Antifungal Powder is available in a 3.0 oz. plastic bottle.
MICATIN Antifungal Spray Liquid is available in a 3.5 oz. aerosol can.

Inactive Ingredients:
MICATIN Antifungal Cream: Benzoic Acid, BHA, Mineral Oil, Peglicol 5 Oleate, Pegoxol 7 Stearate, Purified Water.
MICATIN Antifungal Spray Powder: Alcohol, Propellant A-46, Sorbitan Sesquioleate, Stearalkonium Hectorite, Talc.
MICATIN Antifungal Deodorant Spray Powder: Alcohol, Propellant A-46, Talc, Stearalkonium Hectorite, Sorbitan Sesquioleate, Fragrance.
MICATIN Antifungal Powder: Talc.
MICATIN Antifungal Spray Liquid: Alcohol, Benzyl Alcohol, Cocamide DEA, Propellant A-46, Sorbitan Sesquioleate, Tocopherol.

Storage: Store at room temerature.

Shown in Product Identification Section, page 417

MICATIN®
['mī-kə-tin]
Antifungal For Jock Itch

Description: An antifungal containing the active ingredient miconazole nitrate 2%, clinically proven to cure jock itch.

Indications: Jock itch (tinea cruris).

Actions and Uses: Proven clinically effective in the treatment of jock itch (tinea cruris). For effective relief of the itching, scaling, burning and discomfort that can accompany this condition.

Directions: Cleanse skin with soap and water and dry thoroughly. Apply a thin layer of product over affected area morning and night or as directed by a doctor. Best results are usually obtained within 2 weeks' use of this product. If satisfactory results have not occurred within this time, consult a doctor or pharmacist. Children under 12 years of age should be supervised in the use of this product. This product is not effective on the scalp or nails.

Warnings: Do not use on children under 2 years of age except under the advice and supervision of a doctor. For external use only. If irritation occurs, or if there is no improvement of jock itch within 2 weeks, discontinue use and consult a doctor or pharmacist. Keep this and all drugs out of the reach of children. In case of accidental ingestion, seek professional assistance or contact a Poison Control Center immediately.

How Supplied:
MICATIN® Jock Itch Cream is available in a 0.5 oz. tube.
MICATIN Jock Itch Spray Powder is available in a 3.0 oz. aerosol can.

Inactive Ingredients:
MICATIN Jock Itch Cream: Benzoic Acid, BHA, Mineral Oil, Peglicol 5 Oleate, Pegoxol 7 Stearate, Purified Water.
MICATIN Jock Itch Spray Powder: Alcohol, Propellant A-46, Sorbitan Sesquioleate, Stearalkonium Hectorite, Talc.

Storage: Store at room temperature.

MONISTAT® 7
(miconazole nitrate)
Vaginal Cream, Suppositories

PRODUCT OVERVIEW

Key Facts: Monistat 7 is a vaginal antifungal. Monistat 7 is available in two forms: cream; and soft, emollient vaginal suppositories. The cream form is available with seven disposable cardboard applicators, or one reusable plastic applicator.

Major Uses: 1. For the treatment of **RECURRENT** vulvovaginal candidiasis (moniliasis) when the patient is treating herself, i.e. for women who have been diagnosed by a doctor in the past with vulvovaginal candidiasis, and who recognize the symptoms.
2. For the treatment of vulvovaginal candidiasis (moniliasis) for first-time sufferers **ONLY WHEN THE CONDITION IS DIAGNOSED BY A PHYSICIAN AND THE PHYSICIAN RECOMMENDATION CALLS FOR AN OTC PRODUCT.**

Safety Information:
- Do not use Monistat 7 if the following signs and symptoms are present. If they occur while using Monistat 7, STOP using the product and contact a doctor right away.
  —Fever (Above 100°F orally)
  —Pain in the lower abdomen, back or either shoulder
  —A vaginal discharge that smells bad
- If there is not improvement or if the infection worsens within three days, or complete relief is not felt within seven days, or your symptoms return within two months, then you may have something other than a yeast infection. You should consult your doctor.
- Do not use in girls less than 12 years of age.
- If you are pregnant or think you may be, do not use this product except under the advice and supervision of a doctor.

PRODUCT INFORMATION

Active Ingredients: miconazole nitrate (vaginal cream, 2%; vaginal suppositories, 100 mg each)

Inactive Ingredients: Cream: benzoic acid, BHA, mineral oil, peglicol 5 oleate, pegoxol 7 stearate, purified water. Suppository: hydrogenated vegetable oil base.

Indications:
1. For the treatment of **RECURRENT** vulvovaginal candidiasis (moniliasis) when the patient is treating herself, i.e. for women who have been diagnosed by a doctor in the past with vulvovaginal candidiasis, and who recognize the symptoms.
2. For the treatment of vulvovaginal candidiasis (moniliasis) for first-time sufferers **ONLY WHEN THE CONDITION IS DIAGNOSED BY A PHYSICIAN AND THE PHYSICIAN RECOMMENDATION CALLS FOR AN OTC PRODUCT.**

As Monistat 7 is effective only for candidal vulvovaginitis, the physician diagnosis should be confirmed by KOH smears and/or cultures. Other pathogens commonly associated with vulvovaginitis (*Trichomonas* and *Haemophilus vaginalis* [*Gardnerella*]) should be ruled out by appropriate laboratory methods.

Actions: Monistat 7 exhibits fungicidal activity *in vitro* against the species of the genus *Candida*. The pharmacological mode of action is unknown.

Warnings/Precautions:

- This product is only effective in treating vaginal yeast infection caused by yeast. Do not use in eyes or take by mouth.
- **Do not use Monistat 7 vaginal cream or suppositories if you have any of the following signs and symptoms. Also, if they occur while using Monistat 7, STOP using the product and contact a doctor right away. You may have a more serious illness.**
  Fever (Above 100°F orally)
  Pain in the lower abdomen, back or either shoulder
  A vaginal discharge that smells bad
- If there is no improvement or if the infection worsens within 3 days, or complete relief is not felt within 7 days, or your symptoms return within two months, then you may have something other than a yeast infection. You should consult your doctor.
- Monistat 7 cream contains mineral oil. Monistat 7 suppositories contain hydrogenated vegetable oil. Mineral oil and hydrogenated vegetable oil may weaken latex condoms or diaphragms. Do not rely on condoms or diaphragms to prevent sexually transmitted diseases or pregnancy while using Monistat 7 vaginal cream or suppositories.
- Do not use tampons while using this medication.
- Do not use in girls less than 12 years of age.
- If you are pregnant or think you may be, do not use this product except under the advice and supervision of a doctor.
- Keep this and all drugs out of the reach of children.
- In case of accidental ingestion, seek professional assistance or contact a poison control center immediately.

Dosage and Administration: One applicatorful of cream or one suppository is administered intravaginally once daily at bedtime for seven days. Course of therapy may be repeated after other pathogens have been ruled out by appropriate smears and cultures.

How Supplied: Monistat 7 vaginal cream is available in 1.59 oz. (45 g) tube. The cream is available with seven disposable cardboard applicators (NDC/UPC 0062-5426-02), or one reusable plastic applicator (NDC UPC 0062-5426-01). Monistat 7 vaginal suppositories are available as 100 mg per dose, elliptically-shaped white to off-white suppositories in packages of seven (NDC/UPC 0062-5427-01).

Storage: Store at room temperature.

Shown in Product Identification Section, page 417

P & S Laboratories
210 WEST 131st STREET
LOS ANGELES, CA 90061

See Standard Homeopathic Company.

PRN Laboratories, Inc.
285 NATIONAL PLACE UNIT 127
LONGWOOD, FL 32750

PAIN FREE NATURAL AND PAIN FREE ALOE VERA GEL®

Composition: Aloe gel, carbopol 940, hydantoin, oleoresin of capsicum, DMDM, hydantoin, tetrasodium, germall 115, polysorbate, filtered water, triethanolamine.

Indications: For pain, relief of minor arthritis, bursitis, backache, simple sprains and strains.

Actions: Although the precise mechanism of action is not fully understood, current scientific evidence suggests that capsaicin, a derivative from hot peppers, acts against pain by affecting a brain chemical known as substance P, thought to be a key to the tranmission of pain.

Warnings: FOR EXTERNAL USE ONLY. Keep out of reach of children. *Wash* hands thoroughly after application. Keep this and any analgesic products away from eyes, mouth and other mucous membranes.

Dosage and Administration: Apply a liberal amount (with Pain Free Natural), apply a dime-sized amount (with Pain Free Aloe Gel) to painful muscles and joints and gently massage until the Pain Free is absorbed in. Can be used before and after exercise. Repeat as needed for temporary relief of minor arthritis pain, bursitis pain, strains, sprains and cramps. Additional uses to help relieve pain from shingles and diabetic neuropathy have recently been discovered.

How Supplied: .5 oz trial size
4 oz applicator bottle (P.F. Natural)
4 oz tube—Pain Free Aloe Gel
Gallon jug—(Aloe Gel only)

Products are indexed by product category in the **BLUE SECTION.**

Parke-Davis
Consumer Health Products Group
Division of Warner-Lambert Company
201 TABOR ROAD
MORRIS PLAINS, NJ 07950
(See also Warner-Lambert)

AGORAL® Raspberry
AGORAL® Marshmallow
[*ă 'gō-răl "*]

Description: Each tablespoonful (15 mL) of Agoral Raspberry (pink) or of Agoral Marshmallow (white) contains 4.2 grams mineral oil and 0.2 gram phenolphthalein in a thoroughly homogenized emulsion.
Also contains acacia; agar; benzoic acid; egg albumin; flavors; glycerin; sodium benzoate; tragacanth; citric acid or sodium hydroxide to adjust pH; water. Agoral Raspberry Flavor also contains D&C Red No. 30 Lake and saccharin sodium.

Actions: Agoral, containing mineral oil, facilitates defecation by lubricating the fecal mass and softening the stool. More effective than nonemulsified oil in penetrating the feces, Agoral thereby greatly reduces the possibility of oil leakage at the anal sphincter. Phenolphthalein gently stimulates motor activity of the lower intestinal tract. Agoral's combined lubricating-softening and peristaltic actions can help to restore a normal pattern of evacuation.

Indications: Relief of occasional constipation. This product generally produces bowel movement in 6–8 hours.

Contraindication: Sensitivity to phenolphthalein.

Warning: Do not use laxative products when abdominal pain, nausea, or vomiting are present unless directed by a physician. If you have noticed a sudden change in bowel habits that persists over a period of 2 weeks, consult a physician before using a laxative. Laxative products should not be used for a period longer than 1 week unless directed by a physician. Rectal bleeding or failure to have a bowel movement after use of a laxative may indicate a serious condition. Discontinue use and consult your physician. Do not administer to children under 6 years of age, to pregnant women, to bedridden patients or to persons with difficulty swallowing. As with any drug, if you are nursing a baby, seek the advice of a health professional before using this product. Do not take with meals. If skin

Continued on next page

This product information was prepared in November 1992. On these and other Parke-Davis Products, detailed information may be obtained by addressing PARKE-DAVIS, Consumer Health Products Group, Division of Warner-Lambert Company, Morris Plains, NJ 07950.

Parke-Davis—Cont.

rash appears, do not use this product or any other preparation containing phenolphthalein. Keep this and all drugs out of the reach of children. In case of accidental overdose, seek professional assistance or contact a Poison Control Center immediately. Drug interaction precaution: Do not take this product if you are presently taking a stool softener laxative.

Dosage: Agoral Raspberry and Marshmallow—Adults—½ to 1 tablespoonful at bedtime only, unless other time is advised by physician. Children—Over 6 years, ½ to ¾ teaspoonfuls at bedtime only, unless other time is advised by physician. This product generally produces bowel movement in 6 to 8 hours.

Supplied: Agoral (raspberry flavor), plastic bottles of 16 fl oz. Agoral (marshmallow flavor), plastic bottles of 16 fl oz.
Store between 15°–30° C (59°–86° F). Keep this and all drugs out of the reach of children.
In case of accidental overdose, seek professional assistance or contact a Poison Control Center immediately.

ANUSOL®
[ă′nū-sōl″]
Suppositories/Ointment

Description:
Anusol Suppositories: Active Ingredients: Phenylephrine HCl 0.25% and Hard Fat 88.7%. Also contains: Corn Starch, Methylparaben and Propylparaben.
Anusol Ointment: Active ingredients: Pramoxine HCl 1%, Mineral Oil 46.7% and Zinc Oxide 12.5%. Also contains: Benzyl Benzoate, Calcium Phosphate Dibasic, Cocoa Butter, Glyceryl Monooleate Glyceryl Monostearate, Kaolin, Peruvian Balsam and Polyethylene Wax.

Actions: Anusol Suppositories and Anusol Ointment help to relieve burning, itching and discomfort arising from irritated anorectal tissues. They have a soothing, lubricant action on mucous membranes. Pramoxine Hydrochloride in Anusol Ointment is a rapidly acting local anesthetic for the skin and mucous membranes of the anus and rectum. Pramoxine HCl is also chemically distinct from procaine, cocaine, and dibucaine and can often be used in the patient previously sensitized to other surface anesthetics. Surface analgesia lasts for several hours.

Indications: Anusol Ointment: Temporarily relieves the pain, soreness, and burning of hemorrhoids and other anorectal disorders while it forms a temporary protective coating over inflamed tissues. Anusol Suppositories: Temporarily shrinks the swelling associated with irritated hemorrhoidal tissues, and gives temporary relief from the itching, burning and discomfort of hemorrhoids and other anorectal disorders.

Contraindications: Anusol Suppositories and Anusol Ointment are contraindicated in those patients with a history of hypersensitivity to any of the components of the preparations.

Warnings: Anusol Ointment: Certain persons can develop allergic reactions to ingredients in this product. If the symptom being treated does not subside, if condition worsens or does not improve within 7 days, if redness, irritation, swelling, pain, or other symptoms develop or increase, discontinue use and consult a physician promptly. Do not exceed the recommended daily dosage unless directed by a physician. Do not put this product into the rectum by using fingers or any mechanical device or applicator. Keep this and all drugs out of the reach of children. In case of accidental ingestion seek professional advice or contact a Poison Control Center immediately. Anusol Suppositories: Do not exceed recommended daily dosage unless directed by a physician. Do not use this product if you have heart disease, high blood pressure, thyroid disease, diabetes, or difficulty in urination due to enlargement of the prostate gland unless directed by a physician. It condition worsens or does not improve within 7 days, consult a physician. In case of bleeding, consult a doctor. Keep this and all drugs out of the reach of children. In case of accidental ingestion seek professional advice or contact a Poison Control Center immediately. As with any drug, if you are pregnant or nursing a baby, seek the advice of a health professional before using this product.

Adverse Reactions: Upon application of Anusol Ointment, which contains Pramoxine HCl, a patient may occasionally experience burning, especially if the anoderm is not intact. Sensitivity reactions have been rare; discontinue medication if suspected. Certain persons can develop allergic reactions to ingredients in this product.

Drug Interaction Precaution: Anusol Suppositories: Do not use this product if you are presently taking a prescription drug for high blood pressure or depression without consulting a physician

Directions: Anusol Suppositories: Adults: When practical, cleanse the affected area with Tucks® Hemorrhoidal Pads or mild soap and warm water and rinse thoroughly. Gently dry by patting or blotting with toilet tissue or soft cloth before application of this product. Remove foil wrapper and insert suppository into the anus. Insert one suppository rectally up to four times daily: one in the morning, one in the evening, and one after each bowel movement. Children under 12 years of age: consult a physician.
Anusol Ointment: Adults: When practical, cleanse the affected area with Tucks® Hemorrhoidal Pads or mild soap and warm water and rinse thoroughly. Gently dry by patting or blotting with toilet tissue or soft cloth before application of this product. Apply ointment externally to the affected area up to five (5) times daily. To use dispensing cap, attach it to tube, lubricate well, then gently insert part way into the anus. Squeeze tube to deliver medication. Thoroughly cleanse dispensing cap after use. Children under 12 years of age: Consult a physician.
NOTE: If staining from either of the above products occurs, the stain may be removed from fabric by hand or machine washing with household detergent.

How Supplied: Anusol Suppositories—boxes of 12, 24 and 48; in silver foil strips.
Anusol Ointment—1-oz tubes and 2-oz tubes with plastic applicator.
Store between 15° and 30°C (59° and 86°F).

Shown in Product Identification Section, page 417

ANUSOL HC-1

Active Ingredient: Hydrocortisone Acetate (equivalent to 1% Hydrocortisone).

Inactive Ingredients: Diazolidinyl Urea, Methylparaben, Microcrystalline Wax, Mineral Oil, Propylene Glycol, Propylparaben, Sorbitan Sesquioleate and White Petrolatum.

Indications: Temporarily relieves itch associated with external anal inflammation and irritation. Other uses of this product should be only under the advice and supervision of a physician.

Warnings: For external use only. Avoid contact with the eyes. If condition worsens, or if symptoms persist for more than 7 days or clear up and occur again within a few days, stop use of this product and do not begin use of any other hydrocortisone product unless you have consulted a physician. Do not exceed the recommended daily dosage unless directed by a physician. In case of bleeding, consult a physician promptly. Do not put this product into the rectum by using fingers or any mechanical device or applicator. Do not use for treatment of diaper rash. Consult a physician. Keep this and all drugs out of the reach of children. In case of accidental ingestion seek professional assistance or contact a Poison Control Center immediately.

Dosage and Administration: Adults: when practical cleanse affected area with mild soap and warm water. Rinse thoroughly. Gently dry by patting or blotting with tissue or soft cloth before application. Apply to affected area not more than 3 to 4 times daily. Children under 12 years: do not use, consult a physician.

How Supplied: Anusol HC-1 Ointment in 0.7 oz tube. Store at 59°–86°F.

Shown in Product Identification Section, page 417

BENADRYL Anti-Itch Cream, Regular Strength, 1%
BENADRYL Anti-Itch Cream, Maximum Strength, 2%

Active Ingredients: Regular Strength contains Benadryl® (diphenhydramine hydrochloride USP) 1%; Maximum Strength contains Benadryl® (diphenhydramine hydrochloride USP) 2%.

Inactive Ingredients: Cetyl Alcohol, Methylparaben, Polyethylene Glycol Monostearate, Propylene Glycol and Water, Purified.

Indications: For the temporary relief of itching and pain associated with insect bites, allergic itches, minor skin irritations and rashes due to poison ivy, poison oak or poison sumac.

Actions: Benadryl is the most prescribed topical antihistamine available. It stops the itch at the source by blocking the action of histamine that causes the itch. Benadryl also provides local anesthetic action to soothe the pain. Benadryl gives you the kind of itch and pain relief that you can't get from hydrocortisone. Benadryl cream is soothing and greaseless.

Warnings: For external use only. Do not apply to blistered, raw or oozing areas of the skin. Do not use on chicken pox or measles unless supervised by a physician. Do not use on extensive areas of the skin or for longer than 7 days except as directed by a physician. Avoid contact with the eyes or other mucous membranes. If condition worsens, or if symptoms persist for more than 7 days, or clear up and occur again within a few days, discontinue use of this product and consult a physician. Do not use any other drugs containing diphenhydramine while using this product. KEEP THIS AND ALL DRUGS OUT OF THE REACH OF CHILDREN. In case of accidental ingestion, seek professional assistance or contact a Poison Control Center immediately.

Dosage and Administration: Regular Strength 1%—For adults and children 6 years of age and older: Apply to affected area not more than three to four times daily, or as directed by a physician. For children under 6 years of age: consult a physician.
Maximum Strength 2%—For adults and children 12 years of age and older: Apply to affected area not more than three to four times daily, or as directed by a physician. For children under 12 years of age: consult a physician.

How Supplied: Benadryl Anti-Itch Cream is available in ½ oz. Regular Strength and ½ oz. Maximum Strength tubes.

Shown in Product Identification Section, page 417

BENADRYL®
[bĕ 'nă-drĭl]
Decongestant Elixir

Description: Each teaspoonful (5 mL) contains: Benadryl (diphenhydramine hydrochloride) 12.5 mg; pseudoephedrine hydrochloride 30 mg; alcohol 5%. Also contains: FD&C Yellow No. 6; glucose, liquid; glycerin, USP; flavors; menthol, USP; saccharin sodium, USP; sodium citrate, USP; sucrose, NF; water, purified, USP.

Indications: Temporarily relieves nasal congestion, runny nose, sneezing, itching of the nose or throat, itchy, watery eyes due to hay fever or other upper respiratory allergies, and runny nose, sneezing and nasal congestion of the common cold.

Warnings: Do not exceed recommended dosage because at higher doses nervousness, dizziness, or sleeplessness may occur. Do not take this product for more than 7 days. If symptoms do not improve or are accompanied by fever, consult a physician. Do not take this product if you have high blood pressure, heart disease, diabetes, thyroid disease, asthma, glaucoma, emphysema, chronic pulmonary disease, shortness of breath, difficulty in breathing or difficulty in urination due to enlargement of the prostate gland unless directed by a physician. May cause excitability, especially in children. May cause marked drowsiness; alcohol, sedatives and tranquilizers may increase the drowsiness effect. Avoid driving a motor vehicle or operating machinery or drinking alcoholic beverages while taking this product. Do not take this product if you are taking sedatives or tranquilizers without first consulting your physician. Do not use other products containing diphenhydramine while using this product. As with any drug, if you are pregnant or nursing a baby seek the advice of a health professional before using this product. Keep this and all drugs out of the reach of children. In case of accidental overdose, seek professional assistance or contact a Poison Control Center immediately.

Drug Interaction Precaution: Do not take this product if you are presently taking a prescription drug for high blood pressure or depression without first consulting your physician.

Directions: Children 6 to under 12 years oral dosage is one teaspoonful every 4 to 6 hours not to exceed 4 teaspoonfuls in 24 hours, or as directed by a physician. For children under 6 years of age, consult a physician. Adult oral dosage is two teaspoonfuls every 4 to 6 hours not to exceed 8 teaspoonfuls in 24 hours, or as directed by a physician.

Professional Labeling: The suggested dosage for children age 2 to under 6 years, only when the child is under the care of a physician, is ½ teaspoonful every 4 to 6 hours not to exceed 2 teaspoonfuls in 24 hours.

How Supplied: Benadryl Decongestant Elixir is supplied in 4-oz bottles. Store below 30° C (86°F). Protect from freezing.

Shown in Product Identification Section, page 418

BENADRYL® Decongestant
[bĕ 'nă-drĭl]
Decongestant Tablets and Kapseals®

Active Ingredients: Each tablet/Kapseal® contains: Benadryl® (diphenhydramine hydrochloride USP) 25 mg. and pseudoephedrine hydrochloride 60 mg.

Inactive Ingredients: Each tablet contains: Corn Starch, Croscarmellose Sodium, Dibasic Calcium Phosphate Dihydrate, FD&C Blue No. 1 Aluminum Lake, Hydroxypropyl Methylcellulose, Microcrystalline Cellulose, Polyethylene Glycol, Polysorbate 80, Stearic Acid, Titanium Dioxide and Zinc Stearate.
Each Kapseals® capsule contains: Calcium Stearate, Lactose (Hydrous), Syloid Silica Gel. The Kapseals® capsule shell contains: Artificial colors, Gelatin, Glyceryl Monooleate, PEG-200 Ricinoleate and Titanium Dioxide.

Indications: Temporarily relieves nasal congestion, runny nose, sneezing, itching of the nose or throat, itchy, watery eyes due to hay fever or other upper respiratory allergies, and runny nose, sneezing and nasal congestion of the common cold.

Warning: Do not exceed recommended dosage because at higher doses nervousness, dizziness, or sleeplessness may occur. Do not take this product for more than 7 days. If symptoms do not improve or are accompanied by fever, consult a physician. Do not take this product if you have high blood pressure, heart disease, diabetes, thyroid disease, asthma, glaucoma, emphysema, chronic pulmonary disease, shortness of breath, difficulty in breathing or difficulty in urination due to enlargement of the prostate gland unless directed by a physician. May cause excitability, especially in children. May cause marked drowsiness; alcohol, sedatives and tranquilizers may increase the drowsiness effect. Avoid driving a motor vehicle or operating machinery or drinking alcoholic beverages while taking this product. Do not take this product if you are taking sedatives or tranquilizers without first consulting your physician. Do not use other products containing di-

Continued on next page

This product information was prepared in November 1992. On these and other Parke-Davis Products, detailed information may be obtained by addressing PARKE-DAVIS, Consumer Health Products Group, Division of Warner-Lambert Company, Morris Plains, NJ 07950.

Parke-Davis—Cont.

phenhydramine while using this product. Do not give this product to children under 12 years except under the advice and supervision of a physician. As with any drug, if you are pregnant or nursing a baby seek the advice of a health professional before using this product. Keep this and all drugs out of the reach of children. In case of accidental overdose, seek professional assistance or contact a Poison Control Center immediately.

Drug Interaction Precaution: Do not take this product if you are presently taking a prescription drug for high blood pressure or depression without first consulting your physician.

Directions: Adults and children over 12 years of age: 1 tablet/Kapseal® every 4 to 6 hours not to exceed 4 tablets/Kapseals® in 24 hours. Benadryl Decongestant is not recommended for children under 12 years of age.

How Supplied: Benadryl Decongestant Tablets and Kapseals® are supplied in boxes of 24.
Store at room temperature 15°-30° C (59°-86° F).
Protect from moisture.

Shown in Product Identification Section, page 417

BENADRYL® Elixir

Active Ingredients: Each teaspoonful (5 mL) contains: Benadryl® (diphenhydramine hydrochloride USP) 12.5 mg.

Inactive Ingredients: Also contains: Alcohol 5.6%, Citric Acid, D&C Red No. 33, Disodium edetate, FD&C Red No. 40, Flavors, Glycerin, Polysorbate 20, Propyl Gallate, Sodium Benzoate, Sodium Citrate, Sodium Saccharin, Sugar, Purified Water.

Indications: Temporarily relieves runny nose, sneezing, itching of the nose or throat and itchy, watery eyes due to hay fever or other upper respiratory allergies and runny nose and sneezing associated with the common cold.

Warnings: Do not take this product if you have asthma, glaucoma, emphysema, chronic pulmonary disease, shortness of breath, difficulty in breathing or difficulty in urination due to enlargement of the prostate gland unless directed by a physician. May cause excitability especially in children. May cause marked drowsiness; alcohol, sedatives and tranquilizers may increase the drowsiness effect. Avoid driving a motor vehicle or operating machinery or drinking alcoholic beverages while taking this product. Do not take this product if you are taking sedatives or tranquilizers without first consulting your physician. Do not use other products containing diphenhydramine while using this product. As with any drug if you are pregnant or nursing a baby seek the advice of a health professional before using this product. Keep this and all drugs out of the reach of children. In case of accidental overdose, seek professional assistance or contact a Poison Control Center immediately.

Dosage and Administration: Children 6 to under 12 years of age oral dosage is 12.5 to 25 mg. (1 to 2 teaspoonfuls) every 4 to 6 hours not to exceed 12 teaspoonfuls in 24 hours, or as directed by a physician. For children under 6 years your physician should be contacted for the recommended dosage. Adult oral dosage is 25 mg. (2 teaspoonfuls) to 50 mg. (4 teaspoonfuls) every 4 to 6 hours not to exceed 24 teaspoonfuls in 24 hours, or as directed by a physician.

Professional Labeling: The suggested dosage for children age 2 to under 6 years, only when the child is under the care of a physician, is ½ teaspoonful every 4 to 6 hours not to exceed 3 teaspoonfuls in 24 hours.

How Supplied: Benadryl Elixir is supplied in 4 oz. and 8 oz. bottles.

Shown in Product Identification Section, page 418

BENADRYL® 25
[*bĕ'nă-drĭl*]
Tablets and Kapseals®

Active Ingredient: Each tablet/Kapseal® contains: Benadryl® (diphenhydramine hydrochloride USP) 25 mg.

Inactive Ingredients: Each tablet contains: Corn Starch, Croscarmellose Sodium, Dibasic Calcium Phosphate Dihydrate, D&C Red No. 27 Aluminum Lake, Hydroxypropyl Methylcellulose, Microcrystalline Cellulose, Polyethylene Glycol, Polysorbate 80, Stearic Acid, Titanium Dioxide and Zinc Stearate. Each Kapseal capsule contains: Lactose (Hydrous) and Magnesium Stearate. The Kapseal capsule shell contains: Artificial Colors, Gelatin, Glyceryl Mono-oleate, PEG-200 Ricinoleate and Titanium Dioxide.

Indications: Temporarily relieves runny nose, sneezing, itching of the nose or throat, itchy, watery eyes due to hay fever or other upper respiratory allergies and runny nose and sneezing of the common cold.

Warnings: Do not take this product if you have asthma, glaucoma, emphysema, chronic pulmonary disease, shortness of breath, difficulty in breathing or difficulty in urination due to enlargement of the prostate gland unless directed by physician. May cause excitability, especially in children. May cause marked drowsiness; alcohol, sedatives and tranquilizers may increase the drowsiness effect. Avoid driving a motor vehicle or operating machinery or drinking alcoholic beverages while taking this product. Do not take this product if you are taking sedatives or tranquilizers without first consulting your physician. Do not use other products containing diphenhydramine while using this product. As with any drug if you are pregnant or nursing a baby seek the advice of a health professional before using this product. Keep this and all drugs out of the reach of children. In case of accidental overdose, seek professional assistance or contact a Poison Control Center immediately.

Directions: Adult oral dosage is 25–50 mg (1 to 2 tablets/Kapseals®) every 4 to 6 hours not to exceed 12 tablets/Kapseals® in 24 hours, or as directed by a physician.
Children 6 to under 12 years oral dosage is 12.5 mg* to 25 mg (1 tablet/Kapseal®) every 4 to 6 hours, not to exceed 6 tablets/Kapseals® in 24 hours, or as directed by a physician. For children under 6 years your physician should be contacted for the recommended dosage.

How Supplied: Benadryl 25 Tablets and Kapseals® are supplied in boxes of 24 and 48.
Store at room temperature 15°-30° C (59°-86° F). Protect from moisture.

* This dosage strength is not available in this package. Do not attempt to break tablets/Kapseals®. This dosage is available in pleasant tasting Benadryl Elixir.

Shown in Product Identification Section, page 417

BENADRYL® Allergy Sinus Headache Formula

Active Ingredients: Each caplet contains Benadryl® (diphenhydramine HCl) 12.5 mg, pseudoephedrine HCl 30 mg and acetaminophen 500 mg.

Inactive Ingredients: Candelilla Wax, Carboxymethyl Cellulose, Corn Starch, Croscarmellose Sodium, D&C Yellow No. 10 Aluminum Lake, FD&C Blue No. 1 Aluminum Lake, FD&C Yellow No. 6 Aluminum Lake, Hydroxypropyl Cellulose, Hydroxypropyl Methylcellulose, Microcrystalline Cellulose, Polyethylene Glycol, Polysorbate 80, Stearic Acid, Titanium Dioxide, Zinc Stearate.

Indications: Temporarily relieves runny nose: sneezing; itching of the nose or throat; itchy, watery eyes; nasal congestion; sinus pain/pressure and headache due to hay fever or other upper respiratory allergies.

Action: BENADRYL ALLERGY/SINUS/HEADACHE is specially formulated to provide effective relief of your upper respiratory allergy symptoms complicated by sinus and headache problems. It combines the strength of BENADRYL to relieve your runny nose: sneezing; itchy water eyes; itchy nose or throat with a maximum strength NASAL DECONGESTANT to relieve nasal and sinus congestion and a maximum strength non-aspirin PAIN RELIEVER to relieve sinus pain and headache.

Warnings: Do not take this product for more than 7 days. Do not use any other drug containing diphenhydramine while using this product. Consult a physician promptly if symptoms do not improve or are accompanied by fever that lasts for more than 3 days or if new symptoms occur. Do not exceed recommended dosage because at higher doses nervousness, dizziness, or sleeplessness may occur. May cause marked drowsiness; alcohol, sedatives and tranquilizers may increase the drowsiness effect. Avoid driving a motor vehicle or operating machinery or drinking alcoholic beverages while taking this product. Do not take this product if you are presently taking sedatives or tranquilizers, without first consulting your physician. Do not take this product if you have high blood pressure, heart disease, diabetes, thyroid disease, asthma, glaucoma, emphysema, chronic pulmonary disease shortness of breath, difficulty in breathing, or diffultly in urination due to enlargement of the prostate gland unless directed by a physician. As with any drug, if you are pregnant or nursing a baby, seek the advice of a health professional before using this product. Keep this and all drugs out of the reach of children. In case of accidental overdose seek professional assistance or contact a Poison Control Center immediately.

Directions: Adults and children over 12 years of age: two (2) caplets every 6 hours, not to exceed 8 caplets in a 24 hour period. Benadryl Allergy Sinus Headache Formula is not recommended for children under 12 years of age.

How Supplied: Benadryl Allergy Sinus Headache Formula is available in boxes of 24. Store at room temperature, 15°–30°C (59°–86°F).

Shown in Product Identification Section, page 417

BENADRYL® COLD
Tablets

Active Ingredients: Each tablet contains: Benadryl® (diphenhydramine hydrochloride USP) 12.5 mg., pseudoephedrine hydrochloride 30 mg., and acetaminophen 500 mg.

Inactive Ingredients: Each tablet contains: Carboxymethylcellulose, Croscarmellose Sodium, Hydroxypropyl Cellulose, Hydroxypropyl Methylcellulose, Magnesium Stearate, Microcrystalline Cellulose, Polyethylene Glycol, Propylene Glycol, Starch, Stearic Acid, Titanium Dioxide, and Zinc Stearate.

Indications: Benadryl Cold has been specially formulated to provide fast and effective relief of the symptoms of common colds and flu. Benadryl Cold tablets combine maximum strength ingredients for relief of nasal congestion, body aches and fever, with the trusted relief of Benadryl for runny nose and sneezing.

Warnings: Do not take this product for more than 7 days. Consult a physician promptly for the following: (1) If symptoms do not improve or are accompanied by fever that lasts for more than 3 days or if new symptoms occur; (2) If sore throat is severe, persists for more than 2 days, is accompanied or followed by fever, headache, rash, nausea, or vomiting. Do not exceed recommended dosage because at higher doses nervousness, dizziness, or sleeplessness may occur. May cause excitability, especially in children. May cause marked drowsiness; alcohol, sedatives and tranquilizers may increase the drowsiness effect. Avoid driving a motor vehicle or operating heavy machinery, or drinking alcoholic beverages. Do not take this product if you are presently taking sedatives or tranquilizers without first consulting your physician. Do not use other products containing diphenhydramine while using this product. Do not take this product if you have high blood pressure, heart disease, diabetes, thyroid disease, asthma, glaucoma, emphysema, chronic pulmonary disease, shortness of breath, difficulty in breathing, or difficulty in urination due to enlargement of the prostate gland unless directed by a physician. As with any drug, if you are pregnant or nursing a baby, seek the advice of a health professional before using this product. Keep this and all drugs out of the reach of children. In case of accidental overdose seek professional assistance or contact a Poison Control Center immediately.

Drug Interaction Precaution: Do not take this product if you are presently taking a prescription drug for high blood pressure or depression without consulting your physician.

Directions: Adults (12 years and over): Two tablets every 6 hours, not to exceed 8 tablets in a 24-hour period. Benadryl Cold is not recommended for children under 12 years of age.

How Supplied: Benadryl Cold Tablets are supplied in boxes of 24 and 48. Store at room temperature 15°–30°C (59°–86°F). Protect from moisture.

Shown in Product Identification Section, page 417

BENADRYL® COLD NIGHTTIME FORMULA

Active Ingredients: Each fluid ounce or 2 tablespoons contains: Acetaminophen 1000 mg., diphenhydramine hydrochloride 50 mg., and pseudoephedrine hydrochloride 60 mg.

Inactive Ingredients: Alcohol 10%, citric acid, D&C Yellow No. 10, FD&C Red No. 40, FD&C Green No. 3, disodium edetate, flavoring, glycerin, polyethylene glycol, potassium sorbate, propyl gallate, propylene glycol, sodium benzoate, sodium citrate, sodium saccharin and purified water.

Indications: Benadryl Cold Nighttime Formula has been specially formulated to provide fast and effective relief of colds and flu symptoms to help you rest. Benadryl Cold Nighttime Formula combines maximum strength ingredients for relief of nasal congestion, body aches, fever, runny nose and sneezing in a pleasant honey-lemon flavor.

Warnings: Do not take this product for more than 7 days. Consult a physician promptly for the following: (1) If symptoms do not improve or are accompanied by fever that lasts for more than 3 days or if new symptoms occur; (2) If sore throat is severe, persists for more than 2 days, is accompanied or followed by fever, headache, rash, nausea, or vomiting. Do not exceed recommended dosage because at higher doses nervousness dizziness, or sleeplessness may occur. May cause excitability, especially in children. May cause marked drowsiness; alcohol, sedatives and tranquilizers may increase the drowsiness effect. Avoid driving a motor vehicle or operating heavy machinery, or drinking alcoholic beverages. Do not take this product if you are presently taking sedatives or tranquilizers without first consulting your physician. Do not use other products containing diphenhydramine while using this product. Do not take this product if you have high blood pressure, heart disease, diabetes, thyroid disease, asthma, glaucoma, emphysema, chronic pulmonary disease, shortness of breath, difficulty in breathing, or difficulty in urination due to enlargement of the prostate gland unless directed by a physician. As with any drug, if you are pregnant or nursing a baby, seek the advice of a health professional before using this product. Keep this and all drugs out of the reach of children. In case of accidental overdose seek professional assistance or contact a Poison Control Center immediately.

Drug Interaction Precaution: Do not take this product if you are presently taking a prescription drug for high blood pressure or depression without first consulting your physician.

Directions for Use: Adults take one fluid ounce using dosage cup or two (2) tablespoons at bedtime for nighttime relief. Dosage may be repeated every six (6) hours or as directed by a physician. Do not exceed 4 fluid ounces or eight (8) tablespoons in any 24-hour period. Children under 12 should use only as directed by a physician.

How Supplied: Benadryl Cold Nighttime Formula is supplied in 6 ounce bottles. Store at room temperature, 15°–30°C (59°–86°F).

Continued on next page

This product information was prepared in November 1992. On these and other Parke-Davis Products, detailed information may be obtained by addressing PARKE-DAVIS, Consumer Health Products Group, Division of Warner-Lambert Company, Morris Plains, NJ 07950.

Parke-Davis—Cont.

Questions about Benadryl® Cold Nighttime Formula?
Call us toll free 9 AM to 5 PM EST. Weekdays at 1-800-524-2624. In New Jersey call 1-800-338-0326.

Shown in Product Identification Section, page 418

BENADRYL® Spray Regular Strength 1%
BENADRYL® Spray Maximum Strength 2%

Active Ingredients: Regular Strength contains Benadryl® (diphenhydramine hydrochloride USP) 1%, Zinc Acetate 0.1%; Maximum Strength contains Benadryl® (diphenhydramine hydrochloride USP) 2%, Zinc Acetate 0.1%.

Inactive Ingredients: Alcohol, Aloe Vera, Glycerin, Povidone, Tromethamine, and Water, Purified.

Indications: For the temporary relief of itching and pain associated with insect bites, allergic itches, minor skin irritations and rashes due to poison ivy, poison oak, or poison sumac. Dries the oozing and weeping of poison ivy, poison oak, and poison sumac.

Actions: Benadryl Spray forms a clear, anti-itch "bandage" to protect and relieve affected areas. Benadryl stops the itch at the source by blocking the action of histamine that causes the itch. Benadryl also provides an anesthetic action to soothe the pain and aloe to soothe the skin. The spray feature allows soothing relief without touching or rubbing the affected area. Benadryl spray is clear, won't stain clothing and won't rinse off (can be easily removed with soap and water).

Warnings: FOR EXTERNAL USE ONLY. Do not apply to blistered, raw or oozing areas of the skin. Do not use on chicken pox or measles unless supervised by a physician. Do not use on extensive areas of the skin for longer than 7 days except as directed by a physician. Avoid contact with the eyes or other mucous membranes. If condition worsens or if symptoms persist for more than 7 days or clear up and occur again within a few days, discontinue use of this product and consult a physician. Do not use any other drugs containing diphenhydramine while using this product. KEEP THIS AND ALL DRUGS OUT OF THE REACH OF CHILDREN. In case of accidental ingestion, seek professional assistance or contact a Poison Control Center immediately. Flammable, keep away from fire or flame.

Dosage and Administration: Regular Strength 1%—For adults and children 6 years of age and older: Spray on affected area not more than three to four times daily, or as directed by a physician. For children under 6 years of age: consult a physician. **Maximum Strength 2%**—For adults and children 12 years of age or older: Spray on affected area not more than three to four times daily, or as directed by a physician. For children under 12 years of age: consult a physician.

How Supplied: Benadryl® Spray is available in a 2 oz. pump spray bottle.

Shown in Product Identification Section, page 417

BENYLIN® Cough Syrup

Description: Each teaspoonful (5 mL) contains:

Diphenhydramine Hydrochloride	12.5 mg

Also contains: Alcohol 5%; Ammonium Chloride; Caramel; Citric Acid; D&C Red No. 33; FD&C Red No. 40; Flavor; Glucose Liquid; Glycerin; Menthol; Purified Water; Sodium Citrate; Sodium Saccharin; Sucrose.

Indications: For the temporary relief of cough due to minor throat and bronchial irritation as may occur with the common cold or with inhaled irritants.

Warnings: A persistent cough may be a sign of a serious condition. Do not take this product for persistent or chronic cough such as occurs with smoking, asthma, emphysema, or when cough is accompanied by excessive phlegm (mucus). If cough persists for more than one (1) week, tends to recur, or is accompanied by fever, rash, or persistent headache, consult a physician. May cause excitability, especially in children. Do not take this product if you have glaucoma, or difficulty in urination due to enlargement of the prostate gland except under the advice of a physician. May cause marked drowsiness. Avoid driving a motor vehicle or operating heavy machinery, or drinking alcoholic beverages. Do not give to children under six (6) years of age except under the advice and supervision of a physician. Keep this and all drugs out of the reach of children. In case of accidental overdose, seek professional assistance or contact a Poison Control Center immediately. As with any drug, if you are pregnant or nursing a baby, seek the advice of a health professional before using this product.

Directions for Use:
Adults (12 years and older): Take 2 teaspoonfuls every 4 hours. Do not exceed 12 teaspoonfuls in 24 hours.
Children (6–12 years): Take 1 teaspoonful every 4 hours. Do not exceed 6 teaspoonfuls in 24 hours.
Children (under 6 years): Consult physician for recommended dosage.

How Supplied: Benylin Cough Syrup is supplied in 4-oz and 8-oz bottles. Store at 59°–86°F.

Shown in Product Identification Section, page 418

BENYLIN® DM® Pediatric Cough Formula

Description: Each teaspoonful (5 mL) contains:

Dextromethorphan Hydrobromide	7.5 mg

Also contains: Caramel, Carboxymethyl Sodium Cellulose, Citric Acid, D&C Red No. 33, FD&C Red No. 40, Flavors, Glycerin, Poloxamer 407, Polysorbate 20, Sodium Benzoate, Sodium Citrate, Sodium Saccharin, Sorbitol Solution, Water.

Indications: Non-narcotic cough suppressant for temporary relief of coughs due to minor bronchial irritation as may occur with the common cold or inhaled irritants.

Warnings: A persistent cough may be a sign of a serious condition. If cough persists for more than one week, tends to recur, or is accompanied by fever, rash, or persistent headache, consult a physician. Do not take this product for persistent or chronic cough such as occurs with smoking, asthma, emphysema, or if cough is accompanied by excessive phlegm (mucus) unless directed by a physician. As with any drug, if you are pregnant or nursing a baby, seek the advice of a health professional before using this product. Keep this and all drugs out of reach of children. In case of accidental overdose, seek professional assistance or contact a Poison Control Center immediately.

Drug Interaction Precaution: Do not use this product if you are taking a prescription drug containing a monoamine oxidase inhibitor [(MAOI) (certain drugs for depression or psychiatric or emotional conditions)], without first consulting your physician.

Directions for Use: Follow dosage recommendations below, or use as recommended by your physician. Repeat every 6 to 8 hours. Do not exceed 4 doses in a 24 hour period.
Dosage should be chosen by age or weight.
[See table below.]

How Supplied: 4-oz bottles.

Shown in Product Identification Section, page 418

AGE	WEIGHT	DOSAGE
Under 2 years	Under 24 lbs.	Consult Physician
2 to under 6 years	24 to 47 lbs.	1 teaspoonful
6 to under 12 years	48 to 95 lbs.	2 teaspoonfuls
12 years & older	96 lbs. & over	4 teaspoonfuls

BENYLIN® Decongestant

Description: Each teaspoonful (5 mL) contains:

Diphenhydramine Hydrochloride	12.5 mg
Pseudoephedrine Hydrochloride	30.0 mg

Also contains: Alcohol 5%; FD&C Yellow No. 6 (Sunset Yellow); Flavors; Glucose Liquid; Glycerin; Menthol; Purified Water; Saccharin Sodium; Sodium Citrate; Sucrose.

Indications: For the temporary relief of cough due to minor throat and bronchial irritations as may occur with the common cold or with inhaled irritants; and nasal congestion due to the common cold, hay fever, or other upper respiratory allergies.

Warnings: A persistent cough may be a sign of a serious condition. Do not take this product for persistent or chronic cough such as occurs with smoking, asthma, emphysema, or when cough is accompanied by excessive phlegm (mucus). If cough persists for more than one (1) week, tends to recur, or is accompanied by fever, rash, or persistent headache, consult a physician. May cause excitability, especially in children. Do not take this product if you have high blood pressure, heart disease, diabetes, thyroid disease, glaucoma, or difficulty in urination due to enlargement of the prostate gland except under the advice and supervision of a physician. Do not exceed recommended dosage because at higher doses nervousness, dizziness, or sleeplessness may occur. Do not give to children under six (6) years of age except under the advice and supervision of a physician. May cause marked drowsiness. Avoid driving a motor vehicle or operating heavy machinery, or drinking alcoholic beverages. Keep this and all drugs out of the reach of children. In case of accidental overdose, seek professional assistance or contact a Poison Control Center immediately. As with any drug, if you are pregnant or nursing a baby, seek the advice of a health professional before using this product.

Drug Interaction Precaution: Do not take this product if you are presently taking a prescription drug for high blood pressure or depression without first consulting your doctor.

Directions for Use:
Adults (12 years and older): Take 2 teaspoonfuls every 4 hours. Do not exceed 8 teaspoonfuls in 24 hours.
Children (6–12 years): Take 1 teaspoonful every 4 hours. Do not exceed 4 teaspoonfuls in 24 hours.
Children (under 6 years): Consult physician for recommended dosage.

How Supplied: 4-oz. bottles. Store at 59°–86°F.

Shown in Product Identification Section, page 418

BENYLIN® Expectorant

Description: Each teaspoonful (5 mL) contains:

Dextromethorphan Hydrobromide	5.0 mg
Guaifenesin	100.0 mg

Also contains: Alcohol 5%; Citric Acid; FD&C Red No. 40; Flavors; Glycerin; Purified Water; Saccharin Sodium, Sodium Benzoate, Sodium Citrate; Sucrose.

Indications: Nonnarcotic cough suppressant for the temporary relief of coughs plus an expectorant to relieve upper chest congestion due to minor bronchial irritations as may occur with the common cold, or inhaled irritants. Helps loosen phlegm (mucus) and thin bronchial secretions to rid the bronchial passageways of bothersome mucus.

Warnings: Do not take this product for persistent or chronic cough such as occurs with smoking, asthma, chronic bronchitis, or emphysema, or where cough is accompanied by excessive phlegm (mucus) unless directed by a physician. A persistent cough may be a sign of a serious condition. If cough persists for more than one week, tends to recur, or is accompanied by fever, rash, or persistent headache, consult a physician. Do not give to children under 2 years of age unless directed by a physician. As with any drug, if you are pregnant or nursing a baby, seek the advice of a health professional before using this product. Keep this and all drugs out of the reach of children. In case of accidental overdose, seek professional assistance or contact a Poison Control Center immediately.

Drug Interaction Precaution: Do not use this product if you are taking a prescription drug containing a monoamine oxidase inhibitor [(MAOI) (certain drugs for depression or psychiatric or emotional conditions)], without first consulting your physician.

Directions for Use:
Adults (12 years and older): Take 2–4 teaspoonfuls every 4 hours (or fill dosage cup to the corresponding teaspoon level indicated). Do not exceed 24 teaspoonfuls in 24 hours.
Children (6–12 years): Take 1–2 teaspoonfuls every 4 hours (or fill dosage cup to the corresponding teaspoon level indicated). Do not exceed 12 teaspoonfuls in 24 hours.
Children (2–6 years): Take ½–1 teaspoonful every 4 hours (or fill dosage cup to the corresponding teaspoon level indicated). Do not exceed 6 teaspoonfuls in 24 hours.
Children (under 2 years): Consult your physician for recommended dosage.

How Supplied: Benylin Expectorant is supplied in 4-oz and 8-oz bottles. Store at 59°–86°F.

Shown in Product Identification Section, page 418

CALADRYL® Lotion
[*că 'lă drĭl "*]
CALADRYL Cream
CALADRYL Spray
CALADRYL Clear Lotion

Description: Caladryl Lotion—A drying, calamine-antihistamine lotion containing Calamine 8%, Benadryl® (diphenhydramine hydrochloride), 1%. Also contains: Alcohol 2%; Camphor; Fragrances; Glycerin; Sodium Carboxymethylcellulose; and Water, Purified.
Caladryl Cream—Calamine 8%, Benadryl (diphenhydramine hydrochloride) 1%. Also contains: Camphor; Cetyl Alcohol; Cresin White; Fragrance; Propylene Glycol; Propylparaben; Polysorbate 60; Sorbitan Stearate; Water, Purified.
Caladryl Spray—Calamine 8%, Benadryl (diphenhydramine hydrochloride) 1%. Also contains: Alcohol 9%, Camphor, FD&C Red #40, Fragrance, Isobutane, Quarternium-18 Hectorite, Sorbitan Sesquioleate, and Talc.
Caladryl Clear Lotion—Benadryl (diphenhydramine hydrochloride) 1%, Zinc Oxide 2%. Also contains: Alcohol 2%, Camphor, Chlorophyllin Sodium, Diazolidinyl Urea, Fragrance, Glycerin, Hydroxypropyl Methylcellulose, Methylparaben, Polysorbate 40, Propylene Glycol, Propylparaben, and Water.

Indications: For relief of itching due to mild poison ivy or oak, insect bites, or other minor skin irritations.

Warnings: For external use only. Do not apply to blistered, raw or oozing areas of the skin. Do not use on chicken pox or measles, unless supervised by a doctor. Do not use on extensive areas of the skin or for longer than 7 days except as directed by a doctor. Avoid contact with the eyes or other mucous membranes. Discontinue use if burning sensation or rash develops or condition persists. Remove by washing with soap and water. Do not use any other drugs containing diphenhydramine while using this product. Additional spray warnings: Flammable. Do not use while smoking or near an open flame. Contents under pressure. Do not puncture or incinerate. Do not store at temperatures above 120°F. Intentional misuse by deliberately concentrating and inhaling the contents can be harmful or fatal.
KEEP THIS AND ALL DRUGS OUT OF THE REACH OF CHILDREN. In case of accidental ingestion seek professional assistance or contact a Poison Control Center immediately.

Continued on next page

This product information was prepared in November 1992. On these and other Parke-Davis Products, detailed information may be obtained by addressing PARKE-DAVIS, Consumer Health Products Group, Division of Warner-Lambert Company, Morris Plains, NJ 07950.

Parke-Davis—Cont.

Directions: For adults and children 6 years of age and older: Apply sparingly to the affected area three to four times daily. Before each application cleanse skin with soap and water and dry affected area. Children under 6 years of age: Consult a doctor.

How Supplied: Caladryl Cream—1½-oz tubes.
Caladryl Lotion—6 fl.-oz. bottles.
Caladryl Spray—4 oz. can.
Caladryl Clear Lotion—6 fl.-oz. bottle.
Shown in Product Identification Section, page 418

GELUSIL®
[jĕl 'ū-sĭl ″]
Antacid–Anti-gas
Liquid/Tablets
Sodium Free

Each teaspoonful (5 mL) or tablet contains:
200 mg aluminum hydroxide
200 mg magnesium hydroxide
25 mg simethicone
Also contains: Liquid: Ammonia Solution Strong; Calcium Hypochlorite; Citric Acid; Flavors; Hydroxypropyl Methylcellulose; Menthol; Sodium Saccharin; Sorbitol Solution; Water; Xanthan Gum. Tablets: Flavors; Magnesium Stearate; Mannitol; Sorbitol; Sugar.

Advantages:
- High acid-neutralizing capacity
- Sodium free
- Simethicone for antiflatulent activity
- Good taste for better patient compliance
- Fast dissolution of chewed tablets for prompt relief

Indications: For the relief of heartburn, sour stomach, acid indigestion and to relieve symptoms of gas.

Dosage and Administration: Two or more teaspoonfuls or tablets one hour after meals and at bedtime, or as directed by a physician.
Tablets should be chewed.

Warnings: Do not take more than 12 tablets or teaspoonfuls in a 24-hour period, or use this maximum dosage for more than two weeks, or use this product if you have kidney disease, except under the advice and supervision of a physician.
Keep this and all drugs out of the reach of children.

Professional Warnings: Prolonged use of aluminum-containing antacids in patients with renal failure may result in or worsen dialysis osteomalacia. Elevated tissue aluminum levels contribute to the development of the dialysis encephalopathy and osteomalacia syndromes. Small amounts of aluminum are absorbed from the gastrointestinal tract and renal excretion of aluminum is impaired in renal failure. Aluminum is not well removed by dialysis because it is bound to albumin and transferrin, which do not cross dialysis membranes. As a result, aluminum is deposited in bone, and dialysis osteomalacia may develop when large amounts of aluminum are ingested orally by patients with impaired renal function. Aluminum forms insoluble complexes with phosphate in the gastrointestinal tract, thus decreasing phosphate absorption. Prolonged use of aluminum-containing antacids by normophosphatemic patients may result in hypophosphatemia if phosphate intake is not adequate. In its more severe forms, hypophosphatemia can lead to anorexia, malaise, muscle weakness, and osteomalacia.

Drug Interaction Precaution: Do not take this product if you are presently taking a prescription antibiotic drug containing any form of tetracycline.

How Supplied:
Liquid—In plastic bottles of 12 fl oz.
Tablets—White, embossed Gelusil P-D 034—individual strips of 10 in boxes of 100.
Store at 59°–86°F (15°–30°C).
Shown in Product Identification Section, page 418

MEDI-FLU™ Caplet, Liquid

Composition:
Each Caplet contains: **Active Ingredients**—Pseudoephedrine Hydrochloride 30mg., Chlorpheniramine Maleate 2mg., Dextromethorphan Hydrobromide 15mg., Acetaminophen 500mg.
Inactive Ingredients—Cellulose derivatives, croscarmellose sodium, magnesium stearate, carnauba wax, polyethylene glycol, starch, stearic acid.
Each fluid ounce contains: **Active Ingredients**—Acetaminophen 1000mg., Chlorpheniramine Maleate 4mg., Dextromethorphan Hydrobromide 30mg., and Pseudoephedrine Hydrochloride 60mg. **Inactive Ingredients**—Alcohol (19%), Citric Acid, D&C Red No. 33, FD&C Red No. 40, Flavors, Glycerin, Propylene Glycol, Sodium Citrate, Sodium Chloride, Sodium Saccharin, Sorbitol Solution, Sugar and Water.

Actions: Medi-Flu provides temporary relief of these flu symptoms: Fever, body aches & pains, nasal congestion, runny nose, minor sore throat pain, coughing, sneezing, headache and watery eyes.

Warnings: Do not exceed recommended dosage because at higher doses nervousness, dizziness or sleeplessness may occur. Do not take this product for more than 7 days. If symptoms do not improve or are accompanied by fever for more than 3 days or if fever recurs after 3 days consult a doctor. Do not take this product if you have high blood pressure, heart disease, diabetes, thyroid disease, asthma, glaucoma, emphysema, chronic pulmonary disease, shortness of breath, difficulty in breathing, or difficulty in urination due to an enlargement of the prostate gland unless directed by a doctor. Do not take this product for persistent or chronic cough such as occurs with smoking, or if cough is accompanied by excessive phlegm (mucus) unless directed by a doctor. A persistent cough may be a sign of a serious condition. If cough persists for more than one week, tends to recur, or is accompanied or followed by fever, headache, rash, nausea, or vomiting consult a doctor promptly. May cause drowsiness: alcohol, sedatives, and tranquilizers may increase drowsiness effect. Avoid alcoholic beverages while taking this product. May cause excitability. Do not take this product if you are taking sedatives or tranquilizers without first consulting your doctor. Use caution when driving a motor vehicle or operating machinery. As with any drug if you are pregnant or nursing a baby, seek the advice of a health professional before using this product. KEEP THIS AND ALL DRUGS OUT OF THE REACH OF CHILDREN. In case of accidental overdose, seek professional assistance or contact a Poison Control Center immediately. Do not give this product to children under 12 years of age except under the advice and supervision of a doctor.

Drug Interaction Precaution: Do not take this product if you are presently taking a prescription drug for high blood pressure or depression without first consulting your doctor.

Dosage and Administration:
Caplets: Adults—two caplets every 6 hours, as needed, not to exceed 8 caplets in 24 hours. Under 12 consult a physician.
Liquid: Adults—1 fluid ounce (2 tablespoonfuls) every 6 hours as needed, not to exceed 4 fluid ounces in 24 hours. Under 12 consult a physician.

How Supplied: 16 caplets or 6 fl. oz. liquid
Shown in Product Identification Section, page 418

MEDI-FLU WITHOUT DROWSINESS™

Composition: Each caplet contains:
Active Ingredients: Pseudoephedrine Hydrochloride 30mg, Dextromethorphan Hydrobromide 15mg, Acetaminophen 500mg.
Inactive Ingredients: Candelilla Wax, Corn Starch, Croscarmellose Sodium, D&C Red No. 33 Aluminum Lake, FD&C Red No. 40 Aluminum Lake, Hydroxypropyl Methylcellulose, Microcrystalline Cellulose, Polyethylene Glycol, Polysorbate 80, Titanium Dioxide, Zinc Stearate.

Indications: Medi-Flu provides temporary relief of these flu symptoms: fever, body aches and pains, nasal and sinus congestion, minor sore throat pain, coughing and headache.

Warnings: Do not exceed recommended dosage because at higher doses nervousness, dizziness or sleeplessness may occur. Do not take this product for more than 7 days. If symptoms do not improve or are accompanied by fever for more than 3 days or if fever recurs after 3 days consult a doctor. Do not take this product if you have high blood pressure, heart disease, diabetes, thyroid disease, or difficulty in urination due to an enlargement of the prostate gland unless directed by a doctor. Do not take this product for persistent or chronic cough or chronic cough such as occurs with smoking, or if cough is accompanied by phlegm (mucus) unless directed by a doctor. A persistent cough may be a sign of a serious condition. If cough persists for more than one week, tends to recur, or is accompanied or followed by fever, headache, rash, nausea, or vomiting consult a doctor promptly. As with any drug if you are pregnant or nursing a baby, seek the advise of a health professional before using this product. KEEP THIS AND ALL DRUGS OUT OF THE REACH OF CHILDREN. In case of accidental overdose, seek professional assistance or contact a Poison Control Center immediately. Do not give this product to children under 12 years of age except under the advice and supervision of a doctor.

Drug Interaction Precaution: Do not take this product if you are presently taking a prescription drug for high blood pressure or depression without first consulting your doctor.

Dosage and Administration: Adults: 2 caplets every 6 hours, as needed, not to exceed 8 caplets in 24 hours. Under 12: consult a physician.

How Supplied: 16 caplet box

Shown in Product Identification Section, page 418

MYADEC®
High Potency Multivitamin Multimineral Formula

[See table next column.]

Ingredients: Dicalcium phosphate, magnesium oxide, potassium chloride, ascorbic acid, dl-alpha tocopheryl acetate, ferrous fumarate, modified starch glycolate, starch, cellulose, modified cellulose gum, niacinamide, silica, zinc oxide, polyethylene glycol, d-calcium pantothenate, beta carotene, vitamin A acetate, manganese sulfate, magnesium stearate, pyridoxine hydrochloride, phytonadione, biotin, cupric oxide, riboflavin, thiamine mononitrate, cyanocobalamin, vitamin D, folic acid, potassium iodide, sodium potassium borates, chromium chloride, sodium selenate, sodium molybdate, stannous chloride, sodium metasilicate, sodium metavanadate, nickelous sulfate, pharmaceutical glaze, methylcellulose, polysorbate, titanium dioxide (color), Yellow #6, Red #40, Blue #2, povidone, propylene glycol, hydroxypropylcellulose.

Actions and Uses: High potency vitamin supplement with minerals for adults.

Each Tablet Represents:		% of US Recommended Daily Allowances (US RDA)
VITAMINS		
Vitamin A**	5,000 IU*	100%
Vitamin D	400 IU	100%
Vitamin E	30 IU	100%
Vitamin C	60 mg	100%
Folic Acid	0.4 mg	100%
Vitamin B_1	1.7 mg	113%
Vitamin B_2	2 mg	118%
Niacin	20 mg	100%
Vitamin B_6	3 mg	150%
Vitamin B_{12}	6 mcg	100%
Biotin	30 mcg	10%
Pantothenic Acid	10 mg	100%
Vitamin K	25 mcg	***
MINERALS		
Calcium	162 mg	16%
Phosphorus	125 mg	13%
Iodine	150 mcg	100%
Iron	18 mg	100%
Magnesium	100 mg	25%
Copper	2 mg	100%
Zinc	15 mg	100%
Manganese	2.5 mg	***
Potassium	40 mg	***
Chloride	36.3 mcg	***
Chromium	25 mcg	***
Molybdenum	25 mcg	***
Selenium	25 mcg	***
Nickel	5 mcg	***
Tin	10 mcg	***
Silicon	10 mcg	***
Vanadium	10 mcg	***
Boron	150 mcg	***

* International Units
** as Acetate and Beta Carotene
*** No US Recommended Daily Allowance (US RDA) has been established for this nutrient.

Dosage: One tablet daily with a full meal.

How Supplied: In bottles of 130. Store below 30°C (86°F). Protect from moisture.

Shown in Product Identification Section, page 418

REPLENS® Vaginal Moisturizer
[ree'plenz]

Description: Replens relieves the discomfort of vaginal dryness for days with a single application. Replens non-hormonal vaginal moisturizer provides natural moisture to continuously hydrate vaginal tissue. Replens is non-staining, fragrance free, unflavored, non-greasy and non-irritating.

Actions: When used as directed, Replens provides long-lasting relief from the discomfort of vaginal dryness by providing continuous hydration to the vaginal tissue.

Ingredients: Purified water, glycerin, mineral oil, polycarbophil, Carbomer 934P, hydrogenated palm oil glyceride, and sorbic acid.

Warnings: Keep out of the reach of children. Replens is not a contraceptive. Does not contain spermicide.

Usage: Use as needed. One application every 2 to 3 days is recommended.

How Supplied: Replens is available in boxes containing 3 or 8 pre-filled disposable applicators. Each applicator delivers 2.5 grams.

Shown in Product Identification Section, page 418

SINUTAB® Sinus Medication, Regular Strength Without Drowsiness Formula, Tablets

Indications: Specially formulated to provide fast, temporary relief of sinus pain and congestion due to colds, flu, allergy and hay fever without drowsiness.

Active Ingredients: Each tablet contains: Acetaminophen 325 mg., pseudoephedrine hydrochloride 30 mg.

Inactive Ingredients: Cellulose microcrystalline, croscarmellose sodium, D&C red No. 33, FD&C red No. 40, hydroxypropyl cellulose, hydroxypropyl methylcellulose, magnesium stearate, propylene glycol, simethicone, starch pregelatinized, titanium dioxide, zinc stearate.

Actions: Sinutab® Sinus Medication, Regular Strength Without Drowsiness Formula, Tablets contain an analgesic (acetaminophen) to relieve pain and a decongestant (pseudoephedrine hydrochloride) to reduce congestion of the nasopharyngeal mucosa.
Acetaminophen is both analgesic and antipyretic. Because acetaminophen is not a salicylate, Sinutab® Sinus Medication, Regular Strength Without Drowsiness Formula, Tablets can be used by patients who are allergic to aspirin.
Pseudoephedrine hydrochloride, a sympathomimetic drug, provides vasoconstriction of the nasopharyngeal mucosa resulting in a nasal decongestant effect. The absence of antihistamine in the formula provides the added benefit of reduced likelihood of drowsiness side effects.

Warnings: Do not exceed recommended dosage. If symptoms persist, do not improve within 7 days, or are accompanied by high fever, or if new symptoms occur, see your doctor before continuing use. Do not take this product if you have high blood pressure, heart disease, diabetes, thyroid disease, or difficulty in urination due to an enlarged prostate except

Continued on next page

This product information was prepared in November 1992. On these and other Parke-Davis Products, detailed information may be obtained by addressing PARKE-DAVIS, Consumer Health Products Group, Division of Warner-Lambert Company, Morris Plains, NJ 07950.

Parke-Davis—Cont.

under doctor's supervision. Do not take this product for more than 10 days. As with any drug, if you are pregnant or nursing a baby, seek the advice of a health professional before using this product.

Drug Interaction: Do not take this product if you are presently taking a prescription drug for high blood pressure or depression without first consulting your doctor.

Precaution: Keep this and all drugs out of the reach of children.

Symptoms and Treatment of Oral Overdosage: In case of accidental overdose, seek professional help or contact a Poison Control Center immediately.

Dosage and Administration: Adults 2 tablets every 4 hours, not to exceed 8 tablets in 24 hours, or as directed by physician. Children under 12 should use only as directed by physician.

How Supplied: Sinutab® Sinus Medication, Regular Strength Without Drowsiness Formula, Tablets are pink, coated and scored so that tablets may be split in half. They are supplied in easy-to-open (exempt) blister packs of 24 tablets.

Shown in Product Identification Section, page 418

SINUTAB® Sinus Allergy Medication, Maximum Strength Formula, Tablets and Caplets

Indications: Specially formulated to provide fast, maximum strength relief of sinus pain and congestion. Sinutab Sinus Allergy Medication is a complete allergy and hay fever medication relieving runny nose, itchy watery eyes and sneezing.

Active Ingredients: Each tablet/caplet contains: Acetaminophen 500 mg., chlorpheniramine maleate 2 mg., pseudoephedrine hydrochloride 30 mg.

Inactive Ingredients:
Tablets contain: Carboxymethyl starch, microcrystalline cellulose, corn starch, croscarmellose sodium, hydroxypropyl cellulose, stearic acid, zinc stearate, D&C yellow No. 10 aluminum lake and FD&C yellow No. 6 aluminum lake.
Caplets contain: Microcrystalline cellulose, corn starch, croscarmellose sodium, hydroxypropyl cellulose, hydroxypropyl methylcellulose, magnesium stearate, polyethylene glycol, simethicone, sodium starch glycolate, stearic acid, titanium dioxide, zinc stearate, D&C yellow No. 10 aluminum lake, and FD&C yellow No. 6 aluminum lake.

Actions: Sinutab® Sinus Allergy Medication, Maximum Strength Formula, Tablets and Caplets contain an analgesic (acetaminophen) to relieve pain, a decongestant (pseudoephedrine hydrochloride) to reduce congestion of the nasopharyngeal mucosa, and an antihistamine (chlorpheniramine maleate) to help control allergic symptoms.
Acetaminophen is both analgesic and antipyretic. Because acetaminophen is not a salicylate, Sinutab® Sinus Allergy Medication, Maximum Strength Formula, Tablets and Caplets can be used by patients who are allergic to aspirin.
Pseudoephedrine hydrochloride, a sympathomimetic drug, provides vasoconstriction of the nasopharyngeal mucosa resulting in a nasal decongestant effect.
Chlorpheniramine maleate is an antihistamine incorporated to provide relief of running nose, sneezing, itching of the nose or throat, and itchy and watery eyes as may occur in allergic rhinitis.

Warnings: Do not exceed recommended dosage. If symptoms persist, do not improve within 7 days, or are accompanied by high fever, or if new symptoms occur, see your doctor before continuing use. Do not take this product if you have high blood pressure, heart disease, diabetes, thyroid disease, glaucoma, or difficulty in urination due to an enlarged prostate except under doctor's supervision. Do not take this product for more than 10 days. As with any drug, if you are pregnant or nursing a baby, seek the advice of a health professional before using this product. This product may cause drowsiness. Alcohol, sedatives and tranquilizers may increase the drowsiness effect. Avoid alcoholic beverages while taking this product. Do not take this product if you are taking sedatives or tranquilizers, without first consulting your doctor. Use caution when driving a motor vehicle or operating machinery.

Drug Interaction: Do not take this product if you are presently taking a prescription drug for high blood pressure or depression without first consulting your doctor.

Precaution: Keep this and all drugs out of the reach of children.

Symptoms and Treatment of Oral Overdosage: In case of accidental overdose, seek professional help or contact a Poison Control Center immediately.

Dosage and Administration: Adults 2 tablets or caplets every 6 hours, not to exceed 8 tablets or caplets in 24 hours, or as directed by physician. Children under 12 should use only as directed by physician.

How Supplied: Sinutab® Sinus Allergy Medication, Maximum Strength Formula, Caplets are yellow and coated. The Tablets are yellow and uncoated. They are supplied in child- resistant blister packs in boxes of 24 tablets or caplets.

Shown in Product Identification Section, page 418

SINUTAB® Sinus Medication, Maximum Strength Without Drowsiness Formula, Tablets and Caplets

Indications: Specially formulated to provide fast, maximum strength relief of sinus pain and congestion due to colds, flu and allergies. Sinutab relieves sinus headache and pressure without drowsiness.

Active Ingredients: Each tablet/caplet contains: Acetaminophen 500 mg., pseudoephedrine hydrochloride 30 mg.

Inactive Ingredients:
Tablets contain: Carboxymethyl starch, microcrystalline cellulose, corn starch, croscarmellose sodium, hydroxypropyl cellulose, stearic acid, zinc stearate, D&C yellow No. 10 aluminum lake and FD&C yellow No. 6 aluminum lake.
Caplets contain: Microcrystalline cellulose, corn starch, croscarmellose sodium, hydroxypropyl cellulose, hydroxypropyl methylcellulose, magnesium stearate, polyethylene glycol, simethicone, sodium starch glycolate, stearic acid, titanium dioxide, zinc stearate, D&C yellow No. 10 aluminum lake and FD&C yellow No. 6 aluminum lake.

Actions: Sinutab® Sinus Medication, Maximum Strength Without Drowsiness Formula, Tablets and Caplets contain an analgesic (acetaminophen) to relieve pain, and a decongestant (pseudoephedrine hydrochloride) to reduce congestion of the nasopharyngeal mucosa.
Acetaminophen is both analgesic and antipyretic. Because acetaminophen is not a salicylate, Sinutab® Sinus Medication, Maximum Strength Without Drowsiness Formula, can be used by patients who are allergic to aspirin.
Pseudoephedrine hydrochloride, a sympathomimetic drug, provides vasoconstriction of the nasopharyngeal mucosa resulting in a nasal decongestant effect.
The absence of antihistamine in the formula provides the added benefit of reduced likelihood of drowsiness side effects.

Warnings: Do not exceed recommended dosage. If symptoms persist, do not improve within seven days, or are accompanied by high fever, or if new symptoms occur, see your doctor before continuing use. Do not take this product if you have high blood pressure, heart disease, diabetes, thyroid disease, or difficulty in urination due to an enlarged prostate except under doctor's supervision. Do not take this product for more than 10 days. As with any drug, if you are pregnant or nursing a baby, seek the advice of a health professional before using this product.

Drug Interaction: Do not take this product if you are presently taking a prescription drug for high blood pressure or depression without first consulting your doctor.

Precaution: Keep this and all drugs out of the reach of children.

Symptoms and Treatment of Oral Overdosage: In case of accidental overdose, seek professional help or contact a Poison Control Center immediately.

Dosage and Administration: Adults 2 tablets or caplets every 6 hours, not to exceed 8 tablets or caplets in 24 hours or as directed by physician. Children under 12 should use only as directed by physician.

How Supplied: Sinutab® Sinus Medication, Maximum Strength Without Drowsiness Formula, Caplets are orange and coated. The Tablets are orange and uncoated. They are supplied in child-resistant blister packs in boxes of 24 tablets or caplets and in bottles of 50 caplets with child-resistant caps.

Shown in Product Identification Section, page 419

TUCKS®
Pre-moistened Hemorrhoidal/Vaginal Pads

Indications: For prompt, temporary relief of minor external itching, burning and irritation associated with hemorrhoids.
—Soothe, cool, and comfort itching, burning, and irritation of sensitive rectal and outer vaginal areas.
—As a compress, to help relieve discomfort from rectal/vaginal surgical stitches.
—Effective hygienic wipe to cleanse rectal area of irritation-causing residue.

Directions: For external use only. *As a hemorrhoidal treatment*—Adults: When practical, cleanse the affected area with soap and warm water, and rinse thoroughly. Gently dry by patting or blotting with toilet tissue or soft cloth before each application of this product. Gently apply to affected area by patting and then discard. Can be used up to six times daily or after each bowel movement. Children under 12 years of age: consult a physician.
As a hygienic wipe—Use as a wipe instead of toilet tissue after bowel movement or after napkin or tampon change.
As a moist compress—For soothing relief, fold pad and place in contact with irritated tissue. Leave in place for 5 to 15 minutes. Repeat as needed.

Warnings: If condition worsens or does not improve within 7 days, consult a physician. Do not exceed recommended daily dosage unless directed by a physician. In case of bleeding, consult a physician promptly. Do not put this product in the rectum by using fingers or any mechanical device or applicator. Keep this and all drugs out of the reach of children. In case of accidental ingestion, seek professional assistance or contact a Poison Control Center immediately.

Contains: Soft pads pre-moistened with a solution containing 50% Witch Hazel; also contains: Water, Glycerin, Alcohol 7%, Sodium Citrate, Citric Acid, Methylparaben, and Benzalkonium Citrate.

How Supplied: Jars of 40 and 100. Also available as Tucks Take-Alongs®, individual, foil-wrapped, nonwoven wipes, 12 per box.

Shown in Product Identification Section, page 419

TUCKS® CREAM

Active Ingredient: Witch Hazel (Hamamelis Water) 50%
Also contains: Alcohol 7%, White Petrolatum, Sorbitol Solution, Cetyl Alcohol, Polysorbate 60, Polyethylene Stearate, Anhydrous Lanolin, Glyceryl Oleate, Propylene Glycol and Benzethonium Chloride

Indications: For prompt, temporary relief of minor external ITCHING, BURNING and IRRITATION associated with Hemorrhoids.

Warnings: If condition worsens or does not improve within 7 days, consult a physician. Do not exceed the recommended daily dosage unless directed by a physician. In case of rectal bleeding, consult a physician promptly. Do not put this product into the rectum by using fingers or any other mechanical device or applicator. KEEP THIS AND ALL DRUGS OUT OF THE REACH OF CHILDREN. In case of accidental ingestion, seek professional assistance or contact a Poison Contol Center immediately.

Directions: Adults: When practical, cleanse the affected area with Tucks Hemorrhoidal Pads or mild soap and warm water and rinse thoroughly. Gently dry by patting or blotting with toilet tissue or soft cloth before each application. Remove cap and apply externally to affected area up to 6 times daily or after each bowel movement. Children under 12 years of age: Consult a physician.

How Supplied: Tucks Cream (water-washable) in 1.4 oz. tube with dispensing cap.

IDENTIFICATION PROBLEM?
Consult the
Product Identification Section
where you'll find
products pictured
in full color.

The Parthenon Co., Inc.
**3311 W. 2400 SOUTH
SALT LAKE CITY, UTAH 84119**

DEVROM® CHEWABLE TABLETS

Active Ingredients: Bismuth Subgallate 200 mg/tablet

Indications: Devrom Chewable Tablets are used as an aid to reduce odor from colostomies or ileostomies.

Warnings: This product cannot be expected to be effective in the reduction of odor due to faulty personal hygiene. Keep this and all medication out of the reach of children.
Note: The beneficial ingredient in these tablets may coat the tongue which may also darken in color. This condition is harmless and temporary. Darkening of the stool is also possible and is equally harmless.

Dosage and Administration: Take one to two tablets three times a day with meals or as directed by physician. Chew or swallow whole if desired. Keep bottle tightly closed in cool, dry place. Protect from light.

How Supplied: 100 tablets per bottle.

Perfective Cosmetics, Inc.
**688 HIGH RIDGE ROAD
P.O. BOX 3488
STAMFORD, CT 06905**

PERFECTIVE PREVENTION Cream
Prevention and Treatment for Aging Skin

Description: PERFECTIVE PREVENTION Cream is patented Glycolic Acid cream for Aging Skin. Acts as a skin nourisher.

Indication: This product is useful for reducing fine wrinkles and age spots, smooths over acne scars. When used regularly, it keeps clean acne-prone skin and removes excess skin oil which is one of the causes of acne. It also helps remove and prevent blackheads.

Action: This product gently dissolves dead cells, revealing smoother younger skin.

Warning: For external use only. Avoid use around eyes and mucous membrane. Discontinue use if severe rash or discomfort occurs.

Active Ingredients: GLYCOLIC ACID, VITAMIN A PALMITATE, Vitamin E Acetate.

Other Ingredients: Deionized Water, Stearyl Alcohol, Cetyl Esters Wax, Glycerin, Cetyl Alcohol, Sodium Lauryl Sulfate, Methylparaben, Quaternium 15, Propylparaben.

How Supplied: 2 Oz Plastic Jar.

Pfizer Consumer Health Care Division
Division of Pfizer Inc.
100 JEFFERSON ROAD
PARSIPPANY, NJ 07054

BEN–GAY® External Analgesic Products

Description: Ben-Gay products contain menthol in an alcohol base gel, combinations of methyl salicylate and menthol in cream and ointment bases, as well as a combination of methyl salicylate, menthol and camphor in a non-greasy cream base; all suitable for topical application.
In addition to the Original Formula Pain Relieving Rub (methyl salicylate, 18.3%; menthol, 16%), Ben-Gay is offered as Regular Strength Pain Relieving Rub [formerly Ben-Gay Greaseless/Stainless] (methyl salicylate, 15%; menthol, 10%), an Extra Strength Arthritis Rub (methyl salicylate, 30%; menthol, 8%), a Sports Formula Sports and Exercise Rub [formerly Extra Strength Sports Balm] (methyl salicylate 28%; menthol 10%), an Ultra Strength Pain Relieving Rub (methyl salicylate 30%; menthol 10%; camphor 4%), a Vanishing Scent Sports and Exercise Rub [formerly Ben-Gay SportsGel] (menthol 3%), Daytime Ben-Gay Pain Relieving Gel and Ben-Gay Warming Ice Vanishing Scent Formulas (2.5% menthol in an alcohol base gel).

Action and Uses: Methyl salicylate, menthol and camphor are external analgesics which stimulate sensory receptors of warmth and/or cold. This produces a counter-irritant response which provides temporary relief of minor aches and pains of muscles and joints associated with simple backache, arthritis, strains, bruises and sprains.
Several double-blind clinical studies of Ben-Gay products containing menthol-methyl salicylate have shown the effectiveness of this combination in counteracting minor pain of skeletal muscle stress and arthritis.
Three studies involving a total of 102 normal subjects in which muscle soreness was experimentally induced showed statistically significant beneficial results from use of the active product vs. placebo for lowered Muscle Action Potential (spasms), greater rise in threshold of muscular pain and greater reduction in perceived muscular pain.
Six clinical studies of a total of 207 subjects suffering from minor pain due to osteoarthritis and rheumatoid arthritis showed the active product to give statistically significant beneficial results vs. placebo for greater relief of perceived pain, increased range of motion of the affected joints and increased digital dexterity. In two studies designed to measure the effect of topically applied Ben-Gay vs. Placebo on muscular endurance, discomfort, onset of exercise pain and fatigue, 30 subjects performed a submaximal three-hour run and another 30 subjects performed a maximal treadmill run. Ben-Gay was found to significantly decrease the discomfort during the submaximal and maximal runs, and increase the time before onset of fatigue during the maximal run.
Applied before workouts, Ben-Gay exercise rubs relax tight muscles and increase circulation to make exercising more comfortable, longer.
To help reduce muscle ache and soreness after exercise, a Ben-Gay exercise rub can be applied and allowed to work before taking a shower.

Directions: Apply generously and gently massage into painful area until Ben-Gay disappears. Repeat 3 to 4 times daily.

Warning: Use only as directed. Do not use with a heating pad (may blister skin). Keep away from children to avoid accidental poisoning. Do not swallow. In case of accidental ingestion, seek professional assistance or contact a Poison Control Center immediately. Keep away from eyes, mucous membranes, broken or irritated skin. If skin irritation develops, pain lasts 10 days or more, redness is present, or with arthritis-like conditions in children under 12, call a physician.

BONINE®
(meclizine hydrochloride) Chewable Tablets

Action: BONINE (meclizine) is an H_1 histamine receptor blocker of the piperazine side chain group. It exhibits its action by an effect on the Central Nervous System (CNS), possibly by its ability to block muscarinic receptors in the brain.

Indications: BONINE is effective in the management of nausea, vomiting and dizziness associated with motion sickness.

Contraindications: Asthma, glaucoma, emphysema, chronic pulmonary disease, shortness of breath, difficulty in breathing, or difficulty in urination due to enlargement of the prostate gland unless directed by a doctor.

Warnings: May cause drowsiness; alcohol, sedatives and tranquilizers may increase the drowsiness effect. Avoid alcoholic beverages while taking this product. Do not take this product if you are taking sedatives or tranquilizers without first consulting your doctor. Do not drive or operate dangerous machinery while taking this medication.
Usage in Children: Clinical studies establishing safety and effectiveness in children have not been done; therefore, usage is not recommended in children under 12 years of age.
Usage in Pregnancy: As with any drug, if you are pregnant or nursing a baby, seek advice of a health care professional before taking this product.

Adverse Reactions: Drowsiness, dry mouth, and on rare occasions, blurred vision have been reported.

Dosage and Administration: For motion sickness, take one or two tablets of Bonine once daily, one hour before travel starts, for up to 24 hours of protection against motion sickness. The tablet can be chewed with or without water or swallowed whole with water. Thereafter, the dose may be repeated every 24 hours for the duration of the travel.

How Supplied: BONINE (meclizine hydrochloride) is available in convenient packets of 8 chewable tablets of 25 mg. meclizine hydrochloride.

Inactive Ingredients: FD&C Red No. 40, Lactose, Magnesium Stearate, Purified Siliceous Earth, Raspberry Flavor, Saccharin Sodium, Starch, Talc.

DESITIN® OINTMENT

Description: Desitin Ointment combines Zinc Oxide (40%) with Cod Liver Oil in a petrolatum-lanolin base suitable for topical application. Also contains: BHA, fragrances, methylparaben, talc and water.

Actions and Uses: Desitin Ointment is designed to provide relief of diaper rash, superficial wounds and burns, and other minor skin irritations. It helps prevent incidents of diaper rash, protects against urine and other irritants, and soothes chafed skin.
Relief and protection is afforded by Zinc Oxide and Cod Liver Oil. These ingredients together with the petrolatum-lanolin base provide a physical barrier by forming a protective coating over skin or mucous membranes which serves to reduce further effects of irritants on the affected area and relieves burning, pain or itch produced by them.
Several studies have shown the effectiveness of Desitin Ointment in the relief and prevention of diaper rash.
Two clinical studies involving 90 infants demonstrated the effectiveness of Desitin Ointment in curing diaper rash. The diaper rash area was treated with Desitin Ointment at each diaper change for a period of 24 hours, while the untreated site served as controls. A significant reduction was noted in the severity and area of diaper dermatitis on the treated area.
Ninety-seven (97) babies participated in a 12-week study to show that Desitin Ointment helps prevent diaper rash. Approximately half of the infants (49) were treated with Desitin Ointment on a regular daily basis. The other half (48) received the ointment as necessary to treat any diaper rash which occurred. The incidence as well as the severity of diaper rash was significantly less among the babies using the ointment on a regular daily basis.
In a comparative study of the efficacy of Desitin Ointment vs. a baby powder, forty-five (45) babies were observed for a total of eight (8) weeks. Results support the conclusion that Desitin Ointment is a

better prophylactic against diaper rash than the baby powder.
In another study, Desitin was found to be dramatically more effective in reducing the severity of medically diagnosed diaper rash than a commercially available diaper rash product in which only anhydrous lanolin and petrolatum were listed as ingredients. Fifty (50) infants participated in the study, half of whom were treated with Desitin and half with the other product. In the group (25) treated with Desitin, seventeen (17) infants showed significant improvement within 10 hours which increased to twenty-three improved infants within 24 hours. Of the group (25) treated with the other product, only three showed improvement at ten hours with a total of four improved within twenty-four hours. These results are statistically valid to conclude that Desitin Ointment reduces severity of diaper rash within ten hours.
Several other studies show that Desitin Ointment helps relieve other skin disorders, such as contact dermatitis.

Directions: Prevention: To prevent diaper rash, apply Desitin Ointment to the diaper area—especially at bedtime when exposure to wet diapers may be prolonged.
Treatment: If diaper rash is present, or at the first sign of redness, minor skin irritation or chafing, simply apply Desitin Ointment three or four times daily as needed. In superficial noninfected surface wounds and minor burns, apply a thin layer of Desitin Ointment, using a gauze dressing, if necessary. For external use only.

How Supplied: Desitin Ointment is available in 1 ounce (28g), 2 ounce (57g), and 4 ounce (114g) tubes, and 9 ounce (255g) and 1 lb. (454g) jars.

Shown in Product Identification Section, page 419

RHEABAN® Maximum Strength TABLETS
[rē'ăban]
(attapulgite)

Description: Maximum Strength Rheaban is an anti-diarrheal medication containing activated attapulgite and is offered in tablet form.
Each white Rheaban tablet contains 750 mg. of colloidal activated attapulgite. Rheaban provides the maximum level of medication when taken as directed.
Rheaban contains no narcotics, opiates or other habit-forming drugs.

Actions and Uses: Rheaban is indicated for relief of diarrhea and the cramps and pains associated with it. Attapulgite, which has been activated by thermal treatment, is a highly sorptive substance which absorbs nutrients and digestive enzymes as well as noxious gases, irritants, toxins and some bacteria and viruses that are common causes of diarrhea.
In clinical studies to show the effectiveness in relieving diarrhea and its symptoms, 100 subjects suffering from acute gastroenteritis with diarrhea participated in a double-blind comparison of Rheaban to a placebo. Patients treated with the attapulgite product showed significantly improved relief of diarrhea and its symptoms vs. the placebo.

Dosage and Administration:
TABLETS
Adults—2 tablets after initial bowel movement, 2 tablets after each subsequent bowel movement. For a maximum of 12 tablets in 24 hours.
Children 6 to 12 years—1 tablet after initial bowel movement, 1 tablet after each subsequent bowel movement. For a maximum of 6 tablets in 24 hours, or as directed by a physician.

Warnings: Do not exceed 12 tablets in 24 hours. Swallow tablets with water, do not chew. Do not use for more than two days, or in the presence of high fever. Tablets should not be used for infants or children under 6 years of age unless directed by physician. If diarrhea persists consult a physician.

How Supplied:
Tablets—Boxes of 12 tablets.

Inactive Ingredients: Colloidal Silicon Dioxide, Croscarmellose Sodium, Ethylcellulose, Hydroxypropyl Methylcellulose 2910, Pectin, Pharmaceutical Glaze, Sucrose, Talc, Titanium Dioxide, Zinc Stearate.

RID® Spray
Lice Control Spray

THIS PRODUCT IS NOT FOR USE ON HUMANS OR ANIMALS

Active Ingredient:

*Permethrin	0.50%
INERT INGREDIENTS	99.50%
	100.00%

*(3-phenoxyphenyl) methyl (±) cis,trans 3-(2,2-dichloroethenyl) 2,2-dimethylcyclopropanecarboxylate. Cis, trans ratio: min. 35% (±) cis and max. 65% (±) trans

Actions: A highly active synthetic pyrethroid for the control of lice and louse eggs on garments, bedding, furniture and other inanimate objects.

Warnings: Harmful if swallowed. May be absorbed through skin. Avoid inhalation of spray mist. Avoid contact with skin, eyes or clothing. Wash thoroughly after handling and before smoking or eating. Avoid contamination of feed and foodstuffs. Remove pets and birds and cover fish aquaria before space spraying or surface applications. **This product is not for use on humans or animals.** If lice infestation should occur on humans, use Rid Lice Killing Shampoo. Vacate room after treatment and ventilate before reoccupying. Do not allow children or pets to contact treated areas until surfaces are dry. Do not overspray.

Physical and Chemical Hazards: Contents under pressure. Do not use or store near heat or open flame. Do not puncture or incinerate container. Exposure to temperatures above 130° F may cause bursting.
CAUTION: Avoid spraying in eyes. Avoid breathing spray mist. Use only in well ventilated areas. Avoid contact with skin. In case of contact wash immediately with soap and water. Vacate room after treatment and ventilate before reoccupying.
Statement of Practical Treatment: If inhaled: Remove affected person to fresh air. Apply artificial respiration if indicated.
If in eyes: Flush with plenty of water. Contact physician if irritation persists.
If on skin: Wash affected areas immediately with soap and water.

Direction For Use: It is a violation of Federal law to use this product in a manner inconsistent with its labeling.
Shake well before each use. Remove protective cap. Aim spray opening away from person. Push button to spray.
To kill lice and louse eggs: Spray in an inconspicuous area to test for possible staining or discoloration. Inspect again after drying, then proceed to spray entire area to be treated.
Hold container upright with nozzle away from you. Depress valve and spray from a distance of 8 to 10 inches.
Spray each square foot for 3 seconds. Spray only those garments, parts of bedding, including mattresses and furniture that cannot be either laundered or dry cleaned. Do not overspray.
Allow all sprayed articles to dry thoroughly before use. Repeat treatment as necessary.
Buyer assumes all risks of use, storage or handling of this material not in strict accordance with direction given herewith.
STORAGE AND DISPOSAL
Store in cool, dry area. Do not store below 32°F.
Wrap container in several layers of newspaper and dispose of in trash. Do not incinerate or puncture.

How Supplied: 5 oz. aerosol can.
Also available in combination with RID® Lice Treatment Kit as the RID® Lice Elimination System.

RID®
Lice Killing Shampoo

Description: Rid contains a liquid pediculicide whose active ingredients are: pyrethrins 0.3% and piperonyl butoxide, technical 3.00%, equivalent to 2.4% (butylcarbityl) (6-propylpiperonyl) ether and to 0.6% related compounds. Also contains petroleum distillate 1.20% and benzyl alcohol 2.4%. Inert ingredients 93.1%.

Continued on next page

Pfizer Consumer—Cont.

Actions: RID kills head lice *(Pediculus humanus capitis),* body lice *(Pediculus humanus humanus),* and pubic or crab lice *(Phthirus pubis).*
The pyrethrins act as a contact poison and affect the parasite's nervous system, resulting in paralysis and death. The efficacy of the pyrethrins is enhanced by the synergist, piperonyl butoxide. Rid rinses out completely after treatment.
The active ingredients in RID are poorly absorbed through the skin. Of the relatively minor amounts that are absorbed, they are rapidly metabolized to water-soluble compounds and eliminated from the body without ill-effects.

Indications: RID is indicated for the treatment of infestations of head lice, body lice and pubic (crab) lice, and their eggs.

Warning: RID should be used with caution by ragweed sensitized persons.

Precautions: This product is for external use only. It is harmful if swallowed. If accidentally swallowed, call a physician or Poison Control Center immediately. It should not be inhaled. It should be kept out of the eyes and contact with mucous membranes should be avoided. If accidental contact with eyes occur, flush eyes immediately with plenty of water and call a physician. In the case of infection or skin irritation, discontinue use immediately and consult a physician. Consult a physician before use if infestation of eyebrows or eyelashes occurs. Avoid contamination of feed or foodstuffs.

Storage and Disposal: Do not store below 32°F (0°C). Do not reuse empty container. Wrap in several layers of newspaper and discard in trash.

Dosage and Administration: (1) Shake well. Apply undiluted RID to dry hair and scalp or to any other infested area until entirely wet. Do not use on eyelashes or eyebrows. (2) Allow RID to remain on area for 10 minutes but no longer. (3) Wash thoroughly with warm water and soap or shampoo. (4) Dead lice and eggs should be removed with the special nit comb provided. (5) Repeat treatment in 7 to 10 days to kill any newly hatched lice. Do not exceed two consecutive applications within 24 hours.
Since lice infestations are spread by contact, each family member should be examined carefully. If infested, he or she should be treated promptly to avoid spread or reinfestation of previously treated individuals. Contaminated clothing and other articles, such as hats, etc. should be dry cleaned, boiled or otherwise treated until decontaminated to prevent reinfestation or spread.

How Supplied: In 2, 4 and 8 fl. oz. plastic bottles. Exclusive nit removal comb that removes nits and patient instruction booklet (English and Spanish) are included in each package of RID.
Also available in combination with RID Lice Control Spray as the RID Lice Elimination System.

UNISOM® NIGHTTIME SLEEP AID
[yu 'na-som]
(doxylamine succinate)

Description: Pale blue oval scored tablets containing 25 mg. of doxylamine succinate, 2-[α-(2-dimethylaminoethoxy)α-methylbenzyl] pyridine succinate.

Action and Uses: Doxylamine succinate is an antihistamine of the ethanolamine class, which characteristically shows a high incidence of sedation. In a comparative clinical study of over 20 antihistamines on more than 3000 subjects, doxylamine succinate 25 mg. was one of the three most sedating antihistamines, producing a significantly reduced latency to end of wakefulness and comparing favorably with established hypnotic drugs such as secobarbital and pentobarbital in sedation activity. It was chosen as the antihistamine, based on dosage, causing the earliest onset of sleep. In another clinical study, doxylamine succinate 25 mg. scored better than secobarbital 100 mg. as a nighttime hypnotic. Two additional, identical clinical studies involving a total of 121 subjects demonstrated that doxylamine succinate 25 mg. reduced the sleep latency period by a third, compared to placebo. Duration of sleep was 26.6% longer with doxylamine succinate, and the quality of sleep was rated higher with the drug than with placebo. An EEG study of 6 subjects confirmed the results of these studies. In yet another study, no statistically significant difference was found between doxylamine succinate and flurazepam in the average time required for 200 patients with mild to moderate insomnia to fall asleep over 5 nights following a nightly dose of doxylamine succinate 25 mg. or flurazepam 30 mg., nor was any statistically significant difference found in the total time the 200 patients slept. Patients on doxylamine succinate awoke an average of 1.2 times per night while those on flurazepam awoke an average of 0.9 times per night. In either case the patients awoke rested the following morning. On a rating scale of 1 to 5, doxylamine succinate was given a 3.0, flurazepam a 3.4 by patients rating the degree of restfulness provided by their medication (5 represents "very well rested"). Although statistically significant, the difference between doxylamine succinate 25 mg. and flurazepam 30 mg. in the number of awakenings and degree of restfulness is clinically insignificant.

Administration and Dosage: One tablet 30 minutes before retiring. Not for children under 12 years of age.

Side Effects: Occasional anticholinergic effects may be seen.

Precautions: Unisom® should be taken only at bedtime.

Contraindications: This product should not be taken by pregnant women, or those who are nursing a baby. This product is also contraindicated for asthma, glaucoma, enlargement of the prostate gland.

Warnings: Should be taken with caution if alcohol is being consumed. Product should not be taken if patient is concurrently on any other drug, without prior consultation with physician. Should not be taken for longer than two weeks unless approved by physician.

How Supplied: Boxes of 8, 32 or 48 tablets in child resistant blisters, and in boxes of 16 with non–child resistant packaging.

Inactive Ingredients: Dibasic Calcium Phosphate, FD&C Blue #1 Aluminum Lake, Magnesium Stearate, Microcrystalline Cellulose, Sodium Starch Glycolate.

UNISOM® WITH PAIN RELIEF
(formerly Unisom Dual Relief)
Nighttime Sleep Aid and Pain Reliever

Description: Unisom® With Pain Relief is a pale blue, capsule-shaped, coated tablet.

Active Ingredients: 650 mg. acetaminophen and 50 mg. diphenhydramine HCl per tablet.

Inactive Ingredients: Corn starch, FD&C Blue #1 Aluminum Lake, FD&C Blue #2 Aluminum Lake, hydroxypropyl methylcellulose, magnesium stearate, polyethylene glycol, polysorbate 80, povidone, stearic acid, titanium dioxide.

Indications: Unisom With Pain Relief (diphenhydramine sleep aid formula) is indicated for the temporary relief of occasional headaches and minor aches and pains with accompanying sleeplessness. If there is difficulty in falling asleep, but pain is not being experienced at the same time, regular Unisom sleep aid is indicated which contains doxylamine succinate as its active ingredient.

Administration and Dosage: Adults and children 12 years of age and over: take one tablet 30 minutes before bedtime if needed, or as directed by a physician.

Warnings: Do not take this product if you have asthma, glaucoma, emphysema, chronic pulmonary disease, shortness of breath, difficulty in breathing, or difficulty in urination due to enlargement of the prostate gland unless directed by a doctor. Do not take this product for more than ten days unless directed by a doctor. If symptoms get worse, or if new symptoms occur, or if sleeplessness persists continuously for more than 2 weeks, consult a doctor because these could be signs of a serious underlying medical illness. Avoid alcoholic beverages while taking this product. Do not take this product if you are taking sedatives or tranquilizers without first consulting your doctor. As with any drug, if you are pregnant or nursing a baby, seek the advice of a health professional before using this product. Do not give to children under 12 years of age. Keep this and all medications out of the reach of children. In case of accidental overdose, seek professional assistance or contact a poison control center immediately. Prompt medical attention is critical for adults as well as for children even if you do not notice any signs of symptoms.

Drug Interaction: Monoamine oxidase (MAO) inhibitors prolong and intensify the anticholinergic effects of antihistamines. The CNS depressant effect is heightened by alcohol and other CNS depressant drugs.

Attention: Use only if tablet blister seals are unbroken. Child resistant packaging.

How Supplied: Boxes of 8 and 16 tablets in child resistant blisters.

VISINE®
Tetrahydrozoline Hydrochloride Redness Reliever Eye Drops

Description: Visine is a sterile, isotonic, buffered ophthalmic solution containing tetrahydrozoline hydrochloride 0.05%, boric acid, sodium borate, sodium chloride and water. It is preserved with benzalkonium chloride 0.01% and edetate disodium 0.1%. Visine is a decongestant ophthalmic solution designed to provide symptomatic relief of conjunctival edema and hyperemia secondary to minor irritations, due to conditions such as smoke, dust, other airborne pollutants, swimming etc. and so-called nonspecific or catarrhal conjunctivitis. Relief is afforded by tetrahydrozoline hydrochloride, a sympathomimetic agent, which brings about decongestion by vasoconstriction. Reddened eyes are rapidly whitened by this effective vasoconstrictor, which limits the local vascular response by constricting the small blood vessels. The onset of vasoconstriction becomes apparent within minutes.
The effectiveness of Visine in relieving conjunctival hyperemia has been demonstrated by numerous clinicals, including several double-blind studies, involving more than 2,000 subjects suffering from acute or chronic hyperemia induced by a variety of conditions. Visine was found to be efficacious in providing relief from conjunctival hyperemia.

Indications: Relieves redness of the eye due to minor eye irritations.

Directions: Instill 1 to 2 drops in the affected eye(s) up to four times daily.

Warning: To avoid contamination, do not touch tip of container to any surface. Replace cap after using. If you experience eye pain, changes in vision, continued redness or irritation of the eye, or if the condition worsens or persists for more than 72 hours, discontinue use and consult a doctor. If you have glaucoma, do not use this product except under the advice and supervision of a doctor. Overuse of this product may produce increased redness of the eye. If solution changes color or becomes cloudy, do not use. Remove contact lenses before using.
Parents: Before using with children under 6 years of age, consult your physician. Keep this and all other drugs out of the reach of children. In case of accidental ingestion, seek professional assistance or contact a poison control center immediately.

How Supplied: In 0.5 fl. oz., 0.75 fl. oz., and 1.0 fl. oz. plastic dispenser bottle and 0.5 fl. oz. plastic bottle with dropper.

Shown in Product Identification Section, page 419

VISINE A.C.®
Astringent/Redness Reliever Eye Drops

Description: Visine A.C. is a sterile, isotonic, buffered ophthalmic solution containing tetrahydrozoline hydrochloride 0.05%, zinc sulfate 0.25%, boric acid, sodium chloride, sodium citrate and purified water. It is preserved with benzalkonium chloride 0.01% and edetate disodium 0.1%. Visine A.C. is an ophthalmic solution combining the effects of the vasoconstrictor tetrahydrozoline hydrochloride with the astringent effects of zinc sulfate. The vasoconstrictor provides symptomatic relief of conjunctival edema and hyperemia secondary to minor irritation due to conditions such as dust and airborne pollutants as well as so-called nonspecific or catarrhal conjunctivitis, while zinc sulfate provides relief from burning and itching, symptoms often associated with hay fever, allergies, etc. Beneficial effects include amelioration of burning, irritation, pruritis, and removal of mucus from the eye. Relief is afforded by both ingredients, tetrahydrozoline hydrochloride and zinc sulfate.
Tetrahydrozoline hydrochloride is a sympathomimetic agent, which brings about decongestion by vasoconstriction. Reddened eyes are rapidly whitened by this effective vasoconstrictor, which limits the local vascular response by constricting the small blood vessels. The onset of vasoconstriction becomes apparent within minutes. Zinc sulfate is an ocular astringent which, by precipitating protein, helps to clear mucus from the outer surface of the eye.
The effectiveness of Visine A.C. in relieving conjunctival hyperemia and associated symptoms induced by allergies has been clinically demonstrated. In one double-blind study allergy sufferers experienced acute episodes of minor eye irritation. Visine A.C. produced statistically significant beneficial results versus a placebo of normal saline solution in relieving irritation of bulbar conjunctiva, irritation of palpebral conjunctiva, and mucous build-up. Treatment with Visine A.C. containing zinc sulfate also significantly improved burning and itching symptoms.

Indications: For temporary relief of discomfort and redness due to minor eye irritations.

Directions: Instill 1 to 2 drops in the affected eye(s) up to 4 times daily.

Warning: To avoid contamination, do not touch tip of container to any surface. Replace cap after using. If you experience eye pain, changes in vision, continued redness or irritation of the eye, or if the condition worsens or persists for more than 72 hours, discontinue use and consult a doctor. If you have glaucoma, do not use this product except under the advice and supervision of a doctor. Overuse of this product may produce increased redness of the eye. If solution changes color or becomes cloudy, do not use. Remove contact lenses before using.
Parents: Before using with children under 6 years of age, consult your physician. Keep this and all other drugs out of the reach of children. In case of accidental ingestion, seek professional assistance or contact a poison control center immediately.

How Supplied: In 0.5 fl. oz. and 1.0 fl. oz. plastic dispenser bottle.

Shown in Product Identification Section, page 419

VISINE EXTRA®
Redness Reliever/Lubricant Eye Drops

Description: Visine Extra is a sterile, isotonic, buffered ophthalmic solution containing tetrahydrozoline hydrochloride 0.05%, polyethylene glycol 400 1.0%, boric acid, sodium borate, sodium chloride and water. It is preserved with benzalkonium chloride 0.013% and edetate disodium 0.1%.
Visine Extra is an ophthalmic solution combining the effects of the decongestant tetrahydrozoline hydrochloride with the demulcent effects of polyethylene glycol. It provides symptomatic relief of conjunctival edema and hyperemia secondary to ocular allergies, minor irritations and so-called nonspecific or catarrhal conjunctivitis. Tetrahydrozoline hydrochloride is a sympathomimetic agent, which brings about decongestion by vasoconstriction. Reddened eyes are rapidly whitened by this effective vasoconstrictor, which limits the local vascular response by constricting the small blood vessels. The onset of vasoconstriction becomes apparent within minutes. Additional effects include amelioration of burning, irritation, pruritus, soreness, and excessive lacrimation. Relief is afforded by polyethylene glycol.
Polyethylene glycol is an ophthalmic demulcent which has been shown to be effective for the temporary relief of dis-

Continued on next page

Pfizer Consumer—Cont.

comfort of minor irritations of the eye due to exposure to wind or sun. It is effective as a protectant and lubricant against further irritation or to relieve dryness of the eye.
The effectiveness of tetrahydrozoline hydrochloride in relieving conjunctival hyperemia and associated symptoms has been demonstrated by numerous clinicals, including several double-blind studies, involving more than 2000 subjects suffering from acute or chronic hyperemia induced by a variety of conditions.
Visine Extra is a product that combines the redness relieving effects of a vasoconstrictor and the soothing moisturizing and protective effects of a demulcent.

Indications: Relieves redness of the eye due to minor eye irritations. For use as a protectant against further irritation or to relieve dryness.

Directions: Instill 1 to 2 drops in the affected eye(s) up to 4 times daily.

Warning: To avoid contamination, do not touch tip of container to any surface. Replace cap after using. If you experience eye pain, changes in vision, continued redness or irritation of the eye, or if the condition worsens or persists for more than 72 hours, discontinue use and consult a doctor. If you have glaucoma, do not use this product except under the advice and supervision of a doctor. Overuse of this product may produce increased redness of the eye. If solution changes color or becomes cloudy, do not use. Remove contact lenses before using.
Parents: Before using with children under 6 years of age, consult your physician. Keep this and all other drugs out of the reach of children. In case of accidental ingestion, seek professional assistance or contact a poison control center immediately.

How Supplied: In 0.5 fl. oz. and 1.0 fl. oz. plastic dispenser bottle.

Shown in Product Identification Section, page 419

VISINE L. R.™ EYE DROPS
(oxymetazoline hydrochloride)

Description: Visine L. R. is a sterile, isotonic, buffered ophthalmic solution containing oxymetazoline hydrochloride 0.025%, boric acid, sodium borate, sodium chloride and water. It is preserved with benzalkonium chloride 0.01% and edetate disodium 0.1%.
Visine L. R. is produced by a process that assures sterility.

Indications: Visine L. R. is a decongestant ophthalmic solution designed for the relief of redness of the eye due to minor eye irritations. Visine L. R. is specially formulated to relieve redness of the eye in minutes with effective relief that lasts up to 6 hours.

Directions: *Adults and children 6 years of age and older*—Place 1 or 2 drops in the affected eye(s). This may be repeated as needed every 6 hours or as directed by a physician.

Warning: If you experience eye pain, changes in vision, continued redness or irritation of the eye, or if the condition worsens or persists for more than 72 hours, discontinue use and consult a physician. If you have glaucoma, do not use this product except under the advice and supervision of a physician. As with any medication, if you are pregnant seek the advice of a physician before using this product. Overuse of this product may produce increased redness of the eye. If solution changes color or becomes cloudy, do not use. To avoid contamination of this product, do not touch tip of container to any surface. Replace cap after using. Remove contact lenses before using this product.
Parents: Before using with children under 6 years of age, consult your physician. Keep this and all other medications out of the reach of children. In case of accidental ingestion, seek professional assistance or contact a poison control center immediately.

Caution: Should not be used if Visine-imprinted neckband on bottle is broken or missing.

Storage: Store between 2° and 30°C (36° and 86°F).

How Supplied: In 0.5 fl. oz. and 1 fl. oz. plastic dispenser bottle.

Shown in Product Identification Section, page 419

WART-OFF®
Liquid

Active Ingredient: Salicylic Acid 17% w/w.

Inactive Ingredients: Alcohol, 26.35% w/w, Flexible Collodion, Propylene Glycol Dipelargonate.

Indications: For the removal of common warts and plantar warts on the bottom of the foot. The common wart is easily recognized by the rough "cauliflower-like" appearance of the surface. The plantar wart is recognized by its location only on the bottom of the foot, its tenderness, and the interruption of the footprint pattern.

Warnings: For external use only. Keep this and all medications out of the reach of children to avoid accidental poisoning. In case of accidental ingestion, contact a physician or a Poison Control Center immediately. Do not use this product on irritated skin, on any area that is infected or reddened, if you are a diabetic, or if you have poor blood circulation. Do not use on moles, birthmarks, warts with hair growing from them, genital warts, or warts on the face or mucous membranes. If product gets into the eye, flush with water for 15 minutes. Avoid inhaling vapors. If discomfort persists, see your doctor.
Extremely Flammable—Keep away from fire or flame. Cap bottle tightly and store at room temperature away from heat (59°–86°F).

Instructions For Use: Read warnings and enclosed instructional brochure. Wash affected area. Dry area thoroughly. Using the special pinpoint applicator, apply one drop at a time to sufficiently cover each wart. Apply Wart-Off to warts only—not to surrounding skin. Let dry. Repeat this procedure once or twice daily as needed (until wart is removed) for up to 12 weeks. Replace cap tightly to prevent evaporation.

How Supplied: 0.5 fluid ounce bottle with special pinpoint plastic applicator and instructional brochure.

PolyMedica Pharmaceuticals (U.S.A.), Inc.
2 CONSTITUTION WAY
WOBURN, MA 01801

ALCONEFRIN®
Phenylephrine hydrochloride
Nasal Decongestant

How Supplied:
Drops 1 oz., 0.16%, 0.25%, 0.50%
Spray 1 oz., 0.25%

AZO-STANDARD™
Phenazopyridine hydrochloride
Urinary Tract Analgesic Tablets

Description: Each tablet contains phenazopyridine hydrochloride 95mg.

Indication: An analgesic for use as an aid for the prompt temporary relief of minor pain, urgency, frequency and burning of urination.

Directions: Adults: 2 tablets 3 times a day after meals. Use is only recommended for up to 2 days. For children under 12, consult a physician.

Warnings: Do not administer to children under 12 unless directed by a physician. Individuals with any hepatic or renal trouble should not use this product unless directed by a physician. Do not use for more than two days without consulting a physician. If you are pregnant or nursing a baby, seek the advice of a physician before using this product. Keep out of the reach of children. If symptoms persist, consult a physician.
Store at room temperature.

How Supplied: Cartons of 30 tablets.

NEOPAP®
Acetaminophen, 125mg
Analgesic

How Supplied: Pediatric Suppositories, 12's

Premier, Inc.
GREENWICH OFFICE PARK ONE
GREENWICH, CT 06831

EXACT™
[*Ex-áct*]
Benzoyl Peroxide Acne Medication Vanishing Cream

Active Ingredient: Benzoyl Peroxide 5.0% in a colorless, odorless, and greaseless cream base containing water, acrylates co-polymer, glycerin, sorbitol, cetyl alcohol, glyceryl dilaurate, stearyl alcohol, sodium lauryl sulfate, magnesium aluminum silicates, sodium citrate, silica, citric acid, methylparaben, xanthan gum and propylparaben.

Indications: For the topical treatment of acne vulgaris

Actions: Exact cream contains 5% benzoyl peroxide. The product clears existing pimples and helps prevent new pimples from forming.

Additional Benefits: Exact utilizes a patented Microsponge® delivery system to provide prolonged release of benzoyl peroxide to the skin. This special Microsponge formula was designed for low irritancy and to provide 50% higher oil absorbancy than other benzoyl peroxide medications.

Warning: For external use only. Using other topical acne medications at the same time or immediately following use of this product may increase dryness or irritation of the skin. If this occurs, only one medication should be used unless directed by a doctor. Do not use this medication if you have very sensitive skin or if you are sensitive to benzoyl peroxide. This product may cause irritation, characterized by redness, burning, itching, peeling, or possibly swelling. Mild irritation may be reduced by using the product less frequently or in a lower concentration. If irritation becomes severe, discontinue use; if irritation still continues, consult a doctor. Keep away from eyes, lips, and mouth. This product may bleach hair or dyed fabrics. Store at room temperature. Keep away from flame, fire and heat.
KEEP THIS AND ALL DRUGS OUT OF REACH OF CHILDREN.

Symptoms and Treatment of Ingestion: These symptoms are based upon medical judgement, not on actual experience. Theoretically, ingestion of very large amounts may cause nausea, vomiting, abdominal discomfort and diarrhea. Treatment is symptomatic, with bed rest and observation.

Directions for Use: Cleanse the skin thoroughly before applying medication. Cover the entire affected area with a thin layer one to three times daily. Because excessive drying of the skin may occur, start with one application daily, then gradually increase to two or three times daily if needed or as directed by a doctor. If bothersome dryness or peeling occurs, reduce application to once a day or every other day.

How Supplied: .65 oz. plastic squeeze tubes.

Procter & Gamble
P. O. BOX 5516
CINCINNATI, OH 45201

CHILDREN'S CHLORASEPTIC® LOZENGES
Benzocaine/Oral Anesthetic (Grape Flavor)

Active Ingredient: Benzocaine 5 mg per lozenge.

Inactive Ingredients: Corn syrup, FD&C Blue No. 1, FD&C Red No. 40, flavor, and sucrose.

Indications: For temporary relief of occasional minor mouth irritation and pain, sore mouth and sore throat. Also for pain associated with canker sores.

Directions: Adults and children 2 years of age and older: Allow 1 lozenge to dissolve slowly in mouth. May be repeated every 2 hours as needed or as directed by a physician or dentist. Children under 2 years of age: Consult a physician or a dentist.

WARNINGS: If sore throat is severe, or is accompanied by difficulty in breathing, or persists for more than two days, do not use, and consult a doctor promptly. If sore throat is accompanied or followed by fever, headache, rash, swelling, nausea, or vomiting, consult a doctor promptly. If sore mouth symptoms do not improve in 7 days, or if irritation, pain, or redness persists or worsens, see your doctor promptly. **KEEP THIS AND ALL DRUGS OUT OF THE REACH OF CHILDREN.** In case of accidental overdose seek professional assistance or contact a poison control center immediately. As with any drug, if you are pregnant or nursing a baby, seek the advice of a health professional before using this product.

How Supplied: Cartons of 18.

VICKS® CHILDREN'S CHLORASEPTIC® SPRAY
Phenol/Oral Anesthetic/Antiseptic

Children's Chloraseptic is specially formulated with a reduced concentration of phenol, the active ingredient in Advanced Formula Chloraseptic, to provide fast, effective relief in a great-tasting grape flavor your child will like.
Children can also use great-tasting Children's Chloraseptic lozenges in a pleasant grape flavor.

Active Ingredient: Phenol 0.5%

Inactive Ingredients: FD&C Blue No. 1, FD&C Red No. 40, flavor, glycerin, purified water, saccharin sodium, and sorbitol.

Indications: For temporary relief of your child's occasional minor sore throat pain and sore mouth. Also, for temporary relief of pain due to canker sores, minor irritation or injury of the mouth and gums, minor dental procedures, and orthodontic appliances.

Directions—Children 2 Years of Age and Over: Spray 5 times directly on throat or affected area and swallow. Repeat every two hours or as directed by a physician or dentist. Children under 12 years of age should be supervised in product use.
Children Under 2 Years of Age: Consult a physician or dentist.

WARNINGS: If sore throat is severe, or is accompanied by difficulty in breathing, or persists for more than 2 days, do not use, and consult a doctor promptly. If sore throat is accompanied or followed by fever, headache, rash, swelling, nausea or vomiting, consult a physician promptly. If sore mouth symptoms do not improve in 7 days, or if irritation, pain, or redness persists or worsens, see your doctor promptly. **KEEP THIS AND ALL DRUGS OUT OF THE REACH OF CHILDREN.** In case of accidental overdose, seek professional assistance or contact a poison control center immediately. As with any drug, if you are pregnant or nursing a baby, seek the advice of a health professional before using this product.

How Supplied: Available in 6 FL. OZ. plastic bottles with sprayer.

CHLORASEPTIC®
Phenol/oral anesthetic/antiseptic Cherry, Menthol and Cool Mint Flavors

Active Ingredient: Gargle and Spray—Phenol 1.4%.

Inactive Ingredients: Original Menthol Liquid: D&C Green No. 5, D&C Yellow No. 10, FD&C Green No. 3, flavor, glycerin, purified water, saccharin sodium.
Cherry Liquid: FD&C Red No. 40, flavor, glycerin, purified water, saccharin sodium.
Cool Mint Liquid: FD&C Blue No. 1, flavor, glycerin, purified water, saccharin sodium.

Indications: For temporary relief of occasional minor sore throat pain and sore mouth. Also for the temporary relief of pain due to canker sores, minor irritation or injury of the mouth and gums, minor dental procedures, dentures or orthodontic appliances.

Administration and Dosage: Chloraseptic Spray (Pump): Spray 5 times directly on throat or affected area. Children 2–12 years of age, spray 3 times and swallow. Repeat every 2 hours or as di-

Continued on next page

Procter & Gamble—Cont.

rected by a physician or dentist. Children under 12 years of age should be supervised in product use. Children under 2 years: consult a physician or dentist.
Chloraseptic Gargle: Adults and children 12 years of age and older: Gargle or swish around the mouth for at least 15 seconds and then spit out. Use every 2 hours or as directed by a physician or dentist. Children 6 to under 12 years: Gargle or swish around in mouth 2 teaspoonsful for at least 15 seconds and then spit out. Use every 2 hours or as directed by a physician or dentist. Children under 12 years should be supervised in product use. Children under 6 years: Consult a physician or dentist.

WARNINGS: If sore throat is severe, or is accompanied by difficulty in breathing, or persists for more than 2 days, do not use, and consult a doctor promptly. If sore throat is accompanied or followed by fever, headache, rash, swelling, nausea, or vomiting, consult a doctor promptly. If sore mouth symptoms do not improve in 7 days, or if irritation, pain, or redness persists or worsens, consult your doctor promptly. **KEEP THIS AND ALL DRUGS OUT OF THE REACH OF CHILDREN.** In case of accidental overdose, seek professional assistance or contact a poison control center immediately. As with any drug, if you are pregnant or nursing a baby, seek the advice of a health professional before using this product.

How Supplied: Available in Original Menthol, Cherry, and Cool Mint flavors in 6 FL. OZ. plastic bottles with sprayer. Menthol and Cherry Flavors also available in 12 FL. OZ. gargle.

CHLORASEPTIC® LOZENGES
Cherry, Menthol, and Cool Mint Flavor
Menthol/Benzocaine
Oral Anesthetic

Active Ingredients: Benzocaine 6 mg, Menthol 10 mg

Inactive Ingredients:
Menthol Lozenges: Corn syrup, D&C Yellow No. 10, FD&C Blue No. 1, FD&C Yellow No. 6, flavor and sucrose.
Cherry Lozenges: Corn syrup, FD&C Blue No. 1, FD&C Red No. 40, flavor and sucrose.
Cool Mint Lozenges: Corn syrup, FD&C Blue No. 1, flavor and sucrose.

Indications: For temporary relief of occasional minor mouth irritation and pain, sore mouth and sore throat. Also, for pain associated with canker sores.

Directions:
Adults and children 2 years of age and older: Allow 1 lozenge to dissolve slowly in mouth. May be repeated every 2 hours as needed or as directed by a physician or dentist. Children under 2 years of age: Consult a physician or a dentist.

WARNINGS: If sore throat is severe, or is accompanied by difficulty in breathing, or persists for more than two days, do not use, and consult a doctor promptly. If sore throat is accompanied or followed by fever, headache, rash, swelling, nausea, or vomiting, consult a doctor promptly. If sore mouth symptoms do not improve in 7 days, see your doctor promptly. Do not use this product if you have a history of allergy to local anesthetics such as procaine, butacaine, or other "caine" anesthetics. **KEEP THIS AND ALL DRUGS OUT OF THE REACH OF CHILDREN.** In case of accidental overdose seek professional assistance or contact a poison control center immediately. As with any drug if you are pregnant or nursing a baby, seek the advice of a health professional before using this product.

How Supplied: Available in Cool Mint, Cherry, and Menthol lozenges in packages of 18.

HEAD & SHOULDERS®
Antidandruff Shampoo

Head & Shoulders Shampoo offers effective dandruff control and beautiful hair in a formula that is pleasant to use. Independently conducted clinical testing (double-blind and dermatologist-graded) has proved that Head & Shoulders reduces dandruff flaking. Head & Shoulders is also gentle enough to use every day for clean, manageable hair.

Active Ingredient: 1.0% pyrithione zinc suspended in an anionic detergent system. Cosmetic ingredients are also included.

Indications: For effective control of typical dandruff and seborrheic dermatitis of the scalp.

Actions: Pyrithione zinc is substantive to the scalp and remains after rinsing. Its mechanism of action has not been fully established, but it is believed to control the microorganisms associated with dandruff flaking and itching.

WARNINGS: Not to be taken internally. Keep out of children's reach. Avoid getting shampoo in eyes—if this happens, rinse eyes with water. If scalp condition worsens or does not improve after regular use of this product as directed, consult a doctor.

Dosage and Administration: For best results in controlling dandruff, Head & Shoulders should be used regularly. It is gentle enough to use for every shampoo. In treating seborrheic dermatitis, a minimum of four shampooings are needed to achieve full effectiveness.

Composition:
Lotion—Fine or Oily Hair Formula: Pyrithione zinc in a shampoo base of water, ammonium laureth sulfate, ammonium lauryl sulfate, cocamide MEA, glycol distearate, ammonium xylenesulfonate, fragrance, citric acid, DMDM hydantoin, sodium chloride, citric acid and FD&C Blue No. 1.
Lotion—Normal or Dry Hair Formula: Pyrithione zinc in a shampoo base of water, ammonium laureth sulfate, ammonium lauryl sulfate, cocamide MEA, dimethicone, glycol distearate, ammonium xylenesulfonate, tricetylmonium chloride, fragrance, cetyl aclohol, stearyl alcohol, DMDM hydantoin, sodium chloride and FD&C Blue No. 1.
Lotion 2-in-1 (Complete Dandruff Shampoo plus Conditioner in One) Formula: Pyrithione zinc in a shampoo base of water, ammonium lauryl sulfate, ammonium laureth sulfate, dimethicone, glycol distearate, cocamide MEA, ammonium xylenesulfonate, fragrance, tricetylmonium chloride, cetyl alcohol, stearyl alcohol, sodium chloride, DMDM hydantoin, sodium phosphate, disodium phosphate and FD&C Blue No. 1.
Cream—Normal to Oily Formula: Pyrithione zinc in a shampoo base of water, sodium cocoglyceryl ether sulfonate, sodium chloride, sodium lauroyl sarcosinate, lauramide DEA, cocoyl sarcosine, fragrance, and FD&C Blue No. 1.

How Supplied: Fine/Oily Lotion—32, 28 pump, 15, 11, 7 oz.
Normal to Dry—28 oz. pump, 15, 11, 7 oz.
2 in 1—12.5 oz., 9 oz.
Fine/Oily Conc—5.5 oz.

HEAD & SHOULDERS® DRY SCALP SHAMPOO

Head & Shoulders Dry Scalp Shampoo offers effective control of irritating itching and flaking due to dandruff and dry scalp. Dry Scalp Shampoo is gentle enough to use every day for clean, manageable hair.

Active Ingredient: 1.0% pyrithione zinc suspended in a mild surfactant base. Shampoo also includes mild conditioning agents.

Indications: For effective control of dandruff.

Actions: Mild surfactants' gentle action reduces insult to the scalp, allowing the scalp to maintain its natural moisture balance. Pyrithione zinc is substantive to the scalp, and remains after rinsing.

WARNINGS: Not to be taken internally. Keep out of children's reach. Avoid getting shampoo in eyes—if this happens, rinse eyes with water. If scalp condition worsens or does not improve after regular use of the product as directed, consult a doctor.

Dosage and Administration: For best results in controlling dandruff, dry scalp and dry scalp symptoms, Head & Shoulders Dry Scalp Shampoo should be used regularly. It is gentle enough to use for every shampoo.

Composition:
Lotion—Dry Scalp Regular Formula: Pyrithione zinc in a shampoo base of water, ammonium laureth sulfate, ammonium lauryl sulfate, cocamide MEA, glycol distearate, dimethicone, ammonium xylenesulfonate, fragrance, tricetylmonium chloride, cetyl alcohol, stearyl alcohol, DMDM hydantoin, sodium chloride, FD&C Blue no. 1.
Lotion—Dry Scalp Conditioning Formula: Pyrithione zinc in a shampoo base of water, ammonium laureth sulfate, ammonium lauryl sulfate, cocamide MEA, glycol distearate, dimethicone, ammonium xylenesulfonate, fragrance, tricetylmonium chloride, cetyl alcohol, stearyl alcohol, DMDM hydantoin, sodium chloride, FD&C Blue no. 1.
Lotion—Dry Scalp 2-in-1 (Dry Scalp Shampoo Plus Conditioner in One) Formula: Pyrithione zinc in a shampoo base of water, ammonium laureth sulfate, ammonium lauryl sulfate, cocamide MEA, glycol distearate, dimethicone, ammonium xylenesulfonate, fragrance, tricetylmonium chloride, cetyl alcohol, stearyl alcohol, DMDM hydantoin, sodium chloride, and FD&C Blue no. 1.

How Supplied: Dry Scalp Regular and Conditioning lotions are available in 7.0, 11.0, and 15.0 fl. oz. unbreakable plastic bottles. Dry Scalp 2-in-1 is available in 9.0 and 12.5 fl. oz. unbreakable plastic bottles.

HEAD & SHOULDERS® INTENSIVE TREATMENT DANDRUFF SHAMPOO

Head & Shoulders Intensive Treatment Dandruff Shampoo offers effective control of persistent dandruff, and beautiful hair from a pleasant-to-use formula. Double-blind and expert-graded testing have proven that Intensive Treatment Dandruff Shampoo reduces persistent dandruff. It is also gentle enough to use every day for clean, manageable hair.

Active Ingredient: 1% selenium sulfide suspended in a mild surfactant base. Shampoo also includes mild conditioning agents.

Indications: For effective control of seborrheic dermatitis and dandruff of the scalp.

Actions: Selenium sulfide is substantive to the scalp and remains after rinsing. Its mechanism is believed to be antiproliferative, and to also control the microorganisms associated with persistent dandruff flaking and itching.

WARNINGS: For external use only. Avoid contact with eyes—if this happens, rinse thoroughly with water. If scalp condition worsens, or does not improve, consult a doctor. Keep out of reach of children.

Caution: If used on light, gray, or chemically treated hair, rinse **(VIGOROUSLY)** for 5 minutes.

Dosage and Administration: For best results in controlling persistent dandruff, Head & Shoulders Intensive Treatment Dandruff Shampoo should be used regularly. It is gentle enough to use for every shampoo.

Composition:
Lotion—Intensive Treatment Regular Formula: Ingredients: Selenium sulfide in a shampoo base of water, ammonium laureth sulfate, ammonium lauryl sulfate, cocamide MEA, glycol distearate, ammonium xylenesulfonate, dimethicone, fragrance, tricetylmonium chloride, cetyl alcohol, DMDM hydantoin, sodium chloride, stearyl alcohol, hydroxypropyl methylcellulose, FD&C Red no. 4.
Lotion—Intensive Treatment 2-in-1 (Persistent Dandruff Shampoo plus Conditioner in One) Formula: Selenium sulfide in a shampoo base of water, ammonium laureth sulfate, ammonium lauryl sulfate, cocamide MEA, glycol distearate, dimethicone, ammonium xylenesulfonate, fragrance, tricetylmonium chloride, cetyl alcohol, DMDM hydantoin, sodium chloride, stearyl alcohol, hydroxypropyl methylcellulose, FD&C Red no. 4.

How Supplied: Intensive Treatment Regular Lotion is available in 7.0 and 11.0 fl. oz. unbreakable plastic bottles. Intensive Treatment 2-in-1 is available in 6.0 and 8.9 fl. oz. unbreakable plastic bottles.

METAMUCIL®
[met'uh-mū'sil]
(psyllium hydrophilic mucilloid)

Description: Metamucil is a bulk-forming natural therapeutic fiber for restoring and maintaining regularity as recommended by a physician. It contains hydrophilic mucilloid, a highly efficient dietary fiber derived from the husk of the psyllium seed (*Plantago ovata*). Metamucil contains no chemical stimulants and is nonaddictive. Each dose contains approximately 3.4 grams of psyllium hydrophilic mucilloid. Inactive ingredients, sodium, potassium, calories, carbohydrate, fat and phenylalanine content are shown in Table 1 for all forms and flavors. NutraSweet®* brand sweetener (aspartame) is used in flavored sugar-free Metamucil powdered products. Metamucil Sugar-Free Regular Flavor contains no sugar and no artificial sweeteners; it contains 129 mg of magnesium per dose. Phenylketonurics should be aware that phenylalanine is present in Metamucil products that contain Nutrasweet.

*NutraSweet® is a registered trademark of the NutraSweet Company.

Metamucil in powdered forms is gluten-free.
Wafers contain gluten: Apple Crisp contains 0.7 g/dose, Cinnamon Spice contains 0.5 g/dose.

Actions: The active ingredient in Metamucil is psyllium, a natural fiber which promotes elimination due to its bulking effect in the colon. This bulking effect is due to both the water-holding capacity of undigested fiber and the increased bacterial mass following partial fiber digestion. This results in enlargement of the lumen of the colon, thereby decreasing intraluminal pressure and speeding colonic transit in constipated patients.

Indications: Metamucil is indicated in the management of chronic constipation, in irritable bowel syndrome, as adjunctive therapy in the constipation of diverticular disease, in the bowel management of patients with hemorrhoids, and for constipation during pregnancy, convalescence, and senility.

Contraindications: Intestinal obstruction, fecal impaction.

WARNINGS: Patients are advised they should not use the product without consulting a doctor when abdominal pain, nausea, or vomiting are present, if they have noticed a sudden change in bowel habits that persists over a period of 2 weeks, or rectal bleeding, or if they have been diagnosed with esophageal narrowing or have difficulty in swallowing. Patients are advised to consult a physician if constipation persists for longer than one week, as this may be a sign of a serious medical condition. Psyllium products may cause allergic reaction in people sensitive to inhaled or ingested psyllium. Keep this and all medications out of the reach of children.

Precaution: *Notice to Health Care Professionals:* To minimize the potential for allergic reaction, health care professionals who frequently dispense powdered psyllium products should avoid inhaling airborne dust while dispensing these products. *Handling and Dispensing:* To minimize generating airborne dust, spoon product from the canister into a glass according to label directions.

Dosage and Administration: The usual adult dosage is 1 rounded teaspoonful or 1 rounded tablespoonful depending on product form. Generally the sugar-free products are dosed by the teaspoonful, sucrose-containing products by the tablespoonful. Some forms are available in packets. The appropriate dose should be mixed with 8 oz. of liquid (e.g. cool water, fruit juice, milk) following the labelled instructions. Metamucil wafers should be consumed with 8 oz. of liquid. An additional glass of liquid after each dose is helpful. Metamucil can be taken orally one to three times a day, depend-

Continued on next page

Procter & Gamble—Cont.

TABLE 1

Forms/ Flavors	Inactive Ingredients	Sodium mg/ Dose	Potassium mg/ Dose	Calories per Dose	Carbohydrate g/ Dose	Fat g/ Dose	Phenylalanine mg/Dose	Dosage 1–3 Times Daily. Each Dose Contains 3.4 g Psyllium Hydrophilic Mucilloid	How Supplied
Regular Flavor METAMUCIL Powder	Dextrose	<5	30	14	6	—	—	1 rounded teaspoonful 7 g	Canisters: 13, 19 and 29 ozs.
Orange Flavor METAMUCIL Powder	Citric acid, FD&C Yellow No. 6, Flavoring, Sucrose	<5	35	30	10	—	—	1 rounded tablespoonful 11 g	Canisters: 13, 19 and 29 ozs.
Sugar-Free Lemon-Lime Flavor METAMUCIL Effervescent Powder	Aspartame, Calcium carbonate, Citric acid, Flavoring, Potassium bicarbonate, Silicon dioxide, Sodium bicarbonate	10	280	6	4	—	30	1 packet 5.4 g	Cartons: 30 single-dose packets (OTC), 100 single-dose packets (Institutional)
Sugar-Free Orange-Flavor METAMUCIL Effervescent Powder	Aspartame, Citric acid, FD&C Yellow No. 6, Flavoring, Potassium bicarbonate, Silicon dioxide, Sodium bicarbonate	5	280	6	4	—	28	1 packet 5.2 g	Cartons: 30 single-dose packets (OTC)
Sunrise Smooth Orange Flavor METAMUCIL Powder	Citric acid, D&C Yellow No. 10, FD&C Yellow No. 6, Flavoring, Sucrose	<5	30	35	12	—	—	1 rounded tablespoonful 12 g	Canisters: 13, 19 and 29 ozs.; Cartons: 30 single-dose packets (OTC)
Sunrise Smooth Citrus Flavor METAMUCIL Powder	Citric acid, D&C Yellow No. 10, FD&C Yellow No. 6, Flavoring, Sucrose	<5	40	35	12	—	—	1 rounded tablespoonful 12 g	Canisters: 13, 19 and 29 ozs.; Cartons: 30 single-dose packets (OTC) 100 single-dose packets (Institutional)
Sunrise Smooth Sugar-Free Orange Flavor METAMUCIL Powder	Aspartame, Citric acid, D&C Yellow No. 10, FD&C Yellow No. 6, Flavoring, Maltodextrin	<5	30	10	5	—	25	1 rounded teaspoonful 5.8 g	Canisters: 10, 15 and 23 ozs.; Cartons: 30 single-dose packets (OTC), 100 single-dose packets (Institutional)
Sunrise Smooth Sugar-Free Citrus Flavor METAMUCIL Powder	Aspartame, Citric acid, D&C Yellow No. 10, FD&C Yellow No. 6, Flavoring, Maltodextrin	<5	30	10	5	—	25	1 rounded teaspoonful 5.8 g	Canisters: 10, 15 and 23 ozs.; Cartons: 30 single-dose packets (OTC)
Sunrise Smooth Sugar-Free Regular Flavor METAMUCIL Powder	Citric Acid (less than 1%), Magnesium Sulfate, Maltodextrin	<5	30	10	5	—	—	1 rounded teaspoonful 5.8 g	Canisters: 10, 15 and 23 oz.
Apple Crisp METAMUCIL Wafers	Ascorbic acid, Brown sugar, Cinnamon, Corn oil, Flavors, Fructose, Lecithin, Modified food starch, Molasses, Oat hull fiber, Sodium bicarbonate, Sucrose, Water, Wheat flour	20	50	100	19	5	—	2 wafers 25 g	Cartons: 12 doses; 24 doses
Cinnamon Spice METAMUCIL Wafers	Ascorbic acid, Cinnamon, Corn oil, Flavors, Fructose, Lecithin, Modified food starch, Molasses, Nutmeg, Oat hull fiber, Oats, Sodium bicarbonate, Sucrose, Water, Wheat flour	20	45	100	18	5	—	2 wafers 25 g	Cartons: 12 doses; 24 doses

ing on the need and response. It may require continued use for 2 to 3 days to provide optimal benefit. For children (6 to 12 years old), use ½ the adult dose in/with 8 oz of liquid, 1 to 3 times daily.

New Users:
(Label statement)
Your doctor can recommend the right dosage of Metamucil to best meet your needs. In general, start by taking one dose each day. Gradually increase to three doses per day, if needed or recommended by your doctor. If minor gas or bloating occurs when you increase doses, try slightly reducing the amount you are taking.

How Supplied:
Powder: canisters (OTC) and cartons of single-dose packets (OTC and Institutional).
Wafers: cartons of single-dose packets (OTC). (See Table 1 [on preceding page]).

OIL OF OLAY®—Daily UV Protectant SPF 15 Beauty Fluid—Original and Fragrance Free Versions
(Olay Co., Inc.)

Oil of Olay Daily UV Protectant Beauty Fluid is a light, greaseless lotion that is specially formulated to provide effective moisturization and SPF 15 protection.
Oil of Olay Daily UV Protectant is PABA free. It is non-comedogenic and is suitable for daily use under facial make-up.

Active Ingredients: Ethylhexyl p-Methoxycinnamate, 2-Phenylbenzimidazole-5-Sulfonic Acid.

Inactive Ingredients: Water, Isohexadecane, Butylene Glycol, Triethanolamine, Glycerin, Stearic Acid, Cetyl Alcohol, Cetyl Palmitate, DEA-Cetyl Phosphate, Aluminum Starch Octenylsuccinate, Titanium Dioxide, Imidazolidinyl Urea, Methylparaben, Propylparaben, Carbomer, Acrylates/C10–30 Alkyl Acrylate Crosspolymer, PEG-10 Soya Sterol, Disodium EDTA, Castor Oil, Fragrance, FD&C Red No. 4, FD&C Yellow No. 5.
Available in a both a lightly scented original version and a 100% color free and fragrance-free version.

Indications: Provides SPF 15 UV protection to help protect against skin-aging UV rays in a light, greaseless moisturizer. The liberal and regular use of the product over the years may help reduce the chance of premature skin aging and skin cancer.

Directions: Apply liberally as needed to face, neck and other exposed areas for protection against UV rays and for moisturization.

WARNINGS: For external use only. Not to be swallowed. Avoid contact with eyes. Discontinue use if signs of irritation or rash appear. Use on children under six months of age only with the advice of a physician. **KEEP OUT OF REACH OF CHILDREN.**

How Supplied: Available in 3.5 fl. oz. and 5.25 fl. oz. plastic bottles.

OIL OF OLAY®—Daily UV Protectant SPF 15 Moisture Replenishing Cream—Original and Fragrance Free Versions
(Olay Co., Inc.)

Oil of Olay Daily UV Protectant Moisture Replenishing Cream is an extra-rich cream specially formulated to provide effective moisturization and SPF 15 protection. Oil of Olay Daily UV Protectant is PABA free. It is non-comedogenic and is suitable for daily use under facial make-up.

Active Ingredients: Ethylhexyl p-Methoxycinnamate, 2-Phenylbenzimidazole-5-Sulfonic Acid.

Inactive Ingredients: Water, Isohexadecane, Glycerin, Butylene Glycol, Triethanolamine, Stearic Acid, Cetyl Alcohol, Cetyl Palmitate, DEA-Cetyl Phosphate, Aluminum Starch Octenylsuccinate, Titanium Dioxide, Imidazolidinyl Urea, Methylparaben, Propylparaben, Carbomer, Acrylates/C10–30 Alkyl Acrylate Crosspolymer, PEG-10 Soya Sterol, Disodium EDTA, Castor Oil, Fragrance, FD&C Red No. 4, FD&C Yellow No. 5.
Available in both lightly scented original version and a 100% color and fragrance free version.

Indications: Provides SPF 15 UV protection to help protect against skin-aging UV rays in a light, greaseless moisturizer. The liberal and regular use of the product over the years may help reduce the chance of premature aging of the skin and skin cancer.

Directions: Apply liberally as needed to face, neck and other exposed areas for protection against UV rays and for moisturization.

WARNINGS: For external use only. Not to be swallowed. Avoid contact with eyes. Discontinue use if signs of irritation or rash appear. Use on children under six months of age only with the advice of a physician. **KEEP OUT OF REACH OF CHILDREN.**

How Supplied: Available in 1.7 oz. glass jar.

PEPTO-BISMOL® ORIGINAL LIQUID AND ORIGINAL AND CHERRY TABLETS
For diarrhea, heartburn, indigestion, upset stomach and nausea.

Multi-symptom Pepto-Bismol contains bismuth subsalicylate and is the only leading OTC stomach remedy clinically proven effective for both upper and lower GI symptoms. Pepto-Bismol is in more households than any other stomach remedy, making it a convenient recommendation with a name your patients will know. It has been clinically-proven in double-blind placebo-controlled trials for relief of upset stomach symptoms and diarrhea.

Description: Each Pepto-Bismol Tablet contains 262 mg bismuth subsalicylate and each tablespoonful (15 ml) of Pepto-Bismol Liquid contains 262 mg bismuth subsalicylate. Each tablet contains 102 mg salicylate (99 mg salicylate for Cherry) and each tablespoonful of liquid contains 130 mg salicylate. Liquid and tablets contain no sugar. Tablets are very low in sodium (less than 2 mg/tablet) and Liquid is low in sodium (less than 3 mg/tablespoonful). Inactive ingredients include (Tablets): adipic acid (in Cherry only), calcium carbonate, D&C Red No. 27, FD&C Red No. 40 (in Cherry only), flavors, magnesium stearate, mannitol, povidone, saccharin sodium and talc; (Liquid): benzoic acid, D&C Red No. 22, D&C Red No. 28, flavor, magnesium aluminum silicate, methylcellulose, saccharin sodium, salicylic acid, sodium salicylate, sorbic acid and water.

Indications: Pepto-Bismol controls diarrhea within 24 hours, relieving associated abdominal cramps; soothes heartburn and indigestion without constipating; and relieves nausea and upset stomach.

Actions: For upset stomach symptoms (i.e. heartburn, indigestion, nausea and fullness caused by over-indulgence), the active ingredient is believed to work via a topical effect on the stomach mucosa. For diarrhea, it is believed to work by several mechanisms in the gastro-intestinal tract, including: 1) by normalizing fluid movement via an antisecretory mechanism and 2) by binding bacterial toxins and antimicrobial activity.

WARNINGS: Children and teenagers who have or are recovering from chicken pox or flu should not use this medicine to treat nausea or vomiting. If nausea or vomiting is present, patients are advised

Continued on next page

Procter & Gamble—Cont.

to consult a doctor because this could be an early sign of Reye Syndrome, a rare but serious illness.
This product contains salicylates. If taken with aspirin and ringing in the ears occurs, discontinue use. This product does not contain aspirin, but should not be administered to those patients who have a known allergy to aspirin or salicylates. Caution is advised in the administration to patients taking medication for anticoagulation, diabetes and gout.
If diarrhea is accompanied by a high fever or continues more than 2 days, patients are advised to consult a physician. As with any drug, caution is advised in the administration to pregnant or nursing women.

Note: This medication may cause a temporary and harmless darkening of the tongue and/or stool. Stool darkening should not be confused with melena.

Overdosage: In case of overdose, patients are advised to contact a physician or Poison Control Center. Emesis induced by ipecac syrup is indicated in large ingestions provided ipecac can be administered within one hour of ingestion. Activated charcoal should be administered after gastric emptying. Patients should be evaluated for signs and symptoms of salicylate toxicity.

Dosage and Administration
Tablets:
Adults—Two tablets
Children (according to age)—

9–12 yrs.	1 tablet
6–9 yrs.	⅔ tablet
3–6 yrs.	⅓ tablet

Chew or dissolve in mouth. Repeat every ½ to 1 hour as needed, to a maximum of 8 doses in a 24-hour period. Drink plenty of clear fluids to help prevent dehydration, which may accompany diarrhea.

Liquid: Shake well before using.
Adults—2 tablespoonsful (1 dose cup)
Children (according to age)—

9–12 yrs.	1 tablespoonful (½ dose cup)
6–9 yrs.	2 teaspoonsful (⅓ dose cup)
3–6 yrs.	1 teaspoonful (⅙ dose cup)

Repeat dosage every ½ to 1 hour, if needed, to a maximum of 8 doses in a 24-hour period. Drink plenty of clear fluids to help prevent dehydration which may accompany diarrhea.
For children under 3 years of age, consult physician.

How Supplied: Pepto-Bismol Liquid is available in: 4 fl. oz. bottle, 8 fl. oz. bottle, 12 fl. oz. bottle, 16 fl. oz. bottle. Pepto-Bismol Tablets are pink, round, chewable, tablets imprinted with "Pepto-Bismol" on one side. Tablets are available in: box of 30, box of 48, and roll pack of 12 (cherry only).

PEPTO-BISMOL® MAXIMUM STRENGTH LIQUID
For diarrhea, heartburn, indigestion, upset stomach and nausea.

Multi-symptom Pepto-Bismol contains bismuth subsalicylate and is the only leading OTC stomach remedy clinically proven effective for both upper and lower GI symptoms. Pepto-Bismol is in more households than any other stomach remedy, making it a convenient recommendation with a name your patients will know. It has been clinically-proven in double-blind placebo-controlled trials for relief of upset stomach symptoms and diarrhea.

Description: Each tablespoonful (15 ml) of Maximum Strength Pepto-Bismol Liquid contains 525 mg bismuth subsalicylate (236 mg salicylate). Maximum Strength Pepto-Bismol Liquid contains no sugar and is low in sodium (less than 3 mg/tablespoonful). Inactive ingredients include: benzoic acid, D&C Red No. 22, D&C Red No. 28, flavor, magnesium aluminum silicate, methylcellulose, saccharin sodium, salicylic acid, sodium salicylate, sorbic acid, and water.

Indications: Maximum Strength Pepto-Bismol controls diarrhea within 24 hours, relieving associated abdominal cramps; soothes heartburn and indigestion without constipating; and relieves nausea and upset stomach.

Actions: For upset stomach symptoms (i.e. heartburn, indigestion, nausea and fullness caused by over-indulgence), the active ingredient is believed to work via a topical effect on the stomach mucosa. For diarrhea, it is believed to work by several mechanisms in the gastro-intestinal tract, including: 1) by normalizing fluid movement via an antisecretory mechanism and 2) by binding bacterial toxins and antimicrobial activity.

WARNINGS: Children and teenagers who have or are recovering from chicken pox or flu should NOT use this medicine to treat nausea or vomiting. If nausea or vomiting is present, patients are advised to consult a doctor because this could be an early sign of Reye Syndrome, a rare but serious illness.
This product contains salicylates. If taken with aspirin and ringing in the ears occurs, discontinue use. This product does not contain aspirin, but should not be administered to those patients who have a known allergy to aspirin or salicylates. Caution is advised in the administration to patients taking medication for anticoagulation, diabetes and gout.
If diarrhea is accompanied by a high fever or continues more than 2 days, patients are advised to consult a physician. As with any drug, caution is advised in the administration to pregnant or nursing women.

Note: This medication may cause a temporary and harmless darkening of the tongue and/or stool. Stool darkening should not be confused with melena.

Overdosage: In case of overdose, patients are advised to contact a physician or Poison Control Center. Emesis induced by ipecac syrup is indicated in large ingestions provided ipecac can be administered within one hour of ingestion. Activated charcoal should be administered after gastric emptying. Patients should be evaluated for signs and symptoms of salicylate toxicity.

Dosage and Administration: Shake well before using.
Adults—2 tablespoonfuls (1 dose cup)
Children (according to age)—

9–12 yrs.	1 tablespoonful (½ dose cup)
6–9 yrs.	2 teaspoonfuls (⅓ dose cup)
3–6 yrs.	1 teaspoonful (⅙ dose cup)

Repeat dosage every hour, if needed, to a maximum of 4 doses in a 24-hour period. Drink plenty of clear fluids to help prevent dehydration, which may accompany diarrhea.

How Supplied: Maximum Strength Pepto-Bismol is available in:
4 fl. oz. bottle
8 fl. oz. bottle
12 fl. oz. bottle

PEPTO DIARRHEA CONTROL®
Loperamide Hydrochloride Oral Solution

Description: Each 5 ml (teaspoon) of Pepto Diarrhea Control contains Loperamide Hydrochloride 1 mg. Pepto Diarrhea Control is a non-chalky, cherry flavored, clear liquid.

Actions: Pepto Diarrhea Control contains a clinically proven antidiarrheal medication, Loperamide Hydrochloride, that works in many cases with just one dose. Loperamide Hydrochloride acts by slowing intestinal motility and by affecting water and electrolyte movement through the bowel.

Indication: Pepto Diarrhea Control controls the symptoms of diarrhea.

Directions: A dose cup is provided to accurately measure doses as noted below. Drink plenty of clear fluids to help prevent dehydration, which may accompany diarrhea.

Usual Dosage: Adults and children 12 years of age and older: Take four teaspoonfuls after first loose bowel move-

ment followed by two teaspoonfuls after each subsequent loose bowel movement but not more than eight teaspoonfuls a day for no more than two days.
Children 9–11 years old (60–95 lbs): Two teaspoonfuls after first loose bowel movement, followed by one teaspoonful after each subsequent loose bowel movement. Do not exceed six teaspoonfuls per day.
Children 6–8 years old (48–59 lbs): Two teaspoonfuls after first loose bowel movement, followed by one teaspoonful after each subsequent loose bowel movement. Do not exceed four teaspoonfuls per day.
Professional Dosage Schedule for children 2–5 years old (24–47 lbs): One teaspoon after first loose bowel movement, followed by one after each subsequent loose bowel movement. Do not exceed three teaspoonfuls a day.

WARNINGS: DO NOT USE FOR MORE THAN TWO DAYS UNLESS DIRECTED BY A PHYSICIAN. Do not use if diarrhea is accompanied by high fever (greater than 101°F), or if blood is present in the stool, or if you have had a rash or other allergic reaction to Loperamide Hydrochloride. If you are taking antibiotics or have a history of liver disease, consult a physician before using this product. As with any drug, if you are pregnant or nursing a baby, seek the advice of a health professional before using this product. Keep this and all drugs out of the reach of children. In case of accidental overdose, seek professional assistance or contact a poison control center immediately. Store at room temperature.

Overdosage: Overdosage of Loperamide Hydrochloride in man may result in constipation, CNS depression and nausea. A slurry of activated charcoal administered promptly after ingestion of Loperamide Hydrochloride can reduce the amount of drug which is absorbed. If vomiting occurs spontaneously upon ingestion, a slurry of 100 grams of activated charcoal should be administered orally as soon as fluids can be retained. If vomiting has not occurred, and CNS depression is evident, gastric lavage should be performed followed by administration of 100 gms of the activated charcoal slurry through the gastric tube. In the event of overdosage, patients should be monitored for signs of CNS depression for at least 24 hours. Children may be more sensitive to central nervous system effects than adults. If CNS depression is observed, naloxone may be administered. If responsive to naloxone, vital signs must be monitored carefully for recurrence of symptoms of drug overdose for at least 24 hours after the last dose of naloxone.

Inactive Ingredients: Alcohol (5.25%), citric acid, flavors, glycerin, methylparaben, propylparaben and purified water.

How Supplied: Cherry flavored liquid (clear) 2 fl. oz. and 4 fl. oz. tamper resistant bottles with child resistant safety caps and special dosage cups.

PERCOGESIC®

[pĕrkō-jē 'zĭk]

Analgesic Tablets
Pain Reliever/Fever Reducer

Active Ingredients: Each tablet contains:
Acetaminophen .... 325 mg
Phenyltoloxamine citrate .... 30 mg

Inactive Ingredients: Cellulose, Flavor, FD&C Yellow No. 6, Hydroxypropyl Methylcellulose, Magnesium Stearate, Polyethylene Glycol, Povidone, Silica Gel, Starch, Stearic Acid, Sucrose.

Indications: For temporary relief of minor aches and pains associated with headaches, muscular aches, backaches, premenstrual and menstrual periods, colds, flu, toothaches, as well as for minor arthritis pain, and to reduce fever.

Dosage and Administration: Adults and children (12 years and over)—1 or 2 tablets every four hours. Maximum daily dose—8 tablets.
Children (6 to under 12 years)—1 tablet every 4 hours. Maximum daily dose—4 tablets.
Children under 6 years of age: consult a doctor.

WARNINGS: Don't take this product for pain for more than 10 days (adults) or 5 days (children), and do not take for fever for more than 3 days unless directed by a doctor. If pain or fever persists or worsens, new symptoms occur or redness or swelling is present, consult a doctor as these could be signs of a serious condition. Don't give to children for arthritis pain unless directed by a doctor. May cause excitability especially in children. Do not take this product if you have asthma, glaucoma, emphysema, chronic pulmonary disease, shortness of breath, or difficulty in breathing unless directed by a doctor. May cause drowsiness; alcohol, sedatives, and tranquilizers may increase the drowsiness effect. Avoid alcoholic beverages while taking this product. Do not take this product if you are taking sedatives or tranquilizers without first consulting your doctor. Use caution when driving a motor vehicle or operating machinery. **KEEP THIS AND ALL DRUGS OUT OF THE REACH OF CHILDREN.** In case of accidental overdose, seek professional assistance or contact a poison control center immediately. Prompt medical attention is critical for adults as well as for children even if you do not notice any signs or symptoms. As with any drug, if you are pregnant or nursing a baby, seek the advice of a health professional before using this product.

How Supplied: Light orange tablets engraved with "Percogesic". Child-resistant bottles of 24 and 90 tablets, and non-child-resistant bottles of 50 tablets.

VICKS® CHILDREN'S NYQUIL® NIGHTTIME COLD/COUGH MEDICINE

Antihistamine/Nasal Decongestant/ Cough Suppressant

Children's NyQuil was specially formulated with three effective ingredients to relieve nighttime cough, nasal congestion, and runny nose so children can rest. Children's NyQuil is alcohol free and analgesic free and has a pleasant cherry flavor.

Active Ingredients: Per ½ FL. OZ. dose (1 TBSP.): Chlorpheniramine Maleate 2 mg, Pseudoephedrine HCl 30 mg, Dextromethorphan Hydrobromide 15 mg.

Inactive Ingredients: Citric Acid, FD&C Red No. 40, Flavor, Potassium Sorbate, Propylene Glycol, Purified Water, Sodium Citrate, Sucrose.

Indications: For temporary relief of nasal congestion, runny nose, sneezing, and coughing due to a cold, so your child can rest.

Directions: Take at bedtime as directed. Use medicine cup provided.
If cold symptoms keep your child at home, 4 doses may be given per day, each 6 hours apart, or use as directed by a doctor.

Age	Weight	Dose
Under 6 yrs	Under 48 lbs.	Consult physician*
6–11 yrs	48–95 lbs.	½ FL. OZ. (1 TBSP.)
12 yrs and over	96 lbs. and over	1 FL. OZ. (2 TBSP.)

* **Professional Labeling:** Children under 6 years of age: Use only as directed by a physician.
Suggested doses for children under 6 years of age:

Age	Weight	Dose
* 6–11 mo.	17–21 lbs.	1 tsp. (5 mL)
*12–23 mo.	22–27 lbs.	1¼ tsp. (6.25 mL)
2–5 yrs.	28–47 lbs.	½ TBSP. (7.5 mL)

Repeat every 6 hours, not to exceed 4 doses in 24 hours, or as directed by doctor.

* Based on extrapolation from studies on the safety and efficacy of active ingredients conducted among older children and adults. Use caution in treating children under 2 years of age who were born prematurely.

Continued on next page

Procter & Gamble—Cont.

WARNINGS: Do not exceed recommended dosage because at higher doses nervousness, dizziness or sleeplessness may occur. Do not take this product for more than 7 days. If symptoms do not improve or are accompanied by fever, consult a doctor. Do not take this product if you have heart disease, high blood pressure, thyroid disease, diabetes, or difficulty in urination due to enlargement of the prostate gland unless directed by a doctor. *DRUG INTERACTION PRECAUTION:* Do not take this product if you are presently taking a prescription drug for high blood pressure or depression, without first consulting your doctor. May cause excitability especially in children. Do not take this product if you have asthma, glaucoma, emphysema, chronic pulmonary disease, shortness of breath, or difficulty in breathing unless directed by a doctor. May cause marked drowsiness; alcohol, sedatives, and tranquilizers may increase the drowsiness effect. Avoid alcoholic beverages while taking this product. Do not take this product if you are taking sedatives or tranquilizers, without first consulting your doctor. Use caution when driving a motor vehicle or operating machinery. A persistent cough may be a sign of a serious condition. If cough persists for more than 1 week, tends to recur, or is accompanied by fever, rash, or persistent headache, consult a doctor. Do not take this product for persistent or chronic cough such as occurs with smoking, asthma, emphysema, or if cough is accompanied by excessive phlegm (mucus) unless directed by a doctor.
KEEP THIS AND ALL DRUGS OUT OF THE REACH OF CHILDREN. In case of accidental overdose, seek professional assistance or contact a poison control center immediately. As with any drug, if you are pregnant or nursing a baby, seek the advice of a health professional before using this product.

How Supplied: Available in 4 FL. OZ. and 8 FL. OZ. bottles with child-resistant, tamper-evident cap and a calibrated medicine cup.

VICKS® CHILDREN'S NYQUIL®
Nighttime Allergy/Head Cold Medicine
Antihistamine/Nasal Decongestant

Children's NyQuil Allergy/Head Cold Medicine was specially formulated with two effective ingredients to relieve allergy symptoms and head colds without coughs.

Active Ingredients per ½ FL. OZ. Dose (1 TBSP): Chlorpheniramine Maleate 2 mg, Pseudoephedrine HCl 30 mg

Inactive Ingredients: Citric Acid, FD&C Blue No. 1, FD&C Red No. 40, Flavors, Methylparaben, Potassium Sorbate, Propylene Glycol, Purified Water, Sodium Citrate, Sorbitol and Sucrose.

Indications: For temporary relief of nasal congestion, runny nose, and sneezing due to a cold. Also relieves nasal and sinus congestion, sneezing, runny nose, and itchy, watery eyes due to hay fever or other upper respiratory allergies.

Directions: Take at bedtime as directed. Use medicine cup provided. If symptoms keep your child at home, 4 doses may be given per day, each 6 hours apart, or use as directed by a doctor.

Age	Weight	Dose
Under 6 yrs	Under 48 lbs.	Consult Physician*
6–11 yrs	48–95 lbs.	½ FL. OZ. (1 TBSP.)
12 yrs and over	96 lbs. and over	1 FL. OZ. (2 TBSP.)

***Professional Labeling:** Children under 6 years of age: Use only as directed by a physician. Suggested doses for children under 6 years of age:

Age	Weight	Dose
*6–11 mo.	17–21 lbs.	1 tsp. (5 mL)
*12–23 mo.	22–27 lbs.	1¼ tsp. (6.25 mL)
2–5 yrs.	28–47 lbs.	½ TBSP. (7.5 mL)

Repeat every 6 hours, not to exceed 4 doses in 24 hours, or as directed by doctor.
*Based on extrapolation from studies on the safety and efficacy of active ingredients conducted among older children and adults. Use caution in treating children under 2 years of age who were born prematurely.

WARNINGS: Do not exceed recommended dosage, because at higher doses nervousness, dizziness or sleeplessness may occur. Do not take this product for more than 7 days. If symptoms do not improve or are accompanied by fever, consult a doctor. Do not take this product if you have heart disease, high blood pressure, thyroid disease, diabetes, or difficulty in urination due to enlargement of the prostate gland unless directed by a doctor. *DRUG INTERACTION PRECAUTION:* Do not take this product if you are presently taking a prescription drug for high blood pressure or depression, without first consulting your doctor. May cause excitability especially in children. Do not take this product if you have asthma, glaucoma, emphysema, chronic pulmonary disease, shortness of breath, or difficulty in breathing, unless directed by a doctor. May cause drowsiness; alcohol, sedatives, and tranquilizers may increase the drowsiness effect. Avoid alcoholic beverages while taking this product. Do not take this product if you are taking sedatives or tranquilizers, without first consulting your doctor. Use caution when driving a motor vehicle or operating machinery. **KEEP THIS AND ALL DRUGS OUT OF THE REACH OF CHILDREN.** In case of accidental overdose, seek professional assistance or contact a poison control center immediately. As with any drug, if you are pregnant or nursing a baby, seek the advice of a health professional before using this product.

How Supplied: Available in 4 FL. OZ. bottles with child-resistant, tamper-evident cap and a calibrated medicine cup.

VICKS® COUGH DROPS
Menthol Cough Suppressant/Oral Anesthetic

Flavors: Available in two popular flavors: Menthol and Cherry.

Active Ingredient: Menthol.

Inactive Ingredients:
Menthol Flavor: Benzyl Alcohol, Camphor, Caramel, Corn Syrup, Eucalyptus Oil, Flavor, Sucrose, Tolu Balsam and Thymol.
Cherry Flavor: Citric Acid, Corn Syrup, FD&C Blue No. 1, FD&C Red No. 40, Flavor, Sucrose.

Indications: Temporarily relieves sore throat and coughs due to colds or inhaled irritants.

Directions: Adults and children 3 to 12 years: Allow drop to dissolve slowly in mouth. **Cough:** may be repeated every hour as needed or as directed by a doctor. **Sore Throat:** may be repeated every 2 hours—as needed or as directed by a doctor. Children under 3 years of age, consult a doctor.

WARNINGS: A persistent cough may be a sign of a serious condition. If cough persists for more than 1 week, tends to recur, or is accompanied by fever, rash, or persistent headache, consult a doctor. Do not take this product for persistent or chronic cough such as occurs with smoking, asthma, emphysema, or if cough is accompanied by excessive phlegm (mucus), unless directed by a doctor. If sore throat is severe, or is accompanied by difficulty in breathing, or persists for more than two days, do not use, and consult a doctor promptly. If sore throat is accompanied or followed by fever, headache, rash, swelling, nausea, or vomiting, consult a doctor promptly. **KEEP THIS AND ALL DRUGS OUT OF THE REACH OF CHILDREN.** As with any drug, if you are pregnant or nursing a baby, seek the advice of a health professional before using this product.

How Supplied: Vicks Cough Drops are available in boxes of 14 drops each and bags of 30 drops.

EXTRA STRENGTH VICKS® COUGH DROPS
Menthol Cough Suppressant/Oral Anesthetic

Flavors: Available in Cherry, Menthol, Honey Lemon and Peppermint flavors.

Active Ingredient: Menthol Flavor: Menthol 8.4 mg. Cherry: Menthol 10 mg, Honey Lemon: Menthol 10 mg, Peppermint: Menthol 10 mg.

Inactive Ingredients:
Menthol Flavor: Corn Syrup, FD&C Blue No. 1, Flavor, Sucrose, Cherry Flavor: Corn Syrup, FD&C Red No. 40, FD&C Blue No. 2, Flavor, Sucrose Honey Lemon: Citric Acid, Corn Syrup, D&C Yellow No. 10, FD&C Yellow No. 6, Flavor, Sucrose, Peppermint: Corn Syrup, Flavor, Peppermint Oil, Sucrose.

Indications: Temporarily relieves sore throat and coughs due to colds or inhaled irritants.

Directions: Adults and children 3 to 12 years: Allow drop to dissolve slowly in mouth. Cough: may be repeated every hour as needed or as directed by a doctor. Sore Throat: may be repeated every 2 hours as needed or as directed by a doctor. Children under 3 years of age, consult a doctor.

WARNINGS: A persistent cough may be a sign of a serious condition. If cough persists for more than 1 week, tends to recur, or is accompanied by fever, rash, or persistent headache, consult a doctor. Do not take this product for persistent or chronic cough such as occurs with smoking, asthma, emphysema, or if cough is accompanied by excessive phlegm (mucus), unless directed by a doctor. If sore throat is severe, or is accompanied by difficulty in breathing, or persists for more than two days, do not use, and consult a doctor promptly. If sore throat is accompanied or followed by fever, headache, rash, swelling, nausea, or vomiting, consult a doctor promptly. **KEEP THIS AND ALL DRUGS OUT OF THE REACH OF CHILDREN.** As with any drug, if you are pregnant or nursing a baby, seek the advice of a health professional before using this product.

How Supplied: Extra Strength Vicks Cough Drops are available in single sticks of 9 drops each and bags of 30 drops.

VICKS DAYQUIL® LIQUID
VICKS DAYQUIL® LIQUICAPS®
Non-Drowsy Colds/Flu Medicine
Nasal Decongestant/Pain Reliever—Fever Reducer
Cough Suppressant/Expectorant

Active Ingredients:
LIQUID—per fluid ounce (2 TBSP.) or LIQUICAPS—per two softgels, contains Acetaminophen 650 mg (Liquid) or 500 mg (softgels), Dextromethorphan Hydrobromide 20 mg, Pseudoephedrine Hydrochloride 60 mg, Guaifenesin 200 mg

Inactive Ingredients:
Liquid: Citric Acid, FD&C Yellow No. 6, Flavor, Glycerin, Polyethylene Glycol, Propylene Glycol, Purified Water, Saccharin Sodium, Sodium Citrate, Sucrose.
Softgels: FD&C Red No. 40, FD&C Yellow No. 6, Gelatin, Gelatin Glycerin, Polyethylene Glycol, Povidone, Propylene Glycol, Purified Water. May contain Edible Ink.

Indications: For the temporary relief of minor aches, pains, headache, muscular aches, sore throat and fever associated with a cold or flu. Temporarily relieves nasal congestion and coughing due to a cold. Helps loosen phlegm (mucus) and thin secretions to drain bronchial tubes and make coughs more productive.

Directions: Take as directed.
Adults 12 years and over: one fluid ounce in medicine cup (2 tablespoons), or swallow 2 softgels with water.
Children 6 to under 12 years of age: one half fluid ounce in medicine cup (1 tablespoon), or swallow 1 softgel with water.
Children under 6 years of age: Consult a doctor.
Repeat every 4 hours, not to exceed 4 doses per day, or as directed by a doctor.

WARNINGS: Do not exceed recommended dosage because at higher doses nervousness, dizziness, or sleeplessness may occur. Do not take this product if you have heart disease, high blood pressure, thyroid disease, diabetes, or difficulty in urination due to enlargement of the prostate gland unless directed by a doctor. *DRUG INTERACTION PRECAUTION:* Do not take this product if you are presently taking a prescription drug for high blood pressure or depression, without first consulting your doctor. Do not take this product for persistent or chronic cough such as occurs with smoking, asthma, chronic bronchitis, or emphysema, or if cough is accompanied by excessive phlegm (mucus) unless directed by a doctor. Do not take this product for more than 7 days (for adults) or 5 days (for children). A persistent cough may be a sign of serious condition. If cough persists for more than 7 days, tends to recur, or is accompanied by rash, or persistent headache, consult a doctor. If symptoms do not improve or are accompanied by fever that lasts for more than 3 days, or if new symptoms occur, consult a doctor. If sore throat is severe, persists for more than 2 days, is accompanied or followed by fever, headache, rash, nausea, or vomiting, consult a doctor promptly. **KEEP THIS AND ALL DRUGS OUT OF THE REACH OF CHILDREN.** In case of accidental overdose, seek professional assistance or contact a poison control center immediately. Prompt medical attention is critical for adults as well as for children even if you do not notice any signs or symptoms. As with any drug, if you are pregnant or nursing a baby, seek the advice of a health professional before using this product.

How Supplied: Available in: **LIQUID** 6 FL. OZ. plastic bottles with child-resistant, tamper-evident cap and a calibrated medicine cup.
LIQUICAP in 12-count child-resistant package and 20-count non-child-resistant packages. Each softgel is imprinted: DayQuil

---

VICKS® FORMULA 44® COUGH MEDICINE
Dextromethorphan HBr/ Cough Suppressant

Active Ingredient per 2 tsp. (10 mL.): Dextromethorphan Hydrobromide 30 mg

Inactive Ingredients: Alcohol 10%, Caramel, Carboxymethylcellulose Sodium, Citric Acid, FD&C Red No. 40, Flavor, Invert Sugar, Propylene Glycol, Purified Water, Sodium Citrate.

Indications: VICKS® FORMULA 44® provides temporary relief of coughs due to minor throat and bronchial irritation associated with a cold.

Actions: VICKS® FORMULA 44® COUGH MEDICINE is a cough suppressant.

Directions:

Adults and Children 12 years of age and over:	2 teaspoons
Children 6–11 years of age:	1 teaspoon
Children 2–5 years of age:	½ teaspoon
Children under 2 years of age:	consult a doctor.

Repeat every 6–8 hours. No more than 4 doses per day or as directed by doctor.

WARNINGS: A persistent cough may be a sign of a serious condition. If cough persists for more than 1 week, tends to recur, or is accompanied by fever, rash, or persistent headache, consult a doctor. Do not take this product for persistent or chronic cough such as occurs with smoking, asthma, emphysema, or if cough is accompanied by excessive phlegm (mucus) unless directed by a doctor. **KEEP THIS AND ALL DRUGS OUT OF THE REACH OF CHILDREN.** In case of accidental overdose, seek professional assistance or contact a poison control center immediately. As with any drug, if you are pregnant or nursing a baby, seek the advice of a health professional before using this product.

Continued on next page

Procter & Gamble—Cont.

How Supplied: Available in 4 FL. OZ. and 8 FL. OZ. squeeze bottles with Vicks AccuTip® Dispenser for accurate, easy dosing.

VICKS® FORMULA 44D® COUGH & DECONGESTANT MEDICINE
Cough Suppressant/ Nasal Decongestant

Active Ingredients per 3 tsp. (15 mL):
Dextromethorphan Hydrobromide 30 mg
Pseudoephedrine Hydrochloride 60 mg

Inactive Ingredients: Alcohol 10%, Citric Acid, FD&C Red No. 40, Flavor, Glycerin, Propylene Glycol, Purified Water, Saccharin Sodium, Sodium Citrate, Sucrose.

Indications: VICKS® FORMULA 44D® provides temporary relief of coughs and nasal congestion due to a common cold.

Actions: VICKS® FORMULA 44D® is a cough suppressant and a nasal decongestant.

Dosage Directions:

Adults and children 12 years of age and over:	3 teaspoons
Children 6–11 years of age:	1½ teaspoons
Children 2–5 years of age:	¾ teaspoon

Children under 2 years of age, consult a doctor.
Repeat every 6 hours. No more than 4 doses per day or as directed by a doctor.

WARNINGS: A persistent cough may be a sign of a serious condition. If cough persists for more than 1 week, tends to recur, or is accompanied by fever, rash, or persistent headache, consult a doctor. Do not take this product for persistent or chronic cough such as occurs with smoking, asthma, emphysema, or if cough is accompanied by excessive phlegm (mucus) unless directed by a doctor. Do not exceed recommended dosage because at higher doses nervousness, dizziness, or sleeplessness may occur. Do not take this product for more than 7 days. If symptoms do not improve or are accompanied by fever, consult a doctor. Do not take this product if you have heart disease, high blood pressure, thyroid disease, diabetes, or difficulty in urination due to enlargement of the prostate gland unless directed by a doctor. *DRUG INTERACTION PRECAUTION:* Do not take this product if you are presently taking a prescription drug for high blood pressure or depression, without first consulting your doctor. **KEEP THIS AND ALL DRUGS OUT OF THE REACH OF CHILDREN.** In case of accidental overdose, seek professional assistance or contact a poison control center immediately. As with any drug, if you are pregnant or nursing a baby, seek the advice of a health professional before using this product.

How Supplied: Available in 4 FL. OZ. and 8 FL. OZ. squeeze bottles with Vicks AccuTip® Dispenser for accurate, easy dosing.

VICKS® FORMULA 44E®
Cough & Expectorant Medicine
Cough Suppressant/Expectorant

Active Ingredients per 3 teaspoons (15mL): Dextromethorphan Hydrobromide 20 mg, Guaifenesin 200 mg

Inactive Ingredients: Alcohol 10%, Citric Acid, FD&C Blue No. 1, FD&C Red No. 40, Flavor, Glycerin, Propylene Glycol, Purified Water, Saccharin Sodium, Sodium Citrate, Sucrose.

Indications: VICKS® FORMULA 44E® provides temporary relief of coughs due to the common cold and helps loosen phlegm to make coughs more productive.

Actions: VICKS® FORMULA 44E® is a cough suppressant and expectorant.

Directions:

Adults and Children 12 years of age and over:	3 teaspoons
Children 6–11 years of age:	1½ teaspoons
Children 2–5 years of age:	¾ teaspoon

Children under 2 years of age: consult a doctor.
Repeat every 4 hours. No more than 6 doses per day, or as directed by a doctor.

WARNINGS: A persistent cough may be a sign of a serious condition. If cough persists for more than 1 week, tends to recur, or is accompanied by fever, rash, or persistent headache, consult a doctor. Do not take this product for persistent or chronic cough such as occurs with smoking, asthma, chronic bronchitis, or emphysema, or if cough is accompanied by excessive phlegm (mucus) unless directed by a doctor. **KEEP THIS AND ALL DRUGS OUT OF THE REACH OF CHILDREN.** In case of accidental overdose, seek professional assistance or contact a poison control center immediately. As with any drug, if you are pregnant or nursing a baby, seek the advice of a health professional before using this product.

How Supplied: Available in 4 FL. OZ. and 8 FL. OZ. squeeze bottles with Vicks AccuTip® Dispenser for accurate, easy dosing.

VICKS® FORMULA 44M® MULTI-SYMPTOM COUGH & COLD MEDICINE
Cough Suppressant/Nasal Decongestant/Antihistamine/ Pain Reliever-Fever Reducer

Active Ingredients per 4 tsp. (20 mL):
Dextromethorphan Hydrobromide 30mg
Pseudoephedrine Hydrochloride 60 mg
Chlorpheniramine Maleate 4 mg
Acetaminophen 500 mg

Inactive Ingredients: Alcohol 20%, Citric Acid, FD&C Blue No. 1, FD&C Red No. 40, Flavor, Glycerin, Purified Water, Saccharin Sodium, Sodium Benzoate, Sodium Citrate, Sucrose.

Indications: VICKS® FORMULA 44M® provides temporary relief of coughing, nasal congestion, runny nose, and sneezing due to a cold. Also for temporary relief of headache, fever, muscular aches and sore throat due to a cold or flu.

Actions: VICKS® FORMULA 44M® is a cough suppressant, nasal decongestant, antihistamine and analgesic.

Directions: Adults and children 12 years of age and over: fill cup to top line or 4 teaspoons
Children 6–11 years of age: fill up to bottom line or 2 teaspoons
Children under 6 years of age: consult a doctor
Repeat every 6 hours. No more than 4 doses per day or as directed by a doctor.

WARNINGS: Do not take this product for persistent or chronic cough such as occurs with smoking, asthma, or emphysema, or if cough is accompanied by excessive phlegm (mucus) unless directed by a doctor. Do not exceed recommended dosage because at higher doses nervousness, dizziness, or sleeplessness may occur. Do not take this product if you have heart disease, high blood pressure, thyroid disease, diabetes, or difficulty in urination due to enlargement of the prostate gland unless directed by a doctor. *DRUG INTERACTION PRECAUTION:* Do not take this product if you are presently taking a prescription drug for high blood pressure or depression, without first consulting your doctor. May cause excitability especially in children. Do not take this product if you have asthma, glaucoma, emphysema, chronic pulmonary disease, shortness of breath, or difficulty in breathing unless directed by a doctor. May cause marked drowsiness; alcohol, sedatives, and tranquilizers may increase the drowsiness effect. Avoid alcoholic beverages while taking this product. Do not take this product if you are taking sedatives or tranquilizers, without first consulting your doctor. Use caution when driving a motor vehicle or operating machinery. Do not take this product for more than 7 days (for adults) or 5 days (for children). A persistent cough may be a sign of a serious condition. If cough persists for more than 7 days, tends to recur, or is accompanied by rash, persistent headache, fever that lasts for more than 3 days, or if new symptoms occur, consult a doctor. If symptoms do not improve or are accompanied by fever that lasts for more than 3 days, or if new symptoms occur, consult a doctor. If sore throat is severe, persists for more than 2 days, is accompanied or followed by fever, headache, rash, nausea or vomiting, consult a doctor. **KEEP THIS AND ALL DRUGS OUT OF THE REACH OF CHILDREN.** In case of accidental overdose, seek professional assistance or contact a poison control center immediately. Prompt medical attention is critical for adults as well as for children, even if you do not notice any signs or symptoms. As with any drug, if you are pregnant or nursing a baby, seek the advice of a health professional before using this product.

How Supplied: Available in 4 FL. OZ. and 8 FL. OZ. squeeze bottles with Vicks AccuTip® Dispenser for accurate, easy dosing. A calibrated dose cup accompanies each bottle.

VICKS® INHALER
with decongestant action
l-Desoxyephedrine/Nasal Decongestant

Active Ingredient per inhaler: *l*-Desoxyephedrine 50 mg.

Inactive Ingredients: Special Vicks Vapors (bornyl acetate, camphor, lavender oil, menthol).

Indications: For the temporary relief of nasal congestion due to the common cold, hay fever, upper respiratory allergies or sinusitis.

Actions: Fast relief from nasal congestion due to colds, hay fever, upper respiratory allergies, sinusitis.

Directions: Adults: 2 inhalations in each nostril not more often than every 2 hours.
Children 6 to under 12 years of age (with adult supervision): 1 inhalation in each nostril not more often than every 2 hours. Children under 6 years of age: consult a doctor.

WARNINGS: Do not exceed recommended dosage because burning, stinging, sneezing, or increase of nasal discharge may occur. The use of this container by more than one person may spread infection. Do not use this product for more than 7 days. If symptoms persist, consult a doctor. **KEEP THIS AND ALL DRUGS OUT OF THE REACH OF CHILDREN.** In case of accidental ingestion, seek professional assistance or contact a poison control center immediately.

VICKS INHALER is effective for a minimum of 3 months after first use. Keep tightly closed.

How Supplied: Available as a cylindrical plastic nasal inhaler (net weight: 0.007 OZ).

VICKS® NYQUIL® LIQUICAPS
Adult Nighttime Cold/Flu Medicine
Nasal Decongestant/Antihistamine/ Cough Suppressant/Pain Reliever–Fever Reducer

Active Ingredients (per softgel):
Acetaminophen 250 mg
Pseudoephedrine HCl 30 mg
Dextromethorphan HBr 10 mg
Doxylamine succinate 6.25 mg

Inactive Ingredients: D&C Yellow No. 10, FD&C Blue No. 1, Gelatin, Glycerin, Polyethylene Glycol, Povidone, Propylene Glycol and Purified Water. May contain Edible Ink. Contains no alcohol.

Indications: For the temporary relief of minor aches, pains, headache, muscular aches, sore throat, and fever associated with a cold or flu. Temporarily relieves nasal congestion, cough due to minor throat and bronchial irritations, runny nose and sneezing associated with the common cold.

Actions: Decongestant, antipyretic, antihistamine, antitussive, analgesic. The nighttime sniffling, sneezing, coughing, aching, stuffy head, fever, so you can rest medicine®.

Directions: ADULTS (12 years and over): Swallow two softgels. If your cold or flu symptoms keep you confined to bed or at home a total of 4 doses may be taken per day, each 4 hours apart, or as directed by a doctor. Do not exceed. **NOT RECOMMENDED FOR CHILDREN.**

WARNINGS: Do not exceed recommended dosage because at higher doses nervousness, dizziness or sleeplessness may occur. Do not take this product if you have heart disease, high blood pressure, thyroid disease, diabetes, or difficulty in urination due to enlargement of the prostate gland unless directed by a doctor. *DRUG INTERACTION PRECAUTION:* Do not take this product if you are presently taking a prescription drug for high blood pressure or depression, without first consulting your doctor. Do not take this product for persistent or chronic cough such as occurs with smoking, asthma, emphysema, or if cough is accompanied by excessive phlegm (mucus) unless directed by a doctor. May cause excitability especially in children. Do not take this product if you have asthma, glaucoma, emphysema, chronic pulmonary disease, shortness of breath, or difficulty in breathing unless directed by a doctor. May cause marked drowsiness; alcohol, sedatives, and tranquilizers may increase the drowsiness effect. Avoid alcoholic beverages while taking this product. Do not take this product if you are taking sedatives or tranquilizers, without first consulting your doctor. Use caution when driving a motor vehicle or operating machinery. Do not take this product for more than 7 days. A persistent cough may be a sign of a serious condition. If cough persists for more than 7 days, tends to recur, or is accompanied by rash, persistent headache, consult a doctor. If symptoms do not improve or are accompanied by fever that lasts for more than 3 days, or if new symptoms occur, consult a doctor. If sore throat is severe, persists for more than 2 days, is accompanied or followed by fever, headache, rash, nausea, or vomiting, consult a doctor promptly. **KEEP THIS AND ALL DRUGS OUT OF THE REACH OF CHILDREN.** In case of accidental overdose, seek professional assistance or contact a poison control center immediately. Prompt medical attention is critical for adults as well as for children even if you do not notice any signs or symptoms. As with any drug, if you are pregnant or nursing a baby, seek the advice of a health professional before using this product.

How Supplied: Available in 12-count child-resistant blister packages and 20-count non-child-resistant blister packages. Each softgel is imprinted NyQuil.

VICKS® NYQUIL®
[*nī'quĭl*]
Adult Nighttime Cold/Flu Medicine in oral liquid form.
Original and Cherry Flavor
Nasal Decongestant/Antihistamine/ Cough Suppressant/Pain Reliever–Fever Reducer

Active Ingredients per fluid oz. (2 TBSP.): Acetaminophen 1000 mg, Dextromethorphan Hydrobromide 30 mg, Pseudoephedrine HCl 60 mg, Doxylamine Succinate 7.5 mg
Contains FD&C Yellow No. 5 (tartrazine) as a color additive (Original flavor only).

Inactive Ingredients: Original Flavor: Alcohol 25%, Citric Acid, FD&C Blue No. 1, Flavor, Glycerin, Purified Water, Sodium Benzoate, Sodium Citrate, Sucrose.
Cherry Flavor: Alcohol 25%, Citric Acid, FD&C Blue No. 1, FD&C Red No. 40, Flavor, Glycerin, Purified Water, Saccharin Sodium, Sodium Citrate, Sucrose.

Indications: For the temporary relief of minor aches, pains, headache, muscular aches, sore throat, and fever associated with a cold or flu. Temporarily relieves nasal congestion, cough due to minor throat and bronchial irritations, runny nose and sneezing associated with the common cold.

Actions: Nasal decongestant, antipyretic, antihistamine, antitussive, analgesic. The nighttime, sniffling, sneezing, coughing, aching, stuffy head, fever, so you can rest medicine.®

Directions:
ADULTS (12 years and over): Take one fluid ounce (2 tablespoons) at bedtime in medicine cup provided.
If your cold or flu symptoms keep you confined to bed or at home, a total of 4 doses may be taken per day, each 6 hours apart, or as directed by a doctor.
NOT RECOMMENDED FOR CHILDREN.

Continued on next page

Procter & Gamble—Cont.

WARNINGS: Do not exceed recommended dosage because at higher doses nervousness, dizziness, or sleeplessness may occur. Do not take this product if you have heart disease, high blood pressure, thyroid disease, diabetes, or difficulty in urination due to enlargement of the prostate gland unless directed by a doctor. *DRUG INTERACTION PRECAUTION:* Do not take this product if you are presently taking a prescription drug for high blood pressure or depression, without first consulting your doctor. Do not take this product for persistent or chronic cough such as occurs with smoking, asthma, emphysema, or if cough is accompanied by excessive phlegm (mucus) unless directed by a doctor. May cause excitability especially in children. Do not take this product if you have asthma, glaucoma, emphysema, chronic pulmonary disease, shortness of breath, or difficulty in breathing unless directed by a doctor. May cause marked drowsiness; alcohol, sedatives and tranquilizers may increase the drowsiness effect. Avoid alcoholic beverages while taking this product. Do not take this product if you are taking sedatives or tranquilizers, without first consulting your doctor. Use caution when driving a motor vehicle or operating machinery. Do not take this product for more than 7 days. A persistent cough may be a sign of a serious condition. If cough persists for more than 7 days, tends to recur, or is accompanied by rash, or persistent headache, consult a doctor. If symptoms do not improve or are accompanied by fever that last for more than 3 days, or if new symptoms occur, consult a doctor. If sore throat is severe, persists for more than 2 days, is accompanied or followed by fever, headache, rash, nausea, or vomiting, consult a doctor promptly. **KEEP THIS AND ALL DRUGS OUT OF THE REACH OF CHILDREN.** In case of accidental overdose, seek professional assistance or contact a poison control center immediately. Prompt medical attention is critical for adults as well as for children even if you do not notice any signs or symptoms. As with any drug, if you are pregnant or nursing a baby, seek the advice of a health professional before using this product.

How Supplied: Available in 6, 10, and 14 fl. oz. plastic bottles with child-resistant, tamper-evident cap and calibrated medicine cup.

VICKS® PEDIATRIC FORMULA 44® COUGH MEDICINE
Dextromethorphan HBr/Cough Suppressant

Active Ingredient per 1 TBSP. (15 mL): Dextromethorphan Hydrobromide 15 mg

CONTAINS NO ALCOHOL

Inactive Ingredients: Carboxymethylcellulose Sodium, Cellulose, Citric Acid, FD&C Red No. 40, Flavors, Glycerin, Polysorbate 80, Potassium Sorbate, Propylene Glycol, Purified Water, Sodium Citrate, Sorbitol, Sucrose.

Indications: For the temporary relief of coughs due to the common cold.

Actions: VICKS® PEDIATRIC FORMULA 44® is an alcohol-free cough suppressant.

Administration and Dosage:
Directions: SHAKE WELL BEFORE USING
Squeeze bottle to accurately dispense medicine into dosage cup provided.

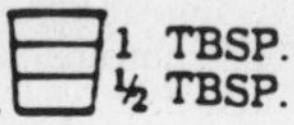

Dosage:

Age	Weight	Dose
Under 2 yrs	Under 28 lbs.	Consult physician*
2–5 yrs	28–47 lbs.	Fill cup to ½ TBSP.
6–11 yrs	48–95 lbs.	Fill cup to 1 TBSP.
12 yrs. and over	96 lbs. and over	2 TBSP. or Try one of the Adult Formula 44® Medicines

Repeat every 6–8 hours, no more than 4 doses in 24 hours, or as directed by a doctor.

Professional Dosage:

*Physicians: Suggested doses for children under 2 years of age.

Age	Weight	Dose
* 6–11 mo.	17–21 lbs.	1 teaspoon (5 mL)
*12–23 mo.	22–27 lbs.	1¼ teaspoon (6.25 mL)

Repeat every 6–8 hours, no more than 4 doses in 24 hours or as directed by doctor.

*Based on extrapolation from studies on the safety and efficacy of active ingredients conducted among older children and adults. Use caution in treating children under 2 years of age who were born prematurely.

WARNINGS: A persistent cough may be a sign of a serious condition. If cough persists for more than 1 week, tends to recur, or is accompanied by fever, rash, or persistent headache, consult a doctor. Do not take this product for persistent or chronic cough such as occurs with smoking, asthma, emphysema, or if cough is accompanied by excessive phlegm (mucus) unless directed by a doctor. **KEEP THIS AND ALL DRUGS OUT OF THE REACH OF CHILDREN.** In case of accidental overdose, seek professional assistance or contact a poison control center immediately. As with any drug, if you are pregnant or nursing a baby, seek the advice of a health professional before using this product.

How Supplied: 4 FL. OZ. squeeze bottles with Vicks® AccuTip® Dispenser for accurate, easy dosing. Calibrated dose cup accompanies each bottle.

VICKS® PEDIATRIC FORMULA 44d® COUGH & DECONGESTANT MEDICINE

Active Ingredients Per 1 TBSP. (15 mL): Dextromethorphan Hydrobromide 15 mg, Pseudoephedrine Hydrochloride 30 mg

CONTAINS NO ALCOHOL

Inactive Ingredients: Carboxymethylcellulose Sodium, Cellulose, Citric Acid, FD&C Red No. 40, Flavor, Glycerin, Polysorbate 80, Potassium Sorbate, Propylene Glycol, Purified Water, Sodium Citrate, Sorbitol, Sucrose.

Indications: For the temporary relief of coughs and nasal congestion due to the common cold.

Actions: VICKS® PEDIATRIC FORMULA 44d® is an alcohol-free suppressant and nasal decongestant.

Administration and Dosage:
Directions: SHAKE WELL BEFORE USING
Squeeze bottle to accurately dispense medicine into dosage cup provided.

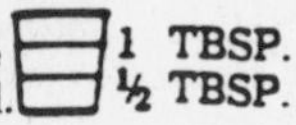

Dosage:

Age	Weight	Dose
Under 2 yrs	Under 28 lbs.	Consult physician*
2–5 yrs	28–47 lbs.	Fill cup to ½ TBSP.
6–11 yrs	48–95 lbs.	Fill cup to 1 TBSP.
12 yrs. and over	96 lbs. and over	2 TBSP. or Try one of the Adult Formula 44® Medicines

Repeat every 6 hours, no more than 4 doses in 24 hours, or as directed by a doctor.

***Professional Dosage:**

Physicians: Suggested doses for children under 2 years of age.

Age	Weight	Dose
* 6–11 mo.	17–21 lbs.	1 teaspoon (5 mL)
*12–23 mo.	22–27 lbs.	1¼ teaspoon (6.25 mL)

Repeat every 6 hours. No more than 4 doses in 24 hours, or as directed by doctor.

*Based on extrapolation from studies on the safety and efficacy of active ingredients conducted among older children

and adults. Use caution in treating children under 2 years who were born prematurely.

WARNINGS: A persistent cough may be a sign of a serious condition. If cough persists for more than 1 week, tends to recur, or is accompanied by fever, rash, or persistent headache, consult a doctor. Do not take this product for persistent or chronic cough such as occurs with smoking, asthma, emphysema, or if cough is accompanied by excessive phlegm (mucus) unless directed by a doctor. Do not exceed recommended dosage because at higher doses nervousness, dizziness, or sleeplessness may occur. Do not take this product for more than 7 days. If symptoms do not improve or are accompanied by fever, consult a doctor. Do not take this product if you have heart disease, high blood pressure, thyroid disease, diabetes, or difficulty in urination due to enlargement of the prostate gland unless directed by a doctor. *DRUG INTERACTION PRECAUTION:* Do not take this product if you are presently taking a prescription drug for high blood pressure or depression, without first consulting your doctor. **KEEP THIS AND ALL DRUGS OUT OF THE REACH OF CHILDREN.** In case of accidental overdose, seek professional assistance or contact a poison control center immediately. As with any drug, if you are pregnant or nursing a baby, seek the advice of a health professional before using this product.

How Supplied: 4 FL. OZ. squeeze bottles with Vicks® AccuTip® Dispenser for accurate, easy dosing. A calibrated dose cup accompanies each bottle.

VICKS® PEDIATRIC FORMULA 44e®
Cough & Expectorant Medicine

Active Ingredients per 1 tablespoon (15 mL):
Dextromethorphan Hydrobromide 10 mg, Guaifenesin 100 mg

CONTAINS NO ALCOHOL

Inactive Ingredients: Carboxymethylcellulose Sodium, Cellulose, Citric Acid, FD&C Red No. 40, Flavor, Glycerin, Polysorbate 80, Potassium Sorbate, Propylene Glycol, Purified Water, Sodium Citrate, Sorbitol, Sucrose.

Indications: For the temporary relief of coughs due to the common cold and helps loosen phlegm to make coughs more productive.

Actions: VICKS® PEDIATRIC 44e® is an alcohol-free cough suppressant and expectorant.

Administration and Dosage:
Directions: (SHAKE WELL BEFORE USING)
Squeeze bottle to accurately dispense medicine into dosage cup provided.

1 TBSP.
½ TBSP.

Dosage:

Age	Weight	Dose
Under 2 yrs	Under 28 lbs.	Consult physician*
2–5 yrs	28–47 lbs.	Fill cup to ½ TBSP.
6–11 yrs	48–95 lbs.	Fill cup to 1 TBSP.
12 yrs. and over	96 lbs. and over	2 TBSP. or Try one of the Adult Formula 44® Medicines

Repeat every 4 hours. No more than 6 doses in 24 hours, or as directed by a doctor.

***Professional Dosage:**

Physicians: Suggested doses for children under 2 years of age.

Age	Weight	Dose
* 6–11 mo.	17–21 lbs.	1 teaspoon (5 mL)
*12–23 mo.	22–27 lbs.	1¼ teaspoon (6.25 mL)

Repeat every 4 hours. No more than 6 doses in 24 hours, or as directed by doctor.

* Based on extrapolation from studies on the safety and efficacy of active ingredients conducted among older children and adults. Use caution in treating children under 2 years who were born prematurely.

WARNINGS: A persistent cough may be a sign of a serious condition. If cough persists for more than 1 week, tends to recur, or is accompanied by fever, rash, or persistent headache, consult a doctor. Do not take this product for persistent or chronic cough such as occurs with smoking, asthma, chronic bronchitis, emphysema, or where cough is accompanied by excessive phlegm (mucus) unless directed by a doctor. **KEEP THIS AND ALL DRUGS OUT OF THE REACH OF CHILDREN.** In case of accidental overdose, seek professional assistance or contact a poison control center immediately. As with any drug, if you are pregnant or nursing a baby, seek the advice of a health professional before using this product.

How Supplied: 4 fl. oz. squeeze bottles with Vicks® AccuTip® Dispenser for accurate, easy dosing. A calibrated dose cup accompanies each bottle.

VICKS® PEDIATRIC FORMULA 44m®
Multi-Symptom COUGH & COLD MEDICINE
Cough Suppressant/Nasal Decongestant/Antihistamine

Active Ingredients Per 1 TBSP. (15 mL):
Dextromethorphan Hydrobromide 15 mg,
Pseudoephedrine Hydrochloride 30 mg,
Chlorpheniramine Maleate 2 mg

CONTAINS NO ALCOHOL

Inactive Ingredients: Carboxymethylcellulose Sodium, Cellulose, Citric Acid, FD&C Red No. 40, Flavors, Glycerin, Polysorbate 80, Potassium Sorbate, Propylene Glycol, Purified Water, Sodium Citrate, Sorbitol, Sucrose.

Indications: For the temporary relief of coughs, nasal congestion, runny nose and sneezing due to the common cold.

Actions: VICKS® PEDIATRIC FORMULA 44m® is an alcohol-free cough suppressant, nasal decongestant and antihistamine.

Administration and Dosage:
Directions: SHAKE WELL BEFORE USING
Squeeze bottle to accurately dispense medicine into dosage cup provided.
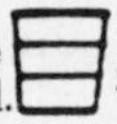
1 TBSP.
½ TBSP.

Dosage:

Age	Weight	Dose
Under 6 yrs	Under 48 lbs.	Consult Physician*
6–11 yrs	48–95 lbs.	Fill cup to 1 TBSP.
12 yrs and over	96 lbs. and over	2 TBSP. or try one of the Adult Formula 44® Medicines

Repeat every 6 hours. No more than 4 doses in 24 hours, or as directed by a doctor.

Professional Dosage:

*Physicians: Suggested doses for children under 6 years of age.

Age	Weight	Dose
* 6–11 mo.	17–21 lbs.	1 teaspoon (5 mL)
*12–23 mo.	22–27 lbs.	1¼ teaspoon (6.25 mL)
2–5 yrs.	28–47 lbs.	½ TBSP. (7.5 mL)

Repeat every 6 hours, no more than 4 doses in 24 hours, or as directed by doctor.

*Based on extrapolation from studies on the safety and efficacy of active ingredients conducted among older children and adults. Use caution in treating children under 2 years of age who were born prematurely.

WARNINGS: A persistent cough may be a sign of a serious condition. If cough persists for more than 1 week, tends to recur, or is accompanied by fever, rash, or persistent headache, consult a doctor. Do not take this product for persistent or chronic cough such as occurs with smoking, asthma, emphysema, or if cough is accompanied by excessive phlegm (mucus) unless directed by a doctor. Do not exceed recommended dosage because at higher doses nervousness, dizziness, or sleeplessness may occur. Do not take this product for more than 7 days. If symptoms do not improve or are accompanied

Continued on next page

Procter & Gamble—Cont.

by fever, consult a doctor. Do not take this product if you have heart disease, high blood pressure, thyroid disease, diabetes, or difficulty in urination due to enlargement of the prostate gland unless directed by a doctor. *DRUG INTERACTION PRECAUTION:* Do not take this product if you are presently taking a prescription drug for high blood pressure or depression, without first consulting your doctor. May cause excitability especially in children. Do not take this product if you have asthma, glaucoma, emphysema, chronic pulmonary disease, shortness of breath, or difficulty in breathing unless directed by a doctor. May cause marked drowsiness; alcohol, sedatives, and tranquilizers may increase the drowsiness effect. Avoid alcoholic beverages while taking this product. Do not take this product if you are taking sedatives or tranquilizers, without first consulting your doctor. Use caution when driving a motor vehicle or operating machinery. **KEEP THIS AND ALL DRUGS OUT OF THE REACH OF CHILDREN.** In case of accidental overdose, seek professional assistance or contact a poison control center immediately. As with any drug, if you are pregnant or nursing a baby, seek the advice of a health professional before using this product.

How Supplied: 4 FL OZ squeeze bottles with Vicks® AccuTip® Dispenser for accurate easy dosing. A calibrated dose cup accompanies each bottle.

VICKS® SINEX® REGULAR

[*sī 'nĕx*]

Decongestant Nasal Spray and Ultra Fine Mist

Active Ingredient: Phenylephrine Hydrochloride 0.5%.

Inactive Ingredients: Aromatic Vapors (Camphor, Eucalyptol, Menthol), Cetylpyridinium Chloride, Potassium Phosphate, Purified Water, Sodium Chloride, Sodium Phosphate, Tyloxapol. Preservative: Thimerosal 0.001%.

Indications: For temporary relief of nasal congestion due to colds, hay fever, upper respiratory allergies or sinusitis.

Actions: Provides fast decongestant relief.

Dosage and Administration: Keep head and dispenser upright. May be used every 4 hours as needed.
Ultra Fine Mist: Remove protective cap. Before using for the first time, prime the pump by firmly depressing its rim several times. Hold container with thumb at base and nozzle between first and second fingers. Without tilting your head, insert nozzle into nostril. Fully depress rim with a firm even stroke and inhale deeply.
Adults and Children—age 12 and over: 2 or 3 sprays in each nostril not more often than every 4 hours. Do not give to children under 12 years of age unless directed by a doctor.
Squeeze Bottle: Adults and Children—age 12 and over: 2 or 3 sprays in each nostril not more often than every 4 hours. Do not give to children under 12 years of age unless directed by a doctor.

WARNINGS: Do not exceed recommended dosage because burning, stinging, sneezing, or increase of nasal discharge may occur. The use of this container by more than one person may spread infection. Do not use this product for more than 3 days. If symptoms persist, consult a doctor. Do not use this product if you have heart disease, high blood pressure, thyroid disease, diabetes, or difficulty in urination due to enlargement of the prostate gland unless directed by a doctor.
KEEP THIS AND ALL DRUGS OUT OF THE REACH OF CHILDREN. In case of accidental ingestion, seek professional assistance or contact a poison control center immediately.

How Supplied: Available in ½ FL. OZ. and 1 FL. OZ. plastic squeeze bottles and ½ FL. OZ. measured dose Ultra Fine mist pump.

VICKS® SINEX® LONG-ACTING

[*sī 'nĕx*]

12-hour Formula Decongestant Nasal Spray and Ultra Fine Mist

Active Ingredient: Oxymetazoline Hydrochloride 0.05%.

Inactive Ingredients: Aromatic Vapors (Camphor, Eucalyptol, Menthol), Potassium Phosphate, Purified Water, Sodium Chloride, Sodium Phosphate, Tyloxapol. Preservatives: Benzalkonium Chloride, Chlorhexidine Gluconate, Disodium EDTA.

Indications: For temporary relief of nasal congestion due to colds, hay fever, upper respiratory allergies or sinusitis.

Actions: Provides fast relief of head and nasal congestion and lasts up to 12 hours.

Dosage and Administration: Keep head and dispenser upright. May be used twice daily (morning and evening) or as directed by a physician.
Ultra Fine Mist: Remove protective cap. Before using for the first time, prime the pump by firmly depressing its rim several times. Hold container with thumb at base and nozzle between first and second fingers. Without tilting head, insert nozzle into nostril. Fully depress rim with a firm even stroke and inhale deeply.
Adults and children 6 years of age and over (with adult supervision): 2 or 3 sprays in each nostril not more often than every 10 to 12 hours. Do not exceed 2 applications in any 24-hour period. Children under 6 years of age: consult a doctor.
Squeeze Bottle: Adults and children 6 years of age and over (with adult supervision): 2 or 3 sprays in each nostril not more often than every 10 to 12 hours. Do not exceed 2 applications in any 24-hour period. Children under 6 years of age: consult a doctor.

WARNINGS: Do not exceed recommended dosage because burning, stinging, sneezing or increase of nasal discharge may occur. The use of this container by more than one person may spread infection. Do not use this product for more than 3 days. If symptoms persist, consult a doctor. Do not use this product if you have heart disease, high blood pressure, thyroid disease, diabetes, or difficulty in urination due to enlargement of the prostate gland unless directed by a doctor.
KEEP THIS AND ALL DRUGS OUT OF THE REACH OF CHILDREN. In case of accidental ingestion, seek professional assistance or contact a poison control center immediately.

How Supplied: Available in ½ FL. OZ. and 1 FL. OZ. plastic squeeze bottles and ½ FL. OZ. measured-dose Ultra Fine mist pump.

VICKS® VAPORUB®

[*vā 'pō-rub*]

Nasal Decongestant/Cough Suppressant

Active Ingredients: Menthol 2.6%, Camphor 4.7%, Eucalyptus Oil 1.2%.

Inactive Ingredients: Cedarleaf Oil, Mineral Oil, Nutmeg Oil, Petrolatum, Spirits of Turpentine, Thymol.

Indications: For the temporary relief of nasal congestion and coughs associated with a cold.

Actions: VICKS VAPORUB has antitussive and nasal decongestant effects.

Directions: Adults and children 2 years of age and older: Rub a thick layer of Vicks VapoRub on chest and throat. If desired, cover with a dry, warm cloth, but keep clothing loose to let vapors rise to the nose and mouth. Repeat up to three times daily, especially at bedtime, or as directed by a doctor. Children under two years of age, consult a doctor.

WARNINGS: For external use only. Do not take by mouth or place in nostrils. Do not heat. Never expose to flame, microwave, or place in any container in which you are heating water. A persistent cough may be a sign of a serious condition. If cough persists for more than 1 week, tends to recur, or is accompanied by fever, rash, or persistent headache, consult a doctor. Do not use this product for persistent or chronic cough such as occurs with smoking, asthma, emphysema, or if cough is accompanied by excessive phlegm (mucus) unless directed by a doctor. **KEEP THIS AND ALL DRUGS OUT OF THE REACH OF CHILDREN.** In case of accidental ingestion, seek professional assistance or contact a poison control center immediately.

How Supplied: Available in 1.5 OZ., 3.0 OZ. and 6.0 OZ. plastic jars.

VICKS® VAPOSTEAM®
[*vā 'pō "stēm*]
Liquid Medication for Hot Steam Vaporizers. Nasal Decongestant/Cough Suppressant

Active Ingredients: Menthol 3.2%, Camphor 6.2%, Eucalyptus Oil 1.5%.

Inactive Ingredients: Alcohol 74%, Cedarleaf Oil, Nutmeg Oil, Poloxamer 124, Polyoxyethylene Dodecanol, Silicone.

Indications: For temporary relief of nasal congestion due to colds, hay fever or other upper respiratory allergies. Temporarily relieves cough occurring with a cold.

Actions: VAPOSTEAM increases the action of steam to help relieve cold symptoms in the following ways: relieves coughs of colds, eases nasal congestion, and moistens dry, irritated breathing passages.

Directions:
Adults and children 2 years of age and older: Use VAPOSTEAM in Hot/Warm Steam vaporizers, washbasin or bowl as described below. Follow directions for use carefully. Breathe in medicated vapors. May be repeated up to 3 times daily or as directed by a doctor.
Children under 2 years of age: consult a doctor.
In Hot/Warm Steam Vaporizers: Add VAPOSTEAM directly to the water in your electric vaporizer. Add one tablespoon of VAPOSTEAM with each quart of water added to the vaporizer. For best performance, vaporizer should be thoroughly cleaned after each use according to manufacturer's instructions. In soft water areas, it may be necessary to add salt or other steaming aid to promote steaming. Follow directions of vaporizer manufacturer for best results.
In Bowl or Washbasin: Pour steaming hot water into bowl or washbasin. Then add 1½ teaspoons of VAPOSTEAM for each pint of water used.
Breathe in medicated vapors.

WARNINGS: For hot/warm steam vaporizers only. Do not use in cold steam vaporizers or humidifiers. **Not to be taken by mouth.** A persistent cough may be sign of a serious condition. If cough persists for more than one week, tends to recur or is accompanied by fever, rash, or persistent headache, consult a doctor. Do not use this product for persistent or chronic cough such as occurs with smoking, asthma, emphysema, or if cough is accompanied by excessive phlegm (mucus) unless directed by a doctor. Store at room temperature and always keep VAPOSTEAM away from open flame or excessive heat. Do not direct steam from vaporizer towards face. Use caution in handling any container of hot water. Do not heat water containing VAPOSTEAM or use in microwave oven. **KEEP THIS AND ALL DRUGS OUT OF THE REACH OF CHILDREN.**

Accidental Ingestion: In case of accidental ingestion, seek professional assistance or contact a poison control center immediately.

How Supplied: Available in 4 FL. OZ. and 6 FL. OZ. bottles.

VICKS® VATRONOL®
[*vātrōnŏl*]
Ephedrine Sulfate/Nasal Decongestant Nose Drops

Active Ingredient: Ephedrine Sulfate 0.5%.

Inactive Ingredients: Camphor, Cedarleaf Oil, Eucalyptol, Menthol, Nutmeg Oil, Potassium Phosphate, Purified Water, Sodium Chloride, Sodium Phosphate, Tyloxapol.
Preservative: Thimerosal 0.001%.

Indications: For temporary relief of nasal congestion due to a cold, hay fever, or other upper respiratory allergies, or associated with sinusitis.

Actions: VICKS VATRONOL helps restore freer breathing by relieving nasal stuffiness. Relieves sinus pressure.

Dosage: Adults: Fill dropper to upper mark. Children 6 to under 12 years of age (with adult supervision): Fill dropper to lower mark. Children under 6 years of age: consult a doctor.
Apply in each nostril, not more often than every four hours.

WARNINGS: Do not exceed recommended dosage because burning, stinging, sneezing, or increase of nasal discharge may occur. The use of this container by more than one person may spread infection. Do not use this product for more than 3 days. If symptoms persist, consult a doctor. Do not use this product if you have heart disease, high blood pressure, thyroid disease, diabetes, or difficulty in urination due to enlargement of the prostate gland unless directed by a doctor. **KEEP THIS AND ALL DRUGS OUT OF THE REACH OF CHILDREN.** In case of accidental ingestion, seek professional assistance or contact a poison control center immediately.

How Supplied: Available in 1 FL. OZ. dropper bottles.

EDUCATIONAL MATERIAL

Journal Reprints for Physicians
Reprints of published journal articles illustrating the effectiveness of bismuth subsalicylate (Pepto-Bismol) for the treatment of diarrhea.

Reed & Carnrick
Division of Block Drug Company, Inc.
257 CORNELISON AVENUE
JERSEY CITY, NJ 07302-9988

PHAZYME® and PHAZYME®-95
[*fay-zime*]
Tablets

Description: Contains simethicone, an antiflatulent to alleviate or relieve the symptoms of gas. It has no known side effects or drug interactions.

Actions: Simethicone minimizes gas formation and relieves gas entrapment in both the stomach and the lower G.I. tract. This action combats the distress due to gastrointestinal gas.

Indication: To alleviate or relieve the symptoms of gas. May also be used for postoperative gas pain.

Warnings: Keep this and all drugs out of the reach of children. If condition persists, consult your physician.
Store at controlled room temperature 59°–86°F (15°–30°C).

PHAZYME®

Active Ingredient: Each tablet contains simethicone 60 mg.

Inactive Ingredients: Acacia, calcium sulfate, carnauba wax, crospovidone, D&C red No. 7 calcium lake, FD&C blue No. 1 aluminum lake, gelatin, lactose, methylparaben, microcrystalline cellulose, polyoxyl-40 stearate, povidone, pregelatinized starch, propylparaben, rice starch, sodium benzoate, sucrose, talc, titanium dioxide, white wax.

Dosage: One tablet four times a day after meals and at bedtime. Do not exceed 8 tablets a day unless directed by a physician.

How Supplied: Pink coated tablet imprinted "Phazyme" in bottles of 100, NDC #0021-1400-01

PHAZYME® 95

Active Ingredient: Each tablet contains simethicone 95 mg.

Inactive Ingredients: Acacia, calcium sulfate, carnauba wax, crospovidone, FD&C yellow No. 6 aluminum lake, FD&C red No. 40 aluminum lake, gelatin, lactose, microcrystalline cellulose, polyoxyl-40 stearate, povidone, pregelatinized starch, sodium benzoate, sucrose, talc, titanium dioxide, white wax.

Dosage: One tablet four times a day after meals and at bedtime. Do not exceed 5 tablets per day unless directed by a physician.

How Supplied: Red coated tablet imprinted "Phazyme 95" in

10 pack,	NDC #0021-1420-02
50's	NDC #0021-1420-50
100's,	NDC #0021-1420-01

Shown in Product Identification Section, page 419

Continued on next page

Reed & Carnrick—Cont.

PHAZYME® DROPS
[fay-zime]

Description:
Active Ingredients: Each 0.6 mL contains simethicone, 40 mg.
Inactive Ingredients: Carbomer 934 P, citric acid, flavor (natural orange), hydroxypropylmethylcellulose, PEG-8 stearate, potassium sorbate, sodium citrate, sodium saccharin, water.

Actions: Simethicone minimizes gas formation and relieves gas entrapment in both the stomach and the lower G.I. tract. This action combats the distress due to gastrointestinal gas.

Indication: To alleviate or relieve the symptoms of gas. May also be used for postoperative gas pain or for use in endoscopic examination.

Warnings: Keep this and all drugs out of the reach of children. If condition persists, consult your physician.
Store at controlled room temperature 59°–86°F (15°–30°C).

Dosage/Administration: Shake well before using.
Infants (under 2 years):
0.3 ml four times daily after meals and at bedtime or as directed by a physician. Can also be mixed with liquids for easier administration.
Children (2 to 12 years):
0.6 ml four times daily after meals and at bedtime or as directed by a physician.
Adults: 1.2 ml (take two 0.6 ml doses) four times daily after meals and at bedtime. Do not take more than six times per day unless directed by a physician.

How Supplied: Dropper bottles of 15 mL (0.5 fl oz) and 30 mL (1 fl oz).
15 mL NDC-0021-4300-33
30 mL NDC-0021-4300-17
Shown in Product Identification Section, page 419

Maximum Strength PHAZYME®-125 Capsules

Description: A red softgel containing the highest dose of simethicone available in a single capsule.
Active Ingredient: Each capsule contains simethicone, 125 mg.
Inactive Ingredients: FD&C red No. 40, gelatin, glycerin, hydrogenated soybean oil, lecithin, methylparaben, polysorbate 80, propylparaben, soybean oil, titanium dioxide, vegetable shortening, yellow wax.

Actions: Simethicone minimizes gas formation and relieves gas entrapment in both the stomach and the lower G.I. tract. This action combats the distress due to gastrointestinal gas.

Indication: To alleviate or relieve the symptoms of gas. May also be used for postoperative gas pain.

Warnings: Keep this and all drugs out of the reach of children. If condition persists, consult your physician.
Store at controlled room temperature 59°–86°F (15°–30°C).

Dosage: One softgel capsule four times a day after meals and at bedtime. Do not exceed 4 softgel capsules per day unless directed by a physician.

How Supplied: Red capsule imprinted rc 125 in bottles of 50, NDC #0021-0450-50 and 10 pack, NDC #0021-0450-02.
Shown in Product Identification Section, page 419

EDUCATIONAL MATERIAL

Brochures
Questions and Answers About Head Lice
Available in English and Spanish to physicians, pharmacists and patients.

The Reese Chemical Co.
10617 FRANK AVENUE
CLEVELAND, OHIO 44106

COLICON® DROPS

Active Ingredient: Simethicone.

Inactive Ingredients: Citric Acid, Carbomer 934P, Hydroxypropyl methylcellulose, Sodium Benzoate, Sodium Saccharin, deionized water and flavor.

Indications: For relief of the painful symptoms of excess gas in the digestive tract.
The defoaming action of Colicon relieves flatulence by dispersing and preventing the formation of mucus-surrounded gas pockets in the gastrointestinal tract. Infants: Colicon drops are also useful for relief of the painful symptoms of excess gas associated with such conditions as colic, lactose intolerance or air swallowing.

Warnings: Keep this and all drugs out of the reach of children. In case of accidental overdose consult a physician immediately.

Dosage and Administration: Adults and children 0.6cc four times a day after meals and at bedtime or as directed by a physician. Infants (under two years) 0.3cc four times a day after meals and at bedtime, or as directed by a physician.

How Supplied: 1 Fl. oz. (30cc) plastic dropper enclosed.
NDC 10956-639-01

REDIACON DX PEDIATRIC DROPS

Active Ingredients: Each ml contains
Phenylpropanolamine HCl 6.25 mg.
Guaifenesin 50 mg.
Dextromethorphan HBr 5 mg.

Indications: For the temporary relief of nasal congestion due to the common cold, hay fever or other respiratory allergies. Helps loosen phlegm and thin bronchial secretions and temporarily quiet cough.

Warnings: Do not exceed recommended dosage because at higher doses nervousness, dizziness, or sleeplessness may occur. Do not give to children who have heart disease, high blood pressure, thyroid disease, or diabetes unless directed by a physician.

Warnings: If cough persists for more than one week, tends to recur or is accompanied by fever, rash or persistent headache, consult a physician. Keep this and all drugs out of the reach of children. In case of accidental overdose, seek professional assistance or contact a Poison Control Center immediately.

Dosage and Administration: Children 2 to 6 years of age; oral dosage is 1 ml every 4 hours, not to exceed 6 doses in 24 hours, or as directed by a physician. Children under 2 years of age; consult a physician.

Professional Labeling: Children under 2 years of age: Dosage should be adjusted to age or weight and be administered every 4 hours as shown in the dosage table, not to exceed 6 doses in 24 hours.

Age	Weight	Dosage
1–3 months	8–12 lb	¼ mL
4–6 months	13–17 lb	½ mL
7–9 months	18–20 lb	¾ mL
10–24 months	21 + lb	1.0 mL

How Supplied: Available in 30 ml (1 fl. oz) plastic bottle with child-resistant cap and graduated dropper.

REESE'S PINWORM MEDICINE
Pyrantel Pamoate

Active Ingredient: Oral suspension—Pyrantel pamoate, 144 mg/cc (the equivalent of 50 mg Pyrantel base per cc).
Caplets—Pyrantel pamoate, 180 mg (the equivalent of 62.5 mg Pyrantel pamate base).

Indications: For the treatment of enterobiasis (pinworm infection).

Warnings: Keep this and all drugs out of the reach of children. In case of accidental overdose, seek professional assistance or contact a poison control center immediately.

Precaution: If you are pregnant or have liver disease, do not take this product unless directed by a doctor.

Dosage and Administration: Adults, children 12 years of age and over, and children 2 years to under 12 years of age

—Oral dosage is a single dose of 5 mg of pyrantel pamoate base per pound of body weight, not to exceed 1 gram.
Read package insert before taking this medicine. Do not administer to children under 2 years of age.

How Supplied: Reese's Pinworm Medicine is available in one-ounce bottles as a pleasant-tasting suspension which contains the equivalent of 50 mg Pyrantel pamoate base per cc. Also available in bottles of 24 caplets. It is supplied with English and Spanish label copy and directions.

Shown in Product Identification Section, page 419

Requa, Inc.

BOX 4008
1 SENECA PLACE
GREENWICH, CT 06830

CHARCOAID
Poison Adsorbent, liquid has sweet, pleasant taste and feel; especially good for young patients.

Active Ingredient: Activated vegetable charcoal U.S.P., 30 g per bottle, suspended in 70% sorbitol solution U.S.P., 110 g.

Indication: For the emergency treatment of acute poisoning.

Action: Adsorbent

Warnings: Before using call a poison control center, emergency room, or a physician for advice. If the patient has been given Ipecac Syrup, do not give activated charcoal until after patient has vomited. Do not use in a semi-conscious or unconscious person.

Precaution: May cause laxation. Careful attention to fluids and electrolytes is important, especially with young children and multiple dose therapy.

Dosage and Administration: Adults: Shake well and drink entire contents (add water if too sweet). To insure a full dose, rinse bottle with water and drink. For children, refer to Poison Control Center.

Professional Labeling: Some dilution may be necessary for administration via lavage tube. Add a small amount of water to bottle and shake.

How Supplied: 5 fl. oz. unit dose bottle, 30 g activated charcoal U.S.P., suspended in 70% sorbitol solution U.S.P., 110 g.
U.S. Patent #4,122,169

CHARCOCAPS®
Digestive Aid
Activated Charcoal Capsules and Caplets

Active Ingredient: Activated vegetable charcoal U.S.P., 260 mg per capsule.

Indications: Relief of intestinal gas, gastrointestinal distress associated with indigestion. Also to aid in the prevention of non-specific pruritus associated with kidney dialysis treatment.

Actions: Adsorbent, detoxicant, soothing agent. Reduces the volume of intestinal gas and allays related discomfort.

Warnings: If symptoms of distress persist, stop this medication and consult your physician. Consults a physician if taking other drugs as this medication may interfere with their effectiveness.

Drug Interaction: Activated Charcoal USP can adsorb medication while they are in the digestive tract.

Precaution: General Guidelines— Take two hours before or one hour after medication including oral contraceptives.

Symptoms and Treatment of Oral Overdosage: Overdosage has not been encountered. Medical evidence indicates that high dosage or prolonged use does not cause side effect or harm the nutritional state of the patient.

Dosage and Administration: Two capsules after meals or at first sign of discomfort. Repeat as needed up to eight doses (16 capsules) per day.

Professional Labeling: None.

How Supplied: Bottles of 8, 36, 100 capsules

EDUCATIONAL MATERIAL

Questions & Answers
Brochure with questions and answers about the use of activated charcoal.
Trial Size
Free professional samples of Charcocaps, which includes coupon for regular size for the patient.

Rhône-Poulenc Rorer Pharmaceuticals Inc.

Consumer Pharmaceutical Products
500 ARCOLA ROAD
P.O. BOX 1200
COLLEGEVILLE, PA 19426-0107

Regular Strength ASCRIPTIN®
[ă″skrĭp′tin]
Analgesic
Aspirin buffered with Maalox®

Active Ingredients: Each tablet contains Aspirin (325 mg), buffered with Maalox (Alumina-Magnesia) and Calcium Carbonate.

Inactive Ingredients: Hydroxypropyl Methylcellulose, Magnesium Stearate, Microcrystalline Cellulose, Starch, Talc, Titanium Dioxide, and other ingredients.

Description: Ascriptin is an excellent analgesic, antipyretic, and anti-inflammatory agent for general use, particularly where there is concern over aspirin-induced gastric distress. Coated tablets make swallowing easy.

Indications: As an analgesic for the relief of pain in such conditions as headache, neuralgia, minor injuries, and dysmenorrhea. As an analgesic and antipyretic in adult colds and influenza. As an analgesic and anti-inflammatory agent in arthritis and other rheumatic diseases. As an inhibitor of platelet aggregation, see MI's and TIA's indications.

Usual Adult Dose: Two or three tablets, four times daily. Do not exceed 12 tablets in a 24-hour period. For children under twelve, consult a doctor.
WARNINGS: Children and teenagers should not use this medicine for chicken pox or flu symptoms before a doctor is consulted about Reye syndrome, a rare but serious illness reported to be associated with aspirin. Keep this and all medicines out of children's reach. If pain persists more than 10 days, redness or swelling is present, fever persists more than 3 days, or symptoms worsen, consult a doctor immediately. If you are under medical care or have a history of stomach, kidney, or bleeding disorders or asthma, consult a doctor before using. Do not use if allergic to aspirin. As with any drug, if you are pregnant or nursing a baby, consult a doctor before using. "**IT IS ESPECIALLY IMPORTANT NOT TO USE**" **(select "ASPIRIN" or "CARBASPIRIN CALCIUM," as appropriate) "DURING THE LAST 3 MONTHS OF PREGNANCY UNLESS SPECIFICALLY DIRECTED TO DO SO BY A DOCTOR BECAUSE IT MAY CAUSE PROBLEMS IN THE UNBORN CHILD OR COMPLICATIONS DURING DELIVERY.**" If ringing in the ears or loss of hearing occurs, consult a doctor before taking any more of this product. In case of accidental overdose, contact a doctor immediately. *Drug Interaction Precaution:* Do not use if taking a prescription drug for anticoagulation (blood thinning), diabetes, gout or arthritis, or a tetracycline antibiotic unless directed by a doctor.

Professional Labeling
Aspirin for Myocardial Infarction

Indication: Aspirin is indicated to reduce the risk of death and/or non-fatal myocardial infarction in patients with a previous infarction or unstable angina pectoris.

Dosage and Administration: Although most of the studies used dosages exceeding 300 mg, two trials used only 300 mg, and pharmacologic data indicate that this dose inhibits platelet function fully. Therefore, 300 mg or a conventional 325-mg aspirin dose is a reasonable, routine dose that would minimize gastrointestinal adverse reactions. This use of aspirin applies to both solid, oral dosage forms (buffered and plain aspirin), and

Continued on next page

Rhône-Poulenc Rorer—Cont.

buffered aspirin in solution. *Note:* Complete information and references available.

ASCRIPTIN FOR RECURRENT TIA's IN MEN

*Clinical Trials:*The indication is supported by the results of a Canadian study (1) in which 585 patients with threatened stroke were followed in a randomized clinical trial for an average of 26 months to determine whether aspirin or sulfinpyrazone, singly or in combination was superior to placebo in preventing transient ischemic attacks, stroke, or death. The study showed that, although sulfinpyrazone had no statistically significant effect, aspirin reduced the risk of continuing transient ischemic attacks, stroke, or death by 19 percent and reduced the risk of stroke or death by 31 percent. Another aspirin study carried out in the United States with 178 patients, showed a statistically significant number of "favorable outcomes" including reduced transient ischemic attacks, stroke, and death (2).

Indications: For reducing the risk of recurrent transient ischemic attacks (TIA's) or stroke in men who have had transient ischemia of the brain due to fibrin platelet emboli. There is inadequate evidence that aspirin or buffered aspirin is effective in reducing TIA's in women at the recommended dosage. There is no evidence that aspirin or buffered aspirin is of benefit in the treatment of completed strokes in men or women.

Precautions: (1) Patients presenting with signs and symptoms of TIA's should have a complete medical and neurologic evaluation. Consideration should be given to other disorders which resemble TIA's. **(2)** Attention should be given to risk factors; it is important to evaluate and treat, if appropriate, other diseases associated with TIA's and stroke such as hypertension and diabetes. **(3)** Concurrent administration of absorbable antacids at therapeutic doses may increase the clearance of salicylates in some individuals. The concurrent administration of nonabsorbable antacids may alter the rate of absorption of aspirin, thereby resulting in a decreased acetylsalicylic acid/salicylate ratio in plasma. The clinical significance on TIA's of these decreases in available aspirin is unknown.

Aspirin at dosages of 1,000 milligrams per day has been associated with small increases in blood pressure, blood urea nitrogen, and serum uric acid levels. It is recommended that patients placed on long-term aspirin treatment be seen at regular intervals to assess changes in these measurements.

Adverse Reactions: At dosages of 1,000 milligrams or higher of aspirin per day, gastrointestinal side effects include stomach pain, heartburn, nausea and/or vomiting, as well as increased rates of gross gastrointestinal bleeding.

Dosage: Adults dosage for men is 1300 mg a day, in divided doses of 650 mg twice a day or 325 mg four times a day.

References

(1) The Canadian Cooperative Study Group. "A Randomized Trial of Aspirin and Sulfinpyrazone in Threatened Stroke," *New England Journal of Medicine,* 299:53–59, 1978.

(2) Fields, W.S., et al., "Controlled Trial of Aspirin in Cerebral Ischemia," *Stroke* 8:301–316, 1977.

How Supplied: Bottles of 60 tablets (0067-0145-60), 100 tablets (0067-0145-68), 160 (0067-0145-30) and 225 tablets (0067-0145-77).

Bottles of 500 tablets (0067-0145-74) without child-resistant closures (for arthritic patients).

Shown in Product Identification Section, page 419

Extra Strength
ASCRIPTIN®
Analgesic
Aspirin Buffered with Maalox®
for Extra Pain Relief
with Stomach Comfort

Active Ingredients: Each coated caplet contains Aspirin (500 mg), buffered with Maalox (Alumina-Magnesia) and Calcium Carbonate.

Inactive Ingredients: Hydroxypropyl Methylcellulose, Magnesium Stearate, Microcrystalline Cellulose, Starch, Talc, Titanium Dioxide, and other ingredients.

Description: Extra Strength Ascriptin contains the maximum dose of aspirin for fast, effective pain relief, and is buffered with Maalox for stomach comfort. Coated caplets make swallowing easy.

Indications: For maximum relief of pain in headache, neuralgia, minor injuries, dysmenorrhea, discomfort and fever of ordinary colds. As an analgesic and anti-inflammatory agent in arthritis and other rheumatic diseases.

Usual Adult Dose: 2 caplets, three or four times daily. Not to exceed a total of 8 tablets in a 24-hour period, or as directed by a physician. For children under 12 at the discretion of physician.

WARNINGS: Children and teenagers should not use this medicine for chicken pox or flu symptoms before a doctor is consulted about Reye syndrome, a rate but serious illness reported to be associated with aspirin. Keep this and all medicines out of children's reach. If pain persists more than 10 days, redness or swelling is present, fever persists more than 3 days, or symptoms worsen, consult a doctor immediately. If you are under medical care or have a history of stomach, kidney, or bleeding disorders or asthma, consult a doctor before using. Do not use if allergic to aspirin. As with any drug, if you are pregnant or nursing a baby, consult a doctor before using. **"IT IS ESPECIALLY IMPORTANT NOT TO USE" (select "ASPIRIN" or "CARBASPIRIN CALCIUM," as appropriate) "DURING THE LAST 3 MONTHS OF PREGNANCY UNLESS SPECIFICALLY DIRECTED TO DO SO BY A DOCTOR BECAUSE IT MAY CAUSE PROBLEMS IN THE UNBORN CHILD OR COMPLICATIONS DURING DELIVERY."** If ringing in the ears or loss of hearing occurs, consult a doctor before taking any more of this product. **In case of accidental overdose, contact a doctor immediately.** *Drug interaction precaution:* Do not use if taking a prescription drug for anticoagulation (blood thinning), diabetes, gout or arthritis, or a tetracycline antibiotic unless directed by a doctor.

Professional Labeling
ASCRIPTIN FOR MYOCARDIAL INFARCTION

Indication: Aspirin is indicated to reduce the risk of death and/or nonfatal myocardial infarction in patients with a previous infarction or unstable angina pectoris.

Dosage and Administration: Although most of the studies used dosages exceeding 300 mg, two trials used only 300 mg, and pharmacologic data indicate that this dose inhibits platelet function fully. Therefore, 300 mg or a conventional 325 mg aspirin dose is a reasonable, routine dose that would minimize gastrointestinal adverse reactions. This use of aspirin applies to both solid, oral dosage forms (buffered and plain aspirin), and buffered aspirin in solution. *Note:* Complete information and references available.

ASCRIPTIN FOR RECURRENT TIA's IN MEN

Clinical Trials: The indication is supported by the results of a Canadian study (1) in which 585 patients with threatened stroke were followed in a randomized clinical trial for an average of 26 months to determine whether aspirin or sulfinpyrazone, singly or in combination was superior to placebo in preventing transient ischemic attacks, stroke, or death. The study showed that, although sulfinpyrazone had no statistically significant effect, aspirin reduced the risk of continuing transient ischemic attacks, stroke, or death by 19 percent and reduced the risk of stroke or death by 31 percent. Another aspirin study carried out in the United States with 178 patients, showed a statistically significant number of "favorable outcomes" including reduced transient ischemic attacks, stroke, and death (2).

Indications: For reducing the risk of recurrent transient ischemic attacks (TIA's) or stroke in men who have had transient ischemia of the brain due to fibrin platelet emboli. There is inadequate evidence that aspirin or buffered aspirin is effective in reducing TIA's in women at the recommended dosage. There is no evidence that aspirin or buffered aspirin is of benefit in the treatment of completed strokes in men or women.

Precautions: (1) Patients presenting with signs and symptoms of TIA's should have a complete medical and neurologic evaluation. Consideration should be given to other disorders which resemble TIA's. (2) Attention should be given to risk factors; it is important to evaluate and treat, if appropriate, other diseases associated with TIA's and stroke such as hypertension and diabetes. (3) Concurrent administration of absorbable antacids at therapeutic doses may increase the clearance of salicylates in some individuals. The concurrent administration of nonabsorbable antacids may alter the rate of absorption of aspirin, thereby resulting in a decreased acetylsalicylic acid/salicylate ratio in plasma. The clinical significance on TIA's of these decreases in available aspirin is unknown. Aspirin at dosages of 1,000 milligrams per day has been associated with small increases in blood pressure, blood urea nitrogen, and serum uric acid levels. It is recommended that patients placed on long-term aspirin treatment be seen at regular intervals to assess changes in these measurements.

Adverse Reactions: At dosages of 1,000 milligrams or higher of aspirin per day, gastrointestinal side effects include stomach pain, heartburn, nausea and/or vomiting, as well as increased rates of gross gastrointestinal bleeding."

Dosage: Adults dosage for men is 1300 mg a day, in divided doses of 650 mg twice a day or 325 mg four times a day.

References

(1) The Canadian Cooperative Study Group. "A Randomized Trial of Aspirin and Sulfinpyrazone in Threatened Stroke," *New England Journal of Medicine*, 299:53–59, 1978.
(2) Fields, W.S., et al., "Controlled Trial of Aspirin in Cerebral Ischemia." *Stroke* 8:301–316, 1977."

How Supplied: Bottles of 36 caplets (0067-0146-63) without child-resistant closure, 50 caplets (0067-0146-50) and 85 caplets (0067-0146-85) both with child-resistant caps.

Shown in Product Identification Section, page 419

ASCRIPTIN® A/D for arthritis pain
Analgesic
Aspirin buffered with extra Maalox® for pain relief with extra stomach comfort

Active Ingredients: Each caplet contains Aspirin (325 mg), buffered with Maalox (Alumina-Magnesia) and Calcium Carbonate.

Inactive Ingredients: Hydroxypropyl Methylcellulose, Magnesium Stearate, Microcrystalline Cellulose, Starch, Talc, Titanium Dioxide, and other ingredients.

Description: Ascriptin A/D is a highly buffered analgesic, anti-inflammatory, and antipyretic agent for use in the treatment of rheumatoid arthritis, osteoarthritis, and other arthritic conditions. It is formulated with 50% more Maalox than Regular Strength Ascriptin to provide increased neutralization of gastric acid thus reducing the likelihood of GI disturbance when large antiarthritic doses of aspirin are used. Coated caplets make swallowing easy.

Indications: As an analgesic, anti-inflammatory, and antipyretic agent in rheumatoid arthritis, osteoarthritis, and other arthritic conditions.

Usual Adult Dose: Two or three caplets, four times daily, or as directed by the physician for arthritis therapy. For children under twelve, at the discretion of the physician.

WARNINGS: Children and teenagers should not use this medicine for chicken pox or flu symptoms before a doctor is consulted about Reye syndrome, a rare but serious illness reported to be associated with aspirin. Keep this and all medicines out of children's reach. If pain persists more than 10 days, redness or swelling is present, fever persists more than 3 days, or symptoms worsen, consult a doctor immediately. If you are under medical care or have a history of stomach, kidney, or bleeding disorders or asthma, consult a doctor before using. Do not use if allergic to aspirin. As with any drug, if you are pregnant or nursing a baby, consult a doctor before using. **IT IS ESPECIALLY IMPORTANT NOT TO USE ASPIRIN DURING THE LAST 3 MONTHS OF PREGNANCY UNLESS SPECIFICALLY DIRECTED TO DO SO BY A DOCTOR BECAUSE IT MAY CAUSE PROBLEMS IN THE UNBORN CHILD OR COMPLICATIONS DURING DELIVERY.** If ringing in the ears or loss of hearing occurs, consult a doctor before taking any more of this product. **In case of accidental overdose, contact a doctor immediately.**

Drug Interaction Precaution: Do not use if taking a prescription drug for anticoagulation (blood thinning), diabetes, gout or arthritis, or a tetracycline antibiotic unless directed by a doctor.

Professional Labeling
ASCRIPTIN FOR MYOCARDIAL INFARCTION

Indication: Aspirin is indicated to reduce the risk of death and/or non-fatal myocardial infarction in patients with a previous infarction or unstable angina pectoris.

Dosage and Administration: Although most of the studies used dosages exceeding 300 mg, two trials used only 300 mg, and pharmacologic data indicate that this dose inhibits platelet function fully. Therefore, 300 mg or a conventional 325-mg aspirin dose is a reasonable, routine dose that would minimize gastrointestinal adverse reactions. This use of aspirin applies to both solid, oral dosage forms (buffered and plan aspirin), and buffered aspirin in solution. *Note:* Complete information and references available.

ASCRIPTIN FOR RECURRENT TIA's IN MEN

Clinical Trials: The indication is supported by the results of a Canadian study (1) in which 585 patients with threatened stroke were followed in a randomized clinical trial for an average of 26 months to determine whether aspirin or sulfinpyrazone, singly or in combination was superior to placebo in preventing transient ischemic attacks, stroke, or death. The study showed that, although sulfinpyrazone had no statistically significant effect, aspirin reduced the risk of continuing transient ischemic attacks, stroke, or death by 19 percent and reduced the risk of stroke or death by 31 percent. Another aspirin study carried out in the United States with 178 patients, showed a statistically significant number of "favorable outcomes" including reduced transient ischemic attacks, stroke, and death (2).

Indications: For reducing the risk of recurrent transient ischemic attacks (TIA's) or stroke in men who have had transient ischemia of the brain due to fibrin platelet emboli. There is inadequate evidence that aspirin or buffered aspirin is effective in reducing TIA's in women at the recommended dosage. There is no evidence that aspirin or buffered aspirin is of benefit in the treatment of completed strokes in men or women.

Precautions: (1) Patients presenting with signs and symptoms of TIA's should have a complete medical and neurologic evaluation. Consideration should be given to other disorders which resemble TIA's. (2) Attention should be given to risk factors; it is important to evaluate and treat, if appropriate, other diseases associated with TIA's and stroke such as hypertension and diabetes. (3) Concurrent administration of absorbable antacids at therapeutic doses may increase the clearance of salicylates in some individuals. The concurrent administration of nonabsorbable antacids may alter the rate of absorption of aspirin, thereby resulting in a decreased acetylsalicylic acid/salicylate ratio in plasma. The clinical significance on TIA's of these decreases in available aspirin is unknown. Aspirin at dosages of 1,000 milligrams per day has been associated with small increases in blood pressure, blood urea nitrogen, and serum uric acid levels. It is recommended that patients placed on long-term aspirin treatment be seen at regular intervals to assess changes in these measurements.

Adverse Reactions: At dosages of 1,000 milligrams or higher of aspirin per day, gastrointestinal side effects include stomach pain, heartburn, nausea and/or vomiting, as well as increased rates of gross gastrointestinal bleeding."

Continued on next page

Rhône-Poulenc Rorer—Cont.

Dosage: Adults dosage for men is 1300 mg a day, in divided doses of 650 mg twice a day or 325 mg four times a day.

References

(1) The Canadian Cooperative Study Group. "A Randomized Trial of Aspirin and Sulfinpyrazone in Threatened Stroke," *New England Journal of Medicine*, 299:53–59, 1978.
(2) Fields, W.S., et al., "Controlled Trial of Aspirin in Cerebral Ischemia." *Stroke* 8:301–316, 1977."

How Supplied: Available in bottles of 60 caplets (0067-0147-60), 100 caplets (0067-0147-68), and 225 caplets (0067-0147-77) with child-resistant caps and in special bottles of 500 caplets (without child-resistant closures) for arthritic patients (0067-0147-74). Military Stock #NSN 6505-00-135-2783, bottles of 500.

Shown in Product Identification Section, page 419

MAALOX® Antacid Caplets Antacid

Description: New Maalox® antacid caplets provide fast, effective relief of acid indigestion, heartburn, and sour stomach. Because they are easy-to-swallow caplets, there is no chalky aftertaste.

Active Ingredients: Each caplet contains 1000 mg calcium carbonate.

Inactive Ingredients: Corn starch, croscarmellose, magnesium stearate and sodium lauryl sulfate.

Minimum Recommended Dosage: Maalox Antacid Caplets	Per 2 tsp. (10 mL)
Acid neutralizing capacity	20.0 mEq
Sodium content	0.4 mg

Indications: For the relief of acid indigestion, heartburn, sour stomach and upset stomach associated with these symptoms.

Directions for Use: Take 1 caplet as needed or as directed by physician.
CAPLETS SHOULD NOT BE CHEWED.

Patient Warnings: Do not take more than 8 caplets in a 24-hour period or use the maximum dosage for more than 2 weeks except under the advice and supervision of a physician. If you have a history of calcium stones or decreased renal function, consult a physician before use. Keep this and all drugs out of the reach of children.

Drug Interaction Precaution: Calcium antacid salts can decrease absorption of beta-adrenergic blockers and Dilantin. Thiazide diuretics can cause hypercalcemia by decreasing renal excretion of calcium antacids. The milk-alkali syndrome can occur with prolonged sodium bicarbonate use and/or homogenized milk containing Vitamin D.

Professional Labeling: Indicated for the symptomatic relief of hyperacidity associated with the diagnosis of peptic ulcer, gastritis, peptic esophagitis, gastric hyperacidity, and hiatal hernia.

How Supplied: Maalox Antacid Caplets are available in blister packs of 24 caplets (0067-0183-24) and plastic bottle of 50 caplets (0067-0183-50).

Storage: Store at room temperature. Protect from moisture.

Shown in Product Identification Section, page 419

MAALOX® HRF Heartburn Relief Formula™ Antacid Tablets

Description: New Maalox HRF tablets are specially formulated to provide fast, effective relief of heartburn. Each tablet contains aluminum hydroxide-magnesium carbonate codried gel 180 mg and magnesium carbonate 160 mg. It is formulated in a pleasant, cool mint flavor.

Inactive Ingredients: Compressible sugar, corn starch, D&C Yellow No. 10, FD&C Blue No. 2, flavors, magnesium alginate, magnesium stearate, potassium bicarbonate.

Minimum Recommended Dosage: Maalox Heartburn Relief Antacid Tablets	Per 2 tablets
Acid neutralizing Capacity	14.7 mEq

Directions for Use: Chew 2–4 tablets thoroughly, after meals and at bedtime, or as directed by physician. For best results, follow with a half glass (4 fl. oz.) of water or other liquid.

Patient Warnings: Do not take more than 16 tablets in a 24-hour period or use the maximum dosage for more than 2 weeks or use if you have kidney disease except under the advice and supervision of a physician.

Drug Interaction Precaution: Do not use if you are taking a prescription antibiotic drug containing any form of tetracycline. As with all aluminum-containing antacids, Maalox® Heartburn Relief Formula™ may prevent the proper absorption of the tetracycline.

Professional Labeling:

Warnings: Prolonged use of aluminum-containing antacids in patients with renal failure may result in or worsen dialysis osteomalacia. Elevated tissue aluminum levels contribute to the development of the dialysis encephalopathy and osteomalacia syndromes. Small amounts of aluminum are absorbed from the gastrointestinal tract and renal excretion of aluminum is impaired in renal failure. Aluminum is not well removed by dialysis because it is bound to albumin and transferrin, which do not cross dialysis membranes. As a result, aluminum is deposited in bone and dialysis osteomalacia may develop when large amounts of aluminum are ingested orally by patients with impaired renal function.
Aluminum forms insoluble complexes with phosphate in the gastrointestinal tract, thus decreasing phosphate absorption. Prolonged use of antacids containing aluminum by normophosphatemic patients may result in hypophosphatemia if phosphate intake is not adequate. In its more severe forms, hypophosphatemia can lead to anorexia, malaise, muscle weakness, and osteomalacia.

How Supplied: Maalox HRF antacid tablets are available in plastic bottles of 30 tablets (0067-0353-30), 60 tablets (0067-0353-60) and blister packs of 12 tablets (0067-0353-12).

Shown in Product Identification Section, page 419

MAALOX® HRF Heartburn Relief Formula™ Suspension

Description: Maalox HRF provides symptomatic relief of heartburn, acid indigestion and/or sour stomach. Each 10 ml (2 teaspoonfuls) contains aluminum hydroxide-magnesium carbonate codried gel 280 mg and magnesium carbonate USP 350 mg. It is formulated in a pleasant, cool mint flavor to help provide a cooling and soothing sensation as it goes down the esophagus.

Inactive Ingredients: Calcium carbonate, calcium saccharin, FD&C Blue No. 1, FD&C Yellow No. 5 (tartrazine) as a color additive, flavors, magnesium alginate, methyl and propyl parabens, potassium bicarbonate, purified water, sorbitol and other ingredients.

Minimum Recommended Dosage: Maalox Heartburn Relief Suspension	Per 2 tsp. (10 mL)
Acid neutralizing capacity	19 mEq
Sodium content	4 mg

Directions for Use: Maalox HRF—two to four teaspoonfuls after meals and at bedtime, or as directed by a physician.

Patient Warnings: Do not take more than 16 teaspoonfuls in a 24-hour period or use the maximum dosage for more than 2 weeks or use if you have kidney disease except under the advice and supervision of a physician. Keep this and all drugs out of the reach of children.

Drug Interaction Precaution: Do not use if you are taking a prescription antibiotic drug containing any form of tetracycline.

Professional Labeling:

Warnings:
Prolonged use of aluminum-containing antacids in patients with renal failure may result in or worsen dialysis osteomalacia. Elevated tissue aluminum levels contribute to the development of the dialysis encephalopathy and osteomalacia syndromes. Small amounts of aluminum are absorbed from the gastrointestinal tract and renal excretion of aluminum is impaired in renal failure. Aluminum is not well removed by dialysis because it is bound to albumin and transferrin, which do not cross dialysis membranes. As a result, aluminum is deposited in bone, and dialysis osteomalacia may develop when large amounts of aluminum are ingested orally by patients with impaired renal function.
Aluminum forms insoluble complexes with phosphate in the gastrointestinal tract, thus decreasing phosphate absorption. Prolonged use of antacids containing aluminum by normophosphatemic patients may result in hypophosphatemia if phosphate intake is not adequate. In its more severe forms, hypophosphatemia can lead to anorexia, malaise, muscle weakness, and osteomalacia.

How Supplied: Maalox HRF is available in a 12 fl oz plastic bottle (0067-0350-71).

Shown in Product Identification Section, page 419

MAALOX®
Magnesia and Alumina Oral Suspension Antacid

Liquids
Mint Flavored
Cherry Creme

Description: Maalox® is used for the relief of acid indigestion, heartburn, sour stomach and upset stomach associated with these symptoms.

Active Ingredients	Maalox Suspension 5 mL teaspoon
Magnesium Hydroxide	200 mg.
Aluminum Hydroxide (equivalent to dried gel, USP)	225 mg.

Inactive Ingredients: Citric acid, natural flavors, methylparaben, propylparaben, saccharin sodium, sorbitol, purified water and other ingredients.

Minimum Recommended Dosage: Maalox Suspension	Per 2 Tsp. (10 mL)
Acid neutralizing capacity	26.6 mEq
Sodium content	.12 mg

Indications: As an antacid for symptomatic relief of hyperacidity associated with the diagnosis of peptic ulcer, gastritis, peptic esophagitis, gastric hyperacidity, heartburn, or hiatal hernia.

Professional Labeling

Warnings: (i) Prolonged use of aluminum-containing antacids in patients with renal failure may result in or worsen dialysis osteomalacia. Elevated tissue aluminum levels contribute to the development of the dialysis encephalopathy and osteomalacia syndromes. Small amounts of aluminum are absorbed from the gastrointestinal tract and renal excretion of aluminum is impaired in renal failure. Aluminum is not well removed by dialysis because it is bound to albumin and trensferrin, which do not cross dialysis membranes. As a result, aluminum is deposited in bone, and dialysis osteomalacia may develop when large amounts of aluminum are ingested orally by patients with impaired renal function. (ii) Aluminum forms insoluble complexes with phosphate in the gastrointestinal tract, thus decreasing phosphate absorption. Prolonged use of aluminum-containing antacids by normophosphatemic patients may result in hypophosphatemia if phosphate intake is not adequate. In its more severe forms, hypophosphatemia can lead to anorexia, malaise, muscle weakness, and osteomalacia.

Directions for Use. Two to four teaspoonfuls, four times a day, taken 20 minutes to 1 hour after meals and at bedtime, or as directed by a physician.

Patient Warnings: Do not take more than 16 teaspoonfuls in a 24-hour period or use the maximum dosage for more than 2 weeks or use if you have kidney disease except under the advice and supervision of a physician. Keep this and all drugs out of the reach of children.

Drug Interaction Precaution: Do not use if you are taking a prescription antibiotic drug containing any form of tetracycline.

How Supplied:
Maalox Mint Flavored Suspension is available in plastic bottles of 12 oz (0067-0330-71) and 26 oz (0067-0330-44).
Maalox Cherry Creme Flavored Suspension is available in plastic bottles of 12 oz (0067-0031-71) and 26 oz (0067-0331-44).

Shown in Product Identification Section, page 420

MAALOX® Plus
Alumina, Magnesia and Simethicone Tablets,
Rhône-Poulenc Rorer
Antacid/Anti-Gas

Tablets
Lemon Swiss Creme
Cherry Creme
... the flavors preferred by the physician and patient.

- ☐ **Physician-proven Maalox® formula for antacid effectiveness.**
- ☐ **Simethicone, at a recognized clinical dose, for antiflatulent action.**

Description: Maalox® Plus, a balanced combination of magnesium and aluminum hydroxides plus simethicone, is a non-constipating antacid/anti-gas which comes in pleasant tasting flavors.

Composition: To provide symptomatic relief of hyperacidity plus alleviation of gas symptoms, each tablet contains:

Active Ingredients	Maalox® Plus Per Tablet
Magnesium Hydroxide	200 mg
Aluminum Hydroxide (equivalent to dried gel, USP)	200 mg
Simethicone	25 mg

Inactive Ingredients: Maalox® Plus Tablets: Citric acid, confectioners' sugar, artificial colors, dextrose, flavors, glycerin, magnesium stearate, mannitol, saccharin sodium, sorbitol, starch, talc and may also contain hydrogenated vegetable oil.
To aid in establishing proper dosage schedules, the following information is provided:

Minimum Recommended Dosage:	Per Tablet
Acid neutralizing capacity	10.65 mEq
Sodium content*	<1 mg
Sugar content	0.57 g
Lactose content	None

*Dietetically insignificant.

Indications: As an antacid for symptomatic relief of hyperacidity associated with the diagnosis of peptic ulcer, gastritis, peptic esophagitis, gastric hyperacidity, heartburn, or hiatal hernia. As an antiflatulent to alleviate the symptoms of gas, including postoperative gas pain.

Continued on next page

Rhône-Poulenc Rorer—Cont.

Professional Labeling

Warnings: Prolonged use of aluminum-containing antacids in patients with renal failure may result in or worsen dialysis osteomalacia. Elevated tissue aluminum levels contribute to the development of the dialysis encephalopathy and osteomalacia syndromes. Small amounts of aluminum are absorbed from the gastrointestinal tract and renal excretion of aluminum is impaired in renal failure. Aluminum is not well removed by dialysis because it is bound to albumin and transferrin, which do not cross dialysis membranes. As a result, aluminum is deposited in bone, and dialysis osteomalacia may develop when large amounts of aluminum are ingested orally by patients with impaired renal function.
Aluminum forms insoluble complexes with phosphate in the gastrointestinal tract, thus decreasing phosphate absorption. Prolonged use of aluminum-containing antacids by normophosphatemic patients may result in hypophosphatemia if phosphate intake is not adequate. In its more severe forms, hypophosphatemia can lead to anorexia, malaise, muscle weakness, and osteomalacia.

Advantages: Maalox® Plus Tablets are uniquely palatable—an important feature which encourages patients to follow your dosage directions. Maalox® Plus Tablets have the time-proven, nonconstipating, sodium-free* Maalox® formula—useful for those patients suffering from the problems associated with hyperacidity. Additionally, Maalox® Plus Tablets contain simethicone to alleviate discomfort associated with entrapped gas.

Directions for Use: One to four tablets, well chewed, four times a day, taken twenty minutes to one hour after meals and at bedtime, or as directed by a physician.

Patient Warnings: Do not take more than 16 tablets in a 24-hour period or use the maximum dosage for more than 2 weeks or use if you have kidney disease except under the advice and supervision of a physician. Keep this and all drugs out of the reach of children.

Drug Interaction Precaution: Do not use with patients taking a prescription antibiotic containing any form of tetracycline. As with all aluminum-containing antacids, Maalox® Plus may prevent the proper absorption of the tetracycline.

How Supplied: Maalox® Plus Lemon Swiss Creme Tablets are available in plastic bottles of 50 tablets (0067-0339-50) and 100 tablets (0067-0339-67), convenience packs of 12 tablets (0067-0339-19), tray of 12 rolls (0067-0339-23), and 3 roll packs of 36 tablets (0067-0339-33).
Maalox Plus Cherry Creme Tablets are available in plastic bottles of 50 tablets (0067-0341-50) and 100 tablets (0067-0341-68), tray of 12 rolls (0067-0341-23) and 3 roll packs of 36 tablets (0067-0341-33).

Shown in Product Identification Section, page 420

EXTRA STRENGTH MAALOX® Plus (Reformulated Maalox Plus)
Alumina, Magnesia and Simethicone Oral Suspension and Tablets, Antacid/Anti-Gas

Liquids	Tablets
☐ **Lemon Swiss Creme**	**Mint Creme**
Cherry Creme	
Mint Creme	

. . . the flavors preferred by the physician and patient.
☐ **Physician-proven Maalox® formula for antacid effectiveness.**
☐ **Simethicone, at a recognized clinical dose, for antiflatulent action.**

Description: Extra Strength Maalox® Plus, a balanced combination of magnesium and aluminum hydroxides plus simethicone, is a non-constipating antacid/anti-gas product to provide symptomatic relief of hyperacidity plus alleviation of gas symptoms. Available in liquid form in Cherry Creme, Mint Creme or Lemon Swiss Creme flavors, and in tablet form in the Mint Creme flavor.

Composition: To provide symptomatic relief of hyperacidity plus alleviation of gas symptoms, each teaspoonful/tablet contains:

Active Ingredients	Extra Strength Maalox® Plus Per Tsp. (5 mL)	Extra Strength Maalox® Plus Per Tablet
Magnesium Hydroxide	450 mg	350 mg
Aluminum Hydroxide (equivalent to dried gel, USP)	500 mg	350 mg
Simethicone	40 mg	30 mg

Inactive Ingredients: Extra Strength Maalox® Plus Suspension: Citric acid, flavors, methylparaben, propylparaben, purified water, saccharin sodium, sorbitol, and other ingredients.
Extra Strength Maalox® Plus Tablets: Citric acid, confectioners' sugar, D&C Yellow No. 10, dextrose, FD&C Blue No. 1, flavors, glycerin, hydrogenated vegetable oil, magnesium stearate, mannitol, saccharin sodium, sorbitol, starch, talc.
To aid in establishing proper dosage schedules, the following information is provided:

Minimum Recommended Dosage: Extra Strength Maalox® Plus

	Per 2 Tsp. (10 mL)	Per Tablet
Acid neutralizing capacity	58.1 mEq	18.6 mEq
Sodium content*	<2.5 mg	<1.7 mg
Sugar content	None	0.72 g
Lactose content	None	None

*Dietetically insignificant.

Indications: As an antacid for symptomatic relief of hyperacidity associated with the diagnosis of peptic ulcer, gastritis, peptic esophagitis, gastric hyperacidity, heartburn, or hiatal hernia. As an antiflatulent to alleviate the symptoms of gas, including postoperative gas pain.

Advantages: Among antacids, Extra Strength Maalox® Plus Suspension and Extra Strength Maalox® Plus Tablets are uniquely palatable—an important feature which encourages patients to follow your dosage directions. Extra Strength Maalox® Plus Suspension and Extra Strength Maalox® Plus Tablets have the time-proven, nonconstipating, sodium-free* Maalox® formula—useful for those patients suffering from the problems associated with hyperacidity. Additionally, Extra Strength Maalox® Plus Suspension and Extra Strength Maalox® Plus Tablets contain simethicone to alleviate discomfort associated with entrapped gas.

Professional Labeling

Warnings:
(i) Prolonged use of aluminum-containing antacids in patients with renal failure may result in or worsen dialysis osteomalacia. Elevated tissue aluminum levels contribute to the development of the dialysis encephalopathy and osteomalacia syndromes. Small amounts of aluminum are absorbed from the gastrointestinal tract and renal excretion of aluminum is impaired in renal failure. Aluminum is not well removed by dialysis because it is bound to albumin and transferrin, which do not cross dialysis membranes. As a result, aluminum is deposited in bone, and dialysis osteomalacia may develop when large amounts of aluminum are ingested orally by patients with impaired renal function.
(ii) Aluminum forms insoluble complexes with phosphate in the gastrointestinal tract, thus decreasing phosphate absorption. Prolonged use of aluminum-containing antacids by normophosphatemic patients may result in hypophosphatemia if phosphate intake is not adequate. In its more severe forms, hypophosphatemia can lead to anorexia, malaise, muscle weakness, and osteomalacia.

Extra Strength Maalox® Plus Suspension

Directions for Use: Two to four teaspoonfuls, four times a day, taken twenty minutes to one hour after meals and at bedtime, or as directed by a physician. Stomach pain and discomfort should always be evaluated by a physician for proper diagnosis.

Patient Warnings: Do not take more than 12 teaspoonfuls in a 24-hour period or use the maximum dosage for more than 2 weeks or use if you have kidney disease except under the advice and supervision of a physician. Keep this and all drugs out of the reach of children.

Extra Strength Maalox® Plus Tablets

Directions for Use: Chew one to three tablets twenty minutes to one hour after meals and at bedtime, or as directed by a physician.

Patient Warnings: Do not take more than 12 tablets in a 24-hour period or use the maximum dosage for more than two weeks or use if you have kidney disease except under the advice and supervision of a physician. Keep this and all drugs out of the reach of children.

Drug Interaction Precaution: Do not use with patients taking a prescription antibiotic containing any form of tetracycline. As with all aluminum-containing antacids, Extra Strength Maalox® Plus may prevent the proper absorption of the tetracycline.

How Supplied:
Extra Strength Maalox® Plus Suspension
Available in Lemon Swiss Creme in the following sizes: 5 fl. oz. (148 mL) (0067-0333-62), 12 fl. oz. (355 mL) (0067-0333-71), and 26 fl. oz. (769 mL) (0067-0333-44).
Cherry Creme is available in plastic bottles of 5 fl. oz. (148 mL) (0067-0336-62, 12 fl. oz. (355 mL) (0067-0336-71), and 26 fl. oz. (769 mL) (0067-0336-44).
Mint Creme is available in plastic bottles of 5 fl. oz. (148 mL) (0067-0338-62), 12 fl. oz. (355 mL) (0067-0338-71) and 26 fl. oz. (769 mL) (0067-0338-44).
Extra Strength Maalox® Plus Mint Creme Tablets are available in flip-top bottles of 38 tablets (0067-0345-38) and 75 tablets (0067-0345-75).

Shown in Product Identification Section, page 420

PERDIEM®
[*pĕr″dē′ŭm*]

Indication: For relief of constipation.

Actions: Perdiem®, with its 100% natural, gentle action provides comfortable relief from constipation. Perdiem® is a unique combination of bulk-forming fiber and natural stimulant. The vegetable mucilages of Perdiem® soften the stool and provide pain-free evacuation of the bowel with no chemical stimulants. Perdiem® is effective as an aid to elimination for the hemorrhoid or fissure patient prior to and following surgery.

Composition: Perdiem® contains as its active ingredients, 82% psyllium (Plantago Hydrocolloid) a natural grain and 18% senna (Cassia Pod Concentrate), a natural vegetable derivative. Each rounded teaspoonful (6.0 g) contains approximately 3.3 g psyllium, 0.74 g senna, 2 mg of sodium, 4.0 mg of potassium, and 4 calories. Perdiem® is "Dye-Free" and contains no artificial sweeteners.

Inactive Ingredients: Acacia, iron oxides, natural flavors, paraffin, sucrose, talc.

Patient Warning: Should not be used in the presence of undiagnosed abdominal pain. Frequent or prolonged use without the direction of a physician is not recommended, as it may lead to laxative dependence. Do not use in patients with a history of psyllium allergy. Psyllium allergy is rare but can be severe. If an allergic reaction occurs, discontinue use and consult a physician immediately. Bulk-forming agents have the potential to obstruct the esophagus, particularly in the presence of esophageal narrowing or when consumed with insufficient fluid. Patients should be made aware of the symptoms of esophageal obstruction, including chest pain/pressure, regurgitation, and difficulty swallowing. Patients experiencing these symptoms should seek immediate medical attention. Patients with esophageal narrowing or dysphagia should not use Perdiem®.
As with any drug, if you are pregnant or nursing a baby, seek the advice of a health professional before using this product. Keep this and all drugs out of the reach of children. In case of accidental overdose, seek professional assistance or contact a poison control center immediately.

Directions for Use: Perdiem must be taken with at least 8 ounces of liquid.
Adults and children 12 years and older: In the evening and/or before breakfast, 1–2 rounded teaspoonfuls of Perdiem® granules (in single or partial teaspoon doses) should be placed in the mouth and swallowed with at least 8 fl oz of cool beverage after the dose. Additional liquid would be helpful. Perdiem® granules should not be chewed.
Children 7 to 11 years: One rounded teaspoon one to two times daily with at least 8 ounces of cool liquid.
Perdiem® generally takes effect within 12 hours. Subsequent doses may be adjusted after adequate laxation is obtained.

Note: It is extremely important that Perdiem® be taken with at least 8 fl oz of cool liquid.

Warning: TAKE THIS PRODUCT WITH AT LEAST 8 OUNCES [A FULL GLASS] OF WATER OR OTHER FLUID. TAKING THIS PRODUCT WITHOUT ADEQUATE FLUID MAY CAUSE IT TO SWELL AND BLOCK YOUR THROAT OR ESOPHAGUS AND MAY CAUSE CHOKING. DO NOT TAKE THIS PRODUCT IF YOU HAVE EVER HAD DIFFICULTY IN SWALLOWING OR HAVE ANY THROAT PROBLEMS. IF YOU EXPERIENCE CHEST PAIN, VOMITING, OR DIFFICULTY IN SWALLOWING OR BREATHING AFTER TAKING THIS PRODUCT, SEEK IMMEDIATE MEDICAL ATTENTION.

In Severe Cases of Constipation: Perdiem® may be taken more frequently, up to 2 rounded teaspoonfuls every 6 hours not to exceed 5 teaspoonfuls in a 24-hour period. In severe cases, 24 to 72 hours may be required for optimal relief.

For Patients Habituated to Strong Purgatives: Two rounded teaspoonfuls of Perdiem® in the morning and evening may be required along with half the usual dose of the purgative being used. The purgative should be discontinued as soon as possible and the dosage of Perdiem® granules reduced when and if bowel tone shows lessened laxative dependence.

For Colostomy Patients: To ensure formed stools, give one to two rounded teaspoonfuls of Perdiem® in the evening.

For Clinical Regulation: For patients confined to bed, for those of inactive habits, and in the presence of cardiovascular disease where straining must be avoided, one rounded teaspoonful of Perdiem® taken once or twice daily will provide regular bowel habits.

How Supplied: Granules: 250-gram (8.8 oz) (0067-0690-70) plastic container, 6 single serving packets 6 gm (0067-0690-16) and 20 single serving packets 6 gm (0067-0690-17).

Shown in Product Identification Section, page 420

PERDIEM® FIBER
[*pĕr″dē′ŭm*]

Indications: Perdiem® Fiber provides gentle relief from simple, chronic, and spastic constipation. In addition, it relieves constipation associated with convalescence, pregnancy, and advanced age. Perdiem® Fiber is also indicated for use in special diets lacking in residue fiber to aid regularity and in the management of constipation associated with irritable bowel syndrome, diverticular disease, hemorrhoids, and anal fissures.

Action: Perdiem® Fiber is a 100% natural bulk-forming fiber that gently helps maintain regularity and prevents constipation. Perdiem® Fiber's unique form is easy to swallow and requires no mixing but must be followed by at least 8 ounces of cool liquid. Perdiem® Fiber contains no chemical stimulants and may be used daily by those who may lack sufficient dietary fiber. When recommended by a doctor, Perdiem Fiber is also useful for the treatment of bowel disorders other than constipation.

Continued on next page

Rhône-Poulenc Rorer—Cont.

Composition: Perdiem® Fiber contains as its active ingredient 100% psyllium (Plantago Hydrocolloid), a natural grain with no chemical stimulants. Each rounded teaspoonful (6.0 g) contains approximately 4 g of psyllium, 2 mg of sodium, 35 mg of potassium and 4 calories. Perdiem® Fiber is "Dye-Free" and contains no artificial sweeteners.

Inactive Ingredients: Acacia, iron oxides, natural flavors, paraffin, sucrose, talc, titanium dioxide.

Directions for Use: Perdiem Fiber must be taken with at least 8 ounces of cool liquid. Additional liquid is helpful.
Adults and children 12 years and older: In the evening and/or before breakfast, 1 to 2 rounded teaspoonfuls (6.0 to 12.0 g) of Perdiem® Fiber granules (in full or partial teaspoon doses) should be placed in the mouth and swallowed with at least 8 fl oz of cool beverage after the dose. Perdiem® Fiber granules should not be chewed.
During Pregnancy: Because of its natural ingredients and bulking action, Perdiem Fiber is effective for expectant mothers—follow directions.
Children 7 to 11 years: One (1) rounded teaspoonful one to two times daily with at least 8 ounces of cool liquid.

Patient Warning: Should not be used in the presence of undiagnosed abdominal pain. Frequent or prolonged use without the direction of a physician is not recommended.
Do not use in patients with a history of psyllium allergy. Psyllium allergy is rare but can be severe. If an allergic reaction occurs, discontinue use.
Bulk-forming agents have the potential to obstruct the esophagus, particularly in the presence of esophageal narrowing or when consumed with insufficient fluid. Patients should be made aware of the symptoms of esophageal obstruction, including chest pain/pressure, regurgitation, and difficulty swallowing. Patients experiencing these symptoms should seek immediate medical attention. Patients with esophageal narrowing or dysphagia should not use Perdiem® Fiber.
Keep this and all drugs out of the reach of children. In case of accidental overdose, seek professional assistance or contact a poison control center immediately.

In Severe Cases of Constipation: Perdiem® Fiber may be taken more frequently, up to 2 rounded teaspoonfuls every 6 hours depending upon need and response not to exceed 5 teaspoonfuls in a 24-hour period. Perdiem Fiber generally takes effect after 24 hours; in severe cases 48 to 72 hours may be required to provide optimal benefit.

Warning: TAKE THIS PRODUCT WITH AT LEAST 8 OUNCES [A FULL GLASS] OF WATER OR OTHER FLUID. TAKING THIS PRODUCT WITHOUT ADEQUATE FLUID MAY CAUSE IT TO SWELL AND BLOCK YOUR THROAT OR ESOPHAGUS AND MAY CAUSE CHOKING. DO NOT TAKE THIS PRODUCT IF YOU HAVE EVER HAD DIFFICULTY IN SWALLOWING OR HAVE ANY THROAT PROBLEMS. IF YOU EXPERIENCE CHEST PAIN, VOMITING, OR DIFFICULTY IN SWALLOWING OR BREATHING AFTER TAKING THIS PRODUCT, SEEK IMMEDIATE MEDICAL ATTENTION.

After Rectal Surgery: The vegetable mucilages of Perdiem® Fiber soften the stool and provide pain-free evacuation of the bowel. Perdiem® Fiber is effective as an aid to elimination for the hemorrhoid or fissure patient prior to and following surgery.

For Clinical Regulation: For patients confined to bed—after an operation for example—and for those of inactive habits, 1 rounded teaspoonful of Perdiem® Fiber taken 1–2 times daily will ensure regular bowel habits.

How Supplied: Granules: 250-gram (8.8 oz) (0067-0795-70) plastic container, 6 single serving packets 6 gm (0067-0795-09) and 20 single serving packets 6 gm (0067-0795-10).

Shown in Product Identification Section, page 420

Richardson-Vicks Inc.
(See Procter & Gamble.)

Roberts Pharmaceutical Corporation
6 INDUSTRIAL WAY WEST
EATONTOWN, NJ 07724

CHERACOL® Nasal Spray Pump
Cherry Scented

Description: CHERACOL® NASAL SPRAY PUMP is a cherry scented long acting topical nasal decongestant. One application lasts up to 12 hours.

Indications: For the temporary relief of a nasal congestion associated with colds ("flu"), hay fever, and sinusitis.

Active Ingredients: Oxymetazoline hydrochloride USP 0.05% (0.5 mg/ml).

Inactive Ingredients: Benzalkonium chloride, glycine, sodium hydroxide, phenylmercuric acetate (0.02 mg/ml), sorbitol, artificial cherry flavor, and purified water.

Dosage and Administration: CHERACOL Nasal Spray has a long duration of action lasting up to 12 hours with each topical application. One application mornings and at bedtime is usually sufficient for round-the-clock action. For adults and children 6 years of age and over: Two or three sprays in each nostril twice daily—morning and bedtime. Remove protective cap. Hold bottle with thumb at base and nozzle between first and second fingers. With head upright, insert metered pump spray nozzle in nostril. Depress pump 2 or 3 times all the way down with a firm even stroke and sniff deeply. Repeat in other nostril. Do not tilt head backward while spraying. Wipe tip clean after each use. Before using the first time, remove the protective cap from the tip and prime the metered pump by depressing pump firmly several times.

Warning: Do not give this product to children under 6 years of age except under the advice and supervision of a physician. Do not exceed recommended dosage because symptoms may occur such as burning, stinging, sneezing or increase of nasal discharge. Do not use this product for more than 3 days. If symptoms persist, consult a physician. The use of this dispenser by more than one person may spread infection. Store at room temperature. Keep this and all medicines out of children's reach.

Overdose: In case of accidental overdose contact a physician or regional poison control center immediately.

How Supplied: Available in 1 fluid ounce bottles fitted with a metered pump (NDC 54092-880-30).

CHERACOL® SINUS
12 Hour Formula

Description: Cheracol® SINUS sustained-action tablets combine a nasal decongestant with an antihistamine in a special continuous-acting timed-release tablet to provide temporary relief of nasal congestion due to the common cold, and associated with sinusitis. Also alleviates running nose and sneezing due to hay fever.

Each Cheracol® SINUS Sustained-Action Tablet Contains: 6 mg of dexbrompheniramine maleate and 120 mg of pseudoephedrine sulfate. Half of the medication is released after the tablet is swallowed and the remaining amount of medication is sustained-release, providing continuous long-lasting relief for 12 hours.

Indications: For temporary relief of nasal congestion due to the common cold, hay fever, or other upper respiratory allergies, and associated with sinusitis. Helps decongest sinus openings, sinus passages. Reduces swelling of nasal passages; shrinks swollen membranes; and temporarily restores freer breathing through the nose. Alleviates running nose, sneezing, itching of the nose or throat, and itchy and watery eyes as may occur in allergic rhinitis (such as hay fever).

Directions: Adults and Children 12 Years and Over—one tablet every 12 hours. Do not exceed two tablets in 24 hours.

Warnings: If symptoms do not improve within 7 days or are accompanied by high fever, consult a physi-

cian before continuing use. May cause drowsiness; alcohol may increase the drowsiness effect. Avoid alcoholic beverages while taking this product. Use caution when driving a motor vehicle or operating machinery. May cause excitability especially in children. Do not exceed recommended dosage, because at higher doses nervousness, dizziness, or sleeplessness may occur. Do not give this product to children under 12 years, except under the advice and supervision of a physician. Do not take this product if you have emphysema, chronic pulmonary disease, shortness of breath, and difficulty in breathing, asthma, glaucoma, difficulty in urination due to enlargement of the prostate gland, high blood pressure, heart disease, diabetes, or thyroid disease except under the advice and supervision of a physician. As with any drug, if you are pregnant or nursing a baby, seek the advice of a health professional before using this product. Keep this and all drugs out of the reach of children. In case of accidental overdose, seek professional assistance or contact a Poison Control Center immediately.

Drug Interaction Precaution: Do not take this product if you are presently taking a prescription drug for high blood pressure or depression, without first consulting your doctor.

Active Ingredients: Dexbrompheniramine Meleate 6 mg, Pseudoephedrine Sulfate 120 mg.

Also Contains: Acacia, Calcium Carbonate, Carnauba Wax, Confectioner's Sugar, D&C Yellow #10, FD&C Blue #1, FD&C Yellow #6, Gelatin, Hydrogenated Castor Oil, Magnesium Stearate, Methylparaben, Povidone, Propylparaben, Shellac, Sodium Benzoate, Sucrose, Talc, Titanium Dioxide.
Use by expiration date printed on package.

Store between 2° and 30°C (36° and 86°F). Protect from excessive moisture.

How Supplied: 10 sustained-action release tablets. NDC 54092-045-10
Manufactured for:
Roberts Laboratories Inc., a subsidiary of
ROBERTS PHARMACEUTICAL CORPORATION
Eatontown, NJ 07724, USA

CHERACOL® Sore Throat Spray
Anesthetic/Antiseptic Liquid

Description: A pleasant tasting cherry flavored liquid spray with anesthetic and antiseptic properties.

Indications: For the temporary relief of occasional minor sore throat pain and irritation. Also for temporary relief of pain associated with sore mouth, canker sores, tonsillitis, pharyngitis and throat infections.

Active Ingredients: Phenol 1.4%.

Inactive Ingredients: Alcohol 12.5%, citric acid, FD&C Red No. 40, flavor, glycerin, propylene glycol, sodium citrate, sodium saccharin, sorbitol and purified water.

Directions For Use: Mouthwash and gargle: Irritated throat: Spray 5 times (children 2–12 years of age, 3 times) and swallow. May be used as a gargle. Repeat every 2 hours or as directed by physician or dentist. Children under 12 years of age should be supervised in the use of this product.

Warning: If sore throat is severe, persists for more than 2 days, is accompanied or followed by fever, headache, rash, nausea or vomiting, consult a doctor promptly. If sore mouth symptoms do not improve in 7 days, see your doctor or dentist promptly. As with any drug, if you are pregnant or nursing a baby, seek the advice of a health professional before using this product. Do not administer to children under 2 years unless directed by a physician or dentist. Keep this and all medicines out of the reach of children.

Overdose: In case of accidental overdose contact a physician or a poison control center immediately.

How Supplied: Available in 6 fluid ounce spray pump bottle (NDC 54092-340-06).

CHERACOL–D® Cough Formula
Maximum Strength Cough Formula

Description: CHERACOL-D® is a nonnarcotic cough formula which combines two important medicines in one safe, fast-acting pleasant tasting liquid:

- The highest level of cough suppressant available without prescription.
- A clinically proven expectorant to help loosen phlegm and drain bronchial tubes.

Indications: CHERACOL-D® cough formula helps quiet dry, hacking coughs, and helps loosen phlegm and mucus. Recommended for adults and children 2 years of age and older.

Active Ingredients: Each teaspoonful (5 ml) contains dextromethorphan hydrobromide, 10 mg; guaifenesin, 100 mg; alcohol, 4.75%. Also contains benzoic acid, FD&C Red #40, flavors, fragrances, fructose, glycerin, propylene glycol, sodium chloride, sucrose, and purified water.

Dosage and Administration: Adults and children 12 years of age and over: 2 teaspoonfuls. Children 6 to 12 years: 1 teaspoonful. Children 2 to 6 years: ½ teaspoonful. May be repeated every 4 hours if necessary. Children under 2 years, consult a physician.

Warnings: Keep this and all drugs out of the reach of children. Do not give this product to children under 2 years of age except under the advice and supervision of a physician. Do not use this product for persistent or chronic cough such as occurs with smoking, asthma, or emphysema or where cough is accompanied by excessive secretions except under the advice and supervision of a physician. As with any drug, if you are pregnant or nursing a baby, seek the advice of a health professional before using this product.

Caution: A persistent cough may be a sign of a serious condition. If cough persists for more than 1 week, tends to recur or is accompanied by high fever, rash or persistent headache, consult a physician.

Overdose: In case of accidental overdose contact a physician or a poison control center immediately.

How Supplied: Available in 2 oz bottle (NDC 54092-400-60), 4 oz bottle (NDC 54092-400-04), and 6 oz bottle (NDC 54092-400-06).

Shown in Product Identification Section, page 420

CHERACOL PLUS® Cough Syrup
Multisymptom cough/cold formula

Description: CHERACOL PLUS® Cough Syrup is a pleasant tasting 3-ingredient non-narcotic liquid formulation.

Indications: Cheracol Plus syrup is an effective 3-ingredient, maximum strength formula for the temporary relief of head cold symptoms and cough (without narcotic side effects).

Active Ingredients: Each tablespoonful (15ml) contains phenylpropanolamine, 25 mg; dextromethorphan hydrobromide, 20 mg; chlorpheniramine maleate, 4 mg; and alcohol, 8%.

Inactive Ingredients: Flavors, glycerin, methylparaben, propylene glycol, propylparaben, FD&C Red No. 40, sodium chloride, sorbitol solution, and purified water.

Dosage and Administration: Adults and children over 12 years of age: 1 tablespoonful (15ml) every 4 hours or as directed by a physician. Do not take more than 6 tablespoonfuls in a 24 hour period. Do not administer to children under 12 years of age.

Uses: Cheracol Plus® multisymptom head cold/cough formula provides cough suppressant and decongestant activity and controls runny nose associated with the common cold ("flu").

Warnings: Do not take this product for persistent or chronic cough such as occurs with smoking, asthma, or emphysema or where cough is accompanied by excessive secretions or if you have high blood pressure, heart or thyroid disease, diabetes, asthma, glaucoma, or difficulty in urination due to enlargement of the prostate gland except under the advice and supervision of a physician. If symp-

Continued on next page

Roberts—Cont.

toms do not improve within 7 days or are accompanied by high fever, consult a physician before continuing use. May cause excitability, especially in children. Do not give this product to children under 12 years except under the advice and supervision of a physician. As with any drug, if you are pregnant or nursing a baby consult a health professional before using this product. Keep out of reach of children.

Drug Interaction Precaution: Do not take this product if you are presently taking antihypertensive or antidepressant medication containing a monoamine oxidase inhibitor except under the advice and supervision of a physician.

Overdose: In case of accidental overdose contact a physician or a poison control center immediately.

How Supplied: Available in 4 oz bottle (NDC 54092-401-04), 6 oz bottle (54092-401-06).

Shown in Product Identification Section, page 420

CITROCARBONATE® Antacid

Active Ingredients: When dissolved, each 3.9 grams (1 teaspoonful) contains approximately: sodium bicarbonate, 0.78 gram and sodium citrate, 1.82 grams. **As derived from (per teaspoonful):** sodium bicarbonate, 2.34 gram; citric acid anhydrous, 1.19 gram; sodium citrate hydrous, 254 mg; calcium lactate pentahydrate, 151 mg; sodium chloride, 79 mg; monobasic sodium phosphate anhydrous, 44 mg; and magnesium sulfate dried, 42 mg. Each 3.9 grams (teaspoonful) contains 30.46 mEq (700.6 mg) of sodium.

Indications: For the relief of heartburn, acid indigestion, and sour stomach; and upset stomach associated with these symptoms.

Dosage and Administration: Adults: 1 to 2 teaspoonfuls (not to exceed 5 level teaspoonfuls per day) in a glass of cold water after meals. Persons 60 years or older: ½ to 1 teaspoonful after meals. Children 6 to 12 years: ¼ to ½ teaspoonful. For children under 6 years: Consult physician.

How Supplied: Available in 5 oz (NDC 54092-900-05) and 10 oz (NDC 54092-900-10) bottles.

CLOCREAM®
Skin Protectant Cream

Description: CLOCREAM® skin protectant cream contains Vitamins A and D in a greaseless vanishing cream base that leaves no residue. Also contains cetylpalmitate, cottonseed oil, glycerin, glyceryl monostearate, fragrance, methylparaben, mineral oil, potassium stearate, propylparaben, sodium citrate, and purified oil. Each ounce of CLOCREAM® contains Vitamins A and D equivalent to 1 ounce of cod liver oil.

Indications: CLOCREAM® is indicated for the temporary relief of chapped skin, diaper rash, wind burn, sunburn and minor non-infected skin irritations. CLOCREAM® promotes epithelization.

Uses: CLOCREAM® may be particularly useful for health care personnel or others who frequently wash their hands and for general patient care to reduce dermal excoriation and breakdown from prolonged bed rest, bedwetting and abrasions. The vanishing action of CLOCREAM skin protectant cream makes it cosmetically acceptable when the skin treated is on an exposed part of the body such as the hands or arms.

Warnings: CLOCREAM® skin protectant cream is for external use only. Avoid contact with the eyes. If condition worsens or if symptoms persist for more than 7 days, discontinue use of this product and consult a physician. Keep this and all medications out of the reach of children. In case of accidental ingestion seek professional assistance or contact a poison control center immediately.

Dosage and Administration: Gently massage or apply liberally to unbroken skin or abraded skin where promotion of epitheliazation is denied. Use as often as desired.

How Supplied: Available in 1 ounce tubes (NDC 54092-300-30).

HALTRAN® Tablets
Ibuprofen/Analgesic
MENSTRUAL CRAMP RELIEVER

WARNING: ASPIRIN SENSITIVE PATIENTS. Do not take this product if you have had a severe allergic reaction to aspirin, eg—asthma, swelling, shock or hives, because even though this product contains no aspirin or salicylates cross-reactions may occur in patients allergic to aspirin.

Indications: For the pain of menstrual cramps and also the temporary relief of minor aches and pains associated with the common cold, headache, toothache, muscular aches, backache, for the minor pain of arthritis and for reduction of fever.

Directions: *Adults:* Take 1 tablet every 4 to 6 hours while symptoms persist. If pain or fever does not respond to 1 tablet, 2 tablets may be used, but do not exceed 6 tablets in 24 hours, unless directed by a doctor. The smallest effective dose should be used. Take with food or milk if occasional and mild heartburn, upset stomach, or stomach pain occurs with use. Consult a doctor if these symptoms are more than mild or if they persist. *Children:* Do not give this product to children under 12 except under the advice and supervision of a doctor.

Warnings: Do not take for pain for more than 10 days or for fever for more than 3 days unless directed by a doctor. If pain or fever persists or gets worse, if new symptoms occur, or if the painful area is red or swollen, consult a doctor. These could be signs of serious illness. If you are under a doctor's care for any serious condition, consult a doctor before taking this product. As with aspirin and acetaminophen, if you have any condition which requires you to take prescription drugs or if you have had any problems or serious side effects from taking any non-prescription pain reliever, do not take HALTRAN Tablets (ibuprofen) without first discussing it with your doctor. If you experience any symptoms which are unusual or seem unrelated to the condition for which you took ibuprofen, consult a doctor before taking any more of it. Although ibuprofen is indicated for the same conditions as aspirin and acetaminophen, it should not be taken with them except under a doctor's direction. Before using any drug, including HALTRAN, you should seek the advice of a health professional if you are pregnant or nursing a baby. IT IS ESPECIALLY IMPORTANT NOT TO USE IBUPROFEN DURING THE LAST 3 MONTHS OF PREGNANCY UNLESS SPECIFICALLY DIRECTED TO DO SO BY A DOCTOR BECAUSE IT MAY CAUSE PROBLEMS IN THE UNBORN CHILD OR COMPLICATIONS DURING DELIVERY. Keep this and all drugs out of the reach of children. In case of accidental overdose, seek professional assistance or contact a poison control center immediately.

Active Ingredient: Each tablet contains ibuprofen USP 200 mg.

Other Ingredients: Carnauba wax, cornstarch, hydroxypropyl methylcellulose, propylene glycol, silicon dioxide, pregelatinized starch, stearic acid, and titanium dioxide.

Store at room temperature. Avoid excessive heat 40°C (104°F).

How Supplied: Available in bottles of 30 (NDC 54092-020-30).

Shown in Product Identification Section, page 420

KASOF® Capsules
[kay 'sof]
High Strength Stool Softener Laxative

Ingredients: Each capsule contains:

Active: docusate potassium, 240 mg.

Inactive: Blue 1, gelatin, glycerin, methylparaben, polyethylene glycol, propylparaben, purified water, Red 40, sorbitol, Yellow 10.

Indications: KASOF provides a highly efficient wetting action to restore moisture to the bowel, thus softening the stool to prevent straining. The action of KASOF does not interfere with normal peristalsis and generally does not cause griping or extreme sensation of urgency. KASOF is sodium-free, containing a unique potassium formulation, without the problems associated with sodium intake. KASOF is especially valuable for the severely constipated, as well as patients with anorectal disorders, such as hemorrhoids and anal fissures. KASOF is ideal for patients with any condition that can be complicated by straining at stool, for example, cardiac patients. The simple, one-a-day dosage helps assure patient compliance in maintaining normal bowel function.

Directions: Adults: One KASOF capsule daily for several days, or until bowel movements are normal and gentle. It is helpful to increase the daily intake of fluids by drinking a glass of water with each dose.
Store in a closed container, protect from freezing and avoid excessive heat (104°F).

Warnings: As with any drug, if you are pregnant or nursing a baby, seek the advice of a health professional before using this product. Keep out of the reach of children.

How Supplied: KASOF is available in bottles of 30, (NDC 54092-050-30) and 60 (NDC 54092-050-60) brown gelatin capsules identified "KASOF".

ORTHOXICOL® Cough Syrup
Multisymptom cough/cold formula

Description: ORTHOXICOL® Cough Syrup is a pleasant tasting 3-ingredient non-narcotic liquid formulation.

Indications: Orthoxicol syrup is an effective 3-ingredient, maximum strength formula for the temporary relief of head cold symptoms and cough (without narcotic side effects).

Active Ingredients: Each tablespoonful (15 ml) contains phenylpropanolamine, 25 mg; dextromethorphan hydrobromide, 20 mg; chlorpheniramine, 4 mg; and alcohol, 8%.

Inactive Ingredients: Flavors, glycerin, methylparaben, propylene glycol, propylparaben, FD&C Red No. 40, sodium chloride, sorbitol solution, and purified water.

Dosage and Administration: Adults and children over 12 years of age: 1 tablespoonful (15 ml) every 4 hours or as directed by a physician. Do not take more than 6 tablespoonfuls in a 24 hour period. Do not administer to children under 12 years of age.

Uses: Orthoxicol multisymptom head cold/cough formula provides cough suppressant and decongestant activity and controls runny nose associated with the common cold ("flu").

Warnings: Do not take this product for persistent or chronic cough such as occurs with smoking, asthma, or emphysema or where cough is accompanied by excessive secretions or if you have high blood pressure, heart or thyroid disease, diabetes, asthma, glaucoma, or difficulty in urination due to enlargement of the prostate gland except under the advice and supervision of a physician. If symptoms do not improve within 7 days or are accompanied by high fever, consult a physician before continuing use. May cause excitability, especially in children. Do not give this product to children under 12 years except under the advice and supervision of a physician. As with any drug, if you are pregnant or nursing a baby consult a health professional before using this product. Keep this and all other drugs out of the reach of children.

Drug Interaction Precaution: Do not take this product if you are presently taking antihypertensive or antidepressant medication containing a monoamine oxidase inhibitor except under the advice and supervision of a physician.

Overdose: In case of accidental overdose contact a physician or a poison control center immediately.

How Supplied: Available in 2 oz bottle (NDC 54092-410-60), 4 oz bottle (NDC 54092-410-04), 16 oz bottle (NDC 54092-410-16).

P-A-C® Analgesic Tablets

Description: A combination tablet formulation providing more pain-relieving ingredients per tablet than conventional tablets.

Indications: P-A-C® tablets are indicated for the temporary relief of occasional minor aches, pains, headache and the reduction of fever.

Active Ingredients: Each tablet contains: aspirin; caffeine anhydrous, 32 mg. Contains non-standard strength of 400 mg (6.17 gr) aspirin per tablet compared to the established standard of 325 mg (5 gr) aspirin per tablet.

Inactive Ingredients: Cellulose, corn starch, croscarmellose sodium, FD&C Blue No. 2, FD&C Yellow No. 5 (tartrazine), sucrose.

Directions for Use: Adults—1 or 2 tablets every 4 hours. Do not exceed 10 tablets in 24 hours. Children under 12 years: consult a doctor. Do not take this product for pain for more than 10 days or for fever for more than 3 days unless directed by a doctor.

Warnings: Children and teenagers should not use this product for chickenpox or flu symptoms before a physician is consulted about Reye Syndrome, a rare but serious illness reported to be associated with aspirin. Do not take this product if you are allergic to aspirin or if you have asthma. As with any drug, if you are pregnant or nursing a baby seek the advice of a health professional before you use this product. **IT IS ESPECIALLY IMPORTANT NOT TO USE ASPIRIN DURING THE LAST 3 MONTHS OF PREGNANCY UNLESS SPECIFICALLY DIRECTED BY A DOCTOR BECAUSE IT MAY CAUSE PROBLEMS IN THE UNBORN CHILD OR COMPLICATIONS DURING DELIVERY.** Do not exceed recommended dosage.

Cautions: Do not take this product if you have stomach distress, ulcers, bleeding problems, are presently taking a prescription drug for anticoagulation (thinning of the blood), diabetes, gout, arthritis, or for the treatment of arthritis. Stop taking this product if ringing of the ears or other symptoms occur. In case of accidental overdose seek professional assistance or contact a poison control center immediately. Keep this and all other drugs out of the reach of children.

How Supplied: Available in bottles of 100 (NDC 54092-010-01), and 1000 (NDC 54092-010-10) tablets.

Shown in Product Identification Section, page 420

PYRROXATE® Capsules
Extra Strength Decongestant/ Antihistamine/ Analgesic Capsules

Description: *Pyrroxate*® provides single-capsule, multisymptom relief for colds, allergies, nasal/sinus congestion, runny nose, sneezing, and watery eyes. Because it contains the non-aspirin analgesic **acetaminophen,** *Pyrroxate* gives temporary relief of occasional minor aches, pains, headache, and helps in the reduction of fever. *Pyrroxate* is caffeine and aspirin-free.

Ingredients: Each *Pyrroxate* Capsule contains: chlorpheniramine maleate, 4 mg; phenylpropanolamine HCl, 25 mg; acetaminophen, 500 mg. Also contains benzyl alcohol, butylparaben, D&C yellow No. 10, erythrosine sodium, FD&C blue No. 1, FD&C yellow No. 6 (sunset yellow) as a color additive, gelatin, glycerin, magnesium stearate, methylparaben, propylparaben, sodium lauryl sulfate, sodium propionate, starch, and talc.

Indications: *Pyrroxate* Capsules are for the temporary relief of runny nose, sneezing, itching of the nose or throat; for the temporary relief of nasal congestion due to the common cold, allergies (hay fever), and sinus congestion; for the temporary relief of occasional minor aches, pains, headache, and for the reduction of fever.

Actions: Chlorpheniramine maleate is an antihistamine effective in controlling runny nose, sneezing, watery eyes, and itching of the nose and throat. Phenylpropanolamine HCl is an oral nasal decongestant effective in relieving nasal/sinus congestion due to the common cold or allergies (hay fever). Acetaminophen is a clinically effective analgesic and antipyretic without aspirin side effects.

Warnings: Do not take this product for more than 7 days. If symptoms persist, do

Continued on next page

Roberts—Cont.

not improve, or new ones occur, or if fever persists for more than 3 days, discontinue use and consult your physician. Do not take this product if you have asthma, glaucoma, difficulty in urination due to the enlargement of the prostate gland, high blood pressure, diabetes, thyroid disease, or if you are presently taking a prescription antihypertensive or antidepressant drug containing a monamine oxidase inhibitor, except under the advice and supervision of a physician. As with any drug, if you are pregnant or nursing a baby, seek the advice of a health professional before using this product. Do not exceed recommended dosage because severe liver damage may occur and at higher doses, nervousness, dizziness or sleeplessness may occur. Do not take other medications containing acetaminophen simultaneously, to avoid the risk of overdosage.

Cautions: Avoid alcoholic beverages, driving a motor vehicle, or operating heavy machinery while taking this product. This product may cause drowsiness or excitability, especially in children.

Keep this and all drugs out of the reach of children. In case of accidental overdose, seek professional assistance or contact a poison control center immediately.

Dosage and Administration: Take 1 capsule every 4 hours or as directed by a physician. Do not take more than 6 capsules in a 24-hour period. Do not administer to children under 12 years of age.

How Supplied: Black/yellow capsules available in bottles of 24 (NDC 54092-040-24) and 500 (NDC 54092-040-05).

Shown in Product Identification Section, page 420

SIGTAB® Tablets
High Potency Vitamin Supplement

Each Tablet Contains:		% U.S. RDA*
Vitamin A	5000 IU	100
Vitamin D	400 IU	100
Vitamin E	15 IU	50
Vitamin C	333 mg	555
Folic Acid	0.4 mg	100
Thiamine	10.3 mg	687
Riboflavin	10 mg	588
Niacin	100 mg	500
Vitamin B_6	6 mg	300
Vitamin B_{12}	18 mcg	300
Pantothenic Acid	20 mg	200

*Percentage of U.S. Recommended Daily Allowance.

Recommended Dosage: 1 tablet daily

Ingredient List: Sucrose, Ascorbic acid (Vit. C), Calcium Sulfate, Niacinamide, Vitamin E Acetate, Calcium Pantothenate, Vitamin A Acetate, Thiamine Mononitrate (B-1), Riboflavin (B-2), Gelatin, Pyridoxine HCl (B-6), Povidone, Lacca, Magnesium Stearate, Silica, Artificial Color, Sodium Benzoate, Folic Acid, Polyethylene Glycol, Cholecalciferol (Vit. D), Carnauba Wax, Cyanocobalamin (B-12), Medical Antifoam, Sesame Seed Oil and Titanium Dioxide.

How Supplied: Available in bottles of 90 (NDC 54092-033-90) and 500 (NDC 54092-033-05).

Shown in Product Identification Section, page 420

SIGTAB®-M Tablets

[See table below.]

How Supplied: Bottle of 100 tablets. NDC 54092-038-01

Recommended dosage for adults: 1 tablet daily.

Warning: Keep out of the reach of children.

Keep container tightly closed. Store at room temperature.

Do not use if seal under cap is broken.

Manufactured for:
Roberts Laboratories Inc., a subsidiary of
ROBERTS PHARMACEUTICAL CORPORATION
Eatontown, NJ 077244, USA

Shown in Product Identification Section, page 420

ZYMACAP® Capsules
High Potency Vitamin Supplement

Description: Dietary multivitamin supplement providing 150% of the RDA for Vitamin B and Vitamin C plus 100% of the RDA for Vitamins A and D.

Each Capsule Contains:		% US RDA*
Vitamin A	5,000 IU	100
Vitamin D	400 IU	100
Vitamin E	15 IU	50
Vitamin C	90 mg	150
Folic Acid	400 mcg	100
Thiamine	2.25 mg	150
Riboflavin	2.6 mg	150
Niacin	30 mg	150
Vitamin B-6	3 mg	150
Vitamin B-12	9 mcg	150
Pantothenic Acid	15 mg	150

*Percentage of U.S. recommended daily allowance.

Recommended Dosage: 1 Capsule daily.

Ingredient List: Soybean oil, ascorbic acid (Vitamin C), gelatin, glycerin, niacinamide, calcium pantothenate, Vitamin E acetate, lecithin, pyridoxine hydrochloride (Vitamin B-6), yellow wax, thiamine mononitrate (Vitamin B-1), ri-

---

Each Tablet Contains:		% U.S. RDA*
Active Ingredients:		
Vitamin A (From Vit. A & Beta Carotene)	6000 Intl. Units	120
Vitamin D3	400 Intl. Units	100
Vitamin E (DL-Alpha Tocopherol Acetate)	45 Intl. Units	150
Vitamin C (Ascorbic Acid)	100 mg	166
Niacinamide	25 mg	125
Thiamine Mononitrate	5 mg	333
Riboflavin	5 mg	294
Pyridoxine (Pyridoxine HCl)	3 mg	150
Folic Acid	400 mcg	100
Pantothenic Acid (D-Calcium Pant.)	15 mcg	150
Vitamin B12	18 mcg	300
Vitamin K1	25 mcg	8
Biotin	45 mcg	15
Calcium	200 mg	20
Phosphorus (Dicalcium Phosphate)	150 mg	15
Iron (Ferrous Fumarate)	18 mg	100
Magnesium (Magnesium Oxide)	100 mg	25
Copper (Copper Oxide)	2 mg	100
Zinc (Zinc Oxide)	15 mg	100
Iodine (Potassium Iodide)	150 mcg	100
Manganese (Manganese Sulfate)	5 mg	**
Potassium (Potassium Chloride)	40 mg	**
Chloride	36.3 mg	**
Selenium (Sodium Selenate)	25 mcg	**
Molybdenum (Sodium Molybdate)	25 mcg	**
Chromium (Chromium Chloride)	25 mcg	**
Nickel	5 mcg	**
Tin	10 mcg	**
Vanadium	10 mcg	**
Silicon	2 mcg	**
Boron	150 mcg	**

Inactive Ingredients:
Microcrystalline Cellulose NF, Stearic Acid NF, Croscarmellose Sodium NF, Magnesium Stearate NF, Hydroxypropyl Methylcellulose NF, Propylene Glycol, USP, FD&C Yellow #6

*Percentage of U.S. Recommended Daily Allowances
**These beneficial minerals are in addition to the Recommended Daily Allowances of the vitamins.

boflavin (Vitamin B-2), Vitamin A palmitate, corn oil, FD&C Red No. 40, folic acid, titanium dioxide, ethyl vanillin, vanilla enhancer, cholecalciferol (Vitamin D), cyanocobalamin (Vitamin B-12).

How Supplied: Available in bottles of 90 capsules (NDC 54092-030-90).

A. H. Robins Company, Inc.

Subsidiary of American Home Products Corporation
CONSUMER PRODUCTS DIVISION
1405 CUMMINGS DRIVE
RICHMOND, VIRGINIA 23220

ALLBEE® WITH C CAPLETS
[all 'bē]
ALLBEE® C-800 TABLETS
ALLBEE® C-800 plus IRON TABLETS

[See Table below for vitamins provided in each formula.]

Ingredients:
Allbee with C Caplets: Niacinamide Ascorbate, Ascorbic Acid, Microcrystalline Cellulose, Corn Starch, Thiamine Mononitrate, Calcium Pantothenate, Riboflavin, Hydroxypropyl Methylcellulose, Pyridoxine Hydrochloride, Magnesium Stearate, Silicon Dioxide, Propylene Glycol, Lactose, Methacrylic Acid, Triethyl Citrate, Titanium Dioxide, Polysorbate 20, Artificial Flavor, Saccharin Sodium, Sodium Sorbate.
Allbee C-800 Tablets: Ascorbic Acid, Niacinamide Ascorbate, Modified Starch, Vitamin E Acetate, Hydrolyzed Protein, Calcium Pantothenate, Hydroxypropyl Methylcellulose, Pyridoxine Hydrochloride, Riboflavin, Stearic Acid, Thiamine Mononitrate, Artificial Color, Silicon Dioxide, Lactose, Magnesium Stearate, Povidone, Polyethylene Glycol 400 or 4000, Vanillin, Gelatin, Polysorbate 20 or 80, Sorbic Acid, Sodium Benzoate, Cyanocobalamin. May also contain: Hydroxypropylcellulose and Propylene Glycol.
Allbee C-800 plus Iron Tablets: Ascorbic Acid, Niacinamide Ascorbate, Ferrous Fumarate, Modified Starch, Vitamin E Acetate, Hydrolyzed Protein, Calcium Pantothenate, Hydroxypropyl Methylcellulose, Pyridoxine Hydrochloride, Riboflavin, Stearic Acid, Thiamine Mononitrate, Povidone, Silicon Dioxide, Artificial Color, Lactose, Magnesium Stearate, Polyethylene Glycol 400 or 4000, Vanillin, Gelatin, Polysorbate 20 or 80, Sorbic Acid, Sodium Benzoate, Cyanocobalamin. May also contain: Hydroxypropylcellulose and Propylene Glycol.

Drug Interaction Precaution: Do not take *Allbee C-800 plus Iron* within two hours of oral tetracycline antibiotics, since oral iron products interfere with absorption of tetracycline. *Allbee C-800 plus Iron* is not intended for the treatment of iron-deficiency anemia.

Adverse Reactions: *Allbee C-800 plus Iron:* Iron-containing medications may occasionally cause gastrointestinal discomfort, nausea, constipation or diarrhea.

Directions: For adults and children twelve or more years of age, one tablet daily. Under the direction and supervision of a physician, the dose and frequency of administration may be increased in accordance with the patient's requirements.

How Supplied: *Allbee with C:* Yellow, capsule-shaped film-coated tablets engraved AHR on one side and ALLBEE C on the other in bottles of 130 (NDC 0031–0673–66) and in Dis-Co® Unit Dose Packs of 100 (NDC 0031–0673–64). *Allbee C-800:* Orange, film-coated, elliptically-shaped tablets engraved AHR on one side and 0677 on the other in bottles of 60 (NDC 0031–0677–62). *Allbee C-800 plus Iron:* Red, film-coated, elliptically-shaped tablets engraved AHR on one side and 0678 on the other in bottles of 60 (NDC 0031–0678–62).
[See table below.]

ALLBEE	ALLBEE C-800		ALLBEE C-800 WITH IRON		ALLBEE WITH C	
	Quantity Per Tablet	% US RDA	Quantity Per Tablet	% US RDA	Quantity Per Caplet	% US RDA
Vitamin E	45 I.U.	150	45 I.U.	150	—	—
Vitamin C	800 mg	1333	800 mg	1333	300 mg	500
Folic Acid	—	—	0.4 mg	100	—	—
Thiamine (Vitamin B_1)	15 mg	1000	15 mg	1000	15 mg	1000
Riboflavin (Vitamin B_2)	17 mg	1000	17 mg	1000	10.2 mg	600
Niacin	100 mg	500	100 mg	500	50 mg	250
Vitamin B_6	25 mg	1250	25 mg	1250	5 mg	250
Vitamin B_{12}	12 mg	200	12 mg	200	—	—
Pantothenic Acid	25 mg	250	25 mg	250	10 mg	100
Iron	—	—	27 mg	150	—	—

ANACIN®
[an 'a-sin]
Coated Caplets
Coated Tablets

Description: Each caplet or tablet contains:

Aspirin	400 mg
Caffeine	32 mg

Inactive Ingredients:
Caplets: Hydroxypropyl Methylcellulose, Iron Oxide, Microcrystalline Cellulose, Polyethylene Glycol, Sodium Lauryl Sulfate, Starch.
Tablets: Hydroxypropyl Methylcellulose, Microcrystalline Cellulose, Polyethylene Glycol, Sodium Lauryl Sulfate, Starch.

Indications: Temporary relief of minor aches and pains from headaches, colds, muscle aches, backache, toothache, premenstrual and menstrual cramps, and minor arthritis pain. Also reduces fever.

Warnings: Children and teenagers should not use this medicine for chicken pox or flu symptoms before a doctor is consulted about Reye Syndrome, a rare but serious illness reported to be associated with aspirin. Patients are warned to consult a physician immediately if pain persists for more than 10 days, or redness is present, or in arthritic or rheumatic conditions affecting children under 12 years of age. As with any drug, women who are pregnant or nursing a baby should seek the advice of a health professional before using this product. Women are also warned that **IT IS ESPECIALLY IMPORTANT NOT TO USE ASPIRIN DURING THE LAST 3 MONTHS OF PREGNANCY UNLESS SPECIFICALLY DIRECTED TO DO SO BY A DOCTOR BECAUSE IT MAY CAUSE PROBLEMS IN THE UNBORN CHILD OR COMPLICATIONS DURING DELIVERY.** Patients

Continued on next page

Prescribing information on A. H. Robins products listed here is based on official labeling in effect November 1, 1992, with Indications, Contraindications, Warnings, Precautions, Adverse Reactions, and Dosage stated in full.

A. H. Robins—Cont.

are also warned to keep this and all drugs out of the reach of children, and that in case of accidental overdose, to seek professional assistance or contact a poison control center immediately.

Directions: Adults: 2 caplets or tablets with water every 4 hours, as needed. Do not exceed 10 caplets or tablets daily. Children 6 to under 12 years of age: half the adult dose.

How Supplied: *Caplets:* coated, white, capsule-shaped tablets monogrammed "ANACIN" in black—bottles of 30 (NDC 0573-0206-20), 50 (NDC 0573-0206-30), and 100 (NDC 0573-0206-40). *Tablets:* coated, white tablets engraved with an arrow on both sides—tins of 12 (NDC 0573-0200-05) and bottles of 30 (NDC 0573-0200-25), 50 (NDC 0573-0200-35), 100 (NDC 0573-0200-45), 200 (NDC 0573-0200-55), and 300 (NDC 0573-0200-65).

Shown in Product Identification Section, page 420

ASPIRIN FREE ANACIN®
[*an 'a-sin*]
Maximum Strength Caplets
Maximum Strength Gel Caplets
Maximum Strength Tablets

Description: Each caplet, gel caplet, or tablet contains:
Acetaminophen .... 500 mg

Inactive Ingredients:
Caplet: Calcium Stearate, Croscarmellose Sodium, D&C Red No. 7 Lake, FD&C Blue No. 1 Lake, Hydroxypropyl Methylcellulose, Polyethylene Glycol, Povidone, Propylene Glycol, Starch, Stearic Acid, Titanium Dioxide.
Gel Caplet: Croscarmellose Sodium, D&C Red No. 27 Lake, Dimethicone, EDTA, FD&C Blue No. 1 Lake, Gelatin, Glycerin, Hydroxypropyl Methylcellulose, Iron Oxide, Lecithin, Pharmaceutical Glaze, Polyethylene Glycol, Povidone, Propylene Glycol, Starch, Stearic Acid, Titanium Dioxide, Triacetin.
Tablet: Croscarmellose Sodium, FD&C Blue No. 1 Lake, Hydroxypropyl Methylcellulose, Polyethylene Glycol, Povidone, Propylene Glycol, Starch, Stearic Acid, Titanium Dioxide.

Indications: For the temporary relief of minor aches and pains of headaches, colds, flu, muscle aches, backache, toothache, menstrual cramps, and minor arthritis pain. Also reduces fever.

Warnings: Patients are warned not to take this product for pain for more than 10 days or for fever for more than 3 days unless directed by a physician. If redness or swelling is present, patients are directed to consult a physician because these could be signs of a serious condition. Patients should not take this product if they are hypersensitive to any of the ingredients. As with any drug, women who are pregnant or nursing a baby should seek the advice of a health professional before using this product. Patients are also warned to keep this and all drugs out of the reach of children, and that in case of accidental overdose, to seek professional assistance or contact a poison control center immediately. Because of the acetaminophen, they are told that prompt medical attention is critical for adults as well as for children even if they do not notice any signs or symptoms.

Directions: Adults and children 12 years of age and older: 2 caplets, gel caplets, or tablets 3 or 4 times a day. Do not exceed 8 caplets, gel caplets, or tablets in 24 hours.

Overdose: Acetaminophen in massive overdosage may cause hepatic toxicity in some patients. In all cases of suspected overdose, immediately call your regional poison control center or the Rocky Mountain Poison Control Center for assistance in diagnosis and for directions in the use of *N*-acetylcysteine as an antidote. In adults, hepatic toxicity has rarely been reported with acute overdoses of less than 10 grams and fatalities with less than 15 grams. Importantly, young children seem to be more resistant than adults to the hepatotoxic effect of an acetaminophen overdose. Despite this, the measures outined below should be initiated in any adult or child suspected of having ingested an acetaminophen overdose.
Early symptoms following a potentially hepatotoxic overdose may include: nausea, vomiting, diaphoresis, and general malaise. Clinical and laboratory evidence of hepatic toxicity may not be apparent until 48 to 72 hours post-ingestion. The stomach should be emptied promptly by lavage or by induction of emesis with syrup of ipecac. Patients' estimates of the quantity of a drug ingested are notoriously unreliable. Therefore, if an acetaminophen overdose is suspected, a serum acetaminophen assay should be obtained as early as possible, but no sooner than four hours following ingestion. Liver function studies should be obtained initially and at 24-hour intervals. The antidote, *N*-acetylcysteine, should be administered as early as possible and within 16 hours of the overdose ingestion for optimal results. Following recovery, there are no residual structural or functional hepatic abnormalities.

How Supplied: *Caplets:* white, capsule-shaped, compressed tablets monogrammed "AF ANACIN" in blue—bottles of 30 (NDC 0573-0330-10), 60 (NDC 0573-0330-20), and 100 (NDC 0573-0330-30). *Gel Caplets:* blue and white gelatin coated, capsule-shaped tablets monogrammed "AF ANACIN" in black—bottles of 24 (NDC 0573-0340-20), 50 (NDC 0573-0340-30), and 100 (NDC 0573-0340-40). *Tablets:* white compressed tablets engraved "A" over "AF" on one side and "500" on the other—tins of 12 (NDC 0573-0310-05) and bottles of 30 (NDC 0573-0310-10), 60 (NDC 0573-0310-20), and 100 (NDC 0573-0310-30).

Shown in Product Identification Section, page 420

ASPIRIN FREE ANACIN® P.M.
[*an 'a-sin*]
Caplets

Description: Each caplet contains:
Acetaminophen .... 500 mg
Diphenhydramine HCl .... 25 mg

Inactive Ingredients: Calcium Stearate, FD&C Blue No. 1 Lake, Hydroxypropyl Methylcellulose, Magnesium Stearate, Microcrystalline Cellulose, Polyethylene Glycol, Povidone, Starch, Stearic Acid, Titanium Dioxide. May also contain: Ammonium Hydroxide, Iron Oxide, Pharmaceutical Glaze, Potassium Hydroxide, Propylene Glycol.

Indications: For the temporary relief of occasional headaches and minor aches and pains with accompanying sleeplessness.

Warnings: Do not give this product to children under 12 years of age. Patients are warned not to take this product for pain for more than 10 days unless directed by a physician. If pain persists or gets worse, if new symptoms occur, or if redness or swelling is present, patients are directed to consult a physician because these could be signs of a serious condition. If sleeplessness persists continuously for more than 2 weeks, patients are directed to consult a physician because insomnia may be a symptom of a serious underlying medical illness. Patients should not take this product if they have asthma, glaucoma, emphysema, chronic pulmonary disease, shortness of breath, difficulty in breathing or difficulty in urination due to enlargement of the prostate gland unless directed by a physician. Patients are told to avoid alcoholic beverages while taking this product and not to take if they are taking sedatives or tranquilizers without first consulting their physician. As with any drug, women who are pregnant or nursing a baby should seek the advice of a health professional before using this product. Patients are also warned to keep this and all drugs out of the reach of children, and that in case of accidental overdose, to seek professional assistance or contact a poison control center immediately. Because of the acetaminophen, they are told that prompt medical attention is critical for adults as well as for children even if they do not notice any signs or symptoms.

Directions: Adults and children 12 years of age and older: 2 caplets at bedtime if needed, or as directed by a doctor.

Overdose: Acetaminophen in massive overdosage may cause hepatic toxicity in some patients. In all cases of suspected overdose, immediately call your regional poison control center or the Rocky Mountain Poison Control Center for assistance in diagnosis and for directions in the use of *N*-acetylcysteine as an antidote. In adults, hepatic toxicity has rarely been reported with acute overdoses of less than 10 grams and fatalities with less than 15 grams. Importantly, young children seem to be more resistant than adults to the hepatotoxic effect of an acetaminophen overdose. Despite this, the measures outlined below should be initiated in any adult or child suspected of having ingested an acetaminophen overdose.

Early symptoms following a potentially hepatotoxic overdose may include: nausea, vomiting, diaphoresis, and general malaise. Clinical and laboratory evidence of hepatic toxicity may not be apparent until 48 to 72 hours post-ingestion. The stomach should be emptied promptly by lavage or by induction of emesis with syrup of ipecac. Patients' estimates of the quantity of drug ingested are notoriously unreliable. Therefore, if an acetaminophen overdose is suspected, a serum acetaminophen assay should be obtained as early as possible, but no sooner than four hours following ingestion. Liver function studies should be obtained initially and at 24-hour intervals. The antidote, *N*-acetylcysteine, should be administered as early as possible and within 16 hours of the overdose ingestion for optimal results. Following recovery, there are no residual structural or functional hepatic abnormalities.

How Supplied: blue caplet engraved "AFPM" on one side—bottles of 20 (NDC 0573-0315-10), and 40 (NDC 0573-315-20).

Shown in Product Identification Section, page 420

MAXIMUM STRENGTH ANACIN®
[an 'a-sin]
Coated Tablets

Description: Each tablet contains:

Aspirin	500 mg
Caffeine	32 mg

Inactive Ingredients: Hydroxypropyl Methylcellulose, Microcrystalline Cellulose, Polyethylene Glycol, Sodium Lauryl Sulfate, Starch.

Indications: Temporary relief of minor aches and pains from headaches, colds, muscle aches, backache, toothache, premenstrual and menstrual cramps, and minor arthritis pain. Also reduces fever.

Warnings: Children and teenagers should not use this medicine for chicken pox or flu symptoms before a doctor is consulted about Reye Syndrome, a rare but serious illness reported to be associated with aspirin. Patients are warned to consult a physician immediately if pain persists for more than 10 days, or redness is present, or in arthritic or rheumatic conditions affecting children under 12 years of age. As with any drug, women who are pregnant or nursing a baby should seek the advice of a health professional before using this product. Women are also warned that **IT IS ESPECIALLY IMPORTANT NOT TO USE ASPIRIN DURING THE LAST 3 MONTHS OF PREGNANCY UNLESS SPECIFICALLY DIRECTED TO DO SO BY A DOCTOR BECAUSE IT MAY CAUSE PROBLEMS IN THE UNBORN CHILD OR COMPLICATIONS DURING DELIVERY.** Patients are also warned to keep this and all drugs out of the reach of children, and that in case of accidental overdose, to seek professional assistance or contact a poison control center immediately.

Directions: Adults: 2 tablets with water 3 or 4 times a day. Do not exceed 8 tablets in any 24-hour period. This product is not recommended for children under 12 years of age.

How Supplied: Coated white tablet engraved with "500" in an arrow on one side and with "500" on the other side—tins of 12 (NDC 0573-0211-05) and bottles of 20 (NDC 0573-0211-10), 40 (NDC 0573-0211-20), 75 (NDC 0573-0211-40), and 150 (NDC 0573-0211-45).

Shown in Product Identification Section, page 420

CHAP STICK® Lip Balm

Active Ingredients: 44% Petrolatums, 1.5% Padimate O.

Inactive Ingredients:
Regular: Contains FD&C Yellow 5 Aluminum Lake (Tartrazine). Also contains: Wax Paraffin, Mineral Oil, 2-Octyl Dodecanol, Arachidyl Propionate, Polyphenylmethylsiloxane 556, Oleyl Alcohol, White Wax, Isopropyl Lanolate, Lanolin, Carnauba Wax, Isopropyl Myristate, Camphor, Cetyl Alcohol, Fragrance, Methylparaben, Propylparaben, Titanium Dioxide, D&C Red 6 Barium Lake.
Cherry: Wax Paraffin, Mineral Oil, 2-Octyl Dodecanol, Arachidyl Propionate, Polyphenylmethylsiloxane 556, Flavors, White Wax, Isopropyl Lanolate, Lanolin, Carnauba Wax, Isopropyl Myristate, Camphor, Cetyl Alcohol, Methylparaben, D&C Red Barium Lake, Propylparaben, Saccharin.
Mint: Contains FD&C Yellow 5 Aluminum Lake (Tartrazine). Also contains: Wax Paraffin, Mineral Oil, 2-Octyl Dodecanol, Arachidyl Propionate, Polyphenylmethylsiloxane 556, Flavors, White Wax, Isopropyl Lanolate, Lanolin, Carnauba Wax, Isopropyl Myristate, Cetyl Alcohol, Methylparaben, Saccharin, Propylparaben, FD&C Blue 1 Aluminum Lake.
Orange: Wax Paraffin, Mineral Oil, 2-Octyl Dodecanol, Arachidyl Propionate, Polyphenylmethylsiloxane 556, Flavors, White Wax, Isopropyl Lanolate, Lanolin, Carnauba Wax, Isopropyl Myristate, Cetyl Alcohol, FD&C Yellow 6 Aluminum Lake, Methylparaben, Propylparaben, Saccharin.
Strawberry: Wax Paraffin, Mineral Oil, 2-Octyl Dodecanol, Arachidyl Propionate, Polyphenylmethylsiloxane 556, Flavors, White Wax, Isopropyl Lanolate, Lanolin, Carnauba Wax, Isopropyl Myristate, Camphor, Cetyl Alcohol, Methylparaben, Saccharin, Propylparaben, D&C Red 6 Barium Lake.

Indications: Helps prevention and healing of dry, chapped, sun and windburned lips.

Actions: A specially designed lipid complex hydrophobic base containing Padimate O which forms a barrier to prevent moisture loss and protect lips from the drying effects of cold weather, wind and sun which cause chapping. The special emollients soften the skin by forming an occlusive film thus inducing hydration, restoring suppleness to the lips, and preventing drying from evaporation of water that diffuses to the surface from the underlying layers of tissue. Chap Stick also protects the skin from the external environment and its sunscreen offers protection from exposure to the sun.

Warning: Patients should consult a physician if condition worsens or does not improve within 7 days.

Symptoms and Treatment of Oral Ingestion: The oral LD_{50} in rats is greater than 5 gm/kg. There have been no reported overdoses in humans. There are no known symptoms of overdosage.

Directions: For dry, chapped lips apply as needed. To help prevent dry, chapped sun or windburned lips, apply to lips as needed before, during and following exposure to sun, wind, water and cold weather.

How Supplied: Available in 4.25 gm sticks in Regular, Mint, Cherry, Orange, and Strawberry flavors.

Shown in Product Identification Section, page 420

CHAP STICK® MEDICATED Lip Balm Stick
CHAP STICK® MEDICATED Lip Balm Tube
CHAP STICK® MEDICATED Lip Balm Jar

Active Ingredients: *Stick:* 41% Petrolatums, 1% Camphor, 0.6% Menthol, 0.5% Phenol.
Tube: 67% Petrolatum, 1% Camphor, 0.6% Menthol, 0.5% Phenol.
Jar: 60% Petrolatums, 1% Camphor, 0.6% Menthol, 0.5% Phenol.

Continued on next page

Prescribing information on A. H. Robins products listed here is based on official labeling in effect November 1, 1992, with Indications, Contraindications, Warnings, Precautions, Adverse Reactions, and Dosage stated in full.

A. H. Robins—Cont.

Inactive Ingredients: *Stick:* Paraffin Wax, Mineral Oil, Cocoa Butter, 2-Octyl Dodecanol, Arachidyl Propionate, Polyphenyl Methylsiloxane 556, White Wax, Oleyl Alcohol, Isopropyl Lanolate, Carnauba Wax, Isopropyl Myristate, Lanolin, Cetyl Alcohol, Fragrance, Methylparaben, Propylparaben.
Tube: Microcrystalline Wax, Mineral Oil, Cocoa Butter, Lanolin, Fragrance, Methylparaben, Propylparaben.
Jar: Microcrystalline Wax, Mineral Oil, Cocoa Butter, Lanolin, Paraffin Wax, Fragrance, Methylparaben, Propylparaben.

Indications: For the temporary relief of pain and itching associated with fever blisters and cold sores. Also helps prevent dry, chapped, sun and windburned lips.

Actions: Camphor, phenol and menthol act as analgesics and anesthetics. At the concentrations provided in these products, camphor relieves itching and burning, menthol stimulates the nerves for perception of cold and depresses those which perceive pain, and phenol provides a slight numbing action. The petrolatums help soften the skin by forming an occlusive film for inducing hydration, restoring suppleness to the lips and preventing drying from evaporation of water that diffuses to the surface from the underlying layers of tissue.

Directions: Apply as needed.

How Supplied: 4.2 gm stick, 10 gm squeezable tube, and 7 gm jar.
Shown in Product Identification Section, page 420

CHAP STICK® SUNBLOCK 15
Lip Balm

Active Ingredients: 44% Petrolatums, 7% Padimate O, 3% Oxybenzone.

Inactive Ingredients: Contains FD&C Yellow 5 Aluminum Lake (Tartrazine). Also contains: Wax Paraffin, Mineral Oil, White Wax, Isopropyl Lanolate, Camphor, Lanolin, Isopropyl Myristate, Cetyl Alcohol, Carnauba Wax, Fragrance, Methylparaben, Propylparaben, Titanium Dioxide, D&C Red 6 Barium Lake.

Indications: Ultra Sunscreen Protection (SPF-15). Helps prevention and healing of dry, chapped, sun and windburned lips. Overexposure to sun may lead to premature aging of skin and lip cancer. Liberal and regular use may help reduce the sun's harmful effects.

Actions: Ultra sunscreen protection for the lips, plus the attributes of Chap Stick® Lip Balm. The emollients in the specially designed lipid complex hydrophobic base soften the lips by forming an occlusive film while the two sunscreens have specific ultraviolet absorption ranges which overlap to offer ultra sunscreen protection (SPF-15).

Warning: Patients should consult a physician if condition worsens or does not improve within 7 days.

Symptoms and Treatment of Oral Ingestion: Toxicity studies indicate this product to be extremely safe. The oral LD_{50} in rats is greater than 5 gm./kg. There are no known symptoms of overdosage.

Directions: For ultra sunscreen protection, apply evenly and liberally to lips before exposure to sun. Reapply as needed. For dry, chapped lips, apply as needed. To help prevent dry, chapped, sun, and windburned lips, apply to lips as needed before, during, and following exposure to sun, wind, water, and cold weather.

How Supplied: 4.25 gm. tube.
Shown in Product Identification Section, page 420

CHAP STICK® PETROLEUM JELLY PLUS

REGULAR:

Active Ingredients: 99% White Petrolatum, USP .

Inactive Ingredients: Aloe, Lanolin, Phenonip®, Butylated Hydroxytoluene, Fragrance.

CHERRY:

Active Ingredients: 98.85% White Petrolatum, USP.

Inactive Ingredients: Lanolin, Aloe, Phenonip®, Flavors, Butylated Hydroxytoluene, Saccharin, D&C Red 6 Barium Lake.

Indications: Helps prevent and protect against dry, chapped, sun and windburned lips.

Actions: White Petrolatum, USP forms a barrier to prevent moisture loss and protect lips from the drying effects of cold weather, wind and sun which cause chapping. White Petrolatum, USP helps soften the skin by forming an occlusive film for inducing hydration, restoring suppleness to the lips and preventing drying from evaporation of water that diffuses to the surface from the underlying layers of tissue.

Warning: Patients should consult a physician if condition worsens or does not improve within 7 days.

Directions: Apply to lips as needed before, during and following exposure to sun, wind, water and cold weather.

How Supplied: Regular and Cherry flavored available in 0.35 oz. (10 grams) squeezable tube.
Shown in Product Identification Section page 420

CHAP STICK® PETROLEUM JELLY PLUS WITH SUNBLOCK 15

Active Ingredients: 89% White Petrolatum, USP, 7% Padimate O, 3% Oxybenzone.

Inactive Ingredients: Aloe, Lanolin, Phenonip®, Butylated Hydroxytoluene, Fragrance.

Indications: Ultra Sunscreen Protection (SPF-15). Helps prevent and protect against dry, chapped, sun and windburned lips. Overexposure to sun may lead to premature aging of skin and skin cancer. Liberal and regular use may help reduce the sun's harmful effects.

Actions: Ultra sunscreen protection for the lips, plus the attributes of Chap Stick® Petroleum Jelly Plus. White Petrolatum, USP forms a barrier to prevent moisture loss and protect lips from the drying effects of wind and sun while two sunscreens, which have specific ultra violet absorption ranges, overlap to provide ultra sunscreen protection (SPF-15).

Warnings: This product is for external use only. Patients are advised to avoid contact with the eyes and to discontinue use if signs of irritation or rash occur.

Dosage and Treatment: For ultra sunscreen protection, apply evenly and liberally to lips before exposure to sun. Reapply as needed. For dry chapped lips, apply as needed. To help prevent dry, chapped, sun and windburned lips, apply to lips as needed before, during and following exposure to sun, wind, water and cold weather.

How Supplied: Available in 0.35 oz (10 grams) squeezable tube.
Shown in Product Identification Section, page 420

DIMETAPP® Cold & Allergy
[*di 'mĕ-tap*]
Chewable Tablets

Description: Each chewable tablet contains:
Brompheniramine Maleate, USP .... 1 mg
Phenylpropanolamine Hydrochloride, USP .... 6.25 mg

Inactive Ingredients: Aspartame, Citric Acid, Crospovidone, D&C Red 30 Aluminum Lake, D&C Red 7 Calcium Lake, FD&C Blue 1 Aluminum Lake, Flavor, Glycine, Magnesium Stearate, Mannitol, Microcrystalline Cellulose, Pregelatinized Starch, Silicon Dioxide, Sorbitol, Stearic Acid.

Indications: For temporary relief of nasal congestion due to the common cold, hay fever, or other upper respiratory allergies or associated with sinusitis. Temporarily relieves runny nose, sneezing, and itchy, watery eyes as may occur in allergic rhinitis (such as hay fever). Temporarily restores freer breathing through the nose.

Warnings: Parents are warned not to give this product to children with the following conditions, unless directed by a physician: asthma, glaucoma, high blood pressure, heart disease, diabetes, or thyroid disease. This product may cause drowsiness, or in some cases, excitability. Sedatives and tranquilizers may increase the drowsiness effect. Parents are warned not to give this product to children who are taking sedatives or tranquilizers without first consulting the child's physician.

Parents are warned not to exceed the recommended dosage, because at higher doses, nervousness, dizziness, or sleeplessness may occur. They are also warned not to give this product to children for more than 7 days. If their child's symptoms do not improve, or are accompanied by a fever, parents are instructed to consult a physician. Children should not be given this product if they are hypersensitive to any of the ingredients. As with any drug, if the person taking the drug is pregnant or nursing a baby, she should seek the advice of a health professional before using this product.

Drug Interaction Precaution: Concomitant administration of phenylpropanolamine with other sympathomimetic agents may produce additive effects and increased toxicity; with monoamine oxidase inhibitors (MAOIs) may produce a hypertensive crisis; with certain antihypertensive agents may diminish their antihypertensive effect.

This and all drugs should be kept out of the reach of children. In case of accidental overdose, professional assistance should be sought, or a poison control center contacted immediately.

Phenylketonurics are advised that this product contains 8 mg of phenylalanine per tablet.

Directions: Children 6 to under 12 years of age: 2 chewable tablets every 4 hours. Children under 6: consult a physician. DO NOT EXCEED 6 DOSES IN A 24-HOUR PERIOD.

Professional Labeling: The suggested dosage for children age 2 to under 6 years, only when the child is under the care of a physician, is 1 tablet every 4 hours, not to exceed 6 doses in a 24-hour period.

How Supplied: Purple tablet scored on one side and engraved with AHR 2290 on the other in bottles of 24 tablets (NDC 0031–2290–54).

Store at Controlled Room Temperature, Between 15°C and 30°C (59°F and 86°F).

Shown in Product Identification Section page 421

DIMETAPP® COLD AND FLU
[*dī' mĕ-tap*]
CAPLETS

Description: Each **Dimetapp® Cold & Flu Caplet** contains:

Acetaminophen, USP	500 mg
Phenylpropanolamine Hydrochloride, USP	12.5 mg
Brompheniramine Maleate, USP	2 mg

Inactive Ingredients: Corn Starch, FD&C Blue 2 Aluminum Lake, Hydroxypropyl Methylcellulose, Magnesium Stearate, Microcrystalline Cellulose, Polysorbate 20, Povidone, Propylene Glycol, Stearic Acid, Titanium Dioxide. May also contain Calcium Phosphate, Hydroxypropyl Cellulose, Methylparaben, Propylparaben.

Indications: For the temporary relief of minor aches, pains, and headache; for the reduction of fever; for the relief of nasal congestion due to the common cold or associated with sinusitis; and for the relief of runny nose, sneezing, itching of the nose or throat and itchy and watery eyes as may occur in allergic rhinitis (such as hay fever). Temporarily restores freer breathing through the nose.

Warnings: Patients with the following conditions are warned not to take this product, unless directed by a physician: asthma, emphysema, chronic pulmonary disease, shortness of breath, difficulty in breathing, high blood pressure, heart disease, diabetes, thyroid disease, glaucoma, or difficulty in urination due to enlargement of the prostate gland.

This product may cause drowsiness; alcohol, sedatives and tranquilizers may increase the drowsiness effect. Patients are told to avoid alcoholic beverages while taking this product and not to take it if they are taking sedatives or tranquilizers without first consulting their physician. Caution should be used when driving a motor vehicle or operating machinery. May cause excitability, especially in children.

Patients are warned not to exceed the recommended dosage because at higher doses, nervousness, dizziness or sleeplessness may occur. They also are told not to take this product for more than 10 days. If symptoms do not improve or are accompanied by fever that lasts for more than 3 days, or if new symptoms occur, patients should consult a physician.

Patients should not take this product if they are hypersensitive to any of the ingredients. As with any drug, women who are pregnant or nursing a baby should seek the advice of a health professional before using this product.

NOTE: Patients are also warned that IN CASE OF ACCIDENTAL OVERDOSE, they should SEEK PROFESSIONAL ASSISTANCE OR CONTACT A POISON CONTROL CENTER IMMEDIATELY. Because of the acetaminophen content, they are told that PROMPT MEDICAL ATTENTION IS CRITICAL FOR ADULTS AS WELL AS FOR CHILDREN, EVEN IF NO SIGNS OR SYMPTOMS ARE NOTED.

Drug Interaction Precaution: Concomitant administration of phenylpropanolamine with other sympathomimetic agents may produce additive effects and increased toxicity; with monoamine oxidase inhibitors (MAOIs) may produce a hypertensive crisis; with certain antihypertensive agents may diminish their antihypertensive effect.

Directions: Adults and children (12 years and over): Two caplets every 6 hours. DO NOT EXCEED 8 CAPLETS IN A 24-HOUR PERIOD.

Not recommended for children under 12 years of age.

Overdose: Acetaminophen in massive overdosage may cause hepatic toxicity in some patients. In all cases of suspected overdose, immediately call your regional poison control center or the Rocky Mountain Poison Control Center for assistance in diagnosis and for directions in the use of *N*-acetylcysteine as an antidote. In adults, hepatic toxicity has rarely been reported with acute overdoses of less than 10 grams and fatalities with less than 15 grams. Importantly, young children seem to be more resistant than adults to the hepatotoxic effect of an acetaminophen overdose. Despite this, the measures outlined below should be initiated in any adult or child suspected of having ingested an acetaminophen overdose.

Early symptoms following a potentially hepatotoxic overdose may include: nausea, vomiting, diaphoresis, and general malaise. Clinical and laboratory evidence of hepatic toxicity may not be apparent until 48 to 72 hours post-ingestion. The stomach should be emptied promptly by lavage or by induction of emesis with syrup of ipecac. Patients' estimates of the quantity of drug ingested are notoriously unreliable. Therefore, if an acetaminophen overdose is suspected, a serum acetaminophen assay should be obtained as early as possible, but no sooner than four hours following ingestion. Liver function studies should be obtained initially and at 24-hour intervals. The antidote, *N*-acetylcysteine, should be administered as early as possible and within 16 hours of the overdose ingestion for optimal results. Following recovery, there are no residual structural or functional hepatic abnormalities.

How Supplied: Dimetapp® Cold & Flu Caplets are supplied as blue capsule-shaped film-coated tablets, engraved AHR on one side and 2280 on the other, in consumer packages of 24 (NDC 0031-2280-54) (individually packaged), and 48 (NDC 0031-2280-59) (bottle).

Continued on next page

Prescribing information on A. H. Robins products listed here is based on official labeling in effect November 1, 1992, with Indications, Contraindications, Warnings, Precautions, Adverse Reactions, and Dosage stated in full.

A. H. Robins—Cont.

Store at Controlled Room Temperature, between 15°C and 30°C (59°F and 86°F).

Shown in Product Identification Section, page 421

DIMETAPP® Elixir

[*dī' mĕ-tap*]

Description: Each 5 mL (1 teaspoonful) contains:

Brompheniramine Maleate, USP ....2 mg
Phenylpropanolamine Hydrochloride, USP ....12.5 mg

Inactive Ingredients: Alcohol 2.3%, Citric Acid, FD&C Blue 1, FD&C Red 40, Flavor, Saccharin Sodium, Sodium Benzoate, Sorbitol, Water.

Indications: For temporary relief of nasal congestion due to the common cold, hay fever or other upper respiratory allergies or associated with sinusitis; temporarily relieves runny nose, sneezing, and itchy and watery eyes as may occur in allergic rhinitis (such as hay fever). Temporarily restores freer breathing through the nose.

Warnings: Patients with the following conditions are warned not to take this product, unless directed by a physician: asthma, emphysema, chronic pulmonary disease, shortness of breath, difficulty in breathing, high blood pressure, heart disease, diabetes, thyroid disease, glaucoma, or difficulty in urination due to enlargement of the prostate gland.

This product may cause drowsiness; alcohol, sedatives and tranquilizers may increase the drowsiness effect. Patients are told to avoid alcoholic beverages while taking this product and not to take it if they are taking sedatives or tranquilizers without first consulting their physician. Caution should be used when driving a motor vehicle or operating machinery. May cause excitability, especially in children.

Patients are warned not to exceed the recommended dosage because at higher doses, nervousness, dizziness or sleeplessness may occur. They also are told not to take this product for more than 7 days. If symptoms do not improve, or are accompanied by fever, patients should consult a physician.

Patients should not take this product if they are hypersensitive to any of the ingredients. As with any drug, women who are pregnant or nursing a baby should seek the advice of a health professional before using this product.

Patients are also warned to keep this and all drugs out of the reach of children, and that in case of accidental overdose, to seek professional assistance or contact a poison control center immediately.

Drug Interaction Precaution: Concomitant administration of phenylpropanolamine with other sympathomimetic agents may produce additive effects and increased toxicity; with monamine oxidase inhibitors (MAOIs) may produce a hypertensive crisis; with certain antihypertensive agents may diminish their antihypertensive effect.

Directions: Adults and children 12 years of age and over: 2 teaspoonfuls every 4 hours; children 6 to under 12 years: 1 teaspoonful every 4 hours; DO NOT EXCEED 6 DOSES IN A 24-HOUR PERIOD. Children under 6 years: use only as directed by a physician.

Professional Labeling: The suggested dosage for children age 2 to under 6 years, only when the child is under the care of a physician, is ½ teaspoonful every 4 hours, not to exceed 6 doses in a 24-hour period. The dosage for children under 2 years should be determined by the physician on the basis of the patients' weight, physical condition, or other appropriate consideration. Dimetapp Elixir is contraindicated in neonates (children under the age of one month).

How Supplied: Purple, grape-flavored liquid in bottles of 4 fl. oz. (NDC 0031-2230-12), 8 fl. oz. (NDC 0031-2230-18), 12 fl. oz. (NDC 0031-2230-22), pints (NDC 0031-2230-25), gallons (NDC 0031-2230-29), and 5 mL Dis-Co® Unit Dose Packs (10 × 10s) (NDC 0031-2230-23).

Store at Controlled Room Temperature, between 15°C and 30°C (59°F and 86°F).

Shown in Product Identification Section, page 421

DIMETAPP® DM ELIXIR

[*dī'mĕ-tap*]

Description: Each 5 mL (1 teaspoonful) contains:

Brompheniramine Maleate, USP .... 2 mg
Phenylpropanolamine Hydrochloride, USP .... 12.5 mg
Dextromethorphan Hydrobromide, USP .... 10.0 mg

Inactive Ingredients: Alcohol 2.3%, Citric Acid, FD&C Blue 1, FD&C Red 40, Flavors, Glycerin, Propylene Glycol, Saccharin Sodium, Sodium Benzoate, Sorbitol, Water.

Indications: Temporarily relieves cough due to minor throat and bronchial irritation as may occur with a cold. For temporary relief of nasal congestion due to the common cold, hay fever or other upper respiratory allergies or associated with sinusitis; temporarily relieves runny nose, sneezing, and itchy and watery eyes as may occur in allergic rhinitis (such as hay fever). Temporarily restores freer breathing through the nose.

Warnings: Patients with the following conditions are warned not to take this product, unless directed by a physician: asthma, emphysema, chronic pulmonary disease, shortness of breath, difficulty in breathing, or other persistent or chronic cough such as occurs with smoking, or cough that is accompanied by excessive phlegm (mucus). Likewise, patients with high blood pressure, heart disease, diabetes, thyroid disease, glaucoma, or difficulty in urination due to enlargement of the prostate gland are warned not to take this product unless directed by a physician.

This product may cause marked drowsiness; alcohol, sedatives and tranquilizers may increase the drowsiness effect. Patients are instructed to avoid alcoholic beverages while taking this product and not to take it if they are taking sedatives or tranquilizers without first consulting their physician. Caution should be used when driving a motor vehicle or operating machinery. May cause excitability, especially in children.

Patients are warned not to exceed the recommended dosage because at higher doses, nervousness, dizziness or sleeplessness may occur. They also are told not to take the product for more than 7 days. A persistent cough may be a sign of a serious condition. If cough or other symptoms persist for more than one week, tend to recur, or are accompanied by fever, rash or persistent headache, patients should consult a physician.

Patients should not take this product if they are hypersensitive to any of the ingredients. As with any drug, women who are pregnant or nursing a baby should seek the advice of a health professional before using this product.

Patients are also warned to keep this and all drugs out of the reach of children, and that in case of accidental overdose, to seek professional assistance or contact a poison control center immediately.

Drug Interaction Precautions: Concomitant administration of phenylpropanolamine with other sympathomimetic agents may produce additive effects and increased toxicity; with monamine oxidase inhibitors (MAOIs) may produce a hypertensive crisis; with certain antihypertensive agents may diminish their antihypertensive effect. Serious toxicity may result if dextromethorphan is used with MAOIs.

Directions: Adults and children 12 years of age and over: Two teaspoonfuls every 4 hours; children 6 to under 12 years: one teaspoonful every 4 hours. **DO NOT EXCEED 6 DOSES IN A 24-HOUR PERIOD.** Children under 6 years: use only as directed by a physician.

Overdose: Symptoms that may be associated with dextromethorphan overdose include ataxia, respiratory depression and convulsions in children, whereas adults may exhibit altered sensory perception, ataxia, slurred speech and dysphoria.

Professional Labeling: The suggested dosage for children age 2 to under 6 years, only when the child is under the care of a physician, is ½ teaspoonful every 4 hours, not to exceed 6 doses in a 24-hour period. The dosage for children under 2 years should be determined by the physician on the basis of the patients' weight, physical condition, or other appropriate consideration. Dimetapp DM Elixir is contraindicated in neonates (children under the age of one month).

How Supplied: Red, grape-flavored liquid in bottles of 4 fl. oz. (NDC 0031-2240-12), 8 fl. oz. (NDC 0031-2240-18), and 12 fl. oz. (NDC 0031-2240-22).
Store at Room Temperature.

Shown in Product Identification Section, page 421

DIMETAPP® Extentabs®
[*dī' mĕ-tap*]

Description: Each **Dimetapp Extentabs®** Tablet contains:

Brompheniramine Maleate, USP	12 mg
Phenylpropanolamine Hydrochloride, USP	75 mg

Inactive Ingredients: Acacia, Acetylated Monoglycerides, Calcium Sulfate, Carnauba Wax, Castor Wax or Oil, Citric Acid, Edible Ink, FD&C Blue 1 and FD&C Blue 2 Aluminum Lake, Gelatin, Magnesium Stearate, Magnesium Trisilicate, Pharmaceutical Glaze, Polysorbates, Povidone, Silicon Dioxide, Stearyl Alcohol, Sucrose, Titanium Dioxide, Wheat Flour, White Wax. May contain FD&C Red 40 and FD&C Yellow 6 Aluminum Lakes.

Indications: For temporary relief of nasal congestion due to the common cold, hay fever or other upper respiratory allergies or associated with sinusitis; temporarily relieves runny nose, sneezing, and itchy and watery eyes as may occur in allergic rhinitis (such as hay fever). Temporarily restores freer breathing through the nose.

Warnings: Patients with the following conditions are warned not to take this product, unless directed by a physician: asthma, emphysema, chronic pulmonary disease, shortness of breath, difficulty in breathing, high blood pressure, heart disease, diabetes, thyroid disease, glaucoma, or difficulty in urination due to enlargement of the prostate gland.
This product may cause drowsiness; alcohol, sedatives and tranquilizers may increase the drowsiness effect. Patients are told to avoid alcoholic beverages while taking this product and not to take it if they are taking sedatives or tranquilizers without first consulting their physician. Caution should be used when driving a motor vehicle or operating machinery. May cause excitability, especially in children.
Patients are warned not to exceed the recommended dosage because at higher doses, nervousness, dizziness or sleeplessness may occur. They also are told not to take this product for more than 7 days. If symptoms do not improve, or are accompanied by fever, patients should consult a physician.
Dimetapp Extentabs should not be given to children under 12 years, except under the advice and supervision of a physician. Patients should not take this product if they are hypersensitive to any of the ingredients. As with any drug, women who are pregnant or nursing a baby should seek the advice of a health professional before using this product.
Patients are also warned to keep this and all drugs out of the reach of children, and that in case of accidental overdose, to seek professional assistance or contact a poison control center immediately.

Drug Interaction Precaution: Concomitant administration of phenylpropanolamine with other sympathomimetic agents may produce additive effects and increased toxicity; with monoamine oxidase inhibitors (MAOIs) may produce a hypertensive crisis; with certain antihypertensive agents may diminish their antihypertensive effect.

Directions: Adults and children 12 years of age and over: one tablet every 12 hours. DO NOT EXCEED 1 TABLET EVERY 12 HOURS OR 2 TABLETS IN A 24-HOUR PERIOD.

How Supplied: Pale blue sugar-coated tablets monogrammed DIMETAPP AHR in bottles of 100 (NDC 0031-2277-63), 500 (NDC 0031-2277-70); Dis-Co® Unit Dose Packs of 100 (NDC 0031-2277-64); and consumer packages of 12 tablets (NDC 0031-2277-46), 24 tablets (NDC 0031-2277-54) and 48 tablets (NDC 0031-2277-59) (individually packaged).
Store at Controlled Room Temperature, between 15°C and 30°C (59°F and 86°F).
Dimetapp Extentabs® Tablets are the A. H. Robins Company's uniquely constructed extended action tablets.

Shown in Product Identification Section, page 421

DIMETAPP® Sinus Caplets
[*di 'mĕ-tap*]

Description: Each Dimetapp Tablet contains:

Ibuprofen	200 mg
Pseudoephedrine HCl	30 mg

Inactive Ingredients: Carnauba or Equivalent Wax, Croscarmellose Sodium, Iron Oxide, Methylparaben, Microcrystalline Cellulose, Propylparaben, Silicon Dioxide, Sodium Benzoate, Sodium Lauryl Sulfate, Starch, Stearic Acid, Sucrose, Titanium Dioxide.

Indications: For temporary relief of symptoms associated with the common cold, sinusitis or flu including nasal congestion, headache, fever, body aches, and pains.

Warnings: Aspirin sensitive patients are warned not to take this product if they have had a severe allergic reaction to aspirin, e.g. - asthma, swelling, shock, or hives because, even though this product contains no aspirin or salicylates, cross-reactions may occur in patients allergic to aspirin.
Patients are warned not to take this product for colds for more than 7 days or for fever for more than 3 days unless directed by a doctor. If the cold or fever persists or gets worse or if new symptoms occur patients are directed to consult a doctor because these could be signs of a serious illness. Patients are directed that as with aspirin and acetaminophen, if they have any condition which requires them to take prescription drugs or if they have had any problems or serious side effects from taking any non-prescription pain reliever, not to take this product without first discussing it with their doctor. They are also directed to consult their doctor IF they EXPERIENCE ANY SYMPTOMS WHICH ARE UNUSUAL OR SEEM UNRELATED TO THE CONDITION FOR WHICH they TOOK THIS PRODUCT BEFORE TAKING ANY MORE OF IT, and to consult a doctor if they are under a doctor's care for any serious condition. Patients are warned not to exceed the recommended dosage because at higher doses nervousness, dizziness or sleeplessness may occur. Patients with the following conditions are warned not to take this product unless directed by a doctor: high blood pressure, heart disease, diabetes, thyroid disease or difficulty in urination due to enlargement of the prostate gland. As with any drug, women who are pregnant or nursing a baby should seek the advice of a health professional before using this product. Women are warned that IT IS ESPECIALLY IMPORTANT NOT TO USE THIS PRODUCT DURING THE LAST 3 MONTHS OF PREGNANCY UNLESS SPECIFICALLY DIRECTED TO DO SO BY A DOCTOR BECAUSE IT MAY CAUSE PROBLEMS IN THE UNBORN CHILD OR COMPLICATIONS DURING DELIVERY. Patients are warned to keep this and all drugs out of the reach of children and that in case of accidental overdose to seek professional assistance or contact a poison control center immediately.

Drug Interaction Precaution: Concomitant administration of pseudoephedrine with other sympathomimetic amines may produce additive effects and increased toxicity; with monoamine oxidase inhibitors (MAOIs) may produce a hypertensive crisis; with certain antihypertensive agents may diminish their antihypertensive effect. Because of these effects patients are advised not to take this product if they are presently taking a prescription drug for high blood pressure or depression without first consulting their doctor. Patients are also instructed not to combine this product with other non-prescription pain relievers or with any other ibuprofen-containing product.

Directions: Adults: 1 caplet every 4 to 6 hours while symptoms persist. If symptoms do not respond to 1 caplet, 2 caplets

Continued on next page

Prescribing information on A. H. Robins products listed here is based on official labeling in effect November 1, 1992, with Indications, Contraindications, Warnings, Precautions, Adverse Reactions, and Dosage stated in full.

A. H. Robins—Cont.

may be used but do not exceed 6 caplets in 24 hours, unless directed by a doctor. The smallest effective dose should be used. Take with food or milk if occasional and mild heartburn, upset stomach, or stomach pain occurs with use. Consult a doctor if these symptoms are more than mild or if they persist. Children: Do not give this product to children under 12 years of age except under the advice and supervision of a doctor.

How Supplied: White coated caplet monogrammed DIMETAPP SINUS in packages of 20 tablets (NDC 0031–2260–52), and bottles of 40 tablets (NDC 0031–2260–56).
Store at room temperture; avoid excessive heat (40°C, 104°F).

Shown in Product Identification Section, page 421

DIMETAPP® Tablets and
[*dī' mĕ-tap*]
Liqui-Gels®

Description: Each **Dimetapp** Tablet or Liquigel® contains:
Brompheniramine Maleate, USP .... 4 mg
Phenylpropanolamine Hydrochloride, USP .... 25 mg

Inactive Ingredients: Tablets: Corn Starch, FD&C Blue 1 Aluminum Lake, Magnesium Stearate, Microcrystalline Cellulose. Liqui-Gels: D&C Red 33, FD&C Blue 1, Gelatin, Glycerin, Mannitol, Pharmaceutical Glaze, Polyethylene Glycol, Povidone, Propylene Glycol, Sorbitan, Sorbitol, Titanium Dioxide, Water.

Indications: For temporary relief of nasal congestion due to the common cold, hay fever or other upper respiratory allergies or associated with sinusitis; temporarily relieves runny nose, sneezing, and itchy and watery eyes as may occur in allergic rhinitis (such as hay fever). Temporarily restores freer breathing through the nose.

Warnings: Patients with the following conditions are warned not to take this product, unless directed by a physician: asthma, emphysema, chronic pulmonary disease, shortness of breath, difficulty in breathing, high blood pressure, heart disease, diabetes, thyroid disease, glaucoma, or difficulty in urination due to enlargement of the prostate gland.
This product may cause drowsiness; alcohol, sedatives and tranquilizers may increase the drowsiness effect. Patients are told to avoid alcoholic beverages while taking this product and not to take it if they are taking sedatives or tranquilizers without first consulting their physician. Caution should be used when driving a motor vehicle or operating machinery. May cause excitability, especially in children. Patients are warned not to exceed the recommended dosage because at higher doses, nervousness, dizziness or sleeplessness may occur. They also are told not to take this product for more than 7 days. If symptoms do not improve, or are accompanied by fever, patients should consult a physician.
Patients should not take this product if they are hypersensitive to any of the ingredients. As with any drug, women who are pregnant or nursing a baby should seek the advice of a health professional before using this product.
Patients are also warned to keep this and all drugs out of the reach of children, and that in case of accidental overdose, to seek professional assistance or contact a poison control center immediately.

Drug Interaction Precaution: Concomitant administration of phenylpropanolamine with other sympathomimetic agents may produce additive effects and increased toxicity; with monoamine oxidase inhibitors (MAOIs) may produce a hypertensive crisis; with certain antihypertensive agents may diminish their antihypertensive effect.

Directions: Tablets: Adults and children 12 years of age and over: one tablet every 4 hours. Children 6 to under 12 years: one-half tablet every 4 hours. DO NOT EXCEED 6 DOSES IN A 24-HOUR PERIOD. Children under 6 years: Use only as directed by a physician. Liqui-Gels: Adults and children 12 years of age and over: one Liquigel® every 4 hours. Children under 12, consult a physician. DO NOT EXCEED 6 Liqui-Gels in a 24-hour period.

How Supplied: Tablets: Blue, scored compressed tablets engraved AHR and 2254 in consumer packages of 24 (NDC 0031-2254-54) (individually packaged).
Liqui-Gels: Purple Liquigel imprinted AHR and 2255 in consumer packages of 12 (NDC 0031-2255-46) and 24 (NDC 0031-2255-54) (individually packaged).
Tablets and Liqui-Gels: Store at Controlled Room Temperature, between 15°C and 30°C (59°F and 86°F).
Liqui-Gels and Liquigel are registered trademarks of R.P. Scherer International Corporation.

Shown in Product Identification Section, page 421

DONNAGEL
Liquid and Chewable Tablets

Donnagel is now a product of Wyeth-Ayerst Laboratories. For complete information please see page 786.

ROBITUSSIN®
[*ro "bĭ-tuss 'ĭn*]
(Guaifenesin Syrup, USP)

Active Ingredients: Each teaspoonful (5 mL) contains:
Guaifenesin, USP .... 100 mg
in a pleasant tasting syrup.

Inactive Ingredients: Alcohol 3.5%, Caramel, Citric Acid, FD&C Red 40, Flavors, Glucose, Glycerin, High Fructose Corn Syrup, Saccharin Sodium, Sodium Benzoate, Water.

Indications: Expectorant action to help loosen phlegm and thin bronchial secretions to make coughs more productive.

Professional Labeling: Helps loosen phlegm and thin bronchial secretions in patients with stable chronic bronchitis.

Warnings: Patients with the following conditions are warned not to take this product, unless directed by a physician: persistent or chronic cough such as occurs with smoking, asthma, chronic bronchitis, emphysema or where cough is accompanied by excessive phlegm (mucus).
A persistent cough may be a sign of a serious condition. If cough persists for more than one week, tends to recur, or is accompanied by fever, rash, or persistent headache, patients should consult a physician.
Patients should not take this product if they are hypersensitive to any of the ingredients. As with any drug, women who are pregnant or nursing a baby should seek the advice of a health professional before using this product.
Note: Guaifenesin has been shown to produce a color interference with certain clinical laboratory determinations of 5-hydroxyindoleacetic acid (5-HIAA) and vanillylmandelic acid (VMA).

Directions: Adults and children 12 years and over: 2–4 teaspoonfuls every 4 hours; children 6 years to under 12 years: 1–2 teaspoonfuls every 4 hours. Children 2 years to under 6 years: ½–1 teaspoonful every 4 hours; children under 2 years—consult your doctor. DO NOT EXCEED RECOMMENDED DOSAGE.

How Supplied: Robitussin (wine-colored) in bottles of 4 fl. oz. (NDC 0031-8624-12), 8 fl. oz. (NDC 0031-8624-18), pint (NDC 0031-8624-25) and gallon (NDC 0031-8624-29).
Robitussin also available in 1 fl. oz. bottles (4 × 25's) (NDC 0031-8624-02) and Dis-Co® Unit Dose Packs of 10 × 10's in 5 mL (NDC 0031-8624-23), 10 mL (NDC 0031-8624-26) and 15 mL (NDC 0031-8624-28).
Store at Controlled Room Temperature, between 15°C and 30°C (59°F and 86°F).

Shown in Product Identification Section, page 421

ROBITUSSIN®-CF
[*ro "bĭ-tuss 'ĭn*]

Active Ingredients: Each teaspoonful (5 mL) contains:
Guaifenesin, USP .... 100 mg
Phenylpropanolamine HCl, USP .... 12.5 mg
Dextromethorphan HBr, USP ... 10 mg
in a pleasant tasting syrup.

Inactive Ingredients: Alcohol 4.75%, Citric Acid, FD&C Red 40, Flavors, Glycerin, Propylene Glycol, Saccharin Sodium, Sodium Benzoate, Sorbitol, Water.

Indications: Temporarily relieves coughs due to minor throat and bronchial irritation and nasal congestion as may occur with a cold. Expectorant action to help loosen phlegm and thin bronchial secretions to make coughs more productive.

Warnings: Patients with the following conditions are warned not to take this product, unless directed by a physician: persistent or chronic cough such as occurs with smoking, asthma, chronic bronchitis, emphysema, or if cough is accompanied by excessive phlegm (mucus). Likewise, patients with heart disease, high blood pressure, thyroid disease, diabetes, or difficulty in urination due to enlargement of the prostate gland are warned not to take this product unless directed by a physician.
Patients are warned not to exceed the recommended dosage because at higher doses, nervousness, dizziness or sleeplessness may occur. They also are told not to take this product for more than 7 days. A persistent cough may be a sign of a serious condition. If cough or other symptoms persist for more than one week, tend to recur, or are accompanied by fever, rash, or persistent headache, patients should consult a physician.
Patients should not take this product if they are hypersensitive to any of the ingredients. As with any drug, women who are pregnant or nursing a baby should seek the advice of a health professional before using this product.
Patients are also warned to keep this and all drugs out of the reach of children, and that in case of accidental overdose, to seek professional assistance or contact a poison control center immediately.

Overdose: Symptoms that may be associated with dextromethorphan overdose include ataxia, respiratory depression and convulsions in children, whereas adults may exhibit altered sensory perception, ataxia, slurred speech and dysphoria.

Note: Guaifenesin has been shown to produce a color interference with certain clinical laboratory determinations of 5-hydroxyindoleacetic acid (5-HIAA) and vanillylmandelic acid (VMA).

Drug Interaction Precautions: Concomitant administration of phenylpropanolamine with other sympathomimetic agents may produce additive effects and increased toxicity; with MAOIs may produce a hypertensive crisis; with certain antihypertensive agents may diminish their antihypertensive effect. Serious toxicity may result if dextromethorphan is used with MAOIs.

Directions: Adults and children 12 years and over, 2 teaspoonfuls every 4 hours; children 6 years to under 12 years, 1 teaspoonful every 4 hours; children 2 years to under 6 years, ½ teaspoonful every 4 hours; children under 2 years —as directed by a physician. DO NOT EXCEED 6 DOSES IN A 24-HOUR PERIOD.

How Supplied: Robitussin-CF (red-colored) in bottles of 4 fl. oz. (NDC 0031-8677-12), 8 fl. oz. (NDC 0031-8677-18), 12 fl. oz. (NDC 0031-8677-22), and one pint (NDC 0031-8677-25).
Store at Controlled Room Temperature, between 15°C and 30°C (59°F and 86°F).

Shown in Product Identification Section, page 421

ROBITUSSIN®-DM
[ro"bĭ-tuss'ĭn]

Active Ingredients: Each teaspoonful (5 mL) contains:
Guaifenesin, USP .... 100 mg
Dextromethorphan HBr, USP .... 10 mg
in a pleasant tasting syrup.

Inactive Ingredients: Citric Acid, FD&C Red 40, Flavors, Glucose, Glycerin, High Fructose Corn Syrup, Saccharin Sodium, Sodium Benzoate, Water.

Indications: Temporarily relieves coughs due to minor throat and bronchial irritation as may occur with a cold. Expectorant action to help loosen phlegm and thin bronchial secretions to make coughs more productive.

Warnings: Patients with the following conditions are warned not to take this product, unless directed by a physician: persistent or chronic cough such as occurs with smoking, asthma, chronic bronchitis, emphysema, or if cough is accompanied by excessive phlegm (mucus). A persistent cough may be a sign of a serious condition. If cough persists for more than one week, tends to recur, or is accompanied by a fever, rash, or persistent headache, patients should consult a physician.
Patients should not take this product if they are hypersensitive to any of the ingredients. As with any drug, women who are pregnant or nursing a baby should seek the advice of a health professional before using this product.
Patients are also warned to keep this and all drugs out of the reach of children, and that in case of accidental overdose, to seek professional assistance or contact a poison control center immediately.

Overdose: Symptoms may include ataxia, respiratory depression and convulsions in children, whereas adults may exhibit altered sensory perception, ataxia, slurred speech and dysphoria.
Note: Guaifenesin has been shown to produce a color interference with certain clinical laboratory determinations of 5-hydroxyindoleacetic acid (5-HIAA) and vanillylmandelic acid (VMA).

Drug Interaction Precaution: Serious toxicity may result if dextromethorphan is used with MAOIs.

Directions: Adults and children 12 years and over, 2 teaspoonfuls every 4 hours; children 6 years to under 12 years, 1 teaspoonful every 4 hours; children 2 years to under 6 years, ½ teaspoonful every 4 hours; children under 2 years—consult your doctor. DO NOT EXCEED 6 DOSES IN A 24-HOUR PERIOD.

How Supplied: Robitussin-DM (cherry-colored) in bottles of 4 fl. oz. (NDC 0031-8685-12), 8 fl. oz. (NDC 0031-8685-18), 12 fl. oz. (NDC 0031-8685-22), single doses: 6 premeasured doses—⅓ fl. oz. each (NDC 0031-8685-06), pint (NDC 0031-8685-25), and gallon (NDC 0031-8685-29).
Robitussin-DM also available in Dis-Co® Unit Dose Packs of 10 × 10's in 5 mL (NDC 0031-8685-23) and 10 mL (NDC 0031-8685-26).
Store at Controlled Room Temperature, between 15°C and 30°C (59°F and 86°F).

Shown in Product Identification Section, page 421

ROBITUSSIN®-PE
[ro"bĭ-tuss'ĭn]

Active Ingredients: Each teaspoonful (5 mL) contains:
Guaifenesin, USP .... 100 mg
Pseudoephedrine HCl, USP ...... 30 mg
in a pleasant tasting syrup.

Inactive Ingredients: Alcohol 1.4%, Citric Acid, FD&C Red 40, Flavors, Glucose, Glycerin, High Fructose Corn Syrup, Saccharin Sodium, Sodium Benzoate, Water.

Indications: Temporarily relieves nasal congestion as may occur with a cold. Expectorant action to help loosen phlegm and thin bronchial secretions to make coughs more productive.

Warnings: Patients with the following conditions are warned not to take this product, unless directed by a physician: persistent or chronic cough such as occurs with smoking, asthma, chronic bronchitis, emphysema, or if cough is accompanied by excessive phlegm (mucus). Likewise, patients with heart disease, high blood pressure, thyroid disease, diabetes, or difficulty in urination due to enlargement of the prostate gland are warned not to take this product unless directed by a physician.
Patients are warned not to exceed the recommended dosage because at higher doses, nervousness, dizziness or sleeplessness may occur. They also are told not to take this product for more than 7 days. A persistent cough may be a sign of a serious condition. If cough or other symptoms persist for more than one week, tend to recur, or are accompanied by fever, rash, or persistent headache, patients should consult a physician.
Patients should not take this product if they are hypersensitive to any of the in-

Continued on next page

Prescribing information on A. H. Robins products listed here is based on official labeling in effect November 1, 1992, with Indications, Contraindications, Warnings, Precautions, Adverse Reactions, and Dosage stated in full.

A. H. Robins—Cont.

gredients. As with any drug, women who are pregnant or nursing a baby should seek the advice of a health professional before using this product.
Patients are also warned to keep this and all drugs out of the reach of children, and that in case of accidental overdose, to seek professional assistance or contact a poison control center immediately.
Note: Guaifenesin has been shown to produce a color interference with certain clinical laboratory determinations of 5-hydroxyindoleacetic acid (5-HIAA) and vanillylmandelic acid (VMA).

Drug Interaction Precautions: Concomitant administration of pseudoephedrine with other sympathomimetic agents may produce additive effects and increased toxicity; with MAOIs may produce a hypertensive crisis; with certain antihypertensive agents may diminish their antihypertensive effect.

Directions: Adults and children 12 years and over, 2 teaspoonfuls every 4 hours; children 6 years to under 12 years, 1 teaspoonful every 4 hours; children 2 years to under 6 years, ½ teaspoonful every 4 hours; children under 2 years —as directed by physician. DO NOT EXCEED 4 DOSES IN A 24-HOUR PERIOD.

How Supplied: Robitussin-PE (orange-red) in bottles of 4 fl. oz. (NDC 0031-8695-12), 8 fl. oz. (NDC 0031-8695-18) and pint (NDC 0031-8695-25).
Store at Controlled Room Temperature, between 15°C and 30°C (59°F and 86°F).

Shown in Product Identification Section, page 421

ROBITUSSIN® COUGH CALMERS

[ro "bi-tuss 'in]

Description: Each lozenge contains:
Dextromethorphan
Hydrobromide, USP .... 5 mg

Inactive Ingredients: Corn Syrup, FD&C Red 40, flavors, glycerin, gum acacia, sucrose.

Indications: Temporarily relieves coughs due to minor throat and bronchial irritation as may occur with a cold.

Warnings: Patients with the following conditions are warned not to take this product unless directed by a physician: persistent or chronic cough such as occurs with smoking, asthma, or emphysema, or if cough is accompanied by excessive phlegm (mucus).
A persistent cough may be a sign of a serious condition. If cough persists for more than one week, tends to recur, or is accompanied by fever, rash, or persistent headache, patients should consult a physician.
Patients should not take this product if they are hypersensitive to any of the ingredients. As with any drug, women who are pregnant or nursing a baby should seek the advice of a health professional before using this product.

Overdose: Symptoms may include ataxia, respiratory depression and convulsions in children; whereas, adults may exhibit altered sensory perception, ataxia, slurred speech and dysphoria.

Drug Interaction Precaution: Serious toxicity may result if dextromethorphan is used with MAOIs.

Directions: Adults and children 12 years and over: Dissolve 2–4 lozenges in mouth every 4 hours as needed.
Children 6 to under 12 years: Dissolve 1–2 lozenges in mouth every 4 hours or as directed by a doctor.
Children 4 to under 6 years: Dissolve one lozenge in mouth every 4 hours or as directed by a doctor.
Do not exceed recommended dosage.

How Supplied: Square, red cherry-flavored lozenge engraved AHR on both sides. Each consumer carton contains 8 tandem-joined pouches containing 2 lozenges each (16 lozenges total). (NDC 0031-8690-49).
Store at Controlled Room Temperature, between 15°C and 30°C (59°F and 86°F).

ROBITUSSIN® COUGH DROPS

[ro "bĭ-tuss 'ĭn]

Menthol Eucalyptus, Cherry, and Honey-Lemon Flavors

Active Ingredients: Each cough drop contains:
Menthol Eucalyptus and *Cherry:*
Menthol .... 7.4 mg
Honey-Lemon:
Menthol .... 10 mg

Inactive Ingredients:
Menthol Eucalyptus: Corn Syrup, Eucalyptus Oil, Sucrose, Titanium Dioxide (coloring). May contain Starch.
Cherry: Corn Syrup, Eucalyptus Oil, FD&C Red 40, Flavors, Sucrose. May contain Starch.
Honey-Lemon: Corn Syrup, D&C Yellow 10, Eucalyptus Oil, FD&C Yellow 6, Flavors, Sucrose. May contain Starch.

Indications: Temporarily relieves coughs and minor throat irritations due to colds or inhaled irritants.

Warnings: Patients with the following conditions are warned not to use these products unless directed by a physician: sore throat that lasts more than 2 days, or persistent or chronic cough such as occurs with smoking, asthma, or emphysema, or if cough is accompanied by excessive phlegm (mucus).
A persistent cough or sore throat may be a sign of a serious condition. Patients are warned to consult a physician if cough persists for more than one week, tends to recur, or is accompanied by fever, rash, or persistent headache, or if sore throat is severe, persistent or accompanied by high fever, headache, nausea, or vomiting.
These products should not be taken by patients who are hypersensitive to any of the ingredients. As with any drug, women who are pregnant or nursing a baby should seek the advice of a health professional before using these products.

Directions: Adults and children 4 years and over: allow cough drop to dissolve slowly in the mouth. May be repeated every hour, as needed, or as directed by a physician. Children under 4 years: as directed by physician.

How Supplied: All 3 flavors of Robitussin Cough Drops are available in bags of 25 drops and sticks of 9 drops:
Menthol Eucalyptus: Bags (NDC 0031-8622-55); Sticks (NDC 0031-8622-44).
Cherry: Bags (NDC 0031-8623-55); Sticks (NDC 0031-8623-44).
Honey-Lemon: Bags (NDC 0031-8621-55); Sticks (NDC 0031-8621-44).

Shown in Product Identification Section, page 421

ROBITUSSIN® MAXIMUM STRENGTH COUGH SUPPRESSANT

[ro "bĭ-tuss 'ĭn]

Description: Each 5 mL (1 teaspoonful) contains:
Dextromethorphan
Hydrobromide, USP .... 15 mg
in a pleasant tasting liquid.

Inactive Ingredients: Citric Acid, FD&C Red 40, Flavors, Glucose, Glycerin, High Fructose Corn Syrup, Saccharin Sodium, Sodium Benzoate, Water.

Indications: Temporarily relieves coughs due to minor throat and bronchial irritation as may occur with a cold.

Warnings: Patients with the following conditions are warned not to take this product unless directed by a physician: persistent or chronic cough such as occurs with smoking, asthma, emphysema, or if cough is accompanied by excessive phlegm (mucus).
A persistent cough may be a sign of a serious condition. If cough persists for more than one week, tends to recur, or is accompanied by fever, rash, or persistent headache, patients should consult a physician.
Patients should not take this product if they are hypersensitive to any of the ingredients. As with any drug, women who are pregnant or nursing a baby should seek the advice of a health professional before using this product.
Patients are also warned to keep this and all drugs out of the reach of children, and that in case of accidental overdose, to seek professional assistance or contact a poison control center immediately.

Overdose: Symptoms may include ataxia, respiratory depression and convulsions in children, whereas adults may exhibit altered sensory perception, ataxia, slurred speech and dysphoria.

Drug Interaction Precaution: Serious toxicity may result if dextromethorphan is used with MAOIs.

Directions: Adults and children 12 years and over: 2 teaspoonfuls every 6–8 hours in medicine cup. Do not exceed 4 doses in a 24-hour period.

Professional Labeling: Children 6 years to under 12 years, 1 teaspoonful every 6–8 hours; children 2 years to under 6 years, ½ teaspoonful every 6–8 hours. Do not exceed 4 doses in a 24-hour period.

How Supplied: Robitussin Maximum Strength (dark red-colored) in bottles of 4 fl. oz. (NDC 0031-8670-12) and 8 fl. oz. (NDC 0031-8670-18).
Store at Controlled Room Temperature, between 15°C and 30°C (59°F and 86°F).

Shown in Product Identification Section, page 421

ROBITUSSIN® MAXIMUM
[*ro "bĭ-tuss 'ĭn*]
STRENGTH COUGH & COLD

Description: Each teaspoonful (5 mL) contains:
Dextromethorphan HBr, USP ... 15 mg
Pseudoephedrine HCl, USP .... 30 mg

Inactive Ingredients: Alcohol 1.4%, Citric Acid, FD&C Red 40, Flavors, Glycerin, Glucose, High Fructose Corn Syrup, Saccharin Sodium, Sodium Benzoate, Water.

Indications: Temporarily relieves coughs due to minor throat and bronchial irritation and nasal congestion as may occur with a cold.

Warnings: Patients with the following conditions are warned not to take this product unless directed by a physician: persistent or chronic cough such as occurs with smoking, asthma, emphysema, or if cough is accompanied by excessive phlegm (mucus). Likewise patients with heart disease, high blood pressure, thyroid disease, diabetes, or difficulty in urination due to enlargement of the prostate gland are warned not to take this product unless directed by a physician. Patients are warned not to exceed the recommended dosage because at higher doses nervousness, dizziness or sleeplessness may occur. They are also told not to take this product for more than 7 days. A persistent cough may be a sign of a serious condition. If cough or other symptoms persist for more than one week without improvement, tend to recur, or are accompanied by fever, rash, or persistent headache, patients should consult a physician. Patients should not take this product if they are hypersensitive to any of the ingredients. As with any drug, women who are pregnant or nursing a baby should seek the advice of a health professional before using this product. Patients are also warned to keep this and all drugs out of the reach of children, and that in case of accidental overdose, to seek professional assistance or contact a poison control center immediately.

Overdose: Symptoms that may be associated with dextromethorphan overdose include ataxia, respiratory depression and convulsions in children, whereas adults may exhibit altered sensory perception, ataxia, slurred speech and dysphoria.

Drug Interaction Precaution: Concomitant administration of pseudoephedrine with other sympathomimetic amines may produce additive effects and increased toxicity; with monoamine oxidase inhibitors (MAOIs) may produce a hypertensive crisis; with certain antihypertensive agents may diminish their antihypertensive effect. Serious toxicity may result if dextromethorphan is used with MAOIs.

Directions: Adults and children 12 years and over: 2 teaspoonfuls every 6 hours, in medicine cup. Children under 12: consult a physician. Do not exceed 4 doses in a 24 hour period.

How Supplied: Red syrup in bottles of 4 fl. oz. (NDC 0031-8671-12) and 8 fl. oz. (NDC-0031-8671-18).
Store at Controlled Room Temperature, Between 15°C and 30°C (59°F and 86°F).

Shown in Product Identification Section, page 421

ROBITUSSIN® NIGHT RELIEF
[*ro "bĭ-tuss 'ĭn*]
COUGH/COLD/FLU FORMULA

Description:
Each fluid ounce contains:
Acetaminophen, USP .... 650 mg
Pseudoephedrine HCl .... 60 mg
Pyrilamine Maleate, USP .... 50 mg
Dextromethorphan
Hydrobromide, USP .... 30 mg

Inactive Ingredients: Citric Acid, FD&C Blue 1, FD&C Red 40, Flavors, Glycerin, Propylene Glycol, Saccharin Sodium, Sodium Benzoate, Sorbitol, Water and other ingredients.

Indications: For the temporary relief of minor aches, pains, headache, muscular aches, sore throat, and fever associated with a cold or flu. Temporarily relieves nasal congestion, cough, runny nose and sneezing associated with the common cold.

Warnings: Patients with any of the following conditions are warned not to take this product, unless directed by a physician: asthma, emphysema, chronic pulmonary disease, shortness of breath, difficulty in breathing, or other persistent or chronic cough such as occurs with smoking, or cough that is accompanied by excessive phlegm (mucus). Likewise, patients with high blood pressure, heart disease, diabetes, thyroid disease, glaucoma, or difficulty in urination due to enlargement of the prostate gland, are warned not to take this product unless directed by a physician.
This product may cause marked drowsiness; alcohol, sedatives and tranquilizers may increase the drowsiness effect. Patients are warned to avoid alcoholic beverages while taking this product and not to take it if they are taking sedatives or tranquilizers without first consulting their physician. Caution should be used when driving a motor vehicle or operating machinery. This product may cause excitability, especially in children.
Patients are told not to exceed the recommended dosage because at higher doses, nervousness, dizziness or sleeplessness may occur. They also are told not to take the product for more than 10 days. A persistent cough may be a sign of a serious condition. If cough or other symptoms persist for more than one week, tend to recur, or are accompanied by rash, persistent headache, fever that lasts more than 3 days, or if new symptoms occur, patients should consult a physician.
If sore throat is severe, persists for more than 2 days, is accompanied or followed by fever, headache, rash, nausea or vomiting, a physician should be consulted promptly.
Patients should not take this product if they are hypersensitive to any of the ingredients. As with any drug, women who are pregnant or nursing a baby should seek the advice of a health professional before using this product.
NOTE: Patients are also warned that IN CASE OF ACCIDENTAL OVERDOSE, they should SEEK PROFESSIONAL ASSISTANCE OR CONTACT A POISON CONTROL CENTER IMMEDIATELY. Because of the acetaminophen content, they are told that PROMPT MEDICAL ATTENTION IS CRITICAL FOR ADULTS AS WELL AS FOR CHILDREN, EVEN IF NO SIGNS OR SYMPTOMS ARE NOTED.

Drug Interaction Precautions: Concomitant administration of pseudoephedrine with other sympathomimetic agents may produce additive effects and increased toxicity; with MAOIs may produce a hypertensive crisis; with certain antihypertensive agents may diminish their antihypertensive effect. Serious toxicity may result if dextromethorphan is used with MAOIs.

Overdose: Acetaminophen in massive overdosage may cause hepatic toxicity in some patients. In all cases of suspected overdose, immediately call your regional poison control center or the Rocky Mountain Poison Control Center for assistance in diagnosis and for directions in the use of *N*-acetylcysteine as an antidote. In adults, hepatic toxicity has rarely been reported with acute overdoses of less than 10 grams and fatalities with less than 15 grams. Importantly, young children seem to be more resistant than adults to the hepatotoxic effect of an ac-

Continued on next page

Prescribing information on A. H. Robins products listed here is based on official labeling in effect November 1, 1992, with Indications, Contraindications, Warnings, Precautions, Adverse Reactions, and Dosage stated in full.

A. H. Robins—Cont.

etaminophen overdose. Despite this, the measures outlined below should be initiated in any adult or child suspected of having ingested an acetaminophen overdose.
Early symptoms following a potentially hepatotoxic overdose may include: nausea, vomiting, diaphoresis, and general malaise. Clinical and laboratory evidence of hepatic toxicity may not be apparent until 48 to 72 hours post-ingestion. The stomach should be emptied promptly by lavage or by induction of emesis with syrup of ipecac. Patients' estimates of the quantity of drug ingested are notoriously unreliable. Therefore, if an acetaminophen overdose is suspected, a serum acetaminophen assay should be obtained as early as possible, but no sooner than four hours following ingestion. Liver function studies should be obtained initially and at 24-hour intervals. The antidote, *N*-acetylcysteine, should be administered as early as possible and within 16 hours of the overdose ingestion for optimal results. Following recovery, there are no residual structural or functional hepatic abnormalities.
Symptoms that may be associated with dextromethorphan overdose include ataxia, respiratory depression and convulsions in children, whereas adults may exhibit altered sensory perception, ataxia, slurred speech and dysphoria.

Directions: Adult dose (12 years and over): 1 fl. oz. in medicine cup at bedtime (2 tablespoonfuls). If cold or flu keeps the patient confined to bed or at home, one dose may be taken every 6 hours, not to exceed 4 doses in a 24-hour period. Children under 12 should use the product only as directed by a physician.

How Supplied: Bottles of 6 fl. oz. (NDC 0031-8649-15) and 10 fl. oz. (NDC 0031-8649-20).
Store at Controlled Room Temperature, between 15°C and 30°C (59°F and 86°F).

Shown in Product Identification Section, page 421

ROBITUSSIN® PEDIATRIC
[ro "bĭ-tuss 'in]
COUGH & COLD FORMULA

Description: Each 5 mL (1 teaspoonful) contains:
Dextromethorphan
Hydrobromide, USP .... 7.5 mg
Pseudoephedrine
Hydrochloride .... 15 mg
in a pleasant tasting nonalcoholic liquid.

Inactive Ingredients: Citric Acid, FD&C Red 40, Flavors, Glycerin, Propylene Glycol, Saccharin Sodium, Sodium Benzoate, Sorbitol, Water.

Indications: Temporarily relieves coughs due to minor throat and bronchial irritation and nasal congestion as may occur with a cold.

Warnings: Patients with the following conditions are warned not to take this product unless directed by a physician: persistent or chronic cough such as occurs with smoking, asthma, or emphysema, or if cough is accompanied by excessive phlegm (mucus). Likewise, patients with heart disease, high blood pressure, thyroid disease, diabetes, or difficulty in urination due to enlargement of the prostate gland are warned not to take this product unless directed by a physician.
Patients are warned not to exceed the recommended dosage because at higher doses, nervousness, dizziness or sleeplessness may occur. They also are told not to take this product for more than 7 days. A persistent cough may be a sign of a serious condition. If cough or other symptoms persist for more than one week, tend to recur, or are accompanied by fever, rash, or persistent headache, patients should consult a physician.
Patients should not take this product if they are hypersensitive to any of the ingredients. As with any drug, women who are pregnant or nursing a baby should seek the advice of a health professional before using this product.
Patients are also warned to keep this and all drugs out of the reach of children, and that in case of accidental overdose, to seek professional assistance or contact a poison control center immediately.

Drug Interaction Precautions: Concomitant administration of pseudoephedrine with other sympathomimetic agents may produce additive effects and increased toxicity; with monoamine oxidase inhibitors (MAOIs) may produce a hypertensive crisis; with certain antihypertensive agents may diminish their antihypertensive effect. Serious toxicity may result if dextromethorphan is used with MAOIs.

Overdose: Symptoms that may be associated with dextromethorphan overdose include ataxia, respiratory depression and convulsions in children, whereas adults may exhibit altered sensory perception, ataxia, slurred speech and dysphoria.

Directions: Patients are instructed to follow recommendations on the bottle or carton (see below) or to use as directed by a physician. Doses may be repeated every 6–8 hours, not to exceed 4 doses in a 24-hour period. Dosage should be chosen by weight, if known; if weight is not known, choose by age.
[See table below.]

Age	Weight	Dose
Under 2 yrs.	Under 24 lbs.	As directed by physician.
2 to under 6 yrs.	24–27 lbs.	1 Teaspoonful
6 to under 12 yrs.	48–95 lbs.	2 Teaspoonfuls
12 yrs. and older	96 lbs. and over	4 Teaspoonfuls

How Supplied: Robitussin Pediatric Cough & Cold formula (bright red) in bottles of 4 fl. oz. (NDC 0031-8609-12) and 8 fl. oz. (NDC 0031-8609-18).
Store at Controlled Room Temperature, between 15°C and 30°C (59°F and 86°F).

Shown in Product Identification Section, page 421

ROBITUSSIN® PEDIATRIC
[ro "bĭ-tuss 'in]
COUGH SUPPRESSANT

Description: Each 5 mL (1 teaspoonful) contains:
Dextromethorphan
Hydrobromide, USP .... 7.5 mg
in a pleasant tasting nonalcoholic liquid.

Inactive Ingredients: Citric Acid, FD&C Red 40, Flavors, Glycerin, Propylene Glycol, Saccharin Sodium, Sodium Benzoate, Sorbitol, Water.

Indications: Temporarily relieves coughs due to minor throat and bronchial irritation as may occur with a cold.

Warnings: Patients with the following conditions are warned not to take this product unless directed by a physician: persistent or chronic cough such as occurs with smoking, asthma, or emphysema, or if cough is accompanied by excessive phlegm (mucus).
A persistent cough may be a sign of a serious condition. If cough persists for more than one week, tends to recur, or is accompanied by fever, rash, or persistent headache, patients should consult a physician.
Patients should not take this product if they are hypersensitive to any of the ingredients. As with any drug, women who are pregnant or nursing a baby should seek the advice of a health professional before using this product.
Patients are also warned to keep this and all drugs out of the reach of children, and that in case of accidental overdose, to seek professional assistance or contact a poison control center immediately.

Overdose: Symptoms may include ataxia, respiratory depression and convulsions in children, whereas adults may exhibit altered sensory perception, ataxia, slurred speech and dysphoria.

Drug Interaction Precaution: Serious toxicity may result if dextromethorphan is used with MAOIs.

Directions: Patients are instructed to follow recommendations on the bottle or carton (see below) or to use as directed by a physician. Doses may be repeated every 6–8 hours, not to exceed 4 doses in a 24-hour period. Dosage should be chosen by weight, if known; if weight is not known, choose by age.
[See table on next page.]

How Supplied: Robitussin Pediatric (cherry-colored) in bottles of 4 fl. oz.

Age	Weight	Dose
Under 2 yrs.	Under 24 lbs.	As directed by physician.
2 to under 6 yrs.	24–27 lbs.	1 Teaspoonful
6 to under 12 yrs.	48–95 lbs.	2 Teaspoonfuls
12 yrs. and older	96 lbs. and over	4 Teaspoonfuls

(NDC 0031-8610-12) and 8 fl. oz. (NDC 0031-8610-18).
Store at Controlled Room Temperature, between 15°C and 30°C (59°F and 86°F).

Shown in Product Identification Section, page 421

Z-BEC® Tablets
[*zē'běk*]

One tablet daily provides:

Vitamin Composition	Percentage of U.S. Recommended Daily Allowance (U.S. RDA)	
Vitamin E	150	45.0 I.U.
Vitamin C	1000	600.0 mg
Thiamine (Vitamin B_1)	1000	15.0 mg
Riboflavin (Vitamin B_2)	600	10.2 mg
Niacin	500	100.0 mg
Vitamin B_6	500	10.0 mg
Vitamin B_{12}	100	6.0 mcg
Pantothenic Acid	250	25.0 mg
Mineral Composition		
Zinc	150	22.5 mg*

*22.5 mg zinc (equivalent to zinc content in 100 mg zinc sulfate, USP)

Ingredients: Niacinamide Ascorbate, Ascorbic Acid, Microcrystalline Cellulose, Vitamin E Acetate, Zinc Sulfate, Calcium Pantothenate, Hydroxypropyl Methylcellulose, Thiamine Mononitrate, Stearic Acid, Pyridoxine Hydrochloride, Riboflavin, Propylene Glycol, Titanium Dioxide, FD&C Blue 1 Aluminum Lake, Methylparaben, Propylparaben, Xanthan Gum, Sodium Citrate, Potassium Sorbate, Silicon Dioxide, Polysorbate 20, Magnesium Stearate, Polyvinylpyrrolidone, Vanillin, Cyanocobalamin.

Precaution: Not intended for the treatment of pernicious anemia.

Dosage: The recommended OTC dosage for adults and children 12 or more years of age is one tablet daily with food or after meals. Under the direction and supervision of a physician, the dose and frequency of administration may be increased in accordance with the patient's requirements.

How Supplied: Green film-coated, capsule-shaped tablets engraved AHR on one side and Z-BEC on the other in bottles of 60 (NDC 0031-0689-62), 500 (NDC 0031-0689-70), and Dis-Co® Unit Dose Packs of 100 (NDC 0031-0689-64).

Products are indexed by generic and chemical names in the **YELLOW SECTION.**

Ross Laboratories
COLUMBUS, OH 43216

PEDIATRIC NUTRITIONAL PRODUCTS

Alimentum® Protein Hydrolysate Formula With Iron

Isomil® Soy Formula With Iron

Isomil® SF Sucrose-Free Soy Protein Formula With Iron

PediaSure® Liquid Nutrition for Children

RCF® Ross Carbohydrate Free Low-Iron Soy Protein Formula Base

Similac® Low-Iron Infant Formula

Similac® PM 60/40 Low-Iron Infant Formula

Similac® Special Care® With Iron 24 Premature Infant Formula

Similac® With Iron Infant Formula

For most current information, refer to product labels.

CLEAR® EYES
[*klēr īz*]
Lubricating Eye Redness Reliever

Description: Clear Eyes is a sterile, isotonic, buffered solution containing the active ingredients naphazoline hydrochloride (0.012%) and glycerin (0.2%). It also contains boric acid, purified water and sodium borate. Edetate disodium and benzalkonium chloride are added as preservatives. Clear Eyes is a lubricating, decongestant ophthalmic solution specially designed for temporary relief of redness and drying due to minor eye irritation caused by dust, smoke, smog, sun glare, wearing contact lenses, allergies or swimming. Clear Eyes contains laboratory-tested and scientifically blended ingredients, including an effective vasoconstrictor which narrows swollen blood vessels and rapidly whitens reddened eyes in a formulation which also contains a lubricant and produces a refreshing, soothing effect. Clear Eyes is a sterile, isotonic solution compatible with the natural fluids of the eye.

Indications: For the temporary relief of redness due to minor eye irritation AND for protection against further irritation or dryness of the eye.

Warnings: To avoid contamination, do not touch tip of container to any surface. Replace cap after using. If you experience eye pain, changes in vision, continued redness or irritation of the eye, or if the condition worsens or persists for more than 72 hours, discontinue use and consult a doctor. If you have glaucoma, do not use this product except under the advice and supervision of a doctor. Overuse of this product may produce increased redness of the eye. If solution changes color or becomes cloudy, do not use. Keep this and all drugs out of the reach of children.

Directions: Instill 1 or 2 drops in the affected eye(s), up to four times daily.

How Supplied: In 0.5-fl-oz and 1.0-fl-oz plastic dropper bottles.
(FAN 2348)

Shown in Product Identification Section, page 421

CLEAR EYES® ACR
[*klēr īz*]
Astringent/Lubricating Eye Redness Reliever Drops

Description: Clear Eyes ACR is a sterile, isotonic buffered solution containing the active ingredients naphazoline hydrochloride (0.012%), zinc sulfate (0.25%) and glycerin (0.2%). It also contains boric acid, purified water, sodium chloride and sodium citrate. Edetate disodium and benzalkonium chloride are added as preservatives. Clear Eyes ACR is a triple-action formula that: (1) has an extra ingredient to clear away mucus buildup and relieve itching associated with allergies and colds, (2) immediately removes redness and (3) moisturizes irritated eyes. Clear Eyes ACR contains laboratory-tested and scientifically blended ingredients, including an effective vasoconstrictor which narrows swollen blood vessels and rapidly whitens reddened eyes in a formulation which also contains a lubricant and produces a refreshing, soothing effect. Clear Eyes ACR also contains an ocular astringent (zinc sulfate) that precipitates the sticky mucus buildup on the eye often associated with hay fever, allergies and colds and this helps clear the mucus from the outer surface of the eye. Clear Eyes ACR is a sterile, isotonic solution compatible with the natural fluids of the eye.

Indications: For the temporary relief of redness due to minor eye irritation AND for protection against further irritation or dryness of the eye.

Warnings: To avoid contamination, do not touch tip of container to any surface. Replace cap after using. If you experience eye pain, changes in vision, continued redness or irritation of the eye, or if the condition worsens or persists for more than 72 hours, discontinue use and consult a doctor. If you have glaucoma, do not use this product except under the advice and supervision of a doctor. Overuse of this product may produce in-

Continued on next page

If desired, additional information on any Ross Product will be provided upon request to Ross Laboratories.

Ross—Cont.

creased redness of the eye. If solution changes color or becomes cloudy, do not use. Keep this and all drugs out of the reach of children.

Directions: Instill 1 or 2 drops in the affected eye(s), up to four times daily.

How Supplied: In 0.5-fl-oz and 1.0-fl-oz plastic dropper bottles.
(FAN 2348)

Shown in Product Identification Section, page 421

EAR DROPS BY MURINE®
[*myūr 'ēn*]
See Murine Ear Wax Removal System/Murine Ear Drops.

Shown in Product Identification Section, page 421

MURINE® EAR WAX REMOVAL SYSTEM/MURINE® EAR DROPS
[*myūr 'ēn*]
Carbamide Peroxide Ear Wax Removal Aid

Description: MURINE EAR DROPS contains the active ingredient carbamide peroxide, 6.5%. It also contains alcohol (6.3%), glycerin, polysorbate 20 and other ingredients. The MURINE EAR WAX REMOVAL SYSTEM includes a 1.0-fl-oz soft bulb ear syringe. This system is a complete medically approved system to safely remove ear wax. Application of carbamide peroxide drops followed by warm-water irrigation is an effective, medically recommended way to help loosen excessive and/or hardened ear wax.

Actions: The carbamide peroxide formula in MURINE EAR DROPS is an aid in the removal of wax from the ear canal. Anhydrous glycerin penetrates and softens wax while the release of oxygen from carbamide peroxide provides a mechanical action resulting in the loosening of the softened wax accumulation. It is usually necessary to remove the loosened wax by gently flushing the ear with warm water, using the soft bulb ear syringe provided.

Indications: The MURINE EAR WAX REMOVAL SYSTEM is indicated for occasional use as an aid to soften, loosen and remove excessive ear wax.

Warnings: DO NOT USE if you have ear drainage or discharge, ear pain, irritation, or rash in the ear or are dizzy; consult a doctor. DO NOT USE if you have an injury or perforation (hole) of the eardrum or after ear surgery, unless directed by a doctor.
DO NOT USE for more than 4 days; if excessive ear wax remains after use of this product, consult a doctor. Avoid contact with the eyes. KEEP THIS AND ALL MEDICINES OUT OF THE REACH OF CHILDREN.

Directions: FOR USE IN THE EAR ONLY. Adults and children over 12 years of age: Tilt head sideways and place 5 to 10 drops in ear. Tip of applicator should not enter ear canal. Keep drops in ear for several minutes by keeping head tilted or placing cotton in the ear. Use twice daily for up to 4 days if needed, or as directed by a doctor. Any wax remaining after treatment may be removed by gently flushing the ear with warm water, using a soft bulb ear syringe. Children under 12 years, consult a doctor.
Note: When the ear canal is irrigated, the tip of the ear syringe should not obstruct the flow of water leaving the ear canal.

How Supplied: The MURINE EAR WAX REMOVAL SYSTEM contains 0.5-fl-oz drops and a 1.0-fl-oz soft bulb ear syringe.
Also available in 0.5-fl-oz drops only, MURINE EAR DROPS.
(FAN 2348)

Shown in Product Identification Section, page 421

MURINE®
[*myūr 'ēn*]
Lubricating Eye Drops

Description: Murine eye lubricant is a sterile buffered solution containing the active ingredients 0.5% polyvinyl alcohol and 0.6% povidone. Also contains benzalkonium chloride, dextrose, disodium edetate, potassium chloride, purified water, sodium bicarbonate, sodium chloride, sodium citrate and sodium phosphate (mono- and dibasic). Murine is a sterile, hypotonic solution formulated to more closely match the natural tear fluid of the eye for gentle, soothing relief from minor eye irritation while moisturizing and relieving dryness. Use as desired to temporarily relieve minor eye irritation, dryness and burning.

Indications: For the temporary relief or prevention of further discomfort due to minor eye irritations and symptoms related to dry eyes.

Warnings: To avoid contamination, do not touch tip of container to any surface. Replace cap after using. If you experience eye pain, changes in vision, continued redness or irritation of the eye, or if the condition worsens or persists for more than 72 hours, discontinue use and consult a doctor. If solution changes color or becomes cloudy, do not use. Keep this and all drugs out of the reach of children.

Directions: Instill 1 or 2 drops in the affected eye(s) as needed.

How Supplied: In 0.5-fl-oz and 1.0-fl-oz plastic dropper bottles.

(FAN 2348)

Shown in Product Identification Section, page 421

MURINE® PLUS
[*myūr 'ēn*]
Lubricating Redness Reliever Eye Drops

Description: Murine Plus is a sterile, non-staining, buffered solution containing the active ingredients 0.5% polyvinyl alcohol, 0.6% povidone and 0.05% tetrahydrozoline hydrochloride. Also contains benzalkonium chloride, dextrose, disodium edetate, potassium chloride, purified water, sodium bicarbonate, sodium chloride, sodium citrate and sodium phosphate (mono- and dibasic). Murine Plus is a sterile, hypotonic, ophthalmic solution formulated to more closely match the natural fluid of the eye. It contains demulcents for gentle, soothing relief from minor eye irritation as well as the sympathomimetic agent, tetrahydrozoline hydrochloride, which produces local vasoconstriction in the eye. Thus, the drug effectively narrows swollen blood vessels locally and provides symptomatic relief of edema and hyperemia of conjunctival tissues due to eye allergies, minor local irritations and conjunctivitis. Use up to four times daily, to remove redness due to minor eye irritation. The effect of Murine Plus is prompt (apparent within minutes) and sustained.

Indications: For the temporary relief or prevention of further discomfort due to minor eye irritations and symptoms related to dry eyes PLUS removal of redness.

Warnings: To avoid contamination, do not touch tip of container to any surface. Replace cap after using. If you experience eye pain, changes in vision, continued redness or irritation of the eye, or if the condition worsens or persists for more than 72 hours, discontinue use and consult a doctor. If you have glaucoma, do not use this product except under the advice and supervision of a doctor. Overuse of this product may produce increased redness of the eye. If solution changes color or becomes cloudy, do not use. Keep this and all drugs out of the reach of children.

Directions: Instill 1 or 2 drops in the affected eye(s), **up to four times daily.**

How Supplied: In 0.5-fl-oz and 1.0-fl-oz plastic dropper bottles.
(FAN 2348)

Shown in Product Identification Section, page 421

PEDIALYTE®
[*pē 'dē-ah-līt "*]
Oral Electrolyte Maintenance Solution

Usage: To restore fluid and minerals lost in diarrhea and vomiting; for maintenance of water and electrolytes following corrective parenteral therapy for severe diarrhea.
Features:
- Ready To Use—no mixing or dilution necessary.

Pedialyte, Rehydralyte Administration Guide

For Infants and Young Children

Age	2 Weeks	3	6 Months	9	1	1½	2	2½ Years	3	3½	4
Approximate Weight[2]											
(lb)	7	13	17	20	23	25	28	30	32	35	38
(kg)	3.2	6.0	7.8	9.2	10.2	11.4	12.6	13.6	14.6	16.0	17.0
PEDIALYTE UNFLAVORED or FRUIT-FLAVORED fl oz/day for maintenance*	13 to 16	28 to 32	34 to 40	38 to 44	41 to 46	45 to 50	48 to 53	51 to 56	54 to 58	56 to 60	57 to 62
REHYDRALYTE fl oz/day for Replacement for 5% Dehydration (including maintenance)*	18 to 21	38 to 42	47 to 53	53 to 59	58 to 63	64 to 69	69 to 74	74 to 79	78 to 82	83 to 87	85 to 90
REHYDRALYTE fl oz/day for Replacement for 10% Dehydration (including maintenance)*	23 to 26	48 to 52	60 to 66	68 to 74	75 to 80	83 to 88	90 to 95	97 to 102	102 to 106	110 to 114	113 to 118

Administration Guide does not apply to infants less than 1 week of age. For children over 4 years, maintenance intakes may exceed 2 liters daily.

1. Extrapolated from Barness L: Nutrition and nutritional disorders, in Behrman RE, Vaughan VC III: *Nelson Textbook of Pediatrics*, ed 12. Philadelphia: WB Saunders Co, 1983, pp 136-138.
2. Weight based on the 50th percentile of weight for age of the National Center for Health Statistics (NCHS) reference data. Hamill PVV, Drizd TA, Johnson CL, et al: Physical growth: National Center for Health Statistics percentiles. *Am J Clin Nutr* 1979; 32:607-629.

* Fluid intakes do not take into account ongoing stool losses. Fluid loss in the stool should be replaced by consumption of an extra amount of Pedialyte or Rehydralyte equal to stool losses in addition to the amounts given in this Administration Guide.

- Balanced electrolytes to replace stool losses and provide maintenance requirements.
- Provides glucose to promote sodium and water absorption.
- Unflavored form available for younger infants; fruit-flavored form available to enhance compliance in older infants and children.
- Plastic liter bottles are resealable and easy to pour.
- No coloring added.
- Widely available in grocery, drug and convenience stores.

Availability:
1 liter (33.8-fl-oz) plastic bottles; 8 per case; Unflavored, No. 336—NDC 0074-6470-32; Fruit-flavored, No. 365—NDC 0074-6471-32.
8-fl-oz bottles; 4 six-packs per case; Unflavored, No. 160—NDC 0074-6470-08. For hospital use, Pedialyte is available in the Ross Hospital Formula System.

Dosage: See Administration Guide to restore fluid and minerals lost in diarrhea and vomiting (Pedialyte Unflavored or Fruit-flavored) and management of mild to moderate dehydration secondary to moderate to severe diarrhea (Rehydralyte® Oral Electrolyte Rehydration Solution).
Pedialyte (Unflavored or Fruit-flavored) or Rehydralyte should be offered frequently in amounts tolerated. Total daily intake should be adjusted to meet individual needs, based on thirst and response to therapy. The suggested intakes for maintenance are based on water requirements for ordinary energy expenditure.[1] The suggested intakes for replacement are based on fluid losses of 5% or 10% of body weight, including maintenance requirement. [See table above.]

Composition: Unflavored Pedialyte (Fruit-flavored Pedialyte has similar composition and nutrient value. For specific information, see product label.)

Ingredients: (Pareve, Ⓤ) Water, dextrose, potassium citrate, sodium chloride and sodium citrate.

Provides:	Per 8 Fl Oz	Per Liter	Per 32 Fl Oz
Sodium (mEq)	10.6	45	42.4
Potassium (mEq)	4.7	20	18.8
Chloride (mEq)	8.3	35	33.2
Citrate (mEq)	7.1	30	28.4
Dextrose (g)	5.9	25	23.6
Calories	24	100	96

(FAN 806-01)

REHYDRALYTE®
[*rē-hī 'drə-līt "*]
Oral Electrolyte Rehydration Solution

Usage: For replacement of water and electrolytes lost during moderate to severe diarrhea.

Features:
- Ready To Use—no mixing or dilution necessary.
- Safe, economical alternative to IV therapy.
- 75 mEq of sodium per liter for effective replacement of fluid deficits.
- 2½% glucose solution to promote sodium and water absorption and provide energy.
- Available in pharmacies.

Availability: 8-fl-oz bottles; 4 six-packs per case; No. 162; NDC 0074-0162-01.

Dosage: (See Administration Guide under Pedialyte®.)

Ingredients: (Pareve, Ⓤ) Water, dextrose, sodium chloride, potassium citrate and sodium citrate.

Provides:	Per 8 Fl Oz	Per Liter
Sodium (mEq)	17.7	75
Potassium (mEq)	4.7	20
Chloride (mEq)	15.4	65
Citrate (mEq)	7.1	30
Dextrose (g)	5.9	25
Calories	24	100

(FAN 564-01)

SELSUN BLUE®
[*sel 'sun blü*]
Dandruff Shampoo
(selenium sulfide lotion, 1%)

Description: Selsun Blue is a non-prescription anti-dandruff shampoo containing the active ingredient selenium sulfide, 1%, in a freshly scented, pH-balanced formula to leave hair clean and manageable. Available in Dry, Oily, Regular, Extra Conditioning and Medicated Treatment formulas.

Inactive Ingredients:
Dry hair formula—Acetylated lanolin alcohol, ammonium laureth sulfate, ammonium lauryl sulfate, cetyl acetate, citric acid, cocamide DEA, cocamidopropyl betaine, DMDM hydantoin, FD&C blue No. 1, fragrance, hydroxypropyl methylcellulose, magnesium aluminum silicate, polysorbate 80, purified water, sodium chloride and titanium dioxide.
Regular hair formula—Ammonium laureth sulfate, ammonium lauryl sulfate, citric acid, cocamide DEA,

Continued on next page

If desired, additional information on any Ross Product will be provided upon request to Ross Laboratories.

Ross—Cont.

cocamidopropyl betaine, DMDM hydantoin, FD&C blue No. 1, fragrance, hydroxypropyl methylcellulose, magnesium aluminum silicate, purified water, sodium chloride and titanium dioxide.

Oily hair formula—Ammonium laureth sulfate, ammonium lauryl sulfate, citric acid, cocamide DEA, cocamidopropyl betaine, DMDM hydantoin, FD&C blue No. 1, fragrance, hydroxypropyl methylcellulose, magnesium aluminum silicate, purified water, sodium chloride and titanium dioxide.

Extra Conditioning formula—Aloe, ammonium laureth sulfate, ammonium lauryl sulfate, citric acid, cocamide DEA, di (hydrogenated) tallow phthalic acid amide, dimethicone, DMDM hydantoin, FD&C blue No. 1, fragrance, hydroxypropyl methylcellulose, purified water, sodium citrate, sodium isostearoyl lactylate and titanium dioxide.

Medicated Treatment formula—Ammonium laureth sulfate, ammonium lauryl sulfate, citric acid, cocamide DEA, cocamidopropyl betaine, DMDM hydantoin, D&C red No. 33, FD&C blue No. 1, fragrance, hydroxypropyl methylcellulose, magnesium aluminum silicate, menthol, purified water, sodium chloride and TEA-lauryl sulfate.

Clinical testing has shown Selsun Blue to be as safe and effective as other leading shampoos in helping control dandruff symptoms with regular use. May be used on color-treated or permed hair, if used as directed.

Directions: Shake well. Shampoo and rinse thoroughly. For best results, use regularly, at least twice a week or as directed by a doctor.

Warnings: For external use only. Avoid contact with the eyes. If contact occurs, rinse eyes thoroughly with water. If condition worsens or does not improve after regular use of this product as directed, consult a doctor. Keep this and all drugs out of the reach of children.

How Supplied: 4-, 7- and 11-fl-oz plastic bottles.
(FAN 2342-02)

Shown in Product Identification Section, page 421

SELSUN GOLD FOR WOMEN™
[sel 'sun gōld]
Dandruff Shampoo (selenium sulfide lotion, 1%)

Description: Selsun Gold for Women allows you to shampoo, condition and control dandruff flaking and itching with one shampoo. This formula contains patented ingredients to leave hair soft, shiny and manageable. You won't need a separate conditioner to have beautiful hair. May be used on color-treated or permed hair, if used as directed.

Inactive Ingredients: Ammonium lauryl sulfate, ammonium laureth sulfate, citric acid, cocamide DEA, di (hydrogenated) tallow phthalic acid amide, dimethicone, DMDM hydantoin, hydroxypropyl methylcellulose, purified water, sodium citrate and fragrance.

Directions: Shake well. Shampoo and rinse thoroughly. For best results, use regularly, at least twice a week or as directed by a doctor.

Warnings: For external use only. Avoid contact with the eyes. If contact occurs, rinse eyes thoroughly with water. If condition worsens or does not improve after regular use of this product as directed, consult a doctor. Keep this and all drugs out of the reach of children.

How Supplied: 4-, 7- and 11-fl-oz plastic bottles.
(FAN 2336-01)

Shown in Product Identification Section, page 422

TRONOLANE®
[tron 'ə-lān]
Anesthetic Cream for Hemorrhoids

Description: The active ingredient in Tronolane cream is the topical anesthetic agent, pramoxine hydrochloride, 1% (chemically unrelated to the benzoate esters of the "caine" type), which is chemically designated as a 4-n-butoxyphenyl gammamor-pholinopropyl-ether hydrochloride. Also contains the following inactive ingredients: A nongreasy cream base containing beeswax, cetyl alcohol, cetyl esters wax, glycerin, methylparaben, propylparaben, sodium lauryl sulfate and zinc oxide.

Tronolane cream contains a rapidly acting topical anesthetic producing analgesia that lasts up to 5 hours. Because the drug is chemically unrelated to other anesthetics, cross-sensitization is unlikely. Patients who are already sensitized to the "caine" anesthetics can generally use Tronolane cream.

The emollient/emulsion base of Tronolane cream provides soothing lubrication. Tronolane cream is in a nondrying base that is nongreasy and nonstaining to undergarments.

Indications: Tronolane cream is indicated for the temporary relief of the pain, burning, itching and discomfort that accompany hemorrhoids.

Warnings: If condition worsens or does not improve within 7 days, consult a doctor. Do not exceed the recommended daily dosage unless directed by a doctor. In case of bleeding, consult a doctor promptly. Do not put this product into the rectum by using fingers or any mechanical device or applicator. Certain persons can develop allergic reactions to ingredients in this product. If the symptom being treated does not subside, or if redness, irritation, swelling, pain or other symptoms develop or increase, discontinue use and consult a doctor. As with any drug, if you are pregnant or nursing a baby, seek the advice of a health care professional before using this product. Keep this and all drugs out of the reach of children.

Dosage and Administration (Directions): Adults—When practical, cleanse the affected area with mild soap and warm water and rinse thoroughly or cleanse by patting or blotting with an appropriate cleansing pad. Gently dry by patting or blotting with toilet tissue or a soft cloth before application of this product. Apply externally to the affected area up to five times daily. Children under 12 years of age—Consult a doctor.

How Supplied: Tronolane cream is available in 1-oz and 2-oz tubes.
(FAN 2348-02)

Shown in Product Identification Section, page 422

TRONOLANE®
[tron 'ə-lān]
Hemorrhoidal Suppositories

Description: The active ingredients in Tronolane suppositories are zinc oxide, 5%, and hard fat, 95%. Zinc oxide (an astringent) and hard fat (a skin protectant) afford temporary relief of hemorrhoidal itching and burning and protect irritated hemorrhoidal areas.

Indications: Tronolane suppositories are indicated for the temporary relief of the itching and burning associated with hemorrhoids and the protection of irritated hemorrhoidal areas.

Warnings: If condition worsens or does not improve within 7 days, consult a doctor. Do not exceed the recommended daily dosage unless directed by a doctor. In case of bleeding, consult a doctor promptly. As with any drug, if you are pregnant or nursing a baby, seek the advice of a health care professional before using this product. **Do not store above 86°F.** Keep this and all drugs out of the reach of children.

Dosage and Administration (Directions): Adults—When practical, cleanse the affected area with mild soap and warm water and rinse thoroughly or cleanse by patting or blotting with an appropriate cleansing pad. Gently dry by patting or blotting with toilet tissue or a soft cloth before application of this product. Remove foil wrapper before inserting into the rectum. Use up to six times daily or after each bowel movement. Children under 12 years of age—Consult a doctor.

How Supplied: Tronolane suppositories are available in 10- and 20-count boxes.
(FAN 2348)

Shown in Product Identification Section, page 422

If desired, additional information on any Ross Product will be provided upon request to Ross Laboratories.

Rydelle Laboratories
Division of S. C. Johnson & Son, Inc.
1525 HOWE STREET
RACINE, WI 53403

AVEENO® ANTI-ITCH
[*ah-ve 'no*]
CREAM AND LOTION
(External analgesic/Skin protectant)

AVEENO® Anti-Itch Cream provides fast temporary relief of the itching and pain associated with many minor skin irritations such as chicken pox rash, poison ivy/oak/sumac, and insect bites. Unlike hydrocortisone products, AVEENO® Anti-Itch Cream contains calamine to dry up weepy rashes, help control further spreading and promote healing. Aveeno's soothing oatmeal-enriched formula is non-greasy and invisible when rubbed into the skin.

Directions: Adults and children 2 years and older: Apply no more than 4 times daily. Children under 2: Consult a physician.

Warnings: For external use only. Avoid contact with eyes. If condition does not improve or recurs within 7 days, discontinue use and consult a physician. Keep out of children's reach. If ingested, contact a physician or poison control center. Store at 59°–86°F.

Active Ingredients: CALAMINE 3.0%, PRAMOXINE HCl 1.0%, CAMPHOR 0.3% IN A BASE OF WATER, GLYCERIN, DISTEARYLDIMONIUM CHLORIDE, PETROLATUM, OATMEAL FLOUR, ISOPROPYL PALMITATE, CETYL ALCOHOL, DIMETHICONE, SODIUM CHLORIDE.

How Supplied: 1 oz. tube of cream and 4 oz. bottle of lotion.

Shown in Product Identification Section, page 422

AVEENO® BATH TREATMENTS
[*ah-ve 'no*]
REGULAR FORMULA AND OILATED FOR DRY SKIN

AVEENO® BATH TREATMENTS contain colloidal oatmeal, a natural oat derivative developed especially for soothing and cleaning itchy, sore, sensitive skin.
AVEENO® BATH TREATMENTS contain no soaps that may be harmful to the skin. They cleanse naturally because of their unique adsorptive properties.
AVEENO® BATH TREATMENTS can be used for prompt temporary relief of itch due to dry skin, rashes, psoriasis, hemorrhoidal and genital irritations, poison ivy/oak, and sunburn. They are safe for use on children and can be used for prompt temporary relief of itch due to chicken pox, diaper rash, prickly heat and hives.

Ingredients: AVEENO® Bath Regular: 100% colloidal oatmeal; AVEENO® Bath Oilated: 43% colloidal oatmeal, mineral oil.

Shown in Product Identification Section, page 422

AVEENO® CLEANSING BAR
[*ah-ve 'no*]
FOR COMBINATION SKIN

AVEENO® Cleansing Bar For Combination Skin is made especially for itchy, sensitive skin that is irritated by ordinary soaps.
More than 50% of this mild skin cleanser is colloidal oatmeal, noted for its soothing and protective qualities.
AVEENO® Cleansing Bar is completely soap-free. It leaves no harsh alkaline film to irritate delicate skin, and it leaves skin feeling soft and comfortable.

Ingredients: AVEENO® Colloidal Oatmeal, 51%; in a sudsing soap-free base containing a mild surfactant.

Shown in Product Identification Section, page 422

AVEENO® CLEANSING BAR
[*ah-ve 'no*]
FOR ACNE-PRONE SKIN

AVEENO® Cleansing Bar For Acne-Prone Skin is a unique soap-free cleanser made with natural oatmeal. It absorbs and removes excess oil that can cause blemishes, but it won't overdry skin.

Ingredients: AVEENO® Colloidal Oatmeal, 51% in a sudsing soap-free base containing a mild surfactant.

Shown in Product Identification Section, page 422

AVEENO® CLEANSING BAR
[*ah-ve 'no*]
FOR DRY SKIN

AVEENO® Cleansing Bar For Dry Skin is a unique, soap-free cleanser for itchy, dry, sensitive skin that is irritated by ordinary soaps. It contains over 15% skin-softening emollients to help replace natural skin oils and 51% colloidal oatmeal, recommended for its soothing and protective qualities.

Ingredients: AVEENO® Colloidal Oatmeal, 51%, in a sudsing soap-free base containing vegetable oils, glycerine, and a mild surfactant.

Shown in Product Identification Section, page 422

AVEENO® MOISTURIZING CREAM
[*ah-ve 'no*]
Soothing Therapy for Dry, Itchy Skin

Aveeno® Moisturizing Cream has been clinically proven to relieve dry skin. The natural colloidal oatmeal in Aveeno Cream allows it to go beyond soothing and moisturizing dry skin to provide prompt temporary relief from persistent itch. Aveeno Cream is noncomedogenic and contains no fragrance, parabens, or lanolin which can cause allergic reactions. Cream formula is especially effective for extra-dry hands, feet and elbows.

Active Ingredient: Colloidal oatmeal 1% in a base of water, glycerin, distearyldimonium chloride, petrolatum, isopropyl palmitate, 1-hexadecanol, dimethicone, sodium chloride, phenylcarbinol.
For External Use Only.

How Supplied: 4 oz. jar.

Shown in Product Identification Section, page 422

AVEENO® MOISTURIZING LOTION
[*ah-ve 'no*]
FOR RELIEF OF DRY, ITCHY SKIN

AVEENO® Moisturizing Lotion has been clinically proven to relieve dry skin. It contains natural colloidal oatmeal to relieve the itch often associated with dry skin. It is noncomedogenic and contains no fragrance, parabens, or lanolin which can cause allergic reactions.

Active Ingredient: Colloidal oatmeal 1%.
Also Contains: Water, glycerin, distearyldimonium chloride, petrolatum, isopropyl palmitate, cetyl alcohol, dimethicone, sodium chloride, phenylcarbinol.

Shown in Product Identification Section, page 422

AVEENO® SHOWER AND BATH OIL
[*ah-ve 'no*]
FOR RELIEF OF DRY, ITCHY SKIN

AVEENO® Shower and Bath Oil combines the lubricating properties of mineral oil with the natural anti-itch benefits of colloidal oatmeal for the relief of dry, itchy skin. It contains no fragrance, parabens or lanolin which can cause allergic reactions.

Active Ingredient: Colloidal oatmeal 4%.
Also contains: Mineral oil, laureth-4, quaternium-18 hectorite, phenylcarbinol, silica, benzaldehyde.

Shown in Product Identification Section, page 422

RHULICREAM®
(External analgesic/Skin protectant)

Rhulicream® works on contact to provide fast, soothing, temporary relief of the itching and pain associated with many minor skin irritations. Apply this non-greasy calamine formula after exposure to poison ivy/oak/sumac to dry oozing and weeping, help to control further spreading and promote healing.

Continued on next page

Rydelle—Cont.

Directions: Adults and children 2 years and older: Apply to affected area no more than 4 times daily. Children under 2: Consult a physician.

Warnings: For external use only. Avoid contact with eyes. If condition does not improve or recurs within 7 days, discontinue use and consult a physician. Keep out of children's reach. If ingested contact a physician or poison control center. Store at 59°–86°F.

Active Ingredients: CALAMINE 3.0%, PRAMOXINE HCl 1.0%, CAMPHOR 0.3% IN A BASE OF WATER, GLYCERIN, DISTEARYLDIMONIUM CHLORIDE, PETROLATUM, ISOPROPYL PALMITATE, CETYL ALCOHOL, DIMETHICONE, SODIUM CHLORIDE.

How Supplied: 2 oz. tube.

Shown in Product Identification Section, page 422

RHULIGEL®
(External analgesic)

Rhuligel® provides fast, cooling, temporary relief of the itching and pain associated with many minor skin irritations, including poison ivy/oak/sumac, insect bites, and sunburn. Clear Rhuligel® is non-greasy and invisible on the skin. Won't stain clothing.

Directions: Adults and children 2 years and older: Apply to affected area no more than 4 times daily. Children under 2: Consult a physician.

Warnings: For external use only. Avoid contact with eyes. If condition does not improve or recurs within 7 days, discontinue use and consult a physician. Keep out of children's reach. If ingested contact a physician or poison control center. Store at 59°–86°F.

Active Ingredients: Benzyl Alcohol 2%, Menthol 0.3%, Camphor 0.3% in a base of SD Alcohol 23A 31% w/w, Purified Water, Propylene Glycol, Carbomer 940, Triethanolamine, Benzophenone-4, EDTA.

How Supplied: 2 oz. tube.

Shown in Product Identification Section, page 422

RHULISPRAY®
(External analgesic/Skin protectant)

Rhulispray® works on contact to provide fast, cooling, temporary relief of the itching and pain associated with many minor skin irritations. Calamine-based formula dries the oozing and weeping of poison ivy/oak/sumac. Convenient spray action eliminates the need to touch delicate inflamed skin.

Directions: Shake well before use. Adults and children 2 years and older: Apply to affected area no more than 4 times daily. Children under 2: Consult a physician.

Warnings: For external use only. Avoid contact with eyes. If condition does not improve or recurs within 7 days, discontinue use and consult a physician. Keep out of children's reach. If ingested contact a physician or poison control center. Store at 59°–86°F.

Caution: Flammable. Contents under pressure. Do not puncture or incinerate. Intentional misuse by deliberately concentrating and inhaling the contents can be harmful or fatal. Do not use near an open flame. May burst at temperatures above 120°F.

Active Ingredients (in concentrate): Calamine 13.8%, Benzocaine 5.0%, Camphor 0.7% in a base of Benzyl Alcohol, Hydrated Silica, Isobutane, Isopropyl Alcohol 70% w/w (concentrate), Oleyl Alcohol, Sorbitan Trioleate.

How Supplied: 4 oz. aerosol.

Shown in Product Identification Section, page 422

Sandoz Pharmaceuticals/ Consumer Division

59 ROUTE 10
EAST HANOVER, NJ 07936

ACID MANTLE® CREME
[ă'sĭd-mănt'l]
Acid pH

Description: A greaseless, water-miscible preparation containing buffered aluminum acetate. Other ingredients: aluminum sulfate, calcium acetate, cetearyl alcohol, glycerin, light mineral oil, methylparaben, purified water, sodium lauryl sulfate, synthetic beeswax, white petrolatum, white potato dextrin. May also contain: ammonium hydroxide, citric acid.

Indications: A vehicle for compatible topical drugs. Restores and maintains protective acidity of the skin. Provides relief of mildly irritated skin due to exposure to soaps, detergents, chemicals, alkalis. Aids in the treatment of bath dermatitis, athlete's foot, anogenital pruritus, acne, winter eczema and dry, rough, scaly skin of varied causes.

Caution: Limited compatibility and stability with Vitamin A, neomycin and other water-sensitive antibiotics. For external use only. Not for ophthalmic use.

Warnings: Keep this and all drugs out of the reach of children. In case of accidental ingestion, seek professional assistance or contact a Poison Control Center immediately.

Directions: Apply several times daily, especially after wet work.

How Supplied: 1 oz tubes; 4 oz and 1 lb jars.

BiCOZENE® Creme External Analgesic
[bī-cō-zēn]

Active Ingredients: Benzocaine 6%, resorcinol 1.67% in a specially prepared cream base.

Inactive Ingredients: Castor Oil, Chlorothymol, Ethanolamine Stearates, Glycerin, Glyceryl Borate, Glyceryl Stearates, Parachlorometaxylenol, Polysorbate 80, Sodium Stearate, Triglycerol Diisostearate, Perfume.

Indications: For the temporary relief of pain and itching associated with minor burns, sunburn, minor cuts, scrapes, insect bites or minor skin irritations.

Actions: Benzocaine is a topical anesthetic and resorcinol is a topical antipruritic, at the concentrations used in BiCozene Creme. Both exert their actions by depressing cutaneous sensory receptors.

Warnings: Do not apply over large areas of the body. Caution: Use only as directed. Keep away from the eyes. Not for prolonged use. If the symptoms persist for more than seven days or clear up and reoccur within a few days, or if a rash or irritation develops, discontinue use and consult a physician. For external use only. **KEEP THIS AND ALL DRUGS OUT OF THE REACH OF CHILDREN.** In case of accidental ingestion, seek professional assistance or contact a Poison Control Center immediately.

Drug Interaction Precautions: No known drug interaction.

Dosage and Administration: Adults and children 2 years of age and older: apply to affected area not more than 3 to 4 times daily. Children under 2 years of age: consult a physician. Apply liberally to affected area as needed, several times a day.

How Supplied: BiCozene Creme is available in 1-ounce tubes.

Shown in Product Identification Section, page 422

CAMA® ARTHRITIS PAIN RELIEVER
[kă'măh]

Description: Each CAMA Inlay-Tab contains: aspirin USP, 500 mg (7.7 grains); magnesium oxide, USP, 150 mg; dried aluminum hydroxide gel, USP, equivalent to 125 mg aluminum hydroxide. Other ingredients: colloidal silicon dioxide, croscarmellose sodium, hydrogenated vegetable oil, methylcellulose, methylparaben, microcrystalline cellulose, polyethylene glycol, povidone, pregelatinized starch, starch, Yellow 6, Yellow 10.

Indications: For the temporary relief of minor arthritic pain.

Warnings: Children and teenagers should not use this medicine for chicken pox or flu symptoms before a doctor is consulted about Reye syndrome, a rare but serious illness reported to be associated with aspirin. If redness or swelling is present, consult a doctor because these could be signs of a serious condition. Do not take this drug if you have asthma unless directed by a doctor. Do not take this product if you have stomach problems (such as heartburn, upset stomach, or stomach pain) that persists or recurs, or if you have ulcers or bleeding problems, unless directed by a doctor. If pain persists for more than 10 days, consult a physician immediately. As with any drug, if you are pregnant or nursing a baby, seek the advice of a health professional before using this product. **IT IS ESPECIALLY IMPORTANT NOT TO USE ASPIRIN DURING THE LAST 3 MONTHS OF PREGNANCY UNLESS SPECIFICALLY DIRECTED TO DO SO BY A DOCTOR BECAUSE IT MAY CAUSE PROBLEMS IN THE UNBORN CHILD OR COMPLICATIONS DURING DELIVERY.** Stop taking this product if ringing in the ears, loss of hearing, or dizziness occur. Do not take this product if you are presently taking a prescription drug for anticoagulation (thinning the blood), diabetes, arthritis, gout or if you have an aspirin allergy unless directed by a doctor. **Keep this and all medicines out of the reach of children. In case of accidental overdose, contact a physician immediately.**

Directions For Use: Adults: 2 tablets with a full glass of water every 6 hours. Not to exceed 8 tablets in 24 hours unless directed by a physician. Do not use in children under 12 years of age except under the advice and supervision of a physician.

How Supplied: CAMA Arthritis Pain Reliever Tablets (white with salmon inlay), imprinted "Cama 500" on one side, "Dorsey" on the other, in bottles of 100.

DORCOL® CHILDREN'S COUGH SYRUP
[door 'call]

Description: Each teaspoonful (5 ml) of DORCOL Children's Cough Syrup contains pseudoephedrine hydrochloride 15 mg, guaifenesin 50 mg, dextromethorphan hydrobromide 5 mg. Other ingredients: benzoic acid, Blue 1, edetate disodium, flavors, glycerin, propylene glycol, purified water, Red 40, sodium hydroxide, sucrose, tartaric acid.

Indications: Temporarily relieves your child's cough due to minor throat and bronchial irritation as may occur with the common cold. Helps loosen phlegm (mucus) and thin bronchial secretions to rid the bronchial passageways of bothersome mucus. Helps drain bronchial tubes and makes coughs more productive. Temporarily relieves nasal stuffiness due to the common cold, hay fever or upper respiratory allergies, and promotes nasal and/or sinus drainage.

Warnings: Keep this and all drugs out of the reach of children. In case of accidental overdose, seek professional assistance or contact a Poison Control Center immediately.
Except under the advice and supervision of a physician: Do not give your child more than the recommended dosage because at higher doses nervousness, dizziness or sleeplessness may occur. Do not give this preparation if your child has high blood pressure, heart disease, diabetes or thyroid disease. Do not give this product for persistent or chronic cough such as occurs with asthma or where cough is accompanied by excessive secretions. A persistent cough may be a sign of a serious condition. If cough or other symptoms persist for more than one week, tend to recur or are accompanied by high fever, rash or persistent headache, consult a physician before continuing use.
Drug Interaction Precaution: Do not give this product to a child who is taking a prescription drug for high blood pressure or depression, without consulting a physician.

Directions For Use: Children under 2 years—consult physician.
By age:
Children 2 to under 6 years: 1 teaspoonful every 4 hours.
Children 6 to under 12 years: 2 teaspoonfuls every 4 hours.
By weight:
Children 25 to 45 pounds: 1 teaspoonful every 4 hours.
Children 46 to 85 pounds: 2 teaspoonfuls every 4 hours.
Unless directed by a physician, do not exceed 4 doses in 24 hours.

Professional Labeling: The suggested dosage for pediatric patients is:

3–12 months	3 drops/Kg of body weight every 4 hours
12–24 months	7 drops (0.2 ml)/Kg of body weight every 4 hours

Maximum 4 doses in 24 hours.

How Supplied: DORCOL Children's Cough Syrup (grape colored), in 4 fl oz and 8 fl oz plastic bottles with tamper-evident band around child-resistant cap.

Shown in Product Identification Section, page 422

DORCOL® CHILDREN'S DECONGESTANT LIQUID
[door 'call]

Description: Each teaspoonful (5 ml) of DORCOL Children's Decongestant Liquid contains pseudoephedrine hydrochloride 15 mg. Other ingredients: benzoic acid, edetate disodium, flavors, purified water, sodium hydroxide, sorbitol, sucrose, Yellow 6, Yellow 10.

Indications: For temporary relief of nasal congestion due to the common cold, hay fever or other upper respiratory allergies, or associated with sinusitis. Reduces swelling of nasal passages; shrinks swollen membranes.

Warnings: Keep this and all drugs out of the reach of children. In case of accidental overdose, seek professional assistance or contact a Poison Control Center immediately. Do not give your child more than the recommended dosage because at higher doses nervousness, dizziness, or sleeplessness may occur. If symptoms do not improve within seven days or are accompanied by high fever, consult a physician before continuing use. Do not give this preparation if your child has high blood pressure, heart disease, diabetes, or thyroid disease unless directed by a doctor.

Directions For Use: Children under 2 years—consult physician.
By age:
Children 2 to under 6 years: 1 teaspoonful every 4 to 6 hours.
Children 6 years and older: 2 teaspoonfuls every 4 to 6 hours.
By weight:
Children 25 to 45 pounds: 1 teaspoonful every 4 to 6 hours.
Children 46 to 85 pounds: 2 teaspoonfuls every 4 to 6 hours.
Unless directed by a physician, do not exceed 4 doses in 24 hours.

Professional Labeling: The suggested dosage for pediatric patients is:

3–12 months	3 drops/Kg of body weight every 4–6 hours
12–24 months	7 drops (0.2 ml)/Kg of body weight every 4–6 hours

Maximum of 4 doses in 24 hours.
Drug Interaction Precaution: Do not give this product to a child who is taking a prescription drug for high blood pressure or depression, without first consulting the child's doctor.

How Supplied: DORCOL Children's Decongestant Liquid (pale orange), in 4 fl oz bottles with tamper-evident band around child-resistant cap.

Shown in Product Identification Section, page 422

DORCOL® CHILDREN'S LIQUID COLD FORMULA
[door 'call]

Description: Each teaspoonful (5 ml) of DORCOL Children's Liquid Cold Formula contains: pseudoephedrine hydrochloride 15 mg and chlorpheniramine maleate 1 mg. Other ingredients: benzoic acid, Blue 1, flavors, purified water, Red 40, sorbitol, sucrose, Yellow 10. May also contain sodium hydroxide.

Indications: For temporary relief of nasal congestion, runny nose and sneezing due to the common cold, hay fever or other upper respiratory allergies. Temporarily relieves itchy, watery eyes or itching of the nose or throat due to hay fever or other upper respiratory allergies.

Continued on next page

Sandoz—Cont.

Warnings: Keep this and all drugs out of the reach of children. In case of accidental overdose, seek professional assistance or contact a Poison Control Center immediately.
Do not give your child more than the recommended dosage because at higher doses nervousness, dizziness, or sleeplessness may occur. Do not give this preparation if your child has high blood pressure, heart disease, diabetes, thyroid disease, asthma or glaucoma unless directed by a doctor. If symptoms do not improve within 7 days or are accompanied by high fever, consult a physician before continuing use. May cause drowsiness. May cause excitability, especially in children.
Drug Interaction Precaution: Do not give this product to a child who is taking a prescription drug for high blood pressure or depression, without first consulting the child's doctor.

Directions For Use: Children under 6 years—consult physician.
By age:
Children 6 to under 12 years: 2 teaspoonfuls every 4 to 6 hours.
By weight:
Children 45 to 85 pounds: 2 teaspoonfuls every 4 to 6 hours.
Unless directed by a physician, do not exceed 4 doses in 24 hours.

Professional Labeling: The suggested dosage for pediatric patients is:

3–12 months	2 drops/Kg of body weight every 4–6 hours
12–24 months	5 drops (0.2 ml)/Kg of body weight every 4–6 hours
2–6 years	1 teaspoonful every 4–6 hours

Maximum of 4 doses in 24 hours.

Caution: Avoid alcoholic beverages or operating a motor vehicle or heavy machinery while taking this product.

How Supplied: DORCOL Children's Liquid Cold Formula (light brown), in 4 fl oz bottles with tamper-evident band around child-resistant cap.

Shown in Product Identification Section, page 422

EX-LAX® Chocolated Laxative Tablets

Active Ingredient: Yellow phenolphthalein, 90 mg. phenolphthalein per tablet.

Inactive Ingredients: Cocoa, Confectioners' Sugar, Hydrogenated Palm Kernel Oil, Lecithin, Nonfat Dry Milk, Vanillin.

Indication: For relief of occasional constipation (irregularity).

Caution: Do not take any laxative when abdominal pain, nausea, or vomiting are present. Frequent or prolonged use of this or any other laxative may result in dependence on laxatives. If skin rash appears, do not use this or any other preparation containing phenolphthalein.

Warnings: Keep this and all drugs out of the reach of children. In case of accidental overdose, seek professional assistance or contact a poison control center immediately. As with any drug, if you are pregnant or nursing a baby, seek the advice of a health care professional before using this product.

Drug Interaction Precautions: No known drug interaction.

Dosage and Administration: Adults and children 12 years old and over: Chew 1 to 2 tablets, preferably at bedtime. Children over 6 years: Chew ½ tablet.

How Supplied: Available in boxes of 6, 18, 48, and 72 chewable chocolate-flavored tablets.

Shown in Product Identification Section, page 422

EX-LAX® Laxative Pills

Regular Strength Ex-Lax® Laxative Pills
Extra Gentle Ex-Lax® Laxative Pills
Maximum Relief Formula Ex-Lax® Laxative Pills
Ex-Lax® Gentle Nature® Laxative Pills

Active Ingredients: Regular Strength Ex-Lax Laxative Pills—Yellow phenolphthalein, 90 mg. phenolphthalein per pill. **Extra Gentle Ex-Lax Laxative Pills**—Docusate sodium, 75 mg. and yellow phenolphthalein, 65 mg. per pill. **Maximum Relief Formula Ex-Lax Laxative Pills**—Yellow phenolphthalein, 135 mg. phenolphthalein per pill. **Ex-Lax Gentle Nature Laxative Pills**—Sennosides, 20 mg. per pill.

Inactive Ingredients: Regular Strength Ex-Lax Laxative Pills—Acacia, Alginic Acid, Carnauba Wax, Colloidal Silicon Dioxide, Dibasic Calcium Phosphate, Iron Oxides, Magnesium Stearate, Microcrystalline Cellulose, Sodium Benzoate, Sodium Lauryl Sulfate, Starch, Stearic Acid, Sucrose, Talc, Titanium Dioxide. **Extra Gentle Ex-Lax Laxative Pills**—Acacia, Croscarmellose Sodium, Dibasic Calcium Phosphate, Colloidal Silicon Dioxide, Magnesium Stearate, Microcrystalline Cellulose, Red 7, Stearic Acid, Sucrose, Talc, Titanium Dioxide. **Maximum Relief Formula Ex-Lax Laxative Pills**—Acacia, Alginic Acid, Blue No. 1, Carnauba Wax, Colloidal Silicon Dioxide, Dibasic Calcium Phosphate, Magnesium Stearate, Microcrystalline Cellulose, Povidone, Sodium Benzoate, Sodium Lauryl Sulfate, Starch, Stearic Acid, Sucrose, Talc, Titanium Dioxide. **Ex-Lax Gentle Nature Laxative Pills**—Alginic Acid, Colloidal Silicon Dioxide, Dibasic Calcium Phosphate, Magnesium Stearate, Microcrystalline Cellulose, Pregelatinized Starch, Sodium Lauryl Sulfate, Stearic Acid.

Indication: For relief of occasional constipation (irregularity).

Caution: Do not take any laxative when abdominal pain, nausea, or vomiting are present. Frequent or prolonged use of this or any other laxative may result in dependence on laxatives. If skin rash appears, do not use this or any other preparation containing phenolphthalein.

Warnings: Keep this and all drugs out of the reach of children. In case of accidental overdose, seek professional assistance or contact a Poison Control Center immediately. As with any drug, if you are pregnant or nursing a baby, seek the advice of a health care professional before using this product.

Drug Interaction Precautions: No known drug interaction.

Dosage and Administration: Regular Strength Ex-Lax Laxative Pills, Extra Gentle Ex-Lax Laxative Pills, and Ex-Lax Gentle Nature Laxative Pills—Adults and children 12 years old and over: Take 1 to 2 pills with a glass of water, preferably at bedtime. Consult with a physician for children under 12 years of age. **Maximum Relief Formula Ex-Lax Laxative Pills**—Adults and children over 12 years of age, take 1 to 2 pills with a glass of water, preferably at bedtime. Consult with a physician for children under 12 years of age.

How Supplied: Extra Strength Ex-Lax Laxative Pills—Available in boxes of 8, 30, and 60 pills. **Extra Gentle Ex-Lax Laxative Pills and Maximum Relief Formula Ex-Lax Laxative Pills**—Available in boxes of 24 pills. **Ex-Lax Gentle Nature Laxative Pills**—Available in boxes of 16 pills.

Shown in Product Identification Section, page 422

GAS-X® AND EXTRA STRENGTH GAS-X® Antiflatulent, Anti-Gas Tablets

Active Ingredients: GAS-X®—Each tablet contains 80 mg. simethicone.
EXTRA STRENGTH GAS-X®—Each tablet contains 125 mg. simethicone.

Inactive Ingredients: calcium phosphates dibasic and tribasic, calcium silicate, colloidal silicon dioxide, compressible sugar, microcrystalline cellulose and talc. GAS-X cherry creme flavored tablets also contain Red 30. Extra Strength GAS-X peppermint creme and Extra Strength GAS-X cherry creme flavored tablets also contain Red 30 and Yellow 10.

Indications: For relief of the pain and pressure symptoms of excess gas in the digestive tract, which is often accompanied by complaints of bloating, distention, fullness, pressure, pain, cramps or excess anal flatus.

Actions: GAS-X acts in the stomach and intestines to disperse and reduce the formation of mucus-trapped gas bubbles. The GAS-X defoaming action reduces the surface tension of gas bubbles so that they are more easily eliminated.

Warning: Keep this and all medicines out of the reach of children.

Drug Interaction Precautions: No known drug interaction.

Dosage and Administration: Adults: Chew thoroughly and swallow one or two tablets as needed after meals and at bedtime. Do not exceed six GAS-X tablets or four EXTRA STRENGTH GAS-X tablets in 24 hours, except under the advice and supervision of a physician.

Professional Labeling: GAS-X may be useful in the alleviation of postoperative gas pain, and for use in endoscopic examination.

How Supplied: GAS-X is available in peppermint creme and cherry creme flavored, chewable, scored tablets in boxes of 36 tablets and convenience packages of 12 tablets.
EXTRA STRENGTH GAS-X is available in peppermint creme and cherry creme flavored, chewable, scored tablets in boxes of 18 tablets and 48 tablets.

Shown in Product Identification Section, pages 422 and 423

TAVIST-1® TABLETS

Description: Each tablet contains: clemastine fumarate, USP, 1.34 mg (equivalent to 1 mg clemastine). Other ingredients: lactose, povidone, starch, stearic acid, and talc.

Indications: Temporarily reduces runny nose and relieves sneezing, itching of the nose or throat, and itchy, watery eyes due to hay fever or other upper respiratory allergies.

Warnings: May cause drowsiness; alcohol, sedatives, and tranquilizers may increase the drowsiness effect. Do not take this product if you are taking sedatives or tranquilizers without first consulting your doctor. Use caution when driving a motor vehicle or operating machinery. May cause excitability especially in children. Do not take this product if you have asthma, glaucoma, emphysema, chronic pulmonary disease, shortness of breath, difficulty in breathing, or difficulty in urination due to enlargement of the prostate gland unless directed by a doctor. As with any drug, if you are pregnant or nursing a baby, seek the advice of a health professional before using this product. Keep this and all drugs out of reach of children. In case of accidental overdose, seek professional assistance or contact a Poison Control Center immediately.

Directions: Adults and children 12 years of age and over: Take one tablet every 12 hours, not to exceed 2 tablets in 24 hours, or as directed by a doctor. Children under 12 years: Consult a doctor.

How Supplied: Tavist-1 tablets (white) imprinted "Tavist-1" on both sides in blister packs of 8 and 16.

Shown in Product Identification Section, page 423

TAVIST-D® TABLETS

Description: Each tablet contains: clemastine fumarate, USP, 1.34 mg (equivalent to 1 mg clemastine) immediate release and 75 mg phenylpropanolamine hydrochloride, USP, extended release. Other ingredients: Colloidal silicon dioxide, dibasic calcium phosphate, lactose, magnesium stearate, methylcellulose, polyethylene glycol, povidone, starch, synthetic polymers, titanium dioxide and Yellow 10.

Indications: For the temporary relief of nasal congestion associated with upper respiratory allergies or sinusitis when accompanied by other symptoms of hay fever or allergies, including runny nose, sneezing, itchy nose or throat or itchy, watery eyes.

Warnings: May cause drowsiness; alcohol, sedatives, and tranquilizers may increase the drowsiness effect. Avoid alcoholic beverages while taking this product. Do not take this product if you are taking sedatives or tranquilizers without first consulting your doctor. Use caution when driving a motor vehicle or operating machinery. May cause excitability especially in children. **Do not exceed recommended dosage because at higher doses nervousness, dizziness, or sleeplessness may occur.** Do not take this product for more than 7 days. If symptoms do not improve or are accompanied by fever, consult a doctor. Do not take this product if you have asthma, diabetes, glaucoma, heart disease, emphysema, chronic pulmonary disease, shortness of breath, difficulty in breathing, or difficulty in urination due to enlargement of the prostate gland unless directed by a doctor. As with any drug, if you are pregnant or nursing a baby, seek the advice of a health professional before using this product. Keep this and all drugs out of reach of children. In case of accidental overdose, seek professional assistance or contact a Poison Control Center immediately.

Drug Interaction Precaution: Do not take this product if you are presently taking a decongestant or prescription drug for high blood pressure or depression, without first consulting your doctor.

Directions: Adults and children 12 years of age and over: Take one tablet swallowed whole every 12 hours, not to exceed 2 tablets in 24 hours, or as directed by a doctor. Children under 12 years: Consult a doctor.

How Supplied: Tavist-D tablets (white) imprinted "Tavist-D" on both sides, in blister packs of 8 and 16.

Shown in Product Identification Section, page 423

THERAFLU®
Flu and Cold Medicine
Flu, Cold & Cough Medicine

Description: Each packet of TheraFlu Flu and Cold Medicine contains: acetaminophen 650 mg, pseudoephedrine hydrochloride 60 mg, and chlorpheniramine maleate 4 mg. Each packet of TheraFlu Flu, Cold & Cough Medicine also contains dextromethorphan hydrobromide 20 mg. Other ingredients: ascorbic acid (vitamin C), citric acid, natural lemon flavors, sodium citrate, sucrose, titanium dioxide, tribasic calcium phosphate, pregelatinized starch, Yellow 6, and Yellow 10.

Indications: Provides temporary relief of the symptoms associated with flu, common cold and other upper respiratory infections including: headache, body-aches, fever, minor sore throat pain, nasal and sinus congestion, runny nose and sneezing. TheraFlu Flu, Cold & Cough Medicine also suppresses coughs due to minor throat and bronchial irritation.

Warnings: Keep this and all drugs out of the reach of children. In case of accidental overdose, seek professional assistance or contact a Poison Control Center immediately. Prompt medical attention is critical for adults as well as children even if you do not notice any signs or symptoms. Unless directed by a doctor, do not take this product if you have heart disease, high blood pressure, thyroid disease, diabetes, asthma, glaucoma, emphysema, chronic pulmonary disease, shortness of breath, difficulty in breathing, difficulty in urination due to enlargement of the prostate gland or are taking a prescription drug for high blood pressure or depression or are taking sedatives or tranquilizers. Do not exceed recommended dosage because at higher doses nervousness, dizziness or sleeplessness may occur. Do not take for more than 7 days. If symptoms persist or new ones occur, or if accompanied by a fever that persists for more than 3 days, or recurs, consult a doctor. May cause excitability, especially in children. May cause marked drowsiness. Alcohol may increase the drowsiness effect. Avoid drinking alcoholic beverages while taking this product. Use caution when driving or operating machinery while taking this product. As with any drug, if you are pregnant or nursing a baby, seek the advice of a health professional before using this product. Do not take the cough formula if cough is accompanied by excessive secretions, for persistent cough such as occurs with smoking, asthma, or emphysema. A persistent cough may be sign of a serious condition. If cough persists for more than 1 week, tends to recur, or is accompanied by fever, rash or persistent headache, consult a doctor.

Dosage and Administration: Adults and children 12 years and over—dissolve

Continued on next page

Sandoz—Cont.

one packet in 6 oz. cup of hot water. Sip while hot. Microwave Heating Instructions: Add contents of packet and 6 oz. of cool water to a microwave safe cup and stir briskly. Microwave on high 1½ minutes or until hot. Do not boil water or overheat and remember to stir liquid between reheatings. Sweeten to taste if desired. May repeat every 4 hours, but not to exceed 4 doses in 24 hours.

How Supplied: TheraFlu Flu and Cold Medicine powder in foil packets, 6 or 12 packets per carton. TheraFlu Flu, Cold & Cough Medicine powder in foil packets, 6 or 12 packets per carton.

Shown in Product Identification Section, page 423

THERAFLU® MAXIMUM STRENGTH NIGHTTIME Flu, Cold & Cough Medicine

Description: Each packet of TheraFlu Maximum Strength Nighttime Flu, Cold & Cough Medicine contains: acetaminophen 1000 mg, dextromethorphan HBr 30 mg, pseudoephedrine HCl 60 mg, and chlorpheniramine maleate 4 mg. Other ingredients: ascorbic acid (Vitamin C), citric acid, natural lemon flavors, maltol, pregelatinized starch, silicon dioxide, sodium citrate, sucrose, titanium dioxide, tribasic calcium phosphate, Yellow 6 and Yellow 10.

Indications: Provides temporary relief of the symptoms associated with flu, common cold and other upper respiratory infections including: headache, body aches, fever, minor sore throat pain, nasal and sinus congestion, runny nose, sneezing, watery and itchy eyes. TheraFlu Maximum Strength Flu, Cold, & Cough Medicine also suppresses coughs due to minor throat and bronchial irritation.

Warnings: Keep this and all drugs out of the reach of children. In case of accidental overdose, seek professional assistance or contact a Poison Control Center immediately. Prompt medical attention is critical for adults as well as children even if you do not notice any signs or symptoms. Unless directed by a doctor, do not take this product: 1) if cough is accompanied by excessive secretions, 2) for persistent cough such as occurs with smoking, asthma or emphysema, or 3) if you have heart disease, high blood pressure, thyroid disease, diabetes, asthma, glaucoma, emphysema, chronic pulmonary disease, shortness of breath, difficulty in breathing, difficulty in urination due to enlargement of the prostate gland or are taking a prescription drug for high blood pressure or depression or are taking sedatives or tranquilizers.
Do not exceed recommended dosage because at higher doses nervousness, dizziness or sleeplessness may occur. Do not take for more than 7 days. If symptoms persist or new ones occur, or if fever persists for more than 3 days, or recurs, consult a doctor. A persistent cough may be a sign of a serious condition. If cough persists for more than 1 week, tends to recur, or is accompanied by fever, rash, or persistent headache, consult a doctor. May cause excitability especially in children. May cause marked drowsiness.
Alcohol may increase the drowsiness effect. Avoid drinking alcoholic beverages while taking this product. Use caution when driving or operating machinery while taking this product. As with any drug, if you are pregnant or nursing a baby, seek the advice of a health professional before using this product.

Directions: Adults and children 12 years and over: Dissolve one packet in 6 oz. cup of hot water. Sip while hot. Microwave Heating Instructions: Add contents of packet and 6 oz. of cool water to a microwave safe cup and stir briskly. Microwave on high 1½ minutes or until water is hot. Do not boil water or overheat and remember to stir liquid between reheatings. Sweeten to taste if desired. May repeat every 6 hours, but not to exceed 4 doses in 24 hours.

How Supplied: TheraFlu Maximum Strength Nighttime Flu, Cold, & Cough Medicine powder in foil packets, 6 or 12 packets per carton.

Shown in Product Identification Section, page 423

TRIAMINIC® ALLERGY TABLETS
[trī"ah-mĭn'ĭc]

Description: Each tablet contains: phenylpropanolamine hydrochloride 25 mg and chlorpheniramine maleate 4 mg. Other ingredients: calcium stearate, calcium sulfate, colloidal silicon dioxide, methylcellulose, methylparaben, microcrystalline cellulose, polyethylene glycol, povidone, pregelatinized starch, titanium dioxide, Yellow 10.

Indications: For the temporary relief of runny nose, nasal congestion, sneezing, itching of the eyes, nose or throat and watery eyes as may occur in hay fever or other upper respiratory allergies (allergic rhinitis).

Warnings: Do not take this product if you have high blood pressure, heart disease, diabetes, thyroid disease, asthma, glaucoma, emphysema, chronic pulmonary disease, shortness of breath, difficulty in breathing or difficulty in urination due to enlargement of the prostate gland or are taking a prescription drug for high blood pressure or depression unless directed by a doctor. Do not exceed the recommended dosage because at higher doses nervousness, dizziness or sleeplessness may occur or take for more than 7 days. This preparation may cause drowsiness; alcohol, sedatives and tranquilizers may increase the drowsiness effect; avoid alcoholic beverages; do not operate machinery or drive a motor vehicle while taking this product; this preparation may cause excitability, especially in children. If symptoms do not improve within seven days or are accompanied by high fever, consult a doctor. As with any drug, if you are pregnant or nursing a baby, seek the advice of a health professional before using this product. Keep this and all drugs out of the reach of children. In case of accidental overdose, seek professional assistance or contact a Poison Control Center immediately.

Directions: Adults and children over 12 years of age—1 tablet every 4 hours. Children 6 to under 12 years, ½ tablet every 4 hours. Unless directed by physician, do not exceed 6 doses in 24 hours or give to children under 6 years.

How Supplied: Triaminic Allergy Tablets (yellow), scored, in blister packs of 24.

TRIAMINIC® CHEWABLES
[trī"ah-mĭn'ĭc]

Description: Each TRIAMINIC Chewable contains: phenylpropanolamine hydrochloride 6.25 mg, chlorpheniramine maleate 0.5 mg. Other ingredients: calcium stearate, citric acid, flavors, magnesium trisilicate, mannitol, microcrystalline cellulose, saccharin sodium, sucrose, Yellow 6, Yellow 10.

Indications: For the temporary relief of children's nasal congestion, runny nose, and sneezing due to the common cold or hay fever.

Warnings: Do not exceed recommended dosage because at higher doses nervousness, dizziness, or sleeplessness may occur. Do not give this product to children for more than 7 days. If symptoms do not improve or are accompanied by fever, consult a doctor. Do not give this product to children who have heart disease, high blood pressure, thyroid disease, diabetes, asthma, emphysema, shortness of breath, chronic pulmonary disease or glaucoma unless directed by a doctor. May cause drowsiness. Sedatives and tranquilizers may increase the drowsiness effect. May cause excitability.
Drug Interaction Precaution: Do not give this product to a child who is taking a prescription drug for high blood pressure or depression, without first consulting the child's doctor. Keep this and all drugs out of the reach of children. In case of accidental overdose, seek professional assistance or contact a Poison Control Center immediately.

Dosage: Children 6 to 12 years—2 tablets every 4 hours. Children under 6, consult your physician.

Professional Labeling: The suggested dosage for children 2 to 6 years is 1 tablet every 4 hours.

How Supplied: TRIAMINIC Chewables (hexagonal, yellow), in blister packs of 24. Orange flavor.

TRIAMINIC® COLD TABLETS
[*trī"ah-mĭn'ĭc*]

Description: Each tablet contains: phenylpropanolamine hydrochloride 12.5 mg and chlorpheniramine maleate 2 mg. Other ingredients: calcium stearate, colloidal silicon dioxide, flavor, lactose, methylcellulose, methylparaben, microcrystalline cellulose, polyethylene glycol, povidone, pregelatinized starch, Red 40, saccharin sodium, titanium dioxide, Yellow 6.

Indications: For the temporary relief of nasal congestion due to the common cold, hay fever or other upper respiratory allergies and associated with sinusitis. Helps decongest sinus openings, sinus passages, promotes nasal and/or sinus drainage, temporarily restores freer breathing through the nose. For temporary relief of runny nose, sneezing, itching of the nose or throat and itchy and watery eyes as may occur in allergic rhinitis (such as hay fever).

Warnings: Do not take this product if you have high blood pressure, heart disease, diabetes, thyroid disease, asthma, glaucoma, emphysema, chronic pulmonary disease, shortness of breath, difficulty in breathing or difficulty in urination due to enlargement of the prostate gland or are taking a prescription drug for high blood pressure or depression unless directed by a doctor. Do not exceed the recommended dosage because at higher doses nervousness, dizziness or sleeplessness may occur or take for more than 7 days. This preparation may cause drowsiness; alcohol, sedatives and tranquilizers may increase the drowsiness effect; avoid alcoholic beverages; do not operate machinery or drive a motor vehicle while taking this product; this preparation may cause excitability, especially in children. If symptoms do not improve within seven days or are accompanied by high fever, consult a doctor. As with any drug, if you are pregnant or nursing a baby, seek the advice of a health professional before using this product. Keep this and all drugs out of the reach of children. In case of accidental overdose, seek professional assistance or contact a Poison Control Center immediately.

Directions: Adults and children 12 years of age and older: 2 tablets every 4 hours. Children 6 to under 12 years, 1 tablet every 4 hours. Unless directed by physician, do not exceed 6 doses in 24 hours or give to children under 6 years.

How Supplied: Triaminic Cold Tablets (orange) imprinted "DORSEY" on one side, "TRIAMINIC" on the other, in blister packs of 24.

Shown in Product Identification Section, page 423

TRIAMINIC® EXPECTORANT
[*trī"ah-mĭn'ĭc*]

Description: Each teaspoonful (5 ml) of TRIAMINIC Expectorant contains: phenylpropanolamine hydrochloride 6.25 mg and guaifenesin 50 mg in a palatable, citrus-flavored alcohol-free liquid. Other ingredients: benzoic acid, edetate disodium, flavors, purified water, saccharin, saccharin sodium, sodium hydroxide, sorbitol, sucrose, Yellow 6, Yellow 10.

Indications: Relieves chest congestion by loosening phlegm to help clear bronchial passageways. Temporarily relieves stuffy nose.

Warnings: Keep this and all drugs out of the reach of children. In case of accidental overdose, seek professional assistance or contact a Poison Control Center immediately.
Do not exceed recommended dosage because at higher doses nervousness, dizziness, or sleeplessness may occur. Do not take for more than 7 days. If syptoms persist, are accompanied by fever, rash or persistent headache, or if cough recurs, consult a doctor. A persistent cough may be a sign of a serious condition. Do not take this product: 1) if cough is accompanied by excessive phlegm (sputum), 2) for persistent or chronic cough such as occurs with smoking, asthma, chronic bronchitis or emphysema, or 3) if you have heart disease, high blood pressure, thyroid disease, diabetes, difficulty in urination due to enlargement of the prostate gland, or are taking a prescription drug for high blood pressure or depression.
As with any drug, if you are pregnant or nursing a baby, seek the advice of a health professional before using this product.

Dosage and Administration: Adults and children 12 and over (96+ lbs)—4 teaspoons every 4 hours. Children 6 to under 12 years (48–95 lbs)—2 teaspoons every 4 hours. Children 2 to under 6 years (24–47 lbs)—1 teaspoon every 4 hours. Unless directed by physician, do not exceed 6 doses in 24 hours or give to children under 2 years of age. For convenience, a True-Dose® dosage cup is provided with each 4 fl. oz. and 8 fl. oz. bottle.

Professional Labeling: The suggested dosage for pediatric patients is:

3–12 months (12–17 lbs)	1.25 ml (1/4 tsp) every 4 hours
12–24 months (18–23 lbs)	2.5 ml (1/2 tsp) every 4 hours

How Supplied: TRIAMINIC Expectorant (yellow), in 4 fl oz and 8 fl oz plastic bottles with tamper-evident band around child-resistant cap. Citrus flavored, Alcohol free.

Shown in Product Identification Section, page 423

TRIAMINIC® NITE LIGHT®
Nighttime Cough and Cold Medicine for Children
[*tri"ah-min'ic*]

Description: Each teaspoonful (5 ml) of Triaminic® Nite Light® contains: Pseudoephedrine hydrochloride 15 mg, chlorpheniramine maleate 1 mg, dextromethorphan hydrobromide 7.5 mg in a palatable, grape-flavored, alcohol-free liquid. Other ingredients: benzoic acid, Blue 1, citric acid, flavors, propylene glycol, purified water, Red 33, dibasic sodium phosphate, sorbitol, sucrose.

Indications: Temporarily relieves cold symptoms, including coughs due to minor throat and bronchial irritation, runny nose, stuffy nose, sneezing, itching nose or throat and itchy, watery eyes.

Warnings: Keep this and all drugs out of the reach of children. In case of accidental overdose, seek professional assistance or contact a Poison Control Center immediately.
Do not exceed recommended dosage because at higher doses nervousness, dizziness, or sleeplessness may occur. Do not take for more than 7 days. If symptoms persist, are accompanied by fever, rash or persistent headache, or if cough recurs, consult a doctor. A persistent cough may be a sign of a serious condition. Do not take this product: 1) if cough is accompanied by excessive phlegm (sputum), 2) for persistent or chronic cough such as occurs with smoking, asthma or emphysema, or 3) if you have heart disease, high blood pressure, thyroid disease, diabetes, asthma, glaucoma, difficulty in breathing, chronic pulmonary disease, shortness of breath, of difficulty in urination due to enlargement of the prostate gland, 4) if you are taking a prescription drug for high blood pressure or depression, or 5) if you are taking sedatives or tranquilizers, unless directed by a doctor. May cause excitability, especially in children. May cause drowsiness. Alcohol, sedatives or tranquilizers may increase drowsiness. Avoid driving or operating machinery while taking this product.
As with any drug, if you are pregnant or nursing a baby, seek the advice of a health professional before using this product.

Dosage and Administration: Adults and children 12 and over (96+ lbs.)—4 teaspoons every 6 hours. Children 6 to under 12 years (48–95 lbs.)—2 teaspoons every 6 hours. Unless directed by physician, do not exceed 4 doses in 24 hours or give to children under 6 years of age. For convenience, a True-Dose® dosage cup is provided with each 4 fl. oz. and 8 fl. oz. bottle.

Professional Labeling: The suggested dosage for pediatric patients is:

3 to under 12 months (12–17 lbs.)	1/4 teaspoon or 1.25 ml
12 months to under 2 years (18–23 lbs.)	1/2 teaspoon or 2.5 ml
2 to under 6 years	1 teaspoon or 5 ml

How Supplied: Triaminic® Nite Light® Nighttime Cough and Cold Medicine for Children (purple), in 4 fl. oz. and 8 fl. oz. plastic bottles packaged in car-

Continued on next page

Sandoz—Cont.

tons with tamper-evident band around child-resistant cap. Grape flavored. Alcohol free.

Shown in Product Identification Section, page 423

TRIAMINIC® SYRUP
[*trī"ah-mĭn'ĭc*]

Description: Each teaspoonful (5 ml) of TRIAMINIC Syrup contains: phenylpropanolamine hydrochloride 6.25 mg and chlorpheniramine maleate 1 mg in a palatable, orange-flavored, alcohol-free liquid. Other ingredients: benzoic acid, edetate disodium, flavors, purified water, sodium hydroxide, sorbitol, sucrose. Contains FD&C Yellow No. 6 as a color additive.

Indications: Temporarily relieves cold and allergy symptoms, including runny nose, stuffy nose, sneezing, itching nose or throat, and itchy, watery eyes.

Warnings: Keep this and all drugs out of the reach of children. In case of accidental overdose, seek professional assistance or contact a Poison Control Center immediately.
Do not exceed recommended dosage because at higher doses nervousness, dizziness or sleeplessness may occur. Do not take for more than 7 days. If symptoms persist or are accompanied by fever, consult a doctor. Do not take this product: 1) if you have heart disease, high blood pressure, thyroid disease, diabetes, asthma, glaucoma, difficulty in breathing, chronic pulmonary disease, shortness of breath, or difficulty in urination due to enlargement of the prostate gland, 2) if you are taking a prescription drug for high blood pressure or depression, or 3) if you are taking sedatives or tranquilizers, unless directed by a doctor. May cause excitability, especially in children. May cause drowsiness. Alcohol, sedatives or tranquilizers may increase drowsiness. Avoid driving or operating machinery while taking this product.
As with any drug, if you are pregnant or nursing a baby, seek the advice of a health professional before using this product.

Dosage and Administration: Adults and children 12 and over (96+ lbs)—4 teaspoons every 4 hours. Children 6 to under 12 years (48–95 lbs)—2 teaspoons every 4 hours. Unless directed by physician, do not exceed 6 doses in 24 hours. Consult physician for dosage under 6 years of age. For convenience, a True-Dose® dosage cup is provided with each 4 fl. oz. and 8 fl. oz. bottle.

Professional Labeling: The suggested dosage for pediatric patients is:

3–12 months (12–17 lbs)	1.25 ml (1/4 tsp) every 4 hours
12–24 months (18–23 lbs)	2.5 ml (1/2 tsp) every 4 hours
2–6 years (24–47 lbs)	5 ml (1 tsp) every 4 hours

How Supplied: TRIAMINIC Syrup (orange), in 4 fl oz and 8 fl oz plastic bottles with tamper-evident band around child-resistant cap. Orange flavored. Alcohol-free.

Shown in Product Identification Section, page 423

TRIAMINIC-DM® SYRUP
[*trī"ah-mĭn'ĭc*]

Description: Each teaspoonful (5 ml) of TRIAMINIC-DM Syrup contains: phenylpropanolamine hydrochloride 6.25 mg and dextromethorphan hydrobromide 5 mg in a palatable, berry-flavored alcohol-free liquid. Other ingredients: benzoic acid, Blue 1, flavors, propylene glycol, purified water, Red 40, sodium chloride, sorbitol, sucrose.

Indications: Temporarily quiets coughs due to minor throat and bronchial irritation, and relieves stuffy nose. The decongestant and antitussive are provided in an alcohol-free and antihistamine-free formula.

Warnings: Keep this and all drugs out of the reach of children. In case of accidental overdose, seek professional assistance or contact a Poison Control Center immediately.
Do not exceed recommended dosage because at higher doses nervousness, dizziness, or sleeplessness may occur. Do not take for more than 7 days. If symptoms persist, are accompanied by fever, rash or persistent headache or if cough recurs, consult a doctor. A persistent cough may be a sign of a serious condition. Do not take this product: 1) if cough is accompanied by excessive phlegm (sputum), 2) for persistent or chronic cough such as occurs with smoking, asthma or emphysema, or 3) if you have heart disease, high blood pressure, thyroid disease, diabetes, difficulty in urination due to enlargement of the prostate gland, or are taking a prescription drug for high blood pressure or depression, unless directed by a doctor.
As with any drug, if you are pregnant or nursing a baby, seek the advice of a health professional before using this product.

Dosage and Administration: Adults and children 12 and over (96+ lbs)—4 teaspoons every 4 hours. Children 6 to under 12 years (48–95 lbs)—2 teaspoons every 4 hours. Children 2 to under 6 years (24–47 lbs) 1 teaspoon every 4 hours. Unless directed by physician, do not exceed 6 doses in 24 hours or give to children under 2 years of age. For convenience, a True-Dose® dosage cup is provided with each 4 fl. oz. and 8 fl. oz. bottle.

Professional Labeling: The suggested dosage for pediatric patients is:

3–12 months (12–17 lbs)	1.25 ml (1/4 tsp) every 4 hours
12–24 months (18–23 lbs)	2.5 ml (1/2 tsp) every 4 hours

How Supplied: TRIAMINIC-DM Syrup (dark red), in 4 fl oz and 8 fl oz plastic bottles with tamper-evident band around child-resistant cap. Berry flavored. Alcohol-free.

Shown in Product Identification Section, page 423

TRIAMINIC-12® TABLETS
[*trī"ah-mĭn'ĭc*]

Description: Each tablet contains: phenylpropanolamine hydrochloride 75 mg and chlorpheniramine maleate 12 mg. Other ingredients: carnauba wax, colloidal silicon dioxide, lactose, methylcellulose, polyethylene glycol, povidone, Red 30, stearic acid, titanium dioxide, Yellow 6. Triaminic-12 Tablets contain the nasal decongestant phenylpropanolamine, and the antihistamine chlorpheniramine, in a formulation providing 12 hours of symptomatic relief.

Indications: For the temporary relief of nasal congestion due to the common cold, hay fever or other upper respiratory allergies and associated with sinusitis. Helps decongest sinus openings, sinus passages; promotes nasal and/or sinus drainage; temporarily restores freer breathing through the nose. For temporary relief of running nose, sneezing, itching of the nose or throat and itchy and watery eyes as may occur in allergic rhinitis (such as hay fever).

Warnings: Do not give this product to children under 12 years except under the advice and supervision of a physician. Do not take this product if you are taking another medication containing phenylpropanolamine. Do not take this preparation if you have high blood pressure, heart disease, diabetes, thyroid disease, asthma, glaucoma, emphysema, chronic pulmonary disease, shortness of breath, difficulty in breathing or difficulty in urination due to enlargement of the prostate gland except under the advice and supervision of a physician. Do not exceed the recommended dosage because at higher doses nervousness, dizziness or sleeplessness may occur. This preparation may cause drowsiness; alcohol may increase the drowsiness effect; this preparation may cause excitability, especially in children. If symptoms do not improve within seven days or are accompanied by high fever, consult a physician before continuing use. As with any drug, if you are pregnant or nursing a baby, seek the advice of a health professional before using this product. Keep this and all drugs out of the reach of children. In case of accidental overdose, seek professional assistance or contact a Poison Control Center immediately.

Caution: Avoid driving a motor vehicle or operating heavy machinery. Avoid alcoholic beverages while taking this product.

Drug Interaction Precaution: Do not take this product if you are presently taking a prescription antihypertensive or antidepressant drug containing a monoamine oxidase inhibitor except under the advice and supervision of a physician.

Directions: Adults and children over 12 years of age—1 tablet swallowed whole every 12 hours. Unless directed by physician, do not exceed 2 tablets in 24 hours.

Note: The nonactive portion of the tablet that supplies the active ingredients may occasionally appear in your stool as a soft mass.

How Supplied: Triaminic-12 Tablets (orange) imprinted "DORSEY" on one side, "TRIAMINIC-12" on the other, in blister packs of 10 and 20.

Shown in Product Identification Section, page 423

TRIAMINICIN® TABLETS

[*trī"ah-mĭn'ĭ-sĭn*]

Description: Each tablet contains: phenylpropanolamine hydrochloride 25 mg and chlorpheniramine maleate 4 mg and acetaminophen 650 mg. Other ingredients: colloidal silicon dioxide, croscarmellose sodium, hydroxypropyl cellulose, lactose, magnesium stearate, methylcellulose, methylparaben, polyethylene glycol, povidone, pregelatinized starch, Red 40, titanium dioxide, Yellow 10.

Indications: Temporarily relieves runny nose, sneezing, itching of the nose or throat, and itchy, watery eyes due to hay fever or other upper respiratory allergies (allergic rhinitis). Temporarily relieves nasal congestion due to hay fever or other upper respiratory allergies or associated with sinusitis. Temporarily relieves nasal congestion, runny nose and sneezing associated with the common cold. For the temporary relief of occasional minor aches, pains, headache and for the reduction of fever associated with the common cold.

Warnings: Do not take this product if you have high blood pressure, heart disease, diabetes, thyroid disease, asthma, glaucoma, emphysema, chronic pulmonary disease, shortness of breath, difficulty in breathing or difficulty in urination due to enlargement of the prostate gland or are taking a prescription drug for high blood pressure or depression unless directed by a doctor. Do not exceed recommended dosage because at higher doses nervousness, dizziness, or sleeplessness may occur. This preparation may cause drowsiness; alcohol, sedatives and tranquilizers may increase the drowsiness effect; avoid alcoholic beverages; do not operate machinery or drive a motor vehicle while taking this product; this preparation may cause excitability, especially in children. Do not take this product for more than 7 days. If symptoms do not improve, new ones occur, or if fever persists for more than 3 days (72 hours) or recurs, consult a doctor. As with any drug, if you are pregnant or nursing a baby, seek the advice of a health professional before using this product. Keep this and all drugs out of the reach of children. In case of accidental overdose, seek professional assistance or contact a Poison Control Center immediately. Prompt medical attention is critical for adults as well as for children even if you do not notice any signs or symptoms.

Directions: Adults and children 12 years and older: Take 1 tablet every 4 hours. Unless directed by a doctor, do not exceed 6 doses in 24 hours or give to children under 12 years.

How Supplied: TRIAMINICIN Tablets (yellow) imprinted "DORSEY" on one side, "TRIAMINICIN" on the other, in blister packs of 12, 24 and 48, and bottles of 100 tablets.

Shown in Product Identification Section, page 423

TRIAMINICOL® MULTI-SYMPTOM COLD TABLETS

[*trī"ah-mĭn'ĭ-call*]

Description: Each tablet contains: phenylpropanolamine hydrochloride 12.5 mg, chlorpheniramine maleate 2 mg and dextromethorphan hydrobromide 10 mg. Other ingredients: calcium stearate, colloidal silicon dioxide, lactose, methylcellulose, methylparaben, microcrystalline cellulose, polyethylene glycol, povidone, pregelatinized starch, Red 40, titanium dioxide.

Indications: For the temporary relief of nasal congestion due to the common cold, hay fever or other upper respiratory allergies and associated with sinusitis. Helps decongest sinus openings, sinus passages, promotes nasal and/or sinus drainage, temporarily restores freer breathing through the nose. For temporary relief of runny nose, sneezing, itching of the nose or throat and itchy and watery eyes as may occur in allergic rhinitis (such as hay fever). For temporary relief of cough due to minor throat and bronchial irritation as may occur with the common cold or with inhaled irritants.

Warnings: Do not take this product: 1) if cough is accompanied by excessive secretions, 2) for persistent cough such as occurs with smoking, asthma or emphysema, or 3) if you have high blood pressure, heart disease, diabetes, thyroid disease, asthma, glaucoma, chronic pulmonary disease, shortness of breath, difficulty in breathing or difficulty in urination due to enlargement of the prostate gland or are taking a prescription drug for high blood pressure or depression unless directed by a doctor. Do not exceed recommended dosage because at higher doses nervousness, dizziness, or sleeplessness may occur or take for more than 7 days. This preparation may cause drowsiness; alcohol, sedatives, and tranquilizers may increase the drowsiness effect; avoid alcoholic beverages; do not operate machinery or drive a motor vehicle while taking this product; this preparation may cause excitability, especially in children. If symptoms do not improve within seven days or are accompanied by fever, rash or persistant headache or if cough recurs, consult a doctor. As with any drug, if you are pregnant or nursing a baby, seek the advice of a health professional before using this product. Keep this and all drugs out of the reach of children. In case of accidental overdose, seek professional assistance or contact a Poison Control Center immediately.

Directions: Adults and children 12 years of age and older: 2 tablets every 4 hours. Children 6 to under 12 years, 1 tablet every 4 hours. Unless directed by physician, do not exceed 6 doses in 24 hours or give to children under 6 years.

How Supplied: Triaminicol Tablets (cherry red) imprinted "DORSEY" on one side, "TRIAMINICOL" on the other, in blister packs of 24.

Shown in Product Identification Section, page 423

TRIAMINICOL® MULTI-SYMPTOM RELIEF

[*trī"ah-mĭn'ĭ-call*]

Description: Each teaspoonful (5 ml) of TRIAMINICOL Multi-Symptom Relief contains: phenylpropanolamine hydrochloride 6.25 mg, chlorpheniramine maleate 1 mg, dextromethorphan hydrobromide 5 mg in a palatable, cherry flavored alcohol-free liquid. Other ingredients: benzoic acid, flavors, propylene glycol, purified water, Red 40, saccharin sodium, sodium chloride, sorbitol, sucrose.

Indications: Temporarily relieves cold symptoms, including coughs due to minor throat and bronchial irritation, runny nose, stuffy nose, sneezing, itching nose or throat and itchy, watery eyes.

Warnings: Keep this and all drugs out of the reach of children. In case of accidental overdose, seek professional assistance or contact a Poison Control Center immediately.

Do not exceed recommended dosage because at higher doses nervousness, dizziness, or sleeplessness may occur. Do not take for more than 7 days. If symptoms persist, are accompanied by fever, rash or persistent headache, or if cough recurs, consult a doctor. A persistent cough may be a sign of a serious condition. Do not take this product: 1) if cough is accompanied by excessive phlegm (sputum), 2) for persistent or chronic cough such as occurs with smoking, asthma or emphysema, or 3) if you have heart disease, high blood pressure, thyroid disease, diabetes, asthma, gluacoma, difficulty in breathing, chronic pulmonary

Continued on next page

Sandoz—Cont.

disease, shortness of breath, or difficulty in urination due to enlargement of the prostate gland, 4) if you are taking a prescription drug for high blood pressure or depression, or 5) if you are taking sedatives or tranquilizers, unless directed by a doctor. May cause excitability, especially in children. May cause drowsiness. Alcohol, sedatives or tranquilizers may increase drowsiness. Avoid driving or operating machinery while taking this product.
As with any drug, if you are pregnant or nursing a baby, seek the advice of a health professional before using this product.

Dosage and Administration: Adults and children 12 and over (96+ lbs)—4 teaspoons every 4 hours. Children 6 to under 12 years (48–95 lbs)—2 teaspoons every 4 hours. Unless directed by physician, do not exceed 6 doses in 24 hours or give to children under 6 years of age. For convenience, a True-Dose® Dosage cup is provided with each 4 fl. oz. and 8 fl. oz. bottle.

Professional Labeling: The suggested dosage for pediatric patients is:

3–12 months	1.25 ml (¼ tsp)
(12–17 lbs)	every 4 hours
12–24 months	2.5 ml (½ tsp)
(18–23 lbs)	every 4 hours
2–6 years	5 ml (1 tsp)
(24–47 lbs)	every 4 hours

How Supplied: TRIAMINICOL Multi-Symptom Relief (red), in 4 fl oz and 8 fl oz plastic bottles with tamper-evident band around child-resistant cap. Cherry flavored. Alcohol-free.

Shown in Product Identification Section, page 423

URSINUS® INLAY-TABS®

[yur″sīgn′us]

Description: Each URSINUS Inlay-Tab contains: pseudoephedrine hydrochloride 30 mg and aspirin (USP) 325 mg. Other ingredients: calcium stearate, lactose, microcrystalline cellulose, pregelatinized starch, sodium starch, Yellow 6, Yellow 10.

Indications: For the temporary relief of nasal congestion due to the common cold, hay fever or associated with sinusitis. For the temporary relief of occasional minor aches, pains and headache and for the reduction of fever associated with the common cold.

Warnings: Children and teenagers should not use this medicine for chicken pox or flu symptoms before a doctor is consulted about Reye syndrome, a rare but serious illness reported to be associated with aspirin. Unless directed by a doctor: 1) Do not take this product if you are allergic to aspirin or if you have asthma, or if you have stomach distress, ulcers or bleeding problems; 2) Do not take this product if you have heart disease, thyroid disease, or difficulty in urination due to enlargement of the prostate gland, and 3) Do not exceed recommended dosage because at higher doses nervousness, dizziness, or sleeplessness may occur. Do not take this product for more than 7 days. If symptoms do not improve, are accompanied by fever, or new symptoms occur, consult a doctor. Stop taking this product if ringing in the ears or other symptoms occur. As with any drug, if you are pregnant or nursing a baby, seek the advice of a health professional before using this product. **IT IS ESPECIALLY IMPORTANT NOT TO USE ASPIRIN DURING THE LAST 3 MONTHS OF PREGNANCY UNLESS SPECIFICALLY DIRECTED TO DO SO BY A DOCTOR BECAUSE IT MAY CAUSE PROBLEMS IN THE UNBORN CHILD OR COMPLICATIONS DURING DELIVERY.**

Drug Interaction Precaution: Do not take this product if you are presently taking a prescription drug for high blood pressure or depression without first consulting your doctor. Do not take this product if you are presently taking a prescription drug for anticoagulation (thinning the blood), diabetes, arthritis or gout unless directed by a doctor. **Keep this and all medicines out of the reach of children. In case of accidental overdose, contact a physician immediately.**

Directions for Use: Adults and children 12 years and older: 2 tablets with a full glass of water every 4 hours while symptoms persist or as directed by a physician. Do not take more than 4 doses in 24 hours. For chicken pox or flu see Warnings.

How Supplied: URSINUS INLAY-TABS (white with yellow inlay), in bottles of 24.

Sanofi Winthrop Pharmaceuticals
90 PARK AVENUE
NEW YORK, NY 10016

BRONKOLIXIR®
Bronchodilator • Decongestant

Description: Each 5 mL teaspoonful contains:

Ephedrine sulfate, USP	12 mg
Guaifenesin, USP	50 mg
Theophylline, USP	15 mg
Phenobarbital, USP	4 mg

(Warning: May be habit forming.)
Also contains: Alcohol 19% (v/v), FD&C Red #40, Flavors, Glycerin, Purified Water, Saccharin Sodium, Sodium Chloride, Sodium Citrate, Sucrose.

Indications: For symptomatic control of bronchial asthma. BRONKOLIXIR is also helpful in overcoming the nonproductive cough often associated with bronchitis or colds.

Warnings: Frequent or prolonged use may cause nervousness, restlessness, or sleeplessness. Phenobarbital may cause drowsiness. Do not use if high blood pressure, heart disease, diabetes, or thyroid disease is present, unless directed by a physician. Ephedrine may cause urinary retention, especially in the presence of partial obstruction, as in prostatism. Keep this and all drugs out of the reach of children. In case of accidental overdose, seek professional assistance or contact a poison control center immediately. As with any drug, if you are pregnant or nursing a baby, seek the advice of a health professional before using this product.

Dosage: *Adults*—2 teaspoons every three or four hours, not to exceed four times daily. *Children*—**over six**—one half the adult dose; **under six**—as directed by physician.

How Supplied: Bottle of 16 fl oz (NDC 0024-1004-16)

BRONKOTABS®
Bronchodilator • Decongestant

Description: Each tablet contains ephedrine sulfate, USP, 24 mg; guaifenesin, USP, 100 mg; theophylline, USP, 100 mg; phenobarbital, USP, 8 mg. (Warning: May be habit forming.)
Also contains: Magnesium Stearate, Magnesium Trisilicate, Microcrystalline Cellulose, Starch.

Indications: For symptomatic control of bronchial asthma.

Warnings: Frequent or prolonged use may cause nervousness, restlessness, or sleeplessness. Phenobarbital may cause drowsiness. Do not use if high blood pressure, heart disease, diabetes, or thyroid disease is present unless directed by a physician. Ephedrine may cause urinary retention, especially in the presence of partial obstruction, as in prostatism. Keep this and all drugs out of the reach of children. In case of accidental overdose, seek professional assistance or contact a poison control center immediately. As with any drug, if you are pregnant or nursing a baby, seek the advice of a health professional before using this product.

Dosage: *Adults* — 1 tablet every three or four hours, four to five times daily. *Children:* **over six** — one half the adult dose; **under six** — as directed by physician.

How Supplied: Bottle of 100 (NDC 0024-1006-10)

DRISDOL®
brand of ergocalciferol oral solution, USP (in propylene glycol)
Vitamin D Supplement

Description: 200 International Units (5 μg) per drop. The dropper supplied delivers 40 drops per mL.

Indication: For the prevention of vitamin D deficiency in infants, children, and adults.

Warnings: Keep this and all drugs out of the reach of children. In case of accidental overdose, seek professional assistance or contact a poison control center immediately.

Dosage: 2 drops daily. This dose provides the US Recommended Daily Allowance for vitamin D for infants, children, and adults.

How Supplied: Bottles of 2 fl oz (NDC 0024-0391-02)

pHisoDerm

(See Sterling Health.)

ZEPHIRAN® CHLORIDE
brand of benzalkonium chloride
ANTISEPTIC
AQUEOUS SOLUTION 1:750
TINTED TINCTURE 1:750
SPRAY—TINTED TINCTURE 1:750

Description: ZEPHIRAN Chloride, brand of benzalkonium chloride, NF, a mixture of alkylbenzyldimethylammonium chlorides, is a cationic quaternary ammonium surface-acting agent. It is very soluble in water, alcohol, and acetone. Aqueous solutions of ZEPHIRAN Chloride are neutral to slightly alkaline, generally colorless, and nonstaining. They have a bitter taste, aromatic odor, and foam when shaken. ZEPHIRAN Chloride Tinted Tincture 1:750 contains alcohol 50 percent and acetone 10 percent by volume. ZEPHIRAN Chloride Spray—Tinted Tincture 1:750 contains alcohol 92 percent. The Tinted Tincture and Spray also contain an orange-red coloring agent.

Clinical Pharmacology: ZEPHIRAN Chloride solutions are rapidly acting anti-infective agents with a moderately long duration of action. They are active against bacteria and some viruses, fungi, and protozoa. Bacterial spores are considered to be resistant. Solutions are bacteriostatic or bactericidal according to their concentration. The exact mechanism of bactericidal action is unknown but is thought to be due to enzyme inactivation. Activity generally increases with increasing temperature and pH. Gram-positive bacteria are more susceptible than gram-negative bacteria (TABLE 1).

TABLE 1
Highest Dilution of ZEPHIRAN Chloride Aqueous Solution Destroying the Organism in 10 but not in 5 Minutes

Organisms	20°C
Streptococcus pyogenes	1:75,000
Staphylococcus aureus	1:52,500
Salmonella typhosa	1:37,500
Escherichia coli	1:10,500

Pseudomonas is the most resistant gram-negative genus. Using the AOAC Use-Dilution Confirmation Method, no growth was obtained when *Staphylococcus aureus, Salmonella choleraesuis,* and *Pseudomonas aeruginosa* (strain PRD-10) were exposed for ten minutes at 20°C to ZEPHIRAN Chloride Aqueous Solution 1:750 and Tinted Tincture 1:750.
ZEPHIRAN Chloride Aqueous Solution 1:750 has been shown to retain its bactericidal activity following autoclaving for 30 minutes at 15 lb pressure, freezing, and then thawing.
The tubercle bacillus may be resistant to aqueous ZEPHIRAN Chloride solutions but is susceptible to the 1:750 tincture (AOAC Method, 10 minutes at 20°C).
ZEPHIRAN Chloride solutions also demonstrate deodorant, wetting, detergent, keratolytic, and emulsifying activity.

Indications and Usage: ZEPHIRAN Chloride aqueous solutions in appropriate dilutions (see Recommended Dilutions) are indicated for the antisepsis of skin, mucous membranes, and wounds. They are used for preoperative preparation of the skin, surgeons' hand and arm soaks, treatment of wounds, preservation of ophthalmic solutions, irrigations of the eye, body cavities, bladder, urethra, and vaginal douching.
ZEPHIRAN Chloride Tinted Tincture 1:750 and Spray are indicated for preoperative preparation of the skin and for treatment of minor skin wounds and abrasions.

Contraindication: The use of ZEPHIRAN Chloride solutions in occlusive dressings, casts, and anal or vaginal packs is inadvisable, as they may produce irritation or chemical burns.

Warnings: Sterile Water for Injection, USP, should be used as diluent in preparing diluted aqueous solutions intended for use on deep wounds or for irrigation of body cavities. Otherwise, freshly distilled water should be used. Tap water, containing metallic ions and organic matter, may reduce antibacterial potency. Resin deionized water should not be used since it may contain pathogenic bacteria.
Organic, inorganic, and synthetic materials and surfaces may adsorb sufficient quantities of ZEPHIRAN Chloride to significantly reduce its antibacterial potency in solutions. This has resulted in serious contamination of solutions of ZEPHIRAN Chloride with viable pathogenic bacteria. Solutions should not be stored in bottles stoppered with cork closures, but rather in those equipped with appropriate screw-caps. Cotton, wool, rayon, and other materials should not be stored in ZEPHIRAN Chloride solutions. Gauze sponges and fiber pledgets used to apply solutions of ZEPHIRAN Chloride to the skin should be sterilized and stored in separate containers. Only immediately prior to application should they be immersed in ZEPHIRAN Chloride solutions.
Since ZEPHIRAN Chloride solutions are inactivated by soaps and anionic detergents, thorough rinsing is necessary if these agents are employed prior to their use.
Antiseptics such as ZEPHIRAN Chloride solutions must not be relied upon to achieve complete sterilization, because they do not destroy bacterial spores and certain viruses, including the etiologic agent of infectious hepatitis, and may not destroy *Mycobacterium tuberculosis* and other rare bacterial strains.
ZEPHIRAN Chloride Tinted Tincture 1:750 and Spray contain flammable organic solvents and should not be used near an open flame or cautery.
If solutions stronger than 1:3000 enter the eyes, irrigate immediately and repeatedly with water. Prompt medical attention should then be obtained. Concentrations greater than 1:5000 should not be used on mucous membranes, with the exception of the vaginal mucosa (see Recommended Dilutions).

Precautions: In preoperative antisepsis of the skin, ZEPHIRAN Chloride solutions should not be permitted to remain in prolonged contact with the patient's skin. Avoid pooling of the solution on the operating table.
ZEPHIRAN Chloride solutions that are used on inflamed or irritated tissues must be more dilute than those used on normal tissues (see Recommended Dilutions). ZEPHIRAN Chloride Tinted Tincture 1:750 and Spray, which contain irritating organic solvents, should be kept away from the eyes or other mucous membranes.
Preoperative periorbital skin or head prep should be performed only before the patient, or eye, is anesthetized.

Adverse Reactions: ZEPHIRAN Chloride solutions in normally used concentrations have low systemic and local toxicity and are generally well tolerated, although a rare individual may exhibit hypersensitivity.

Directions for Use:
General: For most surgical applications, the recommended concentration of ZEPHIRAN Chloride Aqueous Solution or ZEPHIRAN Chloride Tinted Tincture is 1:750 (0.13 percent). Liberal use of the solution is recommended to compensate for any adsorption of ZEPHIRAN Chloride by cotton or other materials.
To use ZEPHIRAN Chloride Spray—Tinted Tincture 1:750, remove protective cap, hold in an UPRIGHT position several inches away from the surgical field or injured area, and apply by spraying freely.

Continued on next page

This product information was effective as of October 31, 1992. Current detailed information may be obtained directly from Sanofi Winthrop Pharmaceuticals by writing to 90 Park Avenue, New York, NY 10016.

Sanofi Winthrop—Cont.

Preoperative preparation of skin: ZEPHIRAN Chloride solutions 1:750 are recommended as an antiseptic for use on unbroken skin in the preoperative preparation of the surgical field. Detergents and soaps should be thoroughly rinsed from the skin before applying ZEPHIRAN Chloride solutions. The detergent action of ZEPHIRAN Chloride solutions, particularly when used alternately with alcohol, leaves the skin smooth and clean. When ZEPHIRAN Chloride solutions are applied by friction (using several changes of sponges), dirt, skin fats, desquamating epithelium, and superficial bacteria are effectively removed, thus exposing the underlying skin to the antiseptic activity of the solutions.

The following procedure has been found satisfactory for preparation of the surgical field. On the day prior to surgery, the operative site is shaved and then scrubbed thoroughly with ZEPHIRAN Chloride Aqueous Solution 1:750. Immediately before surgery, ZEPHIRAN Chloride Tinted Tincture 1:750 or Spray is applied to the site in the usual manner (see Precautions). If the red tinted solution turns yellow during the preparation of patient's skin for surgery, it usually indicates the presence of soap (alkali) residue which is incompatible with ZEPHIRAN solutions. Therefore, rinse thoroughly and reapply the antiseptic. Because ZEPHIRAN Chloride Tinted Tincture 1:750 contains alcohol and acetone, its cleansing action on the skin is particularly effective and it dries more rapidly than the aqueous solution. The Tinted Tincture is recommended when it is desirable to outline the operative site.

Recommended Dilutions: For specific directions, see TABLES 2 and 3.

Surgery

Preoperative preparation of skin: Aqueous solution 1:750 and Tinted Tincture 1:750 or Spray

Surgeons' hand and arm soaks: Aqueous solution 1:750

Treatment of minor wounds and lacerations: Tinted Tincture 1:750 or Spray

Irrigation of deep infected wounds: Aqueous solution 1:3000 to 1:20,000

Denuded skin and mucous membranes: Aqueous solution 1:5000 to 1:10,000

Obstetrics and Gynecology

Preoperative preparation of skin: Aqueous solution 1:750 and Tinted Tincture 1:750 or Spray

Vaginal douche and irrigation: Aqueous solution 1:2000 to 1:5000

Postepisiotomy care: Aqueous solution 1:5000 to 1:10,000

Breast and nipple hygiene: Aqueous solution 1:1000 to 1:2000

Urology

Bladder and urethral irrigation: Aqueous solution 1:5000 to 1:20,000

Bladder retention lavage: Aqueous solution 1:20,000 to 1:40,000

Dermatology

Oozing and open infections: Aqueous solution 1:2000 to 1:5000

Wet dressings by irrigation or open dressing (Use in occlusive dressings is inadvisable.): Aqueous solution 1:5000 or less

Ophthalmology

Eye irrigation: Aqueous solution 1:5000 to 1:10,000

TABLE 2

Correct Use of ZEPHIRAN Chloride

ZEPHIRAN Chloride solutions must be prepared, stored, and used correctly to achieve and maintain their antiseptic action. Serious inactivation and contamination of ZEPHIRAN Chloride solutions may occur with misuse.

CORRECT DILUENTS	INCOMPATIBILITIES	PREFERRED FORM
Sterile Water for Injection is recommended for irrigation of body cavities. *Sterile distilled water* is recommended for irrigating traumatized tissue and in the eye. *Freshly distilled water* is recommended for skin antisepsis. *Resin deionized water* should not be used because the deionizing resins can carry pathogens (especially gram-negative bacteria); they also inactivate quaternary ammonium compounds. *Stored water* is not recommended since it may contain many organisms. *Saline* should not be used since it may decrease the antibacterial potency of ZEPHIRAN Chloride solutions.	Anionic detergents and soaps should be thoroughly rinsed from the skin or other areas prior to use of ZEPHIRAN Chloride solutions because they reduce the antibacterial activity of the solutions. Serum and protein material also decrease the activity of ZEPHIRAN Chloride solutions. Corks should not be used to stopper bottles containing ZEPHIRAN Chloride solutions. Fibers or fabrics when stored in ZEPHIRAN Chloride solutions adsorb ZEPHIRAN from the surrounding liquid. Examples are: Cotton, Gauze sponges, Wool, Rayon, Rubber materials Applicators or sponges, intended for a skin prep, should be stored separately and dipped in ZEPHIRAN Chloride solutions immediately before use. Under certain circumstances the following commonly encountered substances are incompatible with ZEPHIRAN Chloride solutions: Iodine, Aluminum, Silver nitrate, Caramel, Fluorescein, Kaolin, Nitrates, Pine oil, Peroxide, Zinc sulfate, Lanolin, Zinc oxide, Potassium permanganate, Yellow oxide of mercury	ZEPHIRAN Chloride Tinted Tincture 1:750 is recommended for preoperative skin preparation because it contains alcohol and acetone which enhance its cleansing action and promote rapid drying. ZEPHIRAN Chloride Tinted Tincture 1:750, containing acetone, is recommended when it is desirable to outline the operative site. (Aqueous solutions of ZEPHIRAN Chloride used in skin preparation have a tendency to "run off" the skin.) Caution: Because of the flammable organic solvents in ZEPHIRAN Chloride Tinted Tincture 1:750 and Spray, these products should be kept away from open flame or cautery.

Preservation of ophthalmic solutions: Aqueous solution 1:5000 to 1:7500 [See TABLE 2 on preceding page.]

TABLE 3
Dilutions of ZEPHIRAN Chloride Aqueous Solution 1:750

Final Dilution	ZEPHIRAN Chloride Aqueous Solution 1:750 (parts)	Distilled Water (parts)
1:1000	3	1
1:2000	3	5
1:2500	3	7
1:3000	3	9
1:4000	3	13
1:5000	3	17
1:10,000	3	37
1:20,000	3	77
1:40,000	3	157

Accidental Ingestion: If ZEPHIRAN Chloride solution, particularly a concentrated solution, is ingested, marked local irritation of the gastrointestinal tract, manifested by nausea and vomiting, may occur. Signs of systemic toxicity include restlessness, apprehension, weakness, confusion, dyspnea, cyanosis, collapse, convulsions, and coma. Death occurs as a result of paralysis of the respiratory muscles.

Treatment: Immediate administration of several glasses of a mild soap solution, milk, or egg whites beaten in water is recommended. This may be followed by gastric lavage with a mild soap solution. Alcohol should be avoided as it promotes absorption.

To support respiration, the airway should be clear and oxygen should be administered, employing artificial respiration if necessary. If convulsions occur, a short-acting barbiturate may be given parenterally with caution.

How Supplied:

ZEPHIRAN Chloride Aqueous Solution 1:750

Bottles of 8 fl oz (NDC 0024-2521-04) and 1 gallon (NDC 0024-2521-08)

ZEPHIRAN Chloride Tinted Tincture 1:750 (*flammable*)

Bottles of 1 gallon (NDC 0024-2523-08)

ZEPHIRAN Chloride Spray—Tinted Tincture 1:750 (*flammable*)

Bottles of 1 fl oz (NDC 0024-2527-01) and 6 fl oz (NDC 0024-2527-03)

ZW-83-H

Schering-Plough HealthCare Products
LIBERTY CORNER, NJ 07938

A and D® Ointment

Description: An ointment containing the emollients, lanolin and petrolatum. Also contains: Cholecalciferol, Fish Liver Oil, Fragrance, Mineral Oil, Paraffin.

Indications: *Diaper rash*—**A and D Ointment** provides prompt, soothing relief for diaper rash and helps heal baby's tender skin; forms a moisture-proof shield that helps protect against urine and detergent irritants; comforts baby's skin and helps prevent chafing.

Chafed Skin—**A and D Ointment** helps skin retain its vital natural moisture; quickly soothes chafed skin in adults and children and helps prevent abnormal dryness.

Abrasions and Minor Burns—**A and D Ointment** soothes and helps relieve the smarting and pain of abrasions and minor burns, encourages healing and prevents dressings from sticking to the injured area.

Warning: Keep this and all drugs out of the reach of children. In case of accidental ingestion, seek professional assistance or contact a poison control center immediately.

Dosage and Administration: *Diaper Rash*—Simply apply a thin coating of **A and D Ointment** at each diaper change. A modest amount is all that is needed to provide protective and healing action.

Chafed Skin—Gently smooth a small quantity of **A and D Ointment** over the area to be treated.

Abrasions, Minor Burns—Wash with lukewarm water and mild soap. When dry, apply **A and D Ointment** liberally. When a sterile dressing is used, change the dressing daily and apply fresh **A and D Ointment.** If no improvement occurs after 48 to 72 hours or if condition worsens, consult your physician.

How Supplied: A and D Ointment is available in 1½-ounce (42.5 g) and 4-ounce (113 g) tubes and 1-pound (454 g) jars and 2.5 oz. pumps.

Store away from heat.

Shown in Product Identification Section, page 423

AFRIN®
[*a 'frin*]

Nasal Spray 0.05%
Nasal Spray Pump 0.05%
Cherry Scented Nasal Spray 0.05%
Menthol Nasal Spray 0.05%
Nose Drops 0.05%
Children's Strength Nose Drops 0.025%

Description: AFRIN products contain oxymetazoline hydrochloride, the longest acting topical nasal decongestant available. Each ml of AFRIN Nasal Spray, Nasal Spray Pump, and Nose Drops contains Oxymetazoline Hydrochloride, USP 0.5 mg (0.05%); Benzalkonium Chloride, Glycine, Phenylmercuric Acetate (0.002%), Sorbitol, and Water.

Each ml of AFRIN Children's Strength Nose Drops contains Oxymetazoline Hydrochloride, USP 0.25 mg (0.025%); Benzalkonium Chloride, Glycine, Phenylmercuric Acetate (0.002%), Sorbitol, and Water.

AFRIN Menthol Nasal Spray contains cooling aromatic vapors of menthol, eucalyptol, camphor and polysorbate, in addition to the ingredients of AFRIN Nasal Spray.

AFRIN Cherry Scented Nasal Spray contains artificial cherry flavor in addition to the ingredients in regular AFRIN.

Indications: For temporary relief of nasal congestion associated with colds, hay fever and sinusitis.

Actions: The sympathomimetic action of AFRIN products constricts the smaller arterioles of the nasal passages, producing a prolonged, gentle and predictable decongesting effect. In just a few minutes a single dose, as directed, provides prompt, temporary relief of nasal congestion that lasts up to 12 hours. AFRIN products last up to 3 or 4 times longer than most ordinary nasal sprays.

AFRIN products used at bedtime help restore freer nasal breathing through the night.

Warnings: Do not exceed recommended dosage because burning, stinging, sneezing or increase of nasal discharge may occur. Do not use these products for more than 3 days. If nasal congestion persists, consult a physician. As with any drug, if you are pregnant or nursing a baby, seek the advice of a health professional before using this product. The use of the dispensers by more than one person may spread infection. Keep these and all medicines out of the reach of children.

Overdosage: In case of accidental ingestion, seek professional assistance or contact a Poison Control Center immediately.

Dosage and Administration: Because AFRIN has a long duration of action, twice-a-day administration—in the morning and at bedtime—is usually adequate.

AFRIN Nasal Spray, Cherry Scented Nasal Spray and Menthol Nasal Spray, 0.05%—For adults and children 6 years of age and over: With head upright, spray 2 or 3 times into each nostril twice daily—morning and evening. To spray, squeeze bottle quickly and firmly. Do not tilt head backward while spraying. Wipe nozzle clean after use. Not recommended for children under six.

Afrin Nasal Spray Pump, 0.05%—For adults and children 6 years of age and over: Two or three sprays in each nostril twice daily—morning and bedtime. Remove protective cap. Hold bottle with thumb at base and nozzle between first and second fingers. With head upright, insert metered pump spray nozzle in nostril. Depress pump 2 or 3 times, all the

Continued on next page

Information on Schering-Plough HealthCare Products appearing on these pages is effective as of November 1992.

Schering-Plough—Cont.

way down, with a firm even stroke and sniff deeply. Repeat in other nostril. Do not tilt head backward while spraying. Wipe tip clean after each use. Before using the first time, remove the protective cap from the tip and prime the metered pump by depressing pump firmly several times.
AFRIN Nose Drops—For adults and children 6 years of age and over: Tilt head back, apply 2 or 3 drops into each nostril twice daily—morning and evening. Immediately bend head forward toward knees. Hold a few seconds, then return to upright position. Wipe dropper clean after each use. Not recommended for children under six.
AFRIN Children's Strength Nose Drops—Children 2 through 5 years of age: Tilt head back, apply 2 or 3 drops into each nostril twice daily—morning and evening. Promptly move head forward toward knees. Hold a few seconds, then return child to upright position. Wipe dropper clean after each use. For children under 2 years, use only as directed by a physician.

How Supplied: AFRIN Nasal Spray 0.05% (1:2000), 15 ml and 30 ml plastic squeeze bottles.
AFRIN Nasal Spray Pump 0.05% (1:2000), 15 ml spray pump bottles.
AFRIN Cherry Scented Nasal Spray 0.05% (1:2000), 15 ml plastic squeeze bottle.
AFRIN Menthol Nasal Spray 0.05% (1:2000), 15 ml plastic squeeze bottle.
AFRIN Nose Drops, 0.05% (1:2000), 20 ml dropper bottle.
AFRIN Children's Strength Nose Drops, 0.025% (1:4000), 20 ml dropper bottle.
Store all nasal sprays and nose drops between 2° and 30°C (36° and 86°F).

Shown in Product Identification Section, pages 423 and 424

AFRIN®
[a 'frin]
Saline Mist

Ingredients: Water, Sodium Chloride, Disodium Phosphate, Sodium Phosphate, Benzalkonium Chloride, Phenyl Mercuric Acetate (0.002%).

Indications: Provides soothing moisture to dry, inflamed nasal membranes due to colds, allergies, low humidity, and other minor nasal irritations. Afrin Saline Mist loosens and thins mucus secretions to aid removal of mucus from nose and sinuses. Afrin Saline Mist can be used as often as needed, and is safe to use with cold, allergy, and sinus medications.

Directions: For infants, children, and adults, 2 to 6 sprays/drops in each nostril as often as needed or as directed by a physician. For a fine mist, keep bottle upright; for nose drops, keep bottle upside down; for a stream, keep bottle horizontal. Wipe nozzle clean after use.
Keep out of the reach of children. As with any drug, if you are pregnant or nursing a baby, seek the advice of a health professional before using this product.
The use of this dispenser by more than one person may spread infection.
CONTAINS NO ALCOHOL

Shown in Product Identification Section, page 424

AFRIN Tablets
[a 'frin]

Active Ingredients: Each Extended Release Tablet contains: 120 mg pseudoephedrine sulfate. Each tablet also contains: Acacia, Butylparaben, Calcium Sulfate, Carnauba Wax, Corn Starch, FD&C Blue No. 1, Gelatin, Lactose, Magnesium Stearate, Neutral Soap, Oleic Acid, Povidone, Rosin, Sugar, Talc, White Wax, Zein. Half the dose (60 mg) is released after the tablet is swallowed and the other half is released hours later; continuous relief is provided for up to 12 hours . . . without drowsiness.

Indications: For temporary relief of nasal congestion due to the common cold, hay fever or other upper respiratory allergies, and nasal congestion associated with sinusitis.

Actions: Promotes nasal and/or sinus drainage, helps decongest sinus openings, sinus passages.

Warnings: Do not exceed recommended dosage because at higher doses nervousness, dizziness or sleeplessness may occur. Do not take this product if you have high blood pressure, heart disease, diabetes, or thyroid disease, difficulty in urination due to enlargement of the prostate gland or give this product to children under 12 years unless directed by a physician. If symptoms do not improve within 7 days or are accompanied by fever, consult a physician before continuing use. Keep this and all drugs out of the reach of children.
As with any drug, if you are pregnant or nursing a baby, seek the advice of a health professional before using this product.

Drug Interactions: Do not take this product if you are presently taking a prescription drug for high blood pressure or depression, without first consulting your physician.

Overdosage: In case of accidental overdose, seek professional assistance or contact a poison control center immediately.

Dosage and Administration: Adults and children 12 years and over—One tablet every 12 hours. AFRIN Tablets are not recommended for children under 12 years of age.

How Supplied: AFRIN Extended Release Tablets—Boxes of 12 and 24 and bottles of 100.
Store between 2° and 30°C (36° and 86° F).
Protect from excessive moisture.

Shown in Product Identification Section, page 424

AFTATE® Antifungal
Aerosol Liquid
Aerosol Powder
Gel
Powder

Active Ingredient: Tolnaftate 1% (Also contains: Aerosol Spray Liquid-36% alcohol; Aerosol Spray Powder-14% alcohol.)

How Supplied:
AFTATE for Athlete's Foot
Sprinkle Powder—2.25 oz. bottle
Aerosol Spray Powder—3.5 oz can
Gel—.5 oz. tube
Aerosol Spray Liquid—4 oz. can
AFTATE for Jock Itch
Aerosol Spray Powder—3.5 oz. can
Sprinkle Powder—1.5 oz. bottle
Gel—.5 oz. tube

Shown in Product Identification Section, page 424

CHLOR-TRIMETON®
[klor-tri 'mĕ-ton]
Allergy Syrup
Allergy Tablets 4 mg
Long Acting Allergy REPETABS® Tablets 8 mg and 12 mg

Active Ingredients: Each Allergy Tablet contains: 4 mg chlorpheniramine maleate, USP; also contains: Corn Starch, D&C Yellow No. 10 Aluminum Lake, Lactose, Magnesium Stearate. Each REPETABS® Tablet contains: 8 mg or 12 mg chlorpheniramine maleate; 8 mg Repetabs also contains: Acacia, Butylparaben, Calcium Phosphate, Calcium Sulfate, Carnauba Wax, Corn Starch, D&C Yellow No. 10 Aluminum Lake, FD&C Yellow No. 6 Aluminum Lake, FD&C Yellow No. 6, Lactose, Magnesium Stearate, Neutral Soap, Oleic Acid, Potato Starch, Rosin, Sugar, Talc, White Wax, Zein.
12 mg Repetabs also contains: Acacia, Butylparaben, Calcium Phosphate, Calcium Sulfate, Carnauba Wax, Corn Starch, D&C Yellow No. 10 Aluminum Lake, FD&C Blue No. 2 Aluminum Lake, FD&C Yellow No. 6, FD&C Yellow No. 6 Aluminum Lake, Lactose, Magnesium Stearate, Neutral Soap, Oleic Acid, Potato Starch, Rosin, Sugar, Talc, White Wax, Zein. Half the dose is released after the tablet is swallowed, and the other half is released hours later; continuous relief is provided for up to 12 hours.
Each teaspoonful (5 ml) of Allergy Syrup contains: 2 mg chlorpheniramine maleate in a pleasant-tasting syrup containing approximately 5% alcohol. Also contains: Benzaldehyde, FD&C Green No. 3, FD&C Yellow No. 6, Flavor, Glycerin, Menthol, Methylparaben, Propylene Glycol, Propylparaben, Sugar, Vanillin, Water.

Indications: For effective relief of sneezing, itchy, watery eyes, itchy throat, and runny nose due to hay fever and other respiratory allergies.

Actions: The active ingredient in CHLOR-TRIMETON is an antihistamine with anticholinergic (drying) and sedative side effects. Antihistamines appear to compete with histamine for cell receptor sites on effector cells.

Warnings: May cause excitability especially in children. Do not give the 8 mg or 12 mg REPETABS Tablets to children under 12 years, or the Allergy Syrup and 4 mg Tablets to children under 6 years except under the advice and supervision of a physician. Do not take this product if you have asthma, glaucoma, emphysema, chronic pulmonary disease, shortness of breath, difficulty in breathing, or difficulty in urination due to enlargement of the prostate gland unless directed by a physician. May cause drowsiness; alcohol may increase the drowsiness effect. Avoid alcoholic beverages while taking this product. Use caution when driving a motor vehicle or operating machinery. As with any drug, if you are pregnant or nursing a baby, seek the advice of a health professional before using this product. Keep this and all drugs out of the reach of children. In case of accidental overdose, seek professional assistance or contact a Poison Control Center immediately.

Dosage and Administration: Allergy Syrup—Adults and Children 12 years and over: Two teaspoonfuls (4 mg) every 4 to 6 hours, not to exceed 12 teaspoonfuls in 24 hours. Children 6 through 11 years: one teaspoonful (2 mg) every 4 to 6 hours, not to exceed 6 teaspoonfuls in 24 hours. For children under 6 years, consult a physician.

4 mg Allergy Tablets—Adults and Children 12 years and over: One tablet (4 mg) every 4 to 6 hours, not to exceed 6 tablets in 24 hours. Children 6 through 11 years: One half the adult dose (break tablet in half) every 4 to 6 hours, not to exceed 3 whole tablets in 24 hours. For children under 6 years, consult a physician.

8 mg & 12 mg Allergy REPETABS Tablets—Adults and Children 12 years and over: One tablet in the morning and one tablet in the evening, not to exceed 24 mg (3 tablets of 8 mg; 2 tablets of 12 mg) in 24 hours. For children under 12 years, consult a physician.

Professional Labeling: Dosage—Allergy Syrup: Children 2 through 5 years: ½ teaspoonful (1 mg) every 4 to 6 hours; 4 mg Allergy Tablets: Children 2 through 5 years: one-quarter tablet (1 mg) every 4 to 6 hours.

8 mg & 12 mg Allergy REPETABS Tablets—Children 6 to 12 years: One tablet (8 mg) at bedtime or during the day, as indicated.

How Supplied: CHLOR-TRIMETON Allergy Tablets, 4 mg, yellow compressed, scored tablets impressed with the Schering trademark and product identification letters, TW or numbers, 080; box of 24, bottles of 100.

CHLOR-TRIMETON Allergy Syrup: 2 mg per 5 ml, blue-green-colored liquid; 4-fluid ounce (118 ml). Protect from light; however, if color fades potency will not be affected.

CHLOR-TRIMETON Allergy REPETABS Tablets, 8 mg, sugar-coated, yellow tablets branded in red with the Schering trademark and product identification letters, CC or numbers, 374; boxes of 15, bottles of 100.

CHLOR-TRIMETON REPETABS Tablets, 12 mg, sugar coated orange tablets branded in black with Schering trademark and product identification letters AAE or numbers 009; boxes of 10 and 24, bottles of 100.

Store the tablets and syrup between 2° and 30°C (36° and 86°F).

Shown in Product Identification Section, page 424

CHLOR-TRIMETON
Allergy-Sinus Headache

Active Ingredients (per Caplet): 500 mg acetaminophen, 2 mg chlorpheniramine maleate, 12.5 mg phenylpropanolamine hydrochloride. **Also contains:** Carnauba Wax, Cellulose, Hydroxypropyl Methylcellulose, Magnesium Stearate, PEG, Povidone.

Indications: CHLOR-TRIMETON caplets provide effective, temporary relief of sinus pain and nasal congestion, sneezing, itchy, watery eyes, itchy throat, and runny nose due to hay fever and other upper respiratory conditions.

Directions: ADULTS AND CHILDREN 12 YEARS AND OVER—Two caplets every 6 hours, not to exceed 8 caplets in 24 hours, or as directed by a physician. Swallow one caplet at a time.

Warnings: Do not take this product for pain or congestion for more than 7 days, and do not take for fever for more than 3 days unless directed by a physician. If pain or fever persists or gets worse, if new symptoms occur, or if redness or swelling is present, consult your physician because these could be signs of a serious condition. May cause excitability, especially in children. Do not give this product to children under 12 years unless directed by a physican. Do not exceed recommended dosage because at higher doses nervousness, dizziness, or sleeplessness may occur. Do not take this product if you have asthma, glaucoma, emphysema, chronic pulmonary disease, shortness of breath, difficulty in breathing, heart disease, high blood pressure, thyroid disease, diabetes, or difficulty in urination due to the enlargement of the prostate gland unless directed by a physician. May cause drowsiness; alcohol, sedatives, and tranquilizers may increase the drowsiness effect. Avoid alcoholic beverages while taking this product. Use caution when driving a motor vehicle or operating machinery. As with any drug, if you are pregnant or nursing a baby, seek the advice of a health care professional before using this product. Keep this and all drugs out of the reach of children. In case of accidental overdose, seek professional assistance or contact a Poison Control Center immediately. Prompt medical attention is critical for adults as well as for children even if you do not notice any signs or symptoms.

Drug Interaction Precaution: Do not take this product if you are presently taking a prescription drug for high blood pressure or depression, sedatives, tranquilizers, or appetite-controlling medication containing phenylpropanolamine without first consulting your physician.

Store between 2° and 30°C (36° and 86°F).

Protect from excessive moisture.

Shown in Product Identification Section, page 424

CHLOR-TRIMETON®
[klor 'tri 'mĕ-ton]
Antihistamine and Decongestant Tablets
Long Acting CHLOR-TRIMETON® Antihistamine and Decongestant REPETABS® Tablets

Active Ingredients: Each tablet contains: 4 mg chlorpheniramine maleate, USP and 60 mg pseudoephedrine sulfate. Each tablet also contains: Corn Starch, FD&C Blue No. 1, Lactose, Magnesium Stearate, Povidone.

Each REPETABS Tablet contains: 8 mg chlorpheniramine maleate and 120 mg pseudoephedrine sulfate. Each repetab also contains: Acacia, Butylparaben, Calcium Sulfate, Carnauba Wax, Corn Starch, D&C Yellow No. 10 Aluminum Lake, FD&C Blue No. 1 Aluminum Lake, FD&C Yellow No. 6 Aluminum Lake, Gelatin, Lactose, Magnesium Stearate, Neutral Soap, Oleic Acid, Povidone, Rosin, Sugar, Talc, White Wax, Zein. Half the dose of each ingredient is released after the tablet is swallowed and the other half is released hours later providing continuous long-lasting relief up to 12 hours.

Indications: For effective relief of sneezing, itchy, watery eyes, itchy throat, and runny nose due to hay fever and other respiratory allergies. Helps decongest sinus openings and sinus passages.

Actions: The antihistamine, chlorpheniramine maleate, provides temporary relief of running nose, sneezing, itching of the nose or throat, and itchy and watery eyes as may occur in allergic rhinitis (such as hayfever). The decongestant, pseudoephedrine sulfate reduces

Continued on next page

Information on Schering-Plough HealthCare Products appearing on these pages is effective as of November 1992.

Schering-Plough—Cont.

swelling of nasal passages; shrinks swollen membranes; and temporarily restores freer breathing through the nose.

Warnings: If symptoms do not improve within 7 days or are accompanied by fever, consult a physician before continuing use. May cause excitability especially in children. Do not exceed recommended dosage because at higher doses nervousness, dizziness or sleeplessness may occur. Do not take this product if you have asthma, glaucoma, emphysema, chronic pulmonary disease, shortness of breath, difficulty in breathing, heart disease, high blood pressure, thyroid disease, diabetes, or difficulty in urination due to enlargement of the prostate gland unless directed by a physician. Do not give the 4mg Allergy/Decongestant Tablets to children under 6 years or the 12 mg Allergy/Decongestant REPETABS Tablets to children under 12 years unless directed by a physician. May cause drowsiness; alcohol may increase the drowsiness effect. Avoid alcoholic beverages while taking this product. Use caution when driving a motor vehicle or operating machinery. As with any drug, if you are pregnant or nursing a baby, seek the advice of a health professional before using this product. Keep this and all drugs out of the reach of children. In case of accidental overdose, seek professional assistance or contact a Poison Control Center immediately.

Drug Interaction Precaution: Do not take this product if you are presently taking a prescription drug for high blood pressure or depression, without first consulting your doctor.

Dosage and Administration: 4 mg Tablets —ADULTS AND CHILDREN 12 YEARS AND OVER: One tablet every 4 to 6 hours, not to exceed 4 tablets in 24 hours. CHILDREN 6 THROUGH 11 YEARS —One half the adult dose (break tablet in half) every 4 to 6 hours not to exceed 2 whole tablets in 24 hours. For children under 6 years, consult a physician. 12 mg REPETABS Tablets—ADULTS AND CHILDREN 12 YEARS AND OVER: one tablet every 12 hours. Do not exceed 2 tablets in 24 hours.

Professional Labeling: Tablets—Children 2-5 years—one quarter the adult dose every 4 hours, not to exceed 1 tablet in 24 hours.

How Supplied: CHLOR-TRIMETON Decongestant Tablets—boxes of 24. Long Acting CHLOR-TRIMETON Decongestant REPETABS Tablets boxes of 10.
Store these CHLOR-TRIMETON Products between 2° and 30°C (36°and 86°F); and protect from excessive moisture.

Shown in Product Identification Section, page 424

CHLOR-TRIMETON
Non-Drowsy Decongestant
4 Hour

Active Ingredient (per tablet): 60 mg pseudoephedrine sulfate.

Also Contains: Corn Starch, D&C Yellow No. 10 Aluminum Lake, FD&C Blue No. 2 Aluminum Lake, FD&C Yellow No. 6 Aluminum Lake, Lactose, Magnesium Stearate, Povidone.

Indications: CHLOR-TRIMETON NON-DROWSY tablets provide effective, temporary relief of nasal congestion due to hay fever or other upper respiratory allergies, the common cold and nasal congestion associated with sinusitis. Helps decongest sinus openings and sinus passages.

Directions: ADULTS AND CHILDREN 12 YEARS AND OVER—One tablet every 4 to 6 hours, not to exceed 4 tablets in 24 hours. CHILDREN 6 THROUGH 11 YEARS—One half the adult dose (break tablet in half) every 4 to 6 hours, not to exceed 2 whole tablets in 24 hours. For children under 6 years, consult a physician.

Warnings: Do not exceed recommended dosage because at higher doses nervousness, dizziness, or sleeplessness may occur. Do not take this product if you have heart disease, high blood pressure, thyroid disease, diabetes, or difficulty in urination due to the enlargement of the prostate gland unless directed by a physician. If symptoms do not improve within 7 days or are accompanied by fever, consult your physician before continuing use.
As with any drug, if you are pregnant or nursing a baby, seek the advice of a health care professional before using this product. Keep this and all drugs out of the reach of children. In case of accidental overdose, seek professional assistance or contact a Poison Control Center immediately.

Drug Interaction Precaution: Do not take this product if you are presently taking a prescription drug for high blood pressure or depression without first consulting your physician.
Store between 2° and 30°C (36° and 86°F). Protect from excessive moisture.

Shown in Product Identification Section, page 424

CHOOZ® ANTACID GUM

Active Ingredients: 500 mg. of calcium carbonate per tablet.

Inactive Ingredients: Sucrose, gum base, glucose, corn starch, peppermint oil, hydrated silica, gelatin, glycerin, acacia, carnauba wax, beeswax, sodium benzoate.

Indications: For relief from acid indigestion, sour stomach, heartburn, and upset stomach associated with these symptoms. Five tablets provide 100% of the adult U.S. Recommended Daily Allowance for calcium. Chooz Antacid Gum is dietically sodium-free, an important benefit for those watching their sodium and salt consumption.

Warnings: Adults—Do not take more than 14 tablets in a 24-hour period. Do not use the maximum dosage of this product for more than 2 weeks except under the advice and supervision of a physician. Children 6 to 12 years—Do not take more than 8 tablets in a 24-hour period. Keep this and all drugs out of reach of children.

Dosage and Administration: Adults chew 1 to 2 tablets every 2 to 4 hours. Children 6 to 12 years of age chew 1 tablet every 2 to 4 hours. Or take as directed by physician.

How Supplied: Tablets—individually foil-backed safety sealed blister packaging in boxes of 16 tablets.

Shown in Product Identification Section, page 424

COMPLEX 15®
Phospholipid Hand & Body Moisturizing Cream
Formulated For Mild To Severe Dry Skin

Ingredients: Water, Mineral Oil, Glycerin, Squalane, Caprylic/Capric Triglyceride, Dimethicone, Glyceryl Stearate, Glycol Stearate, PEG-50 Stearate Stearic Acid, Cetyl Alcohol, Myristyl Myristate, Lecithin, Diazolidinyl Urea Carbomer , Magnesium Aluminum Silicate, C10–30 Carboxylic Acid Sterol Ester, Sodium Hydroxide, Tetrasodium EDTA, BHT

COMPLEX 15® Hand and Body Cream is formulated for mild to severe dry skin with a system modeled from nature. It contains lecithin, a phospholipid water-binding agent found naturally in the skin. Each phospholipid molecule holds 15 molecules of water, restoring the natural moisture balance. COMPLEX 15 Hand and Body Cream is nongreasy and absorbs quickly into the skin. COMPLEX 15 Hand and Body Cream is unscented, contains no parabens or lanolin. COMPLEX 15 Hand and Body Cream is proven to be hypoallergenic and noncomedogenic.

Directions: Apply to the hands and body as needed or as directed by a physician. Avoid contact with eyes.

FOR EXTERNAL USE ONLY

How Supplied: COMPLEX 15® Hand & Body Moisturizing Cream is available in 4 ounce jars (0085-4151-04).

Shown in Product Identification Section, page 424

COMPLEX 15®
Phospholipid Hand & Body Moisturizing Lotion
Formulated For Mild To Severe Dry Skin

Ingredients: Water, Caprylic/Capric Triglyceride, Glycerin, Glyceryl Stearate, Dimethicone, PEG-50 Stearate, Squalane, Cetyl Alcohol, Glycol Stearate, Myristyl Myristate, Stearic Acid, Lecithin, C10–30 Carboxylic Acid Sterol Ester, Diazolidinyl Urea, Carbomer, Magnesium Aluminum Silicate, Sodium Hydroxide, BHT, Tetrasodium EDTA
COMPLEX 15® Hand and Body Lotion is formulated for mild to severe dry skin with a system modeled from nature. It contains lecithin, a phospholipid water-binding agent found naturally in the skin. Each phospholipid molecule holds 15 molecules of water, restoring the natural moisture balance. COMPLEX 15 Hand and Body Lotion is nongreasy and absorbs quickly into the skin. COMPLEX 15 Hand and Body Lotion is unscented, contains no parabens, lanolin, or mineral oil. COMPLEX 15 Hand and Body Lotion is proven to be hypoallergenic and noncomedogenic.

Directions: Apply to the hands and body as needed, or as directed by a physician. Avoid contact with eyes.
FOR EXTERNAL USE ONLY

How Supplied: COMPLEX 15® Hand and Body Moisturizing Lotion is available in 8 fluid ounce and 4 fluid ounce bottles (0085-4115-08).
Shown in Product Identification Section, page 424

COMPLEX 15®
Phospholipid Moisturizing Face Cream

Ingredients: Water, Caprylic/Capric Triglyceride, Glycerin, Squalane, Glyceryl Stearate, Propylene Glycol, PEG-50 Stearate, Cetyl Alcohol, Dimethicone, Glycol Stearate, Myristyl Myristate, Stearic Acid, Carbomer, Magnesium Aluminum Silicate, Diazolidinyl Urea, Lecithin, Sodium Hydroxide, C10–30 Carboxylic Acid Sterol Ester, BHT, Tetrasodium EDTA
COMPLEX 15® Face Cream is formulated for mild to severe dry skin with a system modeled from nature. It contains lecithin, a phospholipid water-binding agent found naturally in the skin. Each phospholipid molecule holds 15 molecules of water, restoring the natural moisture balance. COMPLEX 15 Face Cream is nongreasy and absorbs quickly into the skin. COMPLEX 15 Face Cream is unscented, contains no parabens, lanolin or mineral oil. COMPLEX 15 Face Cream is proven to be hypoallergenic and noncomedogenic.

Directions: Apply to the face as needed or as directed by a physician. Avoid contact with eyes.
FOR EXTERNAL USE ONLY

How Supplied: COMPLEX 15® Moisturizing Face Cream is available in 2.5 oz. tubes (0085-4100-25).
Shown in Product Identification Section, page 424

CORICIDIN® Tablets
[*kor-a-see 'din*]
CORICIDIN 'D'® Decongestant Tablets

Active Ingredients: CORICIDIN Tablets—2 mg chlorpheniramine maleate, USP; 325 mg (5 gr) acetaminophen.
CORICIDIN 'D' Decongestant Tablets—2 mg chlorpheniramine maleate, USP; 12.5 mg phenylpropanolamine hydrochloride, USP; 325 mg (5 gr) acetaminophen.

Inactive Ingredients: CORICIDIN Tablets—Acacia, Butylparaben, Calcium Sulfate, Carnauba Wax, Cellulose, Corn Starch, FD&C Red No. 40 Aluminum Lake, FD&C Yellow No. 6 Aluminum Lake, Lactose, Magnesium Stearate, Povidone, Sugar, Talc, Titanium Dioxide, White Wax.
CORICIDIN 'D' Decongestant Tablets—Acacia, Butylparaben, Calcium Sulfate, Carnauba Wax, Cellulose, Corn Starch, Magnesium Stearate, Povidone, Sugar, Talc, Titanium Dioxide, White Wax.

Indications: CORICIDIN Tablets—For effective, temporary relief of cold, flu, and allergy symptoms.
CORICIDIN 'D' Decongestant Tablets—For effective, temporary relief of congested cold, flu and sinus symptoms.

Actions: CORICIDIN Tablets relieve annoying cold and flu symptoms such as minor aches and pains, fever, sneezing, runny nose, watery/itchy eyes, and headache.
CORICIDIN 'D' Tablets relieve annoying cold and flu symptoms such as minor aches and pains, fever, sneezing, runny nose, watery/itchy eyes, as well as stuffy nose, sinus pressure and sinus headache.

Warnings: CORICIDIN Tablets: Do not take this product for pain for more than 10 days (for adults) or 5 days (for children 6 years through 11 years), and do not take for fever for more than 3 days unless directed by a physician. If pain or fever persists or gets worse, if new symptoms occur, or if redness or swelling is present, consult a physician because these could be signs of a serious condition. May cause excitability especially in children. Do not take this product if you have asthma, glaucoma, emphysema, chronic pulmonary disease, shortness of breath, difficulty in breathing, difficulty in urination due to enlargement of the prostate gland, or give this product to children under 6 years, unless directed by a physician. May cause drowsiness; alcohol, sedatives, and tranquilizers may increase the drowsiness effect. Avoid alcoholic beverages while taking this product. Do not take this product if you are taking sedatives or tranquilizers, without first consulting your physician. Use caution when driving a motor vehicle or operating machinery. Keep this and all drugs out of the reach of children. In case of accidental overdose, seek professional assistance or contact a Poison Control Center immediately. Prompt medical attention is critical for adults as well as for children even if you do not notice any signs or symptoms. As with any drug, if you are pregnant or nursing a baby, seek the advice of a health professional before using this product.
CORICIDIN 'D' Decongestant Tablets: Do not take this product for pain or congestion for more than 7 days (adults) or 5 days (children 6 through 11 years), and do not take for fever for more than 3 days unless directed by a physician. If pain or fever persists or gets worse, if new symptoms occur, or if redness or swelling is present, consult your physician because these could be signs of a serious condition. May cause excitability, especially in children. Do not exceed recommended dosage because at higher doses nervousness, dizziness, or sleeplessness may occur. Do not take this product if you have asthma, glaucoma, emphysema, chronic pulmonary disease, shortness of breath, difficulty in breathing, heart disease, high blood pressure, thyroid disease, diabetes, difficulty in urination due to enlargement of the prostate gland, or give this product to children under 6 years unless directed by a physician. May cause drowsiness; alcohol, sedatives, and tranquilizers may increase the drowsiness effect. Avoid alcoholic beverages while taking this product. Use caution when driving a motor vehicle or operating machinery. Keep this and all drugs out of the reach of children. In case of accidental overdose, seek professional assistance or contact a Poison Control Center immediately. Proper medical attention is critical for adults and children even if you do not notice any signs or symptoms. As with any drug, if you are pregnant or nursing a baby, seek the advice of a health care professional before using this product. *Drug Interaction Precaution:* Do not take this product if you are presently taking a prescription drug for high blood pressure or depression, sedatives, tranquilizers or appetite-controlling medication containing phenylpropanolamine without first consulting your physician.

Dosage and Administration: CORICIDIN Tablets—Adults and children 12 years and over—2 tablets every 4 hours not to exceed 12 tablets in 24 hours. Children 6 through 11 years: 1 tablet every 4 hours not to exceed 5 tablets in 24 hours.

Continued on next page

Information on Schering-Plough HealthCare Products appearing on these pages is effective as of November 1992.

Schering-Plough—Cont.

CORICIDIN 'D' Decongestant Tablets—Adults and children 12 years and over: 2 tablets every 4 hours not to exceed 12 tablets in 24 hours. Children 6 through 11 years: 1 tablet every 4 hours not to exceed 5 tablets in 24 hours.

How Supplied: CORICIDIN Tablets—12, 48, and 100, blisters of 24.
CORICIDIN 'D' Decongestant Tablets—12, 48, and 100, blisters of 24.
Store the tablets between 2° and 30°C (36° and 86°F).

Shown in Product Identification Section, page 424

CORRECTOL®
Laxative
Tablets

Active Ingredients: Tablets—Yellow phenolphthalein, 65 mg. and docusate sodium, 100 mg. per tablet.

Inactive Ingredients: Butylparaben, calcium gluconate, calcium sulfate, carnauba wax, D&C Red No. 7 calcium lake, gelatin, magnesium stearate, sugar, talc, titanium dioxide, wheat flour, white wax, and other ingredients.

Indications: For relief of occasional constipation or irregularity. CORRECTOL generally produces bowel movement in 6 to 8 hours.

Actions: Yellow phenolphthalein—stimulant laxative; docusate sodium—fecal softener.

Warnings: Not to be taken in case of nausea, vomiting, abdominal pain, or signs of appendicitis. Take only as needed —as frequent or continued use of laxatives may result in dependence on them. If skin rash appears, do not use this or any other preparation containing phenolphthalein. As with any drug, if you are pregnant or nursing a baby, seek the advice of a health professional before using this product. Keep out of children's reach.

Dosage and Administration
Dosage: Adults—1 or 2 tablets daily as needed, at bedtime or on arising.
Children over 6 years—1 tablet daily as needed.

How Supplied: Tablets—Individual foil-backed safety sealed blister packaging in boxes of 15, 30, 60 and 90 tablets.

Shown in Product Identification Section, page 425

CORRECTOL® EXTRA GENTLE
Stool Softener

Active Ingredient: Docusate sodium 100 mg. per soft gel.
Also Contains—D&C Red No. 33, FD&C Red No. 40, FD&C Yellow No. 6, gelatin, glycerin, polyethylene glycol 400, propylene glycol, sorbitol.

Indications: For relief of constipation without cramps for sensitive systems. Correctol Extra Gentle will work gradually to return you to regularity in 1 to 3 days.

Warning: Keep out of reach of children.

Directions: Adults: For gradual relief of constipation, take 2 soft gels daily, as needed. Children 6–12: Take 1 daily, as needed.

How Supplied: Tablets—individual foil-backed safety sealed blister packaging in boxes of 30 tablets.
Store below 86°F. Protect from freezing.

Shown in Product Identification Section, page 425

DI–GEL®
Antacid · Anti-Gas
Tablets/Liquid

DI-GEL Tablets: Active Ingredients: (Per Tablet)—Simethicone 20 mg., Calcium Carbonate 280 mg., Magnesium Hydroxide 128 mg. **Inactive Ingredients:** D & C yellow No. 10 aluminum lake, dextrin, FD&C yellow No. 6 aluminum lake, flavor, magnesium stearate, mannitol, povidone, stearic acid, sucrose, talc.
Dietetically sodium free, calcium rich.

DI-GEL Liquid: Active Ingredients—per teaspoonful (5 ml): Simethicone 20 mg., aluminum hydroxide (equivalent to aluminum hydroxide dried gel USP) 200 mg., magnesium hydroxide 200 mg. **Also contains:** Flavor, hydroxypropyl methylcellulose, methylcellulose, methylparaben, propylparaben, sodium saccharin, sorbitol, water.
Dietetically sodium free.

Indications: For fast, temporary relief of acid indigestion, heartburn, sour stomach and accompanying painful gas symptoms.

Actions: The antacid system in DI-GEL relieves and soothes acid indigestion, heartburn and sour stomach. At the same time, the simethicone "defoamers" eliminate gas.
When air becomes entrapped in the stomach, heartburn and acid indigestion can result, along with sensations of fullness, pressure and bloating.

Warnings: Do not take more than 20 teaspoonfuls or 24 tablets in a 24 hour period, or use the maximum dosage of this product for more than 2 weeks, except under the advice and supervision of a physician. If you have kidney disease do not use this product except under the advice and supervision of a physician. May cause constipation or have a laxative effect. Keep this and all drugs out of the reach of children.

Drug Interaction: (Liquid Only) This product should not be taken if patient is presently taking a prescription antibiotic drug containing any form of tetracycline.

Dosage and Administration: Two teaspoonfuls or tablets every 2 hours, or after or between meals and at bedtime, not to exceed 20 teaspoonfuls or 24 tablets per day, or as directed by a physician.

How Supplied:
DI-GEL Liquid in Mint Flavor - 6 and 12 fl. oz. bottles, safety sealed and Lemon/Orange Flavors - 12 fl. oz. bottles, safety sealed.
DI-GEL Tablets in Mint and Lemon/Orange Flavors - In boxes of 30 and 90 in handy portable safety sealed blister packaging. Also available in Mint 60-tablet bottles.

Shown in Product Identification Section, page 425

DRIXORAL®
[*dricks-or 'al*]
Antihistamine/Nasal Decongestant
Syrup

Description: Each 5 ml (1 teaspoonful) of DRIXORAL Syrup contains 2 mg brompheniramine maleate and 30 mg pseudoephedrine sulfate; also contains Citric Acid, D&C Red No. 33, FD&C Yellow No. 6, Flavor, Propylene Glycol, Sodium Benzoate, Sodium Citrate, Sorbitol, Sugar, Water. Drixoral Syrup is alcohol-free.

Indications: DRIXORAL Syrup combines a nasal decongestant with an antihistamine in a pleasant-tasting wild cherry flavor to provide temporary relief of nasal congestion due to the common cold, hay fever or other upper respiratory allergies. Helps decongest sinus openings, sinus passages. Alleviates running nose, sneezing, itching of the nose or throat, and itchy and watery eyes due to hay fever. DRIXORAL Syrup is ideal for adults and children who prefer a syrup instead of tablets or capsules.

Warnings: If symptoms do not improve within 7 days or are accompanied by fever, consult a physician before continuing use. May cause drowsiness. May cause excitability especially in children. Do not exceed recommended dosage because at higher doses nervousness, dizziness, or sleeplessness may occur. Do not give this product to children under 6 years except under the advice and supervision of a physician. Do not take this product if you have asthma, glaucoma, emphysema, chronic pulmonary disease, shortness of breath, difficulty in breathing, difficulty in urination due to enlargement of the prostate gland, high blood pressure, heart disease, diabetes, or thyroid disease except under the advice and supervision of a physician. As with any drug, if you are pregnant or nursing a baby, seek the advice of a health professional before using this product. CAUTION: Avoid driving a motor vehicle or operating heavy machinery. Avoid alcoholic beverages while taking this product. Keep this and all drugs out of the reach of children. In case of accidental overdose, seek professional assistance or contact a Poison Control Center immediately.

Drug Interaction Precaution: Do not take this product if you are presently taking a prescription drug for high blood pressure or depression, without first consulting your doctor.

Directions: Adults and children 12 years of age and over: two teaspoonfuls every 4–6 hours. Children 6 to under 12 years of age: 1 teaspoonful every 4–6 hours. Do not exceed 4 doses in 24 hours. Children under 6 years of age, consult a physician.
Store between 2° and 30°C (36° and 86°F).

Overdosage: In case of accidental overdose, seek professional assistance or contact a Poison Control Center immediately.

How Supplied: DRIXORAL Syrup is available in 4 fl. oz. (118 ml) bottles.

DRIXORAL® COLD & ALLERGY
[dricks-or 'al]
Sustained-Action Tablets

Description: EACH DRIXORAL COLD & ALLERGY SUSTAINED-ACTION TABLET CONTAINS: 120 mg of pseudoephedrine sulfate and 6 mg of dexbrompheniramine maleate. Half of the medication is released after the tablet is swallowed and the remaining amount of medication is released hours later providing continuous long-lasting relief for 12 hours. Also contains: Acacia, Butylparaben, Calcium Sulfate, Carnauba Wax, Corn Starch, D&C Yellow No. 10 Aluminum Lake, FD&C Blue No. 1 Aluminum Lake, FD&C Yellow No. 6 Aluminum Lake, Gelatin, Lactose, Magnesium Stearate, Neutral Soap, Oleic Acid, Povidone, Rosin, Sugar, Talc, White Wax, Zein.

Indications: For temporary relief of nasal congestion due to the common cold, hay fever, or other upper respiratory allergies, and associated with sinusitis. Helps decongest sinus openings, sinus passages. Reduces swelling of nasal passages; shrinks swollen membranes; and temporarily restores freer breathing through the nose. Alleviates running nose, sneezing, itching of the nose or throat, and itchy and watery eyes as may occur in allergic rhinitis (such as hay fever).

Actions: The antihistamine, dexbrompheniramine maleate, provides temporary relief of sneezing; watery, itchy eyes; running nose due to hay fever and other upper respiratory allergies. The decongestant, pseudoephedrine sulfate, temporarily restores freer breathing through the nose and promotes sinus drainage.

Warnings: If symptoms do not improve within 7 days or are accompanied by fever, consult a physician before continuing use. May cause excitability especially in children. Do not exceed recommended dosage because at higher doses nervousness, dizziness, or sleeplessness may occur. Do not take this product if you have asthma, glaucoma, emphysema, chronic pulmonary disease, high blood pressure, thyroid disease, diabetes, or difficulty in urination due to enlargement of the prostate gland or give this product to children under 12 years, unless directed by a physician. May cause drowsiness; alcohol may increase the drowsiness effect. Avoid alcoholic beverages while taking this product. Use caution when driving a motor vehicle or operating machinery. Keep this and all drugs out of the reach of children. In case of accidental overdose, seek professional assistance or contact a Poison Control Center immediately. As with any drug, if you are pregnant or nursing a baby, seek the advice of a health professional before using this product.

Drug Interaction Precaution: Do not take this product if you are presently taking a prescription drug for high blood pressure or depression, without first consulting your physician.

Dosage and Administration: ADULTS AND CHILDREN 12 YEARS AND OVER—one tablet every 12 hours. Do not exceed two tablets in 24 hours.

How Supplied: DRIXORAL Cold & Allergy Sustained-Action Tablets, green, sugar-coated tablets branded in black with the product name, boxes of 10, 20, and 40, bottle of 100.
Store between 2° and 25°C (36° and 77°F).

Shown in Product Identification Section, page 425

DRIXORAL® NON-DROWSY FORMULA
[dricks-or 'al]
Long-Acting Nasal Decongestant

DRIXORAL NON-DROWSY FORMULA Long-Acting Nasal Decongestant Tablets contain pseudoephedrine sulfate, a nasal decongestant, in a special timed-release tablet providing up to 12 hours of continuous relief . . . without drowsiness.

Indications: For temporary relief of nasal congestion due to the common cold, hay fever or other upper respiratory allergies, and nasal congestion associated with sinusitis. Helps decongest sinus openings and sinus passages.

Directions: Adults and Children 12 Years and Over—One tablet every 12 hours. Do not exceed two tablets in 24 hours. DRIXORAL NON-DROWSY FORMULA is not recommended for children under 12 years of age.

Each Extended-Release Tablet Contains: 120 mg pseudoephedrine sulfate. Half the dose is released after the tablet is swallowed and the other half is released hours later, providing continuous relief for up to 12 hours.

Warnings: Do not exceed recommended dosage because at higher doses, nervousness, dizziness, or sleeplessness may occur. Do not take this product if you have heart disease, high blood pressure, thyroid disease, diabetes, difficulty in urination due to enlargement of the prostate gland, or give this product to children under 12 years unless directed by a physician. If symptoms do not improve within 7 days or are accompanied by fever, consult your physician before continuing use. Keep this and all drugs out of the reach of children. In case of accidental overdose, seek professional assistance or contact a Poison Control Center immediately. As with any drug, if you are pregnant or nursing a baby, seek the advice of a health professional before using this product.

Drug Interaction Precautions: Do not take this product if you are presently taking a prescription drug for high blood pressure or depression, without first consulting your physician.

Active Ingredients: Pseudoephedrine Sulfate

Also Contains: Acacia, Butylparaben, Calcium Sulfate, Carnauba Wax, Corn Starch, FD&C Blue No. 1 Aluminum Lake, Gelatin, Lactose, Magnesium Stearate, Neutral Soap, Oleic Acid, Povidone, Rosin, Sugar, Talc, White Wax, Zein.
Store between 2° and 25°C (36° and 77°F).
Protect from excessive moisture.

Shown in Product Identification Section, page 425

DRIXORAL® COLD & FLU
[dricks-or 'al]
Extended-Release Tablets

Active Ingredients: Acetaminophen, Dexbrompheniramine Maleate, Pseudoephedrine Sulfate.

Also Contains: Calcium Phosphate, Carnauba Wax, D&C Yellow No. 10 Aluminum Lake, FD&C Blue No. 1 Aluminum Lake, FD&C Yellow No. 6 Alumium Lake, Hydroxypropyl Methylcellulose, Magnesium Stearate, Methylparaben, PEG, Propylparaben, Stearic Acid.
DRIXORAL® COLD & FLU Extended-Release Tablets combine a nasal decongestant and an antihistamine with a nonaspirin analgesic in a special 12-hour continuous-acting timed-release tablet.

Indications: The *decongestant* temporarily relieves nasal congestion due to the common cold, hay fever or other upper respiratory allergies, and associated with sinusitis. Reduces swelling of nasal passages; shrinks swollen membranes; and temporarily restores freer breathing

Continued on next page

Information on Schering-Plough HealthCare Products appearing on these pages is effective as of November 1992.

Schering-Plough—Cont.

through the nose. Also helps decongest sinus openings, sinus passages. The *non-aspirin analgesic* temporarily relieves occasional minor aches, pains, and headache and reduces fever due to the common cold. The *antihistamine* alleviates running nose, sneezing, itching of the nose or throat, and itchy and watery eyes as may occur in allergic rhinitis (such as hay fever).

EACH DRIXORAL COLD & FLU EXTENDED-RELEASE TABLET CONTAINS: 60 mg of pseudoephedrine sulfate, 3 mg of dexbrompheniramine maleate and 500 mg of acetaminophen. These ingredients are released continuously, providing long-lasting relief for 12 hours.

Directions: ADULTS AND CHILDREN 12 YEARS AND OVER—two tablets every 12 hours. Do not exceed four tablets in 24 hours. Children under 12 years of age: consult a doctor.

Warnings: Do not take this product for more than 7 days. If symptoms do not improve, or are accompanied by fever that lasts for more than three days (72 hours) or recurs, or if new symptoms occur, consult a physician before continuing use. If pain or fever persists or gets worse, or if redness or swelling is present, consult a physician because these could be signs of a serious condition. May cause excitability especially in children. Do not exceed recommended dosage because at higher doses nervousness, dizziness, or sleeplessness may occur. Do not take this product if you have asthma, glaucoma, emphysema, chronic pulmonary disease, shortness of breath, difficulty in breathing, heart disease, high blood pressure, thyroid disease, diabetes difficulty in urination due to enlargement of the prostate gland, or give this product to children under 12 years unless directed by a physician. May cause drowsiness; alcohol, sedatives, and tranquilizers may increase the drowsiness effect. Avoid alcoholic beverages while taking this product. Use caution when driving a motor vehicle or operating machinery. Keep this and all drugs out of the reach of children. In case of accidental overdose, seek professional assistance or contact a Poison Control Center immediately. Prompt medical attention is critical for adults as well as for children even if you do not notice any signs or symptoms. As with any drug, if you are pregnant or nursing a baby, seek the advice of a health professional before using this product.

Drug Interaction Precaution: Do not take this product if you are presently taking a prescription drug for high blood pressure or depression, sedatives or tranquilizers, without first consulting your physician.

How Supplied: DRIXORAL COLD & FLU Extended-Release Tablets are available in boxes of 12's and 24's and bottles of 48.

Store between 2° and 25°C (36° and 77°F).

Protect from excessive moisture.

Shown in Product Identification Section, page 425

DRIXORAL® SINUS

[*dricks-or 'al*]

Nasal decongestant/Pain reliever/ Antihistamine

DRIXORAL® SINUS Extended-Release Tablets combine a nasal decongestant, and a non-aspirin analgesic, with an antihistamine in a special 12-hour continuous-acting timed-release tablet.

Indications: The *decongestant* temporarily relieves nasal congestion due to sinusitis, the common cold, and hay fever or other upper respiratory allergies. Helps decongest sinus openings, sinus passages; relieves sinus pressure. Reduces swelling of nasal passages; shrinks swollen membranes; and temporarily restores freer breathing through the nose. The *non-aspirin analgesic* temporarily relieves occasional headaches, minor aches and pains, and reduces fever due to the common cold. The *antihistamine* alleviates runny nose, sneezing, itching of the nose or throat, and itchy and watery eyes as may occur in allergic rhinitis (such as hay fever).

Each Drixoral Sinus Extended-Release Tablet Contains: 60 mg of pseudoephedrine sulfate, 3 mg of dexbrompheniramine maleate, and 500 mg of acetaminophen. These ingredients are released continuously, providing long-lasting relief for 12 hours.

Directions: ADULTS AND CHILDREN 12 YEARS AND OVER—two tablets every 12 hours. Do not exceed four tablets in 24 hours. Children under 12 years of age: consult a physician.

Store between 2° and 25°C (36° and 77°F).

Warnings: Do not take this product for more than 7 days. If symptoms do not improve, or are accompanied by fever that lasts for more than three days (72 hours) or recurs, or if new symptoms occur, consult a physician before continuing use. If pain or fever persists or gets worse, or if redness or swelling is present, consult a physician because these could be signs of a serious condition. May cause excitability especially in children. Do not exceed recommended dosage because at higher doses nervousness, dizziness, or sleeplessness may occur. Do not take this product if you have asthma, glaucoma, emphysema, chronic pulmonary disease, shortness of breath, difficulty in breathing, heart disease, high blood pressure, thyroid disease, diabetes, difficulty in urination due to enlargement of the prostate gland, or give this product to children under 12 years unless directed by a physician. May cause drowsiness; alcohol, sedatives, and tranquilizers may increase the drowsiness effect. Avoid alcoholic beverages while taking this product. Use caution when driving a motor vehicle or operating machinery. Keep this and all drugs out of the reach of children. In case of accidental overdose, seek professional assistance or contact a Poison Control Center immediately. Prompt medical attention is critical for adults as well as for children even if you do not notice any signs or symptoms. As with any drug, if you are pregnant or nursing a baby, seek the advice of a health care professional before using this product.

Drug Interaction Precaution: Do not take this product if you are presently taking a prescription drug for high blood pressure or depression, sedatives, or tranqullizers, without first consulting your physician.

Shown in Product Identification, Section, page 425

DUOFILM® LIQUID

Active Ingredient: Salicylic Acid 17% (w/w).

Inactive Ingredients: Alcohol 15.8% w/w, castor oil, ether 42.6% w/w, ethyl lactate, and polybutene in flexible collodion.

Indications: For the removal of common and plantar warts. Common warts can be easily recognized by the rough, cauliflower-like appearance of the surface. Plantar warts are found on the bottom of the foot.

Warnings: For external use only. Do not use this product on irritated skin, on any area that is infected or reddened, if you are a diabetic, or if you have poor blood circulation. If discomfort persists, see your doctor. Do not use on moles, birthmarks, warts with hair growing from them, genital warts, or warts on the face or mucous membranes. Keep out of reach of children. If DuoFilm Liquid gets in eyes, flush with water for 15 minutes. Avoid inhaling vapors. DuoFilm Liquid is extremely flammable. Keep away from fire or flame. Cap bottle tightly when not in use. Store at room temperature away from heat.

Directions: Wash affected area. Soak wart in warm water for five minutes. Dry area thoroughly with a clean towel. Apply a thin layer of DuoFilm Liquid directly to wart with the brush applicator. Let dry. Cover treated area with adhesive bandage. Repeat procedure once or twice daily as needed (until wart is removed) for up to 12 weeks.

How Supplied: DuoFilm Liquid is available in ½ fluid oz. spill-resistant bottles with brush applicator for pinpoint application.

Shown in Product Identification Section, page 425

DUOFILM® PATCH

Active Ingredient: Salicylic Acid 40% in a rubber-based vehicle.

Indications: For the concealment and removal of common warts. Common warts can be easily recognized by the rough, cauliflower-like appearance of the surface.

Warnings: For external use only. Do not use this product on irritated skin, on any area that is infected or reddened, if you are a diabetic, or if you have poor blood circulation. If discomfort persists, see your doctor. Do not use on moles, birthmarks, warts with hair growing from them, genital warts, or warts on the face or mucous membranes. Keep out of reach from children.

Directions: Wash affected area. Soak in warm water for five minutes. Dry area thoroughly with a clean towel. Select a Medicated Patch from packet A that matches the size of the wart (trim patch if necessary), then place on wart beige side up. Apply a self-adhesive Cover-Up Patch from packet B over Medicated Patch and wart. Repeat procedure every 48 hours as needed (until wart is removed) for up to 12 weeks. Visible improvement will normally occur within the first one to two weeks of therapy. Removal should be complete within four to twelve weeks of drug use.

How Supplied: DuoFilm Patch includes 54 Medicated Patches of varying sizes, with 20 self-adhesive Cover-Up patches for concealment while treatment is ongoing.

Shown in Product Identification Section, page 425

DUOPLANT® GEL

Active Ingredient: Salicylic Acid 17% (w/w).

Inactive Ingredients: Alcohol 57.6% w/w, ether 16.42% w/w, ethyl lactate, hydroxypropyl cellulose, and polybutene in flexible collodion, USP.

Indications: For the removal of plantar and common warts. Plantar warts are found on the bottom of the foot. Common warts can be easily recognized by the rough, cauliflower-like appearance of the surface.

Warnings: For external use only. Do not use this product on irritated skin, on any area that is infected or reddened, if you are a diabetic, or if you have poor blood circulation. If discomfort persists, see your doctor. Do not use on moles, birthmarks, warts with hair growing from them, genital warts, or warts on the face or mucous membranes. Keep out of reach of children. If DuoPlant Gel gets in eyes, flush with water for 15 minutes. Avoid inhaling vapors. DuoPlant Gel is extremely flammable. Keep away from fire or flame. Keep tube tightly capped when not in use. Store at room temperature away from heat.

Directions: Wash affected area. Soak wart in warm water for five minutes. Dry area thoroughly with a clean towel. Apply a thin layer of DuoPlant Gel directly to wart. Let dry. Cover treated area with adhesive tape. Repeat procedure once or twice daily as needed (until wart is removed) for up to 12 weeks.

How Supplied: DuoPlant Gel is available in ½ oz. tubes with applicator tip for pinpoint application.

Shown in Product Identification Section, page 425

DURATION
12 Hour Nasal Spray 0.05%
12 Hour Nasal Spray Pump 0.05%

Description: DURATION products contain oxymetazoline hydrochloride, the longest acting topical nasal decongestant available. Each ml of DURATION Nasal Spray and Nasal Spray Pump contains Oxymetazoline Hydrochloride, USP 0.5 mg (0.05%), Benzalkonium Chloride, Glycine, Phenylmercuric Acetate (0.002%), Sorbitol and Water.

Indications: Immediate relief for up to 12 hours of nasal congestion due to colds, hay fever and sinusitis.

Actions: The sympathomimetic action of DURATION products constricts the smaller arterioles of the nasal passages, producing a prolonged, gentle and predictable decongesting effect. In just a few minutes a single dose, as directed, provides prompt, temporary relief of nasal congestion that lasts up to 12 hours. DURATION products last up to 3 to 4 times longer than most ordinary nasal sprays.

Warnings: Do not exceed recommended dosage because symptoms may occur such as burning, stinging, sneezing or increase of nasal discharge. Do not use this product for more than three days. If symptoms persist, consult a physician. As with any drug, if you are pregnant or nursing a baby, seek the advice of a health professional before using this product. The use of the dispenser by more than one person may spread infection. Keep this and all medications out of the reach of children. In case of accidental ingestion, seek professional assistance or contact a Poison Control Center immediately.

Dosage and Administration: DURATION 12 Hour Nasal Spray, 0.05%—For adults and children 6 years of age and over: With head upright, spray 2 or 3 times into each nostril twice daily—morning and evening. To spray, squeeze bottle quickly and firmly. Do not tilt head backward while spraying. Wipe nozzle clean after use. Not recommended for children under six.
DURATION Nasal Spray Pump, 0.05%—For adults six years of age and over: Before using first time, remove protective cap. Prime the metered pump by depressing several times. Hold bottle with thumb at base and nozzle between first and second fingers. With head upright (do not tilt backward), insert metered pump-spray nozzle into nostril. Depress pump completely 2 or 3 times. Sniff deeply. Repeat in other nostril. Wipe tip clean after each use. Not recommended for children under six.
Store between 2° and 30°C (36° and 86°F).

How Supplied: DURATION 12 Hour Nasal Spray 0.05%—½ oz and 1 oz plastic squeeze bottles
DURATION 12 Hour Nasal Spray Pump—½ oz metered dose pump spray bottle

Shown in Product Identification Section, page 425

FEEN-A-MINT®
Laxative Gum/Pills

Active Ingredients: Gum—yellow phenolphthalein 97.2 mg. per tablet. Pills—yellow phenolphthalein 65 mg., and docusate sodium 100 mg. per pill.

Indications: For relief of occasional constipation or irregularity. FEEN-A-MINT generally produces bowel movement in 6 to 8 hours.

Inactive Ingredients: Gum—Acacia, butylated hydroxyanisole, carnauba wax, corn starch, gelatin, glucose, glycerin gum base, peppermint oil, sodium benzoate, sugar, water, white wax.
Pills—Butylparaben, calcium gluconate, calcium sulfate, carnauba wax, gelatin, magnesium stearate, sugar, talc, titanium dioxide, wheat flour, white wax and other ingredients.

How Supplied: Gum—Individual foil-backed safety sealed blister packaging in boxes of 5 and 16 tablets.
Pills—Safety sealed boxes of 15, 30, and 60 tablets.

Shown in Product Identification Section, page 425

GYNE–LOTRIMIN®
Clotrimazole
Vaginal Cream
Antifungal

Active Ingredient: Clotrimazole 1%

Inactive Ingredients: Benzyl alcohol, cetearyl alcohol, cetyl esters wax, octyldodecanol, polysorbate 60, purified water, sorbitan monostearate.

Indications: Gyne-Lotrimin® will cure most recurrent vaginal yeast (Candida) infections. Gyne-Lotrimin® usually starts to relieve the itching and other symptoms of vaginal yeast infection within 3 days. If the patient does not im-

Continued on next page

Information on Schering-Plough HealthCare Products appearing on these pages is effective as of November 1992.

Schering-Plough—Cont.

prove in 3 days or if the patient does not get well in 7 days, a condition other than yeast infection may exist. The patient should discontinue use of the product and consult a doctor. Also, if symptoms recur within a 2-month period, patient should consult a doctor.

Important: In order to kill the yeast completely, GYNE-LOTRIMIN must be used the full seven days, even if symptoms are relieved sooner.

Warnings:

- Do not use if you have abdominal pain, fever, or a foul-smelling vaginal discharge. You may have a condition which is more serious than a yeast infection. Contact your doctor immediately.
- Do not use if this is your first experience with vaginal itch and discomfort. See your doctor.
- If there is no improvement within 3 days, you may have a condition other than a yeast infection. Stop using this product and see your doctor.
- If you may have been exposed to the human immunodeficiency virus (HIV, the virus that causes AIDS) and are now having recurrent vaginal infections, especially infections that don't clear up easily with proper treatment, see your doctor promptly to determine the cause of your symptoms and to receive proper medical care.
- If your symptoms return within two months or if you have infections that do not clear up easily with proper treatment, consult your doctor. You could be pregnant or there could be a serious underlying medical cause for your infections, including diabetes or a damaged immune system (including damage from infection with HIV—the virus that causes AIDS). (PLEASE READ EDUCATIONAL PAMPHLET FOUND INSIDE PACKAGE.)
- Do not use during pregnancy except under the advice and supervision of a doctor.
- This medication is for vaginal use only. It is not for use in the mouth or the eyes. In case accidentally swallowed, seek professional assistance or contact a Poison Control Center immediately.
- Keep this and all drugs out of reach of children. This product is not to be used on children less than 12 years of age.

Dosage: Fill the applicator with the cream and then insert one applicatorful of cream into the vagina every day, preferably at bedtime. Repeat this procedure for seven consecutive days.
Cream also available with 7 disposable applicators.

Shown in Product Identification Section, page 425

GYNE-LOTRIMIN®
Clotrimazole
Vaginal Inserts
Antifungal

Active Ingredient: Each insert contains Clotrimazole 100 mg.

Inactive Ingredients: Corn starch, lactose, magnesium stearate, povidone.

Indications: Gyne-Lotrimin® will cure most vaginal yeast (Candida) infections. Gyne-Lotrimin® usually starts to relieve the itching and other symptoms of vaginal yeast infection within 3 days. If the patient does not improve in 3 days or if the patient does not get well in 7 days, a condition other than yeast infection may exist. The patient should discontinue use of the product and consult a doctor. Also, if symptoms recur within a 2-month period, patient should consult a doctor.

Important: In order to kill the yeast completely, GYNE-LOTRIMIN must be used the full seven days, even if symptoms are relieved sooner.

Warnings:

- Do not use if you have abdominal pain, fever, or a foul-smelling vaginal discharge. You may have a condition which is more serious than a yeast infection. Contact your doctor immediately.
- Do not use if this is your first experience with vaginal itch and discomfort. See your doctor.
- If there is no improvement within 3 days, you may have a condition other than a yeast infection. Stop using this product and see your doctor.
- If you may have been exposed to the human immunodeficiency virus (HIV, the virus that causes AIDS) and are now having recurrent vaginal infections, especially infections that don't clear up easily with proper treatment, see your doctor promptly to determine the cause of your symptoms and to receive proper medical care.
- If your symptoms return within two months or if you have infections that do not clear up easily with proper treatment, consult your doctor. You could be pregnant or there could be a serious underlying medical cause for your infections, including diabetes or a damaged immune system (including damage from infection with HIV—the virus that causes AIDS). (PLEASE READ EDUCATIONAL PAMPHLET FOUND INSIDE PACKAGE.)
- Do not use during pregnancy except under the advice and supervision of a doctor.
- This medication is for vaginal use only. It is not for use in the mouth or the eyes. In case accidentally swallowed, seek professional assistance or contact a Poison Control Center immediately.
- Keep this and all drugs out of reach of children. This product is not to be used on children less than 12 years of age.

Dosage: Using the applicator, place one insert into the vagina, preferably at bedtime. Repeat this procedure for seven consecutive days.

Shown in Product Identification Section, page 425

GYNE-MOISTRIN™
Vaginal Moisturizing Gel

Description: Gyne-Moistrin Vaginal Moisturizing Gel was specially developed to soothe and relieve vaginal dryness. Gyne-Moistrin provides natural feeling moisture and lubrication. It is clear, colorless, odorless and proven to be non-irritating. Gyne-Moistrin is water-based, greaseless and non-staining; and it contains no hormones or medication, so it can be used as often as needed.

Actions: When used as directed, Gyne-Moistrin will relieve vaginal dryness. Gyne-Moistrin forms a non-occlusive layer of moisture over the vaginal epithelium, gradually hydrating a dry irritated area. Gyne-Moistrin can be used as often as needed.
Externally, in the vulvar area, Gyne-Moistrin will also moisturize tissues.

Ingredients: Polyglycerylmethacrylate, water, propylene glycol, methylparaben, propylparaben.

Warnings: Gyne-Moistrin is not a contraceptive. Does not harm condoms.

Directions: Gyne-Moistrin may be applied externally and internally according to personal preference using fingertip application or the reusable applicator.
FOR FINGERTIP APPLICATION: Squeeze out small amount of gel to cover fingertip and apply to the vaginal opening and external area as needed. Actual amount applied may be increased or decreased according to personal preference.
FOR INTERNAL USE: Remove reusable applicator from sealed wrapper. Fill with gel to line on applicator. Gently insert front end well into vagina; push end of applicator to fully release gel; remove applicator. Actual amount used may be increased or decreased according to personal preference. Wash applicator in warm soapy water then thoroughly rinse and dry before and after each use.
Store at room temperature.

How Supplied: Gyne-Moistrin is available in 1.5 oz. and 2.5 oz. tubes.

Shown in Product Identification Section, page 425

LOTRIMIN® AF ANTIFUNGAL
[lo-tre-min]
Cream 1%
Solution 1%
Lotion 1%

Description: Lotrimin® AF Cream 1% is a white fully vanishing homogeneous cream containing 1% clotrimazole. The cream contains no sensitizing parabens and is totally grease free and non-staining.

Lotrimin® AF Solution 1% is a non-aqueous liquid, containing polyethylene glycol.
Lotrimin® AF Lotion 1% is light penetrating buffered emulsion also containing no common sensitizing agents and is greaseless and nonstaining.

Indications: Lotrimin® AF Cream, Solution and Lotion contain 1% clotrimazole, a synthetic broad-spectrum antifungal agent. Clotrimazole is used for the treatment of dermal infections caused by a variety of pathogenic dermatophytes, yeasts and *Malassezia furfur*. The primary action of clotrimazole is against dividing and growing organisms. Lotrimin® AF was first made available as an over-the-counter drug in 1990 and is indicated for superficial dermatophyte infections: athlete's foot (tinea pedis), jock itch (tinea cruris) and ringworm (tinea corporis). Lotrimin® remains on prescription for topical candidiasis due to *Candida albicans* and tinea versicolor due to *Malassezia furfur*.

Directions: Cleanse skin with soap and water and dry thoroughly. Apply a thin layer over affected area morning and evening or as directed by a physician. For athlete's foot, pay special attention to the spaces between the toes. It is also helpful to wear well-fitting, ventilated shoes and to change shoes and socks at least once daily. Best results in athlete's foot and ringworm are usually obtained with 4 weeks use of this product, and in jock itch, with 2 weeks use. If satisfactory results have not occurred within these times, consult a physician or pharmacist. Children under 12 years of age should be supervised in the use of this product. This product is not effective on the scalp or nails.

How Supplied: Lotrimin® AF Antifungal Cream is available in a 0.42 oz. tube (12 grams) and a 0.84 oz. tube (24 grams).
Inactive ingredients include: benzyl alcohol, cetearyl alcohol, cetyl esters wax, octyldodecanol, polysorbate, sorbitan monostearate and water.
Lotrimin® AF Antifungal Solution is available in a 0.33 fl. oz. (10 milliliters) bottle. Inactive ingredients include PEG.
Lotrimin® AF Antifungal Lotion is available in a 0.66 fl. oz. (20 milliliters) bottle. Inactive ingredients include benzyl alcohol, cetearyl alcohol, cetyl esters wax, octyldodecanol, polysorbate, sodium biphosphate, sodium phosphate dibasic, sorbitan monostearate and water.

Storage: Keep Lotrimin® AF products between 2° and 30°C (36° and 86°F).

Shown in Product Identification Section, page 425

ST. JOSEPH®
ADULT CHEWABLE ASPIRIN
Low Strength Caplets (81 mg. each)

Active Ingredient: Each St. Joseph Adult Chewable Aspirin caplet contains 81 mg. (1.25 grains) aspirin in a chewable, pleasant citrus-flavored form.

Inactive Ingredients: D&C yellow No. 10 aluminum lake, FD&C yellow No. 6 aluminum lake, flavor, hydrogenated vegetable oil, maltodextrin, mannitol, saccharin, corn starch.

Indications: For safe, effective, temporary relief from: headache, muscular aches, minor aches and pain associated with overexertion, sprains, menstrual cramps, neuralgia, bursitis, and discomforts of fever due to colds.

Actions: Analgesic/Antipyretic.

Warnings: Children and teenagers should not use this medicine for chicken pox or flu symptoms before a doctor is consulted about Reye syndrome, a rare but serious illness reported to be associated with aspirin. As with any drug, if you are pregnant or nursing a baby, seek the advice of a health professional before using this product. **IT IS ESPECIALLY IMPORTANT NOT TO USE ASPIRIN DURING THE LAST 3 MONTHS OF PREGNANCY UNLESS SPECIFICALLY DIRECTED TO DO SO BY A DOCTOR BECAUSE IT MAY CAUSE PROBLEMS IN THE UNBORN CHILD OR COMPLICATIONS DURING DELIVERY.** If symptoms persist, or new ones occur, consult your doctor. NOTE: SEVERE OR PERSISTENT SORE THROAT, HIGH FEVER, HEADACHE, NAUSEA OR VOMITING, MAY BE SERIOUS, DISCONTINUE USE AND CONSULT YOUR DOCTOR IF NOT RELIEVED IN 24 HOURS. Do not take this product for more than five days unless directed by your doctor. Keep out of reach of children. In case of an accidental overdose, seek professional assistance or contact a poison control center immediately.

Dosage and Administration: Adult Dose—Analgesic/Antipyretic Indication: Take from 4 to 8 caplets (325 mg. to 650 mg.) every 4 hours as needed. Do not exceed 48 caplets in 24 hours. For professional dosage see below.

IN MYOCARDIAL INFARCTION PROPHYLAXIS

Indication: Aspirin is indicated to reduce the risk of death and/or nonfatal myocardial infarction in patients with a previous infarction or unstable angina pectoris.

Advantages of Product Form: Four St. Joseph Adult Chewable Aspirin caplets give patients the appropriate dosage (325 mg.) of aspirin to help prevent secondary MI. Because they're chewable, they can be taken anytime and anyplace. And they have a pleasant-tasting citrus flavor.

Clinical Trials: The indication is supported by the results of six, large, randomized, multicenter, placebo-controlled studies[1–7] involving 10,816, predominantly male, post–myocardial infarction (MI) patients and one randomized placebo-controlled study of 1,266 men with unstable angina. Therapy with aspirin was begun at intervals after the onset of acute MI varying from less than 3 days to more than 5 years and continued for periods of from less than 1 year to 4 years. In the unstable angina study, treatment was started within 1 month after the onset of unstable angina and continued for 12 weeks; complicating conditions, such as congestive heart failure were not included in the study.
Aspirin therapy in MI patients was associated with about a 20% reduction in the risk of subsequent death and/or nonfatal reinfarction, a median absolute decrease of 3% from the 12 to 22% event rates in the placebo groups. In aspirin-treated unstable angina patients the reduction in risk was about 50%, a reduction in event rate of 5% from the 10% rate in the placebo group over the 12 weeks of the study.
Daily dosage of aspirin in the post–myocardial infarction studies was 300 mg. in one study and 900 to 1500 mg. in five studies. A dose of 325 mg. was used in the study of unstable angina.

Adverse Reactions: Gastrointestinal Reactions—Doses of 1000 mg. per day of aspirin caused gastrointestinal symptoms and bleeding that in some cases were clinically significant. In the largest postinfarction study, the Aspirin Myocardial Infarction Study (AMIS) trial with 4,500 people, the percentage incidences of gastrointestinal symptoms for the aspirin (1000 mg. of a standard, solid-tablet formulation) and placebo-treated subjects, respectively, were: stomach pain (14.3%; 4.4%); heartburn (11.9%; 4.3%); nausea and/or vomiting (7.3%; 2.1%); hospitalization for GI disorder (4.9%; 3.3%). In the AMIS and other trials, aspirin-treated patients had increased rates of gross gastrointestinal bleeding.

Cardiovascular and Biochemical: In the AMIS trial, the dosage of 1000 mg. per day of aspirin was associated with small increases in systolic blood pressure (BP) (average 1.5 to 2.1 mm) and diastolic BP (0.5 to 0.6 mm), depending upon whether maximal or last available readings were used. Blood urea nitrogen and uric acid levels were also increased, but by less than 1.0 mg.%. Subjects with marked hypertension or renal insufficiency had been excluded from the trial so that the clinical importance of these observations for such subjects or for any subjects treated over more prolonged periods is not known. It is recommended that patients placed on long-term aspirin treatment, even at doses of 300 mg. per day, be seen at regular intervals to assess changes in these measurements.

Dosage and Administration: Although most of the studies used dosages exceed-

Continued on next page

Information on Schering-Plough HealthCare Products appearing on these pages is effective as of November 1992.

Schering-Plough—Cont.

ing 300 mg., two trials used only 300 mg. daily, and pharmacologic data indicate that this dose inhibits platelet function fully. Therefore, 300 mg. or a conventional 325 mg. aspirin dose daily is a reasonable routine dose that would minimize gastrointestinal adverse reactions.

How Supplied: Chewable citrus-flavored caplets in plastic bottles of 36 caplets each.

References: (1) Elwood, P.C., et al.: A Randomized Controlled Trial of Acetylsalicylic Acid in the Secondary Prevention of Mortality from Myocardial Infarction, *British Medical Journal,* 1:436–440, 1974. (2) The Coronary Drug Project Research Group: "Aspirin in Coronary Heart Disease," *Journal of Chronic Disease,* 29:625–642, 1976. (3) Breddin, K., et al.: "Secondary Prevention of Myocardial Infarction: A Comparison of Acetylsalicylic Acid, Placebo and Phenprocoumon, *Homeostasis,* 9:325–344, 1980. (4) Aspirin Myocardial Infarction Study Research Group, "A Randomized, Controlled Trial of Aspirin in Persons Recovered from Myocardial Infarction," *Journal American Medical Association,* 245:661–669, 1980. (5) Elwood, P.C., and Sweetnam, P.M., "Aspirin and Secondary Mortality After Myocardial Infarction," *Lancet,* pp. 1313–1315, December 22–29, 1979. (6) The Persantine-Aspirin Reinfarction Study Research Group, "Persantine and Aspirin in Coronary Heart Disease," *Circulation,* 62: 449–460, 1980. (7) Lewis, H.D., et al., "Protective Effects of Aspirin Against Acute Myocardial Infarction and Death in Men with Unstable Angina. Results of a Veterans Administration Cooperative Study," *New England Journal of Medicine,* 309:396–403, 1983.

ST. JOSEPH® Aspirin-Free Fever Reducer for Children Chewable Tablets

Active Ingredient: Each Children's St. Joseph Aspirin-Free Chewable Tablet contains 80 mg. acetaminophen in a fruit-flavored tablet.

Inactive Ingredients: Tablets: Cellulose, D&C red No. 7 calcium lake, D&C red No. 30 aluminum lake, flavor, mannitol, silicon dioxide, sodium saccharin, zinc stearate.

Indications: For temporary reduction of fever, relief of minor aches and pains of colds and flu.

Actions: Analgesic/Antipyretic

Warnings: Do not administer this product for more than 5 days. If symptoms persist or new ones occur, consult physician. If fever persists for more than three days, or recurs, consult physician. When using St. Joseph Aspirin-Free products do not give other medications containing acetaminophen unless directed by your physician. NOTE: SEVERE OR PERSISTENT SORE THROAT, HIGH FEVER, HEADACHES, NAUSEA OR VOMITING MAY BE SERIOUS. DISCONTINUE USE AND CONSULT PHYSICIAN IF NOT RELIEVED IN 24 HOURS. Do not exceed recommended dosage because severe liver damage may occur. As with any drug, if you are pregnant or nursing a baby, seek the advice of a health professional before using this product. Keep this and all drugs out of the reach of children. In case of accidental overdose, seek professional assistance or contact a Poison Control Center immediately.

Dosage and Administration: [See table below.]
ST. JOSEPH Aspirin-Free Fever Reducer Tablets for Children may be given one of three ways. Always follow with ½ glass of water, milk or fruit juice.
1. Chewed, followed by liquid.
2. Crushed or dissolved in a teaspoon of liquid (for younger children).
3. Powdered for infant use, when so directed by physician.

How Supplied: Chewable fruit flavored tablets in plastic bottles of 30 tablets.
All packages have child resistant safety caps and safety sealed packaging.

ST. JOSEPH® Cold Tablets for Children

Active Ingredients: Per tablet: Acetaminophen 80 mg and phenylpropanolamine hydrochloride 3.125 mg.

Inactive Ingredients: Cellulose, FD&C Yellow No. 6 aluminum lake, flavor, mannitol, silica, sodium saccharin, zinc stearate.

Indications: ST. JOSEPH Cold Tablets combine acetaminophen with a gentle nasal decongestant to relieve congestion, runny nose, difficult breathing, and fever which accompany colds in children. (1) Acetaminophen is widely recommended by pediatricians to reduce fever fast and relieve the aches and pains of cold and flu without causing stomach upset or irritation. (2) The gentle nasal decongestant quickly relieves a stuffy nose and helps restore easier breathing without causing drowsiness. ST. JOSEPH Cold Tablets are sugar-free and fruit-flavored.

DOSAGE BY AGE AND WEIGHT
To be administered under adult supervision

Age (Years)	Weight (lbs.)	Dosage
Under 2...	below 27	As directed by physician.
2–3	27–35	2 tablets
4–5	36–45	3 tablets
6–8	46–65	4 tablets
9–10	66–76	5 tablets
11	77–83	6 tablets
12+	84 & over	8 tablets

May be repeated every 4 hours, but do not exceed 4 doses daily, unless prescribed by your doctor.
ST. JOSEPH Cold Tablets for Children may be dissolved on the child's tongue, chewed or swallowed whole. Always follow immediately with liquid. For younger children crush and dissolve in spoon of liquid.
Each tablet contains: Acetaminophen 80 mg. and phenylpropanolamine hydrochloride 3.125 mg.

Warning: Do not take this product for more than five days. If symptoms persist, or new ones occur, consult your physician. If fever persists for more than three days, or recurs, consult your physician. Do not exceed recommended dosage because severe liver damage may occur. When using ST. JOSEPH Cold Tablets do not give other medications containing acetaminophen unless directed by your physician. NOTE: SEVERE OR PERSISTENT SORE THROAT, HIGH FEVER, HEADACHE, NAUSEA OR VOMITING MAY BE SERIOUS. DISCONTINUE USE AND CONSULT PHYSICIAN IF NOT RELIEVED IN 24 HOURS. As with any drug, if you are pregnant or nursing a baby, seek the advice of a health professional before using this product. Keep this and all drugs out of the reach of chil-

ST. JOSEPH® Aspirin-Free Fever Reducer for Children

ST. JOSEPH CHILDREN'S DOSAGE CHART

Age	0–3 (months)	4–11 (months)	12–23 (months)	2–3 (years)	4–5 (years)	6–8 (years)	9–10 (years)	11 (years)	12+ (years)
Weight (lbs.)	7–12	13–21	22–26	27–35	36–45	46–65	66–76	77–83	84+
Chewable Tablets Acetaminophen (80 mg. each)	—	—	1½	2	3	4	5	6	8

All dosages may be repeated every 4 hours, but do not exceed 5 dosages daily.
Note: Since St. Joseph pediatric products are available without prescription, parents are advised on the package label to consult a physician for use in children under two years.

dren. In case of accidental overdose, seek professional assistance or contact a Poison Control center immediately.

How Supplied: In bottle with 30 fruit flavored chewable tablets.

ST. JOSEPH® Cough Suppressant for Children
Pediatric
Antitussive Suppressant

Active Ingredient: Dextromethorphan hydrobromide 7.5 mg. per 5 ml. (teaspoonful)

Inactive Ingredients: Caramel, citric acid, flavor, glycerin, methylparaben, propylparaben, sodium benzoate, sodium citrate, sucrose, water.

Indications: Temporarily relieves cough associated with a common cold or inhaled irritants. Quiets coughing to help you and your child get needed sleep. The non-narcotic SUPPRESSIN* formula gives advantages of codeine without its side effects.

Dose

Age (yrs.)	WT. (lbs.)	Dosage
Under 2	Below 27	As directed by physician.
2–6	27–45	1 teaspoon every 6 to 8 hours (not to exceed 4 tsp. daily)
6–12	46–83	2 teaspoons every 6 to 8 hours (not to exceed 8 tsp. daily)
12+	84+	4 teaspoons every 6 to 8 hours (not to exceed 16 tsp. daily)

Do not exceed 4 doses per day.

Warnings: Do not give this product to children under 2 years except under the advice and supervision of a physician. Do not take this product for persistent or chronic cough such as occurs with smoking, asthma, or emphysema, or where cough is accompanied by excessive mucus unless directed by a doctor. As with any drug, if you are pregnant or nursing a baby, seek the advice of a health professional before using this product.

Caution: A persistent cough may be a sign of serious condition. If cough persists for more than 1 week, tends to recur or is accompanied by high fever, rash or persistent headache, consult a physician. Keep this and all drugs out of the reach of children. In case of accidental overdose, seek professional assistance or contact a Poison Control Center immediately.

How Supplied: Alcohol-Free Cherry tasting suppressant in plastic bottle of 2 fl. ozs. In safety sealed packaging.

*Dextromethorphan Hydrobromide

TINACTIN® Antifungal
[tin-ak'tin]
Cream 1%
Solution 1%
Powder 1%
Powder (1%) Aerosol
Liquid (1%) Aerosol
Deodorant Powder Aerosol 1%
Jock Itch Cream 1%
Jock Itch Spray Powder 1%

Description: TINACTIN Cream 1% is a white homogeneous, nonaqueous preparation containing the highly active synthetic fungicidal agent, tolnaftate. Each gram contains 10 mg tolnaftate solubilized in BHT, Carbomer, Monoamylamine, PEG-8, Propylene Glycol, and Titanium Dioxide.

TINACTIN Jock Itch Cream 1% is a smooth white homogeneous cream containing the highly active synthetic fungicidal agent, tolnaftate. Each gram contains 10 mg tolnaftate finely dispersed in a water-washable emulsion containing: Cetearyl Alcohol, Ceteareth-30, Chlorocresol, Mineral Oil, Petrolatum, Propylene Glycol, Sodium Phosphate and Water. Phosphoric acid and sodium hydroxide used to adjust pH.

TINACTIN Solution 1% contains in each ml tolnaftate 10 mg, BHT, and PEG. The solution solidifies at low temperatures but liquefies readily when warmed, retaining its potency.

TINACTIN Liquid Aerosol contains 91 mg tolnaftate in a vehicle of Alcohol SD-40-2 (36% w/w), BHT and PPG-12 Buteth-16. The spray deposits solution containing a concentration of 1% tolnaftate.

Each gram of **TINACTIN Powder 1%** contains tolnaftate 10 mg in a vehicle of corn starch and talc.

TINACTIN Powder Aerosol contains 91 mg tolnaftate in a vehicle of Alcohol SD-40-2 (14% w/w), BHT, Hydrocarbon Propellant, PPG-12 Buteth-16 and Talc. The spray deposits a white clinging powder containing a concentration of 1% tolnaftate.

TINACTIN Deodorant Powder Aerosol contains tolnaftate in a vehicle of SD Alcohol 40 (14% w/w), talc, PPG-12-Buteth-16, starch/acrylates/acrylamide copolymer, fragrance, BHT. The spray deposits a white clinging powder containing a concentration of 1% tolnaftate.

TINACTIN Jock Itch Spray Powder contains 91 mg tolnaftate in a vehicle of Alcohol SD-40-2 (14% w/w), BHT, Hydrocarbon Propellant, PPG-12 Buteth-16, Talc. The spray deposits a white clinging powder containing a concentration of 1% tolnaftate.

Indications: TINACTIN Cream, Solution, Liquid Aerosol and **TINACTIN Jock Itch Cream** are highly active antifungal agents that are effective in killing superficial fungi of the skin which cause tinea pedis (athlete's foot), tinea cruris (jock itch) and tinea corporis (body ringworm).

TINACTIN Powder, Powder Aerosol, Deodorant Powder Aerosol and **TINACTIN Jock Itch Spray Powder** are effective in killing superficial fungi of the skin which cause tinea cruris (jock itch) and/or tinea pedis (athlete's foot). All forms begin to relieve burning, itching and soreness quickly. The powder and powder aerosol forms aid the drying of naturally moist areas. The deodorant powder aerosol provides additional protection against odor and wetness.

Actions: The active ingredient in TINACTIN, tolnaftate, is a highly active synthetic fungicidal agent that is effective in the treatment of superficial fungous infections of the skin. It is inactive systemically, virtually nonsensitizing, and does not ordinarily sting or irritate intact or broken skin, even in the presence of acute inflammatory reactions.

TINACTIN products are odorless, greaseless, and do not stain or discolor the skin, hair, or nails.

Warnings: Keep these and all drugs out of the reach of children. Do not use in children under 2 years of age except under the advice and supervision of a physician.

TINACTIN Powder Aerosol, Deodorant Powder Aerosol and **Liquid Aerosol:** Avoid spraying in eyes. Contents under pressure. Do not puncture or incinerate. Flammable mixture, do not use or store near heat or open flame. Exposure to temperatures above 120°F may cause bursting. Never throw container into fire or incinerator. Use only as directed. Intentional misuse by deliberately concentrating and inhaling the contents can be harmful or fatal.

Precautions: If irritation occurs or symptoms do not improve within 10 days, discontinue use and consult your physician or podiatrist.

TINACTIN products are for external use only. Keep out of eyes.

TINACTIN is not effective on nail or scalp infections.

Overdosage: In case of accidental ingestion, seek professional assistance or contact a Poison Control Center immediately.

Dosage and Administration: Children under 12 years of age should be supervised in the use of TINACTIN.

TINACTIN Cream and **TINACTIN Jock Itch Cream**—Wash and dry infected area. Then apply a thin layer of cream and massage gently.

Best results in athlete's foot and body ringworm are usually obtained with 4 weeks use of this product and in jock itch, with 2 weeks use. To help prevent recurrence of athlete's foot, continue treatment for two weeks after disappearance of all symptoms.

Continued on next page

Information on Schering-Plough HealthCare Products appearing on these pages is effective as of November 1992.

Schering-Plough—Cont.

TINACTIN Solution—Wash and dry infected area morning and evening. Then apply two or three drops, and massage gently to cover the infected area. Best results in athlete's foot and body ringworm are usually obtained with 4 weeks use of this product and in jock itch, with 2 weeks use. To help prevent recurrence of athlete's foot, continue treatment for two weeks after disappearance of all symptoms.

TINACTIN Liquid Aerosol—Wash and dry infected area. Spray from a distance of 6 to 10 inches morning and evening or as directed by a doctor. For athlete's foot, spray between toes and on feet. For jock itch, spray infected area. Best results in athlete's foot are usually obtained with 4 weeks use of this product and in jock itch, with 2 weeks use. Continue treatment for two weeks after symptoms disappear. To help prevent reinfection of athlete's foot, bathe daily, dry carefully and apply **TINACTIN Powder** daily.

TINACTIN Powder—Wash and dry infected area. Sprinkle powder liberally on all areas of infection and in shoes or socks morning and evening or as directed by a doctor. Best results in athlete's foot are usually obtained with 4 weeks use of this product and in jock itch, with 2 weeks use. Continue treatment for two weeks after symptoms disappear. To prevent recurrence of athlete's foot, bathe daily, dry carefully and apply **TINACTIN Powder.**

TINACTIN Powder Aerosol, Deodorant Powder Aerosol and **TINACTIN Jock Itch Spray Powder**—Wash and dry infected area. Shake container well before using. Spray liberally from a distance of 6 to 10 inches onto affected area morning and night or as directed by a doctor. Best results in athlete's foot are usually obtained with 4 weeks use of this product and in jock itch, with 2 weeks use. To help prevent recurrence of athlete's foot, bathe daily, dry carefully and apply **TINACTIN Powder Aerosol or TINACTIN Deodorant Powder Aerosol.**

How Supplied: TINACTIN Antifungal Cream 1%, 15 g (½ oz) and 30 g (1 oz) collapsible tube with dispensing tip. **TINACTIN Antifungal Solution 1%,** 10 ml (⅓ oz) plastic squeeze bottle. **TINACTIN Antifungal Liquid (1%) Aerosol,** 113 g (4 oz) spray can. **TINACTIN Antifungal Powder 1%,** 45 g (1.5 oz) and 90 g (3.0 oz) plastic containers. **TINACTIN Antifungal Powder (1%) Aerosol,** 100 g (3.5 oz) and 150 g (5.0 oz) spray containers. TINACTIN Antifungal Deodorant Powder Aerosol 100 g (3.5 oz.) spray container. **TINACTIN Antifungal Jock Itch Cream 1%,** 15 g (½ oz) collapsible tube with dispensing tip. **TINACTIN Antifungal Jock Itch Spray Powder (1%),** 100 g (3.5 oz) spray can.

Store TINACTIN products between 36° and 86°F (2° and 30°C).

Shown in Product Identification Section, pages 425 and 426

Scot-Tussin Pharmacal Co., Inc.
P.O. BOX 8217
CRANSTON, RI 02920-0217

The following SCOT-TUSSIN® may be taken by individuals with diabetes, heart condition and/or high blood pressure:

SCOT-TUSSIN SUGAR-FREE DM
Antitussive-Antihistaminic
Dextromethorphan
Chlorpheniramine Maleate

(Dextromethorphan 15 mg/5 ml, chlorpheniramine maleate 2 mg/5 ml).
No alcohol, sorbitol, saccharin, or decongestant.
#036

SCOT-TUSSIN® SUGAR-FREE ALLERGY RELIEF FORMULA
Antihistaminic
Diphenhydramine HCl

(Diphenhydramine HCl 12.5 mg/5 ml).
No alcohol, sorbitol, saccharin, dye.
#047-04

SCOT-TUSSIN® SUGAR-FREE COUGH CHASERS Lozenges
Antitussive
Dextromethorphan

No sodium, dye. DM 2.5 mg/lozenge.
#044-20

SCOT-TUSSIN® SUGAR-FREE EXPECTORANT
Guaifenesin

(Guaifenesin 100 mg/5 ml, 3.5% alcohol).
No sorbitol, sodium, dye, saccharin.
#006-04

VITALIZE™ SUGAR-FREE STRESS FORMULA WITH IRON
B Complex, B_{12}, Iron

No sugar, alcohol, sorbitol, dye, saccharin.
#021-04; -16

Products are
indexed alphabetically
in the
PINK SECTION.

SmithKline Beecham Consumer Brands
Unit of SmithKline Beecham, Inc.
POST OFFICE BOX 1467
PITTSBURGH, PA 15230

A-200®[1]
Pediculicide Shampoo Concentrate

Description: Active Ingredients: Pyrethrins 0.30% and piperonyl butoxide, technical 3.00%, equivalent to 2.4% (butylcarbityl) (6-propylpiperonyl) ether and to 0.6.% related compounds. Also contains petroleum distillate 1.20% and benzyl alcohol 2.4% and remaining inert ingredients 93.1%.

Indications: A-200 is indicated for the treatment of head lice, body lice, and pubic (crab) lice.

Actions: A-200 is an effective pediculicide to kill head lice (pediculus humanus capitis), body lice (pediculus humanus corporis), and pubic (crab) lice (phthirus pubis).

Warning: A-200 should be used with caution by ragweed sensitized-persons.

Precautions: This product is for external use on humans only. It is harmful if swallowed. If accidently swallowed, call a physician or Poison Control Center immediately. It should not be inhaled. It should be kept out of the eyes and contact with mucous membranes should be avoided. If accidental contact with eyes occurs, flush eyes immediately with plenty of water. Call a physician if eye irritation persists. In case of infection or skin irritation, discontinue use immediately and consult a physician. Consult a physician before using this product if infestation of eyebrows or eyelashes occurs. Avoid contamination of feed or foodstuffs. Keep out of reach of children.

Storage and Disposal: Do not contaminate water, food or feed by storage or disposal. Do not transport or store below 32°F. Do not reuse empty container. Wrap in several layers of newspaper and discard in trash.

Directions for Use: It is a violation of Federal law to use the product in a manner inconsistent with its labeling. 1. Shake well. Apply undiluted A-200 to dry hair and scalp or any other infested areas and wet entirely. Do not use on eyelashes or eyebrows. 2. Allow A-200 shampoo to remain on area for 10 minutes before washing thoroughly with warm water and soap or regular shampoo. 3. Dead lice and eggs should be removed with special A-200 precision comb provided. 4. Repeat treatment in 7–10 days to kill any newly hatched lice. Do not exceed two consecutive applications within 24 hours.
Since lice infestations are spread by contact, it is important that each family member be examined carefully. If infested, they should be treated promptly to avoid spread or reinfestation of previously treated individuals. To eliminate infestation, all personal head gear,

scarfs, coats, and bed linen should be laundered in hot water or dry cleaned. Carpets, upholstery, and mattresses should be vacuumed thoroughly. Combs and brushes should be soaked in hot water (above 130°) for 5 to 10 minutes.

How Supplied: In 2 and 4 fl. oz. unbreakable plastic bottles. An A-200 precision comb that removes nits and patient instruction booklet in English and Spanish are included in each carton. Also available in combination with A-200 Lice Treatment Kit.

Shown in Product Identification Section, page 426

CĒPACOL®/CĒPACOL MINT
[sē 'pə-cŏl]
Mouthwash/Gargle

Description: Cēpacol Mouthwash contains: Ceepryn® (cetylpyridinium chloride) 0.05%. Also contains: Alcohol 14%, Edetate Disodium, FD&C Yellow No. 5 (tartrazine) as a color additive, Flavors, Glycerin, Polysorbate 80, Saccharin, Sodium Biphosphate, Sodium Phosphate, and Water.
Cēpacol Mint Mouthwash contains: Ceepryn® (cetylpyridinium chloride) 0.05%. Also contains: Alcohol 14.5%, D&C Yellow No. 10, FD&C Green No. 3, Flavor, Glucono Delta-Lactone, Glycerin, Poloxamer 407, Saccharin Sodium, Sodium Gluconate, and Water.

Actions: Cēpacol/Cēpacol Mint is a soothing, pleasant-tasting mouthwash/gargle. It kills germs that cause bad breath for a fresher, cleaner mouth.
Cēpacol/Cēpacol Mint has a low surface tension, approximately ½ that of water. This property is the basis of the spreading action in the oral cavity as well as its foaming action. Cēpacol/Cēpacol Mint leaves the mouth feeling fresh and clean and helps provide soothing, temporary relief of dryness and minor mouth irritations.

Uses: Recommended as a mouthwash and gargle for daily oral care; as an aromatic mouth freshener to provide a clean feeling in the mouth; as a soothing, foaming rinse to freshen the mouth.
Used routinely before dental procedures, helps give patient confidence of not offending with mouth odor. Often employed as a foaming and refreshing rinse before, during, and after instrumentation and dental prophylaxis. Convenient as a mouth-freshening agent after taking dental impressions. Helpful in reducing the unpleasant taste and odor in the mouth following gingivectomy.
Used in hospitals as a mouthwash and gargle for daily oral care. Also used to refresh and soothe the mouth following emesis, inhalation therapy, and intubations, and for swabbing the mouths of patients incapable of personal care.

Warning: Keep out of the reach of children.

Directions for Use: Rinse vigorously before or after brushing or any time to freshen the mouth. Particularly useful after meals or before social engagements. Cēpacol/Cēpacol Mint leaves the mouth feeling refreshingly clean.
Use full strength every two or three hours as a soothing, foaming gargle, or as directed by a physician or dentist. May also be mixed with warm water.
Product label directions are as follows: Use full strength. Rinse mouth thoroughly before or after brushing or whenever desired or use as directed by a physician or dentist.

How Supplied:
Cēpacol Mouthwash: 12 oz, 18 oz, 24 oz, and 32 oz. 4 oz trial size.

Shown in Product Identification Section, page 426

CĒPACOL®
[sē 'pə-cŏl]
Dry Throat Lozenges
Cherry Flavor

Description: Each lozenge contains Menthol 3.6 mg. Also contains: Benzyl Alcohol, Cetylpyridinium Chloride, D&C Red No. 33, FD&C Red No. 40, Flavor, Liquid Glucose, and Sucrose.

Actions: Menthol provides a cooling sensation to aid in symptomatic relief of minor throat irritations.

Indications: Cēpacol Cherry Flavor Lozenges provide temporary relief of occasional dry, scratchy throat.

Warnings: If sore throat is severe, persists for more than 2 days, is accompanied or followed by fever, headache, rash, nausea, or vomiting, consult a physician promptly. If sore mouth symptoms do not improve in 7 days, see your dentist or physician promptly. Do not administer to children under 6 years of age unless directed by physician or dentist. Keep this and all drugs out of the reach of children. In case of accidental overdose, seek professional assistance or contact a Poison Control Center immediately. As with any drug, if you are pregnant or nursing a baby, seek the advice of a health professional before using this product.

Dosage and Administration: Adults and children 6 years of age and older: Allow product to dissolve slowly in the mouth. May be repeated every 2 hours as needed or as directed by a dentist or physician. Do not exceed 10 lozenges per day.

How Supplied:
18 lozenges in 2 pocket packs of 9 each. Store at room temperature, below 86°F (30°C). Protect contents from humidity.

Shown in Product Identification Section, page 426

CĒPACOL®
[sē-pə-cŏl]
Dry Throat Lozenges
Honey-Lemon Flavor

Description: Each lozenge contains Menthol 3.6 mg. Also contains: Benzyl Alcohol, Caramel, Cetylpyridinium Chloride, FD&C Yellow No. 6, D&C Yellow No. 10, Flavors, Liquid Glucose, and Sucrose.

Actions: Menthol provides a cooling sensation to aid in symptomatic relief of minor throat irritations.

Indications: Cēpacol Honey-Lemon Flavor Lozenges provide temporary relief of occasional dry, scratchy throat.

Warnings: If sore throat is severe, persists for more than 2 days, is accompanied or followed by fever, headache, rash, nausea, or vomiting, consult a physician promptly. If sore mouth symptoms do not improve in 7 days, see your dentist or physician promptly. Do not administer to children under 6 years of age unless directed by physician or dentist. Keep this and all drugs out of the reach of children. In case of accidental overdose, seek professional assistance or contact a Poison Control Center immediately. As with any drug, if you are pregnant or nursing a baby, seek the advice of a health professional before using this product.

Dosage and Administration: Adults and children 6 years of age and older: Allow product to dissolve slowly in the mouth. May be repeated every 2 hours as needed or as directed by a dentist or physician.

How Supplied:
18 lozenges in 2 pocket packs of 9 each. Store at room temperature, below 86°F (30°C). Protect contents from humidity.

Shown in Product Identification Section, page 426

CĒPACOL®
[sē-pə-cŏl]
Dry Throat Lozenges
Menthol-Eucalyptus Flavor

Description: Each lozenge contains Menthol 5.0 mg. Also contains: Benzyl Alcohol, Cetylpyridinium Chloride, Eucalyptol, Liquid Glucose, and Sucrose.

Actions: Menthol provides a cooling sensation to aid in symptomatic relief of minor throat irritations.

Indications: Cēpacol Menthol-Eucalyptus Flavor Lozenges provide temporary relief of occasional dry, scratchy throat.

Warnings: If sore throat is severe, persists for more than 2 days, is accompanied or followed by fever, headache, rash, nausea, or vomiting, consult a physician promptly. If sore mouth symptoms do not improve in 7 days, see your dentist or physician promptly. Do not administer to children under 6 years of age unless di-

Continued on next page

SmithKline Beecham—Cont.

rected by physician or dentist. Keep this and all drugs out of the reach of children. In case of accidental overdose, seek professional assistance or contact a Poison Control Center immediately. As with any drug, if you are pregnant or nursing a baby, seek the advice of a health professional before using this product.

Dosage and Administration: Adults and children 6 years of age and older: Allow product to dissolve slowly in the mouth. May be repeated every 2 hours as needed or as directed by a dentist or physician.

How Supplied:
18 lozenges in 2 pocket packs of 9 each.
Store at room temperature, below 86°F (30°C). Protect contents from humidity.

Shown in Product Identification Section, page 426

CĒPACOL®
[*sē'pə-cŏl*]
Dry Throat Lozenges
Original Flavor

Description: Each lozenge contains Ceepryn® (cetylpyridinium chloride) 0.07%, Benzyl Alcohol 0.3%. Also contains: FD&C Yellow No. 5 (tartrazine) as a color additive, Flavor, Glucose, and Sucrose.

Actions: Cetylpyridinium chloride (Ceepryn) is a cationic quaternary ammonium compound, which is a surface-active agent. Aqueous solutions of cetylpyridinium chloride have a surface tension lower than that of water.
Cetylpyridinium chloride in the concentration used in Cēpacol is nonirritating to tissues.

Indications: For soothing, temporary relief of dryness of the mouth and throat.

Warnings: Severe sore throat or sore throat accompanied by high fever, headache, nausea, or vomiting, or any sore throat or mouth irritations persisting more than 2 days may be serious. Consult a physician promptly. Persons with a high fever or persistent cough should not use this preparation unless directed by a physician. Do not administer to children under 6 years of age unless directed by a physician or dentist. If sensitive to any of the ingredients, do not use. Keep this and all drugs out of the reach of children. In case of accidental overdose, seek professional assistance or contact a Poison Control Center immediately. As with any drug, if you are pregnant or nursing a baby, seek the advice of a health professional before using this product.

Dosage and Administration: Adults and children 6 years and older, dissolve 1 lozenge in the mouth every 2 hours, if needed. For children under 6 years, consult a physician or dentist.

How Supplied:
Trade Package: 18 lozenges in 2 pocket packs of 9 each.
Professional Package: 648 lozenges in 72 blisters of 9 each.
Store at room temperature, below 86°F (30°C). Protect contents from humidity.

Shown in Product Identification Section, page 426

CĒPACOL®
[*sē'pə-cŏl*]
Anesthetic Lozenges (Troches)

Description: Each lozenge contains Benzocaine 10 mg, Ceepryn® (cetylpyridinium chloride) 0.07%. Also contains: FD&C Blue No. 1, FD&C Yellow No. 5 (tartrazine) as a color additive, Flavors, Glucose, and Sucrose.

Actions: Cetylpyridinium chloride (Ceepryn) is a cationic quaternary ammonium compound, which is a surface-active agent. Aqueous solutions of cetylpyridinium chloride have a surface tension lower than that of water.
Cetylpyridinium chloride in the concentration used in Cēpacol is nonirritating to tissues.
Cēpacol Anesthetic Lozenges stimulate salivation to relieve dryness of the mouth and provide a mild anesthetic effect for pain relief.

Indications: For fast, temporary relief of minor sore throat pain. For temporary relief of minor pain and discomfort associated with tonsillitis and pharyngitis.

Warnings: If sore throat is severe, persists for more than 2 days, is accompanied or followed by fever, headache, rash, nausea, or vomiting, consult a physician promptly. Keep this and all drugs out of the reach of children. In case of accidental overdose, seek professional assistance or contact a Poison Control Center immediately. As with any drug, if you are pregnant or nursing a baby, seek the advice of a health professional before using this product.

Dosage and Administration: Adults and children 6 years and older, dissolve 1 lozenge in the mouth every 2 hours, if needed. For children under 6 years, consult a physician or dentist.

How Supplied:
Trade Package: 18 lozenges in 2 pocket packs of 9 each.
Professional Package: 324 lozenges in 36 blisters of 9 each.
Store at room temperature, below 86°F (30°C). Protect contents from humidity.

Shown in Product Identification Section, page 426

CĒPASTAT®
[*sē'pə-stăt*]
Sore Throat Lozenges
Cherry Flavor and Extra Strength

Description: Each Cherry Flavor lozenge contains: Phenol 14.5 mg. Also contains: Antifoam Emulsion, D&C Red No. 33, FD&C Yellow No. 6, Flavor, Gum Crystal, Mannitol, Menthol, Saccharin Sodium, and Sorbitol.
Each Extra Strength lozenge contains: Phenol 29 mg. Also contains: Antifoam Emulsion, Caramel, Eucalyptus Oil, Gum Crystal, Mannitol, Menthol, Saccharin Sodium, and Sorbitol.

Actions: Phenol is a recognized topical anesthetic. The sugar-free formula should not promote tooth decay as sugar-based lozenges can.

Indications: For fast, temporary relief of minor sore throat pain.

Warnings: If sore throat is severe, persists for more than 2 days, is accompanied or followed by fever, headache, rash, nausea, or vomiting, consult a physician promptly. If sore mouth symptoms do not improve in 7 days, see your dentist or physician promptly. Keep this and all drugs out of the reach of children. In case of accidental overdose, seek professional assistance or contact a Poison Control Center immediately. As with any drug, if you are pregnant or nursing a baby, seek the advice of a health professional before using this product.

Note to Diabetics: Each lozenge contributes approximately 8 calories from 2 grams of sorbitol.

Dosage and Administration:
Lozenges–Cherry Flavor
Adults and children 12 years of age and older: Allow the lozenge to dissolve slowly in the mouth. May be repeated every 2 hours, or as directed by a dentist or physician. Children 6 to under 12 years of age: Allow lozenge to dissolve slowly in the mouth. May be repeated every 2 hours, not to exceed 10 lozenges per day, or as directed by a dentist or physician. Children under 6 years of age: Consult a dentist or physician.
Lozenges–Extra Strength
Adults and children 12 years of age and older: Allow the lozenge to dissolve slowly in the mouth. May be repeated every 2 hours, or as directed by a dentist or physician. Children 6 to under 12 years of age: Allow lozenge to dissolve slowly in the mouth. May be repeated every 2 hours, not to exceed 10 lozenges per day, or as directed by a dentist or physician. Children under 6 years of age: Consult a dentist or physician.

How Supplied:
Lozenges–Cherry Flavor
Trade package: Boxes of 18 lozenges as 2 pocket packs of 9 lozenges each.
Professional package: 648 lozenges in 72 blisters of 9 lozenges each.
Lozenges–Extra Strength
Trade package: Boxes of 18 lozenges as 2 pocket packs of 9 lozenges each.
Professional package: 648 lozenges in 72 blisters of 9 lozenges each.
Store at room temperature, below 86°F (30°C). Protect contents from humidity.

Shown in Product Identification Section, page 426

Orange Flavor
CITRUCEL®
[*sĭt 'rə-sĕl*]
(Methylcellulose)
Bulk-forming Fiber Laxative

Description: Each 19 g adult dose (approximately one heaping measuring tablespoonful) contains Methylcellulose 2 g. Each 9.5 g child's dose (one-half the adult dose) contains Methylcellulose 1 g. Methylcellulose is a nonallergenic fiber. Also contains: Citric Acid, FD&C Yellow No. 6, Orange Flavors (natural and artificial), Potassium Citrate, Riboflavin, Sucrose, and other ingredients. Each adult dose contains approximately 3 mg of sodium, 105 mg of potassium, and contributes 60 calories from Sucrose.

Actions: Promotes elimination by providing additional fiber (bulk) to the diet. This product generally produces bowel movement in 12 to 72 hours.

Indications: For relief of constipation (irregularity). May also be used for relief of constipation associated with other bowel disorders such as irritable bowel syndrome, diverticular disease, and hemorrhoids as well as for bowel management during postpartum, postsurgical, and convalescent periods when recommended by a physician.

Contraindications: Intestinal obstruction, fecal impaction, known hypersensitivity to formula ingredients.

Precautions: Patients should be instructed to consult their physician before using any laxative if they have noticed a sudden change in bowel habits which persists for two weeks. Unless directed by a physician, patients should be advised not to use laxative products when abdominal pain, nausea, or vomiting is present. Patients should also be advised to discontinue use and consult a physician if rectal bleeding or failure to have a bowel movement occurs after use of any laxative product.

Dosage and Administration: Adults and children older than 12 years of age: *one heaping measuring* tablespoonful stirred briskly into 8 ounces of cold water one to three times a day at the first sign of constipation. Children 6 to under 12 years: *one-half the adult dose stirred briskly into 4 ounces of cold water, one to three times a day. The mixture should be administered promptly and drinking additional water is helpful. Children under 6 years: use only as directed by a physician.* Continued use for two or three days may be necessary for full benefit.

How Supplied:
16 oz, 24 oz, and 30 oz containers.
Boxes of 20 single-dose packets.
Store below 86°F (30°C). Protect contents from humidity; keep tightly closed.

Shown in Product Identification Section, page 426

Sugar Free Orange Flavor
CITRUCEL®
[*sĭt 'rə-sĕl*]
(Methylcellulose)
Bulk-forming Fiber Laxative

Description: Each 10.2 g adult dose (approximately one rounded measuring tablespoonful) contains Methylcellulose 2 g. Each 5.1 g child's dose (one-half the adult dose) contains Methylcellulose 1 g. Methylcellulose is a nonallergenic fiber. Also contains: Aspartame*, Dibasic Calcium Phosphate, FD&C Yellow No. 6, Malic Acid, Maltodextrin, Orange Flavors (natural and artificial), Potassium Citrate and Riboflavin. Each 10.2 g dose contributes 24 calories from Maltodextrin.

Actions: Promotes elimination by providing additional fiber (bulk) to the diet. This product generally produces bowel movement in 12 to 72 hours.

Indications: For relief of constipation (irregularity). May also be used for relief of constipation associated with other bowel disorders such as irritable bowel syndrome, diverticular disease, and hemorrhoids as well as for bowel management during postpartum, postsurgical, and convalescent periods when recommended by a physician.

Contraindications: Intestinal obstruction, fecal impaction, known hypersensitivity to formula ingredients.

Warning: Individuals with phenylketonuria and other individuals who must restrict their intake of phenylalanine should be warned that each 10.2 g adult dose contains aspartame which provides 52 mg of phenylalanine.

Precautions: Patients should be instructed to consult their physician before using any laxative if they have noticed a sudden change in bowel habits which persists for two weeks. Unless directed by a physician, patients should be advised not to use laxative products when abdominal pain, nausea, or vomiting is present. Patients should also be advised to discontinue use and consult a physician if rectal bleeding or failure to have a bowel movement occurs after use of any laxative product.

Dosage and Administration: Adults and children older than 12 years of age: one rounded measuring tablespoonful stirred briskly into 8 ounces of cold water, one to three times a day at the first sign of constipation. Children 6 to 12 years of age: one-half the adult dose stirred briskly into 4 ounces of cold water one to three times a day. The mixture should be administered promptly and drinking additional water is helpful. Continued use for two or more days may be necessary for full benefit.

*NutraSweet and the NutraSweet symbol are trademarks of the NutraSweet Company.

How Supplied:
8.6 oz and 16.9 oz containers.
Store below 86°F (30°C). Protect contents from humidity; keep tightly closed.

Shown in Product Identification Section, page 426

CLEAR BY DESIGN®
Medicated Acne Gel for Sensitive Skin

Product Information: CLEAR BY DESIGN contains benzoyl peroxide, an effective anti-acne agent available without a prescription in a lower 2.5% strength. CLEAR BY DESIGN is as effective as 10% benzoyl peroxide but with less of the irritation and redness that you may get with the higher strengths. Greaseless, colorless CLEAR BY DESIGN is invisible while it works fast. Helps prevent new acne pimples and blackheads from forming.

Directions: Wash problem areas thoroughly but gently and dry well. Using fingertips, apply CLEAR BY DESIGN to all affected and surrounding areas of face, neck, and body. Apply one or two times a day or as directed by a physician.

Warnings: Persons with a known allergy to benzoyl peroxide should not use this medication. To test for an allergy, apply CLEAR BY DESIGN on a small affected area once a day for two days. If discomforting irritation or undue dryness occurs during treatment, reduce frequency of use or amount. If excessive itching, redness, burning, swelling, irritation or dryness occurs, discontinue use and consult a physician. Avoid contact with eyes, lips and mouth. May bleach hair or dyed fabrics. Keep tightly closed. Keep this and all drugs out of reach of children. Store at controlled room temperature (59°–86°F). Avoid excessive heat. FOR EXTERNAL USE ONLY

Formula: Active Ingredient: Benzoyl Peroxide, 2.5% in a gel base. Inactive Ingredients: Purified water, carbomer 940, dioctyl sodium sulfosuccinate, sodium hydroxide, and edetate disodium.

How Supplied: Available in 1.5 oz. tubes.

Shown in Product Identification Section, page 426

CONTAC®
DAY & NIGHT COLD & FLU
Day Caplets

Indications: For temporary relief of nasal congestion, fever, coughs, minor aches and pains due to the common cold and flu.

Directions: Adults and children 12 and older: Take one yellow Day caplet every 6 hours. Children under 12, use only as directed by a doctor.
DO NOT EXCEED A TOTAL OF 4 CAPLETS (whether all Day or all Night

Continued on next page

SmithKline Beecham—Cont.

or combination of each) **IN 24 HOURS. ALL CAPLETS SHOULD BE TAKEN AT LEAST 6 HOURS APART.**

Warnings: Do not exceed recommended dosage because at higher doses, dizziness, sleeplessness, or nervousness may occur. A persistent cough may be a sign of a serious condition. Do not use this product if: cough or other symptoms do not improve within 7 days, worsen, recur, or are accompanied by fever, rash, redness, swelling or persistent headache; fever lasts for more than 3 days; you have high blood pressure, heart disease, diabetes, thyroid disease, or difficulty in urination due to an enlarged prostate gland; you have persistent or chronic cough such as occurs with smoking, asthma, emphysema or if cough is accompanied by excessive phlegm (mucus), unless directed by a doctor.

Drug Interaction Precaution: Do not take if you are presently taking a prescription drug for high blood pressure or depression, without first consulting a doctor. Do not use this product if you are taking a prescription drug containing a monoamine oxidose inhibitor (MAOI) (certain drugs for depression or psychiatric or emotional conditions), without first consulting your doctor. If you are uncertain whether your prescription drug contains an MAOI, consult a health professional before taking this product.

Active Ingredients: Each caplet contains:
Acetaminophen 650 mg.,
Pseudoephedrine Hydrochloride 60 mg.,
Dextromethorphan Hydrobromide 30mg.

Inactive Ingredients: Carnauba Wax, D&C Yellow 10 FD&C Yellow 6, Hydroxypropyl Methylcellulose, Magnesium Stearate, Microcrystalline Cellulose, Polyethylene Glycol, Polysorbate 80, Silicon Dioxide, Starch, Stearic Acid, Titanium Dioxide, White Wax.

How Supplied: Consumer package of 15 caplets.

Note: There are other CONTAC products. Make sure this is the one you are interested in.

Shown in Product Identification Section, page 426

CONTAC®
Day & Night Cold & Flu Night Caplets

Indications: For temporary relief of nasal congestion, fever, minor aches and pains, runny nose, and sneezing, due to the common cold and flu.

Directions: Adults and children 12 and older: Take one blue Night caplet every 6 hours. Children under 12, use only as directed by a doctor. DO NOT EXCEED A TOTAL OF 4 CAPLETS (whether all Day or all Night or combination of each) IN 24 HOURS. ALL CAPLETS SHOULD BE TAKEN AT LEAST 6 HOURS APART.

Warnings: Do not exceed recommended dosage, because at higher doses, dizziness, sleeplessness, or nervousness may occur. Do not use this product if: cough or other symptoms do not improve within 7 days, worsen, recur, or are accompanied by fever, redness, swelling; fever lasts more than three days; you have chronic pulmonary disease, high blood pressure, asthma, heart disease, diabetes, thyroid disease, glaucoma, shortness of breath, difficulty in breathing, emphysema, or difficulty in urination due to an enlarged prostate gland. May cause marked drowsiness; use caution when driving a motor vehicle or operating machinery. Alcohol, sedatives or tranquilizers will increase drowsiness; avoid alcoholic beverages. May cause excitability especially in children.

Drug Interaction Precaution: Do not take if you are presently taking a prescription drug for high blood pressure or depression, without first consulting a doctor.

Active Ingredients: Each caplet contains:
Acetaminophen 650 mg.,
Pseudoephedrine Hydrochloride 60 mg.,
Diphenhydramine Hydrochloride 50 mg.

Inactive Ingredients: Carnauba Wax, FD&C Blue 1, Hydroxypropyl Methylcellulose, Magnesium Stearate, Microcrystalline Cellulose, Polyethylene Glycol, Polysorbate 80, Silicon Dioxide, Starch, Stearic Acid, Titanium Dioxide, White Wax.

How Supplied: Consumer package of 5 caplets.

Note: There are other CONTAC products. Make sure this is the one you are interested in.

Shown in Product Identification Section, page 426

CONTAC®
MAXIMUM STRENGTH
Continuous Action Nasal Decongestant/Antihistamine Caplets

Composition: [See table on next page.]

Product Information: Each CONTAC Maximum Strength continuous action caplet provides up to 12 hours of relief. Part of the caplet goes to work right away for fast relief; the rest is released gradually to provide up to 12 hours of prolonged relief. With just *one* caplet in the morning and *one* at bedtime, you feel better all day, sleep better at night, breathing freely without congestion. CONTAC Maximum Strength provides:

- A NASAL DECONGESTANT which helps clear nasal passages, shrinks swollen membranes and helps decongest sinus openings.
- AN ANTIHISTAMINE at the maximum level to help relieve itchy, watery eyes, sneezing, and runny nose.

Indications: For temporary relief of nasal congestion due to the common cold, hay fever or other upper respiratory allergies, and nasal congestion associated with sinusitis.

Directions: One caplet every 12 hours. Do not exceed 2 caplets in 24 hours.

NOTE: The nonactive portion of the caplet that supplies the active ingredients may occasionally appear in your stool as a soft mass.

This carton is protected by a clear overwrap printed with "safety-sealed"; do not use if overwrap is missing or broken.

TAMPER-RESISTANT PACKAGING FEATURES FOR YOUR PROTECTION:

- Each caplet is encased in a plastic cell with a foil back; do not use if cell or foil is broken.
- The name CONTAC appears on each caplet; do not use this product if the CONTAC name is missing.

Warnings: Do not give this product to children under 12 years except under the advice and supervision of a physician. Do not exceed recommended dosage because at higher doses nervousness, dizziness, or sleeplessness may occur. Do not take this product if you have high blood pressure, heart disease, diabetes or thyroid disease except under the advice and supervision of a physician. If symptoms do not improve within 7 days or are accompanied by high fever, consult a physician before continuing use. Do not take this product if you have asthma, glaucoma or difficulty in urination due to enlargement of the prostate gland except under the advice and supervision of a physician. Do not take this product if you are taking another medication containing phenylpropanolamine. Avoid alcoholic beverages while taking this product. Do not drive or operate heavy machinery. May cause drowsiness. May cause excitability, especially in children. Keep this and all drugs out of reach of children. In case of accidental overdose, seek professional assistance or contact a poison control center immediately. As with any drug, if you are pregnant or nursing a baby, seek the advice of a health professional before using this product. Store at controlled room temperature (59°–86°F).

Drug Interaction Precaution: Do not take this product if you are presently taking a prescription antihypertensive or antidepressant drug containing monoamine oxidase inhibitor except under the advice and supervision of a physician.

Formula: Active Ingredients: Each Maximum Strength caplet contains Phenylpropanolamine Hydrochloride 75 mg.; Chlorpheniramine Maleate 12 mg. (which is a higher dose of antihistamine than CONTAC capsules). **Inactive Ingredients (listed for individuals with specific allergies):** Acetylated Monoglycerides, Carnauba Wax, Colloidal Silicon Dioxide, Ethylcellulose, Hydroxypropyl

CONTAC	CONTAC Maximum Strength Continuous Action Decongestant Caplets	CONTAC Continuous Action Decongestant Capsules	CONTAC Severe Cold and Flu Formula Caplets (each 2 caplet dose)	CONTAC Severe Cold and Flu Hot Medicine Drink (each Packet dose)	CONTAC Severe Cold and Flu Nighttime Liquid (each fluid dose)	CONTAC Day & Night Cold & Flu Day Caplets	CONTAC Day & Night Cold & Flu Night Caplets
Phenylpropanolamine HCl	75.0 mg	75.0 mg	25.0 mg	—	—	60.0 mg	60.0 mg
Chlorpheniramine Maleate	12.0 mg	8.0 mg	4.0 mg	4.0 mg	4.0 mg	—	—
Pseudoephedrine HCl				60.0 mg	60.0 mg	—	—
Acetaminophen	—	—	1000.0 mg	650.0 mg	1000.0 mg	650.0 mg	650.0 mg
Dextromethorphan Hydrobromide	—	—	30.0 mg	20.0 mg	30.0 mg	30.0 mg	—
Alcohol					18.5% by volume		
Diphenhydramine HCl							60.0 mg

Methylcellulose, Lactose, Stearic Acid, Titanium Dioxide.

How Supplied: Consumer packages of 10, 20 and 40 caplets.

Note: There are other CONTAC products. Make sure this is the one you are interested in.

Shown in Product Identification Section, page 426

CONTAC®
Continuous Action Nasal Decongestant/Antihistamine Capsules

Composition: [See table above.]

Product Information: Each CONTAC continuous action capsule contains over 600 "tiny time pills." Some go to work right away. The rest are scientifically timed to dissolve slowly to give up to 12 hours of relief. With just *one* capsule in the morning and *one* at bedtime, you feel better all day, sleep better at night, breathing freely without congestion. CONTAC provides:

- A NASAL DECONGESTANT which helps clear nasal passages, shrinks swollen membranes and helps decongest sinus openings.
- AN ANTIHISTAMINE to help relieve itchy, watery eyes, sneezing, and runny nose.

Indications: For temporary relief of nasal congestion due to the common cold, hay fever or other upper respiratory allergies, and nasal congestion associated with sinusitis.

Directions: One capsule every 12 hours. Do not exceed 2 capsules in 24 hours.
This carton is protected by a clear overwrap printed with "safety-sealed"; do not use if overwrap is missing or broken.

TAMPER-RESISTANT PACKAGING FEATURES FOR YOUR PROTECTION:

- Each capsule is encased in a plastic cell with a foil back; do not use if cell or foil is broken.
- Each CONTAC capsule is protected by a red Perma-Seal™ band which bonds the two capsule halves together; do not use if capsule or band is broken.

Warnings: Do not give this product to children under 12 years except under the advice and supervision of a physician. Do not exceed recommended dosage because at higher doses nervousness, dizziness, or sleeplessness may occur. Do not take this product if you have high blood pressure, heart disease, diabetes or thyroid disease except under the advice and supervision of a physician. If symptoms do not improve within 7 days or are accompanied by a high fever, consult a physician before continuing use. Do not take this product if you have asthma, glaucoma or difficulty in urination due to enlargement of the prostate gland except under the advice and supervision of a physician. Do not take this product if you are taking another medication containing phenylpropanolamine. Avoid alcoholic beverages while taking this product. Do not drive or operate heavy machinery. May cause drowsiness. May cause excitability, especially in children. Keep this and all drugs out of reach of children. In case of accidental overdose, seek professional assistance or contact a poison control center immediately. As with any drug, if you are pregnant or nursing a baby, seek the advice of a health professional before using this product. Store at controlled room temperature (59°–86°F). Protect against excess moisture.

Drug Interaction Precaution: Do not take this product if you are presently taking a prescription antihypertensive or antidepressant drug containing monoamine oxidase inhibitor except under the advice and supervision of a physician.

Each Capsule Contains: Phenylpropanolamine Hydrochloride 75 mg. and Chlorpheniramine Maleate 8 mg. Also Contains: Benzyl Alcohol, Butylparaben, Carboxymethylcellulose Sodium, D&C Red No. 33, D&C Red 27, D&C Red 30, D&C Yellow No. 10, Edetate Calcium Disodium, FD&C Red No. 3, FD&C Red 40, FD&C Yellow No. 6, Gelatin, Methylparaben, Pharmaceutical Glaze, Polysorbate 80, Propylparaben, Sodium Lauryl Sulfate, Sodium Propionate, Starch, Sucrose and other ingredients.

How Supplied: Consumer packages of 10, 20 and 40 capsules.

Note: There are other CONTAC products. Make sure this is the one you are interested in.

Shown in Product Identification Section, page 426

CONTAC®
Severe Cold and Flu Formula Caplets
Analgesic • Decongestant Antihistamine • Cough Suppressant

Composition: [See table above.]

Product Information: Two caplets every 6 hours to help relieve the discomforts of severe colds with flu-like symptoms.

Product Benefits: CONTAC Severe Cold and Flu Formula contains a non-aspirin analgesic, a decongestant, an antihistamine and a cough suppressant. These safe and effective ingredients provide temporary relief from these major cold symptoms: fever, body aches and pains, minor sore throat pain, headache, runny nose, postnasal drip, sneezing, itchy, watery eyes, nasal and sinus congestion, and temporarily relieves cough due to the common cold.

Directions: Adults (12 years and over): Two caplets every 6 hours, not to exceed 8 caplets in any 24 hour period.
This carton is protected by a clear overwrap printed with "safety-sealed". Do not use if overwrap is missing or broken.

TAMPER-RESISTANT PACKAGING FEATURES FOR YOUR PROTECTION:

- Caplets are encased in a plastic cell with a foil back; do not use if cell or foil is broken.
- The letters SCF appear on each caplet; do not use this product if these letters are missing.

Warnings: Do not administer to children under 12. Do not take this product for more than 7 days or for fever for more than 3 days unless directed by a doctor. If symptoms do not improve or are accompanied by fever, consult a doctor. A persistent cough may be a sign of a serious condition. If cough persists for more than one week, tends to recur or is accompanied by fever, rash, or persistent headache, consult a doctor. Do not take this product for persistent or chronic coughs such as occurs with smoking, asthma, emphysema, or if cough is accompanied by excessive phlegm (mucus), unless directed by a doctor. Do not exceed recommended dosage because at higher doses

Continued on next page

SmithKline Beecham—Cont.

nervousness, dizziness, or sleeplessness may occur. May cause excitability, especially in children. Do not take this product if you have asthma, glaucoma, heart disease, high blood pressure, emphysema, chronic pulmonary disease, shortness of breath, difficulty in breathing, diabetes, thyroid disease, or difficulty in urination due to enlargement of the prostate gland unless directed by a doctor. Do not take this product if you are taking another medication containing phenylpropanolamine. May cause marked drowsiness. Alcohol may increase the drowsiness effect. Avoid alcoholic beverages while taking this product. Use caution when driving a motor vehicle or operating machinery. Keep this and all medication out of the reach of children. As with any drug, if you are pregnant or nursing a baby, seek the advice of a health professional before using this product. In case of accidental overdose, contact a physician or poison control center immediately. Prompt medical attention is critical for adults as well as for children even if you do not notice any signs or symptoms.

Drug Interaction Precaution: Do not take this product if you are presently taking a prescription drug for high blood pressure or depression without first consulting your doctor.

Formula: Active Ingredients: Each caplet contains Acetaminophen, 500 mg., Dextromethorphan Hydrobromide, 15 mg.; Phenylpropanolamine Hydrochloride, 12.5 mg.; Chlorpheniramine Maleate, 2 mg. **Inactive Ingredients (listed for individuals with specific allergies):** Cellulose, FD&C Blue 1, Hydroxypropyl Methylcellulose, Polyethylene Glycol, Polysorbate 80, Povidone, Sodium Starch Glycolate, Starch, Stearic Acid, Titanium Dioxide.

How Supplied: Consumer packages of 10, 20 and 40 caplets.

Note: There are other CONTAC products. Make sure this is the one you are interested in.

Shown in Product Identification Section, page 426

CONTAC®
SEVERE COLD & FLU NIGHTTIME
Antihistamine • Analgesic
Cough Suppressant • Nasal Decongestant

Composition: [See table on page 717.]

Product Information: CONTAC Severe Cold & Flu Nighttime:

- Provides temporary relief from nasal and sinus congestion, runny nose, coughing, postnasal drip, sneezing, itchy, watery eyes and minor aches and pains associated with the common cold, sore throat, and flu, so you can get the rest you need.
- Contains a non-aspirin analgesic and fever reducer, a cough suppressant, a nasal decongestant and an antihistamine.

Directions: Adults and children 12 years and older: Take 2 Tbsps. every 6 hours in dosage cup provided. May be repeated every 6 hours as needed, not to exceed 8 Tbsps. in 24 hours.

TAMPER RESISTANT PACKAGE FEATURE: DO NOT USE IF PRINTED SEAL AROUND BOTTLE CAP IS MISSING OR BROKEN.

Warnings: Do not administer to children under 12. Do not take this product for more than 7 days or for fever for more than 3 days unless directed by a doctor. If symptoms do not improve or are accompanied by fever, consult a doctor. A persistent cough may be a sign of a serious condition. If cough persists for more than one week, tends to recur or is accompanied by fever, rash, or persistent headache, consult a doctor. Do not take this product for persistent or chronic coughs such as occurs with smoking, asthma, emphysema, or if cough is accompanied by excessive phlegm (mucus) unless directed by a doctor. Do not exceed recommended dosage because at higher doses nervousness, dizziness, or sleeplessness may occur. May cause excitability, especially in children. Do not take this product if you have asthma, glaucoma, heart disease, high blood pressure, emphysema, chronic pulmonary disease, shortness of breath, difficulty in breathing, diabetes, thyroid disease, or difficulty in urination due to enlargement of the prostate gland unless directed by a doctor. May cause drowsiness. Alcohol may increase the drowsiness effect. Avoid alcoholic beverages while taking this product. Use caution when driving a motor vehicle or operating machinery.
Keep this and all medication out of the reach of children. As with any drug, if you are pregnant or nursing a baby, seek the advice of a health professional before using this product. In case of accidental overdose, contact a physician or poison control center immediately. Prompt medical attention is critical for adults as well as children even if you do not notice any signs or symptoms.

Drug Interaction Precaution: Do not take this product if you are presently taking a prescription drug for high blood pressure or depression without first consulting your doctor.

Active Ingredients: Per dose (2 Tbsps.):
Acetaminophen 1000 mg
Pseudoephedrine Hydrochloride 60 mg
Dextromethorphan Hydrobromide 30 mg
Chlorpheniramine Maleate 4 mg
Alcohol content: 18.5% by volume.
Contains no sugar or aspirin.

Inactive Ingredients: Alcohol, FD&C Blue 1, Dibasic Sodium Phosphate, Flavors, Glycerin, Hydrogenated Glucose Syrup, Phosphoric Acid, Potassium Sorbate, Povidone, D&C Red 33, FD&C Red 40, Saccharin Sodium, Sorbitol, Water.

How Supplied: In 6 fl. oz. bottles.

Note: There are other CONTAC products. Make sure this is the one you are interested in.

DEBROX® Drops

Description: Carbamide peroxide 6.5%. Also contains citric acid, glycerin, propylene glycol, sodium stannate, water, and other ingredients.

Actions: DEBROX®, used as directed, cleanses the ear with sustained microfoam. DEBROX Drops foam on contact with earwax due to the release of oxygen.

Indications: DEBROX Drops provide a safe, nonirritating method of softening and removing earwax.

Directions: FOR USE IN THE EAR ONLY. Adults and children over 12 years of age: tilt head sideways and place 5 to 10 drops into ear. Tip of applicator should not enter ear canal. Keep drops in ear for several minutes by keeping head tilted or placing cotton in the ear. Use twice daily for up to four days if needed, or as directed by a doctor. Any wax remaining after treatment may be removed by gently flushing the ear with warm water, using a soft rubber bulb ear syringe. Children under 12 years of age: consult a doctor.

Warnings: Do not use if you have ear drainage or discharge, ear pain, irritation or rash in the ear, or are dizzy, unless directed by a physician. Do not use if you have an injury or perforation (hole) of the eardrum or after ear surgery unless directed by a physician. Do not use for more than four consecutive days. If excessive earwax remains after use of this product, consult a physician. Consult a physician prior to use in children under 12.

Cautions: Avoid exposing bottle to excessive heat and direct sunlight. Keep tip on bottle when not in use. Avoid contact with eyes. Keep this and all drugs out of the reach of children. In case of accidental ingestion, seek professional assistance or contact a poison control center immediately.

How Supplied: DEBROX Drops are available in ½- or 1-fl-oz plastic squeeze bottles with applicator spouts.

Shown in Product Identification Section, page 426

ECOTRIN®
Enteric-Coated Aspirin
Antiarthritic, Antiplatelet

Description: 'Ecotrin' is enteric-coated aspirin (acetylsalicylic acid, ASA) available in tablet and caplet forms in 325 mg and 500 mg dosage units.
The enteric coating covers a core of aspirin and is designed to resist disintegra-

tion in the stomach, dissolving in the more neutral-to-alkaline environment of the duodenum. Such action helps to protect the stomach from injury that may result from ingestion of plain, buffered or highly buffered aspirin (see SAFETY).

Indications: 'Ecotrin' is indicated for:

- conditions requiring chronic or long-term aspirin therapy for pain and/or inflammation, e.g., rheumatoid arthritis, juvenile rheumatoid arthritis, systemic lupus erythematosus, osteoarthritis (degenerative joint disease), ankylosing spondylitis, psoriatic arthritis, Reiter's syndrome and fibrositis,
- antiplatelet indications of aspirin (see the ANTIPLATELET-EFFECT section) and
- situations in which compliance with aspirin therapy may be affected because of the gastrointestinal side effects of plain, i.e., non-enteric-coated, or buffered aspirin.

Dosage: For analgesic or anti-inflammatory indications, the OTC maximum dosage for aspirin is 4000 mg per day in divided doses, i.e., up to 650 mg every 4 hours or 1000 mg every 6 hours.

For antiplatelet effect dosage: see the ANTIPLATELET EFFECT section.

Under a physician's direction, the dosage can be increased or otherwise modified as appropriate to the clinical situation. When 'Ecotrin' is used for anti-inflammatory effect, the physician should be attentive to plasma salicylate levels, and may also caution the patient to be alert to the development of tinnitus as an indicator of elevated salicylate levels. It should be noted that patients with a high frequency hearing loss (such as may occur in older individuals) may have difficulty perceiving the tinnitus. Tinnitus would then not be a reliable indicator in such individuals.

Inactive Ingredients: Cellulose, Cellulose Acetate Phthalate, D&C Yellow 10, Diethyl Phthalate, FD&C Yellow 6, Pregelatinized Starch, Silicon Dioxide, Sodium Starch Glycolate, Stearic Acid, Titanium Dioxide, and trace amounts of other inactive ingredients.

Bioavailability: The bioavailability of aspirin from 'Ecotrin' has been demonstrated in a number of salicylate excretion studies. The studies show levels of salicylate (and metabolites) in urine excreted over 48 hours for 'Ecotrin' do not differ statistically from plain, i.e., non-enteric-coated, aspirin.

Plasma studies, in which 'Ecotrin' has been compared with plain aspirin in steady-state studies over eight days, also demonstrate that 'Ecotrin' provides plasma salicylate levels not statistically different from plain aspirin.

Information regarding salicylate levels over a range of doses was generated in a study in which 24 healthy volunteers (12 male and 12 female) took daily (divided) doses of either 2600 mg, 3900 mg, or 5200 mg of 'Ecotrin'. Plasma salicylate levels generally acknowledged to be anti-inflammatory (15 mg/dL.) were attained at daily doses of 5200 mg, on Day 2 by females and Day 3 by males. At 3900 mg, anti-inflammatory levels were attained at Day 3 by females and Day 4 by males. Dissolution of the enteric coating occurs at a neutral-to-basic pH and is therefore dependent on gastric emptying into the duodenum. With continued dosing, appropriate plasma levels are maintained.

Safety: The safety of 'Ecotrin' has been demonstrated in a number of endoscopic studies comparing 'Ecotrin', plain aspirin, buffered aspirin and highly buffered aspirin preparations. In these studies, all forms of aspirin were dosed to the OTC maximum (3900–4000 mg per day) for up to 14 days. The normal healthy volunteers participating in these studies were gastroscoped before and after the courses of treatment and 14-day drug-free periods followed active drug. Compared to all the other preparations, there was less gastric damage at a statistically significant level during the 'Ecotrin' courses. There was also statistically less duodenal damage when compared with the plain, i.e., non-enteric-coated, aspirin.

Details of studies demonstrating the safety and bioavailability of 'Ecotrin' are available to health care professionals. Write: Professional Services Department, SmithKline Beecham Consumer Brands, P.O. Box 1467, Pittsburgh, Pa. 15230.

Warning:

Consumer Warning: Children and teenagers should not use this medicine for chicken pox or flu symptoms before a doctor is consulted about Reye syndrome, a rare but serious illness. Do not take this product for pain for more than 10 days unless directed by a physician. If pain persists or gets worse, if new symptoms occur, or if redness or swelling is present, consult a physician because these could be signs of a serious condition. Also, consult a physician before using this medicine to treat arthritic or rheumatic conditions affecting children under 12. Discontinue use if dizziness occurs. Do not take this product if you are allergic to aspirin, have asthma, or if you have ulcers or bleeding problems unless directed by a physician. If ringing in the ears or a loss of hearing occurs, consult a physician before taking any more of this product. If you experience persistent or unexplained stomach upset, consult a physician. Keep this and all drugs out of children's reach. In case of accidental overdose, seek professional assistance or contact a poison control center immediately. As with any medicine, if you are pregnant or nursing a baby, seek the advice of a health professional before using this product. **IT IS ESPECIALLY IMPORTANT NOT TO USE ASPIRIN DURING THE LAST 3 MONTHS OF PREGNANCY UNLESS SPECIFICALLY DIRECTED TO DO SO BY A DOCTOR, BECAUSE IT MAY CAUSE PROBLEMS IN THE UNBORN CHILD OR COMPLICATIONS DURING DELIVERY.** Store at controlled room temperature (59°–86°F).

Drug Interaction Precaution: Do not take this product if you are taking a prescription drug for anticoagulation (thinning of the blood), diabetes, gout, or arthritis unless directed by a physician.

Professional Warning: There have been occasional reports in the literature concerning individuals with impaired gastric emptying in whom there may be retention of one or more 'Ecotrin' tablets over time. This unusual phenomenon may occur as a result of outlet obstruction from ulcer disease alone or combined with hypotonic gastric peristalsis. Because of the integrity of the enteric coating in an acidic environment, these tablets may accumulate and form a bezoar in the stomach. Individuals with this condition may present with complaints of early satiety or of vague upper abdominal distress. Diagnosis may be made by endoscopy or by abdominal films which show opacities suggestive of a mass of small tablets *(Ref.: Bogacz, K. and Caldron, P.: Enteric-coated Aspirin Bezoar: Elevation of Serum Salicylate Level by Barium Study. Amer. J. Med. 1987:83, 783–6.).* Management may vary according to the condition of the patient. Options include: gastrotomy and alternating slightly basic and neutral lavage *(Ref.: Baum, J.: Enteric-Coated Aspirin and the Problem of Gastric Retention. J. Rheum., 1984:11, 250–1.).* While there have been no clinical reports, it has been suggested that such individuals may also be treated with parenteral cimetidine (to reduce acid secretion) and then given sips of slightly basic liquids to effect gradual dissolution of the enteric coating. Progress may be followed with plasma salicylate levels or via recognition of tinnitus by the patient.

It should be kept in mind that individuals with a history of partial or complete gastrectomy may produce reduced amounts of acid and therefore have less acidic gastric pH. Under these circumstances, the benefits offered by the acid-resistant enteric coating may not exist.

Antiplatelet Effect: Aspirin may be recommended to reduce the risk of death and/or nonfatal myocardial infarction (MI) in patients with a previous infarction or unstable angina pectoris and its use in reducing the risk of transient ischemic attacks in men.

Labeling for both indications follows:

ASPIRIN FOR MYOCARDIAL INFARCTION

Indication: Aspirin is indicated to reduce the risk of death and/or nonfatal myocardial infarction in patients with a previous infarction or unstable angina pectoris.

Clinical Trials: The indication is supported by the results of six, large, randomized multicenter, placebo-controlled studies involving 10,816 predominantly male, post-myocardial infarction (MI) patients and one randomized placebo-controlled study of 1,266 men with unstable angina.[1–7] Therapy with aspirin was

Continued on next page

SmithKline Beecham—Cont.

begun at intervals after the onset of acute MI varying from less than three days to more than five years and continued for periods of from less than one year to four years. In the unstable angina study, treatment was started within one month after the onset of unstable angina and continued for 12 weeks, and patients with complicating conditions such as congestive heart failure were not included in the study.
Aspirin therapy in MI patients was associated with about a 20 percent reduction in the risk of subsequent death and/or nonfatal reinfarction, a median absolute decrease of 3 percent from the 12 to 22 percent event rates in the placebo groups. In aspirin-treated unstable angina patients, the reduction in risk was about 50 percent, a reduction in event rate to 5% from the 10% in the placebo group over the 12 weeks of the study.
Daily dosage of aspirin in the post-myocardial infarction studies was 300 mg in one study and 900 to 1500 mg in five studies. A dose of 325 mg was used in the study of unstable angina.

Adverse Reactions:
Gastrointestinal Reactions: Doses of 1000 mg per day of plain aspirin caused gastrointestinal symptoms and bleeding that in some cases were clinically significant. In the largest postinfarction study (the Aspirin Myocardial Infarction Study [AMIS] with 4,500 people), the percentage incidences of gastrointestinal symptoms of a standard, solid-tablet formulation and placebo-treated subjects, respectively, were: stomach pain (14.5%; 4.4%); heartburn (11.9%; 4.8%); nausea and/or vomiting (7.6%; 2.1%); hospitalization for gastrointestinal disorder (4.9%; 3.5%). In the AMIS and other trials, plain aspirin-treated patients had increased rates of gross gastrointestinal bleeding. Symptoms and signs of gastrointestinal irritation were not significantly increased in subjects treated for unstable angina with buffered aspirin in solution.

Cardiovascular and Biochemical: In the AMIS trial, the dosage of 1000 mg per day of plain aspirin was associated with small increases in systolic blood pressure (BP) (average 1.5 to 2.1 mmHg) and diastolic BP (0.5 to 0.6 mmHg), depending upon whether maximal or last available readings were used. Blood urea nitrogen and uric acid levels were also increased, but by less than 1.0 mg%. Subjects with marked hypertension or renal insufficiency had been excluded from the trial so that the clinical importance of these observations for such subjects or for any subjects treated over more prolonged periods is not known. It is recommended that patients placed on long-term aspirin treatment, even at doses of 300 mg per day, be seen at regular intervals to assess changes in these measurements.

Sodium in Buffered Aspirin for Solution Formulations: One tablet daily of buffered aspirin in solution adds 553 mg of sodium to that in the diet and may not be tolerated by patients with active sodium-retaining states such as congestive heart or renal failure. This amount of sodium adds about 30 percent to the 70 to 90 meq intake suggested as appropriate for dietary hypertension in the 1984 Report of the Joint National Committee on Detection, Evaluation, and Treatment of High Blood Pressure.[8]

Dosage and Administration: Although most of the studies used dosages exceeding 300 mg daily, two trials used only 300 mg and pharmacologic data indicate that this dose inhibits platelet function fully. Therefore, 300 mg or a conventional 325 mg aspirin dose daily is a reasonable, routine dose that would minimize gastrointestinal adverse reactions for both solid oral dosage forms (buffered and plain aspirin) and buffered aspirin in solution.

References:
1. Elwood, P.C., et al.: A Randomized Controlled Trial of Acetylsalicylic Acid in the Secondary Prevention of Mortality from Myocardial Infarction, *Br. Med. J.* 1:436–440, 1974.
2. The Coronary Drug Project Research Group: Aspirin in Coronary Heart Disease, *J. Chronic Dis.* 29:625–642, 1976.
3. Breddin, K., et al.: Secondary Prevention of Myocardial Infarction: A Comparison of Acetylsalicylic Acid, Phenprocoumon or Placebo, *Homeostasis* 470:263–268, 1979.
4. Aspirin Myocardial Infarction Study Research Group: A Randomized Controlled Trial of Aspirin in Persons Recovered from Myocardial Infarction, *J.A.M.A.* 243:661–669, 1980.
5. Elwood, P.C., and Sweetnam, P.M.: Aspirin and Secondary Mortality After Myocardial Infarction, *Lancet* pp. 1313–1315, Dec. 22–29, 1979.
6. The Persantine-Aspirin Reinfarction Study Research Group, Persantine and Aspirin in Coronary Heart Disease, *Circulation* 62: 449–469, 1980.
7. Lewis, H.D., et al.: Protective Effects of Aspirin Against Acute Myocardial Infarction and Death in Men with Unstable Angina, Results of a Veterans Administration Cooperative Study, *N. Engl. J. Med.* 309:396–403, 1983.
8. 1984 Report of the Joint National Committee on Detection, Evaluation, and Treatment of High Blood Pressure, U.S. Department of Health and Human Services and U.S. Public Health Service, National Institutes of Health. NIH Pub. No. 84–1088.

ASPIRIN FOR TRANSIENT ISCHEMIC ATTACKS

Indication For reducing the risk of recurrent transient ischemic attacks (TIAs) or stroke in men who have had transient ischemia of the brain due to fibrin platelet emboli. There is inadequate evidence that aspirin or buffered aspirin is effective in reducing TIAs in women at the recommended dosage. There is no evidence that aspirin or buffered aspirin is of benefit in the treatment of completed strokes in men or women.
Clinical Trials: The indication is supported by the results of a Canadian study[1] in which 585 patients with threatened stroke were followed in a randomized clinical trial for an average of 26 months to determine whether aspirin or sulfinpyrazone, singly or in combination, was superior to placebo in preventing transient ischemic attacks, stroke or death. The study showed that, although sulfinpyrazone had no statistically significant effect, aspirin reduced the risk of continuing transient ischemic attacks, stroke or death by 19 percent and reduced the risk of stroke or death by 31 percent. Another aspirin study carried out in the United States with 178 patients showed a statistically significant number of "favorable outcomes," including reduced transient ischemic attacks, stroke and death.[2]
Precautions: Patients presenting with signs and/or symptoms of TIAs should have a complete medical and neurologic evaluation. Consideration should be given to other disorders that resemble TIAs. Attention should be given to risk factors: it is important to evaluate and treat, if appropriate, other diseases associated with TIAs and stroke, such as hypertension and diabetes.
Concurrent administration of absorbable antacids at therapeutic doses may increase the clearance of salicylates in some individuals. The concurrent administration of nonabsorbable antacids may alter the rate of absorption of aspirin, thereby resulting in a decreased acetylsalicylic acid/salicylate ratio in plasma. The clinical significance of these decreases in available aspirin is unknown.
Aspirin at dosages of 1,000 mg per day has been associated with small increases in blood pressure, blood urea nitrogen, and serum uric acid levels. It is recommended that patients placed on long-term aspirin treatment be seen at regular intervals to assess changes in these measurements.

Adverse Reactions: At dosages of 1,000 mg or higher of aspirin per day, gastrointestinal side effects include stomach pain, heartburn, nausea and/or vomiting, as well as increased rates of gross gastrointestinal bleeding.

Dosage and Administration: Adult dosage for men is 1,300 mg a day, in divided doses of 650 mg twice a day or 325 mg four times a day.

References:
1. The Canadian Cooperative Study Group: Randomized Trial of Aspirin and Sulfinpyrazone in Threatened Stroke, *N. Engl. J. Med.* 299:53, 1978.
2. Fields, W. S., et al.: Controlled Trial of Aspirin in Cerebral Ischemia, *Stroke* 8:301–316, 1980.

How Supplied:
'Ecotrin' Tablets
325 mg in bottles of 100*, 250, 500 and 1000.
500 mg in bottles of 60*, 150 and 300.
'Ecotrin' Caplets
325 mg in bottles of 100.
500 mg in bottles of 60.
* Without child-resistant caps.

TAMPER-RESISTANT PACKAGE FEATURES FOR YOUR PROTECTION:
- Bottle has imprinted seal under cap.
- The words ECOTRIN REG or ECOTRIN MAX appear on each tablet or caplet (see product illustration printed on carton).
- **DO NOT USE THIS PRODUCT IF ANY OF THESE TAMPER-RESISTANT FEATURES ARE MISSING OR BROKEN.**

Comments or Questions? Call Toll-Free 800-245-1040 weekdays.

Shown in Product Identification Section, page 426

FEOSOL® CAPSULES
Hematinic

Product Information: FEOSOL capsules provide the body with ferrous sulfate, iron in its most efficient form, for iron deficiency and iron-deficiency anemia when the need for such therapy has been determined by a physician.
The special targeted-release capsule is formulated to reduce stomach upset, a common problem with iron.

Directions: *Adults:* 1 or 2 capsules daily or as directed by a physician. *Children:* As directed by a physician.
- The carton is protected by a clear overwrap printed with "safety sealed"; do not use if overwrap is missing or broken.

TAMPER-RESISTANT PACKAGING FEATURES FOR YOUR PROTECTION:
- Each capsule is encased in a plastic cell with a foil back; do not use if cell or foil is broken.
- Each FEOSOL capsule is protected by a red Perma-Seal™ band which bonds the two capsule halves together; do not use if capsule is broken or band is missing or broken.

Warnings: Do not exceed recommended dosage. The treatment of any anemic condition should be under the advice and supervision of a physician. Iron-containing medication may occasionally cause constipation or diarrhea. Since oral iron products interfere with absorption of oral tetracycline antibiotics, these products should not be taken within two hours of each other. Keep this and all drugs out of reach of children. In case of accidental overdose, seek professional assistance or contact a poison control center immediately. As with any drug, if you are pregnant or nursing a baby, seek the advice of a health professional before using this product.
Store at controlled room temperature (59°–86°F).

Formula: Active Ingredients: Each capsule contains 159 mg. of dried ferrous sulfate USP (50 mg. of elemental iron), equivalent to 250 mg. of ferrous sulfate USP. **Inactive Ingredients (listed for individuals with specific allergies):** Benzyl Alcohol, Cetylpyridinium Chloride, D&C Red 33, Yellow 10, FD&C Blue 1, D&C Red #7, Red 40, Gelatin, Glyceryl Stearates, Iron Oxide, Polyethylene Glycol, Povidone, Sodium Lauryl Sulfate, Starch, Sucrose, White Wax and trace amounts of other inactive ingredients.

How Supplied: Packages of 30 and 60 capsules, bottles of 500; in Single Unit Packages of 100 capsules (intended for institutional use only).
Also available in Tablets and Elixir.

Note: There are other FEOSOL products. Make sure this is the one you are interested in.

Shown in Product Identification Section, page 427

FEOSOL® ELIXIR
Hematinic

Product Information: FEOSOL Elixir, an unusually palatable iron elixir, provides the body with ferrous sulfate—iron in its most efficient form. The standard elixir for simple iron deficiency and iron-deficiency anemia when the need for such therapy has been determined by a physician.

Directions: Adults: 1 to 2 teaspoonfuls three times daily. Children: ½ to 1 teaspoonful three times daily preferably between meals. Infants: as directed by physician. Mix with water or fruit juice to avoid temporary staining of teeth; do not mix with milk or wine-based vehicles.

TAMPER-RESISTANT PACKAGE FEATURE: Imprinted seal around top of bottle; do not use if seal is missing.

Warnings: The treatment of any anemic condition should be under the advice and supervision of a physician. Since oral iron products interfere with absorption of oral tetracycline antibiotics, these products should not be taken within two hours of each other. Occasional gastrointestinal discomfort (such as nausea) may be minimized by taking with meals and by beginning with one teaspoonful the first day, two the second, etc. until the recommended dosage is reached. Iron-containing medication may occasionally cause constipation or diarrhea, and liquids may cause temporary staining of the teeth (this is less likely when diluted). Keep this and all drugs out of reach of children. In case of accidental overdose, seek professional assistance or contact a poison control center immediately.
As with any drug, if you are pregnant or nursing a baby, seek the advice of a health professional before using this product.
Store at controlled room temperature (59°–86°F).

Formula: Each 5 ml. (1 teaspoonful) contains ferrous sulfate USP, 220 mg. (44 mg. of elemental iron); alcohol, 5%. **Inactive Ingredients (listed for individuals with specific allergies):** Citric Acid, FD&C Yellow 6 (Sunset Yellow) as a color additive, Flavors, Glucose, Saccharin Sodium, Sucrose, Purified Water.

How Supplied: A clear orange liquid in 16 fl. oz. bottles.
Also available in Tablets and Capsules.

Note: There are other FEOSOL products. Make sure this is the one you are interested in.

Shown in Product Identification Section, page 427

FEOSOL® TABLETS
Hematinic

Product Information: FEOSOL Tablets provide the body with ferrous sulfate, iron in its most efficient form, for iron deficiency and iron-deficiency anemia when the need for such therapy has been determined by a physician. The distinctive triangular-shaped tablet has a coating to prevent oxidation and improve palatability.

Directions: *Adults*—one tablet 3 to 4 times daily after meals and upon retiring or as directed by a physician. *Children 6 to 12 years*—one tablet three times a day after meals. *Children under 6 and infants*—use Feosol® Elixir.
- The carton has been sealed at the factory with a clear overwrap printed with "safety sealed."

TAMPER-RESISTANT PACKAGE FEATURES FOR YOUR PROTECTION:
- Bottle has imprinted "SKCP" seal under cap.
- FEOSOL Tablets are triangular shaped (see product illustration printed on carton).
- **DO NOT USE THIS PRODUCT IF ANY OF THESE TAMPER-RESISTANT FEATURES ARE MISSING OR BROKEN.**

Comments or Questions? Call Toll-Free 800-245-1040 Weekdays.

Warnings: Do not exceed recommended dosage. The treatment of any anemic condition should be under the advice and supervision of a physician. Since oral iron products interfere with absorption of oral tetracycline antibiotics, these products should not be taken within two hours of each other.
Occasional gastrointestinal discomfort (such as nausea) may be minimized by taking with meals and by beginning with one tablet the first day, two the second, etc. until the recommended dosage is reached. Iron-containing medication may occasionally cause constipation or diarrhea.
Keep this and all drugs out of reach of children. In case of accidental overdose, seek professional assistance or contact a poison control center immediately.
As with any drug, if you are pregnant or nursing a baby, seek the advice of a

Continued on next page

SmithKline Beecham—Cont.

health professional before using this product.
Store at controlled room temperature (59°–86°F).

Formula: Active Ingredients: Each tablet contains 200 mg. of dried ferrous sulfate USP (65 mg. of elemental iron), equivalent to 325 mg. (5 grains) of ferrous sulfate USP. **Inactive Ingredients (listed for individuals with specific allergies):** Calcium Sulfate, D&C Yellow 10, FD&C Blue 2, Glucose, Hydroxypropyl Methylcellulose, Mineral Oil, Polyethylene Glycol, Sodium Lauryl Sulfate, Starch, Stearic Acid, Talc, Titanium Dioxide, and trace amounts of other inactive ingredients.

How Supplied: Bottles of 100 and 1000 tablets; in Single Unit Packages of 100 tablets (intended for institutional use only).
Also available in Capsules and Elixir.

Note: There are other FEOSOL products. Make sure this is the one you are interested in.

Shown in Product Identification Section, page 427

GAVISCON® Antacid Tablets

[*găv 'ĭs-kŏn*]

Composition: Each chewable tablet contains the following active ingredients:

Aluminum hydroxide dried gel	80 mg
Magnesium trisilicate	20 mg

and the following inactive ingredients: alginic acid, calcium stearate, flavor, sodium bicarbonate, starch (may contain cornstarch), and sucrose.

Actions: Unique formulation produces soothing foam which floats on stomach contents. Foam containing antacid precedes stomach contents into the esophagus when reflux occurs to help protect the sensitive mucosa from further irritation. GAVISCON® acts locally without neutralizing entire stomach contents to help maintain integrity of the digestive process. Endoscopic studies indicate that GAVISCON Antacid Tablets are equally as effective in the erect or supine patient.

Indications: GAVISCON is specifically formulated for the temporary relief of heartburn (acid indigestion) due to acid reflux. GAVISCON is not indicated for the treatment of peptic ulcers.

Directions: Chew two to four tablets four times a day or as directed by a physician. Tablets should be taken after meals and at bedtime or as needed. For best results follow by a half glass of water or other liquid. DO NOT SWALLOW WHOLE.

Warnings: Do not take more than 16 tablets in a 24-hour period or 16 tablets daily for more than 2 weeks, except under the advice and supervision of a physician. Do not use this product except under the advice and supervision of a physician if you are on a sodium-restricted diet. Each GAVISCON Tablet contains approximately 0.8 mEq sodium.

Drug Interaction Precautions: Do not take this product if you are presently taking a prescription antibiotic drug containing any form of tetracycline.
Store at a controlled room temperature in a dry place.
Keep this and all drugs out of the reach of children. In case of accidental overdose, seek professional assistance or contact a poison control center immediately.

How Supplied: Available in bottles of 100 tablets and in foil-wrapped 2s in boxes of 30 tablets.

Issued 2/87

Shown in Product Identification Section, page 427

GAVISCON® EXTRA STRENGTH RELIEF FORMULA Antacid Tablets

[*găv 'ĭs-kŏn*]

Composition: Each chewable tablet contains the following active ingredients:

Aluminum hydroxide	160 mg
Magnesium carbonate	105 mg

and the following inactive ingredients: alginic acid, calcium stearate, flavor, mannitol, sodium bicarbonate, stearic acid, and sucrose.

Directions: Chew 2 to 4 tablets four times a day or as directed by a physician. Tablets should be taken after meals and at bedtime or as needed. For best results follow by a half glass of water or other liquid. DO NOT SWALLOW WHOLE.

> **FDA Approved Uses:** For the relief of heartburn, sour stomach, and/or acid indigestion, and upset stomach associated with heartburn, sour stomach, and/or acid indigestion.

Warnings: Do not take more than 16 tablets in a 24-hour period or 16 tablets daily for more than 2 weeks, except under the advice and supervision of a physician. Do not use this product except under the advice and supervision of a physician if you are on a sodium-restricted diet. Each tablet contains approximately 1.3 mEq sodium.

Drug Interaction Precautions: Do not take this product if you are presently taking a prescription antibiotic drug containing any form of tetracycline.
Store at a controlled room temperature in a dry place.
Keep this and all drugs out of the reach of children.
In case of accidental overdose, seek professional assistance or contact a poison control center immediately.

How Supplied: Available in bottles of 100 tablets and in foil-wrapped 2s in boxes of 30.

Shown in Product Identification Section, page 427

GAVISCON® EXTRA STRENGTH RELIEF FORMULA Liquid Antacid

[*găv 'ĭs-kŏn*]

Composition: Each 2 teaspoonfuls (10 mL) contains the following active ingredients:

Aluminum hydroxide	508 mg
Magnesium carbonate	475 mg

And the following inactive ingredients: butylparaben, edetate disodium, flavor, glycerin, propylparaben, saccharin sodium, simethicone emulsion, sodium alginate, sorbitol solution, water, and xanthan gum.

> **FDA Approved Uses:** For the relief of heartburn, sour stomach and/or acid indigestion, and upset stomach associated with heartburn, sour stomach and/or acid indigestion.

Directions: **SHAKE WELL BEFORE USING.** Take 2 to 4 teaspoonfuls four times a day or as directed by a physician. GAVISCON Extra Strength Relief Formula Liquid should be taken after meals and at bedtime, followed by half a glass of water. Dispense product only by spoon or other measuring device.

Warnings: Except under the advice and supervision of a physician, do not take more than 16 teaspoonfuls in a 24-hour period or 16 teaspoonfuls daily for more than 2 weeks. May have laxative effect. Do not use this product if you have a kidney disease; do not use this product if you are on a sodium-restricted diet. Each teaspoonful contains approximately 0.9 mEq sodium.

Drug Interaction Precautions: Do not take this product if you are presently taking a prescription antibiotic drug containing any form of tetracycline.
Keep tightly closed. Avoid freezing. Store at a controlled room temperature.
Keep this and all drugs out of the reach of children.
In case of accidental overdose, seek professional assistance or contact a poison control center immediately.

How Supplied: Available in 12 fl oz (355 mL) bottles.

Shown in Product Identification Section, page 427

GAVISCON® Liquid Antacid

[*găv 'ĭs-kŏn*]

Composition: Each tablespoonful (15 ml) contains the following active ingredients:

Aluminum hydroxide	95 mg
Magnesium carbonate	358 mg

And the following inactive ingredients: D&C Yellow #10, edetate disodium, FD&C Blue #1, flavor, glycerin, paraben preservatives, saccharin sodium, sodium alginate, sorbitol solution, water, and xanthan gum.

FDA Approved Uses: For the relief of heartburn, sour stomach and/or acid indigestion, and upset stomach associated with heartburn, sour stomach and/or acid indigestion.

Directions: SHAKE WELL BEFORE USING. Take 1 or 2 tablespoonfuls four times a day or as directed by a physician. GAVISCON Liquid should be taken after meals and at bedtime, followed by half a glass of water. Dispense product only by spoon or other measuring device.

Warnings: Except under the advice and supervision of a physician, do not take more than 8 tablespoonfuls in a 24-hour period or 8 tablespoonfuls daily for more than 2 weeks. May have laxative effect. Do not use this product if you have a kidney disease; do not use this product if you are on a sodium-restricted diet. Each tablespoonful of GAVISCON Liquid contains approximately 1.7 mEq sodium.

Drug Interaction Precautions: Do not take this product if you are presently taking a prescription antibiotic drug containing any form of tetracycline.
Keep tightly closed. Avoid freezing. Store at a controlled room temperature.
Keep this and all drugs out of the reach of children.
In case of accidental overdose, seek professional assistance or contact a poison control center immediately.

How Supplied: Bottles of 12 fluid ounce (355 ml) and 6 fluid ounce (177 ml).

Shown in Product Identification Section, page 427

GAVISCON®-2 Antacid Tablets

[*găv 'ĭs-kŏn*]

Composition: Each chewable tablet contains the following active ingredients:
Aluminum hydroxide dried gel...160 mg
Magnesium trisilicate .... 40 mg
and the following inactive ingredients: alginic acid, calcium stearate, flavor, sodium bicarbonate, starch (may contain cornstarch), and sucrose.

Indications: GAVISCON® is specifically formulated for the temporary relief of heartburn (acid indigestion) due to acid reflux. GAVISCON is not indicated for the treatment of peptic ulcers.

Directions: Chew one to two tablets four times a day or as directed by a physician. Tablets should be taken after meals and at bedtime or as needed. For best results follow by a half glass of water or other liquid. DO NOT SWALLOW WHOLE.

Warnings: Do not take more than eight tablets in a 24-hour period or eight tablets daily for more than 2 weeks, except under the advice and supervision of a physician. Do not use this product except under the advice and supervision of a physician if you are on a sodium-restricted diet. Each GAVISCON-2 Tablet contains approximately 1.6 mEq sodium.

Drug Interaction Precautions: Do not take this product if you are presently taking a prescription antibiotic drug containing any form of tetracycline.
Store at a controlled room temperature in a dry place.
Keep this and all drugs out of the reach of children. In case of accidental overdose, seek professional assistance or contact a poison control center immediately.

How Supplied: Boxes of 48 foil-wrapped tablets.

Issued 2/87

Shown in Product Identification Section, page 427

GERITOL COMPLETE™ Tablets

[*jer 'e-tol*]

The High Iron Multi-Vitamin/Mineral

Active Ingredients (Per Tablet): Vitamin A (6000 IU as Beta Carotene); Vitamin E (30 IU); Vitamin C (60 mg.); Folic Acid (400 mcg.); Vitamin B_1 (1.5 mg.); Vitamin B_2 (1.7 mg.); Niacin (20 mg.); Vitamin B_6 (2 mg.); Vitamin B_{12} (6 mcg.); Vitamin D (400 IU); Biotin (45 mcg.); Pantothenic Acid (10 mg.); Vitamin K (25 mcg.); Calcium (162 mg.); Phosphorus (125 mg.); Iodine (150 mcg.); Iron (50 mg.); Magnesium (100 mg.); Copper (2 mg.); Manganese (2.5 mg.); Potassium (37.5 mg.); Chloride (34 mg.); Chromium (15 mcg.); Molybdenum (15 mcg.); Selenium (15 mcg.); Zinc (15 mg.); Nickel (5 mcg.); Silicon (80 mcg.); Tin (10 mcg); Vanadium (10 mcg).

Inactive Ingredients: Carnauba wax, Crospovidone, Flavors, Gelatin, Glycerides of Stearic and Palmitic acids, Hydroxypropyl cellulose, Hydroxypropyl methylcellulose, Magnesium stearate, Microcrystalline cellulose, Polyethylene glycol, Silicon dioxide, Stearic acid, White wax, FD&C Red #40, FD&C Blue #2, FD&C Yellow #6, Titanium dioxide.

Indications: For use as a dietary supplement.

Actions: Help treat and prevent iron deficiency.

Warnings: Keep out of reach of children.

Precaution: Alcoholics and individuals with chronic liver or pancreatic disease may have enhanced iron absorption with the potential for iron overload.
NOTE: Unabsorbed iron may cause some darkening of the stool.

Symptoms and Treatment of Oral Overdose: Toxicity and symptoms are primarily due to iron overdose. Abdominal pain, nausea, vomiting and diarrhea may occur, with possible subsequent acidosis and cardiovascular collapse with severe poisoning. If an overdose is suspected, immediately seek professional assistance by contacting your physician, the local poison control center, or the Rocky Mt. Poison Control Center at 303-592-1710 (Collect), 24 hours a day.

Dosage and Administration (Adults): One (1) tablet daily after mealtime.

How Supplied: Bottles of 14, 40, 100, and 180 tablets.

GERITOL EXTEND™ Tablets or Caplets

Nutritional Supplement

Active Ingredients (per tablet): Vitamin A (3333 IU, including 1250 IU from Beta Carotene); Vitamin D (200 IU); Vitamin E (15 IU); Vitamin C (60 mg); Folic Acid (0.2 mg); Vitamin B_1 (1.2 mg); Vitamin B_2 (1.4 mg); Niacin (15 mg); Vitamin B_6 (2.0 mg); Vitamin B_{12} (2 mcg); Vitamin K (80 mcg); Calcium (130 mg); Phosphorus (100 mg); Magnesium (35 mg); Zinc (15 mg); Iodine (150 mcg); Iron (10 mg); Selenium (70 mcg)

Inactive Ingredients: Carnauba Wax, Croscarmelose Sodium, Flavors, Gelatin, Glycerides of Stearic and Palmitic Acids, Hydroxypropyl Methylcellulose, Magnesium Stearate, Microcrystalline Cellulose, Polyethylene Glycol, Silicon Dioxide, Stearic Acid, White Wax, FD&C Red #40, FD&C Blue #2, Titanium Dioxide.

Indications: For use as a dietary supplement. Recommended for active adults over 50.

Actions: Help treat and prevent iron deficiency.

Warnings: Keep out of reach of children.

Precaution: Alcoholics and individuals with chronic liver or pancreatic disease may have enhanced iron absorption with the potential for iron overload.
NOTE: Unabsorbed iron may cause some darkening of the stool.

Symptoms and Treatment of Oral Overdose: Toxicity and symptoms are primarily due to iron overdose. Abdominal pain, nausea, vomiting, and diarrhea may occur with possible subsequent acidosis and cardiovascular collapse with severe poisoning. If an overdose is suspected, immediately seek professional assistance by contacting your physician, the local poison control center, or the Rocky Mountain Poison Control Center at 303-592-1710 (collect), 24 hours a day.

Dosage and Administration (Adults 50+): One (1) tablet/caplet daily after mealtime.

How Supplied: Bottles of 40 and 100 tablets or caplets in blister-pack cartons.

GERITOL® Liquid

[*jer 'e-tol*]

High Potency Iron & Vitamin Tonic

Active Ingredients Per Dose (½ fluid ounce): Iron (as ferric ammonium citrate) 50 mg; Thiamine (B_1) 2.5 mg; Riboflavin (B_2) 2.5 mg; Niacinamide 50 mg;

Continued on next page

SmithKline Beecham—Cont.

Panthenol 2 mg; Pyridoxine (B_6) 0.5 mg; Cyanocobalamin (B_{12}) 0.75 mcg; Methionine 25 mg; Choline Bitartrate 50 mg.

Inactive Ingredients: Alcohol, Benzoic acid, Caramel color, Citric acid, Invert sugar, Sucrose, Water, Flavors.

Indications: For use as a dietary supplement.

Actions: Help treat and prevent iron deficiency.

Warnings: Keep out of reach of children.

Precaution: Alcohol accelerates absorption of ferric iron. Alcoholics and individuals with chronic liver or pancreatic disease may have enhanced iron absorption with the potential for iron overload.
NOTE: Unabsorbed iron may cause some darkening of the stool.

Symptoms and Treatment of Oral Overdose: Toxicity and symptoms are primarily due to iron overdose. Abdominal pain, nausea, vomiting and diarrhea may occur, with possible subsequent acidosis and cardiovascular collapse with severe poisoning. If an overdose is suspected, immediately seek professional assistance by contacting your physician, the local poison control center, or the Rocky Mt. Poison Control Center at 303-592-1710 (Collect), 24 hours a day.

Dosage and Administration (Adults): As an iron supplement and for normal menstrual needs: One (1) tablespoonful (0.5 fl. oz.) daily at mealtime. For iron deficiency: One (1) tablespoonful (0.5 fl. oz.) three times daily at mealtime or as directed by a physician.

How Supplied: Bottles of 4 oz. and 12 oz.
7001M
11/14/83

GLY-OXIDE® Liquid

Description: GLY-OXIDE® Liquid contains carbamide peroxide 10%. Also contains citric acid, flavor, glycerin, propylene glycol, sodium stannate, water, and other ingredients.

Actions: GLY-OXIDE® Liquid has an oxygen-rich formula that works to relieve the pain of canker sores by cleaning and debriding damaged tissue so natural healing can occur.

Administration: Do not dilute. Apply directly from bottle. Replace tip on bottle when not in use.

Indications: For local treatment and hygienic prevention of minor oral inflammation such as canker sores, denture irritation, and postdental procedure irritation. Place several drops on affected area four times daily, after meals and at bedtime, or as directed by a dentist or physician; expectorate after two or three minutes. Or place 10 drops onto tongue, mix with saliva, swish for several minutes, and expectorate.
As an adjunct to oral hygiene (orthodontics, dental appliances) after regular brushing, swish 10 or more drops vigorously. Continue for two to three minutes; expectorate.
When normal oral hygiene is inadequate or impossible (total care geriatrics, etc), swish 10 or more drops vigorously after meals and expectorate.

Precautions: Severe or persistent oral inflammation, denture irritation, or gingivitis may be serious. If these conditions or unexpected side effects occur, consult a dentist or physician immediately.
Avoid contact with eyes. Protect from heat and direct light. Keep this and all drugs out of the reach of children. In case of accidental overdose, seek professional assistance or contact a poison control center immediately.

How Supplied: GLY-OXIDE® Liquid is available in ½-fl-oz and 2-fl-oz nonspill, plastic squeeze bottles with applicator spouts.

Shown in Product Identification Section, page 427

MASSENGILL® Douches
[mas 'sen-gil]

PRODUCT OVERVIEW

Key Facts
Massengill is the brand name for a line of douches which are recommended for routine cleansing and for temporary relief of vaginal itching and irritation. Massengill Disposable douches are available in two Vinegar & Water formulas (Extra Mild and Extra Cleansing), a Baking Soda formula, four Cosmetic solutions (Country Flowers, Fresh Baby Powder Scent (formerly Belle Mai), Mountain Breeze and Spring Rain Freshness) and a Medicated formula (with povidone-iodine). Massengill also is available in a Medicated liquid concentrate (povidone-iodine) and a Non-Medicated liquid concentrate and powder form.

Major Uses: Massengill's Vinegar & Water, Baking Soda & Water, Fragrance-Free, and Cosmetic douches are recommended for routine douching, or for cleansing following menstruation, prescribed use of vaginal medication or use of contraceptives. Massengill Medicated is recommended in a seven day regimen for the symptomatic relief of minor itching and irritation associated with vaginitis due to Candida albicans, Trichomonas vaginalis, and Gardnerella vaginalis.

Safety Information: Do not douche during pregnancy unless directed by a physician. Douching does not prevent pregnancy. Do not use this product and consult your physician if you are experiencing any of the following symptoms: unusual vaginal discharge, painful and/or frequent urination, lower abdominal pain, or you or your sex partner has genital sores or ulcers.
Massengill Vinegar & Water, Baking Soda & Water, and Cosmetic Douches—If irritation occurs, discontinue use.
Massengill Medicated — Women with iodine-sensitivity should not use this product. If symptoms persist after seven days, or if redness, swelling or pain develop, consult a physician. Do not use while nursing unless directed by a physician.

PRODUCT INFORMATION

MASSENGILL®
[mas 'sen-gil]
Disposable Douches
MASSENGILL®
Liquid Concentrate
MASSENGILL® Powder

Ingredients:
DISPOSABLES: Extra Mild Vinegar and Water—Water and Vinegar.
Extra Cleansing Vinegar and Water—Water, Vinegar, Puraclean™ (Cetylpyridinium Chloride), Diazolidinyl Urea, Disodium EDTA.
Baking Soda and Water—Sanitized Water, Sodium Bicarbonate (Baking Soda).
Fresh Baby Powder Scent (formerly Belle-Mai Powder) Water, SD Alcohol 40, Lactic Acid, Sodium Lactate, Octoxynol-9, Cetylpyridinium Chloride, Propylene Glycol (and) Diazolidinyl Urea (and) Methyl Paraben (and) Propyl Paraben, Disodium EDTA, Fragrance, FD&C Blue #1.
Country Flowers—Water, SD Alcohol 40, Lactic Acid, Sodium Lactate, Octoxynol-9, Cetylpyridinium Chloride, Propylene Glycol (and) Diazolidinyl Urea (and), Methyl Paraben (and) Propyl Paraben, Disodium EDTA, Fragrance, D&C Red #28, FD&C Blue #1.
Mountain Breeze—Water, SD Alcohol 40, Lactic Acid, Sodium Lactate, Octoxynol-9, Cetylpyridinium Chloride, Propylene Glycol (and) Diazolidinyl Urea (and) Methyl Paraben (and) Propyl Paraben, Disodium EDTA, Fragrance, D&C Yellow #10, FD&C Blue #1.
Spring Rain freshness—Water, SD Alcohol 40, Lactic Acid, Sodium Lactate, Octoxynol-9, Cetylpyridinium Chloride, Propylene Glycol (and) Diazolidinyl Urea (and) Methylparaben (and) Propylparaben, Disodium EDTA, fragrance.
LIQUID CONCENTRATE: Water, SD Alcohol 40, Lactic Acid, Sodium Bicarbonate, Octoxynol-9, Methyl Salicylate, Liquid Menthol, Eucalyptol, Thymol, D&C Yellow #10, FD&C Yellow #6 (Sunset Yellow).
POWDER: Sodium Chloride, Ammonium alum, PEG-8, Phenol, Methyl Salicylate, Eucalyptus Oil, Menthol, Thymol, D&C Yellow #10, FD&C Yellow #6 (Sunset Yellow).
FLORAL POWDER: Sodium Chloride, Ammonium alum, Octoxynol-9, SD Alcohol 23-A, Fragrance, and FD&C Yellow #6 (Sunset Yellow).

Indications: Recommended for routine cleansing at the end of menstruation, after use of contraceptive creams or jellies (check the contraceptive package instructions first) or to rinse out the residue of prescribed vaginal medication (as directed by physician).

Actions: The buffered acid solutions of Massengill Douches are valuable adjuncts to specific vaginal therapy following the prescribed use of vaginal medication or contraceptives and in feminine hygiene.

Directions:
DISPOSABLES: Twist off flat, wing-shaped tab from bottle containing premixed solution, attach nozzle supplied and use. The unit is completely disposable.
LIQUID CONCENTRATE: Fill cap 3/4 full, to measuring line, and pour contents into douche bag containing 1 quart of warm water. Mix thoroughly.
POWDER: Dissolve two rounded teaspoonfuls in a douche bag containing 1 quart of warm water. Mix thoroughly.

Warning: Douching does not prevent pregnancy. If vaginal dryness or irritation occurs discontinue use. Do not use during pregnancy except under the advice and supervision of your physician. If you are experiencing vaginal discharge of an unusual amount, color, or odor, or painful and/or frequent urination, lower abdominal pain or genital sores or ulcers, or have had sex with a partner who has genital symptoms, you may have a serious condition. Do not use this product and contact your doctor immediately.
Use this product only as directed for routine cleansing. You should douche no more than twice a week except on the advice of your doctor.
An association has been reported between frequent douching and pelvic inflammatory disease (PID), a serious infection of the reproductive system, which can lead to sterility and/or ectopic (tubal) pregnancy. PID requires immediate medical attention.
PID's most common symptoms are pain and/or tenderness in the lower part of the abdomen and pelvis. You may also experience a vaginal discharge, vaginal bleeding, nausea or fever. Douches should not be used for self-treatment of any sexually transmitted diseases or PID. If you suspect you have one of these infections, stop using this product and see your doctor immediately.
Keep out of reach of children. In case of accidental ingestion, seek professional assistance by contacting your physician, the local poison control center, or the Rocky Mt. Poison Control Center at 303-592-1710 (collect), 24 hours a day.

How Supplied:
Disposable—6 oz. disposable plastic bottle.
Liquid Concentrate—4 oz., 8 oz., plastic bottles.
Powder—4 oz., 8 oz., 16 oz., Packettes —10's, 12's.

MASSENGILL® Medicated
[mas 'sen-gil]
Disposable Douche
MASSENGILL® Medicated
Liquid Concentrate

Active Ingredient:
DISPOSABLE: Cepticin™ (povidone-iodine)
LIQUID CONCENTRATE: Cepticin™ (povidone-iodine)

Indications: For symptomatic relief of minor vaginal irritation or itching associated with vaginitis due to Candida albicans, Trichomonas vaginalis, and Gardnerella vaginalis.

Action: Povidone-iodine is widely recognized as an effective broad spectrum microbicide against both gram negative and gram positive bacteria, fungi, yeasts and protozoa. While remaining active in the presence of blood, serum or bodily secretions, it possesses virtually none of the irritating properties of iodine.

Warnings: Douching does not prevent pregnancy. Do not use during pregnancy or while nursing except under the advice and supervision of your physician. If vaginal dryness or irritation occurs discontinue use. If you are experiencing vaginal discharge of an unusual amount, color, or odor or painful and/ or frequent urination, lower abdominal pain or genital sores or ulcers, or have had sex with a partner who has genital symptoms, you may have a serious condition. Do not use this product and contact your doctor immediately.
Use this product only as directed. Do not use this product for routine cleansing.
An association has been reported between frequent douching and pelvic inflammatory disease (PID), a serious infection of the reproductive system, which can lead to sterility and/or ectopic (tubal) pregnancy. PID requires immediate medical attention.
PID's most common symptoms are pain and/or tenderness in the lower part of the abdomen and pelvis. You may also experience and vaginal discharge, vaginal bleeding, nausea or fever. Douches should not be used for self-treatment of any sexually transmitted diseases or PID. If you suspect you have one of these infections, stop using this product and see your doctor immediately. Women with iodine sensitivity should not use this product. Keep out of the reach of children. In case of accidental ingestion, seek professional assistance by contacting your physician, the local poison control center, or the Rocky Mt. Poison Control Center at 303-592-1710 (Collect), 24 hours a day.

Dosage and Administration:
DISPOSABLE: Dosage is provided as a single unit concentrate to be added to 6 oz. of sanitized water supplied in a disposable bottle. A specially designed nozzle is provided. After use, the unit is discarded. Use one bottle a day. Although symptoms may be relieved earlier, for maximum relief, use for seven days.
LIQUID CONCENTRATE: Pour one capful into douche bag containing one quart of water. Mix thoroughly. Use once daily. Although symptoms may be relieved earlier, for maximum relief, use for seven days.

How Supplied:
Disposable—6 oz. bottle of sanitized water with 0.17 oz. vial of povidone-iodine and nozzle.
Liquid Concentrate—4 oz., 8 oz. plastic bottles.

Shown in Product Identification Section, page 427

MASSENGILL®
[mas 'sen-gil]
Unscented Soft Cloth Towelette

Inactive Ingredients: Water, Octoxynol-9, Lactic Acid, Sodium Lactate, Potassium Sorbate, Disodium EDTA, and Cetylpyridinium Chloride.

Indications: For cleansing and refreshing the external vaginal area.

Actions: Massengill Unscented Soft Cloth Towelettes safely cleanse the external vaginal area and do not contain fragrance. The towelette delivery system makes the application soft and gentle.

Warnings: For external use only. Avoid contact with eyes.

Directions: Remove towelette from foil packet, unfold, and gently wipe. Throw away towelette after it has been used once.

How Supplied: Sixteen individually wrapped, disposable towelettes per carton.

MASSENGILL® Medicated
[mas 'sen-gil]
Soft Cloth Towelette

Active Ingredient: Hydrocortisone (0.5%).
Inactive Ingredients: Diazolidinyl Urea, DMDM Hydantoin, Isopropyl Myristate, Methylparaben, Polysorbate 60, Propylene Glycol, Propylparaben, Sorbitan Stearate, Steareth-2, Steareth-21, Water.
Tamper Resistant: If foil packet is torn or broken, do not use.
Also available in non-medicated Baby Powder Scent and Unscented formulas to freshen and cleanse the external vaginal area.

Indications: Massengill Medicated Towelettes provide temporary soothing relief of minor external feminine itching associated with irritations. They can also be used for the temporary relief of itching associated with skin rashes. Other uses of this product should be only under the advice and supervision of a physician.

Continued on next page

SmithKline Beecham—Cont.

Action: Massengill Medicated Soft Cloth Towelettes contain hydrocortisone, a proven anti-inflammatory, anti-pruritic ingredient. The towelette delivery system makes the application soothing, soft, and gentle.

Warnings: For external use only. Avoid contact with eyes. if condition worsens, symptoms persist for more than 7 days, or symptoms recur within a few days, do not use this or any other hydrocortisone product unless you have consulted a physician. Do not use if you are experiencing a vaginal discharge—see a physician. Do not use this towelette for the treatment of diaper rash. See a physician.
Keep this and all drugs out of the reach of children. As with any drug, if you are pregnant or nursing a baby, seek the advice of a health professional before using this product. In case of accidental ingestion, seek professional assistance or contact a Poison Control Center immediately.
Avoid storing at extreme temperatures (below 40°F or greater than 100°F).

Directions: For adults and children two years of age and older. Remove towelette from foil packet and gently wipe. Throw away towelette after it has been used once. Apply to the affected area not more than 3 to 4 times daily. Children under 2 years of age: DO NOT USE, consult a physician.

How Supplied: Ten individually wrapped, disposable towelettes per carton.

NATURE'S REMEDY®
Natural Vegetable Laxative

Active Ingredients: Cascara Sagrada 150 mg, Aloe 100 mg.

Inactive Ingredients: Calcium Stearate, Cellulose, Lactose, Coating, Colors (contains FD&C Yellow No. 6).

Indications: For gentle, overnight relief of constipation.

Actions: Nature's Remedy has two natural active ingredients that give gentle, overnight relief of constipation. These ingredients, Cascara Sagrada and Aloe, gently stimulate the body's natural function.

Dosage and Administration: Adults, swallow two tablets daily along with a full glass of water; children (8–15 yrs.), one tablet daily; or as directed by a physician.

Warnings: Do not take any laxative when nausea, vomiting, abdominal pain, or other symptoms of appendicitis are present. Frequent or prolonged use of laxatives may result in dependence on them. As with any drug, if you are pregnant or nursing a baby, seek the advice of a health professional before using this product.
KEEP OUT OF THE REACH OF CHILDREN.

Symptoms and Treatment of Oral Overdosage: If an overdose is suspected, immediately seek professional assistance by contacting your physician, local poison control center, or the Rocky Mountain Poison Control Center at 303-592-1710 (Collect) 24 hours a day.

How Supplied: Beige, film-coated tablets with foil-backed blister packaging in boxes of 12s, 30s and 60s.

Shown in Product Identification Section, page 427

N'ICE® Medicated Sugarless Sore Throat and Cough Lozenges
[*nis*]

Active Ingredient: Cherry—Each lozenge contains 5.0 mg. menthol in a sorbitol base. Citrus—Each lozenge contains 5.0 mg. menthol in a sorbitol base. Menthol Eucalyptus—Each lozenge contains 5.0 mg. menthol in a sorbitol base. Menthol Mint—Each lozenge contains 5.0 mg. menthol in a sorbitol base.

Inactive Ingredients: Cherry—Flavors, Red 33, Sorbitol, Tartaric Acid, Yellow 6, Citrus—Citric Acid, Flavors, Saccharin Sodium, Sodium Citrate, Sorbitol, Yellow 10. Menthol Eucalyptus—Citric Acid, Flavors, Sorbitol. Menthol Mint—Blue 1, Flavor, Hydrogenated Glucose Syrup, Sorbitol, Yellow 10.

Indications: Temporarily suppresses cough due to minor throat and bronchial irritation associated with a cold or inhaled irritants. Temporarily relieves minor sore throat pain.

Warnings: Do not administer to children under six years of age unless directed by a physician. Severe or persistent sore throat or sore throat accompanied by high fever, headache, nausea, and vomiting may be serious. Consult a physician in such case, or if sore throat persists for more than two days. A persistent cough may be a sign of a serious condition. If cough persists for more than one week, tends to recur, or is accompanied by fever, rash, or persistent headache, consult a physician. Do not take this product for persistent or chronic cough such as occurs with smoking, asthma, emphysema, or if cough is accompanied by excessive phlegm, unless directed by a physician.
Keep this and all medicines out of the reach of children.

Drug Interaction: No known drug interaction.

Dosage and Administration: Cherry, Citrus, Menthol Eucalyptus, Menthol Mint—Let lozenge dissolve slowly in the mouth. Repeat as needed, up to 10 lozenges per day.

Professional Labeling: For the temporary relief of pain associated with tonsillitis, pharyngitis, throat infections or stomatitis.

How Supplied: Available in packages of 2, 8 and 16 lozenges.

NOVAHISTINE® DMX
[*nō″vă-hĭs′tēn*]
Cough/Cold Formula & Decongestant

Description: Each 5 mL teaspoonful of NOVAHISTINE DMX contains: Dextromethorphan Hydrobromide 10 mg, Guaifenesin 100 mg, Pseudoephedrine Hydrochloride 30 mg. Also contains: Alcohol 10%, FD&C Red No. 40, FD&C Yellow No. 6, Flavors, Glycerin, Hydrochloric Acid, Invert Sugar, Saccharin Sodium, Sodium Chloride, Sorbitol, and Water.
Dextromethorphan hydrobromide, a synthetic nonnarcotic antitussive, is the dextrorotatory isomer of 3-methoxy-*N*-methylmorphinan. Guaifenesin is the glyceryl ether of guaiacol. Pseudoephedrine hydrochloride is the salt of a pharmacologically active stereoisomer of ephedrine (1-phenyl-2-methylamino-1-propanol).

Actions: Dextromethorphan hydrobromide suppresses the cough reflex by a direct effect on the cough center in the medulla of the brain. Although it is chemically related to morphine, it produces no analgesia or addiction. Its antitussive activity is about equal to that of codeine.
Pseudoephedrine hydrochloride is an orally effective nasal decongestant. It is a sympathomimetic amine with peripheral effects similar to epinephrine and central effects similar to, but less intense than, amphetamines. Therefore, it has the potential for excitatory side effects.
Pseudoephedrine hydrochloride at the recommended oral dosage has little or no pressor effect in normotensive adults. Patients taking pseudoephedrine orally have not been reported to experience the rebound congestion sometimes experienced with frequent, repeated use of topical decongestants. Pseudoephedrine is not known to produce drowsiness.
Guaifenesin acts as an expectorant by increasing respiratory tract fluid which reduces the viscosity of tenacious secretions, thus making expectoration easier.

Indications: NOVAHISTINE DMX is indicated for temporary relief of cough and nasal congestion; helps loosen phlegm and bronchial secretions. It is useful when exhausting, nonproductive cough accompanies respiratory tract congestion and in the symptomatic relief of upper respiratory congestion associated with the common cold, influenza, bronchitis, and sinusitis.

Contraindications: NOVAHISTINE DMX is contraindicated in patients with severe hypertension, severe coronary artery disease, and in patients on MAO inhibitor therapy. Patient idiosyncrasy to adrenergic agents may be manifested by insomnia, dizziness, weakness, tremor, or arrhythmias.

Nursing mothers: Pseudoephedrine is contraindicated in nursing mothers

because of the higher than usual risk for infants from sympathomimetic amines.
Hypersensitivity: NOVAHISTINE DMX is contraindicated in patients with hypersensitivity or idiosyncrasy to sympathomimetic amines, dextromethorphan, or to other formula ingredients.

Warnings: At dosages higher than the recommended dose, nervousness, dizziness, sleeplessness, nausea, or headache may occur. Do not take for more than 7 days. A persistent cough may be a sign of a serious condition. If symptoms do not improve, recur, or are accompanied by fever, rash, or persistent headache, patients should be advised to consult their physician before continuing use. Do not use for persistent or chronic cough such as occurs with smoking, asthma, chronic bronchitis or emphysema, or where cough is accompanied by excessive phlegm (sputum) unless directed by a physician. Sympathomimetic amines should be used judiciously and sparingly in patients with hypertension, diabetes mellitus, cardiovascular disease (e.g. ischemic heart disease), increased intraocular pressure, hyperthyroidism, or prostatic hypertrophy. Sympathomimetics may produce central nervous system stimulation with convulsions or cardiovascular collapse with accompanying hypotension. See Contraindications.
Use in elderly: The elderly (60 years and older) are more likely to have adverse reactions to sympathomimetics. Overdosage of sympathomimetics in this age group may cause hallucinations, convulsions, CNS depression, and death.
Use in children: NOVAHISTINE DMX should not be used in children under 2 years except under the advice and supervision of a physician.
Use in pregnancy: Safety for use during pregnancy has not been established. As with any drug, if you are pregnant or nursing a baby, seek the advice of a health professional before using this product.
If sensitive to any of the ingredients, do not use.
Keep this and all drugs out of the reach of children. In case of accidental overdose, seek professional assistance or contact a Poison Control Center immediately.

Adverse Reactions: Adverse reactions occur infrequently with usual oral doses of NOVAHISTINE DMX. When they occur, adverse reactions may include gastrointestinal upset and nausea. Because of the pseudoephedrine in NOVAHISTINE DMX, hyperreactive individuals may display ephedrine-like reactions such as tachycardia, palpitations, headache, dizziness or nausea. Sympathomimetic drugs have been associated with certain untoward reactions including fear, anxiety, tenseness, restlessness, tremor, weakness, pallor, respiratory difficulty, dysuria, insomnia, hallucinations, convulsions, CNS depression, arrhythmias, and cardiovascular collapse with hypotension.
Note: Guaifenesin interferes with the colorimetric determination of 5-hydroxyindoleacetic acid (5-HIAA) and vanillylmandelic acid (VMA).

Drug Interactions: NOVAHISTINE DMX should not be used in patients taking a prescription drug for hypertension or depression without the advice of a physician. MAO inhibitors and beta-adrenergic blockers increase the effects of pseudoephedrine (sympathomimetics). Sympathomimetics may reduce the antihypertensive effects of methyldopa, mecamylamine, reserpine, and veratrum alkaloids.

Dosage and Administration: Adults and children 12 years and over, 2 teaspoonfuls every 4 hours. Children 6 to under 12 years, 1 teaspoonful every 4 hours. Children 2 to under 6 years, ½ teaspoonful every 4 hours. Not more than 4 doses every 24 hours. For children under 2 years of age, give only as directed by a physician.

How Supplied: As a red syrup in 4 fluid ounce bottles.
Keep tightly closed. Protect from excessive heat and light. Avoid freezing.

Shown in Product Identification Section, page 427

NOVAHISTINE® Elixir
[*nō″vă-hĭs′tēn*]
Cold & Hay Fever Formula

Description: Each 5 mL teaspoonful of NOVAHISTINE Elixir contains: Chlorpheniramine Maleate 2 mg, Phenylephrine Hydrochloride 5 mg. Also contains: Alcohol 5%, D&C Yellow No. 10, FD&C Blue No. 1, Flavors, Glycerin, Sodium Chloride, Sorbitol, and Water. Although considered sugar-free, each 5 mL contributes approximately 7 calories from sorbitol.

Actions: Phenylephrine is a nasal decongestant. Its effects are similar to epinephrine, but it is less potent on a weight basis, and has a longer duration of action. Phenylèphrine produces peripheral effects similar to epinephrine, but has little or no central nervous system stimulation. After oral administration, nasal decongestion may occur within 15 or 20 minutes and persist for 2 to 4 hours.
Chlorpheniramine maleate, an antihistaminic effective for the symptomatic relief of allergic rhinitis, possesses anticholinergic and sedative effects. Chlorpheniramine antagonizes many of the pharmacologic actions of histamine. It prevents released histamine from dilating capillaries and causing edema of the respiratory mucosa.

Indications: For the temporary relief of nasal congestion and eustachian tube congestion associated with the common cold, sinusitis, and hay fever (allergic rhinitis). Also provides temporary relief of runny nose, sneezing, itching of nose or throat, and itchy, watery eyes due to the common cold, hay fever (allergic rhinitis) or other upper respiratory allergies. May be given concomitantly, when indicated, with analgesics and antibiotics.

Contraindications: NOVAHISTINE Elixir is contraindicated in patients with severe hypertension, severe coronary artery disease, and in patients on MAO inhibitor therapy. Patient idiosyncrasy to adrenergic agents may be manifested by insomnia, dizziness, weakness, tremor, or arrhythmias.
NOVAHISTINE Elixir is also contraindicated in patients with narrow-angle glaucoma, urinary retention, peptic ulcer, asthma, emphysema, chronic pulmonary disease, shortness of breath, or difficulty in breathing.
Nursing mothers: Phenylephrine is contraindicated in nursing mothers.
Hypersensitivity: NOVAHISTINE Elixir is also contraindicated in patients with hypersensitivity or idiosyncrasy to sympathomimetic amines, antihistamines or to other formula ingredients.

Warnings: At dosages higher than the recommended dose, nervousness, dizziness, or sleeplessness may occur. If symptoms do not improve within 7 days or are accompanied by high fever, patients should be advised to consult their physician before continuing use. Sympathomimetic amines should be used judiciously and sparingly in patients with hypertension, diabetes mellitus, cardiovascular disease (e.g. ischemic heart disease), increased intraocular pressure, hyperthyroidism, or prostatic hypertrophy. Sympathomimetics may produce central nervous system stimulation with convulsions or cardiovascular collapse with accompanying hypotension. See Contraindications.
Use in elderly: The elderly (60 years and older) are more likely to have adverse reactions to sympathomimetics. Overdosage of sympathomimetics in this age group may cause hallucinations, convulsions, CNS depression, and death.
Use in children: May cause excitability. NOVAHISTINE Elixir should not be used in children under 6 years except under the advice and supervision of a physician.
Use in pregnancy: Safety for use during pregnancy has not been established. As with any drug, if you are pregnant or nursing a baby, seek the advice of a health professional before using this product.
If sensitive to any of the ingredients, do not use.
Keep this and all drugs out of the reach of children. In case of accidental overdose, seek professional assistance or contact a Poison Control Center immediately.

Precautions: The antihistamine may cause drowsiness, and ambulatory patients who operate machinery or motor vehicles should be cautioned accordingly.

Continued on next page

SmithKline Beecham—Cont.

Adverse Reactions: Drugs containing sympathomimetic amines have been associated with certain untoward reactions, including fear, anxiety, tenseness, restlessness, tremor, weakness, pallor, respiratory difficulty, dysuria, insomnia, hallucinations, convulsions, CNS depression, arrhythmias, and cardiovascular collapse with hypotension. Individuals hyperreactive to phenylephrine may display ephedrine-like reactions such as tachycardia, palpitation, headache, dizziness, or nausea.

Phenylephrine is considered safe and relatively free of unpleasant side effects when taken at recommended dosage.

Patients sensitive to antihistamine drugs may experience mild sedation. Other side effects from antihistamines may include dry mouth, dizziness, weakness, anorexia, nausea, vomiting, headache, nervousness, polyuria, heartburn, diplopia, dysuria, and, very rarely, dermatitis.

Drug Interactions: NOVAHISTINE Elixir should not be used in patients taking a prescription drug for hypertension or depression without the advice of a physician. MAO inhibitors and beta-adrenergic blockers increase the effects of sympathomimetics. Sympathomimetics may reduce the antihypertensive effects of methyldopa, mecamylamine, reserpine, and veratrum alkaloids. Antihistamines have been shown to enhance one or more of the effects of tricyclic antidepressants, barbiturates, alcohol, and other central nervous system depressants.

Dosage and Administration: Adults and children 12 years and older, 2 teaspoonfuls every 4 hours; children 6 to under 12 years, 1 teaspoonful every 4 hours; children 2 to under 6 years, ½ teaspoonful every 4 hours.

For children under 2 years, at the discretion of the physician.

Product label dosage is as follows: Adults and children 12 years and older, 2 teaspoonfuls every 4 hours. Children 6 to under 12 years, 1 teaspoonful every 4 hours. Not more than 6 doses every 24 hours. For children under 6 years, give only as directed by a physician.

How Supplied: NOVAHISTINE Elixir, as a green liquid in 4 fluid ounce bottles. Keep tightly closed. Protect from excessive heat and light. Avoid freezing.

Shown in Product Identification Section, page 427

OS-CAL® 500 Chewable Tablets
[*ăhs 'kăl*]
(calcium supplement)

Each Tablet Contains: 1,250 mg of calcium carbonate.
Elemental calcium .... 500 mg
Ingredients: calcium carbonate, dextrose monohydrate, maltodextrin, microcrystalline cellulose, magnesium stearate, Bavarian cream flavor, sodium chloride, and coconut cream flavor.

Directions: One tablet two to three times a day with meals, or as recommended by your physician.

Two Tablets Provide: 1,000 mg calcium, 100% of U.S. RDA for adults and children 12 or more years of age.

Three Tablets Provide: 1,500 mg calcium, 115% of U.S. RDA for pregnant and lactating women.

Store at room temperature. Keep out of reach of children.

How Supplied: OS-CAL® 500 Chewable Tablets is available in bottles of 60 tablets.

Issued 5/91

Shown in Product Identification Section, page 427

OS-CAL® 500 Tablets
[*ăhs 'kăl*]
(calcium supplement)

Each Tablet Contains: 1,250 mg of calcium carbonate from oyster shell, an organic calcium source.
Elemental calcium .... 500 mg
Ingredients: oyster shell powder, corn syrup solids, talc, hydroxypropyl methylcellulose, cornstarch, sodium starch glycolate, calcium stearate, polysorbate 80, pharmaceutical glaze, titanium dioxide, methyl propyl paraben, polyethylene glycol, polyvinylpyrrolidone, carnauba wax, D&C Yellow #10, acetylated monoglyceride, edetate disodium, FD&C Blue #1, and simethicone emulsion.

Directions: One tablet two or three times a day with meals, or as recommended by your physician.

Two Tablets Provide: 1,000 mg calcium, 100% of U.S. RDA for adults and children 12 or more years of age.

Three Tablets Provide: 1,500 mg calcium, 115% of U.S. RDA for pregnant and lactating women.

Store at room temperature. Keep out of reach of children.

How Supplied: OS-CAL® 500 is available in bottles of 60 and 120 tablets.

Issued 10/87

Shown in Product Identification Section, page 427

OS-CAL® 250+D Tablets
[*ăhs 'kăl*]
(calcium supplement with vitamin D)

Each Tablet Contains: 625 mg of calcium carbonate from oyster shell, an organic calcium source.
Elemental calcium .... 250 mg
Vitamin D .... 125 USP Units

Ingredients: oyster shell powder, corn syrup solids, talc, cornstarch, hydroxypropyl methylcellulose, calcium stearate, polysorbate 80, titanium dioxide, methyl propyl paraben, polyethylene glycol, pharmaceutical glaze, vitamin D, polyvinylpyrrolidone, carnauba wax, D&C Yellow #10, acetylated monoglyceride, edetate disodium, FD&C Blue #1, simethicone emulsion, and edible gray ink.

Directions: One tablet three times a day with meals, or as recommended by your physician.

Three Tablets Provide:

		% U.S. RDA for Adults
Calcium	750 mg	75%
Vitamin D	375 Units	94%

Store at room temperature. Keep out of reach of children.

How Supplied: OS-CAL® 250+D is available in bottles of 100 and 240.

Issued 10/87

Shown in Product Identification Section, page 427

OS-CAL® 500+D Tablets
[*ăhs 'kăl*]
(calcium supplement with vitamin D)

Each Tablet Contains: 1,250 mg of calcium carbonate from oyster shell, an organic calcium source.
Elemental calcium .... 500 mg
Vitamin D .... 125 USP Units

Ingredients: oyster shell powder, corn syrup solids, talc, hydroxypropyl methylcellulose, cornstarch, sodium starch glycolate, calcium stearate, polysorbate 80, pharmaceutical glaze, titanium dioxide, methyl propyl paraben, polyethylene glycol, polyvinylpyrrolidone, vitamin D, carnauba wax, D&C Yellow #10, acetylated monoglyceride, edetate disodium, FD&C Blue #1, and simethicone emulsion.

Directions: One tablet two or three times a day with meals, or as recommended by your physician.

Two Tablets Provide: 1,000 mg calcium, 100% of U.S. RDA for adults and children 12 or more years of age and 64% of vitamin D.

Three Tablets Provide: 1,500 mg calcium, 115% of U.S. RDA for pregnant and lactating women and 94% of vitamin D.

Store at room temperature. Keep out of reach of children.

How Supplied: OS-CAL® 500+D is available in bottles of 60 and 120.

Issued 10/87

Shown in Product Identification Section, page 427

OS–CAL® FORTIFIED Tablets
[*ăhs 'kăl*]
(multivitamin and minerals supplement with added calcium)

[See table top of next page]

Ingredients: oyster shell powder, ascorbic acid, corn syrup solids, niacinamide, D&C Yellow #10 Aluminum Lake, ferrous fumarate, calcium stearate, FD&C

Each Tablet Contains:

Vitamin A (palmitate)	1668 USP Units
Vitamin D	125 USP Units
Thiamine mononitrate (vitamin B_1)	1.7 mg
Riboflavin (vitamin B_2)	1.7 mg
Pyridoxine hydrochloride (vitamin B_6)	2.0 mg
Ascorbic acid (vitamin C)	50.0 mg
dl-alpha-tocopherol acetate (vitamin E)	0.8 IU
Niacinamide	15.0 mg
Calcium (from oyster shell)	250.0 mg
Iron (as ferrous fumarate)	5.0 mg
Magnesium (as oxide)	1.6 mg
Manganese (as sulfate)	0.3 mg
Zinc (as sulfate)	0.5 mg

Blue #1 Aluminum Lake, cornstarch, vitamin A palmitate, polysorbate 80, magnesium oxide, pyridoxine, thiamine, riboflavin, vitamin E, pharmaceutical glaze, methyl paraben, zinc sulfate, manganese sulfate, propylparaben, povidone, vitamin D, hydroxypropyl methylcellulose, carnauba wax, titanium dioxide, ethylcellulose, and acetylated monoglyceride.

Indication: Multivitamin and mineral supplement with added calcium.

Dosage: One tablet three times daily with meals or as directed by physician. In case of accidental overdose, seek professional assistance or contact a poison control center immediately.

Keep out of reach of children.
Store at room temperature.

How Supplied: Bottles of 100 tablets.
Issued 6/89

Shown in Product Identification Section, page 428

OS-CAL® PLUS Tablets

[*ăhs 'kăl*]

(multivitamin and multimineral supplement)

Each Tablet Contains:

Elemental calcium (from oyster shell)	250	mg
Vitamin D	125 USP	Units
Vitamin A (palmitate)	1666 USP	Units
Vitamin C (ascorbic acid)	33.0	mg
Vitamin B_2 (riboflavin)	0.66	mg
Vitamin B_1 (thiamine mononitrate)	0.5	mg
Vitamin B_6 (pyridoxine HCl)	0.5	mg
Niacinamide	3.33	mg
Iron (as ferrous fumarate)	16.6	mg
Zinc (as the sulfate)	0.75	mg
Manganese (as the sulfate)	0.75	mg

Ingredients: oyster shell powder, corn syrup solids, ferrous fumarate, ascorbic acid, calcium stearate, cornstarch, hydroxypropyl methylcellulose, polysorbate 80, titanium dioxide, vitamin A palmitate, niacinamide, ethylcellulose, manganese sulfate, methyl propyl paraben, zinc sulfate, pharmaceutical glaze, acetylated monoglyceride, riboflavin, thiamine mononitrate, pyridoxine hydrochloride, povidone, vitamin D, carnauba wax, and D&C Red #33.

Indications: As a multivitamin and multimineral supplement.

Dosage: One (1) tablet three times a day before meals or as directed by a physician. For children under 4 years of age, consult a physician.
Store at room temperature.
Keep out of reach of children. In case of accidental overdose, seek professional assistance or contact a poison control center immediately.

How Supplied: Bottles of 100 tablets.
Issued 1/91

Shown in Product Identification Section, page 428

OXY ACNE MEDICATIONS
OXY–5® and OXY–10® with SORBOXYL®

Benzoyl peroxide lotion 5% and 10% with silica oil absorber
Vanishing and Tinted Formulas

Description: Active Ingredient: Oxy-5: Benzoyl peroxide 5%. Oxy-10: Benzoyl peroxide 10%.

Inactive Ingredients: Oxy-5 Vanishing: Cetyl alcohol, citric acid, methylparaben, propylene glycol, propylparaben, silica (Sorboxyl®), sodium lauryl sulfate, sodium PCA, and water.
Oxy-5 Tinted: Cetyl alcohol, citric acid, iron oxides, methylparaben, propylene glycol, propylparaben, silica (Sorboxyl®), sodium lauryl sulfate, stearyl alcohol, sodium PCA, titanium dioxide and water.
Oxy-10 Vanishing: Cetyl alcohol, citric acid, methylparaben, propylene glycol, propylparaben, silica (Sorboxyl®), sodium citrate, sodium lauryl sulfate, and water.
Oxy-10 Tinted: Cetyl alcohol, citric acid, glyceryl stearate, iron oxides, methylparaben, propylene glycol, propylparaben, silica (Sorboxyl®), sodium citrate, sodium lauryl sulfate, stearic acid, titanium dioxide and water.

Indications: Topical medications for the treatment of acne vulgaris.

Action: Provides antibacterial activity against Propionibacterium acnes.

Additional Benefits: Absorbs excess skin oil up to 12 hours.
Vanishing formulas are colorless, odorless, greaseless lotions that vanish upon application. Tinted formulas are flesh tone, odorless, greaseless lotions.

Directions: Wash skin thoroughly and dry well. Shake well before using. Dab on Oxy 5 or Oxy 10, smoothing it into acne pimple areas of face, neck, and body (see Warnings). Apply once a day initially, then two or three times a day, or as directed by a physician.

Warnings: FOR EXTERNAL USE ONLY. Using other topical acne medications at the same time or immediately following use of this product may increase dryness or irritation of the skin. If this occurs only one medication should be used unless directed by a doctor. Do not use this medication if you have very sensitive skin or if you are sensitive to benzoyl peroxide. To test for sensitivity, apply to a small affected area once a day for two days. Follow label instructions and continue use if no discomfort or burning occurs. This product may cause irritation, characterized by redness, burning, itching, peeling, or possibly swelling. More frequent use or higher concentrations may aggrevate such irritation. Mild irritation may be reduced by using the product less frequently or in lower concentration. If irritation becomes severe, discontinue use. If irritation still continues, consult a doctor. Keep away from eyes, lips, and mouth. Keep this and all drugs out of reach of children. This product may bleach hair or dyed fabrics, including clothing and carpeting. Keep tightly closed. Store at room temperature, avoid excessive heat.

Symptoms and Treatment of Ingestion: These symptoms are based upon medical judgment, not on actual experience. Theoretically, ingestion of very large amounts may cause nausea, vomiting, abdominal discomfort, and diarrhea. If an oral overdose is suspected, contact a physician, the local poison control center, or the Rocky Mountain Poison Control Center at 303-592-1710 (Collect) 24 hours a day.

How Supplied: 1 fl. oz. plastic bottles.

Shown in Product Identification Section, page 428

OXY®
Medicated Cleanser and Medicated Soap

Active Ingredient: Oxy® Medicated Cleanser: Salicylic Acid* 0.5%.
Oxy® Medicated Soap: Triclosan 1.0%.

Inactive Ingredients:
Oxy® Medicated Cleanser: Citric acid, menthol, propylene glycol, sodium lauryl sulfate, and water. Also contains Alcohol 40%.
Oxy® Medicated Soap: Bentonite, cocoamphodipropionate, fragrance, glycerin, iron oxides, magnesium silicate, sodium borohydride, sodium chloride, sodium cocoate, sodium tallowate, talc, tetrasodium EDTA, titanium dioxide, trisodium HEDTA, water.

Indications: These skin care products are useful for removing excess dirt and oil. Also helps remove and prevent blackheads.

Additional Benefits: When used regularly cleanses acne-prone skin and removes dirt, grime and excess skin oil. For a complete anti-acne program, after using Oxy® Cleansing Products follow use with Oxy-5® Tinted and Vanishing, or Oxy-10® Tinted and Vanishing acne pimple medications.

*Salicylic Acid (2-Hydroxybenzoic Acid).

Continued on next page

SmithKline Beecham—Cont.

Warning (Oxy® Medicated Cleanser and Soap): FOR EXTERNAL USE ONLY. Using other topical acne medications at the same time or immediately following use of this product may increase dryness or irritation of the skin. If this occurs, only one medication should be used unless directed by a doctor. Do not leave pad on skin for an extended period of time. Keep away from eyes, lips and mouth. If contact occurs, flush thoroughly with water. Keep this and all drugs out of reach of children. Keep tightly closed. Store at room temperature. Avoid high temperature greater than 86°F. Protect from freezing. Flammable. Keep away from flame, fire and heat.

Warning (Oxy Medicated Soap): Do not use this product on infants under six months of age.

Symptoms and Treatment of Ingestion: If large amounts are ingested, nausea, vomiting, or gastrointestinal irritation may develop. If an oral overdose is suspected, contact a physician, the local poison control center, or the Rocky Mountain Poison Control Center at 303-592-1710 (Collect) 24 hours a day.

Dosage and Administration: See labeling instructions for use.

How Supplied:
Medicated Liquid Cleanser—4 fl. oz.
Medicated Soap—3.25 oz. soap bar.

OXY® MEDICATED PADS
Regular, Sensitive Skin, and Maximum Strength

Active Ingredient:
Oxy® Medicated Pads Regular Strength: Salicylic Acid* 0.5%.
Oxy® Medicated Pads Sensitive Skin: Salicylic Acid* 0.5%.
Oxy® Medicated Pads Maximum Strength: Salicylic Acid* 2.0%.

Inactive Ingredients:
Oxy® Medicated Pads Regular Strength: Citric acid, fragrance, menthol, propylene glycol, sodium lauryl sulfate, water. Also contains Alcohol 40%.
Oxy® Medicated Pads Sensitive Skin: Disodium lauryl sulfosuccinate, fragrance, menthol, PEG-4, sodium lauroyl sarcosinate, sodium PCA, trisodium EDTA, water. Also contains Alcohol 22%.
Oxy® Medicated Pads Maximum Strength: Citric acid, fragrance, menthol, PEG-8, propylene glycol, sodium lauryl sulfate, water. Also contains Alcohol 50%.

Indications: These medicated pad products are useful for removing excess dirt and oil. Also helps remove and prevent blackheads.

Additional Benefits: When used regularly cleanses acne-prone skin and removes dirt, grime and excess skin oil.

Warnings: FOR EXTERNAL USE ONLY. Using other topical acne medications at the same time or immediately following use of this product may increase dryness or irritation of the skin. If this occurs, only one medication should be used unless directed by a doctor. Do not leave pad on skin for an extended period of time. Keep away from eyes, lips and mouth. If contact occurs, flush thoroughly with water. Keep this and all drugs out of reach of children. Keep tightly closed. Store at room temperature. Avoid high temperature greater than 86°F. Protect from freezing. Flammable. Keep away from flame, fire and heat.

Symptoms and Treatment of Ingestion: If large amounts are ingested, nausea, vomiting, or gastrointestinal irritation may develop. If an oral overdose is suspected, contact a physician, the local poison control center, or the Rocky Mountain Poison Control Center at 303-592-1710 (Collect) 24 hours a day.

Dosage and Administration: See labeling instructions for use.

How Supplied:
Medicated Pads Regular Strength—Plastic Jar/50 pads or 90 pads
Medicated Pads Sensitive Skin—Plastic Jar/50 pads or 90 pads
Medicated Pads Maximum Strength—Plastic Jar/50 pads or 90 pads

---

OXY NIGHT WATCH™
Maximum Strength and Sensitive Skin Formulas

Active Ingredient:
Oxy Night Watch™ Maximum Strength: Salicylic Acid (2-Hydroxybenzoic Acid) 2.0%.
Oxy Night Watch™ Sensitive Skin: Salicylic Acid (2-Hydroxybenzoic Acid) 1.0%.

Inactive Ingredients: Cetyl alcohol, disodium EDTA, methylparaben, propylene glycol, propylparaben, silica (Sorboxyl®), sodium lauryl sulfate, stearyl alcohol, and water.

Indications: These medicated skin products penetrate pores to help treat pimples and blackheads before they form.

Additional Benefits: Absorbs excess skin oil up to 12 hours.
Stays on all night to treat and help prevent acne pimples and blackheads.

Directions:
Before Using: At bedtime, wash your face gently using a non-abrasive soap. Rinse thoroughly and pat dry.
Usage: Squeeze out a small amount of lotion. Smooth a thin layer evenly over your entire face, avoiding eyes, lips, and mouth. Do not wash off. OXY NIGHT WATCH works best when left on overnight. The next morning, wash your face and pat dry.

Warnings: FOR EXTERNAL USE ONLY. Some skin types may experience sensitivity to this medication. To test sensitivity, apply to a small facial area once a night for two nights. If skin irritation, excessive drying, or discomfort develops, use less frequently or discontinue use. Using other topical acne medications at the same time or immediately following use of this product may increase dryness or irritation of the skin. If this occurs, only one medication should be used unless directed by a doctor. Keep away from eyes, lips and mouth. If contact occurs, flush thoroughly with water. Keep this and all drugs out of reach of children. Keep tightly closed. Store at room temperature. Flammable. Keep away from flame, fire and heat.

How Supplied: 2.0 oz. plastic tubes.

OXY 10® BENZOYL PEROXIDE WASH

Active Ingredient: Benzoyl peroxide 10%.

Inactive Ingredients: Citric acid, cocamidopropyl betaine, diazolidinyl urea, methylparaben, propylparaben, sodium citrate, sodium cocoyl isethionate, sodium lauroyl sarcosinate, water, and xanthan gum.

Indications: Antibacterial skin wash used as an aid in the treatment of acne vulgaris.

Actions: Promotes antibacterial activity against Propionibacterium acnes.

Additional Benefits: When used instead of regular soap, cleanses acne-prone skin and removes dirt, grime and excess skin oil.

Directions: Shake well. Wet area to be washed. Apply Oxy 10 Benzoyl Peroxide Wash and work into lather, massaging gently for 1 to 2 minutes. Rinse thoroughly. Use 2 to 3 times daily or as directed by a physician.

Warnings: FOR EXTERNAL USE ONLY. Using other topical acne medications at the same time or immediately following use of this product may increase dryness or irritation of the skin. If this occurs, only one medication should be used unless directed by a doctor. Do not use this medication if you have very sensitive skin or if you are sensitive to benzoyl peroxide. To test for sensitivity, apply to a small affected area once a day for two days. Follow label instructions and continue use if no discomfort or burning occurs. This product may cause irritation, characterized by redness, burning, itching, peeling, or possibly swelling. More frequent use or higher concentrations may aggravate such irritation. Mild irritation may be reduced by using the product less frequently or in a lower concentration. If irritation becomes severe, discontinue use; if irrita-

---

*Salicylic Acid (2-Hydroxybenzoic Acid).

tion still continues, consult a doctor. Keep away from eyes, lips, and mouth. Keep this and all drugs out of reach of children. This product may bleach hair or dyed fabrics, including clothing and carpeting. Keep tightly closed. Store at room temperature; avoid excessive heat.

Symptoms and Treatment of Ingestion: These symptoms are based upon medical judgment, not on actual experience. Theoretically, ingestion of very large amounts may cause nausea, vomiting, abdominal discomfort, and diarrhea. If an oral overdose is suspected, contact a physician, the local poison control center, or the Rocky Mountain Poison Control Center at 303-592-1710 (Collect) 24 hours a day.

How supplied: 4 fl. oz. plastic bottles.

Shown in Product Identification Section, page 428

SINE–OFF® Maximum Strength No Drowsiness Formula Caplets

Composition: [See table below.]

Product Information: SINE-OFF Maximum Strength No Drowsiness Formula provides maximum strength relief from headache and sinus pain. Relieves pressure and congestion due to sinusitis, allergic sinusitis or the common cold. This formula contains acetaminophen, a non-aspirin pain reliever.

NO ANTIHISTAMINE DROWSINESS

Product Benefits: Eases headache, pain and pressure • Promotes sinus drainage • Shrinks swollen membranes to relieve congestion.

Directions: Adults and children over 12 years of age: 2 caplets every 6 hours, not to exceed 8 caplets in any 24-hour period. Children under 12 should use only as directed by physician.

TAMPER-RESISTANT PACKAGE FEATURES FOR YOUR PROTECTION:

- Each caplet is encased in a clear plastic cell with a foil back.
- The name SINE-OFF appears on each caplet (see product illustration on front of carton).
- **DO NOT USE THIS PRODUCT IF ANY OF THESE TAMPER-RESISTANT FEATURES ARE MISSING OR BROKEN.**

Comments or Questions? Call Toll-Free 800-245-1040 Weekdays.

For maximum strength relief of headache and sinus pain, without antihistamine drowsiness. Relieves pressure and congestion due to sinusitis, or the common cold. This formula contains acetaminophen, a non-aspirin pain reliever.

Directions: Adults and children over 12 years of age: 2 caplets every 6 hours, not to exceed 8 caplets in 24 hours. Children under 12 should use only as directed by physician.

Warnings: Do not exceed recommended dosage because dizziness, sleeplessness, or nervousness may occur. Do not take this product for more than 10 days. If symptoms do not improve or are accompanied by fever that lasts more than 3 days, or if new symptoms occur, consult a physician. Do not take this product if you have heart disease, high blood pressure, diabetes, thyroid disease, or difficulty in urination due to enlargement of the prostate gland unless directed by a physician. Keep this and all drugs out of reach of children. In case of accidental overdose, seek professional assistance or contact a poison control center immediately. Prompt medical attention is critical for adults as well as children even if you do not notice any signs or symptoms. As with any drug, if you are pregnant or nursing a baby, seek the advice of a health professional before using this product.

Drug Interaction Precaution: Do not take this product if you are presently taking a prescription drug for high blood pressure or depression, without first consulting your physician.

Avoid storing at high temperatures (greater than 100°F).

Active Ingredients: Each caplet contains: 30 mg. Pseudoephedrine Hydrochloride, 500 mg. Acetaminophen (500 mg. is a non-standard dosage of acetaminophen, as compared to the standard of 325 mg.).

Inactive Ingredients: Crospovidone, Hydroxypropyl Methylcellulose, Magnesium Stearate, Microcrystalline Cellulose, Polyethylene Glycol, Polysorbate 80, Povidone, FD&C Red 40, Starch, Titanium Dioxide.

How Supplied: Consumer packages of 24 caplets.

Note: There are other SINE-OFF products. Make sure this is the one you are interested in.

Also Available:

SINE-OFF® Tablets with Aspirin

SINE-OFF® Maximum Strength Allergy/Sinus Formula Caplets

Shown in Product Identification Section, page 428

SINE–OFF® Sinus Medicine Tablets–Aspirin Formula Relieves sinus headache and congestion.

Composition: [See table below.]

Product Information: SINE-OFF relieves headache, pain, pressure and congestion due to sinusitis, allergic sinusitis, or the common cold.

Product Benefits: Eases headache, pain and pressure • Promotes sinus drainage • Shrinks swollen membranes to relieve congestion • Relieves postnasal drip.

Directions: Adults: 2 tablets every 4 hours, not to exceed 8 tablets in any 24-hour period. Children (6–12) one-half the adult dosage. Children under 6 years should use only as directed by a physician.

TAMPER-RESISTANT PACKAGE FEATURES FOR YOUR PROTECTION:

- Each tablet is encased in a clear plastic cell with a foil back.
- The name SINE-OFF appears on each tablet (see product illustration on front of carton).
- **DO NOT USE THIS PRODUCT IF ANY OF THESE TAMPER-RESISTANT FEATURES ARE MISSING OR BROKEN.**

Comments or Questions? Call Toll-Free 800-245-1040 Weekdays.

Warnings: Children and teenagers should not use this medicine for chicken pox or flu symptoms before a doctor is consulted about Reye Syndrome, a rare but serious illness. Do not take this product for more than 10 days. If symptoms do not improve or are accompanied by fever that lasts for more than 3 days, or if new symptoms occur, consult a doctor. Do not take this product if you have asthma, glaucoma, heart disease, high blood pressure, thyroid disease, diabetes, emphysema, chronic pulmonary disease, shortness of breath, difficulty in breathing or difficulty in urination due to en-

Continued on next page

SINE-OFF

Each tablet/ caplet contains:	SINE-OFF Tablets—Aspirin Formula	SINE-OFF Maximum Strength No Drowsiness Formula Caplets
Chlorpheniramine maleate	2.0 mg	—
Phenylpropanolamine HCl	12.5 mg	—
Aspirin	325.0 mg	—
Acetaminophen	—	500.0 mg
Pseudoephedrine HCl	—	30.0 mg

SmithKline Beecham—Cont.

largement of the prostate gland unless directed by a doctor. Do not take this product if you are allergic to aspirin, have stomach problems, ulcers or bleeding problems unless directed by a doctor. Do not exceed recommended dosage. At higher doses nervousness, dizziness or sleeplessness may occur. May cause excitability, especially in children. May cause drowsiness. Avoid alcoholic beverages while taking this product. Do not drive or operate heavy machinery. Keep this and all drugs out of reach of children. In case of accidental overdose, seek professional assistance or contact a poison control center immediately. As with any drug, if you are pregnant or nursing a baby, seek the advice of a health professional before using this product. **IT IS ESPECIALLY IMPORTANT NOT TO USE ASPIRIN DURING THE LAST 3 MONTHS OF PREGNANCY UNLESS SPECIFICALLY DIRECTED TO DO SO BY A DOCTOR BECAUSE IT MAY CAUSE PROBLEMS IN THE UNBORN CHILD OR COMPLICATIONS DURING DELIVERY.**

Drug Interaction Precaution: Do not take this product if you are taking a prescription drug for anticoagulation (thinning the blood), high blood pressure, depression, diabetes, gout or arthritis unless directed by a doctor.
Store at controlled room temperature (59°–86°F.).

Each tablet contains: Active Ingredients: Aspirin, 325 mg.; Chlorpheniramine Maleate, 2 mg.; Phenylpropanolamine Hydrochloride, 12.5 mg.

Inactive Ingredients: Acacia, Calcium Sulfate, Carnauba Wax, D&C Yellow 10, Ethylcellulose, FD&C Yellow 6, Gelatin, Guar Gum, Polysorbate 80, Silicon Dioxide, Starch, Sucrose, Titanium Dioxide, and trace amounts of other inactive ingredients.

How Supplied: Consumer packages of 24, 48 and 100 tablets.

Note: There are other SINE-OFF products. Make sure this is the one you are interested in.

Also Available: SINE-OFF® Maximum Strength Allergy/Sinus Formula Caplets 24's. SINE-OFF® Maximum Strength No Drowsiness Formula Caplets 24's.

Shown in Product Identification Section, page 428

SINGLET® For Adults
Decongestant/Antihistamine/ Analgesic (pain reliever)/Antipyretic (fever reducer)

Description: Each pink Singlet tablet contains Pseudoephedrine Hydrochloride 60 mg, Chlorpheniramine Maleate 4 mg, and Acetaminophen 650 mg. Also contains: D&C Red No. 27, D&C Yellow No. 10, FD&C Blue No. 1, Hydroxypropyl Cellulose, Hydroxypropyl Methylcellulose 2910, Magnesium Stearate, Microcrystalline Cellulose, Polyethylene Glycol 8000, Pregelatinized Corn Starch, Sodium Starch Glycolate, Sucrose, and Titanium Dioxide.

Indications: For the temporary relief of nasal congestion, runny nose, occasional sinus headache, fever, sneezing, watery eyes or itching of the nose, throat, and eyes due to colds, hay fever, or other upper respiratory allergies.

Warnings: Do not take this product for more than 7 days. Unless directed by a physician, do not take this product if you have asthma, glaucoma, emphysema, chronic pulmonary disease, heart disease, high blood pressure, thyroid disease, diabetes, shortness of breath, difficulty in breathing, difficulty in urination due to enlargement of the prostate gland, or if you are presently taking a prescription drug for high blood pressure or depression. Do not exceed recommended dosage because severe liver damage, nervousness, dizziness, or sleeplessness may occur. May cause excitability. Consult your physician if symptoms persist, if new symptoms occur, or if redness or swelling is present, because these could be signs of a serious condition. Consult your physician if fever persists for more than 3 days (72 hours) or recurs. May cause drowsiness; alcohol, sedatives, and tranquilizers may increase the drowsiness effect. Avoid alcoholic beverages while taking this product. Do not take this product if you are taking sedatives or tranquilizers without first consulting your physician. Use caution when driving a motor vehicle or operating machinery. If sensitive to any of the ingredients, do not use.
As with any drug, if you are pregnant or nursing a baby, seek the advice of a health professional before using this product. KEEP THIS AND ALL DRUGS OUT OF THE REACH OF CHILDREN. In case of accidental overdose, seek professional assistance or contact a Poison Control Center immediately. Prompt medical attention is critical for adults as well as for children even if you do not notice any signs or symptoms.

Dosage and Administration: Adults and children 12 years and older: one tablet 3 to 4 times a day, taken with water, while symptoms persist. Do not take more than 1 tablet within a 4-hour period. Do not exceed 4 tablets in 24 hours. Children under 12 years of age: consult a physician.

Storage: Protect from excessive heat and moisture.

How Supplied: Bottles of 100.

SOMINEX®
[som 'in-ex]
Tablets and Caplets

Active Ingredients: Each tablet contains Diphenhydramine HCl, 25 mg. Each caplet contains Diphenhydramine HCl, 50 mg.

Inactive Ingredients Tablets: Dibasic Calcium Phosphate, Magnesium Stearate, Microcrystalline Cellulose, Silicon Dioxide, Starch, FD&C Blue #1.

Inactive Ingredients Caplets: Carnauba Wax, Crospovidone, Dibasic Calcium Phosphate, Hydroxypropyl Methylcellulose, Magnesium Stearate, Microcrystalline Cellulose, Polyethylene Glycol, Polysorbate 80, Silicon Dioxide, Starch, Titanium Dioxide, White Wax, FD&C Blue #1.

Indications: Helps to reduce difficulty falling asleep.

Action: An antihistamine with anticholinergic and sedative effects.

Directions: Take 50 mg. (2 tablets or 1 caplet) at bedtime if needed, or as directed by a doctor.

Warnings: Do not give to children under 12 years of age. If sleeplessness persists continuously for more than two weeks, consult your doctor. Insomnia may be a symptom of serious underlying medical illness. Avoid alcoholic beverages while taking this product. Do not take this product if you are taking sedatives or tranquilizers, without first consulting your doctor. Do not take this product if you have asthma, glaucoma, emphysema, chronic pulmonary disease, shortness of breath, difficulty in breathing, or difficulty in urination due to enlargement of the prostate gland unless directed by a doctor. As with any drug, if you are pregnant or nursing a baby, seek the advice of a health professional before using this product. Keep this and all drugs out of the reach of children. In case of accidental overdose, seek professional assistance or contact a poison control center immediately or the Rocky Mountain Poison Control Center at 303-592-1710 (Collect) 24 hours a day.

Drug Interaction: Monoamine oxidase (MAO) inhibitors prolong and intensify the anticholinergic effects of antihistamines. The CNS depressant effect is heightened by alcohol and other CNS depressant drugs.

Symptoms and Treatment of Oral Overdosage: Antihistamine overdosage reactions may vary from central nervous system depression to stimulation. Stimulation is particularly likely in children. Atropine-like signs and symptoms, such as dry mouth, fixed and dilated pupils, flushing, and gastrointestinal symptoms, may also occur.

How Supplied Tablets: Available in blister packs of 16, 32, and 72.

How Supplied Caplets: Available in blister packs of 8, 16, and 32.

Shown in Product Identification Section, page 428

SOMINEX® Pain Relief Formula
[*som 'in-ex*]

Active Ingredients: Each tablet contains 500 mg. Acetaminophen and 25 mg. Diphenhydramine HCl.

Inactive Ingredients: Crospovidone, Povidone, Silicon Dioxide, Starch, Stearic Acid, FD&C Blue #1.

Indications: For sleeplessness with accompanying occasional minor aches, pains, or headache.

Action: An antihistamine with sedative effects combined with an internal analgesic.

Directions: Take two tablets thirty minutes before bedtime, or as directed by a physician.

Warnings: Do not give to children under 12 years of age. If symptoms persist continuously for more than 10 days, or if new ones occur, consult your physician. Do not exceed recommended dosage because severe liver damage may occur. Insomnia may be a symptom of serious underlying medical illness. Take this product with caution if alcohol is being consumed. Do not take this product for the treatment of arthritis, except under the advice and supervision of a physician. As with any drug, if you are pregnant or nursing a baby, seek the advice of a health professional before using this product. Keep this and all drugs out of the reach of children. In case of accidental overdose, seek professional assistance by contacting your physician, the local poison control center, or the Rocky Mountain Poison Control Center at 303-592-1710 (Collect), 24 hours a day.

DO NOT TAKE THIS PRODUCT IF YOU HAVE ASTHMA, GLAUCOMA OR ENLARGEMENT OF THE PROSTATE GLAND, EXCEPT UNDER THE ADVICE AND SUPERVISION OF A PHYSICIAN.

Drug Interaction: Monoamine oxidase (MAO) inhibitors prolong and intensify the anticholinergic effects of antihistamines. The CNS depressant effect is heightened by alcohol and other CNS depressant drugs.

Symptoms and Treatment of Oral Overdosage: Antihistamine overdosage reactions may vary from central nervous system depression to stimulation. Stimulation is particularly likely in children. Atropine-like signs and symptoms, such as dry mouth, fixed and dilated pupils, flushing, and gastrointestinal symptoms, may also occur.

How Supplied: Available in blister packs of 16 tablets and bottles of 32 tablets.

Shown in Product Identification Section, page 428

SUCRETS® Maximum Strength Wintergreen
SUCRETS® Wild Cherry Regular Strength
SUCRETS® Children's Cherry Flavored
Sore Throat Lozenges
[*su 'krets*]

Active Ingredient: Maximum Strength Wintergreen: Dyclonine Hydrochloride 3.0 mg. per lozenge. Wild Cherry, Regular Strength: Dyclonine Hydrochloride 2.0 mg. per lozenge. Children's Cherry: Dyclonine Hydrochloride 1.2 mg. per lozenge.

Inactive Ingredients: Maximum StrengthWintergreen: Citric Acid, Corn Syrup, Silicon Dioxide, Sucrose, Yellow 10. Wild Cherry Regular Strength: Blue 1, Corn Syrup, Flavor, Red 40, Silicon Dioxide, Sucrose, Tartaric Acid. Children's Cherry: Blue 1, Citric Acid, Corn Syrup, Red 40, Silicon Dioxide, Sucrose.

Indications: For temporary relief of occasional minor sore throat pain and mouth irritations.

Actions: Dyclonine Hydrochloride's soothing anesthetic action relieves minor throat irritations.

Warnings: If sore throat is severe, persists more than 2 days, is accompanied or followed by fever, headache, rash, nausea, or vomiting, consult a doctor promptly. If sore mouth symptoms do not improve in 7 days, see your dentist or doctor promptly. KEEP THIS AND ALL MEDICINES OUT OF THE REACH OF CHILDREN.

Drug Interaction: No known drug interaction.

Symptoms and Treatment of Oral Overdosage: Reactions due to large overdosage are systemic and involve the central nervous system and cardiovascular system. Central nervous system reactions are characterized by excitation and/or depression. Nervousness, dizziness, blurred vision or tremors may occur. Reactions involving the cardiovascular system include depression of the myocardium, hypotension or bradycardia. Should a large overdose be suspected seek professional assistance. Call your physician, local poison control center or the Rocky Mountain Poison Control Center at 303-592-1710 (Collect), 24 hours a day.

Dosage and Administration: Adults and children 2 years of age or older: Allow to dissolve slowly in the mouth. Repeat every two hours as needed. Do not administer to children under 2 years of age unless directed by a doctor.

Professional Labeling: For the temporary relief of pain associated with tonsillitis, pharyngitis, throat infections or stomatitis.

How Supplied: Available in tins of 24 lozenges.

TELDRIN®
Chlorpheniramine Maleate
Timed-Release Allergy Capsules
Maximum Strength 12 mg.

Product Information: Hay fever and allergies are caused by grass and tree pollen, dust and pollution. TELDRIN provides up to 12 hours of relief from hay fever/upper respiratory allergy symptoms: sneezing, runny nose, itchy, watery eyes. TELDRIN is formulated to release some medication initially and the rest gradually over a prolonged period.

Directions: Adults and children over 12: Just one capsule in the morning, and one in the evening. Do not give to children under 12 without the advice and consent of a physician. Not to exceed 24 mg. (2 capsules) in 24 hours.

- The carton is protected by a clear overwrap printed with "safety sealed"; do not use if overwrap is missing or broken.

TAMPER-RESISTANT PACKAGING FEATURES FOR YOUR PROTECTION:

- Each capsule is encased in a plastic cell with a foil back; do not use if the cell or foil is broken.
- Each TELDRIN capsule is protected by a green PERMA-SEAL™ band which bonds the two capsule halves together; do not use if capsule or band is broken.

Warnings: Do not take this product if you have asthma, glaucoma, or difficulty in urination due to enlargement of the prostate gland, except under the advice and supervision of a physician. Do not drive or operate heavy machinery. May cause drowsiness. Avoid alcoholic beverages while taking this product. May cause excitability, especially in children. Keep this and all drugs out of the reach of children. In case of accidental overdose, seek professional assistance or contact a poison control center immediately. As with any drug, if you are pregnant or nursing a baby, seek the advice of a health professional before using this product.

Formula:
Active Ingredient: Each capsule contains Chlorpheniramine Maleate, 12 mg. Inactive Ingredients (listed for individuals with specific allergies): Benzyl Alcohol, Cetylpyridinium Chloride, D&C Red 27, FD&C Red 30, D&C Red 33, Ethylcellulose, FD&C Green 3, FD&C Red 40, FD&C Yellow 6, Gelatin, Hydrogenated Castor Oil, Silicon Dioxide, Sodium Lauryl Sulfate, Starch, Sucrose, and trace amounts of other inactive ingredients.
Store at controlled room temperature (59°–86°F).

How Supplied: Maximum Strength 12 mg. Timed-Release capsules in packages of 12, 24 and 48 capsules.

Shown in Product Identification Section, page 428

Continued on next page

SmithKline Beecham—Cont.

THROAT DISCS® Throat Lozenges

Description: Each lozenge contains sucrose, starch (may contain cornstarch), acacia, glycyrrhiza extract (licorice), gum tragacanth, anethole, linseed, cubeb oleoresin, anise oil, peppermint oil, capsicum, and mineral oil.

Indications: Effective for soothing, temporary relief of minor throat irritations from hoarseness and coughs due to colds.

Precautions: For severe or persistent cough or sore throat, or sore throat accompanied by high fever, headache, nausea, and vomiting, consult physician promptly. Not recommended for children under 3 years of age.

Directions: Allow lozenge to dissolve slowly in mouth. One or two should give the desired relief.

How Supplied: Boxes of 60 lozenges.

Shown in Product Identification Section, page 428

TUMS® Antacid Tablets
TUMS E-X® Antacid Tablets

Description: Tums: Active Ingredient: Calcium Carbonate, precipitated U.S.P. 500 mg.

Tums Original Flavor: Inactive Ingredients: Flavor, mineral oil, sodium polyphosphate, starch, sucrose, talc.

Tums Assorted Flavors: Inactive Ingredients: Adipic acid, colors (contains FD&C Yellow No. 6), flavors, mineral oil, sodium polyphosphate, starch, sucrose, talc.

An antacid composition providing liquid effectiveness in a low-cost, pleasant-tasting tablet. Tums tablets are free of the chalky aftertaste usually associated with calcium carbonate therapy and remain pleasant tasting even during long-term therapy. Each TUMS tablet contains not more than 2 mg of sodium and is considered to be dietetically sodium free. Non-laxative/ non-constipating.

Tums E-X: Active Ingredient: Calcium Carbonate, 750 mg.

Tums E-X Wintergreen Flavor Inactive Ingredients: Colors (contains FD&C Yellow No. 6), flavor, mineral oil, sodium polyphosphate, starch, sucrose, talc.

Tums E-X Cherry Flavor Inactive Ingredients: Adipic acid, color, flavor, mineral oil, sodium polyphosphate, starch, sucrose, talc.

Tums E-X Peppermint Flavor Inactive Ingredients: Flavor, mineral oil, sodium polyphosphate, starch, sucrose, talc.

Tums E-X Assorted Flavors Inactive Ingredients: Adipic acid, colors (contains FD&C Yellow No. 6), flavors, mineral oil, sodium polyphosphate, starch, sucrose, talc.

Each tablet contains not more than 2 mg of sodium and is considered to be dietetically sodium free. Non-laxative/ non-constipating.

Indications: For fast relief of acid indigestion, heartburn, sour stomach and upset stomach associated with these symptoms.

Actions: Tums lowers the upper limit of the pH range without affecting the innate antacid efficiency of calcium carbonate. One tablet, when tested *in vitro* according to the *Federal Register* procedure (*Fed. Reg.* 39-19862, June 4, 1974), neutralizes 10 mEq of 0.1N HCl. This high neutralization capacity combined with a rapid rate of reaction makes Tums an ideal antacid for management of conditions associated with hyperacidity. It effectively neutralizes free acid yet does not cause systemic alkalosis in the presence of normal renal function. A double-blind placebo-controlled clinical study demonstrated that calcium carbonate taken at a dosage of 16 Tums tablets daily for a two-week period was non-constipating/non-laxative.

Warnings: Tums: Do not take more than 16 tablets in a 24-hour period or use the maximum dosage of this product for more than 2 weeks, except under the advice and supervision of a physician.

Tums E-X: Do not take more than 10 tablets in a 24-hour period or use the maximum dosage of this product for more than two weeks, except under the advice and supervision of a physician. Keep this and all drugs out of the reach of children.

Dosage and Administration: Chew 1 or 2 TUMS tablets as symptoms occur. Repeat hourly if symptoms return, or as directed by a physician. No water is required. Simulated Drip Method: The pleasant-tasting TUMS tablet may be kept between the gum and cheek and allowed to dissolve gradually by continuous sucking to prolong the effective relief time.

Important Dietary Information—As a Source of Extra Calcium—Chew 1 or 2 tablets after meals or as directed by a physician.

Tums Original and Assorted Flavors:- The 500 mg of calcium carbonate in each tablet provide 200 mg of elemental calcium which is 20% of the adult U.S. RDA for calcium. Five tablets provide 100% of the daily calcium needs for adults.

Tums E-X: The 750 mg of calcium carbonate in each tablet provide 300 mg of elemental calcium which is 30% of the adult U.S. RDA for calcium. Four tablets provide 120% of the daily calcium needs for adults.

Professional Labeling: Indicated for the symptomatic relief of hyperacidity associated with the diagnosis of peptic ulcer, gastritis, peptic esophagitis, gastric hyperacidity, and hiatal hernia.

How Supplied: Tums: Peppermint and Assorted Flavors of Cherry, Lemon, Orange and Lime are available in 12-tablet rolls, 3-roll wraps, and bottles of 75 and 150 tablets. **Tums E-X Wintergreen, E-X Cherry, E-X Peppermint, and Assorted Flavors of Cherry, Lemon, Lime and Orange:** 8-tablet rolls, 3-roll wraps and bottles of 48 and 96 tablets.

Shown in Product Identification Section, page 428

TUMS Anti-gas /Antacid Formula

Active Ingredients: 500 mg of calcium carbonate and 20 mg of simethicone per tablet.

Tums Anti-gas/Antacid formula Assorted Fruit Flavor Inactive Ingredients: Adipic Acid, Corn Syrup, D&C Red 27, D&C Red 30, D&C Yellow 10, FD&C Blue 1, FD&C Yellow 6, Flavors, Microcrystalline Cellulose, Mineral Oil, Sodium Polyphosphate, Starch, Sucrose, Talc, Triglycerol Monooleate.

Each tablet contains not more than 2 mg of sodium and is considered dietetically sodium free.

The 500 mg of calcium carbonate in each tablet provide 200 mg of elemental calcium.

Non-laxative/non-constipating.

Indications: For fast relief of acid indigestion, heartburn, and sour stomach accompanied by gas and upset stomach associated with these symptoms.

Actions: Calcium carbonate in Tums anti-gas/antacid formula lowers the upper limit of the pH range without affecting the innate antacid efficiency of calcium carbonate. Calcium carbonate, when tested in vitro according to the Federal Register procedure (Fed. Reg. 39-19862, June 4, 1974), neutralizes 10 mEq of 0.1N HCl. This high neutralization capacity combined with a rapid rate of reaction makes calcium carbonate an ideal antacid for management of conditions associated with hyperacidity. It effectively neutralizes free acid yet does not cause systemic alkalosis in the presence of normal renal function.

Warnings: Do not take more than 16 tablets in a 24-hour period or use the maximum dosage of this product for more than 2 weeks, except under the advice and supervision of a doctor. Keep this and all drugs out of the reach of children.

Dosage and Administration: Chew 1 or 2 tablets as symptoms occur. Repeat hourly if symptoms return, or as directed by a doctor. No water is required. Simulated Drip Method: The pleasant-tasting Tums Anti-gas/Antacid formula tablets may be kept between the gum and cheek and allowed to dissolve gradually by continually sucking to prolong the effective relief time.

Professional Labeling: Indicated for the symptomatic relief of hyperacidity associated with the diagnosis of peptic ulcer, gastritis, peptic esophagitis, gastric hyperacidity, and hiatal hernia.

How Supplied: 60 tablet bottles 4770D

Shown in Product Identification Section, page 428

VIVARIN® Stimulant Tablets and Caplets
[*vi 'va-rin*]

Active Ingredient: Each tablet/caplet contains 200 mg. Caffeine Alkaloid.

Inactive Ingredients Tablets: Dextrose, Magnesium Stearate, Microcrystalline Cellulose, Powdered Cellulose, Silicon Dioxide, Starch, FD&C Yellow #6, D&C Yellow #10.

Inactive Ingredients Caplets: Carnauba Wax, Dextrose, Hydroxypropyl Methylcellulose, Magnesium Stearate, Microcrystalline Cellulose, Polyethylene Glycol, Polysorbate 80, Powdered Cellulose, Silicon Dioxide, Starch, Titanium Dioxide, White Wax, FD&C Yellow #6, D&C Yellow #10.

Indications: Helps restore mental alertness or wakefulness when experiencing fatigue or drowsiness.

Actions: Stimulates cerebrocortical areas involved with active mental processes.

Directions: Adults and children 12 years of age and over: Oral dosage is 1 tablet or caplet (200 mg) not more often than every 3 to 4 hours.

Warnings: The recommended dose of this product contains about as much caffeine as two cups of coffee. Limit the use of caffeine containing medications, foods, or beverages while taking this product because too much caffeine may cause nervousness, irritability, sleeplessness, and, occasionally, rapid heart beat. For occasional use only. Not intended for use as a substitute for sleep. If fatigue or drowsiness persists or continues to recur, consult a doctor. Do not give to children under 12 years of age. As with any drug, if you are pregnant or nursing a baby, seek the advice of a health professional before using this product. In case of accidental overdose, seek professional assistance or contact a poison control center immediately. Keep this and all drugs out of the reach of children.

Drug Interaction: Use of caffeine should be lowered or avoided if drugs are being used to treat cardiovascular ailments, psychological problems, or kidney trouble.

Precaution: Higher blood glucose levels may result from caffeine use.

Symptoms and Treatment of Oral Overdosage: Convulsions may occur if caffeine is consumed in doses larger than 10 g. Emesis should be induced to empty the stomach. In case of accidental overdose, seek professional assistance by contacting your physician, the local poison control center, or the Rocky Mt. Poison Control Center at 303-592-1710 (Collect), 24 hours a day.

How Supplied Tablets: Available in packages of 16, 40 and 80 tablets.

How Supplied Caplets: Available in packages of 24 and 48.

EDUCATIONAL MATERIAL

Booklets:
"A Personal Guide to Feminine Freshness"
A 16 page illustrated booklet on vaginal infections, feminine hygiene and douching. Free to physicians, pharmacists and patients in limited quantities by writing SmithKline Beecham Consumer Brands or calling 800-233-2426.
"Myths and Truths About STDS: An Easy Guide For Women"
A 16 page booklet on the common types of STDs and prevention. Free to physicians, pharmacists and patients in limited quantities by sending a SASE to: SmithKline Beecham Consumer Brands or calling 800-233-2426.
Film, Video:
"Feminine Hygiene and You"
This 14 minute color film begins with a simple explanation of how a woman's body works (reproductive system, menstrual cycle, and vaginal secretions) then explains douching. Free loan to physicians, pharmacists and clinics. Available in 16mm, and VHS by writing SmithKline Beecham Consumer Brands or calling 800-233-2426.

Standard Homeopathic Company
210 WEST 131st STREET
BOX 61067
LOS ANGELES, CA 90061

HYLAND'S ARNICAID™ TABLETS
100% natural temporary relief of symptoms of pain and soreness from muscle overexertion or injury.

Indications: Hyland's Arnicaid Tablets are a homeopathic product indicated for the control and symptomatic relief of acute bruising and soreness due to falls, blows, and muscle strain. Arnicaid provides a 100% natural relief for children and adults. Use after minor accidents or after sports workouts. Arnicaid contains no sucrose, dextrose or fillers. Like all homeopathic products, Arnicaid has no known contraindications or side effects.

Directions: Adults—1–2 tablets every 4 hours, or as needed.
Children over 3 years of age—½ adult dose.

Active Ingredients: Arnica Montana 30X HPUS in a base of lactose USP.

Warnings: Do not use if cap band is broken or missing. If symptoms persist for more than seven days or worsen, contact a licensed health care professional. Do not use in children under three years of age without consulting a licensed health care professional. As with any drug, if you are pregnant or nursing a baby, seek the advice of a licensed health care professional before using this product. Keep this and all medications out of reach of children. In case of accidental overdose, contact a poison control center or the manufacturer at the number provided below.
P&S Laboratories
Los Angeles, CA 90061
Questions? Call us: 800/624-9659
MADE IN USA
Arnicaid and Hyland's are trademarks of Standard Homeopathic Co.

HYLAND'S BED WETTING TABLETS

Active Ingredients: *Equisetum hyemale* (Scouring Rush) 2X HPUS, *Rhus aromatica* (Fragrant Sumac) 3X HPUS, *Belladonna* 3X HPUS (0.0003% Alkaloids).

Inactive Ingredients: Lactose USP.

Indications: A homeopathic combination for the temporary relief of involuntary urination (common bed wetting) in children.

Directions: Children 3 to 12 years: 2 to 3 tablets before meals and at bedtime, or as directed by a licensed health care practitioner. Children over 12 years: double the above recommended dose.

Warnings: If symptoms persist for more than seven days or worsen, consult a Health Care Professional. As with any drug, if you are pregnant or nursing a baby, seek the advice of a health professional before using this product. Keep this and all medication out of the reach of children.

How Supplied: Bottles of 125—one grain sublingual tablets (NDC 54973-7501-01). Store at room temperature.

HYLAND'S CALMS FORTÉ TABLETS

Active Ingredients: *Passiflora* (Passion Flower) 1X triple strength HPUS, *Avena sativa* (Oat) 1X triple strength HPUS, *Humulus lupulus* (Hops) 1X double strength HPUS, *Chamomilla* (Chamomile) 2X HPUS, *Calcarea Phosphorica* (Calcium Phosphate) 3X HPUS, *Ferrum Phosphorica* (Iron Phosphate) 3X HPUS, *Kali Phosphoricum* (Potassium Phosphate) 3X HPUS, *Natrum Phosphoricum* (Sodium Phosphate) 3X HPUS, *Magnesia Phosphoricum* (Magnesium Phosphate) 3X HPUS.

Inactive Ingredients: Lactose USP.

Indications: Temporary symptomatic relief of simple nervous tension and insomnia.

Continued on next page

Standard Homeopathic—Cont.

Directions: Adults, As a relaxant: 1 to 2 tablets as needed or 3 times daily between meals. In insomnia: 1 to 3 tablets ½ to 1 hour before retiring. Repeat as needed without danger of side effects. Children, As a relaxant: 1 tablet as needed or 3 times daily before meals. In insomnia: 1 to 2 tablets 1 hour before retiring. Non-habit-forming.

Warnings: If symptoms persist for more than seven days or worsen, consult a Health Care Professional. As with any drug, if you are pregnant or nursing a baby, seek the advice of a health professional before using this product. Keep this and all medication out of the reach of children.

How Supplied: Bottles of 100 four grain tablets (NDC 54973-1121-02). Store at room temperature. Bottles of 50 four grain tablets (NDC 54973-1121-01). Store at room temperature.

HYLAND'S CLEARAC™ TABLETS

All natural ClearAc helps clear up acne, pimples, and acne blemishes.

Indications: Hyland's ClearAc Tablets are a homeopathic combination indicated for the management and symptomatic relief of symptoms of pimples, blackheads, and blemishes associated with common acne (acne vulgaris). ClearAc Tablets provide a 100% natural approach. Like all homeopathic products, ClearAc Tablets have no known contraindications or side effects. Use in conjunction with a high-quality skin cleanser, such as 100% Natural Hyland's ClearAc Cleanser with Calendula.

Directions: Adults—2–3 tablets every 4 hours, or as needed.

Active Ingredients: Echinacea Ang. 6X HPUS, Berberis Vulg. 6X HPUS, Sulphur Iod. 6X HPUS, Hepar Sulph. 6X HPUS in a base of lactose USP.

Warnings: Do not use if cap band is broken or missing. If symptoms persist or worsen, contact a licensed health care professional. As with any drug, if you are pregnant or nursing a baby, seek the advice of a licensed health care professional before using this product. Keep this and all medications out of reach of children. In case of accidental overdose, contact a poison control center or the manufacturer at the number provided below.
P&S Laboratories
Los Angeles, CA 90061
Questions? Call us: 800/624-9659
MADE IN USA
ClearAc and Hyland's are trademarks of Standard Homeopathic Co.

HYLAND'S COLIC TABLETS

Active Ingredients: *Disocorea* (Wild Yam) 2X HPUS, *Chamomilla* (Chamomile) 3X HPUS, *Colocynth* (Bitter Apple) 3X HPUS.

Inactive Ingredients: Lactose USP.

Indications: A homeopathic combination for the temporary relief of colic and gas pains caused by irritating food, feeding too quickly, swallowing air and similar conditions during teething, colds and other minor upset periods in children.

Directions: For children to 2 years of age: administer 2 tablets dissolved in a teaspoon of water or on the tongue every 15 minutes until relieved; then every 2 hours as required. Children over 2 years: 3 tablets dissolved on the tongue as above; or as recommended by a licensed health care practitioner.

Warnings: If symptoms persist for more than seven days or worsen, consult a Health Care Professional. Keep this and all medication out of the reach of children.

How Supplied: Bottles of 125—one grain sublingual tablets (NDC 54973-7502-01). Store at room temperature.

HYLAND'S COUGH SYRUP WITH HONEY™

Active Ingredients: Each fluid ounce contains: *Ipecacuanha* (Ipecac) 3X HPUS, *Aconitum napellus* (Aconite) 3X HPUS, *Spongia Tosta* (Sponge) 3X HPUS, *Antimonium Tartaricum* (Potassium Antimony Tartrate) 6X HPUS.

Inactive Ingredients: Simple syrup and honey.

Indications: A homeopathic combination for the temporary relief of symptoms of simple, dry, tight or tickling coughs due to colds in children.

Directions: Children 1 to 12 years: 1 to 3 teaspoonfuls as required. Children over 12 years and adults: 3 to 4 teaspoonfuls as required. May be taken with or without water. Repeat as often as necessary to relieve symptoms. For children under 1 year of age, consult a licensed health care practitioner.

Warnings: Do not use this product for persistent or chronic cough such as occurs with asthma, smoking or emphysema; or if cough is accompanied with excessive mucus, unless directed by a licensed health care practitioner. If symptoms persist for more than seven days, tend to recur, or are accompanied by a high fever, rash, or persistent headache, consult a Health Care Professional. As with any drug, if you are pregnant or nursing a baby, seek the advice of a health professional before using this product. Keep this and all medication out of the reach of children.

How Supplied: Bottles of 4 fluid ounces (120 ml) (NDC 54973-7503-02). Store at room temperature.

HYLAND'S C-PLUS™ COLD TABLETS

Active Ingredients: *Eupatorium perfoliatum* (Boneset) 2X HPUS, *Euphrasia officinalis* (Eyebright) 2X HPUS, *Gelsemium sempervirens* (Yellow Jasmine) 3X HPUS, *Kali Iodatum* (Potassium Iodide) 3X HPUS.

Inactive Ingredients: Lactose USP, Natural Raspberry Flavor.

Indications: A homeopathic combination for the temporary relief of symptoms of runny nose and sneezing due to common head colds in children.

Directions: Children 1 to 3 years: 2 tablets every 15 minutes for 4 doses, then hourly until relieved. For children 3 to 6 years: 3 tablets as above; for children 6 and older: 6 tablets as above or as directed by a licensed health care practitioner.

Warnings: If symptoms persist for more than seven days or worsen, consult a Health Care Professional. As with any drug, if you are pregnant or nursing a baby, seek the advice of a health professional before using this product. Keep this and all medication out of the reach of children.

How Supplied: Bottles of 125—one grain sublingual tablets (NDC 54973-7505-01). Store at room temperature.

HYLAND'S DIARREX™ TABLETS

100% natural temporary relief of symptoms of acute gastrointestinal distress associated with nonspecific diarrhea.

Indications: Hyland's Diarrex Tablets are a homeopathic combination indicated for the temporary control and symptomatic relief of acute nonspecific diarrhea. Diarrex provides a 100% natural approach which aids in relief of symptoms of loose stools and associated gastric symptoms. Like all homeopathic products, Diarrex has no known contraindications or side effects.

Directions: Adults—2–3 tablets every 4 hours, or as needed. Children over 3 years of age—½ adult dose.

Active Ingredients: Arsenicum Alb. 6X HPUS, Podophyllum Pelt. 6X HPUS, Chamomilla 6X HPUS, Phosphorus 6X HPUS, Mercurius Viv. 6X HPUS in a base of lactose USP.

Warnings: Do not use if cap band is broken or missing. If symptoms persist for more than two days or worsen, contact a licensed health care professional. Do not use in children under three years of age without consulting a licensed health care professional. Discontinue use if diarrhea is accompanied by a high fever (greater than 101°F), or if blood is present in the stool and contact a licensed health care professional. As with any drug, if you are pregnant or nursing a baby, seek the advice of a licensed

health care professional before using this product. Keep this and all medication out of reach of children. In case of accidental overdose, contact a poison control center or the manufacturer at the number provided below.
P&S Laboratories
Los Angeles, CA 90061
Questions? Call us: 800/624-9659
MADE IN USA
Diarrex and Hyland's are trademarks of Standard Homeopathic Co.

HYLAND'S ENURAID™ TABLETS
100% natural temporary relief of symptoms of common incontinence in adults.

Indications: Hyland's EnurAid Tablets are a homeopathic combination indicated for the control and symptomatic relief of involuntary urination (common incontinence) in adults. EnurAid provides a 100% natural approach which aids in relief of symptoms of bladder control and related symptoms. Like all homeopathic products, EnurAid has no known contraindications or side effects.

Directions: Adults—2–3 tablets every 4 hours, or as needed.

Active Ingredients: Belladonna 6X HPUS, Cantharis 6X HPUS, Apis Mell. 6X HPUS, Arnica Mont. 6X HPUS, Allium Cepa 6X HPUS, Rhus Arom. 6X HPUS, Equisetum Hyem. 6X HPUS in a base of lactose USP.

Warnings: Do not use if cap band is broken or missing. If symptoms persist for more than seven days or worsen, contact a licensed health care professional. Discontinue use if symptoms are accompanied by a high fever (greater than 101°F), or if blood is present in urine and contact a licensed health care professional. As with any drug, if you are pregnant or nursing a baby, seek the advice of a licensed health care professional before using this product. Keep this and all medications out of reach of children. In case of accidental overdose, contact a poison control center or the manufacturer at the number provided below.
P&S Laboratories
Los Angeles, CA 90061
Questions? Call us: 800/624-9659
MADE IN USA
EnurAid and Hyland's are trademarks of Standard Homeopathic Co.

HYLAND'S TEETHING TABLETS

Active Ingredients: *Calcarea Phosphorica* (Calcium Phosphate) 3X HPUS, *Chamomilla* (Chamomile) 3X HPUS, *Coffea Cruda* (Coffee) 3X HPUS, *Belladonna* 3X HPUS (Alkaloids 0.0003%).

Inactive Ingredients: Lactose USP.

Indications: A homeopathic combination for the temporary relief of symptoms of simple restlessness and wakeful irritability due to cutting of teeth.

Directions: 2 to 3 tablets in a teaspoon of water or on the tongue, 4 times per day. If the child is restless or wakeful, 2 tablets every hour for 6 doses or as directed by a licensed health care practitioner.

Warnings: If symptoms persist for more than seven days or worsen, consult a Health Care Professional. As with any drug, if you are pregnant or nursing a baby, seek the advice of a health professional before using this product. Keep this and all medication out of the reach of children.

How Supplied: Bottles of 125—one grain sublingual tablets (NDC 54973-7504-01). Store at room temperature.

HYLAND'S VITAMIN C FOR CHILDREN™

Active Ingredients: 25 mg Vitamin C as Sodium Ascorbate (30 mg).

Inactive Ingredients: Lactose USP, Natural Lemon Flavor.

Indications: Each tablet provides children with 55% of the daily recommended requirement of Vitamin C. Sodium Ascorbate is preferred to Ascorbic Acid when gastric irritation may result from free acid.

Directions: Children 2 years and older: 1 to 2 tablets on the tongue or as directed by a licensed health care practitioner.

Warning: Keep this and all medication out of the reach of children.

How Supplied: Bottles of 125—one grain sublingual tablets (NDC 54973-7506-01). Store at room temperature. Tablets may turn brown in color with exposure to light. Color change does not affect potency.

EDUCATIONAL MATERIAL

Booklets—Brochures
"Homeopathy—What it is, How it Works," A Consumer's Guide to Homeopathic Medicine, Free
"Homeopathy—A Guide for Pharmacists," An ACPE (0.2 CEU) program on the basic principles of homeopathy.

Products are indexed by generic and chemical names in the **YELLOW SECTION.**

Stellar Pharmacal Corp.
Div./Star Pharmaceuticals, Inc.
1990 N.W. 44TH STREET
POMPANO BEACH, FL
33064-8712

STAR-OPTIC® EYE WASH
[*star op'tik*]
STERILE, ISOTONIC, BUFFERED SOLUTION

Description: STAR-OPTIC Eye Wash is specially formulated to soothe irritating 'Swimmers Eye'™ by bathing (washing) the eye providing cooling, refreshing relief. STAR-OPTIC Eye Wash is a sterile, isotonic buffered solution containing sodium chloride, sodium phosphate monobasic and sodium phosphate dibasic, preserved with edetate disodium and benzalkonium chloride in purified water, USP. CONTAINS NO BORIC ACID or THIMEROSAL (MERCURY).

Indications: For irrigating the eye to help relieve irritation, discomfort, burning, stinging or itching by removing loose foreign material, air pollutants (smog or pollen) or CHLORINATED WATER.

Directions: If eye cup is used, rinse cup with STAR-OPTIC Eye Wash or clean water immediately before and after each use. Avoid contamination of rim and inside surfaces of cup. Fill cup one-half full with STAR-OPTIC Eye Wash. Apply cup tightly to the affected eye to prevent leakage and tilt head backward. Open eyelids wide and rotate eyeball to ensure thorough bathing with the wash.
Note: Enclosed eye cup is sterile if package is intact. If cup is not used, flush affected eye by controlling the rate of flow of solution by pressure on the bottle.

Warnings: To avoid contamination, do not touch tip of container to any surface. Replace cap after using. If you experience eye pain, changes in vision, continued redness or irritation of the eye or if the condition worsens or persists, consult a physician. Obtain immediate medical treatment for all open wounds in or near the eyes. If solution changes color or becomes cloudy, do not use.
Keep out of the reach of children. Not for use with contact lenses. DO NOT USE IF IMPRINTED SAFETY SEAL ON CAP IS BROKEN OR MISSING AT TIME OF PURCHASE.
Store at room temperature. Use before expiration date marked on bottle and carton.

How Supplied: Bottles of 4 fl. oz. (118 ml) with eye cup.
Shown in Product Identification Section, page 428

STAR-OTIC® EAR SOLUTION
Antibacterial, Antifungal, Nonaqueous Ear Solution

Active Ingredients: Acetic acid nonaqueous, Burow's solution, Boric acid, in

Continued on next page

Stellar Pharmacal—Cont.

a propylene glycol vehicle, with an acid pH and a low surface tension.

Indications: For the prevention of otitis externa, commonly called "Swimmer's Ear".

Actions: Star-Otic Ear Solution is antibacterial, antifungal, hydrophilic, has an acid pH and a low surface tension. Acetic acid and boric acid inhibit the rapid multiplication of microorganisms and help maintain the lining mantle of the ear canal in its normal acid state. Burow's solution (aluminum acetate) is a mild astringent. Propylene glycol reduces moisture in the ear canal.

Warning: Do not use in ear if tympanic membrane (ear drum) is perforated or punctured.

Symptoms and Treatment of Overdosage: Discontinue use if undue irritation or sensitivity occurs.

Dosage and Administration: Adults and Children: To help restore normal pH to the outer ear canal. In susceptible persons, instill 3–5 drops of Star-Otic Ear Solution in each ear before and after swimming or bathing, or as directed by physician.

Professional Labeling: Same as those outlined under Indications.

How Supplied: Available in ½ oz measured drop, safety tip, plastic bottle.

Shown in Product Identification Section, page 428

EDUCATIONAL MATERIAL

First Aid Prevention of Swimmer's Ear
Public health information on cause and care of preventing swimmer's ear.

Star-Otic Patient Instruction Pads
Instructions for patients on use of Star-Otic antibacterial-antifungal ear solution.

Sterling Health

Division of Sterling Winthrop Inc.
90 PARK AVENUE
NEW YORK, NY 10016

BAYER® Children's Chewable Aspirin
Aspirin (Acetylsalicylic Acid)

Active Ingredients: Bayer Children's Chewable Aspirin—Aspirin 1¼ grains (81 mg) per orange flavored chewable tablet.

Inactive Ingredients: Dextrose excipient, FD&C Yellow No. 6, flavor, Saccharin Sodium, Starch.

Indications: Analgesic, antipyretic, anti-inflammatory. For effective, gentle relief of painful discomforts, sore throat; fever of colds; headache; teething pain, toothache; and other minor aches and pains.

Directions: The following dosages are those provided in the packaging, as appropriate for self-medication.

Children's Dose: To be administered only under adult supervision. For children under 2 consult physician.

Age (Years)	Weight (lb)	Dosage
2 up to 4	32 to 35	2 tablets
4 up to 6	36 to 45	3 tablets
6 up to 9	46 to 65	4 tablets
9 up to 11	66 to 76	5 tablets
11 up to 12	77 to 83	6 tablets
12 and over	84 and over	8 tablets

Indicated dosage may be repeated every four hours up to but not more than five times a day. Larger dosage may be prescribed by a physician.

Ways to Administer: CHEW, then follow with a half glass of water, milk or fruit juice.
SWALLOW WHOLE with a half a glass of water, milk or fruit juice.
DISSOLVE ON TONGUE, follow with a half a glass of water, milk or fruit juice.
DISSOLVE TABLET in a little water, milk or fruit juice and drink the solution.
CRUSHED in a teaspoonful of water—followed with part of a glass of water.

Warnings: Children and teenagers should not use this medicine for chicken pox or flu symptoms before a doctor is consulted about Reye syndrome, a rare but serious illness reported to be associated with aspirin. Keep this out of the reach of children. In case of accidental overdose, contact a doctor immediately. As with any drug, if you are pregnant or nursing a baby, seek the advice of a health professional before using this product. IT IS ESPECIALLY IMPORTANT NOT TO USE ASPIRIN DURING THE LAST 3 MONTHS OF PREGNANCY UNLESS SPECIFICALLY DIRECTED TO DO SO BY A DOCTOR BECAUSE IT MAY CAUSE PROBLEMS IN THE UNBORN CHILD OR COMPLICATIONS DURING DELIVERY. Do not take for pain for more than 10 days (for adults) or 5 days (for children) or for fever for more than 3 days unless directed by a doctor. If pain or fever persists or gets worse, if new symptoms occur, or if redness or swelling is present, consult a doctor because these could be signs of a serious condition. Do not give this product to children for the pain of arthritis unless directed by a doctor. If sore throat is severe, persists for more than 2 days, is accompanied or followed by fever, headache, rash, nausea, or vomiting, consult a doctor promptly. Do not take this product for at least 7 days after tonsillectomy or oral surgery unless directed by a doctor. Do not take if: allergic to aspirin, have asthma, have stomach problems (such as heartburn, upset stomach or stomach pain) that persist or recur, or have ulcers or bleeding problems, unless directed by a doctor. If ringing in the ears or loss of hearing occurs, consult a doctor before taking again.

Drug Interaction Precaution: Do not take this product if taking a prescription drug for anticoagulation (thinning of the blood), diabetes, gout or arthritis unless directed by a doctor.

How Supplied: Bayer Children's Chewable Aspirin 1¼ grains (81 mg) is supplied in bottles of 36 tablets with child-resistant safety closure.

Shown in Product Identification Section, page 429

Genuine BAYER® Aspirin
Aspirin (Acetylsalicylic Acid)
Tablets and Caplets

Active Ingredients: Each Genuine Bayer Aspirin contains aspirin 5 grains (325 mg) in a thin, inert, hydroxypropyl methylcellulose coating for easier swallowing. This is not an enteric coating and does not alter the onset of action of Genuine Bayer Aspirin.

Inactive Ingredients: Starch and Triacetin.

Indications: Analgesic, antipyretic, anti-inflammatory. For relief of headache; painful discomfort and fever of colds and flu; sore throats; muscular aches and pains; temporary relief of minor pains of arthritis, rheumatism, bursitis, lumbago, sciatica; toothache, and pain following dental procedures; neuralgia and neuritic pain; functional menstrual pain; painful discomfort and fever accompanying immunizations.

Directions: The following dosages are those provided in the packaging, as appropriate for self-medication. Larger or more frequent dosage may be necessary as appropriate to the condition or needs of the patient. The hydroxypropyl methylcellulose coating makes Genuine Bayer Aspirin particularly appropriate for those who have difficulty in swallowing uncoated tablets and caplets.
Usual Adult Dose: One or two tablets/caplets with water. May be repeated every four hours as necessary up to 12 tablets/caplets a day or as directed by a doctor. Do not give to children under 12 unless directed by a doctor.

Warnings: Children and teenagers should not use this medicine for chicken pox or flu symptoms before a doctor is consulted about Reye syndrome, a rare but serious illness reported to be associated with aspirin. Do not take for pain for more than 10 days or for fever for more than 3 days unless directed by a doctor. If pain or fever persists or gets worse, if new symptoms occur, or if redness or swelling is present consult a doctor because these could be signs of a serious condition. Do not take this product if you are allergic to aspirin, have asthma, stomach problems that persist or recur, gastric ulcers or bleeding problems unless directed by a doctor. If ringing in the ears or loss of hearing occurs, consult a doctor before taking any more of this product. Keep this and all drugs out of the reach of children. In case of accidental overdose, seek professional assistance or contact a poison control center immediately. As with any drug, if you are pregnant or nursing a baby, seek the advice of a health professional before using this product. **IT IS ESPECIALLY IMPORTANT NOT TO USE ASPIRIN DURING THE LAST 3 MONTHS OF PREGNANCY UNLESS SPECIFICALLY DIRECTED TO DO SO BY A DOCTOR BECAUSE IT MAY CAUSE PROBLEMS IN THE UNBORN CHILD OR COMPLICATIONS DURING DELIVERY.**

Drug Interaction Precaution: Do not take this product if you are taking a prescription drug for anticoagulation (thinning of the blood), diabetes, gout, or arthritis unless directed by doctor.

Professional Labeling:

ANTIARTHRITIC EFFECT

Indication: Conditions requiring chronic or long-term aspirin therapy for pain and/or inflammation, e.g., rheumatoid arthritis, juvenile rheumatoid arthritis, systemic lupus erythematosus, osteoarthritis (degenerative joint disease), ankylosing spondylitis, psortatic arthritis, Reiter's syndrome, and fibrositis.

ANTIPLATELET EFFECT

In MI Prophylaxis:

Indication: Aspirin is indicated to reduce the risk of death and/or nonfatal myocardial infarction in patients with a previous infarction or unstable angina pectoris.

Clinical Trials: The indication is supported by the results of six large randomized, multicenter, placebo-controlled studies[1–7] involving 10,816 predominantly male post-myocardial infarction (MI) patients and one randomized placebo-controlled study of 1,266 men with unstable angina. Therapy with aspirin was begun at intervals after the onset of acute MI varying from less than three days to more than five years and continuing for periods of from less than one year to four years. In the unstable angina study, treatment was started within one month after the onset of unstable angina and continued for 12 weeks, and complicating conditions, such as congestive heart failure, were not included in the study. Aspirin therapy in MI patients was associated with about a 20% reduction in the risk of subsequent death and/or nonfatal reinfarction, a median absolute decrease of 3% from the 12% to 22% event rates in the placebo groups. In the aspirin-treated unstable angina patients, the reduction in risk was about 50%, a reduction in the event rate of 5% from the 10% rate in the placebo group ovcr the 12 weeks of study.

Daily dosage of aspirin in the post-myocardial infarction studies was 300 mg in one study and 900–1,500 mg in five studies. A dose of 325 mg was used in the study of unstable angina.

Adverse Reactions: Gastrointestinal reactions: Doses of 1,000 mg per day of aspirin caused gastrointestinal symptoms and bleeding that, in some cases, were clinically significant. In the largest postinfarction study (the Aspirin Myocardial Infarction Study [AMIS] with 4,500 people), the percentage of incidences of gastrointestinal symptoms for the aspirin (1,000 mg of a standard, solid-tablet formulation) and placebo-treated subjects, respectively, were stomach pain (14.5%, 4.4%), heartburn (11.9%, 4.8%), nausea and/or vomiting (7.6%, 2.1%), hospitalization for Gl disorder (4.9%, 3.5%). In the AMIS and other trials, aspirin-treated patients had increased rates of gross gastrointestinal bleeding. Symptoms and signs of gastrointestinal irritation were not significantly increased in subjects treated for unstable angina with buffered aspirin in solution.

Cardiovascular and Biochemical: In the AMIS trial, the dosage of 1,000 mg per day of aspirin was associated with small increases in systolic blood pressure (BP) (average 1.5 to 2.1 mm) and diastolic BP (0.5 to 0.6 mm), depending upon whether maximal or last available readings were used. Blood urea nitrogen and uric acid levels were also increased but by less than 1.0 mg percent. Subjects with marked hypertension or renal insufficiency had been excluded from the trial so that the clinical importance of these observations for such subjects or for any subjects treated over more prolonged periods is not known. It is recommended that patients placed on long-term aspirin treatment, even at doses of 300 mg per day, be seen at regular intervals to assess changes in these measurements.

Sodium in Buffered Aspirin for Solution Formulations: One tablet daily of buffered aspirin in solution adds 553 mg of sodium to that in the diet and may not be tolerated by patients with active sodium-retaining states, such as congestive heart or renal failure. This amount of sodium adds about 30% to the 70 to 90 meq intake suggested as appropriate for dietary treatment of essential hypertension in the 1984 Report of the Joint National Committee on Detection, Evaluation and Treatment of High Blood Pressure.[8]

Dosage and Administration: Although most of the studies used dosages exceeding 300 mg, two trials used only 300 mg daily and pharmacologic data indicate that this dose inhibits platelet function fully. Therefore, 300 mg or a conventional 325 mg aspirin dose daily is a reasonable routine dose that would minimize gastrointestinal adverse reactions. This use of aspirin applies to both solid oral dosage forms (buffered and plain aspirin) and buffered aspirin in solution.

In Transient Ischemic Attacks:

Indication: Aspririn is indicated for reducing the risk of recurrent transient ischemic attacks (TIAs) or stroke in men who have transient ischemia of the brain due to fibrin emboli. There is no evidence that aspirin is effective in reducing TIAs in women, or is of benefit in the treatment of completed strokes in men or women.

Clinical Trials: The indication is supported by the results of a Canadian study[9] in which 585 patients with threatened stroke were followed in a randomized clinical trial for an average of 28 months to determine whether aspirin or sulfinpyrazone, singly or in combination, was superior to placebo in preventing transient ischemic attacks, stroke, or death. The study showed that, although sulfinpyrazone had no statistically significant effect, aspirin reduced the risk of continuing transient ischemic attacks, stroke, or death by 19 percent and reduced the risk of stroke or death by 31 percent. Another aspirin study carried out in the United States with 178 patients showed a statistically significant number of "favorable outcomes," including reduced transient ischemic attacks, stroke, and death.[10]

Precautions: Patients presenting with signs and/or symptoms of TIAs should have a complete medical and neurologic evaluation. Consideration should be given to other disorders which may resemble TIAs. It is important to evaluate and treat, if appropriate, diseases associated with TIAs and stroke, such as hypertension and diabetes.

Dosage: The recommended dosage for this new indication is 1,300 mg per day (650 mg b.i.d. or 325 mg q.i.d).

References: 1. Elwood PC, et al: A randomized controlled trial of acetylsalicylic acid in the secondary prevention of mortality from myocardial infarction. *Br Med J* 1974;1:436–440. 2. The Coronary Drug Project Research Group: Aspirin in coronary heart disease. *J Chronic Dis* 1976;29:625–642. 3. Breddin K, et al: Secondary prevention of myocardial infarction: A comparison of acetylsalicylic acid, phenprocoumon or placebo. *Homeostasis* 1979;470:263–268. 4. Aspirin Myocardial Infarction Study Research Group: A randomized, controlled trial of aspirin in persons recovered from myocardial infarction. *JAMA* 1980;245:661–669. 5. Elwood PC, Sweetnam PM: Aspirin and secondary mortality after myocardial infarction. *Lancet*, December 22–29, 1979, pp 1313–1315. 6. The Persantine-Aspirin Reinfarction Study Research Group: Persantine and aspirin in coronary heart disease. *Circulation* 1980;62:449–460. 7. Lewis, HD, et al: Protective effects of aspirin against acute myocardial infarction and death in men with unstable angina: Results of a Veterans Administration Cooperative Study.

Continued on next page

This product information was effective as of November 1, 1992. Current information may be obtained directly from Sterling Health, by writing to 90 Park Avenue, New York, NY 10016.

Sterling Health—Cont.

N Engl J Med 1983;309:396–403. 8. *1984 Report of the Joint National Committee on Detection, Evaluation and Treatment of High Blood Pressure,* US Dept of Health and Human Services and US Public Health Service, National Institutes of Health. 9. The Canadian Cooperative Study Group: A randomized trial of aspirin and sulfinpyrazone in threatened stroke. *N Engl J Med* 1978;299:53–59. 10. Fields WS, et al: Controlled trial of aspirin in cerebral ischemia. *Stroke* 1977;8:301–316.

How Supplied:
Genuine Bayer Aspirin 5 grains (325 mg) is supplied in packs of 12 tablets, bottles of 24, 50, 100, 200 and 300 tablets, and bottles of 50, 100 and 200 caplets.
Child-resistant safety closures on 12s, 24s, 50s, 200s, 300s tablets and 50s and 200s caplets. Bottles of 100s tablets and caplets available without safety closure for households without small children.

Shown in Product Identification Section, page 428

Maximum BAYER® Aspirin Aspirin (Acetylsalicylic Acid) Tablets and Caplets

Active Ingredients: Maximum Bayer Aspirin—Aspirin 500 mg (7.7 grains) contains a thin, inert, Hydroxypropyl Methylcellulose coating for easier swallowing. This is not an enteric coating and does not alter the onset of action of Bayer Aspirin.

Inactive Ingredients: Starch and Triacetin.

Indications: Analgesic, antipyretic, anti-inflammatory. For relief of headache; painful discomfort and fever of colds and flu; sore throats; muscular aches and pains; temporary relief of minor pains of arthritis, rheumatism, bursitis, lumbago, sciatica; toothache, and pain following dental procedures; neuralgia and neuritic pain; functional menstrual pain; painful discomfort and fever accompanying immunizations.

Directions: The following dosages are those provided on the packaging, as appropriate for self- medication. Larger or more frequent dosage may be necessary as appropriate for the condition or needs of the patient. The hydroxypropyl methylcellulose coating makes Maximum Bayer Aspirin particularly appropriate for those who have difficulty in swallowing uncoated tablets/caplets.
Maximum Bayer Aspirin—500 mg (7.7 grains) tablets/caplets.
Usual Adult Dose: One or two tablets/caplets with water. May be repeated every four hours as necessary up to 8 tablets/caplets a day. Do not give to children under 12 unless directed by a doctor.

Warnings: Children and teenagers should not use this medicine for chicken pox or flu symptoms before a doctor is consulted about Reye syndrome, a rare but serious illness reported to be associated with aspirin. Do not take for pain for more than 10 days or for fever for more than 3 days unless directed by a doctor. If pain or fever persists or gets worse, if new symptoms occur, or if redness or swelling is present consult a doctor because these could be signs of a serious condition. Do not take this product if you are allergic to aspirin, have asthma, stomach problems that persist or recur, gastric ulcers or bleeding problems unless directed by a doctor. If ringing in the ears or loss of hearing occurs, consult a doctor before taking any more of this product. Keep this and all drugs out of the reach of children. In case of accidental overdose, seek professional assistance or contact a poison control center immediately. As with any drug, if you are pregnant or nursing a baby, seek the advice of a health professional before using this product. **IT IS ESPECIALLY IMPORTANT NOT TO USE ASPIRIN DURING THE LAST 3 MONTHS OF PREGNANCY UNLESS SPECIFICALLY DIRECTED TO DO SO BY A DOCTOR BECAUSE IT MAY CAUSE PROBLEMS IN THE UNBORN CHILD OR COMPLICATIONS DURING DELIVERY.**

Drug Interaction Precaution: Do not take this product if you are taking a prescription drug for anticoagulation (thinning of the blood), diabetes, gout, or arthritis unless directed by a doctor.

How Supplied:
Maximum Bayer Aspirin 500 mg (7.7 grains) is available in bottles of 30, 60 and 100 tablets, and bottles of 30 and 60 caplets.
Child-resistant safety closures on 30s bottles of tablets and caplets, 60s, bottles of caplets, and 100s bottles of tablets. Bottle of 60s tablets available without safety closure for households without young children.

Shown in Product Identification Section, page 428

Extended-Release BAYER® 8-Hour Aspirin Aspirin (acetylsalicylic acid)

Active Ingredients: Each oblong white scored caplet contains 10 grains (650 mg) of aspirin in microencapsulated form.

Inactive Ingredients: Guar Gum, Microcrystalline Cellulose, Starch and other ingredients.

Indications: Extended-Release BAYER 8-Hour Aspirin is indicated for the temporary relief of low-grade pain amenable to relief with salicylates, such as in rheumatoid arthritis, osteoarthritis, spondylitis, bursitis and other forms of rheumatism, as well as in many common musculoskeletal disorders. It possesses the same advantages for other types of prolonged aches and pains, such as minor injuries, dental pain and dysmenorrhea. Its long-lasting effectiveness should also make it valuable as an analgesic in simple headache, colds, grippe, flu and other similar conditions in which aspirin is indicated for symptomatic relief, either by itself or as an adjunct to specific therapy.

Directions: Two Extended-Release BAYER 8-Hour Aspirin caplets q. 8 h. provide effective long-lasting pain relief. This two-caplet (20 grain or 1300 mg) dose of extended-release aspirin promptly produces salicylate blood levels greater than those achieved by a 10-grain (650 mg) dose of regular aspirin, and in the second 4-hour period produces a salicylate blood level curve which approximates that of two successive 10-grain (650 mg) doses of regular aspirin at 4-hour intervals. The 10-grain (650 mg) scored Extended-Release BAYER 8-Hour Aspirin caplets permit administration of aspirin in multiples of 5 grains (325 mg) allowing individualization of dosage to meet the specific needs of the patient. For the convenience of patients on a regular aspirin dosage schedule, two 10-grain (650 mg) Extended-Release BAYER 8-Hour Aspirin caplets may be administered with water every 8 hours. Whenever necessary, two caplets (20 grains or 1300 mg) should be given before retiring to provide effective analgesic and anti-inflammatory action—for relief of pain throughout the night and lessening of stiffness upon arising. Do not exceed 6 caplets in 24 hours. Extended-Release BAYER 8-Hour Aspirin has been made in a special caplet to permit easy swallowing. However, for patients who do have difficulty, Extended-Release BAYER 8-Hour Aspirin caplets may be gently crumbled in the mouth and swallowed with water without loss of timed-release effect. There is no bitter "aspirin" taste. For children under 12, consult physician.

Warnings: Children and teenagers should not use this medicine for chicken pox or flu symptoms before a doctor is consulted about Reye syndrome, a rare but serious illness reported to be associated with aspirin. Do not take for pain for more than 10 days or for fever for more than 3 days unless directed by a doctor. If pain or fever persists or gets worse, if new symptoms occur, or if redness or swelling is present consult a doctor because these could be signs of a serious condition. Do not take this product if you are allergic to aspirin, have asthma, stomach problems that persist or recur, gastric ulcers or bleeding problems unless directed by a doctor. If ringing in the ears or loss of hearing occurs, consult a doctor before taking any more of this product. Keep this and all drugs out of the reach of children. In case of accidental overdose, seek professional assistance or contact a poison control center immediately. As with any drug, if you are pregnant or nursing a baby, seek the advice of a health professional before using this product. **IT IS ESPECIALLY IMPORTANT NOT TO USE ASPIRIN DURING THE LAST 3 MONTHS OF PREGNANCY UNLESS SPECIFICALLY DIRECTED TO DO SO BY A DOCTOR BECAUSE IT MAY CAUSE PROBLEMS IN THE UNBORN CHILD OR COMPLICATIONS DURING DELIVERY.**

Drug Interaction Precaution: Do not take this product if you are taking a prescription drug for anticoagulation (thinning of the blood), diabetes, gout, or arthritis unless directed by a doctor.

How Supplied: Extended-Release Bayer 8-Hour Aspirin 650 mg (10 grains) is supplied in bottles of 72 and 125 caplets.
The 72s size, without a child-resistant safety closure, is recommended for households without young children.

Shown in Product Identification Section, page 429

BAYER® ENTERIC Aspirin
Delayed-Release Enteric Aspirin Regular Strength (325 mg) and Adult Low Strength (81 mg) (Acetylsalicylic Acid) Caplets

Composition: BAYER Enteric is enteric-coated aspirin. The enteric coating prevents disintegration in the stomach and promotes dissolution in the duodenum, where there is a more neutral-to-alkaline environment. This action aids in protecting the stomach against injuries that may occur as a result of ingesting non-enteric-coated aspirin (see **Safety**).

Inactive Ingredients: Regular Strength—D&C Yellow No. 10, FD&C Yellow No. 6, Hydroxypropyl Methylcellulose, Methacrylic Acid Co-polymer, Starch, Titanium Dioxide, Triacetin.
Adult Low Strength—Croscarmellose Sodium, D&C Yellow No. 10, FD&C Yellow No. 6, Hydroxypropyl Methylcellulose, Iron Oxide, Lactose, Methacrylic Acid, Microcrystalline Cellulose, Polysorbate 80, Sodium Lauryl Sulfate, Starch, Titanium Dioxide, Triacetin.

Indications: BAYER ENTERIC is an anti-inflammatory, analgesic, and antiplatelet agent indicated for the relief of painful discomfort and muscular aches and pains associated with conditions requiring long-term aspirin therapy, e.g., arthritis or rheumatism and for situations where compliance with aspirin is hindered by the gastrointestinal side effects of non-enteric-coated or buffered aspirin.

Dosage: For analgesic or anti-inflammatory indications, the OTC maximum dosage for aspirin is 4,000 mg per day in divided doses, i.e., one or two 325 mg caplets every 4 hours, four to eight 81 mg tablets every 4 hours. For antiplatelet effect dosage, see the **Antiplatelet Effect** section.

Warnings: Children and teenagers should not use this medicine for chicken pox or flu symptoms before a doctor is consulted about Reye syndrome, a rare but serious illness reported to be associated with aspirin. Do not take for pain for more than 10 days or for fever for more than 3 days unless directed by a doctor. If pain or fever persists or gets worse, if new symptoms occur, or if redness or swelling is present, consult a doctor because these could be signs of a serious condition. Do not take this product if you are allergic to aspirin, have asthma, have stomach problems (such as heartburn, upset stomach or stomach pain) that persist or recur, or if you have gastric ulcers or bleeding problems unless directed by a doctor. If ringing in the ears or loss of hearing occurs, consult a doctor before taking any more of this product. Keep out of reach of children. In case of accidental overdose, contact a doctor immediately. As with any drug, if you are pregnant or nursing a baby, seek the advice of a health professional before using this product. **IT IS ESPECIALLY IMPORTANT NOT TO USE ASPIRIN DURING THE LAST 3 MONTHS OF PREGNANCY UNLESS SPECIFICALLY DIRECTED TO DO SO BY A DOCTOR BECAUSE IT MAY CAUSE PROBLEMS IN THE UNBORN CHILD OR COMPLICATIONS DURING DELIVERY.**

Drug Interaction Precaution: Do not take this product if you are taking a prescription drug for anticoagulation (thinning of the blood), diabetes, gout, or arthritis unless directed by a doctor.

Professional Labeling

Professional Warning: Occasional reports have documented individuals with impaired gastric emptying in whom there may be retention of one or more enteric-coated aspirin caplets over time. This phenomenon may occur as a result of outlet obstruction from ulcer disease alone or combined with hypotonic gastric peristalsis. Because of the integrity of the enteric coating in an acidic environment, these caplets may accumulate and form a bezoar in the stomach. Individuals with this condition may present with complaints of early satiety or of vague upper abdominal distress. Diagnosis may be made by endoscopy or by abdominal films, which show opacities suggestive of a mass of small caplets.[1] Management may vary according to the condition of the patient. Options include gastrotomy and alternating slightly basic and neutral lavage.[2] While there have been no clinical reports, it has been suggested that such individuals may also be treated with parenteral cimetidine (to reduce acid secretion) and then given sips of slightly basic liquids to effect gradual dissolution of the enteric coating. Progress may be followed with plasma salicylate levels or via recognition of tinnitus by the patient.
It should be kept in mind that individuals with a history of partial or complete gastrectomy may produce reduced amounts of acid and therefore have less acidic gastric pH. Under these circumstances, the benefits offered by the acid-resistant enteric coating may not exist.

Safety: The safety of enteric-coated aspirin has been demonstrated in a number of endoscopic studies comparing enteric-coated aspirin and plain aspirin, as well as plain buffered and "arthritis-strength" preparations. In these studies, endoscopies were performed in healthy volunteers before and after either two-day or 14-day administration of aspirin doses of 3,900 or 4,000 mg per day. Compared to all the other preparations, the enteric-coated aspirin produced significantly less damage to the gastric mucosa. There was also statistically less duodenal damage when compared with the plain, i.e., non-enteric-coated, aspirin.

Bioavailability: The bioavailability of aspirin from BAYER® Enteric has been confirmed. In single-dose studies[3] in which plasma acetylsalicylic acid and salicylic acid levels were measured, maximum concentrations were achieved at approximately five hours postdosing. BAYER® Enteric, when compared with plain aspirin, achieves maximum plasma salicylate levels not significantly different from plain, i.e., non-enteric-coated aspirin. Dissolution of the enteric coating occurs at a neutral-to-basic pH and is therefore dependent on gastric emptying into the duodenum. With continued dosing, appropriate therapeutic plasma levels are maintained.

ANTIARTHRITIC EFFECT

Indication: Conditions requiring chronic or long-term aspirin therapy for pain and/or inflammation, e.g., rheumatoid arthritis, juvenile rheumatoid arthritis, systemic lupus erythematosus, osteoarthritis (degenerative joint disease), ankylosing spondylitis, psoriatic arthritis, Reiter's syndrome, and fibrositis.

ANTIPLATELET EFFECT

In MI Prophylaxis:

Indication: Aspirin is indicated to reduce the risk of death and/or nonfatal myocardial infarction in patients with a previous infarction or unstable angina pectoris.

Clinical Trials: The indication is supported by the results of six large randomized, multicenter, placebo-controlled studies[4–10] involving 10,816 predominantly male post–myocardial infarction (MI) patients and one randomized placebo-controlled study of 1,266 men with unstable angina. Therapy with aspirin was begun at intervals after the onset of acute MI varying from less than three days to more than five years and continuing for periods of from less than one year to four years. In the unstable angina study, treatment was started within one

Continued on next page

This product information was effective as of November 1, 1992. Current information may be obtained directly from Sterling Health, by writing to 90 Park Avenue, New York, NY 10016.

Sterling Health—Cont.

month after the onset of unstable angina and continued for 12 weeks, and complicating conditions, such as congestive heart failure, were not included in the study. Aspirin therapy in MI patients was associated with about a 20% reduction in the risk of subsequent death and/or nonfatal reinfarction, a median absolute decrease of 3% from the 12% to 22% event rates in the placebo groups. In the aspirin-treated unstable angina patients, the reduction in risk was about 50%, a reduction in event rate of 5% from the 10% rate in the placebo group over the 12 weeks of the study.

Daily dosage of aspirin in the post-myocardial infarction studies was 300 mg in one study and 900–1,500 mg in five studies. A dose of 325 mg was used in the study of unstable angina.

Adverse Reactions: Gastrointestinal reactions: Doses of 1,000 mg per day of aspirin caused gastrointestinal symptoms and bleeding that, in some cases, were clinically significant. In the largest postinfarction study (the Aspirin Myocardial Infarction Study [AMIS] with 4,500 people), the percentage of incidences of gastrointestinal symptoms for the aspirin (1,000 mg of a standard, solid-tablet formulation) and placebo-treated subjects, respectively, were: stomach pain (14.5%, 4.4%), heartburn (11.9%, 4.8%), nausea and/or vomiting (7.6%, 2.1%), and hospitalization for GI disorder (4.9%, 3.5%). In the AMIS and other trials, aspirin-treated patients had increased rates of gross gastrointestinal bleeding. Symptoms and signs of gastrointestinal irritation were not significantly increased in subjects treated for unstable angina with buffered aspirin in solution.

Cardiovascular and Biochemical: In the AMIS trial, the dosage of 1,000 mg per day of aspirin was associated with small increases in systolic blood pressure (BP) (average 1.5 to 2.1 mm) and diastolic BP (0.5 to 0.6 mm), depending upon whether maximal or last available readings were used. Blood urea nitrogen and uric acid levels were also increased but by less than 1.0 mg percent. Subjects with marked hypertension or renal insufficiency had been excluded from the trial so that the clinical importance of these observations for such subjects or for any subjects treated over more prolonged periods is not known. It is recommended that patients placed on long-term aspirin treatment, even at doses of 300 mg per day, be seen at regular intervals to assess changes in these measurements.

Sodium in Buffered Aspirin for Solution Formulations: One tablet daily of buffered aspirin in solution adds 553 mg of sodium to that in the diet and may not be tolerated by patients with active sodium-retaining states, such as congestive heart or renal failure. This amount of sodium adds about 30% to the 70 to 90 meq intake suggested as appropriate for dietary treatment of essential hypertension in the 1984 Report of the Joint National Committee on Detection, Evaluation and Treatment of High Blood Pressure.[11]

Dosage and Administration: Although most of the studies used dosages exceeding 300 mg, two trials used only 300 mg daily and pharmacologic data indicate that this dose inhibits platelet function fully. Therefore, 300 mg or a conventional 325 mg aspirin dose daily is a reasonable routine dose that would minimize gastrointestinal adverse reactions. This use of aspirin applies to both solid oral dosage forms (buffered and plain aspirin) and buffered aspirin in solution.

In Transient Ischemic Attacks:

Indication: Aspirin is indicated for reducing the risk of recurrent transient ischemic attacks (TIAs) or stroke in men who have transient ischemia of the brain due to fibrin emboli. There is no evidence that aspirin is effective in reducing TIAs in women, or is of benefit in the treatment of completed strokes in men or women.

Clinical Trials: The indication is supported by the results of a Canadian study[12] in which 585 patients with threatened stroke were followed in a randomized clinical trial for an average of 28 months to determine whether aspirin or sulfinpyrazone, singly or in combination, was superior to placebo in preventing transient ischemic attacks, stroke, or death. The study showed that, although sulfinpyrazone had no statistically significant effect, aspirin reduced the risk of continuing transient ischemic attacks, stroke, or death by 19 percent and reduced the risk of stroke or death by 31 percent. Another aspirin study carried out in the United States with 178 patients showed a statistically significant number of "favorable outcomes," including reduced transient ischemic attacks, stroke, and death.[13]

Precautions: Patients presenting with signs and/or symptoms of TIAs should have a complete medical and neurologic evaluation. Consideration should be given to other disorders which may resemble TIAs. It is important to evaluate and treat, if appropriate, diseases associated with TIAs and stroke, such as hypertension and diabetes.

Dosage: The recommended dosage for this new indication is 1,300 mg per day (650 mg b.i.d. or 325 mg q.i.d.).

References: 1. Bogacz K, Caldron P: Enteric-coated aspirin bezoar: Elevation of serum salicylate level by barium study. *Am J Med* 1987;83:783–786. 2. Baum J: Enteric-coated aspirin and the problem of gastric retention. *J Rheumatol* 1984; 11:250–251. 3. Data on file, Sterling Health. 4. Elwood PC, et al: A randomized controlled trial of acetylsalicylic acid in the secondary prevention of mortality from myocardial infarction. *Br Med J* 1974;1:436–440. 5. The Coronary Drug Project Research Group: Aspirin in coronary heart disease. *J Chronic Dis* 1976;29:625–642. 6. Breddin K, et al: Secondary prevention of myocardial infarction: A comparison of acetylsalicylic acid, phenprocoumon or placebo. *Homeostasis* 1979;470:263–268. 7. Aspirin Myocardial Infarction Study Research Group: A randomized, controlled trial of aspirin in persons recovered from myocardial infarction. *JAMA* 1980;245:661–669. 8. Elwood PC, Sweetnam PM: Aspirin and secondary mortality after myocardial infarction. *Lancet,* December 22–29, 1979, pp 1313–1315. 9. The Persantine-Aspirin Reinfarction Study Research Group: Persantine and aspirin in coronary heart disease. *Circulation* 1980;62:449–460. 10. Lewis HD, et al: Protective effects of aspirin against acute myocardial infarction and death in men with unstable angina: Results of a Veterans Administration Cooperative Study. *N Eng J Med* 1983;309:396–403. 11. *1984 Report of the Joint National Committee on Detection, Evaluation and Treatment of High Blood Pressure,* U.S. Dept of Health and Human Services and US Public Health Service, National Institutes of Health. 12. The Canadian Cooperative Study Group: A randomized trial of aspirin and sulfinpyrazone in treatened stroke. *N Engl J Med* 1978;299:53–59. 13. Fields WS, et al: Controlled trial of aspirin in cerebral ischemia. *Stroke* 1977;8:301, 316.

How Supplied: Regular Strength BAYER Enteric 325 mg caplets in bottles of 50, 100. Child-resistant safety closure on 50s caplets. Bottles of 100s caplets available without safety closure for households without small children.

Adult Low Strength BAYER Enteric 81 mg tablets in bottles of 120 with child resistent safety closure.

Shown in Product Identification Section, page 429

BAYER® PLUS
Buffered Aspirin

Active Ingredients: Each Bayer Plus contains Aspirin (325 mg), in a formulation buffered with Calcium Carbonate, Magnesium Carbonate, and Magnesium Oxide.

Inactive Ingredients: Corn Starch, Ethylcellulose, FD&C Blue #2, Hydroxypropyl Methylcellulose, Microcrystalline Cellulose, Pharmaceutical Glaze, Sodium Starch Glycolate, Talc, Zinc Stearate.

Indications: Analgesic, antipyretic, anti-inflammatory. For relief of headache; painful discomfort and fever of colds and flu; muscular aches and pains; temporary relief of minor pains of arthritis, rheumatism, bursitis, lumbago, sciatica; toothache, and pain following dental procedures; neuralgia and neuritic pain; functional menstrual pain; painful discomfort and fever accompanying immunizations.

Directions: The following dosages are those provided in the packaging, as appropriate for self-medication. Larger or more frequent dosage may be necessary as appropriate to the condition or needs of the patient. The addition of buffering agents makes Bayer® Plus particularly appropriate for those who must take frequent doses of aspirin. The hydroxypropyl methylcellulose coating benefits aspirin users who have difficulty in swallowing uncoated tablets and caplets.

Usual Adult Dose: One or two tablets with water. May be repeated every four hours as necessary up to 12 tablets a day or as directed by a doctor. Do not give to children under 12 unless directed by a doctor.

Warnings: Children and teenagers should not use this medicine for chicken pox or flu symptoms before a doctor is consulted about Reye syndrome, a rare but serious illness reported to be associated with aspirin. Do not take for pain for more than 10 days or for fever for more than 3 days unless directed by a doctor. If pain or fever persists or gets worse, if new symptoms occur, or if redness or swelling is present consult a doctor because these could be signs of a serious condition. Do not take this product if you are allergic to aspirin, have asthma, stomach problems that persist or recur, gastric ulcers or bleeding problems unless directed by a doctor. If ringing in the ears or loss of hearing occurs, consult a doctor before taking any more of this product. Keep this and all drugs out of the reach of children. In case of accidental overdose, seek professional assistance or contact a poison control center immediately. As with any drug, if you are pregnant or nursing a baby, seek the advice of a health professional before using this product. **IT IS ESPECIALLY IMPORTANT NOT TO USE ASPIRIN DURING THE LAST 3 MONTHS OF PREGNANCY UNLESS SPECIFICALLY DIRECTED TO DO SO BY A DOCTOR BECAUSE IT MAY CAUSE PROBLEMS IN THE UNBORN CHILD OR COMPLICATIONS DURING DELIVERY.**

Drug Interaction Precaution: Do not take this product if you are taking a prescription drug for anticoagulation (thinning of the blood), diabetes, gout, or arthritis unless directed by a doctor.

Professional Labeling

ANTIARTHRITIC EFFECT

Indication: Conditions requiring chronic or long-term aspirin therapy for pain and/or inflammation, e.g., rheumatoid arthritis, juvenile rheumatoid arthritis, systemic lupus erythematosus, osteoarthritis (degenerative joint disease), ankylosing spondylitis, psoriatic arthritis, Reiter's syndrome, and fibrositis.

ANTIPLATELET EFFECT

In MI Prophylaxis:

Indication: Aspirin is indicated to reduce the risk of death and/or nonfatal myocardial infarction in patients with a previous infarction or unstable angina pectoris.

Clinical Trials: The indication is supported by the results of six large randomized, multicenter, placebo-controlled studies.[1–7] involving 10,816 predominantly male post-myocardial infarction (MI) patients and one randomized placebo-controlled study of 1,266 men with unstable angina. Therapy with aspirin was begun at intervals after the onset of acute MI varying from less than three days to more than five years and continuing for periods of from less than one year to four years. In the unstable angina study, treatment was started within one month after the onset of unstable angina and continued for 12 weeks, and complicating conditions, such as congestive heart failure, were not included in the study. Aspirin therapy in MI patients was associated with about a 20% reduction in the risk of subsequent death and/or nonfatal reinfarction, a median absolute decrease of 3% from the 12% to 22% event rates in the placebo groups. In the aspirin-treated unstable angina patients, the reduction in risk was about 50%, a reduction in the event rate of 5% from the 10% rate in the placebo group over the 12 weeks of the study.

Daily dosage of aspirin in the postmyocardial infarction studies was 300 mg in one study and 900–1,500 mg in five studies. A dose of 325 mg was used in the study of unstable angina.

Adverse Reactions: Gastrointestinal reactions: Doses of 1,000 mg per day of aspirin caused gastrointestinal symptoms and bleeding that, in some cases, were clinically significant. In the largest postinfarction study (the Aspirin Myocardial Infarction Study [AMIS] with 4,500 people), the percentage of incidences of gastrointestinal symptoms for the aspirin (1,000 mg of a standard, solid-tablet formulation) and placebo-treated subjects, respectively, were stomach pain (14.5%, 4.4%), heartburn (11.9%, 4.8%), nausea and/or vomiting (7.6%, 2.1%), and hospitalization for GI disorder (4.9%, 3.5%). In the AMIS and other trials, aspirin-treated patients had increased rates of gross gastrointestinal bleeding., Symptoms and signs of gastrointestinal irritation were not significantly increased in subjects treated for unstable angina with buffered aspirin in solution.

Cardiovascular and Biochemical: In the AMIS trial, the dosage of 1,000 mg per day of aspirin was associated with small increases in systolic blood pressure (BP) (average 1.5 to 2.1 mm) and diastolic BP (0.5 to 0.6 mm), depending upon whether maximal or last available readings were used. Blood urea nitrogen and uric acid levels were also increased but by less than 1.0 mg percent. Subjects with marked hypertension or renal insufficiency had been excluded from the trial so that the clinical importance of these observations for such subjects or for any subjects treated over more prolonged periods is not known. It is recommended that patients placed on long-term aspirin treatment, even at doses of 300 mg per day, be seen at regular intervals to assess changes in these measurements.

Sodium in Buffered Aspirin for Solution Formulations: One tablet daily of buffered aspirin in solution adds 553 mg of sodium to that in the diet and may not be tolerated by patients with active sodium-retaining states, such as congestive heart or renal failure. This amount of sodium adds about 30% to the 70 to 90 meq intake suggested as appropriate for dietary treatment of essential hypertension in the 1984 Report of the Joint National Committee on Detection, Evaluation and Treatment of High Blood Pressure[8].

Dosage and Administration: Although most of the studies used dosages exceeding 300 mg, two trials used only 300 mg daily and pharmacologic data indicate that this dose inhibits platelet function fully. Therefore, 300 mg or a conventional 325 mg aspirin dose daily is a reasonable routine dose that would minimize gastrointestinal adverse reactions. This use of aspirin applies to both solid oral dosage forms (buffered and plain aspirin) and buffered aspirin in solution.

In Transient Ischemic Attacks:

Indication: Aspirin is indicated for reducing the risk of recurrent transient ischemic attacks (TIAs) or stroke in men who have transient ischemia of the brain due to fibrin emboli. There is no evidence that aspirin is effective in reducing TIAs in women, or is of benefit in the treatment of completed strokes in men or women.

Clinical Trials: The indication is supported by the results of a Canadian study[9] in which 585 patients with threatened stroke were followed in a randomized clinical trial for an average of 28 months to determine whether aspirin or sulfinpyrazone, singly or in combination, was superior to placebo in preventing transient ischemic attacks, stroke, or death. The study showed that, although sulfinpyrazone had no statistically significant effect, aspirin reduced the risk of continuing transient ischemic attacks, stroke, or death by 19 percent and reduced the risk of stroke or death by 31 percent. Another aspirin study carried out in the United States with 178 patients showed a statistically significant number of "favorable outcomes," including reduced transient ischemic attacks, stroke, and death.[10]

Precautions: Patients presenting with signs and/or symptoms of TIAs should have a complete medical and neurologic evaluation. Consideration should be given to other disorders which may resemble TIAs. It is important to evaluate and treat, if appropriate, diseases associ-

Continued on next page

This product information was effective as of November 1, 1992. Current information may be obtained directly from Sterling Health, by writing to 90 Park Avenue, New York, NY 10016.

ated with TIAs and stroke, such as hypertension and diabetes.

Dosage: The recommended dosage for this new indication is 1,300 mg per day (650 mg b.i.d. or 325 mg q.i.d.).

References: 1. Elwood PC, et al: A randomized controlled trial of acetylsalicylic acid in the secondary prevention of mortality from myocardial infarction. *Br Med J* 1974;1:436-440. 2. The Coronary Drug Project Research Group: Aspirin in coronary heart disease. *J Chronic Dis* 1976;29:625–642. 3. Breddin K, et al: Secondary prevention of myocardial infarction: A comparison of acetylsalicylic acid, phenprocoumon or placebo. *Homeostasis* 1979;470:263–268. 4. Aspirin Myocardial Infarction Study Research Group: A randomized, controlled trial of aspirin in persons recovered from myocardial infarction. *JAMA* 1980;245:661–669. 5. Elwood PC, Sweetnam PM: Aspirin and secondary mortality after myocardial infarction. *Lancet,* December 22–29, 1979, pp 1313–1315. 6. The Persantine-Aspirin Reinfarction Study Research Group: Persantine and aspirin in coronary heart disease. *Circulation* 1980;62:449–460. 7. Lewis HD, et al: Protective effects of aspirin against acute myocardial infarction and death in men with unstable angina: Results of a Veterans Administration Cooperative Study. *N. Engl J Med* 1983;309:396–403. 8. *1984 Report of the Joint National Committee on Detection, Evaluation and Treatment of High Blood Pressure,* US Dept of Health and Human Services and US Public Health Service, National Institute of Health. 9. The Canadian Cooperative Study Group: A randomized trial of aspirin and sulfinpyrazone in threatened stroke. *N. Engl J Med* 1978;299:53–59. 10. Fields WS, et al: Controlled trial of aspirin in cerebral ischemia. *Stroke* 1977;8:301–316.

How Supplied: Bayer® Plus Aspirin (325 mg) is available in bottles of 8, 24, 50, and 100 tablets.

Child resistant closures on 8s, 24s and 50s tablets. Bottles of 100s tablets available without safety closure for households without young children.

Shown in Product Identification Section, page 429

Extra Strength BAYER® PLUS Buffered Aspirin

Active Ingredients: Each Extra Strength Bayer Plus contains Aspirin (500 mg), in a formulation buffered with Calcium Carbonate, Magnesium Carbonate, and Magnesium Oxide.

Inactive Ingredients: Corn Starch, FD&C Blue #2, Hydroxypropyl Cellulose, Hydroxypropyl Methylcellulose, Methylparaben, Microcrystalline Cellulose, Propylene Glycol, Propylparaben, Sodium Starch Glycolate, Zinc Stearate.

Indications: Analgesic, antipyretic, anti-inflammatory. For relief of headache; painful discomfort and fever of colds and flu; muscular aches and pains; temporary relief of minor pains of arthritis, rheumatism, bursitis, lumbago, sciatica; toothache, and pain following dental procedures; neuralgia and neuritic pain; functional menstrual pain; painful discomfort and fever accompanying immunizations.

Directions: The following dosages are those provided in the packaging, as appropriate for self-medication. Larger or more frequent dosage may be necessary as appropriate to the condition or needs of the patient. The addition of buffering agents makes Extra Strength Bayer® Plus particularly appropriate for those who must take frequent doses of aspirin. The hydroxypropyl methylcellulose coating benefits aspirin users who have difficulty in swallowing uncoated tablets and caplets.

Usual Adult Dose: One or two caplets with water. May be repeated every four to 6 hours as necessary up to 8 caplets a day, or as directed by a doctor. Do not give to children under 12 unless directed by a doctor.

Warnings: Children and teenagers should not use this medicine for chicken pox or flu symptoms before a doctor is consulted about Reye syndrome, a rare but serious illness reported to be associated with aspirin. Do not take for pain for more than 10 days or for fever for more than 3 days unless directed by a doctor. If pain or fever persists or gets worse, if new symptoms occur, or if redness or swelling is present consult a doctor because these could be signs of a serious condition. Do not take this product if you are allergic to aspirin, have asthma, stomach problems that persist or recur, gastric ulcers or bleeding problems unless directed by a doctor. If ringing in the ears or loss of hearing occurs, consult a doctor before taking any more of this product. Keep this and all drugs out of the reach of children. In case of accidental overdose, seek professional assistance or contact a poison control center immediately. As with any drug, if you are pregnant or nursing a baby, seek the advice of a health professional before using this product. **IT IS ESPECIALLY IMPORTANT NOT TO USE ASPIRIN DURING THE LAST 3 MONTHS OF PREGNANCY UNLESS SPECIFICALLY DIRECTED TO DO SO BY A DOCTOR BECAUSE IT MAY CAUSE PROBLEMS IN THE UNBORN CHILD OR COMPLICATIONS DURING DELIVERY.**

Drug Interaction Precaution: Do not take this product if you are taking a prescription drug for anticoagulation (thinning of the blood), diabetes, gout, or arthritis unless directed by a doctor.

How Supplied: Extra Strength Bayer® Plus Aspirin (500 mg) is available in bottles of 30 and 60 caplets. Child resistant closure on 30s caplets. Bottles of 60s caplets available without safety closure for households without young children.

Shown in Product Identification Section, page 429

BAYER® SELECT™ IBUPROFEN Pain Relief Formula Pain Reliever/Fever Reducer

Warning: ASPIRIN SENSITIVE PATIENTS. Do not take this product if you have had a severe allergic reaction to aspirin, e.g.-asthma, swelling, shock or hives, because even though this product contains no aspirin or salicylates, cross-reactions may occur in patients allergic to aspirin.

Active Ingredient: 200 mg Ibuprofen USP per caplet

Inactive Ingredients: Calcium Phosphate, Cellulose, Magnesium Stearate, Silicon Dioxide, Sodium Lauryl Sulfate, Sodium Starch Glycolate, Stearic Acid, Titanium Dioxide.

Indications: For the temporary relief of minor aches and pains associated with the common cold, headache, toothache, muscular aches, backache, for the minor pain of arthritis, for the pain of menstrual cramps and for reduction of fever.

Directions: ADULTS: Take 1 caplet every 4 to 6 hours while symptoms persist. If pain or fever does not respond to 1 caplet, 2 caplets may be used but do not exceed 6 caplets in 24 hours, unless directed by a doctor. The smallest effective dose should be used. Take with food or milk if occasional and mild heartburn, upset stomach, or stomach pain occurs with use. Consult a doctor if these symptoms are more than mild or if they persist. CHILDREN: Do not give this product to children under 12 except under the advice and supervision of a doctor.

Warnings: Do not take for pain for more than 10 days or for fever for more than 3 days unless directed by a doctor. If pain or fever persists or gets worse, if new symptoms occur, or if the painful area is red or swollen, consult a doctor. These could be signs of a serious illness. If you are under a doctor's care for any serious condition, consult a doctor before taking this product. As with aspirin and acetaminophen, if you have any condition which requires you to take prescription drugs or if you have had any problems or serious side effects from taking any non-prescription pain reliever, do not take this product without first discussing it with your doctor. If you experience any symptoms which are unusual or seem unrelated to the condition for which you took ibuprofen, consult a doctor before taking any more of it. Although ibuprofen is indicated for the same conditions as aspirin and acetaminophen, it should not be taken with them except under a doctor's direction. Do not combine this product with any other ibuprofen containing product. As with any drug if you are pregnant or nursing a baby, seek the advice of a health professional before using this product. IT IS ESPECIALLY IMPORTANT NOT TO USE IBUPROFEN DURING THE LAST 3 MONTHS OF PREGNANCY UNLESS SPECIFICALLY DIRECTED TO DO SO BY A DOCTOR BECAUSE IT MAY CAUSE PROBLEMS IN THE UNBORN CHILD OR COMPLICATIONS DURING DELIVERY. Keep this and all drugs out of the reach of children. In case of accidental overdose, seek professional assistance or contact a poison control center immediately.

How Supplied: BAYER® SELECT™ IBUPROFEN Pain Relief Formula is available in 24, 50 and 100 count bottles.

Shown in Product Identification Section, page 429

BAYER® SELECT™
Maximum Strength HEADACHE
Pain Relief Formula
Aspirin-Free

Active Ingredients: Acetaminophen 500 mg and Caffeine 65 mg per caplet.

Inactive Ingredients: Croscarmellose Sodium, FD&C Blue #2, Hydroxypropyl Methylcellulose, Magnesium Stearate, Microcrystalline Cellulose, Polyethylene Glycol, Potassium Sorbate, Starch, Titanium Dioxide, Xanthan Gum.

Indications: BAYER® SELECT™ HEADACHE Pain Relief Formula contains a specially chosen combination of safe, aspirin-free ingredients in a maximum dosage form for strong, fast, temporary relief of HEADACHES.

Directions: Adults: Take 2 caplets with water every 4 hours, as needed, up to a maximum of 8 caplets per 24 hours. **Children under 12 years of age:** Consult a doctor.

Warnings: Do not take this product for pain for more than 10 days or fever for more than 3 days unless directed by a doctor. If pain is severe or recurrent, or fever persists or gets worse, if new symptoms occur, or if redness or swelling is present, consult a doctor because these could be signs of a serious condition. Keep out of reach of children. In case of accidental overdose, prompt medical attention is essential for adults as well as for children even if you do not notice any signs or symptoms. Contact a doctor immediately. As with any drug, if you are pregnant or nursing a baby, seek the advice of a health professional before using this product.

How Supplied: BAYER® SELECT™ Maximum Strength HEADACHE Pain Relief Formula is available in 24, 50 and 100 count bottles.

Shown in Product Identification Section, page 429

BAYER® SELECT™
Maximum Strength MENSTRUAL
Multi-Symptom Formula
Aspirin-Free

Active Ingredients: Acetaminophen 500 mg and Pamabrom 25 mg per caplet.

Inactive Ingredients: Croscarmellose Sodium, D&C Red #27, Hydroxypropyl Methylcellulose, Iron Oxide, Magnesium Stearate, Microcrystalline Cellulose, Polyethylene Glycol, Polysorbate 80, Starch, Titanium Dioxide.

Indications: BAYER® SELECT™ MENSTRUAL Multi-Symptom Formula contains a specially chosen combination of safe, aspirin-free, caffeine-free ingredients that is not found in any ordinary pain reliever to provide temporary relief of the following symptoms associated with PREMENSTRUAL and MENSTRUAL pain and discomfort:

- Cramps
- Bloating
- Backache
- Water-weight gain
- Headache
- Muscular aches and pains

Directions: Adults: Take 2 caplets with water every 4 hours, as needed, up to a maximum of 8 caplets per 24 hours. **Children under 12 years of age:** Consult a doctor.

Warnings: Do not take for pain for more than 10 days unless directed by a doctor. Consult a doctor if pain is severe or recurrent, as this may be a sign of serious illness. Keep out of reach of children. In case of accidental overdose, prompt medical attention is essential for adults as well as for children even if you do not notice any signs or symptoms. As with any drug, if you are pregnant or nursing a baby, seek the advice of a health professional before using this product.

How Supplied: BAYER® SELECT™ Maximum Strength MENSTRUAL Multi-Symptom Formula is available in 24 and 50 count bottles.

Shown in Product Identification Section, page 429

BAYER® SELECT™
Maximum Strength
NIGHT TIME PAIN RELIEF
Analgesic/Sleep Aid Formula
Aspirin-Free

Active Ingredients: Acetaminophen 500 mg and Diphenhydramine HCl 25 mg per caplet.

Inactive Ingredients: FD&C Blue #1 and #2, Hydroxypropyl Methylcellulose, Polyethylene Glycol, Polysorbate 80, Potassium Sorbate, Povidone, Starch, Stearic Acid, Talc, Titanium Dioxide.

Indications: BAYER® SELECT™ NIGHT TIME PAIN RELIEF Formula contains a specially chosen combination of safe, aspirin-free, caffeine-free ingredients in a maximum dosage form to provide temporary relief of minor aches and NIGHT TIME PAIN while helping you fall asleep safely and gently.

Directions: Adults: Take 2 caplets at bedtime if needed or as directed by a doctor. Do not exceed recommended dosage.

Warnings: Do not give this product to children under 12 years of age or use for more than 10 days unless directed by a doctor. Consult a doctor if pain is severe, recurrent, persists or gets worse, if new symptoms occur, or if sleeplessness persists continuously for more than 2 weeks. These may be symptoms of a serious underlying medical illness. Do not take this product if you have asthma, glaucoma, emphysema, chronic pulmonary disease, shortness of breath, difficulty in breathing, or difficulty in urination due to enlargement of the prostate gland unless directed by a doctor. Avoid alcoholic beverages while taking this product. Do not take this product if you are taking sedatives or tranquilizers without first consulting your doctor. Keep out of reach of children. In case of accidental overdose, prompt medical attention is essential for adults as well as for children even if you do not notice any signs or symptoms. Contact a doctor immediately. As with any drug, if you are pregnant or nursing a baby, seek the advice of a health professional before using this product.

How Supplied: BAYER® SELECT™ Maximum Strength NIGHT TIME PAIN RELIEF FORMULA is available in 24 and 50 count bottles.

Shown in Product Identification Section, page 429

BAYER® SELECT™
Maximum Strength
SINUS PAIN RELIEF
Analgesic/Decongestant Formula
Aspirin-Free

Active Ingredients: Acetaminophen 500 mg and Pseudoephedrine HCl 30 mg per caplet.

Inactive Ingredients: Colloidal Silicon Dioxide, D&C Yellow #10, FD&C Blue #1, FD&C Yellow #6, Hydroxypropyl Methylcellulose, Iron Oxide, Magnesium Stearate, Microcrystalline Cellulose, Polyethylene Glycol, Polysorbate 80, Povidone, Starch, Titanium Dioxide.

Indications: BAYER® SELECT™ SINUS PAIN RELIEF Formula contains a specially chosen combination of safe, aspirin-free, caffeine-free ingredients in a maximum dosage to provide temporary relief of the following SINUS symptoms without making you drowsy:

Continued on next page

This product information was effective as of November 1, 1992. Current information may be obtained directly from Sterling Health, by writing to 90 Park Avenue, New York, NY 10016.

Sterling Health—Cont.

- Sinus headache pain and pressure
- Swollen nasal passages
- Nasal congestion due to the common cold, hay fever, other respiratory allergies or associated with sinusitis.

Directions: Adults: Take 2 caplets with water every 4-6 hours, up to a maximum of 8 caplets per 24 hours. **Children under 12 years of age:** Consult your doctor.

Warnings: Do not exceed recommended dosage because at higher doses nervousness, dizziness, or sleeplessness may occur. Do not take this product for more than 7 days unless directed by a doctor. If symptoms do not improve, are severe or recurrent, or are accompanied by fever, consult a doctor. Do not take this product if you have heart disease, high blood pressure, thyroid disease, diabetes, or difficulty in urination due to enlargement of the prostate gland unless directed by a doctor. Keep out of reach of children. In case of accidental overdose, prompt medical attention is essential for adults as well as for children even if you do not notice any signs or symptoms. Contact a doctor immediately. As with any drug, if you are pregnant or nursing a baby, seek the advice of a health professional before using this product.

Drug Interaction Precaution: Do not take this product if you are presently taking a prescription drug for high blood pressure or depression without first consulting your doctor.

How Supplied: BAYER® SELECT™ Maximum Strength SINUS PAIN RELIEF FORMULA is available in 24 and 50 count bottles.

Shown in Product Identification Section, page 429

BRONKAID® Mist
(Epinephrine)
Bronchodilator

Description: BRONKAID Mist, brand of Epinephrine inhalation aerosol. Contains: Epinephrine, USP, 0.5% (w/w) (as nitrate and hydrochloric salts). Also contains: Alcohol 33% (w/w), Ascorbic Acid Dichlorodifluoromethane, Dichlorotetrafluoroethane, Purified water. Each spray delivers 0.25 mg Epinephrine. Contains no sulfites.

Indication: For temporary relief of shortness of breath, tightness of chest and wheezing due to bronchial asthma.

Warnings: FOR ORAL INHALATION ONLY. Do not use this product unless a diagnosis of asthma has been made by a doctor, or if you have heart disease, high blood pressure, thyroid disease, diabetes, or difficulty in urination due to enlargement of the prostate gland, if you have ever been hospitalized for asthma or if you are taking any prescription drug for asthma. **Do not use this product more frequently or at higher doses than recommended, unless directed by a doctor.** Keep this and all drugs out of the reach of children. In case of accidental overdose, seek professional assistance or contact a poison control center immediately. As with any drug, if you are pregnant or nursing a baby, seek the advice of a health professional before using this product.
Excessive use may cause nervousness and rapid heart beat, and, possibly, adverse effects on the heart. **Do not continue to use this product, but seek medical assistance immediately if symptoms are not relieved within 20 minutes or become worse.**

Drug Interaction Precaution: Do not use this product if you are presently taking a prescription drug for high blood pressure or depression, without first consulting your doctor.

Warnings: Avoid spraying in eyes. Contents under pressure. Do not break or incinerate. Using or storing near open flame or heating above 120°F may cause bursting.

Dosage: Inhalation dosage for adults and children 4 years of age and older. Start with one inhalation, then wait at least one (1) minute. If not relieved, use once more. Do not use again for at least 3 hours. The use of this product by children should be supervised by an adult. Children under 4 years of age, consult a doctor.

Directions for Use:

1. Remove cap and mouthpiece from bottle.
2. Remove cap from mouthpiece.
3. Turn mouthpiece sideways and fit metal stem of nebulizer into hole in flattened end of mouthpiece.
4. Exhale, as completely as possible. Now, hold bottle **upside down** between thumb and forefinger and close lips loosely around end of mouthpiece.
5. Inhale deeply while pressing down firmly on bottle, once only.
6. Remove mouthpiece and hold your breath a moment to allow for maximum absorption of medication. Then exhale slowly through nearly closed lips.

After use, remove mouthpiece from bottle and replace cap. Slide mouthpiece over bottle for protection. When possible rinse mouthpiece with tap water immediately after use. Soap and water will not hurt it. A clean mouthpiece always works better.

How Supplied: Bottles of ½ fl oz (15 mL) with actuator. Also available—refills (no mouthpiece) in 15 mL (½ fl oz) and 22.5 mL (¾ fl oz).

Shown in Product Identification Section, page 429

BRONKAID® Mist Suspension
(Epinephrine Bitartrate)
Bronchodilator

Active Ingredients: Each spray delivers 0.3 mg Epinephrine Bitartrate equivalent to 0.16 mg Epinephrine base. Contains Epinephrine Bitartrate 7.0 mg per cc. Also contains: Cetylpyridinium Chloride, Dichlorodifluoromethane, Dichlorotetrafluoroethane, Sorbitan Trioleate, Trichloromonofluoromethane. Contains no sulfites.

Indication: Provides temporary relief of shortness of breath, tightness of chest, and wheezing due to bronchial asthma.

Warnings: FOR ORAL INHALATION ONLY. Do not use this product unless a diagnosis of asthma has been made by a doctor, or if you have heart disease, high blood pressure, thyroid disease, diabetes, or difficulty in urination due to enlargement of the prostate gland, if you have ever been hospitalized for asthma or if you are taking any prescription drug for asthma. **Do not use this product more frequently or at higher doses than recommended, unless directed by a doctor.** Keep this and all drugs out of the reach of children. In case of accidental overdose, seek professional assistance or contact a poison control center immediately. As with any drug, if you are pregnant or nursing a baby, seek the advice of a health professional before using this product.
Excessive use may cause nervousness and rapid heart beat, and, possibly, adverse effects on the heart. **Do not continue to use this product, but seek medical assistance immediately if symptoms are not relieved within 20 minutes or become worse.**

Drug Interaction Precaution: Do not use this product if you are presently taking a prescription drug for high blood pressure or depression, without first consulting your doctor.

Warning: Avoid spraying in eyes. Contents under pressure. Do not break or incinerate. Using or storing near open flame or heating above 120°F may cause bursting.

Administration:

1. SHAKE WELL.
2. HOLD INHALER WITH NOZZLE DOWN WHILE USING. Empty the lungs as completely as possible by exhaling.
3. Purse the lips as in saying the letter "O" and hold the nozzle up to the lips, keeping the tongue flat. As you start to take a deep breath, squeeze nozzle and can together, releasing one full application. Complete taking deep breath, drawing medication into your lungs.
4. Hold breath for as long as comfortable. This distributes the medication in the lungs. Then exhale slowly keeping the lips nearly closed.
5. Rinse nozzle daily with soap and hot water after removing from vial. Dry with clean cloth.

Before each use, remove dust cap and inspect mouthpiece for foreign objects. Replace dust cap after each use.

Dosage: Inhalation dosage for adults and children 4 years of age and older. Start with one inhalation, then wait at least one (1) minute. If not relieved, use once more. Do not use again for at least 3 hours. The use of this product by children should be supervised by an adult. Children under 4 years of age; consult a doctor.

Professional Labeling: Same as stated under Indication.

How Supplied:
⅓ fl oz (10 cc) pocketsize aerosol inhaler, with actuator.

Shown in Product Identification Section, page 429

BRONKAID® Tablets
Bronchodilator and Expectorant

Description: Each tablet contains Ephedrine Sulfate 24 mg, Guaifenesin 100 mg, and Theophylline 100 mg. Also contains: Magnesium Stearate, Magnesium Trisilicate, Microcrystalline Cellulose, Starch.

Indication: For symptomatic control of bronchial congestion and bronchial asthma. Clears bronchial passages. Helps relieve shortness of breath, plus helps loosen phlegm.

Warnings: Do not use this product unless a diagnosis of asthma has been made by a doctor, or if you have heart disease, high blood pressure, thyroid disease, diabetes, difficulty in urination due to enlargement of the prostate gland, if you have ever been hospitalized for asthma or if you are taking any prescription drug for asthma unless directed by a doctor. Do not continue to use this product, but seek medical assistance immediately if symptoms are not relieved within an hour or become worse. Some users of this product may experience nervousness, tremor, sleeplessness, nausea, and loss of appetite. If these symptoms persist or become worse, consult your doctor.

Drug Interaction Precaution: Do not use this product if you are presently taking a prescription drug for high blood pressure or depression. Do not exceed recommended dosage unless directed by a physician.

Warnings: As with any drug, if you are pregnant or nursing a baby, seek the advice of a health professional before using this product. Keep this and all drugs out of the reach of children. In case of accidental overdose, seek professional assistance or contact a poison control center immediately.

Dosage and Administration: *Adult Dosage:* 1 tablet every four hours. Do not take more than 5 tablets in a 24-hour period. Swallow tablets whole with water. *Children under 12 years of age:* Consult a doctor. *Morning Dose:* An early dose of 1 tablet (for adults) can relieve the coughing and wheezing caused by the night's accumulation of mucus, and can help you start the day with better breathing capacity. *Before an Attack:* Many persons feel an attack of asthma coming on. One BRONKAID tablet beforehand may stop the attack before it starts. *During the Day:* The precise dose of BRONKAID tablets can be varied to meet your individual needs as you gain experience with this product. It is advisable to take 1 tablet before going to bed, for nighttime relief. However, be sure not to exceed recommended daily dosage.

How Supplied:
Boxes of 24 and 60.

Shown in Product Identification Section, page 429

CAMPHO-PHENIQUE®
[kam 'fo-finēk]
COLD SORE GEL
Analgesic/Antiseptic

Description: Contains phenol 4.7% (w/w) and camphor 10.8% (w/w). Also contains: colloidal silicon dioxide, eucalyptus oil, glycerin, light mineral oil.
Use at the first sign of cold sore, fever blister and sun blister symptoms (tingling, pain, itching).

Indications: For relief of pain and itching due to cold sores and fever blisters. To combat infection from minor injuries and skin lesions.
Also effective for:
Minor skin injuries: abrasions, cuts, scrapes, burns, razor nicks and chafed or irritated skin.
Insect bites: mosquitoes, black flies, sandfleas, chiggers.

Warnings: Do not use longer than 1 week unless directed by a doctor. Not to be used on large areas. In case of deep or puncture wounds, serious burns, or persisting redness, swelling or pain, or if rash or infection develops, discontinue use and consult physician. Do not bandage.
Avoid using near eyes. If product gets into the eye, flush thoroughly with water and obtain medical attention. Keep this and all drugs out of the reach of children. In case of accidental ingestion, seek professional assistance or contact a poison control center immediately.

Directions for Use: For external use. Apply directly to cold sore, fever blister or injury three or four times a day.

How Supplied: Tubes of 0.23 oz (6.5 g) and 0.50 oz (14 g).

Shown in Product Identification Section, page 429

CAMPHO-PHENIQUE® Liquid
[kam 'fo-finēk]
ANTISEPTIC LIQUID

Description: Contains phenol 4.7% (w/w) and camphor 10.8% (w/w). Also contains: Eucalyptus oil, light mineral oil.

Actions: Pain-relieving antiseptic for scrapes, cuts, burns, insect bites, fever blisters, and cold sores.

Indications: For relief of pain and to combat infection from minor injuries and skin lesions.

Warnings: Do not use longer than 1 week unless directed by a doctor. Not to be used on large areas or in or near the eyes. In case of deep or puncture wounds, serious burns, or persisting redness, swelling or pain, or if rash or infection develops, discontinue use and consult physician. Do not bandage.
Keep this and all drugs out of the reach of children. In case of accidental ingestion, seek professional assistance or contact a poison control center immediately.

Directions for Use: For external use. Apply with cotton three or four times daily.
4 oz size only: Do not use more than ½ the contents of the 4 fl oz bottle in any 24-hour period.

How Supplied:
Bottles of ¾, 1½ and 4 fl oz.

Shown in Product Identification Section, page 429

CAMPHO-PHENIQUE™
[kam 'fo-finēk]
TRIPLE ANTIBIOTIC OINTMENT PLUS PAIN RELIEVER

Description: Each gram contains bacitracin zinc 500 units, neomycin sulfate 5 mg (equiv to 3.5 mg neomycin base), polymyxin B sulfate 5000 units, lidocaine HCl 40 mg (Pain Reliever). Also contains white petrolatum.

Actions: Pain-relieving triple antibiotic with anesthetic to help prevent infection in minor cuts, scrapes, burns and other minor wounds.

Indications: Helps prevent infections in minor cuts, burns, and other minor wounds. Provides soothing, nonstinging temporary relief of pain and itching associated with these conditions.

Warnings: For external use only. In case of deep or puncture wounds, animal bites or serious burns, consult physician. If redness, irritation, swelling or pain persists or increases, if a rash or other allergic reaction develops, or if infection occurs, discontinue use and consult physician. Do not use in eyes or over large areas of the body. Do not use longer than 1 week unless directed by doctor. Keep

Continued on next page

This product information was effective as of November 1, 1992. Current information may be obtained directly from Sterling Health, by writing to 90 Park Avenue, New York, NY 10016.

Sterling Health—Cont.

this and all drugs out of the reach of children. In case of accidental ingestion seek professional assistance or contact a poison control center immediately.

Directions: Clean the affected area. Apply a small amount (an amount equal to the surface area of the tip of a finger) on the area 1 to 3 times daily. May be covered.

How Supplied: Tubes of 0.50 oz and 1.0 oz.

Shown in Product Identification Section, page 429

DAIRY EASE® Tablets/Caplets Natural Lactase Enzyme Supplement

Ingredients: Each Tablet/Caplet contains 3000 FCC Lactase units (derived from Aspergillus Oryzae). Other ingredients are: (Tablets) Dibasic Calcium Phosphate, Mannitol, Colloidal Silicon Dioxide, Magnesium Stearate. (Caplets): Colloidal Silicon Dioxide, Dibasic Calcium Phosphate, FD&C Blue No. 2, Hydroxypropyl Methylcellulose, Magnesium Stearate, Microcrystalline Cellulose, Polyethylene Glycol, Potassium Sorbate, Pregelatinized Starch, Titanium Dioxide and Xanthan Gum.

Indications: Lactase insufficiency, suspected from gastrointestinal disturbances after consumption of milk or milk-containing products (i.e., Gas, Bloating, Flatulence, Cramps and Diarrhea) or identified by a lactose intolerance test.

Action: Lactase enzyme converts, by hydrolysis, the lactose into its simple sugar components: glucose and galactose.

Product Uses: Dairy Ease is a natural lactase enzyme which supplements the natural level of lactase in the body and helps make lactose more easily digestible. The most common products where lactose can be found are milk, cheese, ice cream & chocolate and it is also found in some vitamins and medications. Dairy Ease can be used with all foods which contain lactose such as pizza, hot dogs, pancakes, creamed salad dressings and soups, instant cocoa mix, puddings and other foods where milk, milk solids, whey, whey protein concentrate, casein or cheese are listed on the ingredient panel.

Dosage: Recommended dosage is 2–3 chewable tablets/swallowable caplets along with or immediately following dairy food consumption. However, since natural lactase levels vary, actual dosage may differ from person to person.

Toxicity: None.

Drug Interactions: None. Dairy Ease tablets and caplets are classified as food products.

Warnings: Do not use if you have had an allergic reaction to products containing lactase enzyme. If symptoms persist consult a doctor about a possible food allergy or other digestive disorder.

Precautions: Diabetics should be aware that the milk sugar will now be metabolically available and must be taken into account (17.5 gm glucose and 17.5 gm galactose per quart at 70% hydrolysis). No reports received of any diabetics' reactions. Galactosemics may not have milk in any form, lactase enzyme modified or not.

Note: Possible adverse reactions are mainly gastrointestinal in nature, sometimes mimicking the symptoms of lactose intolerance and sometimes involving vomiting. Skin rashes possibly due to allergic reactions have been reported. Persons sensitive to penicillin and other molds may be particularly susceptible. Discontinue use of tablets/caplets immediately and consult a physician.

How Supplied: Dairy Ease Chewable Tablets are available in 12, 36, 60 and 100 counts. Dairy Ease Swallowable Caplets are available in a 40 count bottle.

Shown in Product Identification Section, pages 429 and 430

DAIRY EASE® Drops Natural Lactase Enzyme

Ingredients: Water, Glycerol, Lactase Enzyme (derived from Kluyveromyces Lactis). One ml contains no less than 5400 Neutral Lactase units.

Indications: Lactase insufficiency, suspected from gastrointestinal disturbances after consumption of milk or milk-containing products (i.e., Gas, Bloating, Flatulence, Cramps and Diarrhea) or identified by a lactose tolerance test.

Product Uses: Dairy Ease drops are a natural lactase enzyme in liquid form which when added to milk, make it more easily digestible. Dairy Ease drops can be used in any kind of milk including: whole, 1%, 2%, nonfat, canned, powdered and chocolate. Also, cream, baby formulas containing milk and high protein diet formulas. The treated milk can be used for cooking, on cereal or directly from the carton.

Action: Lactase enzyme converts, by hydrolysis, the lactose into its simple sugar components: glucose and galactose.

Dosage: Add Dairy Ease drops to a quart of milk, shake gently and refrigerate for 24 hours. Five drops will remove 70% of the lactose, 10 drops, 90% and 15 drops, 97+%. Since the degree of natural lactase levels varies, each person may have to adjust the number of drops that work best.

Toxicity: None.

Drug Interactions: None. Dairy Ease drops are classified as food products.

Warnings: Do not use if you have had an allergic reaction to products containing lactase enzyme. If symptoms persist consult a doctor about a possible food allergy or other digestive disorder.

Precautions: Diabetics should be aware that the milk sugar will now be metabolically available and must be taken into account (17.5 gm glucose and 17.5 gm galactose per quart at 70% hydrolysis). No reports received of any diabetics' reactions. Galactosemics may not have milk in any form, lactase enzyme modified or not.

Adverse Reactions: No reactions of any kind have been observed from Dairy Ease liquid drops.

How Supplied: Dairy Ease drops are available in a 7ml bottle which will treat up to 32 quarts of milk.

Shown in Product Identification Section, page 430

DAIRY EASE® Real Milk Lactose Reduced Milk

Dairy Ease is also available in Real Milk which is 70% lactose reduced and contains vitamins A & D. A one quart size in three varieties is available: Nonfat, 1% lowfat, and 2% lowfat. Dairy Ease Real Milk can be used for cooking, on cereal or directly from the carton.

Shown in Product Identification Section, page 430

FERGON® Iron Supplement Tablets
[fur-gone]
brand of ferrous gluconate

Each FERGON Iron Supplement tablet contains 320 mg (5 grains) Ferrous Gluconate equal to approximately 36 mg elemental iron. Also contains: Acacia, Carnauba Wax, Dextrose Excipient, FD&C Red #40, D&C Yellow #10, FD&C Blue #1 as color additives. Gelatin, Kaolin, Magnesium Stearate, Parabens, Povidone, Precipitated Calcium Carbonate, Sodium Benzoate, Starch, Sucrose, Talc, Titanium Dioxide, Yellow Wax.

Action and Uses: For use as a dietary supplement.

Warnings: **KEEP IRON CONTAINING DIETARY SUPPLEMENTS OUT OF THE REACH OF CHILDREN.** If you are pregnant or nursing a baby, seek the advice of a health professional before using this product. In case of accidental overdose, seek professional assistance or contact a poison control center immediately.

AVOID EXCESSIVE HEAT

Dosage and Administration: Adults —One FERGON tablet daily.

How Supplied: FERGON Tablets of 320 mg (5 grains) bottle of 100.

Shown in Product Identification Section, page 430

HALEY'S M-O®
Lubricant/Saline Laxative

Active Ingredients: A suspension of Magnesium Hydroxide in purified water plus mineral oil. Haley's M-O contains 301 mg (flavored: 300 mg) of Magnesium Hydroxide and 1.25 mL of mineral oil per teaspoon (5 mL).

Inactive Ingredients: Purified Water. For flavored Haley's M-O only, D&C Red No. 28, flavor, Purified Water, Saccharin Sodium.

Indications: For the relief of occasional constipation or irregularity accompanied by hemorrhoids. This product generally produces bowel movement in 6-8 hrs.

Action at Laxative Dosage: Haley's M-O is a mild saline laxative which acts by drawing water into the gut, increasing intraluminal pressure, and increasing intestinal motility.

Directions:

ADULTS and CHILDREN 12 years and over: 2 to 4 tablespoons at bedtime or upon arising, followed by a full glass (8 oz.) of liquid.**

CHILDREN 6 to 11 years: 1 teaspoonful to 1 tablespoonful at bedtime or upon arising, followed by a full glass (8 oz.) of liquid.**

CHILDREN UNDER 6 YEARS: Consult a doctor.

Warnings: Do not use laxative products when abdominal pain, nausea, vomiting, sudden change in bowel habits persisting for over 2 weeks, or kidney disease are present unless directed by a doctor. Laxative products should not be used for a period longer than 1 week, unless directed by a doctor. Rectal bleeding or failure to have a bowel movement after use may indicate a serious condition. Discontinue and consult a doctor. Do not administer to children under 6 years of age, to pregnant women, to bedridden patients, or to persons with difficulty in swallowing. Do not take with meals. Keep this and all drugs out of the reach of children. In case of accidental overdose, seek professional assistance or contact a poison control center immediately. As with any drug, if you are nursing a baby, seek the advice of a health professional before using this product.

Drug Interaction Precaution: Do not take this product if you are presently taking a stool softener laxative unless directed by a doctor.

How Supplied: Haley's M-O is available in regular and flavored 12 oz, and flavored 26 oz bottles.

** As bowel function improves, reduce dose gradually.

Shown in Product Identification Section, page 430

Regular Strength
Multi-Symptom Formula
MIDOL®
Menstrual Formula

Indications: Relieves cramps, headaches, backaches and muscular aches and pains.

- Provides effective relief of painful menstrual symptoms.
- Contains aspirin-free, caffeine-free ingredients.

Directions: Adults and children 12 years and over: Take 2 caplets with water. Repeat every 4 hours, as needed, up to a maximum of 12 caplets per day. Under age 12: Consult your doctor.

Warnings: If pain persists for more than 10 days, consult a doctor immediately. May cause drowsiness. Use caution when driving or operating machinery. Do not take this product if you have asthma, glaucoma, emphysema, chronic pulmonary disease, shortness of breath, difficulty in breathing, or difficulty in urination due to enlargement of the prostate gland unless directed by a doctor. Alcohol, sedatives or tranquilizers may increase drowsiness. Keep out of reach of children. In case of accidental overdose, immediate medical attention is essential for adults as well as for children even if you do not notice any signs or symptoms. As with any drug, if you are pregnant or nursing a baby, seek the advice of a health professional before using this product.

Active Ingredients: Each caplet contains Acetaminophen 325 mg and Pyrilamine Maleate 12.5 mg.

Inactive Ingredients: Croscarmellose Sodium, Hydroxypropyl Methylcellulose, Magnesium Stearate, Microcrystalline Cellulose, Pregelatinized Starch and Triacetin.

How Supplied: White capsule-shaped caplets available in packages of 2 blisters of 8 caplets each and bottles of 32 caplets. Child-resistant safety closure on bottles of 32 caplets.

Shown in Product Identification Section, page 430

PMS
Multi-Symptom Formula
MIDOL®
Menstrual Formula

Indications: Contains maximum strength medication for all these PMS symptoms: bloating, water-weight gain, cramps, headaches and backaches.

- Provides maximum strength relief of the physical symptoms of Premenstrual Syndrome so you can feel like yourself again.
- Contains a combination of aspirin-free ingredients which is not found in any ordinary pain reliever, a diuretic to alleviate water retention and an analgesic for pain.

Directions: Adults and children 12 years and over: Take 2 caplets with water. Repeat every 4 hours, as needed, up to a maximum of 8 caplets per day. Under age 12: Consult your doctor.

Warnings: If pain persists for more than 10 days, consult a doctor immediately. May cause drowsiness. Use caution when driving or operating machinery. Alcohol, sedatives or tranquilizers may increase drowsiness. Do not take this product if you have asthma, glaucoma, emphysema, chronic pulmonary disease, shortness of breath, difficulty in breathing, or difficulty in urination due to enlargement of the prostate gland unless directed by a doctor. Keep out of reach of children. In case of accidental overdose, immediate medical attention is essential for adults as well as for children even if you do not notice any signs or symptoms. As with any drug, if you are pregnant or nursing a baby, seek the advice of a health professional before using this product.

Active Ingredients: Each caplet contains Acetaminophen 500 mg, Pamabrom 25 mg and Pyrilamine Maleate 15 mg.

Inactive Ingredients: Croscarmellose Sodium, Hydroxypropyl Methylcellulose, Magnesium Stearate, Microcrystalline Cellulose, Pregelatinized Starch and Triacetin.

How Supplied: White capsule-shaped caplets available in packages of 2 blisters of 8 caplets each and bottles of 32 caplets. Child-resistant safety closure on bottles of 32 caplets.

Shown in Product Identification Section, page 430

CRAMP RELIEF FORMULA
MIDOL ® IB
Ibuprofen Tablets, USP 200 mg
Menstrual Pain/Cramp Reliever

Warning: Aspirin-Sensitive Patients—Do not take this product if you have had a severe allergic reaction to aspirin, eg, asthma, swelling, shock or hives, because even though this product contains no aspirin or salicylates, cross-reactions may occur in patients allergic to aspirin.

Indications: For the temporary relief of painful menstrual cramps (dysmenorrhea); also headaches, backaches and muscular aches and pains associated with Premenstrual Syndrome.

Continued on next page

This product information was effective as of November 1, 1992. Current information may be obtained directly from Sterling Health, by writing to 90 Park Avenue, New York, NY 10016.

Sterling Health—Cont.

Directions:
Adults: Take 1 tablet every 4 to 6 hours at the onset of menstrual symptoms and while pain persists. If pain does not respond to 1 tablet, 2 tablets may be used but do not exceed 6 tablets in 24 hours, unless directed by a doctor. The smallest effective dose should be used. Take with food or milk if occasional and mild heartburn, upset stomach, or stomach pain occurs with use. Consult a doctor if these symptoms are more than mild or if they persist. *Children:* Do not give this product to children under 12 except under the advice and supervision of a doctor.

Warnings: Do not take for pain for more than 10 days unless directed by a doctor. If pain persists or gets worse, or if new symptoms occur, consult a doctor. These could be signs of serious illness. If you are under a doctor's care for any serious condition, consult a doctor before taking this product. As with aspirin and acetaminophen, if you have any condition which requires you to take prescription drugs or if you have had any problems or serious side effects from taking any nonprescription pain reliever, do not take this product without first discussing it with your doctor. If you experience any symptoms which are unusual or seem unrelated to the condition for which you took ibuprofen, consult a doctor before taking any more of it. Although ibuprofen is indicated for the same conditions as aspirin and acetaminophen, it should not be taken with them except under a doctor's direction. Do not combine this product with any other ibuprofen-containing product. As with any drug, if you are pregnant or nursing a baby, seek the advice of a health professional before using this product. **IT IS ESPECIALLY IMPORTANT NOT TO USE IBUPROFEN DURING THE LAST 3 MONTHS OF PREGNANCY UNLESS SPECIFICALLY DIRECTED TO DO SO BY A DOCTOR BECAUSE IT MAY CAUSE PROBLEMS IN THE UNBORN CHILD OR COMPLICATIONS DURING DELIVERY.** Keep this and all drugs out of the reach of children. In case of accidental overdose, seek professional assistance or contact a poison control center immediately.

Action and Uses: Ibuprofen is used for the relief of painful menstrual cramps and the pain associated with Premenstrual Syndrome. Ibuprofen has been proven more effective in relieving menstrual pain and cramps than aspirin and is gentler on the stomach. Ibuprofen had been widely prescribed for years and is now available in nonprescription strength.

Active Ingredient: Each tablet contains ibuprofen USP 200 mg.

Inactive Ingredients: Calcium phosphate, cellulose, magnesium stearate, silicon dioxide, sodium lauryl sulfate, sodium starch glycolate, stearic acid, titanium dioxide.
Store at room temperature; avoid excessive heat 40°C (104°F).

How Supplied:
White tablets in bottles of 16 and 32 tablets.
Child-resistant safety closure on bottles of 32 tablets.

Shown in Product Identification Section, page 430

Maximum Strength Multi-Symptom Formula MIDOL® Menstrual Formula

Indications: Relieves all of these physical menstrual symptoms: cramps, bloating, water-weight gain, headaches, backaches and muscular aches.

- Provides maximum strength relief of painful physical symptoms suffered during your menstrual cycle.
- Contains a combination of maximum strength, aspirin-free ingredients which is not found in any ordinary pain reliever.

Directions: Adults and children 12 years and over: Take 2 caplets with water. Repeat every 4 hours, as needed, up to a maximum of 8 caplets per day. Under age 12: Consult your doctor.

Warnings: If pain persists for more than 10 days, consult a doctor immediately. May cause drowsiness. Use caution when driving or operating machinery. Alcohol, sedatives or tranquilizers may increase drowsiness. The recommended dose of this product contains about as much caffeine as a cup of coffee. Limit the use of caffeine-containing medications, foods, or beverages while taking this product because too much caffeine may cause nervousness, irritability, sleeplessness, and occasionally, rapid heartbeat. Keep out of reach of children. In case of accidental overdose, immediate medical attention is essential for adults as well as for children even if you do not notice any signs or symptoms. As with any drug, if you are pregnant or nursing a baby, seek the advice of a health professional before using this product.

Active Ingredients: Each caplet contains Acetaminophen 500 mg, Caffeine 60 mg and Pyrilamine Maleate 15 mg.

Inactive Ingredients: Croscarmellose Sodium, Hydroxypropyl Methylcellulose, Magnesium Stearate, Microcrystalline Cellulose, Pregelatinized Starch and Triacetin.

How Supplied: White capsule-shaped caplets available in 2-caplet packets for sample use, bottles of 8 and 32 caplets, and packages of 2 blisters of 8 caplets each. Child-resistant safety closures on bottles of 8 and 32 caplets.

Shown in Product Identification Section, page 430

Night Time Formula MIDOL® PM Pain Reliever/Sleep Aid

Active Ingredients: Each caplet contains Acetaminophen 500 mg, Diphenhydramine HCl 25 mg

Inactive Ingredients: FD&C Blue #1 & #2, Hydroxypropyl Methylcellulose, Polyethylene Glycol, Potassium Sorbate, Povidone, Pregelatinized Starch,.Stearic Acid, Talc and Titanium Dioxide.

Indications: For the temporary relief of occasional headaches, minor aches, pains and cramps with accompanying sleeplessness.

Directions: Adults and children 12 years and over: Take two caplets at bedtime if needed or as directed by a doctor. Do not exceed recommended dosage. Under age 12: Consult your doctor.

Warnings: Keep out of reach of children. In case of accidental overdose, immediate medical attention is essential for adults as well as for children even if you do not notice any signs or symptoms. As with any drug, if you are pregnant or nursing a baby, seek the advice of a health professional before using this product. Do not give this product to children under 12 years of age or use for more than 10 days unless directed by a doctor. Consult a doctor if symptoms persist, get worse, if new ones occur, or if sleeplessness persists continuously for more than 2 weeks. These may be symptoms of a serious underlying medical illness. Do not take this product if you have asthma, glaucoma, emphysema, chronic pulmonary disease, shortness of breath, difficulty in breathing or difficulty in urination due to enlargement of the prostate gland unless directed by a doctor. Avoid alcohol beverages while taking this product. Do not take this product if you have been taking sedatives or tranquilizers without first consulting your doctor.

How Supplied: Blue capsule shaped caplets available in packages of 2 blisters of 8 caplets each and bottles of 32 caplets. Child-resistant safety closures on bottles of 32 caplets.

Shown in Product Identification Section; page 430

Teen Multi-Symptom Formula MIDOL® Menstrual Formula

Indications: Relieves cramps, bloating, water-weight gain, headaches, backaches and muscular aches and pains.

- Provides effective relief of painful menstrual symptoms so you can get on with your life.
- Contains a special combination of safe, aspirin-free, caffeine-free ingredients which is not found in any ordinary pain reliever.
- Non-drowsy formula won't slow you down!

Directions: Adults and children 12 years and over: Take 2 caplets with water. Repeat every 4 hours, as needed, up to a maximum of 8 caplets per day. Under age 12: Consult your doctor.

Warnings: If pain persists for more than 10 days, consult a doctor immediately. Keep out of reach of children. In case of accidental overdose, immediate medical attention is essential for adults as well as for children even if you do not notice any signs or symptoms. As with any drug, if you are pregnant or nursing a baby, seek the advice of a health professional before using this product.

Active Ingredients: Each caplet contains Acetaminophen 400 mg and Pamabrom 25 mg.

Inactive Ingredients: Croscarmellose Sodium, Hydroxpropyl Methylcellulose, Magnesium Stearate, Microcrystaline Cellulose, Pregelatinized Starch and Triacetin.

How Supplied: White capsule-shaped caplets available in packages of 2 blisters of 8 caplets each and bottles of 32 caplets. Child-resistant safety closure on bottles of 32 caplets.

Shown in Product Identification Section, page 430

NaSal™ Moisturizer AF
Saline (buffered)
0.65% Sodium chloride
Nasal Spray and Drops

Description: The nasal spray and nose drops contain Sodium Chloride 0.65%. Also contains: Benzalkonium Chloride and Thimerosal 0.001% as preservative, Mono- and Dibasic Sodium Phosphates as buffers, Purified Water.
Contains No Alcohol.

Actions: Immediate relief for dry nose. Formulated to match the pH of normal nasal secretions to help prevent stinging or burning.

Indications: Provides gentle relief for dry, irritated nasal passages due to colds, low humidity, air travel, allergies, minor nose bleeds, crusting, overuse of decongestant sprays/drops and other nasal irritations. As an ideal moisturizer, it can be used with cold, allergy, and sinus medications.

Adverse Reactions: No associated side effects.

Dosage and Administration: Spray: Spray twice in each nostril as often as needed or as directed by doctor.
Drops: For infants, children and adults, 2 to 6 drops in each nostril as often as needed or as directed by doctor.

How Supplied: Nasal Spray—plastic squeeze bottles of 30 mL (1 fl. oz.).
Nose Drops—MonoDrop® bottles of 15 mL (½ fl. oz.).

Shown in Product Identification Section, page 430

NEO-SYNEPHRINE®
Pediatric Formula, Mild Formula, Regular Strength, and Extra Strength.
phenylephrine hydrochloride

Description: This line of Nasal Sprays, Drops and Spray Pumps contains Phenylephrine Hydrochloride in strengths ranging from 0.125% (drops only) to 1%. Also contains: Benzalkonium Chloride and Thimerosal 0.001% as preservatives, Citric Acid, Purified Water, Sodium Chloride, Sodium Citrate.

Action: Rapid-acting nasal decongestant.

Directions: Adults and children 12 years and over: May use 0.25%, 0.5% or 1.0%
Adults and children 6 years and over: May use 0.25%
Children 2 to under 6 years: Use 0.125%

2 or 3 sprays (drops) in each nostril not more often than every 4 hours.

Indications: For temporary relief of nasal congestion due to common cold, hay fever, sinusitis, or other upper respiratory allergies.

Warnings: Do not exceed recommended dosage because symptoms may occur such as burning, stinging, sneezing or increased nasal discharge. Do not use this product for more than 3 days. If symptoms persist, consult a doctor. Frequent and continued usage of the higher concentrations (especially the 1% solution) occasionally may cause a rebound congestion of the nose. Therefore, long-term or frequent use of this solution is not recommended without the advice of a physician.
Prolonged exposure to air or strong light will cause oxidation and some loss of potency. Do not use if brown in color or contains a precipitate.
Keep these and all drugs out of the reach of children. In case of accidental ingestion seek professional assistance or contact a poison control center immediately. The use of the dispenser by more than one person may spread infection.
Do not use this product if you have heart disease, high blood pressure, thyroid disease, diabetes, or difficulty in urination due to enlargement of the prostate gland unless directed by a doctor.

Adverse Reactions: Generally very well tolerated; systemic side effects such as tremor, insomnia, or palpitation rarely occur at recommended dosages.

How Supplied: Pediatric Formula (0.125%) in 15 mL drops. Mild Formula (0.25%) in 15 mL drops and spray. Regular Strength (0.5%) in 15 mL drops and spray. Extra Strength (1.0%) in 15 mL drops and spray.

Shown in Product Identification Section, page 430

NEO-SYNEPHRINE®
Maximum Strength 12 Hour oxymetazoline hydrochloride
Nasal Spray 0.05%

Description: *Adult Strength Nasal Spray* and *Nasal Spray Pump* contain: Oxymetazoline Hydrochloride 0.05%. Also contain: Benzalkonium Chloride and Phenylmercuric Acetate 0.002% as preservatives, Glycine, Purified Water, Sorbitol, may also contain Sodium Chloride.

Action: 12 HOUR Nasal Decongestant.

Indications: Provides temporary relief, for up to 12 HOURS, of nasal congestion due to colds, hay fever, sinusitis, or other upper respiratory allergies. NEO-SYNEPHRINE MAXIMUM STRENGTH 12-HOUR Nasal Spray and Pump contain oxymetazoline which provides the longest-lasting relief of nasal congestion available.

Warnings: Do not exceed recommended dosage because symptoms may occur such as burning, stinging, sneezing, or increase of nasal discharge. Do not use these products for more than 3 days. If symptoms persist, consult a doctor. The use of the dispenser by more than one person may spread infection.
Do not use this product if you have heart disease, high blood pressure, thyroid disease, diabetes, or difficulty in urination due to enlargement of the prostate gland unless directed by a doctor.
Keep this and all drugs out of the reach of children. In case of accidental ingestion, seek professional assistance or contact a poison control center immediately.

Directions: *Adult Strength Nasal Spray*—For adults and children 6 years of age and over (with adult supervision): 2 or 3 sprays in each nostril not more often than every 10 to 12 hours. Do not exceed 2 applications in any 24-hour period. Children under 6 years of age: consult a doctor. To administer, hold head upright, spray 2 or 3 times in each nostril twice daily—morning and evening. To spray, squeeze bottle quickly and firmly.
Nasal Spray Pump—For adults and children 6 years of age and over (with adult supervision): 2 or 3 sprays in each nostril not more often than every 10–12 hours. Do not exceed 2 applications in any 24 hour period. Children under 6 years of age: consult a doctor. Hold bottle with thumb at base and nozzle between first and second fingers. To administer, hold head upright and insert spray nozzle in nostril. Depress pump 2 or 3 times, all the way down, with a firm even stroke

Continued on next page

This product information was effective as of November 1, 1992. Current information may be obtained directly from Sterling Health, by writing to 90 Park Avenue, New York, NY 10016.

Sterling Health—Cont.

and sniff deeply. Repeat in other nostril. Do not tilt head backward while spraying.

How Supplied: *Nasal Spray Adult Strength* — plastic squeeze bottles of 15 ml (½ fl. oz.); *Nasal Spray Pump* —15 ml bottle (½ fl. oz.).

Shown in Product Identification Section, page 430

NTZ®
Long Acting
Oxymetazoline hydrochloride
Nasal Spray 0.05%
Nose Drops 0.05%

Description: Both the nasal spray and nose drops contain Oxymetazoline Hydrochloride 0.05%. Also contain: Benzalkonium Chloride and Phenylmercuric Acetate 0.002% as preservatives, Glycine, Purified Water, Sorbitol, and may also contain Sodium Chloride.

Actions: 12 Hour Nasal Decongestant.

Indications: Provides temporary relief, for up to 12 hours, of nasal congestion due to colds, hay fever, sinusitis, or allergies. Oxymetazoline hydrochloride provides the longest-lasting relief of nasal congestion available. It decongests nasal passages up to 12 hours, reduces swelling of nasal passages, and temporarily restores freer breathing through the nose.

Warnings: Not recommended for children under six. Do not exceed recommended dosage because symptoms may occur such as burning, stinging, sneezing, or increase of nasal discharge. Do not use these products for more than 3 days. If symptoms persist, consult a physician. The use of the dispenser by more than one person may spread infection. Do not use this product if you have heart disease, high blood pressure, thyroid disease, diabetes, or difficulty in urination due to enlargement of the prostate gland unless directed by a doctor. Keep these and all drugs out of the reach of children. In case of accidental ingestion seek professional assistance or contact a poison control center immediately.

Directions: Intranasally by spray and dropper. *Nasal Spray*—For adults and children 6 years of age and over: With head upright, spray 2 or 3 times in each nostril twice daily—morning and evening. To spray, squeeze bottle quickly and firmly. *Nose Drops* —For adults and children 6 years of age and over: 2 or 3 drops in each nostril twice daily—morning and evening.

How Supplied: *Nasal Spray*—plastic squeeze bottles of 15 ml (½ fl. oz.). *Nose Drops* —bottles of 15 ml (½ fl. oz.) with dropper.

Children's PANADOL®
Acetaminophen Chewable Tablets, Liquid, Drops

Description: Each Children's PANADOL Chewable Tablet contains 80 mg acetaminophen in a fruit-flavored sugar-free tablet. Children's PANADOL Acetaminophen Liquid is fruit-flavored, red in color, and is alcohol-free, sugar-free and aspirin-free. Each ½ teaspoonful contains 80 mg of acetaminophen. Infant's PANADOL Drops are fruit-flavored, red in color, and are alcohol-free, sugar-free and aspirin-free. Each 0.8 mL (one calibrated dropperful) contains 80 mg acetaminophen.

Indications: Acetaminophen, the active ingredient in Children's PANADOL, is the analgesic/antipyretic most widely recommended by pediatricians for fast, effective relief of children's fevers. It also relieves the aches and pains of colds and flu, earaches, headaches, teething, immunizations, tonsillectomy, and childhood illnesses.
Children's PANADOL Tablets, Liquid, and Drops are aspirin-free and contain no alcohol or sugar. The pleasant-tasting formulations are not likely to upset or irritate children's stomachs.

Usual Dosage: Dosing is based on single doses in the range of 10–15 mg/kg body weight. Doses may be repeated every four hours up to 4 or 5 times daily, but not to exceed 5 doses in 24 hours. To be administered to children under 2 years only on advice of a physician.
Children's PANADOL Chewable Tablets: 2–3 yr, 24–35 lb, 2 tablets; 4–5 yr, 36–47 lb, 3 tablets; 6–8 yr, 48–59 lb, 4 tablets; 9–10 yr, 60–71 lb, 5 tablets; 11 yr, 72–95 lb, 6 tablets. May be repeated every 4 hours, up to 5 times in a 24-hour period.
Children's PANADOL Liquid: 0–3 mo, 6–11 lb, ¼ teaspoonful; 4–11 mo, 12–17 lb, ½ teaspoonful; 12–23 mo, 18–23 lb, ¾ teaspoonful; 2–3 yr, 24–35 lb, 1 teaspoonful; 4–5 yr, 36–47 lb, 1½ teaspoonfuls; 6–8 yr, 48–59 lb, 2 teaspoonfuls; 9–10 yr, 60–71 lb, 2½ teaspoonfuls; 11 yr, 72–95 lb, 3 teaspoonfuls. May be repeated every 4 hours up to 5 times in a 24-hour period. May be administered alone or mixed with formula, milk, juice, cereal, etc.
Infant's PANADOL Drops: 0–3 mo, 6–11 lb, ½ dropperful (0.4 mL); 4–11 mo, 12–17 lb, 1 dropperful (0.8 mL); 12–23 mo, 18–23 lb, 1½ dropperfuls (1.2 mL); 2–3 yr, 24–35 lb, 2 dropperfuls (1.6 mL); 4–5 yr, 36–47 lb, 3 dropperfuls (2.4 mL); 6–8 yr, 48–59 lb, 4 dropperfuls (3.2 mL). May be repeated every 4 hours, up to 5 times in a 24-hour period. May be administered alone or mixed with formula, milk, juice, cereal, etc.

Warnings: Since Children's PANADOL Acetaminophen Chewable Tablets, Liquid, and Drops are available without a prescription as an analgesic/antipyretic, the following appears on the package labels: "**WARNINGS:** Do not give this product for pain for more than 5 days or for fever for more than 3 days unless directed by a doctor. If symptoms persist or new ones occur, consult a doctor. Keep this and all drugs out of the reach of children. In case of accidental overdose, immediate medical attention is essential even if you do not notice any sign or symptoms."
Tamper Resistant: Children's PANADOL Acetaminophen Chewable Tablets packaging provides tamper-resistant features on both the outer carton and bottle. The following copy appears on the end flaps of this carton—"Purchase only if carton end flaps are sealed." "Use only if seal under bottle cap with white G/W print is intact. The outer carton of the liquid and drops contain the following copy: "Purchase only if overwrap printed with red Panda bears is intact."
Children's PANADOL Liquid and Drops provide tamper-resistant features on the carton. The following copy appears on the carton—"Purchase only if Red Tear Tape and Plastic Overwrap are intact," and bottle—"Use only if Carton Overwrap and Red Tear Tape Are Intact."

Composition:
Tablets: Active Ingredient: Acetaminophen. Inactive Ingredients: FD&C Red No. 28, FD&C Red No. 40, flavor, Mannitol, Saccharin Sodium, Starch, Stearic Acid and other ingredients.
Liquid: Active Ingredient: Acetaminophen. Inactive Ingredients: Benzoic acid, FD&C Red No. 40, Flavor, Glycerin, Polyethylene Glycol, Potassium Sorbate, Propylene Glycol, Purified Water, Saccharin Sodium, Sorbitol solution. May also contain Sodium Chloride or Sodium Hydroxide.
Drops: Active Ingredient: Acetaminophen. Inactive Ingredients: Citric Acid, FD&C Red No. 40, Flavors, Glycerin, Parabens, Polyethylene Glycol, Propylene Glycol, Purified Water, Saccharin Sodium, Sodium Chloride, Sodium Citrate.

How Supplied: Chewable Tablets (colored pink and scored)—bottles of 30. Liquid (colored red)—bottles of 2 fl. oz. and 4 fl. oz. Drops (colored red)—bottles of ½ oz. (15 mL).
All packages listed above have child-resistant safety caps and tamper-resistant features.

Shown in Product Identification Section, page 431

Junior Strength PANADOL®
Acetaminophen Caplets

Description: Each Junior Strength PANADOL® Caplet contains 160 mg of acetaminophen.

Indications: Acetaminophen, the active ingredient in Junior Strength PANADOL®, is the analgesic/antipyretic most widely recommended by pediatricians for fast, effective relief of children's fevers. It also relieves the aches and pains of colds and flu, earaches, headaches, teething, immunizations, tonsillectomy,

menstrual discomfort, and childhood illness.
Junior Strength PANADOL® Caplets are aspirin-free, sugar-free.

Usual Dosage: Dosing is based on single doses in the range of 10–15 mg/kg body weight. Doses may be repeated every 4 hours up to 4 or 5 times daily, but not to exceed 5 doses in 24 hours. To be administered to children under 2 years only on the advice of a physician.
2–3 yr, 24–35 lb, 1 caplet; 4–5 yr, 36–47 lb, 1½ caplets; 6–8 yr, 48–59 lb, 2 caplets; 9–10 yr, 60–71 lb, 2½ caplets; 11 yr, 72–95 lb, 3 caplets. 12 yr and over, 96 lb and over, 4 caplets. Dosage may be repeated every 4 hours, up to 5 times in a 24-hour period.

Inactive Ingredients: Hydroxypropyl Methylcellulose, Potassium Sorbate, Povidone, Pregelatinized Starch, Starch, Stearic Acid, Talc, Triacetin.

Warnings: Do not give this product for pain for more than 5 days or for fever for more than 3 days unless directed by a doctor. If symptoms persist or new ones occur, consult a doctor. Keep this and all drugs out of the reach of children. In case of accidental overdose, immediate medical attention is essential even if you do not notice any sign or symptoms.

How Supplied: Swallowable caplets (white)—blister-pack of 30. Package has child-resistant and tamper-resistant features.

Shown in Product Identification Section, page 431

Maximum Strength PANADOL® Tablets and Caplets Acetaminophen

Active Ingredients: Each Maximum Strength PANADOL micro-thin coated tablet and caplet contains acetaminophen 500 mg.

Inactive Ingredients: Hydroxypropyl Methylcellulose, Potassium Sorbate, Povidone, Pregelatinized Starch, Starch, Stearic Acid, Talc, Triacetin.

Actions: PANADOL acetaminophen has been clinically proven as a fast, effective analgesic (pain reliever) and antipyretic (fever reducer). PANADOL acetaminophen is a nonaspirin product designed to provide relief without stomach upset. Its patented micro-thin coating makes each 500 mg tablet or caplet easy to swallow.

Indications: For the temporary relief from pain of headaches, colds or flu, sinusitis, backaches, muscle aches, and menstrual discomfort. Also to reduce fever and for temporary relief of minor arthritis pain and toothache.

Directions: *Adults:* Two tablets or caplets every 4 hours as needed. Do not exceed 8 tablets or caplets in 24 hours unless directed by a physician. *Children under 12:* Consult a doctor.

Warnings: Do not take this product for pain for more than 10 days or for fever for more than 3 days unless directed by a doctor. If pain or fever persists or gets worse, if new symptoms occur, or if redness or swelling is present, consult a doctor because these could be signs of a serious condition. Keep this and all drugs out of the reach of children. In case of accidental overdose, immediate medical attention is essential for adults as well as for children even if you do not notice any sign or symptoms. As with any drug, if you are pregnant or nursing a baby, seek the advice of a health professional before using this product.

How Supplied: Tablets and caplets (white, micro-thin coated, imprinted "PANADOL" and "500"). Tablets packaged in tamper-evident bottles of 30 and 60. Caplets packaged in tamper-evident bottles of 24.

Shown in Product Identification Section, page 431

PHILLIPS'® GELCAPS Laxative plus Stool Softener

Active Ingredients: A combination of phenolphthalein (90 mg) and docusate sodium (83 mg) per gelcap.

Inactive Ingredients: FD&C Blue # 2, gelatin, glycerin, PEG 400 and 3350, propylene glycol, sorbitol, and titanium dioxide.

Indications: For relief of occasional constipation (irregularity). This product generally produces bowel movement in 6 to 12 hours.

Action: Phenolphthalein is a stimulant laxative which increases the peristaltic activity of the intestine. Docusate sodium is a stool softener which allows easier passage of the stool.

Directions: Adults and children 12 and over take one (1) or two (2) gelcaps daily with a full glass (8 oz) of liquid, or as directed by a doctor. For children under 12, consult your doctor.

Warnings: Do not take any laxative if abdominal pain, nausea, vomiting, change in bowel habits persisting for over 2 weeks, rectal bleeding or kidney disease is present. Laxative products should not be used for a period longer than one week, unless directed by a physician. If there is a failure to have a bowel movement after use, discontinue and consult your doctor. If a skin rash appears do not take this or any other preparation which contains phenolphthalein. Keep this and all drugs out of the reach of children. In case of accidental overdose, seek professional assistance or contact a Poison Control Center immediately. As with any drug, if you are pregnant or nursing a baby, seek the advice of a health professional before using this product.

How Supplied: Blister packs of 30 and 60 gelcaps.

Shown in Product Identification Section, page 430

PHILLIPS'® MILK OF MAGNESIA Laxative/Antacid

Active Ingredients: A suspension of magnesium hydroxide in purified water meeting all USP specifications. Phillips' Milk of Magnesia contains 400 mg per teaspoon (5 mL) of magnesium hydroxide.

Inactive Ingredients: Original—Purified water. Mint—Carboxymethylcellulose Sodium, Citric Acid, Flavor, Glycerin, Microcrystalline Cellulose, Propylene Glycol, Purified water, Sorbitol, Sucrose, Xanthan Gum.
Cherry—(same as mint), D&C Red #28.

Indications: For relief of occasional constipation (irregularity), relief of acid indigestion, sour stomach and heartburn. The laxative dosage generally produces bowel movement in ½ to 6 hours.

Action at Laxative Dosage: Phillips' Milk of Magnesia is a mild saline laxative which acts by drawing water into the gut, increasing intraluminal pressure, and increasing intestinal motility.

Action at Antacid Dosage: Phillips' Milk of Magnesia is an effective acid neutralizer.

Directions: As a laxative, adults and children 12 years and older, 2–4 tbsp; children 6–11 years, 1–2 tbsp; children 2–5 years, 1–3 tsp followed by a full glass (8 oz) of liquid. Children under 2, consult a doctor.
As an antacid, adults & children 12 & older, 1–3 tsp with a little water, up to four times a day, or as directed by your doctor.

Drug Interaction Precaution: Antacids may interact with certain prescription drugs. If you are taking a prescription drug do not take this product without checking with your doctor.

Laxative Warnings: Do not take any laxative if abdominal pain, nausea, vomiting, change in bowel habits persisting for over 2 weeks, rectal bleeding, or kidney disease is present. Laxative products should not be used for a period longer than 1 week, unless directed by a doctor. If there is a failure to have a bowel movement after use, discontinue and consult your doctor.

Antacid Warnings: Do not take more than the maximum recommended daily dosage in a 24-hour period (see Directions), or use the maximum dosage of this product for more than two weeks, or use this product if you have kidney disease, except under the advice and supervision of a doctor. May have laxative effect.

Continued on next page

This product information was effective as of November 1, 1992. Current information may be obtained directly from Sterling Health, by writing to 90 Park Avenue, New York, NY 10016.

Sterling Health—Cont.

General Warnings: As with any drug, if you are pregnant or nursing a baby, seek the advice of a health professional before using this product. Keep this and all drugs out of reach of children. In case of accidental overdose, seek professional assistance or contact a poison control center immediately.

How Supplied: Phillips' Milk of Magnesia is available in original and mint flavor in 4, 12 and 26 fl oz bottles. Cherry flavor available in 12 and 26 fl oz bottles. Also available in tablet form and concentrated liquid form.

Shown in Product Identification Section, page 430

Concentrated PHILLIPS'® MILK OF MAGNESIA
Laxative/Antacid

Active Ingredients: A suspension of magnesium hydroxide in purified water meeting all USP specifications. Concentrated Phillips' Milk of Magnesia contains 800 mg per teaspoon (5 ml) of magnesium hydroxide.

Inactive Ingredients: Carboxymethylcellulose Sodium, Citric Acid, D&C Red #28 or FD&C Yellow #6, Flavor, Glycerin, Microcrystalline Cellulose, Propylene Glycol, Purified Water, Sorbitol, Sucrose, Xanthan Gum.

Indications: For relief of occasional constipation (irregularity), relief of acid indigestion, sour stomach and heartburn. The laxative dosage generally produces bowel movement in ½ to 6 hours.

Action at Laxative Dosage: Concentrated Phillips' Milk of Magnesia is a mild saline laxative which acts by drawing water into the gut, increasing intraluminal pressure, and increasing intestinal motility.

Action at Antacid Dosage: Concentrated Phillips' Milk of Magnesia is an effective acid neutralizer.

Directions: As a laxative, adults and children 12 years and older, 1–2 tbsp.; children 6–11 years, ½–1 tbsp.; children 2–5 years, ½ to 1½ tsp. followed by a full glass (8 oz.) of liquid. Children under 2, consult a doctor.
As an antacid, adults and children 12 years and older, ½ to 1½ tsp. with a little water, up to four times a day or as directed by a doctor.

Laxative Warnings: Do not take any laxative if abdominal pain, nausea, vomiting, change in bowel habits (that persists for over two weeks), rectal bleeding, or kidney disease are present. Laxative products should not be used for a period longer than 1 week, unless directed by a doctor. If there is a failure to have a bowel movement after use, discontinue and consult a doctor.

Antacid Warnings: Do not take more than the maximum recommended daily dosage in a 24 hour period (see directions), or use the maximum dosage of this product for more than two weeks, or use this product if you have kidney disease, except under the advice and supervision of a doctor. May have laxative effect.

General Warnings: As with any drug, if you are pregnant or nursing a baby, seek the advice of a health professional before using this product. Keep this and all drugs out of reach of children. In case of accidental overdose seek professional assistance or contact a poison control center immediately.

Drug Interaction: Antacids may interact with certain prescription drugs. If you are presently taking a prescription drug, do not take this product without checking with your doctor.

How Supplied: Concentrated Phillips' Milk of Magnesia is available in strawberry creme and orange vanilla creme flavors in bottles of 8 fl. oz.

Shown in Product Identification Section, page 430

PHILLIPS'® CHEWABLE TABLETS
Antacid/Laxative

Active Ingredients: Each Tablet contains 311 mg of magnesium hydroxide.

Inactive Ingredients: Flavor, starch, sucrose.

Indications: For relief of acid indigestion, sour stomach, heartburn and occasional constipation (irregularity). The laxative dosage generally produces bowel movement in ½ to 6 hours.

Action at Antacid Dosage: Phillips' Chewable Tablets are effective acid neutralizers.

Action at Laxative Dosage: Phillips' Chewable Tablets offer the same mild saline laxative ingredient as liquid Phillips' Milk of Magnesia in a convenient, chewable tablet form. It acts by drawing water into the gut, increasing intraluminal pressure, and increasing intestinal motility.

Directions:
As an Antacid —Adults chew thoroughly 2 to 4 tablets up to 4 times a day. Children 7 to 14 years, chew thoroughly 1 tablet up to 4 times a day or as directed by a doctor.
As a Laxative —Adults and children 12 years of age and older, 6 to 8 tablets. Children 6 to 11 years, 3 to 4 tablets; children 2 to 5 years, 1 to 2 tablets. Tablet should be chewed thoroughly, preferably before bedtime and follow with a full glass (8 oz) of liquid. Children under 2, consult a doctor.

Antacid Warnings: Do not take more than the maximum recommended daily dosage in a 24-hour period (see Directions), or use the maximum dosage of this product for more than two weeks, or use this product if you have kidney disease, except under the advice and supervision of a physician. May have laxative effect.

Laxative Warnings: Do not take any laxative if abdominal pain, nausea, vomiting, change in bowel habits (that persists for over 2 weeks), rectal bleeding, or kidney disease are present. Laxative products should not be used for a period longer than 1 week, unless directed by a doctor. If there is a failure to have a bowel movement after use, discontinue and consult your doctor.

General Warnings: As with any drug, if you are pregnant or nursing a baby, seek the advice of a health professional before using this product. Keep this and *all* drugs out of reach of children. In case of accidental overdose, seek professional assistance or contact a poison control center immediately.

How Supplied: Phillips' Chewable Tablets are available in a mint flavored chewable tablet in bottles of 100 and 200. Also available in liquid form.

Shown in Product Identification Section, page 431

---

pHisoDerm®
[fi-zo-derm]
Skin Cleanser and Conditioner

Description: pHisoDerm, a nonsoap emollient skin cleanser, is a unique liquid emulsion containing sodium octoxynol-2 ethane sulfonate solution, water, petrolatum, octoxynol-3, mineral oil (with lanolin alcohol and oleyl alcohol), cocamide MEA, imidazolidinyl urea, sodium benzoate, tetrasodium EDTA, and methylcellulose. Adjusted to normal skin pH with hydrochloric acid. Contains no hexachlorophene. pHisoDerm contains no soap, perfumes, or irritating alkali. Its pH value, unlike that of soap, lies within the pH range of normal skin. pHisoDerm Lightly Scented contains fragrance.

Actions: pHisoDerm is well tolerated and can be used frequently by those persons whose skin may be irritated by the use of soap or other alkaline cleansers, or by those who are sensitive to the fatty acids contained in soap. pHisoDerm contains an effective detergent for removing soil and acts as an active emulsifier of all types of oil—animal, vegetable, and mineral.
pHisoDerm produces suds when used with any kind of water—hard or soft, hot or cold (even cold seawater)—at any temperature and under acid, alkaline, or neutral conditions.
pHisoDerm deposits a fine film of lanolin components and petrolatum on the skin during the washing process and, thereby, helps protect against the dryness that soap can cause.

Indications: A sudsing emollient cleanser for use on skin of infants, children, and adults.
Useful for removal of ointments and cosmetics from the skin.

Directions: For external use only.
HANDS. Squeeze a few drops of pHisoDerm into the palm, add a little water, and work up a lather. Rinse thoroughly.
FACE. After washing your hands, squeeze a small amount of pHisoDerm into the palm or onto a small sponge or washcloth, and work up a lather by adding a little water. Massage the suds onto the face for approximately one minute. Rinse thoroughly. Avoid getting suds into the eyes.
BATHING. First wet the body. Work a small amount of pHisoDerm into a lather with hands or a soft wet sponge, gradually adding small amounts of water to make more lather. Rinse thoroughly.

Caution: pHisoDerm suds that get into the eyes accidentally during washing should be rinsed out promptly with a sufficient amount of water.
pHisoDerm is intended for external use only. pHisoDerm should not be poured into measuring cups, medicine bottles, or similar containers since it may be mistaken for baby formula or medications. If swallowed, pHisoDerm may cause gastrointestinal irritation.
pHisoDerm should not be used on persons with sensitivity to any of its components.

How Supplied: pHisoDerm is supplied in three formulations: Regular Formula Unscented, Regular Formula Lightly Scented and Oily Skin Formula Unscented. It is packaged in sanitary squeeze bottles of 5 and 16 ounces. The Regular Unscented and Lightly Scented Formulas are also supplied in squeeze bottles of 9 ounces.

Shown in Product Identification Section, page 431

---

pHisoDerm®
Cleansing Bar

Description: pHisoDerm Cleansing Bar, is a unique cleansing bar containing sodium tallowate, coconut oil, water, glycerin, petrolatum, lanolin, sodium chloride, BHT, trisodium HEDTA, and titanium dioxide.

Actions: pHisoDerm Cleansing Bar is formulated to clean thoroughly, removing dirt and oil. Special emollients leave skin feeling soft and smooth, not tight and dry. pHisoDerm Cleansing Bar contains no detergents or harsh ingredients which could irritate delicate skin.

Administration: Use every time you wash. First wet area to be washed. Using hands, sponge or washcloth, mix with water and work up a creamy lather. Massage the suds onto the area to be washed for approximately one minute. Rinse thoroughly. Avoid getting suds into the eyes.

Precautions: pHisoDerm Cleansing Bar suds that get into the eyes accidentally during washing should be rinsed out promptly with a sufficient amount of water. pHisoDerm Cleansing Bar is intended for external use only. It should not be used on persons with sensitivity to any of its components.

How Supplied: pHisoDerm Cleansing Bar is supplied in an Unscented and Lightly Scented formula. It is packaged in specially coated cardboard cartons containing a 3.3 oz. bar.

Shown in Product Identification Section, page 431

---

pHisoDerm® FOR BABY
[fi 'zo-derm]
Skin Cleanser

Description: pHisoDerm FOR BABY, a nonsoap emollient skin cleanser, is a unique liquid emulsion containing sodium octoxynol-2 ethane sulfonate solution, water, petrolatum, octoxynol-3, mineral oil (with lanolin alcohol and oleyl alcohol), cocamide MEA, fragrance, imidazolidinyl urea, sodium benzoate, tetrasodium EDTA, and methylcellulose. Adjusted to normal skin pH with hydrochloric acid. Contains no hexachlorophene or irritating alkali. Its pH value, unlike that of soap, lies within the pH range of normal skin.

Actions: pHisoDerm FOR BABY gently cleans babies' delicate skin without irritating. Petrolatum and lanolin leave skin soft and smooth and protect against dryness.
pHisoDerm FOR BABY rinses easily without leaving a soapy film. The powder fragrance leaves skin smelling fresh and clean.

Precautions: pHisoDerm FOR BABY suds that get into babies' eyes accidentally during washing should be rinsed out promptly with a sufficient amount of water.
pHisoDerm FOR BABY is intended for external use only. It should not be poured into measuring cups, medicine bottles, or similar containers since it may be mistaken for baby formula or medications. If swallowed, pHisoDerm FOR BABY may cause gastrointestinal irritation.
pHisoDerm FOR BABY should not be used on babies with sensitivity to any of its components.

Administration: First wet the baby's body. Work a small amount of pHisoDerm FOR BABY into a lather with hands or a soft wet sponge, gradually adding small amounts of water to make more lather. Spread the lather over all parts of the baby's body, including the head. Avoid getting suds into the baby's eyes. Wash the diaper area last. Be sure to carefully cleanse all folds and creases. Rinse thoroughly. Pat the baby dry with a soft towel.

How Supplied: pHisoDerm FOR BABY is packaged in soft plastic, sanitary, squeeze bottles of 5 and 9 ounces and can be opened and closed with one hand.

Shown in Product Identification Section, page 431

---

pHisoPUFF®
[fi-zo-puf]
Nonmedicated Cleansing Sponge

Description: pHisoPUFF is a nonmedicated cleansing sponge with a special dual layer construction combining a white polyester fiber side and a green sponge side.

Actions: pHisoPUFF cleanses two ways: (1) white fiber side for extra thorough cleansing to gently remove the top layer of dead skin cells, free dirt, debris, and oil trapped in this layer and reveal new, fresh skin cells and (2) green sponge side works to cleanse and rinse skin clean. Using this side will help apply your cleanser or soap more evenly. Also good for removing eye makeup.

Precautions: Do not use pHisoPUFF fiber side on skin that is irritated, sunburned, windburned, damaged, broken, or infected. Do not use on skin which is prone to rashes or itching.

Administration: For the green sponge side: Wet pHisoPUFF with warm water, apply pHisoDerm® or another skin cleanser of your choice, and develop a lather. Glide sponge over your face up and down, back and forth, or in a circle; whatever is the easiest for you. Rinse face and dry.
For the white fiber side: Wet pHisoPUFF with warm water, apply pHisoDerm or another skin cleanser of your choice, and develop a lather. Try pHisoPUFF on the back of your hand before using it on your face. Experiment by changing the pressure and speed with which you move it. Now move pHisoPUFF gently and slowly over your face. Use no more than a few seconds on each area. You can move it in any direction, whichever comes natural to you. Rinse face and dry. As you use this fiber side more often, usage and pressure may be increased to best fit your skin sensitivity. Always rinse your pHisoPUFF thoroughly each time you use it. Hold under running water, let it drain, then give it a few quick shakes.

How Supplied: Box of 1 pHisoPUFF.

Shown in Product Identification Section, page 431

Continued on next page

This product information was effective as of November 1, 1992. Current information may be obtained directly from Sterling Health, by writing to 90 Park Avenue, New York, NY 10016.

Sterling Health—Cont.

STRI-DEX® DUAL TEXTURED PADS
Regular Strength
STRI-DEX® DUAL TEXTURED PADS
Maximum Strength
STRI-DEX® DUAL TEXTURED PADS
Sensitive Skin
STRI-DEX® SUPER SCRUB PADS
Oil Fighting Formula
STRI-DEX® SINGLE TEXTURED PADS
Maximum Strength
STRI-DEX® ANTIBACTERIAL CLEANSING BAR

Active Ingredients:
Stri-Dex® Regular Strength: Salicylic Acid 0.5%.
Stri-Dex® Maximum Strength: Salicylic Acid 2.0%.
Stri-Dex® Sensitive Skin: Salicylic Acid 0.5%.
Stri-Dex® Super Scrub: Salicylic Acid 2.0%.
Stri-Dex® Single Textured Maximum Strength: Salicylic Acid 2.0%.
Stri-Dex® Antibacterial Cleansing Bar: Triclosan 1%.

Inactive Ingredients:
Stri-Dex® Regular Strength: Purified Water, SD Alcohol 28%, Sodium Xylenesulfonate, Sodium Dodecylbenzenesulfonate, Citric Acid, Sodium Carbonate, Fragrance, Menthol, Simethicone Emulsion.
Stri-Dex® Maximum Strength: Purified Water, SD Alcohol 44%, Ammonium Xylenesulfonate, Sodium Dodecylbenzenesulfonate, Citric Acid, Sodium Carbonate, Fragrance, Menthol, Simethicone Emulsion.
Stri-Dex® Sensitive Skin: Purified Water, SD Alcohol 28%, Aloe Vera Gel, Sodium Xylenesulfonate, Sodium Dodecylbenzenesulfonate, Citric Acid, Sodium Carbonate, Fragrance, Menthol, Simethicone Emulsion.
Stri-Dex® Super Scrub: SD Alcohol 54%, Purified Water, Ammonium Xylenesulfonate, Sodium Dodecylbenzenesulfonate, Citric Acid, Sodium Lauroyl Sarcosinate, Sodium Carbonate, Menthol, Fragrance, Simethicone Emulsion.
Stri-Dex® Single Textured: Purified Water, SD Alcohol 44%, Ammonium Xylenesulfonate, Sodium Dodecylbenzenesulfonate, Citric Acid, Sodium Carbonate, Fragrance, Simethicone Emulsion.
Stri-Dex® Antibacterial Cleansing Bar: Sodium Tallowate, Sodium Cocoate and/or Sodium Palm Kernelate, Water, Glycerin, Sucrose, Potassium Cyclocarboxypropyloleate, Bentonite, Cetyl Acetate, Acetylated Lanolin Alcohol, Pentasodium Pentetate, Tetrasodium Etidronate, D&C Yellow #10, D&C Orange #4.

Indications: Stri-Dex® Pads for the treatment of acne. Reduces the number of acne pimples and blackheads, and allows the skin to heal. Helps prevent new acne pimples from forming.
Stri-Dex® Antibacterial Cleansing Bar: Antibacterial Soap.

Directions:
Stri-Dex® Pads. Cleanse the skin thoroughly before using all varieties of Stri-Dex medicated pads. Use the pad to open pores and loosen the oil and dirt that can clog them. Then wipe away oil and dirt and leave behind a tough pimple fighting medicine that will treat pimples and help prevent new ones from forming. Use the pad to wipe the entire affected area one to three times daily. Because excessive drying of the skin may occur, start with one application daily, then gradually increase to two or three times daily if needed or as directed by a doctor.
Stri-Dex Bar. Use Stri-Dex® Antibacterial Cleansing Bar in place of ordinary soap. For best results use three times daily. Work up an abundant lather with warm water and massage into the skin. Rinse thoroughly and pat dry with a towel. Use Stri-Dex® Antibacterial Cleansing Bar for facial cleansing as well as in the bath.
After deep cleaning the skin with Stri-Dex® Antibacterial Cleansing Bar, continue on acne treatment program with Stri-Dex® Medicated Acne Pads.

Warnings: Stri-Dex Pads : FOR EXTERNAL USE ONLY: Using other topical acne medications at the same time or immediately following use of this product may increase dryness or irritation of the skin. If this occurs, only one medication should be used unless directed by a doctor. Persons with very sensitive skin or known allergy to salicylic acid should not use this medication. If irritation or excessive dryness and/or peeling occurs, reduce frequency of use or dosage. If excessive itching, dryness, redness, or swelling occurs, discontinue use. If these symptoms persist, consult a physician promptly. Keep away from eyes, lips, and other mucous membranes. Keep this and all drugs out of reach of children. In the case of accidental ingestion, seek professional assistance or contact a Poison control center immediately.
Stri-Dex Antibacterial Cleansing Bar: Do not use this product on infants under 6 months of age. For external use only. Do not get in eyes.

How Supplied:
Stri-Dex Regular Strength is available in packages of 32 and 50 pads.
Stri-Dex Maximum Strength is available in packages of 32 and 50 pads.
Stri-Dex Sensitive Skin is available in a package of 32 pads.
Stri-Dex Super Scrub is available in a package of 32 pads.
Stri-Dex Single Textured is available in a package of 55 pads.
Stri-Dex Antibacterial Cleansing Bar is available in a 3.5 ounce package.

Shown in Product Identification Section, page 431

VANQUISH® Analgesic Caplets

Active Ingredients: Each caplet contains aspirin 227 mg, acetaminophen 194 mg, caffeine 33 mg, dried aluminum hydroxide gel 25 mg, magnesium hydroxide 50 mg.

Inactive Ingredients: Acacia, colloidal silicon dioxide, hydrogenated vegetable oil, microcrystalline cellulose, powdered cellulose, sodium lauryl sulfate, starch, talc.

Indications: A buffered analgesic, antipyretic for relief of headache; muscular aches and pains; neuralgia and neuritic pain; toothache; pain following dental procedures; for painful discomforts and fever of colds and flu; functional menstrual pain, headache and pain due to cramps; temporary relief from minor pains of arthritis, rheumatism, bursitis, lumbago, sciatica.

Directions: Adults and children 12 years and over: Two caplets with water. May be repeated every four hours if necessary up to 12 caplets per day. Larger or more frequent doses may be prescribed by doctor if necessary.

Warnings: Children and teenagers should not use this medicine for chicken pox or flu symptoms before a doctor is consulted about Reye syndrome, a rare but serious illness reported to be associated with aspirin. Do not take for pain for more than 10 days or for fever for more than 3 days unless directed by a doctor. If pain or fever persists or gets worse, if new symptoms occur, or if redness or swelling is present consult a doctor immediately. Do not take this product if you are allergic to aspirin, have asthma, stomach problems that persist or recur, gastric ulcers or bleeding problems unless directed by a doctor. If ringing in the ears or loss of hearing occurs, consult a doctor before taking any more of this product. Keep this and all drugs out of the reach of children. In case of accidental overdose, immediate medical attention is essential for adults as well as for children even if you do not notice any sign or symptoms. As with any drug, if you are pregnant or nursing a baby, seek the advice of a health professional before using this product. **IT IS ESPECIALLY IMPORTANT NOT TO USE ASPIRIN DURING THE LAST 3 MONTHS OF PREGNANCY UNLESS SPECIFICALLY DIRECTED TO DO SO BY A DOCTOR BECAUSE IT MAY CAUSE PROBLEMS IN THE UNBORN CHILD OR COMPLICATIONS DURING DELIVERY.**

Drug Interaction Precaution: Do not take this product if you are taking a prescription drug for anticoagulation (thinning of the blood), diabetes, gout, or arthritis unless directed by a doctor.

How Supplied:
White, capsule-shaped caplets in bottles of 30, 60 and 100 caplets.

Shown in Product Identification Section, page 431

WinGel®
[win 'jel]
Liquid Antacid

Active Ingredients: Each teaspoon (5 mL) of liquid contains a specially processed, short polymer, hexitol-stabilized aluminum-magnesium hydroxide equivalent to 180 mg of aluminum hydroxide and 160 mg of magnesium hydroxide.

Inactive ingredients: benzoic acid, flavor, methylcellulose, purified water, red ferric oxide, saccharin sodium, sodium hypochlorite solution, sorbitol solution.

Action: Antacid.

Indications: An antacid for the relief of acid indigestion, heartburn, and sour stomach. Nonconstipating. For the symptomatic relief of hyperacidity associated with the diagnosis of peptic ulcer, gastritis, peptic esophagitis, gastric hyperacidity, and hiatal hernia.

Directions: *Adults and children over 6*—1 to 2 teaspoonfuls up to four times daily, or as directed by a physician.

Warnings: Do not take more than eight teaspoonfuls in a 24-hour period or use the maximum dosage of the product for more than 2 weeks, except under the advice and supervision of a physician.
Keep this and all drugs out of the reach of children. In case of accidental overdose, seek professional assistance or contact a poison control center immediately.

Drug Interaction Precautions: Antacids may react with certain prescription drugs. Do not take this product if you are presently taking a prescription antibiotic drug containing any form of tetracycline. If the patient is presently taking a prescription drug, this product should not be taken without checking with the physician.
Acid Neutralization: The acid neutralization capacity of WinGel liquid is not less than 10 mEq/5 ml.

How Supplied: WinGel liquid is supplied in a 12 fl oz bottle.

Syntex Laboratories, Inc

3401 HILLVIEW AVENUE
PALO ALTO, CA 94304

CARMOL® 10
10% urea lotion
for total body
dry skin care.

Active Ingredient: Urea 10% in a scented lotion of purified water, carbomer 940, cetyl alcohol, isopropyl palmitate, PEG-8 dioleate, PEG-8 distearate, propylene glycol, propylene glycol dipelargonate, stearic acid, sodium laureth sulfate, trolamine, and xanthan gum.

Indications: For total body dry skin care.

Actions: Keratolytic CARMOL 10 is non-occlusive, contains no mineral oil or petrolatum. CARMOL 10 is hypoallergenic; contains no lanolin, parabens or other preservatives.

Precautions: For external use only. Discontinue use if irritation occurs. Keep out of the reach of children. In case of accidental ingestion, seek professional assistance or contact a poison control center immediately.

Dosage and Administration: Rub in gently on hands, face or body. Repeat as necessary.

How Supplied: 6 fl. oz. bottle.

Thompson Medical Company, Inc.

222 LAKEVIEW AVENUE
WEST PALM BEACH
FLORIDA 33401

ASPERCREME®
[ăs-per-crēme]
External Analgesic Rub

Description: ASPERCREME® is available as an odor-free creme and lotion for use as a topical massage rub that temporarily relieves minor muscle aches and pains without stomach upset.
Aspercreme does not contain aspirin.

Active Ingredients: Salycin® 10% (Thompson Medical's brand of Trolamine Salicylate).

Other Ingredients: Creme: Cetyl Alcohol, Glycerin, Methylparaben, Mineral Oil, Potassium Phosphate, Propylparaben, Stearic Acid, Triethanolamine, Water. Lotion: Cetyl Alcohol, Fragrance, Glyceryl Stearate, Isopropyl Palmitate, Lanolin, Methylparaben, Potassium Phosphate, Propylene Glycol, Propylparaben, Sodium Lauryl Sulfate, Stearic Acid, Water.

Actions: External analgesic rub.

Indications: Analgesic rub for temporary relief of minor aches and pains of muscles associated with simple strains and sprains. **Aspercreme contains no aspirin.**

Warnings: Use only as directed. If prone to allergic reaction from aspirin or salicylate, consult your doctor before using. If redness is present or condition worsens, or if pain persists for more than 7 days or clears up and occurs again within a few days, discontinue use and consult a doctor. Do not use on children under 10 years of age. Do not apply if skin is irritated or if irritation develops. As with any drug, if you are pregnant or nursing a baby, seek the advice of a health professional before using this product. For external use only. Avoid contact with eyes. Keep this and all medicines out of the reach of children. In case of accidental ingestion seek professional assistance or contact a Poison Control Center immediately.

Dosage and Administration: Apply generously directly to affected area. Massage into painful area until thoroughly absorbed into skin, repeat as necessary, especially before retiring but not more than 4 times daily.

How to Store: Store at controlled room temperature 59°–86°F (15°–30°C).

How Supplied: Creme: 1¼ oz., 3 oz. and 5 oz. tubes. Lotion: 6 oz. bottle.

CORTIZONE–5®
Cream, Ointment, and Wipes
CORTIZONE FOR KIDS™ Cream
Anti-itch
(0.5% hydrocortisone)

Description: CORTIZONE-5® cream, ointment, and wipes are topical anti-itch preparations.

Active Ingredient: Hydrocortisone 0.5%.

Other Ingredients: Cream: Aluminum Sulfate, Calcium Acetate, Glycerin, Light Mineral Oil, Methylparaben, Potato Dextrin, Purified Water, Sodium Lauryl Sulfate, White Petroleum. May Also Contain: Cetearyl Alcohol, Propylparaben, Sodium C_{12-15} Alcohols Sulfate, Synthetic Beeswax, White Wax. CORTIZONE for Kids additionally contains Aloe Vera gel.
Ointment: White Petrolatum.
Wipes: Methylparaben, Octoxynol 9, Propylene Glycol, Propylparaben, Purified Water.

Indications: CORTIZONE-5® is recommended for the temporary relief of itching associated with minor skin irritations, inflammations and rashes due to: eczema, insect bites, poison ivy, oak, sumac, soaps, detergents, cosmetics, jewelry, seborrheic dermatitis, psoriasis, external anal and genital itching. Other uses of this product should be only under the advice and supervision of a physician.

Warnings: For external use only. Avoid contact with the eyes. If condition worsens, or if symptoms persist for more than 7 days or clear up and occur again within a few days, stop use of this product and do not begin use of any hydrocortisone product unless you have consulted a physician. Do not use in genital area if you have a vaginal discharge. Consult a physician. Do not use for the treatment of diaper rash. Consult a physician.
Warnings For External Anal Itching Users: Do not exceed the recommended daily dosage unless directed by a physician. In case of bleeding, consult a physician promptly. Do not put this product into the rectum by using fingers or any mechanical device or applicator.
KEEP THIS AND ALL MEDICINES OUT OF THE REACH OF CHILDREN. In case of accidental ingestion, seek pro-

Continued on next page

Thompson Medical—Cont.

fessional assistance or contact a poison control center immediately.

Dosage and Administration: Adults and children 2 years of age and older: Apply to affected area not more than 3 to 4 times daily. Children under 2 years of age: Do not use, consult a physician. Directions For External Anal Itching Users: Adults: When practical, cleanse the affected area with mild soap and warm water and rinse thoroughly. Gently dry by patting or blotting with toilet tissue or a soft cloth before application of this product. Children under 12 years of age: Consult a physician.

How to Store: Store at controlled room temperature 15°–30°C (59°–86°F).

How Supplied: CORTIZONE-5 cream: 1 oz. and 2 oz. tubes. CORTIZONE for Kids™ cream: ½ oz. and 1 oz. tubes. CORTIZONE-5 ointment: 1 oz. tube. CORTIZONE-5 wipes: carton containing 14 individual packets.

CORTIZONE–10™
Cream and Ointment

CORTIZONE-10™ EXTERNAL ANAL ITCH RELIEF Cream

CORTIZONE-10™ SCALP ITCH FORMULA™ Liquid
Anti-itch
(1.0% hydrocortisone)

Description: CORTIZONE-10™ cream, ointment and liquid are topical anti-itch preparations. Maximum Strength available without a prescription.

Active Ingredient: Hydrocortisone 1.0%.

Other Ingredients: Cream: Aluminum Sulfate, Calcium Acetate, Cetearyl Alcohol, Glycerin, Light Mineral Oil, Methylparaben, Potato Dextrin, Sodium Lauryl Sulfate, Water, White Petroleum, White Wax. **May Also Contain:** Aloe Vera Gel, Sodium C12–15 Alcohols Sulfate, Propylparaben.
Ointment: White Petrolatum.
Liquid: Benzyl Alcohol, Propylene Glycol, Purified Water, SD Alcohol 40-2 (60% v/v)

Indications: Cortizone-10™ is recommended for the temporary relief of itching associated with minor skin irritations, inflammation and rashes due to: eczema, insect bites, poison ivy, oak, sumac, soaps, detergents, cosmetics, jewelry, seborrheic dermatitis, psoriasis, external anal and genital itching. Other uses of this product should be only under the advice and supervision of a physician.

Warnings: For external use only. Avoid contact with the eyes. If condition worsens, or if symptoms persist for more than 7 days or clear up and occur again within a few days, stop use of this product and do not begin use of any hydrocortisone product unless you have consulted a physician. Do not use in genital area if you have a vaginal discharge. Consult a physician. Do not use for the treatment of diaper rash. Consult a physician. **Warnings For External Anal Itching Users:** Do not exceed the recommended daily dosage unless directed by a physician. In case of bleeding, consult a physician promptly. Do not put this product into the rectum by using fingers or any mechanical device or applicator.
KEEP THIS AND ALL MEDICINES OUT OF THE REACH OF CHILDREN. In case of accidental ingestion, seek professional assistance or contact a poison control center immediately.

Dosage and Administration: Adults and children 2 years of age and older: Apply to affected area not more than 3 to 4 times daily. Children under 2 years of age: Do not use, consult a physician.

Directions For External Anal Itching Users: Adults: When practical, cleanse the affected area with mild soap and warm water and rinse thoroughly. Gently dry by patting or blotting with toilet tissue or a soft cloth before application of this product. Children under 12 years of age: consult a physician.

How to Store: Store at controlled room temperature 15°–30°C (59°–86°F).

How Supplied: CORTIZONE-10 cream: 1 oz. and 2 oz. tubes. CORTIZONE-10 ointment: 1 oz. tube. CORTIZONE-10™ External Anal Itch Relief cream: 1 oz. tube. CORTIZONE-10™ Scalp Itch Formula™ liquid: 1.5 fl. oz.

Shown in Product Identification Section, page 431

DEXATRIM® Capsules, Caplets, and Tablets
[*dĕx-a-trĭm*]
Prolonged action anorectic for weight control

DEXATRIM® Maximum Strength Plus Vitamin C/Caffeine-Free Capsules and Caffeine-Free Capsules
phenylpropanolamine HCl 75mg (time release)
(180 mg Vitamin C, immediate release, added for nutritional supplementation)

DEXATRIM® Maximum Strength Plus Vitamin C/Caffeine-Free Caplets and Caffeine-Free Caplets
phenylpropanolamine HCl 75mg (time release)
(180 mg Vitamin C, immediate release, added for nutritional supplementation)

DEXATRIM® Maximum Strength Extended Duration Time Tablets
phenylpropanolamine HCl 75mg (time release)

Indication: DEXATRIM® is an aid for effective appetite control to assist weight reduction. It is available in a time release dosage form.

Caution: READ BEFORE USING. FOR ADULT USE ONLY. Do not give this product to children under 12 years of age. Persons between the ages of 12 and 18 or over 60 are advised to consult their physician or pharmacist before using this or any drug. If nervousness, dizziness, headaches, rapid pulse, palpitations, sleeplessness, or other symptoms occur, stop using and consult your physician.

Warning: DO NOT EXCEED RECOMMENDED DOSAGE. Taking more of this or any drug than is recommended can cause untoward health complications. It is sensible to check your blood pressure regularly. Do not use if you have high blood pressure, diabetes, heart, thyroid, kidney, or other disease or are being treated for high blood pressure or depression except under the advice and supervision of a physician. If you are taking a cough/cold allergy medication containing any form of phenylpropanolamine, do not take this product. As with any drug if you are pregnant or nursing a baby, seek the advice of a health professional before using this product. Do not use continuously for more than 3 months. When you have reached your desired weight or are able to control your appetite by yourself, use DEXATRIM only as needed.

Drug Interaction Precaution: Do not take if you are presently taking another medication containing phenylpropanolamine, or any type of nasal decongestant, or a prescription drug for high blood pressure or depression, or any other type of prescription medication except under the advice and supervision of a physician.
KEEP THIS AND ALL MEDICATION OUT OF THE REACH OF CHILDREN. In case of accidental overdose seek professional assistance or contact a Poison Control Center immediately.

Dosage and Administration:
Capsule Dosage Forms: DEXATRIM® Maximum Strength Plus Vitamin C, DEXATRIM® Maximum Strength/Caffeine-Free.
Caplet Dosage Forms: DEXATRIM® Maximum Strength Plus Vitamin C, DEXATRIM® Maximum Strength/Caffeine-Free.
Tablet Dosage Form: DEXATRIM® Maximum Strength Extended Duration Time Tablets.
Administration: One capsule or caplet at midmorning (10 am) with a full glass of water.

How Supplied: All Dexatrim products are supplied in tamper-evident blister packages. Do not use if individual seals are broken.
DEXATRIM® Maximum Strength Plus Vitamin C/Caffeine-Free Capsules: Packages of 10, 20 and 40 with 1250 calorie DEXATRIM Diet Plan.
DEXATRIM® Maximum Strength Plus Vitamin C/Caffeine-Free Caplets: Packages of 20 and 40 with 1250 calorie DEXATRIM Diet Plan.

DEXATRIM® Maximum Strength Extended Duration Time Tablets: Packages of 20 and 40 with 1250 calorie DEXATRIM Diet Plan.

References: Altschuler, S., and Frazer, D.L., Double-Blind Clinical Evaluation of the Anorectic Activity of Phenylpropanolamine Hydrochloride Drops and Placebo Drops in the Treatment of Exogenous Obesity. *Current Therapeutic Research,* 40(1), 211–217, July 1986.
Altschuler, S., et. al., Three Controlled Trials of Weight Loss with Phenylpropanolamine, *Int J Obesity,* 1982;6:549–556.
Blackburn, G.L., et. al., Determinants of the Pressor Effect of Phenylpropanolamine in Healthy Subjects. *JAMA,* 1989; 261:3267–3272.
Morgan, J.P., et. al., Subjective Profile of Phenylpropanolamine: Absence of Stimulant or Euphorigenic Effects at Recommended Dose Levels. *J Clin Psychopharm,* 1989;9(1):33–38.
Lasagna, L., *Phenylpropanolamine—A Review,* New York, John Wiley and Sons, 1988.
All referenced materials available on request.

Shown in Product Identification Section, page 431

ENCARE®

[en'kar]

Vaginal Contraceptive Suppositories

Description: Encare is a safe and effective contraceptive in a convenient vaginal suppository form available without a prescription. Encare is reliable because it offers two-way protection: (1) Encare kills sperm on contact by releasing a precise dose of nonoxynol 9, the spermicide most recommended by doctors. (2) Encare gently disperses a physical barrier of protection against the cervix to help prevent pregnancy.
Encare is colorless and odorless; it is as pleasant to use as it is effective.
Encare is an effective contraceptive in vaginal suppository form.

Active Ingredient: Each Suppository contains 100 mg Nonoxynol 9.

Other Ingredients: Polyethylene Glycols, Sodium Bicarbonate, Sodium Citrate, Tartaric Acid.

Indications: Encare is effective in the prevention of pregnancy.

Action: Encare is 100% free of hormones and free of the serious side effects associated with oral contraceptives.
Encare is convenient and easy to use. Women like Encare because each insert is individually wrapped and can be easily carried in a pocket or purse. Encare is approximately as effective as vaginal foam contraceptives in actual use, yet there is no applicator, so there is nothing to fill, remove, or clean. In addition, women may find Encare convenient to use in conjunction with other contraceptive methods, such as a condom or as a second application with a diaphragm.
Because Encare can be inserted as much as an hour before intercourse, it does not interfere with spontaneity or ruin the mood. Many men are not even aware a woman is using Encare. Encare has been used successfully by millions of women throughout Europe and America.

Special Warning: Spermicidal contraceptives should not be used during pregnancy. Some experts believe that there may be an increased risk of birth defects occurring in children whose mothers used a spermicidal contraceptive at the time of conception or during pregnancy. If you have used a spermicidal contraceptive after becoming pregnant, or used a spermicidal contraceptive when you became pregnant, discuss this issue with your doctor.

Cautions: If your doctor has told you that you should not become pregnant, consult your doctor as to which method, including Encare, is best for you.
If you or your partner experience irritation, discontinue use. If irritation persists, consult your doctor.
Do not take orally. **KEEP THIS AND ALL DRUGS OUT OF THE REACH OF CHILDREN.** In case of accidental ingestion, call a Poison Control Center, emergency medical facility or a doctor immediately.
Keep away from excessive heat and moisture. Store at controlled room temperature: 15°C–30°C (59°–86°F).

Dosage and Administration: For best protection against pregnancy, it is essential to follow package instructions. At least 10 minutes before intercourse, place one Encare insert with your fingertip as far as possible into the vagina, towards the small of your back. Best protection will occur when Encare is placed deep into the vagina. You may feel a pleasant sensation of warmth as Encare effervesces and distributes the spermicide, nonoxynol 9, within the vagina. This is a natural attribute of the active ingredient.
IMPORTANT: It is essential to insert Encare at least 10 minutes before intercourse. If one chooses, Encare can be inserted up to one hour before intercourse. If intercourse has not taken place within one hour after insertion, use a new Encare insert. Use a new Encare insert each time intercourse is repeated. Encare can be used safely as frequently as needed.
Douching after use of Encare is not required; however, should you desire to do so, wait at least six hours after intercourse.

How Supplied: Boxes of 12.

References: Barwin, B., Encare Oval: A Clinical Study, *Contraceptive Delivery System,* 4, 331–334, 1983. Masters, W., In Vivo Evaluation of an Effervescent Intravaginal Contraceptive Inserted by Simulated Coital Activity, *Fertility and Sterility,* 32, 161–165, 1979.

SLEEPINAL®

Night-time Sleep Aid Capsules
Medicated Night Tea Packets
(Diphenhydramine HCl)

Description: SLEEPINAL is a night-time sleep aid. Sleepinal Medicated Night Tea is a night-time sleep aid in a flavored powder that mixes with hot water. When taken prior to bedtime, it helps to relieve sleeplessness and aids in falling asleep.

Active Ingredient: Diphenhydramine HCl 50 mg.

Other Ingredients: Capsules: FD&C Blue No. 1, Gelatin, Lactose, Magnesium Stearate, Povidone, Talc.
Medicated Night Tea Packet: Aspartame, Citric Acid, Colloidal Silicon Dioxide, D&C Yellow No. 10, FD&C Blue No. 1, FD&C Red No. 40, Flavors, Lactose, Polyethylene Glycol, Povidone, Sodium Chloride, Sodium Citrate.

Indications: For relief of occasional sleeplessness.

Action: SLEEPINAL is an antihistamine with anticholinergic and sedative action.

Warnings: **Read before using.** Do not exceed recommended dosage. Do not give to children under 12 years of age. If sleeplessness persists continuously for more than 2 weeks, consult a physician. Insomnia may be a symptom of serious underlying medical illness. Do not take this product if you have asthma, glaucoma, emphysema, chronic pulmonary disease, shortness of breath, difficulty in breathing, or difficulty in urination due to enlargement of the prostate gland unless directed by a physician. Avoid alcoholic beverages while taking this product. Do not take this product if you are taking sedatives or tranquilizers, without first consulting your physician. As with any drug, if you are pregnant or nursing a baby, seek the advice of a health professional before using this product.
KEEP THIS AND ALL MEDICATIONS OUT OF THE REACH OF CHILDREN.
In the case of accidental overdose, seek professional assistance or contact a Poison Control Center immediately. Medicated Night Tea Packet: Phenylketonurics: Contains Phenylalanine 16.8 mg. per packet.

Dosage and Administration: Capsules: Adults and children 12 years of age and over: Oral dosage, one capsule at bedtime if needed, or as directed by a physician.
Medicated Night Tea Packet: Adults and children 12 years of age and over. To open, cut along dotted line, pour contents and dissolve one packet into 8 ounces of hot water. Sip while hot at bedtime, if needed, or as directed by a physician.

How to Store: Store in a dry place at controlled room temperature 15° C–30° C (59° F–86° F).

Continued on next page

Thompson Medical—Cont.

How Supplied: Capsules: Sleepinal is supplied in tamper-evident blister packages. Do not use if individual seals are broken. Packages of 16 and 32 capsules. Medicated Night Tea: is supplied in packages containing single-dose packets. Do not use if foil packet is torn or broken. Packages contain 8 or 16 packets.

Shown in Product Identification Section, page 431

SPORTSCREME
[*spŏrts-crēme*]
External Analgesic Rub Products

Description: Sportscreme External Analgesic Rub Products are available in a fresh scent, 10% Trolamine Salicylate lotion and cream formulation, as well as a 2% Menthol ice.

Actions and Uses: These products were formulated for hours of relief of aches, strains, and minor muscle pain of the arms, legs, shoulders, and back. The ice formulation also provides temporary relief of minor arthritis pain.

Directions: Apply generously. Massage into painful area until completely absorbed into skin. Repeat as needed not more than 4 times daily.

Warnings: For external use only as directed. Avoid contact with eyes. Do not apply if skin is irritated. Keep this and all medicines out of the reach of children. In case of accidental ingestion, seek professional assistance or contact a poison control center immediately. If redness is present or condition worsens, or if pain persists for more than 7 days or clears up and occurs again within a few days, discontinue use and consult a doctor.
Cream and lotion: If prone to allergic reaction from aspirin or salicylate, consult your doctor before using. Do not use on children under 10 years of age. Do not apply if skin is irritated or if irritation develops. As with any drug, if you are pregnant or nursing a baby, seek the advice of a health professional before using this product.
Ice: Avoid contact with mucous membranes, broken or irritated skin. Do not bandage tightly. Do not use on children under 2 years of age except under the advice and supervision of a doctor.

How to Store: Store at controlled room temperature 59°–86°F (15°–30°C).

How Supplied: Cream: 1¼ oz., 3 oz., and 5 oz tubes. Lotion: 6 oz bottle. Ice: 8 oz jar.

Shown in Product Identification Section, page 431

TEMPO
[*tem-pō*]
Soft Antacid

Description: Tempo is a unique, chewable soft antacid that provides fast, effective relief from acid indigestion, heartburn, and gas. Tempo has 75% more acid relieving medicine than the leading tablet, so you need just one. Tempo is pleasant tasting, not chalky or gritty.

Active Ingredients: Each drop contains Calcium Carbonate 414 mg., Aluminum Hydroxide 133 mg., Magnesium Hydroxide 81 mg., Simethicone 20 mg.

Other Ingredients: Corn Syrup, Deionized Water, FD&C Blue No. 1, Flavor, Sorbitol, Soy Protein, Starch, Titanium Dioxide, 3.0 mg. Sodium per drop (dietetically sodium free).

Indication: For the relief of heartburn, sour stomach, acid indigestion, gas, and upset stomach associated with these symptoms.

Warnings: Do not take more than 12 drops in a 24-hour period or use the maximum dosage for more than two weeks except under the advice and supervision of a doctor. Keep this and all drugs out of the reach of children. **Drug Interaction Precaution:** Do not take this product if you are presently taking a prescription antibiotic drug containing any form of tetracycline.

Dosage and Administration: One tablet dosage. Not to exceed more than 12 tablets in a 24-hour period.

How to Store: Store at controlled room temperature 15°–30°C (59°–86°F).

How Supplied: 10, 30, and 60 Pieces

Shown in Product Identification Section, page 431

Triton Consumer Products, Inc.
561 W. GOLF ROAD
ARLINGTON HEIGHTS, IL 60005

MG 217® PSORIASIS/DANDRUFF MEDICATION
Skin Care: Ointment and Lotion
Scalp: Shampoo

Active Ingredients: Ointment—Coal Tar Solution USP 10%. **Lotion**—Coal Tar Solution USP 5%. **Tar Shampoo**—Coal Tar Solution USP 15%. **Tar-Free Shampoo**—Sulfur 5% and salicylic acid 3%.

Action/Uses: Relief for itching, scaling and flaking of psoriasis, seborrheic dermatitis and/or dandruff.

Warnings: For external use only. Keep out of the reach of children. Avoid contact with eyes. If undue skin irritation occurs, discontinue use.

Administration: Ointment or Lotion—Apply to affected area one to four times daily. **Shampoo**—Shake well before using. Wet hair, then massage liberal amount of MG 217 into scalp and leave on for several minutes. Rinse thoroughly. For best results, use at least twice a week or as directed by a physician.

How Supplied: Ointment—3.8 oz. jars. **Lotion**—4 oz. bottles. **Shampoo**—4 oz. and 8 oz. bottles.

UAS Laboratories
9201 PENN AVENUE SOUTH #10
MINNEAPOLIS, MN 55431

DDS–ACIDOPHILUS
Capsule, Tablet & Powder free of dairy products, corn, soy, and preservatives

Description: DDS-Acidophilus is the source of a special strain of Lactobacillus acidophilus free of dairy products, corn, soy and preservatives. Each capsule or tablet contains one billion viable DDS-1 L.acidophilus at the time of manufacturing. One gram of powder contains two billion viable DDS-1 L.acidophilus.

Indications and Usages: An aid in implanting the gut with beneficial Lactobacillus acidophilus under conditions of digestive disorders, acne, yeast infections, and following antibiotic therapy.

Administration: One to two capsules or tablets twice daily before meals. One-fourth teaspoon powder can be substituted for two capsules or tablets.

How Supplied: Bottles of 100 capsules or tablets. 12 bottles per case. Powder is available in 2 oz. bottle; 12 bottles per case.

Storage: Keep refrigerated under 40°F.

EDUCATIONAL MATERIAL

DDS-Acidophilus
Booklet describing superior-strain Acidophilus without dairy products, corn, soy, or preservatives. Two billion viable DDS-L. acidophilus per gram.

IDENTIFICATION PROBLEM?
Consult the
Product Identification Section
where you'll find
products pictured
in full color.

The Upjohn Company
KALAMAZOO, MI 49001

CORTAID®
Maximum Strength and Regular Strength
Cream, Ointment and Spray (hydrocortisone 1% and ½%)
Anti-itch products

Description: Maximum Strength and Regular Strength CORTAID provide safe, effective relief of many different types of itches and rashes and is the brand recommended most by physicians and pharmacists. Maximum Strength CORTAID is the same strength and form of hydrocortisone relief formerly available only with a prescription. Both strengths are available in 1) a greaseless, odorless vanishing cream that leaves no residue; 2) a soothing, lubricating ointment; 3) a quick-drying non-staining, non-aerosol spray. Regular Strength is also available in a greaseless, odorless vanishing lotion.

Active Ingredients: CORTAID Cream, CORTAID Ointment, and CORTAID Lotion: hydrocortisone acetate (equivalent to 1% or ½% hydrocortisone).
CORTAID Spray: hydrocortisone 1% or ½%.

Other Ingredients:
Maximum Strength Products:
Maximum Strength Cream: butylparaben, cetyl alcohol, glycerin, methylparaben, sodium lauryl sulfate, stearic acid, stearyl alcohol, purified water, and white petrolatum.
Maximum Strength Ointment: butylparaben, cholesterol, methylparaben, microcrystalline wax, mineral oil, and white petrolatum.
Maximum Strength Spray: alcohol, glycerin, methylparaben, and purified water.
Regular Strength Products:
Regular Strength Cream: aloe vera, butylparaben, cetyl palmitate, glyceryl stearate, methylparaben, polyethylene glycol, stearamidoethyl diethylamine, and purified water.
Regular Strength Ointment: aloe vera, butylparaben, cholesterol, methylparaben, mineral oil, white petrolatum, and microcrystalline wax.
Regular Strength Spray: alcohol, glycerin, methylparaben, and purified water.
Regular Strength Lotion: butylparaben, cetyl palmitate, glyceryl monostearate, methylparaben, polysorbate 80, propylene glycol, stearamidoethyl diethylamine, and purified water.

Indications: Use CORTAID for the temporary relief of itching associated with minor skin irritations, inflammation, and rashes due to eczema, psoriasis, seborrheic dermatitis, poison ivy, poison oak, or poison sumac, insect bites, soaps, detergents, cosmetics, jewelry, and for external feminine and anal itching. Other uses of this product should be only under the advice and supervision of a physician.

Uses: The vanishing action of CORTAID Cream makes it cosmetically acceptable when the skin itch or rash treated is on exposed parts of the body such as the hands or arms. CORTAID Ointment is best used where protection, lubrication and soothing of dry and scaly lesions is required. The ointment is also recommended for treating itchy genital and anal areas. CORTAID Spray is a quick-drying, non-staining formulation suitable for covering large areas of the skin. CORTAID Lotion is a free-flowing Lotion and is especially suitable for hairy body areas such as the scalp or arms.

Warnings: For external use only. Avoid contact with the eyes. If condition worsens, or if symptoms persist for more than 7 days or clear up and occur again within a few days, stop use of this product and do not begin use of any other hydrocortisone product unless you have consulted a physician. Do not use for the treatment of diaper rash. Consult a physician. For external feminine itching, do not use if you have a vaginal discharge. Consult a physician. For external anal itching, do not exceed the recommended daily dosage unless directed by a physician. In case of bleeding, consult a physician promptly. Do not put this product into the rectum by using fingers or any mechanical device or applicator.
Keep this and all drugs out of the reach of children. In case of accidental ingestion, seek professional assistance or contact a poison control center immediately.

Dosage and Administration: *Adults and children 2 years of age and older:* Apply to affected area not more than 3 to 4 times daily. *Children under 2 years of age:* Do not use, consult a physician. *Adults:* For external anal itching, when practical, cleanse the affected area with mild soap and warm water and rinse thoroughly by patting or blotting with an appropriate cleansing pad. Gently dry by patting or blotting with toilet tissue or a soft cloth before application of this product. *Children under 12 years of age:* For external anal itching, consult a physician.

How Supplied:
Cream: ½ oz. and 1 oz. tubes
Ointment: ½ oz. and 1 oz. tubes
Non-Aerosol Spray: 1.5 fluid oz.
Lotion: 1 oz. bottle

Shown in Product Identification Section, page 432

DOXIDAN® LIQUI-GELS®
Stimulant/Stool Softener Laxative

Active Ingredients: Each soft gelatin capsule contains 65 mg yellow phenolphthalein and 60 mg docusate calcium.

Inactive Ingredients: Alcohol up to 1.5% (w/w), corn oil, FD&C Blue #1 and Red #40, gelatin, glycerin, hydrogenated vegetable oil, lecithin, parabens, sorbitol, titanium dioxide, vegetable shortening, yellow wax, and other ingredients.

Indications: DOXIDAN is a safe, reliable laxative for the relief of occasional constipation. The combination of a stimulant/stool softener laxative allows positive laxative action on a softened stool for gentle evacuation without straining. DOXIDAN generally produces a bowel movement in 6 to 12 hours.

Dosage and Administration: Adults and children 12 years of age and over: one or two capsules by mouth daily. For use in children under 12, consult a physician.

Warnings: Do not use laxative products when abdominal pain, nausea, or vomiting are present unless directed by a doctor. If you have noticed a sudden change in bowel habits that persists over a period of 2 weeks, consult a doctor before using a laxative. Laxative products should not be used for a period longer than 1 week unless directed by a doctor. Rectal bleeding or failure to have a bowel movement after use of a laxative may indicate a serious condition. Discontinue use and consult your doctor. If skin rash appears, do not use this product or any other preparation containing phenolphthalein. Keep this and all drugs out of the reach of children. In case of accidental overdose, seek professional assistance or contact a poison control center immediately. As with any drug, if you are pregnant or nursing a baby, seek the advice of a health professional before using this product.

How Supplied: Packages of 10, 30, 100 and 1,000 maroon soft gelatin capsules, and Unit Dose 100s (10 × 10 strips).
LIQUI-GELS® Reg TM R P Scherer Corp

Shown in Product Identification Section, page 432

DRAMAMINE® Tablets (dimenhydrinate USP)
DRAMAMINE® Chewable Tablets (dimenhydrinate USP)
DRAMAMINE® Children's (dimenhydrinate syrup USP)

Description: Dimenhydrinate is the chlorotheophylline salt of the antihistaminic agent diphenhydramine. Dimenhydrinate contains not less than 53% and not more than 56% of diphenhydramine, and not less than 44% and not more than 47% of 8-chlorotheophylline, calculated on the dried basis.

Active Ingredients:
DRAMAMINE Tablets and Chewable Tablets: Dimenhydrinate 50 mg.
DRAMAMINE Children's: Dimenhydrinate 12.5 mg. per 5 ml, Alcohol 5%.

Inactive Ingredients:
DRAMAMINE Tablets: Acacia, Carboxymethylcellulose Sodium, Corn

Continued on next page

Upjohn—Cont.

Starch, Magnesium Stearate, and Sodium Sulfate.
DRAMAMINE Children's: FD&C Red No. 40, Flavor, Glycerin, Methylparaben, Sucrose, and Water.
DRAMAMINE Chewable Tablets: Aspartame, Citric Acid, FD&C Yellow No. 6, Flavor, Magnesium Stearate, Methacrylic Acid Copolymer, Sorbitol.
Phenylketonurics: Contains Phenylalanine 1.5 mg per tablet.
Contains FD&C Yellow No. 5 (tartrazine) as a color additive.

Actions: While the precise mode of action of dimenhydrinate is not known, it has a depressant action on hyperstimulated labyrinthine function.

Indications: For the prevention and treatment of the nausea, vomiting, or dizziness associated with motion sickness.

Directions:
DRAMAMINE Tablets and Chewable Tablets: To prevent motion sickness, the first dose should be taken one half to one hour before starting activity.
ADULTS: 1 to 2 tablets every 4 to 6 hours, not to exceed 8 tablets in 24 hours or as directed by a doctor.
CHILDREN 6 TO UNDER 12: ½ to 1 tablet every 6 to 8 hours, not to exceed 3 tablets in 24 hours or as directed by a doctor.
CHILDREN 2 to UNDER 6: ¼ to ½ tablet every 6 to 8 hours not to exceed 1½ tablets in 24 hours or as directed by a doctor.
Children may also be given DRAMAMINE Cherry Flavored Liquid in accordance with directions for use.
DRAMAMINE Children's: To prevent motion sickness, the first dose should be taken one half to one hour before starting activity. CHILDREN 2 TO UNDER 6: 1 to 2 teaspoonfuls every 6 to 8 hours not to exceed 6 teaspoonfuls in 24 hours or as directed by a doctor. Use of a measuring device is recommended for all liquid medication. CHILDREN 6 TO UNDER 12: 2 to 4 teaspoonfuls every 6 to 8 hours, not to exceed 12 teaspoonfuls in 24 hours or as directed by a doctor. CHILDREN 12 YEARS OR OLDER: 4 to 8 teaspoons (5 ml per teaspoonful) every 4 to 6 hours, not to exceed 32 teaspoonfuls in 24 hours or as directed by a doctor.

Warnings: Do not take this product if you have asthma, glaucoma, emphysema, chronic pulmonary disease, shortness of breath, difficulty in breathing, or difficulty in urination due to enlargement of the prostate gland unless directed by a doctor. Do not give to children under 2 years of age unless directed by a doctor. May cause marked drowsiness; alcohol, sedatives, and tranquilizers may increase the drowsiness effect. Avoid alcoholic beverages while taking this product. Do not take this product if you are taking sedatives or tranquilizers, without first consulting your doctor. Use caution when driving a motor vehicle or operating machinery. Not for frequent or prolonged use except on advice of a doctor. Do not exceed recommended dosage. Keep this and all drugs out of the reach of children. In case of accidental overdose, seek professional assistance or contact a poison control center immediately. As with any drug, if you are pregnant or nursing a baby, seek the advice of a health professional before using this product.

How Supplied: *Tablets*—scored, white tablets available in packets of 12 and 36 and bottles of 100 (OTC); *Liquid*—Available in bottles of 4 fl oz (OTC); *Chewables*—scored, orange tablets available in packets of 8 and 24 (OTC).

Shown in Product Identification Section, page 432

DRAMAMINE II™
(Meclizine hydrochloride)

Description: Meclizine hydrochloride is an antihistamine of the piperazine class with antiemetic action.

Actions: While the precise mode of action of meclizine hydrochloride is not known, it has a depressant action on hyperstimulated labyrinthine function.

Indications: For the prevention and treatment of the nausea, vomiting, or dizziness associated with motion sickness.

Active Ingredients: Each tablet contains 25 mg. meclizine hydrochloride.

Inactive Ingredients: Colloidal silicon dioxide, croscarmellose sodium, dibasic calcium phosphate, D&C yellow no. 10 aluminum lake, microcrystalline cellulose, magnesium stearate.

Directions: To prevent motion sickness, the first dose should be taken one hour before starting your activity. **Adults:** Take 1 to 2 tablets daily or as directed by a doctor. Do not exceed 2 tablets in 24 hours.

Warnings: Do not take this product if you have asthma, glaucoma, emphysema, chronic pulmonary disease, shortness of breath, difficulty in breathing, or difficulty in urination due to enlargement of the prostate gland unless directed by a doctor. Do not give to children under 12 years of age unless directed by a doctor. May cause drowsiness; alcohol, sedatives, and tranquilizers may increase the drowsiness effect. Avoid alcoholic beverages while taking this product. Do not take this product if you are taking sedatives or tranquilizers without first consulting your doctor. Use caution when driving a motor vehicle or operating machinery. Do not exceed recommended dosage. Keep this and all drugs out of reach of children. In case of accidental overdose, seek professional assistance or contact a poison control center immediately. As with any drug, if you are pregnant or nursing a baby, seek the advice of a health professional before using this product.

How Supplied: Dramamine II is supplied as a yellow tablet in packages of 8 (OTC).

Shown in Product Identification Section, page 432

KAOPECTATE®
Concentrated Anti-Diarrheal, Peppermint Flavor and Regular Flavor

Active Ingredient: Each tablespoon contains 600 mg attapulgite.

Inactive Ingredients: Flavors, glucono-delta-lactone, magnesium aluminum silicate, methylparaben, sorbic acid, sucrose, titanium dioxide, xanthan gum and purified water; Peppermint flavor contains FD&C Red #40.

Indications: For the fast relief of diarrhea and cramping.

Dosage and Administration: For best results, take full recommended dose at first sign of diarrhea and after each subsequent bowel movement. (Maximum 7 times in 24 hours.) Adults and children 12 years of age and over: 2 tablespoons. Children 6 to under 12 years of age: 1 tablespoon. Children 3 to under 6 years of age: ½ tablespoon.

Warnings: Unless directed by a physician, do not use in infants and children under 3 years of age or for more than two days or in the presence of high fever. Keep this and all drugs out of the reach of children. In case of accidental overdose, seek professional assistance or contact a poison control center immediately.

How Supplied: Regular flavor available in 8 oz, 12 oz and 16 oz bottles. Peppermint flavor available in 8 oz and 12 oz bottles.

Shown in Product Identification Section, page 432

KAOPECTATE® Children's Liquid and Chewable Tablets, Anti-Diarrheal

Active Ingredient: Each ½ tablespoon of liquid or chewable tablet contains 300 mg attapulgite.

Inactive Ingredients: Children's Liquid includes FD&C Red #40, flavors, glucono-delta-lactone, magnesium aluminum silicate, methylparaben, sorbic acid, sucrose, titanium dioxide, xanthan gum, and purified water. Children's Chewable Tablets include cornstarch, dextrins, dextrose, D&C Red #27, D&C Red #30, flavor, magnesium stearate, sucrose and titanium dioxide.

Indications: For the fast relief of diarrhea and cramping; in good-tasting, easy-to-take forms. Especially formulated to meet the needs of children age 3 and up.

Dosage and Administration: For best results, take full recommended dose at first sign of diarrhea and after each subsequent bowel movement (maximum 7 times in 24 hours). Liquid—Children 3 to under 6 years of age: ½ tablespoon; Children 6 to under 12 years of age: 1 tablespoon; children (and adults) 12 years of age and older: 2 tablespoons. Chewable Tablets—Children 3 to under 6 years of age: 1 tablet; Children 6 to under 12 years of age: 2 tablets; Children (and adults) 12 years of age and over: 4 tablets.

Warnings: Unless directed by a physician, do not use in infants and children under 3 years of age or for more than two days or in the presence of high fever. Keep this and all drugs out of the reach of children. In case of accidental overdose, seek professional assistance or contact a poison control center immediately.

How Supplied: Available in 6 oz bottles (liquid) and blister packs of 16 chewable tablets.

Shown in Product Identification Section, page 432

KAOPECTATE® Maximum Strength Caplets
Anti-Diarrheal

Active Ingredient: Each caplet contains 750 mg attapulgite.

Inactive Ingredients: Croscarmellose sodium, hydroxypropyl cellulose, hydroxypropyl methylcellulose, methylparaben, pectin, propylene glycol, propylparaben, sucrose, titanium dioxide and zinc stearate.

Indications: For the fast relief of diarrhea and cramping.

Dosage and Administration: Swallow whole caplets with water; do not chew. For best results, take full recommended dose.
Adults: Take 2 caplets after the initial bowel movement and 2 caplets after each subsequent bowel movement, not to exceed 12 caplets in 24 hours. Children 6 to 12 years of age: Take 1 caplet after the initial bowel movement and 1 caplet after each subsequent bowel movement, not to exceed 6 caplets in 24 hours.
Children 3 to under 6 years of age: Use Cherry Flavor Children's Liquid or Chewable Tablets, or Advanced Formula KAOPECTATE Liquid.

Warnings: Unless directed by a physician, do not use in infants and children under 6 years of age or for more than two days or in the presence of high fever. Keep this and all drugs out of the reach of children. In case of accidental overdose, seek professional assistance or contact a poison control center immediately.

How Supplied: Available in blister packs of 12 and 20 caplets.

Shown in Product Identification Section, page 432

MOTRIN® IB
Caplets or Tablets
(ibuprofen, USP)
Pain Reliever/Fever Reducer

WARNING: ASPIRIN-SENSITIVE PATIENTS. Do not take this product if you have had a severe allergic reaction to aspirin, eg—asthma, swelling, shock or hives because even though this product contains no aspirin or salicylates, cross-reactions may occur in patients allergic to aspirin.

Indications: For the temporary relief of headache, muscular aches, minor pain of arthritis, toothache, backache, minor aches and pains associated with the common cold, pain of menstrual cramps, and for reduction of fever.

Directions: Adults: Take 1 caplet or tablet every 4 to 6 hours while symptoms persist. If pain or fever does not respond to 1 caplet or tablet, 2 caplets or tablets may be used, but do not exceed 6 caplets or tablets in 24 hours, unless directed by a doctor. The smallest effective dose should be used. Take with food or milk, if occasional and mild heartburn, upset stomach or stomach pain occurs with use. Consult a doctor if these symptoms are more than mild or if they persist. Children: Do not give this product to children under 12 except under the advice and supervision of a doctor.

Warnings: Do not take for pain for more than 10 days or for fever for more than 3 days unless directed by a doctor. If pain or fever persists or gets worse, if new symptoms occur, or if the painful area is red or swollen, consult a doctor. These could be signs of serious illness. If you are under a doctor's care for any serious condition, consult a doctor before taking this product. As with aspirin and acetaminophen, if you have any condition which requires you to take prescription drugs or if you have had any problems or serious side effects from taking any nonprescription pain reliever, do not take MOTRIN® IB without first discussing it with your doctor. If you experience any symptoms which are unusual or seem unrelated to the condition for which you took ibuprofen, consult a doctor before taking any more of it. Although ibuprofen is indicated for the same conditions as aspirin and acetaminophen, it should not be taken with them except under a doctor's direction. Do not combine this product with any other ibuprofen-containing product. As with any drug, if you are pregnant or nursing a baby, seek the advice of a health professional before using this product. IT IS ESPECIALLY IMPORTANT NOT TO USE IBUPROFEN DURING THE LAST 3 MONTHS OF PREGNANCY UNLESS SPECIFICALLY DIRECTED TO DO SO BY A DOCTOR BECAUSE IT MAY CAUSE PROBLEMS IN THE UNBORN CHILD OR COMPLICATIONS DURING DELIVERY. Keep this and all drugs out of the reach of children. In case of accidental overdose, seek professional assistance or contact a poison control center immediately. **Store at room temperature. Avoid excessive heat 40°C (104°F).**

Active Ingredient: Each caplet or tablet contains ibuprofen 200 mg.

Other Ingredients: Carnauba wax, cornstarch, hydroxypropyl methylcellulose, propylene glycol, silicon dioxide, pregelatinized starch, stearic acid, titanium dioxide.

How Supplied: Bottles of 24, 50, 100, and 165 Caplets or Tablets. Vial of 8 caplets.

Shown in Product Identification Section, page 432

Maximum Strength
MYCITRACIN®
Triple Antibiotic First Aid Ointment
MYCITRACIN® Plus Pain Reliever

Description: MYCITRACIN combines three topical antibiotics in a soothing, non-irritating petrolatum base that does not sting, aids healing, and helps prevent infection. MYCITRACIN Plus Pain Reliever also temporarily relieves pain.

Indications: Maximum Strength MYCITRACIN and MYCITRACIN Plus Pain Reliever are first aid ointments to help prevent infection in minor burns, cuts, nicks, scrapes, scratches and abrasions. MYCITRACIN Plus Pain Reliever also temporarily relieves pain.

Directions: *For adults and children (all ages):* Clean the affected area. Apply a small amount of MYCITRACIN (an amount equal to the surface area of the tip of a finger) on the affected area 1 to 3 times daily. If desired, cover the affected area with a sterile bandage.

Warnings: For external use only. Do not use in the eyes or apply over large areas of the body. In case of deep or puncture wounds, animal bites, or serious burns, consult a physician. Stop use and consult a physician if the condition persists or gets worse. Do not use longer than 1 week unless directed by a physician. Keep this and all medications out of the reach of children. In case of accidental ingestion, seek professional assistance or contact a poison control center immediately.

Active Ingredients:
Maximum Strength MYCITRACIN: Each gram contains bacitracin, 500 units; neomycin sulfate equiv. to 3.5 mg neomycin; polymyxin B sulfate, 5,000 units.
MYCITRACIN Plus Pain Reliever: Each gram contains bacitracin, 500 units; neomycin sulfate equiv. to 3.5 mg neomycin; polymyxin B sulfate, 5000 units; lidocaine, 40 mg.

Other Ingredients:
Maximum Strength MYCITRACIN: butylparaben, cholesterol, methylparaben, microcrystalline wax, mineral oil, and white petrolatum.

Continued on next page

Upjohn—Cont.

MYCITRACIN Plus Pain Reliever: butylparaben, cholesterol, methylparaben, microcrystalline wax, mineral oil, and white petrolatum.

How Supplied:
½ oz. tubes, 1 oz. tubes and 1/32 oz. foil packets (144 per carton)
Shown in Product Identification Section, page 432

PROGAINE®
Shampoo for Thinning Hair

Description: PROGAINE Shampoo has been scientifically formulated to clean delicate thinning hair without damaging while adding body and manageability. PROGAINE is also an ideal shampoo for the user of thinning hair treatments. The exclusive, patented formula for PROGAINE Shampoo has been dermatologist tested on over 1000 adults in 31 medical clinics and proven safe for delicate thinning hair. PROGAINE Shampoo is different from many other shampoos in that PROGAINE contains none of the commonly used coating ingredients such as oils, waxes, silicones, proteins, quaternary ammonium salts, or cationic polymers which may leave a deposit on hair and scalp. PROGAINE is also hypoallergenic; it contains no harsh detergents or additives such as dyes, added formaldehydes, or parabens, commonly found in other shampoos, which may irritate sensitive scalps. PROGAINE Shampoo is pH balanced, ranging from 5.4 to 5.7, and will not affect the scalp's normal pH.

Ingredients:
Normal-to-Oily formula: Water, TEA lauryl sulfate, sodium laureth sulfate, cocamide DEA, cocamidopropyl betaine, propylene glycol, citric acid, disodium EDTA, fragrance, and sodium chloride.
Normal-to-Dry formula: Water, sodium laureth sulfate, TEA lauryl sulfate, cocamide DEA, cocamidopropyl betaine, acetamide MEA, citric acid, disodium EDTA, fragrance, sodium chloride.

Directions: PROGAINE Shampoo is gentle enough to use for every shampoo. For best results, wet hair and scalp, apply PROGAINE Shampoo, bring to a lather, then rinse. Repeat if desired.

How Supplied: Both the Normal-to-Oily and Normal-to-Dry formulas are available in 5 oz. and 8 oz. bottles.

SURFAK® LIQUI-GELS®
Stool Softener Laxative

Active Ingredients: Each soft gelatin capsule contains 240 mg docusate calcium.

Inactive Ingredients: Alcohol up to 3% (w/w), corn oil, FD&C Blue #1 and Red #40, gelatin, glycerin, parabens, sorbitol, and other ingredients.

Indications: SURFAK is indicated for the relief of occasional constipation. SURFAK generally produces a bowel movement in 12 to 72 hours. SURFAK is useful when only stool softening (without propulsive action) is required to relieve constipation.

Dosage and Administration: Adults and children 12 years of age and over: one capsule by mouth daily for several days or until bowel movements are normal. For use in children under 12, consult a physician.

Warnings: Do not use laxative products when abdominal pain, nausea, or vomiting are present unless directed by a doctor. If you have noticed a sudden change in bowel habits that persists over a period of 2 weeks, consult a doctor before using a laxative. Laxative products should not be used for a period longer than 1 week unless directed by a doctor. Rectal bleeding or failure to have a bowel movement after use of a laxative may indicate a serious condition. Discontinue use and consult your doctor. Keep this and all drugs out of the reach of children. In case of accidental overdose, seek professional assistance or contact a poison control center immediately. As with any drug, if you are pregnant or nursing a baby, seek the advice of a health professional before using this product.

How Supplied: Packages of 10, 30, 100 and 500 red soft gelatin capsules and Unit Dose 100s (10 × 10 strips).
LIQUI-GELS® Reg TM R P Scherer Corp
Shown in Product Identification Section, page 432

UNICAP® Capsules/Tablets
Multivitamin Supplement
100% RDA of Essential Vitamins in Easy to Swallow Capsule
Sugar and Sodium Free Tablet

Indications: Dietary multivitamin supplement of ten essential vitamins for health-conscious families (adults and children 4 or more years of age).
Each capsule contains:

		% U.S. RDA*
Vitamin A	5000 Int. Units	100
Vitamin D	400 Int. Units	100
Vitamin E	30 Int. Units	100
Vitamin C	60 mg	100
Folic Acid	400 mcg	100
Thiamine	1.5 mg	100
Riboflavin	1.7 mg	100
Niacin	20 mg	100
Vitamin B_6	2 mg	100
Vitamin B_{12}	6 mcg	100

Each tablet has same content except:

Vitamin E	15 Int. Units	50

*Percentage of U.S. Recommended Daily Allowance.

Ingredient List:
Capsules: Gelatin, Ascorbic Acid (Vit. C), Soybean Oil, Glycerin, Vitamin E Acetate, Niacinamide, Yellow Wax, Lecithin, Pyridoxine Hydrochloride (B-6), Thiamine Mononitrate (B-1), Riboflavin (B-2), Vitamin A Palmitate, Titanium Dioxide, Corn Oil, Folic Acid, FD&C Yellow No. 5, Ethyl Vanillin, Vanilla Enhancer, FD&C Yellow No. 6, Cholecaliciferol (Vit. D), Cyanocobalamin (B-12).
Tablets: Calcium Phosphate, Ascorbic Acid (Vit. C), Vitamin E Acetate, Hydroxypropyl Methylcellulose, Niacinamide, Artificial Color, Vitamin A Acetate, Magnesium Stearate, Pyridoxine Hydrochloride (B-6), Riboflavin (B-2), Silica Gel, Thiamine Mononitrate (B-1), FD&C Yellow No. 5, Folic Acid, Artificial Flavor, Cholecalciferol (Vit. D), Carnauba Wax, Cyanocobalamin (B-12).

Recommended Dosage: 1 capsule or tablet daily.

How Supplied: Available in bottles of 120 capsules or tablets.
Shown in Product Identification Section, page 432

UNICAP Jr.® Chewable Tablets
Good-tasting, Orange-flavored Chewable Tablet

Indications: Dietary multivitamin supplement providing up to 100% of the RDA of essential vitamins. For **children** 4 or more years of age.

Each tablet contains:		% U.S. RDA*
Vitamin A	5000 Int. Units	100
Vitamin D	400 Int. Units	100
Vitamin E	15 Int. Units	50
Vitamin C	60 mg	100
Folic Acid	400 mcg	100
Thiamine	1.5 mg	100
Riboflavin	1.7 mg	100
Niacin	20 mg	100
Vitamin B_6	2 mg	100
Vitamin B_{12}	6 mcg	100

*Percentage of U.S. Recommended Daily Allowance.

Ingredient List: Sucrose, Mannitol, Sodium Ascorbate (Vit C), Lactose, Cornstarch, Niacinamide, Citric Acid, Vitamin E Acetate, Povidone, Artificial Flavor, Dextrins, Silica, Calcium Stearate, Pyridoxine HCl (B-6), Artificial Color, Vitamin A Acetate, Thiamine Mononitrate (B-1), Riboflavin (B-2), Folic Acid, Cyanocobalamin (B-12), Cholecalciferol (Vit D).

Recommended Dosage: 1 tablet daily.

How Supplied: Available in bottles of 120 tablets.

UNICAP M® Tablets
Multivitamins and Minerals
Sugar Free and Sodium Free

Indications: Dietary supplement providing up to 100% of the RDA for essential vitamins and minerals, including vitamin C and B-complex vitamins your body cannot store.

Each tablet contains:		% U.S. RDA
Vitamin A	5000 Int. Units	100
Vitamin D	400 Int. Units	100
Vitamin E	30 Int. Units	100
Vitamin C	60 mg	100
Folic Acid	400 mcg	100
Thiamine	1.5 mg	100
Riboflavin	1.7 mg	100
Niacin	20 mg	100
Vitamin B_6	2 mg	100
Vitamin B_{12}	6 mcg	100
Pantothenic Acid	10 mg	100
Iodine	150 mcg	100
Iron	18 mg	100
Copper	2 mg	100
Zinc	15 mg	100
Calcium	60 mg	6
Phosphorus	45 mg	5
Manganese	1 mg	+
Potassium	5 mg	+

+Recognized as essential in human nutrition, but no U.S. Recommended Daily Allowance (U.S. RDA) has been established.

Ingredient List: Calcium Phosphate, Ascorbic Acid (Vit C), Vitamin E Acetate, Ferrous Fumarate, Cellulose, Niacinamide, Artificial Color, Zinc Oxide, Calcium Pantothenate, Vitamin A Acetate, Potassium Sulfate, Magnesium Stearate, Cupric Sulfate, Silica Gel, Manganese Sulfate, Pyridoxine Hydrochloride, Riboflavin (B-2), Thiamine Mononitrate (B-1), FD&C Yellow No. 5, Folic Acid, Artificial Flavor, Cholecalciferol (Vit D), Potassium Iodide, Carnauba Wax, Cyanocobalamin (B-12).

Recommended Dosage: 1 tablet daily.

How Supplied: Available in bottles of 120 and 500 tablets.

Shown in Product Identification Section, page 432

UNICAP® Plus Iron Tablets
Multivitamin Supplement With 100% of the U.S. RDA of Essential Vitamins Plus Calcium and Extra Iron
Sugar Free and Sodium Free

Indications: Dietary multivitamin supplement providing essential vitamins. 125% of the RDA of Iron plus Calcium for women 12 or more years of age.

Each tablet contains: [See table top of next column.]

		% U.S. RDA*
Vitamins		
Vitamin A	5000 Int. Units	100
Vitamin D	400 Int. Units	100
Vitamin E	30 Int. Units	100
Vitamin C	60 mg	100
Folic Acid	400 mcg	100
Thiamine	1.5 mg	100
Riboflavin	1.7 mg	100
Niacin	20 mg	100
Vitamin B_6	2 mg	100
Vitamin B_{12}	6 mcg	100
Pantothenic Acid	10 mg	100
Minerals		
Iron	22.5 mg	125
Calcium	100 mg	10

*Percentage of U.S. Recommended Daily Allowance.

Ingredient List: Calcium Phosphate, Cellulose, Ascorbic Acid (Vit C), Ferrous Fumarate, Vitamin E Acetate, Artificial Color, Niacinamide, Vitamin A Acetate, Calcium Pantothenate, Magnesium Stearate, Silica Gel, Pyridoxine HCl (B-6), Riboflavin (B-2), Thiamine Mononitrate (B-1), Folic Acid, Artificial Flavor, Cholecalciferol (Vit D), Carnauba Wax, Cyanocobalamin (B-12).

Recommended Dosage: 1 tablet daily.

How Supplied: Available in bottles of 120 tablets.

UNICAP Sr.® Tablets
Vitamins and Minerals for Adults 50+ Based on the National Academy of Sciences–National Research Council Recommendations
Sugar Free and Sodium Free

Indications: Dietary supplement of essential vitamins and minerals formulated for the nutritional needs of adults 50+.

Each tablet contains:

		% U.S.* RDA
Vitamin A (as Acetate and Beta Carotene)	5000 Int. Units	100
Vitamin D	200 Int. Units	50
Vitamin E	15 Int. Units	50
Vitamin C	60 mg	100
Folic Acid	400 mcg	100
Thiamine	1.2 mg	80
Riboflavin	1.4 mg	82
Niacin	16 mg	80
Vitamin B_6	2.2 mg	110
Vitamin B_{12}	3 mcg	50
Pantothenic Acid	10 mg	100
Iodine	150 mcg	100
Iron	10 mg	56
Copper	2 mg	100
Zinc	15 mg	100
Calcium	100 mg	10
Phosphorus	77 mg	8
Magnesium	30 mg	8
Manganese	1 mg	+
Potassium	5 mg	+

* U.S. Recommended Daily Allowance for Adults.

+Recognized as essential in human nutrition, but no U.S. Recommended Daily Allowance (U.S. RDA) has been established.

Ingredient List: Calcium Phosphate, Cellulose, Ascorbic Acid (Vit C), Magnesium Oxide, Vitamin E Acetate, Ferrous Fumarate, Artificial Color, Zinc Oxide, Niacinamide, Calcium Pantothenate, Vitamin A Acetate, Magnesium Stearate, Potassium Sulfate, Cupric Sulfate, Silica Gel, Beta-Carotene, Manganese Sulfate, Pyridoxine Hydrochloride (B-6), Riboflavin (B-2), Thiamine Mononitrate (B-1), Folic Acid, Artificial Flavor, Cholecalciferol (Vit D), Potassium Iodide, Carnauba Wax, Cyanocobalamin (B-12).

Recommended Dosage: 1 tablet daily.

How Supplied: Available in bottles of 120 tablets.

Shown in Product Identification Section, page 432

UNICAP T® Tablets
Stress Formula
A More Complete Vitamin and Mineral Supplement
Sugar Free and Sodium Free

Indications: Dietary supplement offering higher levels of vitamin C and B-complex vitamins essential for the return to, and maintenance of good health.

Each tablet contains:		% U.S. RDA
Vitamin A	5000 Int. Units	100
Vitamin D	400 Int. Units	100
Vitamin E	30 Int. Units	100
Vitamin C	500 mg	833
Folic Acid	400 mcg	100
Thiamine	10 mg	667
Riboflavin	10 mg	588
Niacin	100 mg	500
Vitamin B_6	6 mg	300
Vitamin B_{12}	18 mcg	300
Pantothenic Acid	25 mg	250
Iodine	150 mcg	100
Iron	18 mg	100
Copper	2 mg	100
Zinc	15 mg	100
Manganese	1 mg	+
Potassium	5 mg	+
Selenium	10 mcg	+

+Recognized as essential in human nutrition, but no U.S. Recommended Daily Allowance (U.S. RDA) has been established.

Ingredient List: Ascorbic Acid (Vit C), Niacinamide, Cellulose, Hydroxypropyl Methylcellulose, Vitamin E Acetate, Ferrous Fumarate, Artificial Color, Calcium Pantothenate, Calcium Phosphate, Zinc Oxide, Vitamin A Acetate, Magnesium Stearate, Potassium Sulfate, Thiamine Mononitrate (B-1), Riboflavin (B-2), Selenium Yeast, Pyridoxine Hydrochloride (B-6), Cupric Sulfate, Silica Gel, Manganese Sulfate, FD&C Yellow No. 5, Folic Acid, Artificial Flavor, Cholecalciferol (Vit D), Potassium Iodide, Carnauba Wax, Cyanocobalamin (B-12).

Recommended Dosage: 1 tablet daily.

How Supplied: Available in bottles of 60 tablets.

Shown in Product Identification Section, page 432

Continued on next page

Vision Pharmaceuticals, Inc.

1022 N. MAIN STREET
MITCHELL, SD 57301

VIVA-DROPS™
Lubricant Eye Drops

Description: VIVA-DROPS™ is a preservative-free, non-oily, sterile ophthalmic lubricant for relief from irritation due to dryness of the eye or discomfort caused by exposure to wind, sun or dry air. The patented formulation of VIVA-DROPS™ includes antioxidants that protect the active ingredient from autoxidation.

Contains: Active: polysorbate 80. **Inactives:** sodium chloride, citric acid, edetate disodium, purified water, with retinyl palmitate, mannitol, sodium citrate, and pyruvate as antioxidants.

FDA APPROVED USES

Indications: FOR USE AS A LUBRICANT TO PREVENT FURTHER IRRITATION OR TO RELIEVE DRYNESS OF THE EYE.

Warnings: If you experience eye pain, changes in vision, continued redness or irritation of the eye, or if the condition persists for more than 72 hours, discontinue use and consult a doctor. If solution changes color or becomes cloudy, do not use. Keep this and all drugs out of the reach of children.

Directions: Instill 1 or 2 drops in the affected eye(s) as needed.

How Supplied: In 10mL (NDC 54891-001-02) and 15mL (NDC 54891-001-01) bottles.
Store at room temperature.
U.S. Patent No. 5,032,392

Wakunaga of America Co., Ltd.

Subsidiary of Wakunaga Pharmaceutical Co., Ltd.
23501 MADERO
MISSION VIEJO, CA 92691

KYOLIC®
Odor Modified Garlic

Active Ingredient: Aged Garlic Extract.™

Indications: Dietary Supplement.

Suggested Use: Average serving, four capsules or tablets a day during or after meals.

How Supplied: Liquid—Kyolic-Aged Garlic Extract Flavor and Odor Modified Enriched with Vitamin B_1 and B_{12} (and empty gelatine capsules) 2 fl oz (62 capsules) and 4 fl oz (124 capsules). Kyolic-Aged Garlic Extract Flavor and Odor Modified Plain (and empty gelatine capsules) 2 fl oz (62 capsules) and 4 fl oz (124 capsules).

Tablets and Capsules—Ingredients per Tablet or Capsule:
Kyolic—Super Formula 100 Tablets: Aged Garlic Extract Powder (300 mg), Whey (168 mg) blended with natural vegetable sources: Cellulose and Algin, bottles of 100 and 200 tablets.
Kyolic—Super Formula 100 Capsules: Aged Garlic Extract Powder (300 mg), Whey (168 mg), bottles of 100 and 200 capsules.
Kyolic—Super Formula 101 Garlic Plus® Tablets: Aged Garlic Extract Powder (270 mg) blended with Brewer's Yeast (27 mg), Kelp (9 mg), bottles of 100 and 200 tablets.
Kyolic—Super Formula 101 Garlic Plus® Capsules: Aged Garlic Extract Powder (270 mg) blended with Brewer's Yeast (27 mg), Kelp (9 mg), bottles of 50, 100 and 200 capsules.
Kyolic—Super Formula 102 Tablets: Aged Garlic Extract Powder (350 mg), "Kyolic Enzyme Complex™" [Amylase, Protease, Cellulase and Lipase] (30 mg), bottles of 100 and 200 tablets.
Kyolic—Super Formula 102 Capsules: Aged Garlic Extract Powder (350 mg), "Kyolic Enzyme Complex™" [Amylase, Protease, Cellulase and Lipase] (30 mg), bottles of 100 and 200 tablets.
Kyolic—Super Formula 103 Capsules: Aged Garlic Extract Powder (220 mg), Ester C® [Calcium Ascorbate] (150 mg), Astragulus membranaceous (100 mg), Calcium citrate (80 mg), bottles of 100 and 200 capsules.
Kyolic—Super Formula 104 Capsules: Aged Garlic Extract Powder (300 mg), Lecithin (200 mg), bottles of 100 and 200 capsules.
Kyolic—Super Formula 105 Capsules: Aged Garlic Extract Powder (250 mg), Beta-Carotene (37.5 mg) *d*-Alpha-Tocopheryl Acid Succinate [Vitamin E] (50 mg) in a base of Alfalfa and Parsley, bottles of 100 capsules.
Kyolic—Super Formula 106 Capsules: Aged Garlic Extract Powder (300 mg), *d*-Alpha Tocopheryl Succinate [Vitamin E] (90 mg), Hawthorn Berry (50 mg), Cayenne Pepper (10 mg), bottles of 50 and 100 capsules.

Professional label "SGP" is available in Aged Garlic Extract powder forms.

Shown in Product Identification Section, page 432

EDUCATIONAL MATERIAL

From Soil to Shelf
Brochure describing our company, garlic fields, aging tanks and factory, plus our product line.

Walker Pharmacal Company

4200 LACLEDE AVENUE
ST. LOUIS, MO 63108

PRID SALVE
(Smile's PRID Salve)
Drawing Salve and Anti-infectant

Active Ingredients: Ichthammol (Ammonium Ichthosulfonate) Phenol (Carbolic Acid) Lead Oleate, Rosin, Bees Wax, Lard.

Description: PRID has a very stiff consistency and is almost black in color.

Indication: PRID is an anti-infective salve, which also serves as a skin protective ointment. As a drawing salve, PRID softens the skin around the foreign body, and assists the natural rejection. PRID also helps to prevent the spread of infection. PRID aids in relieving the discomfort of minor skin irritations, superficial cuts, scratches and wounds. PRID is also helpful in the treatment of boils and carbuncles. PRID has been used with some success in the treatment of acne and furunculosis as well as other skin disorders.

Warning: When applied to fingers or toes, do not use a bandage; use loose gauze so as to not interfere with circulation. Apply according to directions for use and in no case to large areas of the body without a physician's direction. Keep out of eyes.

Caution: If PRID salve is not effective in 10 days, see your physician.

Directions For Use: Wash affected parts thoroughly with hot water; dry and apply PRID at least twice daily on a clean bandage or gauze. After irritation subsides, repeat application once a day for several days. DO NOT irritate by squeezing or pressing skin area.

How Supplied: PRID is packaged in a telescoping orange metal can containing 20 grams of PRID salve.

Wallace Laboratories

P.O. BOX 1001
HALF ACRE ROAD
CRANBURY, NJ 08512

MALTSUPEX®
(malt soup extract)
Powder, Liquid, Tablets

Composition: 'Maltsupex' is a nondiastatic extract from barley malt, which is available in powder, liquid, and tablet form. 'Maltsupex' has a gentle laxative action and promotes soft, easily passed stools. Each Tablet contains 750 mg of 'Maltsupex' and approximately 0.15 to 0.25 mEq of potassium. Tablet Ingredients: acetylated monoglycerides, FD&C Yellow #5, FD&C Yellow #6, flavor (artificial), hydroxypropyl methylcellulose,

AGE	CORRECTIVE*	MAINTENANCE
12 years to ADULTS	Up to 4 scoops twice a day (Take a full glass [8 oz.] of liquid with each dose.)	2 to 4 scoops at bedtime
CHILDREN 6–12 years of age	Up to 2 scoops twice a day (Take a full glass [8 oz.] of liquid with each dose.)	
CHILDREN 2–6 years of age	1 scoop twice a day (Take a full glass [8 oz.] of liquid with each dose.)	
BOTTLE FED INFANTS (Over 1 month)	1 to 2 scoops per day in formula	½ to 1 scoop per day in formula
BREAST FED INFANTS (Over 1 month)	½ scoop in 2–4 oz. of water or fruit juice twice a day	

* Full corrective dosage should be used for 3 or 4 days or until relief is noted. Then continue on maintenance dosage as needed. Use a clean, dry scoop to remove powder. Replace cover tightly to keep out moisture.

polyethylene glycol, povidone, stearic acid, talc, titanium dioxide.
Powder: Each level scoop provides approximately 8 g of Malt Soup Extract.

Other Ingredients: Potassium Hydroxide.
Liquid: Each tablespoonful (½ fl. oz.) contains approximately the equivalent of 16 g Malt Soup Extract Powder. Other ingredients: Sodium propionate and potassium sorbate.

EFFECTIVE, NON-HABIT FORMING

Indications: For relief of occasional constipation. This product generally produces bowel movement in 12 to 72 hours.

Warnings: Do not use laxative products when abdominal pain, nausea or vomiting are present unless directed by a physician. If constipation persists, consult a physician.
If you have noticed a sudden change in bowel habits that persists over a period of 2 weeks, consult a physician before using a laxative.
Keep this and all medications out of the reach of children.
Laxative products should not be used for a period longer than one week unless directed by a physician. Rectal bleeding or failure to have a bowel movement after use of a laxative may indicate a serious condition. Discontinue use and consult with a physician.
'Maltsupex' Powder and Liquid only—Do not use these products except under the advice and supervision of a physician if you have kidney disease.

AGE	CORRECTIVE*	MAINTENANCE
12 years to ADULTS	2 tablespoonfuls twice a day (Take a full glass [8 oz.] of liquid with each dose.)	1 to 2 tablespoonfuls at bedtime
CHILDREN 6–12 years of age	1 to 2 tablespoonfuls once or twice a day (Take a full glass [8 oz.] of liquid with each dose.)	
CHILDREN 2–6 years of age	½ tablespoonful twice a day (Take a full glass [8 oz.] of liquid with each dose.)	
BOTTLE FED INFANTS (Over 1 month)	½ to 2 tablespoonfuls per day in formula	1 to 2 teaspoonfuls per day in formula
BREAST FED INFANTS (Over 1 month)	1 to 2 teaspoonfuls in 2 to 4 oz. water or fruit juice once or twice a day	

* Full corrective dosage should be used for 3 or 4 days or until relief is noted. Then continue on maintenance dosage as needed. Use a clean, dry scoop to remove the liquid. Replace cover tightly after use.

As with any drug, if you are pregnant or nursing a baby, seek the advice of a health professional before using this product.

Precautions: Allow for carbohydrate content in diabetic diets and infant formulas.
Liquid: (67%, 14 g/tablespoon, or 56 calories/tablespoon)
Powder: (83%, 6 g or 24 calories per scoop)
Tablets: 0.6 g per tablet or 3 calories.
Maltsupex **Liquid** contains approximately 23 mg of sodium per tablespoonful. Each scoop of **Powder** contains the equivalent of 8 g of Malt Soup Extract Powder and 1.5 to 2.75 mEq of potassium.
Tablets only: This product contains FD&C Yellow No. 5 (tartrazine) which may cause allergic-type reactions (including bronchial asthma) in certain susceptible individuals. Although the overall incidence of FD&C Yellow No. 5 (tartrazine) sensitivity in the general population is low, it is frequently seen in patients who also have aspirin hypersensitivity.

Directions: General—Drink a full glass (8 ounces) of liquid with each dose. The recommended daily dosage of 'Maltsupex' may vary. Use the smallest dose that is effective and lower dosage as improvement occurs.
'Maltsupex' **Powder**—Each bottle contains a scoop. Each scoopful (which is the equivalent to a standard measuring tablespoon) should be levelled with a knife.

Usual Dosage—Powder:
[See table above.]
Usual Dosage—Liquid:
[See table below.]
Maltsupex **Tablets:** Adult Dosage: The recommended daily dosage of Maltsupex may vary from 12 to 64 g. Start with four tablets (3 g) four times daily (with meals and at bedtime) and adjust dosage according to response. Drink a full glass of (8 oz.) of liquid with each dose.
Preparation Tips: Powder—Add dosage to milk, water, or fruit juice and stir until dissolved. Mixing is easier if added to warm milk or warm water. May be flavored with vanilla or cocoa to make "malteds."
Excellent with hot milk at bedtime. Also available in tablet and liquid forms.
Note: Although shade, texture, taste, and height of contents may vary between bottles, action remains the same.
Liquid: Mixing is easier if Maltsupex Liquid is added to an ounce or two of warm water and stirred. Then add milk, water, or fruit juice and stir until dissolved. May be flavored with vanilla or cocoa to make "malteds." Excellent with hot milk at bedtime. Also available in tablet and powder forms.

How Supplied: 'Maltsupex' is supplied in 8 ounce (NDC 0037-9101-12) and 16 ounce (NDC 0037-9101-08) jars of

Continued on next page

Wallace—Cont.

'Maltsupex' Powder; 8 fluid ounce (NDC 0037-9051-12) and 1 pint (NDC 0037-9051-08) bottles of 'Maltsupex' Liquid; and in bottles of 100 'Maltsupex' Tablets (NDC 0037-9201-01).
'Maltsupex' **Powder** and **Liquid** are Distributed by
WALLACE LABORATORIES
Division of
CARTER-WALLACE, INC.
Cranbury, New Jersey 08512
'Maltsupex' **Tablets** are Manufactured by
WALLACE LABORATORIES
Division of
CARTER-WALLACE, INC.
Cranbury, New Jersey 08512
Rev. 9/92
Shown in Product Identification Section, page 432

RYNA®
(Liquid)
RYNA-C® ©
(Liquid)
RYNA-CX® ©
(Liquid)

Description:
RYNA Liquid—Each 5 mL (one teaspoonful) contains:
Chlorpheniramine maleate .... 2 mg
Pseudoephedrine hydrochloride....30 mg
Other ingredients: flavor (artificial), glycerin, malic acid, sodium benzoate, sorbitol, purified water, in a clear, slightly yellow colored, lemon-vanilla flavored demulcent base containing no sugar, dyes, or alcohol.
RYNA-C Liquid—Each 5 mL (one teaspoonful) contains, in addition:
Codeine phosphate ....10 mg
(WARNING: May be habit-forming)
Other ingredients: flavor (artificial), glycerin, malic acid, purified water, saccharin sodium, sodium benzoate, sorbitol, in a clear, colorless to slightly yellow, cinnamon-flavored, demulcent base containing no sugar, dyes, or alcohol.
RYNA-CX Liquid—Each 5 mL (one teaspoonful) contains:
Codeine phosphate ....10 mg
(WARNING: May be habit-forming)
Pseudoephedrine hydrochloride....30 mg
Guaifenesin ....100 mg
Other ingredients: flavors (artificial), glycerin, glycine, malic acid, povidone, propylene glycol, purified water, saccharin sodium, sorbitol, in a clear, colorless, cherry-vanilla-menthol flavored demulcent base containing no sugar, dyes, or alcohol.

Actions:
Chlorpheniramine maleate in RYNA and RYNA-C is an antihistamine that antagonizes the effects of histamine.
Codeine phosphate in RYNA-C and RYNA-CX is a centrally-acting antitussive that relieves cough.
Pseudoephedrine hydrochloride in RYNA, RYNA-C and RYNA-CX is a sympathomimetic nasal decongestant that acts to shrink swollen mucosa of the respiratory tract.
Guaifenesin in RYNA-CX is an expectorant that increases mucus flow to help prevent dryness and relieve irritated respiratory tract membranes.

Indications:
RYNA: For the temporary relief of nasal congestion due to the common cold, hay fever or other upper respiratory allergies. Temporarily relieves runny nose, sneezing, itching of the nose or throat, and itchy, watery eyes due to hay fever or other respiratory allergies such as allergic rhinitis.
RYNA-C: Temporarily relieves cough, nasal congestion, runny nose and sneezing as may occur with the common cold.
RYNA-CX: Temporarily relieves cough and nasal congestion as may occur with the common cold. Relieves irritated membranes in the respiratory passageways by preventing dryness through increased mucus flow.

Warnings:
For RYNA:
Do not give this product to children taking other medication or to children under 6 years except under the advice and supervision of a physician. Do not exceed recommended dosage because nervousness, dizziness or sleeplessness may occur. Do not take this product for more than 7 days. If symptoms do not improve or are accompanied by fever, consult a doctor. Do not take this product except under the advice and supervision of a physician if you have any of the following symptoms or conditions: high blood pressure; heart disease; thyroid disease; diabetes; asthma; glaucoma; emphysema; chronic pulmonary disease; shortness of breath; difficulty in breathing; or difficulty in urination due to enlargement of the prostate.
For RYNA-C and RYNA-CX:
Adults and children who have a chronic pulmonary disease or shortness of breath, or children who are taking other drugs, should not take these products unless directed by a physician. Do not give these products to children under 6 years of age except under the advice and supervision of a physician. A persistent cough may be a sign of a serious condition. If cough persists for more than one week, tends to recur, or is accompanied by fever, rash or persistent headache, consult a physician. Do not take these products for persistent or chronic cough such as occurs with smoking, asthma, emphysema, or if cough is accompanied by excessive phlegm (mucus) unless directed by a physician. Do not take these products if you have glaucoma, asthma, emphysema, difficulty in breathing, difficulty in urination due to enlargement of the prostate gland, heart disease, high blood pressure, thyroid disease, or diabetes unless directed by a physician. May cause or aggravate constipation.
Do not take these products or give to children for more than 7 days. If symptoms do not improve or are accompanied by fever, consult a physician. Unless directed by a physician, do not exceed recommended dosage because nervousness, dizziness or sleeplessness may occur at higher doses.
For RYNA and RYNA-C:
These products contain an antihistamine which may cause excitability, especially in children, or may cause drowsiness. Alcohol may increase the drowsiness effect. Do not drive motor vehicles, operate machinery, or drink alcoholic beverages while taking these products.
As with any drug, if you are pregnant or nursing a baby, seek the advice of a health professional before using these products.

Drug Interaction Precaution: Do not use these products if you are presently taking a prescription drug for high blood pressure or depression without first consulting your doctor.

Dosage and Administration:
Adults: 2 teaspoonfuls every 6 hours
Children 6 to under 12 years: 1 teaspoonful every 6 hours.
Children under 6 years: Do not take except under the advice and supervision of a physician.
DO NOT EXCEED 4 DOSES IN 24 HOURS.
Ryna-C and Ryna-CX:
A special measuring device should be used to give an accurate dose of these products to children under 6 years of age. Giving a higher dose than recommended by a physician could result in serious side effects for the child.

How Supplied:
RYNA: bottles of 4 fl oz (NDC 0037-0638-66) and one pint (NDC 0037-0638-68).
RYNA-C: bottles of 4 fl oz (NDC 0037-0522-66) and one pint (NDC 0037-0522-68).
RYNA-CX: bottles of 4 fl oz (NDC 0037-0801-66) and one pint (NDC 0037-0801-68).
TAMPER-RESISTANT BAND ON CAP, PRINTED "WALLACE LABORATORIES". DO NOT USE IF BAND IS MISSING OR BROKEN.

Storage:
RYNA: Store below 30°C (86°F).
RYNA-C and RYNA-CX: Store at controlled room temperature. Protect from excessive heat and freezing.
KEEP THESE AND ALL DRUGS OUT OF THE REACH OF CHILDREN. IN CASE OF ACCIDENTAL OVERDOSE, SEEK PROFESSIONAL ASSISTANCE OR CONTACT A POISON CONTROL CENTER IMMEDIATELY.
WALLACE LABORATORIES
Division of
CARTER-WALLACE, Inc.
Cranbury, New Jersey 08512
Rev. 4/91
Shown in Product Identification Section, pages 432 and 433

SYLLACT®
(Psyllium Hydrophilic Mucilloid for Oral Suspension, U.S.P.)
(Powdered Psyllium Seed Husks)

Description: Each rounded teaspoonful of fruit-flavored **Syllact** contains approximately 3.3 g of powdered psyllium seed husks and an equal amount of dextrose as a dispersing agent, and provides about 14 calories. Potassium sorbate, methyl and propylparaben are added as preservatives. Other ingredients: citric acid, dextrose, FD&C Red #40, flavor (artificial), and saccharin sodium.

Actions: The active ingredient in 'Syllact' is hydrophilic mucilloid, nonabsorbable dietary fiber derived from the powdered husks of natural psyllium seed, which acts by increasing the water content and bulk volume of stools. It gives 'Syllact' a bland, non-irritating, laxative action and promotes physiologic evacuation of the bowel.

Indications: 'Syllact' is indicated for the relief of occasional constipation. This product generally produces bowel movement in 12 to 72 hours.

Warnings: Do not use laxative products when abdominal pain, nausea or vomiting are present unless directed by a physician. If you have noticed a sudden change in bowel habits that persists over a period of 2 weeks, consult a physician before using a laxative. Laxative products should not be used for a period longer than 1 week unless directed by a physician. Rectal bleeding or failure to have a bowel movement after use of a laxative may indicate a serious condition. Discontinue use and consult a physician. Bulk-forming agents should not be swallowed dry. They should not be used if impaction or gross intestinal pathology is present.
WARNING: MIX THIS PRODUCT WITH AT LEAST 8 OUNCES (A FULL GLASS) OF WATER OR OTHER FLUID. TAKING THIS PRODUCT WITHOUT ADEQUATE FLUID MAY CAUSE IT TO SWELL AND TO BLOCK YOUR THROAT OR ESOPHAGUS AND MAY CAUSE CHOKING. DO NOT TAKE THIS PRODUCT IF YOU HAVE EVER HAD DIFFICULTY IN SWALLOWING OR HAVE ANY THROAT PROBLEMS.
IF YOU EXPERIENCE CHEST PAIN, VOMITING, OR DIFFICULTY IN SWALLOWING OR BREATHING AFTER TAKING THIS PRODUCT, SEEK IMMEDIATE MEDICAL ATTENTION.
Keep this and all medications out of the reach of children. This product may cause allergic reactions in people sensitive to inhaled or ingested psyllium powder. As with any drug, if you are pregnant or nursing a baby, seek the advice of a health professional before using this product.

Dosage and Administration: Drink a full glass (8 ounces) of liquid with each dose. Do not swallow dry. Use the smallest dose that is effective and lower the dosage as improvement occurs. Use a dry spoon to measure powder. Tighten lid to keep out moisture.
Adults and children 12 years of age and over: Oral dosage is 1 rounded teaspoonful in a full glass of liquid, one to three times daily, before or after meals.
Children 6 to under 12 years of age: ½ to 1 rounded teaspoonful in a full glass of liquid, one to three times daily.
Children under 6 years of age: Consult a physician.
For best results, place powder in a dry glass, add about ½ inch of liquid and stir briskly. Add remainder of liquid, stir and drink immediately. Follow with an additional glass of water if desired.

How Supplied: 'Syllact' Powder—in 10 oz jars (NDC 0037-9501-13).

Rev. 2/91

WALLACE LABORATORIES
Division of
CARTER-WALLACE, INC.
Cranbury, New Jersey 08512

Shown in Product Identification Section, page 433

Warner-Lambert Company
Consumer Health Products Group
201 TABOR ROAD
MORRIS PLAINS, NJ 07950

HALLS® MENTHO-LYPTUS®
Cough Suppressant Tablets

Active Ingredients: Each tablet contains eucalyptus oil and menthol.

Inactive Ingredients: Glucose Syrup, Flavoring, Sugar and Artificial Colors.

Indications: For temporary relief of minor throat irritation and coughs due to colds or inhaled irritants. Makes nasal passages feel clearer.

Warning: A persistent cough or sore throat may be a sign of a serious condition. If cough persists for more than 1 week, tends to recur, or is accompanied by fever, rash or persistent headache, or if sore throat is severe, persistent or accompanied by high fever, headache, nausea, and vomiting, consult a doctor. Do not take this product for sore throat lasting more than 2 days or persistent or chronic cough such as occurs with smoking, asthma, emphysema, or if cough is accompanied by excessive phlegm (mucus) unless directed by a doctor. Keep this and all drugs out of the reach of children.

Dosage and Administration: Adults and children 5 years and over: dissolve one tablet slowly in mouth. Repeat every hour as needed or as directed by a doctor. Children under 5 years: consult a doctor.

How Supplied: Halls Mentho-Lyptus Cough Suppressant Tablets are available in single sticks of 9 tablets each, in 5-stick packs, and in bags of 30 tablets. They are available in five flavors: Regular, Cherry, Honey-Lemon, Ice Blue–Peppermint, and Spearmint.

Shown in Product Identification Section, page 433

HALLS® PLUS
Cough Suppressant Tablets

Active Ingredients: Each centerfilled tablet contains menthol.

Inactive Ingredients: Glucose Syrup, Flavoring, Glycerin, High Fructose Corn Syrup, Sugar and Artificial Colors

Indications: For temporary relief of minor throat irritation and coughs due to colds or inhaled irritants. Makes nasal passages feel clearer.

Warnings: A persistent cough or sore throat may be a sign of a serious condition. If cough persists for more than 1 week, tends to recur, or is accompanied by fever, rash or persistent headache or if sore throat is severe, persistent or accompanied by high fever, headache, nausea, and vomiting, consult a doctor. Do not take this product for sore throat lasting more than 2 days or persistent or chronic cough such as occurs with smoking, asthma, emphysema, or if cough is accompanied by excessive phlegm (mucus) unless directed by a doctor. Keep this and all drugs out of the reach of children.

Dosage and Administration: Adults and children 5 years and over dissolve one centerfilled tablet slowly in mouth. Repeat every hour as needed or as directed by a doctor. Children under 5 years: consult a doctor.

How Supplied: Halls Plus Cough Suppressant Tablets are available in single sticks of 10 tablets each and in bags of 25 tablets. They are available in three flavors: Regular, Cherry and Honey-Lemon.

Shown in Product Identification Section, page 433

HALLS® Vitamin C Drops

Description: Halls Vitamin C Drops are a delicious way to get 100% of the U.S. Recommended Daily Allowance of Vitamin C. Each drop provides 60 mg. of Vitamin C (100% U.S. RDA).

Ingredients: Sugar, Glucose Syrup, Sodium Ascorbate, Citric Acid, Ascorbic Acid, Natural Flavoring and Artificial Color (Including Yellow 5 and Yellow 6).

Indication: Dietary Supplementation.

How Supplied: Halls Vitamin C Drops are available in single sticks of 9 drops each and in bags of 30 drops. They are available in 2 great-tasting assortments: All-natural citrus flavors (tangerine, lemon, sweet grapefruit, lime and orange) and berry flavors (grape, cherry, strawberry and raspberry).

Shown in Product Identification Section, page 433

Continued on next page

Warner-Lambert—Cont.

LISTERINE® Antiseptic

Active Ingredients: Thymol .06%, Eucalyptol .09%, Methyl Salicylate .06% and Menthol .04%. Also contains: Water, Alcohol 26.9%, Benzoic Acid, Poloxamer 407 and Caramel.

Indications: To help prevent and reduce supragingival plaque and gingivitis; for general oral hygiene and bad breath.

Actions: Listerine Antiseptic has been shown to help prevent and reduce supragingival plaque and gingivitis when used in a conscientiously applied program of daily oral hygiene and regular professional care. Its effect on periodontitis has not been determined. Listerine is the only leading nonprescription mouthrinse that has received the American Dental Association's Council on Dental Therapeutics Seal of Acceptance for helping to prevent and reduce plaque above the gumline and gingivitis.

Directions: Rinse full strength for 30 seconds with ⅔ ounce (4 teaspoonfuls) morning and night. If bad breath persists, see your dentist.

How Supplied: Listerine Antiseptic is supplied in 3, 6, 12, 18, 24, 32, 48, 58 fl. oz. bottles, and available to professionals in 3 and 48 fl. oz. bottles and in gallons.

Shown in Product Identification Section, page 433

COOL MINT LISTERINE™

Active Ingredients: Thymol 0.06%, Eucalyptol 0.09%, Methyl Salicylate 0.06%, and Menthol 0.04%.

Inactive Ingredients: Water, Sorbitol Solution, Alcohol 21.6%, Poloxamer 407, Benzoic Acid, Flavoring, Sodium Saccharin, Sodium Citrate, Citric Acid and FD&C Green #3.

Indications: To help prevent and reduce supragingival plaque and gingivitis; for general oral hygiene and bad breath.

Actions: Cool Mint Listerine Antiseptic has been shown to help prevent and reduce supragingival plaque and gingivitis when used in a conscientiously applied program of daily oral hygiene and regular professional care. Its effect on periodontitis has not been determined. Listerine is the only leading nonprescription mouthrinse that has received the American Dental Association's Council on Dental Therapeutics Seal of Acceptance for helping to prevent and reduce plaque above the gumline and gingivitis.

Directions: Rinse full strength for 30 seconds with ⅔ ounce (4 teaspoonfuls) morning and night. If bad breath persists, see your dentist.

How Supplied: Cool Mint Listerine Antiseptic is supplied in 3, 6, 12, 18, 24, 32, 48, 58 fl. oz. bottles, and available to professionals in 3 and 48 fl. oz. bottles and in gallons.

Shown in Product Indentification Section, page 433

LISTERMINT®
Mouthwash with Fluoride

Active Ingredient: Sodium Fluoride (0.02%). Also contains: Water, SD alcohol 38-B (6.65%), glycerin, poloxamer 407, sodium lauryl sulfate, sodium citrate, flavoring, sodium saccharin, zinc chloride, citric acid, D&C Yellow No. 10, FD&C Green No. 3.

Indications: Aids in prevention of dental cavities and freshens breath.

Directions: Adults and children 6 years of age and older: Use twice a day after brushing teeth with toothpaste. Vigorously swish 10 ml. (2 teaspoonfuls) of rinse between teeth for 1 minute and spit out. Do not swallow the rinse. Do not eat or drink for 30 minutes after rinsing.

Warnings: Children under 12 years of age should be supervised in the use of this product. Consult a dentist or physician for use in children under 6 years of age. Developing teeth of children under 6 years of age may become permanently discolored if excessive amounts of fluoride are repeatedly swallowed. This is not a dentifrice and should not be used as a substitute for regular toothbrushing. Keep this and all drugs out of reach of children.

How Supplied: Listermint with Fluoride is supplied to consumers in 6, 12, 18, 24 and 32 fl. oz. bottles and available to professionals in 3 fl. oz. bottles and in gallons.

Shown in Product Identification Section, page 433

LUBRIDERM® LOTION
Skin Lubricant Moisturizer

Composition:
Scented—Contains Water, Mineral Oil, Petrolatum, Sorbitol, Lanolin, Lanolin Alcohol, Stearic Acid, Triethanolamine, Cetyl Alcohol, Fragrance, Butylparaben, Methylparaben, Propylparaben, Sodium Chloride.
Fragrance Free—Contains Water, Mineral Oil, Petrolatum, Sorbitol, Lanolin, Lanolin Alcohol, Stearic Acid, Triethanolamine, Cetyl Alcohol, Butylparaben, Methylparaben, Propylparaben, Sodium Chloride.

Actions and Uses: Lubriderm Lotion is an oil-in-water emulsion indicated for use in softening, soothing and moisturizing dry chapped skin. Lubriderm relieves the roughness, tightness and discomfort associated with dry or chapped skin and helps protect the skin from further drying.
Lubriderm's formula smoothes easily into skin without leaving a greasy feeling.

Administration and Dosage: Apply as often as needed to hands and body to restore and maintain the skin's natural suppleness.

Precautions: For external use only.

How Supplied:
Scented: Available in 1, 4, 8, 12 and 16 fl. oz. plastic bottles, and a 2.5 ounce tube.
Fragrance Free: Available in 1, 8, 12 and 16 fl. oz. plastic bottles, and a 2.5 ounce tube.

Shown in Product Identification Section, page 433

LUBRIDERM® BATH OIL
Skin Conditioning Oil

Composition: Contains Mineral Oil, PPG-15 Stearyl Ether, Oleth-2, Nonoxynol-5, Fragrance, D&C Green No. 6.

Actions and Uses: Lubriderm Skin Conditioning Oil is a lanolin-free, mineral oil–based, bath oil designed for softening and soothing dry skin during the bath. The formula disperses into countless droplets of oil that coat the skin and help lubricate and soften. It is equally effective in hard or soft water and provides an excellent way to moisturize the skin and help counterbalance the drying effects of harsh soaps and hot water.

Administration and Dosage: One to two capfuls in bath, or apply with hand or moistened cloth in shower and rinse. For use as a skin cleanser, rub into wet skin and rinse.

Precautions: Avoid getting in eyes; if this occurs, flush with clear water. When using any bath oil, take precautions against slipping. For external use only.

How Supplied: Available in 8 fl. oz. plastic bottles.

ROLAIDS® Antacid Tablets

Active Ingredient: Dihydroxyaluminum Sodium Carbonate 300 mg.

Inactive Ingredients: Corn Starch, Corn Syrup, Flavoring, Magnesium Stearate and Sugar. May also contain pregelatinized starch. Contains 50 mg. sodium per tablet.

Indications: For the relief of heartburn, sour stomach or acid indigestion and upset stomach associated with these symptoms.

Actions: Rolaids® provides rapid neutralization of stomach acid. Each tablet has acid-neutralizing capacity of 75–80 ml. of 0.1N hydrochloric acid and the ability to maintain the pH of the stomach contents close to 3.5 for a significant period of time.
Due to the relatively low solubility and other physical and chemical properties of dihydroxyaluminum sodium carbonate (DASC), it is for the most part nonabsorbed.

Although sodium is present in DASC, the sodium is available for absorption only when the antacid reacts with stomach acid. When Rolaids are consumed in excess of the amount of acid present in the stomach, this sodium is unavailable for absorption and the active ingredient is passed through the digestive system unchanged, with no sodium released.

Warnings: Keep this and all drugs out of the reach of children. Do not take more than 24 tablets in a 24-hour period, nor use the maximum dosage of this product for more than two weeks, nor use this product if you are on a sodium-restricted diet, except under the advice and supervision of a physician.

Professional Warnings: Prolonged use of aluminum-containing antacids in patients with renal failure may result in or worsen dialysis osteomalacia. Elevated tissue aluminum levels contribute to the development of the dialysis encephalopathy and osteomalacia syndromes. Small amounts of aluminum are absorbed from the gastrointestinal tract and renal excretion of aluminum is impaired in renal failure. Aluminum is not well removed by dialysis because it is bound to albumin and transferrin, which do not cross dialysis membranes. As a result, aluminum is deposited in bone, and dialysis osteomalacia may develop when large amounts of aluminum are ingested orally by patients with impaired renal function. Aluminum forms insoluble complexes with phosphate in the gastrointestinal tract, thus decreasing phosphate absorption. Prolonged use of aluminum-containing antacids by normophosphatemic patients may result in hypophosphatemia if phosphate intake is not adequate. In its more severe forms, hypophosphatemia can lead to anorexia, malaise, muscle weakness, and osteomalacia.

Drug Interaction Precaution: Do not take this product if you are presently taking a prescription antibiotic drug containing any form of tetracycline.

Dosage and Administration: Chew 1 or 2 tablets as symptoms occur. Repeat hourly if symptoms return or as directed by a physician.

How Supplied: Rolaids is available in Original (Peppermint), Spearmint and Wintergreen Flavors. One roll contains 12 tablets; 3-pack contains three 12-tablet rolls; one bottle contains 75 tablets; one bottle contains 150 tablets.

Shown in Product Identification Section, page 433

CALCIUM RICH/SODIUM FREE ROLAIDS® Antacid Tablets

Active Ingredient: Calcium Carbonate 550 mg. per tablet.

Inactive Ingredients:
Cherry Flavor: Colors (Red 27 and Titanium Dioxide), Corn Starch, Flavoring, Light Mineral Oil, Magnesium Stearate, Mannitol, Pregelatinized Starch, Silicon Dioxide and Sucrose.
Assorted Fruit Flavors: Colors (Blue 1, Red 27, Red 40, Titanium Dioxide, Yellow 5 [Tartrazine] and Yellow 6), Corn Starch, Flavoring, Light Mineral Oil, Magnesium Stearate, Mannitol, Pregelatinized Starch, Silicon Dioxide and Sucrose.
Peppermint Flavor: Corn Starch, Flavoring, Light Mineral Oil, Magnesium Stearate, Mannitol, Pregelatinized Starch, Silicon Dioxide and Sucrose.

Indications: For the relief of heartburn, sour stomach or acid indigestion and upset stomach associated with these symptoms.

Actions: Calcium Rich/Sodium Free Rolaids provides rapid neutralization of stomach acid. Each tablet has an acid neutralizing capacity of 110 ml of 0.1N hydrochloric acid and the ability to maintain the pH of the stomach contents at 3.5 or greater for a significant period of time. Each tablet contains less than 0.4 mg of sodium and provides 22% of the Adult U.S. RDA for calcium.

Warnings: Do not take more than 14 tablets in a 24-hour period or use the maximum dosage of this product for more than 2 weeks except under the advice and supervision of a physician. Keep this and all drugs out of the reach of children.

Dosage and Administration: Chew 1 or 2 tablets as symptoms occur. Repeat hourly if symptoms return or as directed by a physician.

How Supplied: Calcium Rich/Sodium Free Rolaids is available in Peppermint, Cherry and Assorted Fruit Flavors. One roll contains 12 tablets: 3-pack contains three 12-tablet rolls; one bottle contains 75 tablets; one bottle contains 150 tablets.

Shown in Product Identification Section, page 433

EXTRA STRENGTH ROLAIDS®
Antacid Plus Anti-Gas Tablets

Active Ingredient: Calcium Carbonate 1000 mg. and Simethicone 25 mg. per tablet.

Inactive Ingredients: Acesulfame Potassium, Colors (FD&C Blue No. 1, FD&C Yellow No. 5 [Tartrazine] and Titanium Dioxide), Corn Syrup, Dextrose, Flavoring, Glyceryl Monostearate, Pregelatinized Starch, Sucrose and Triglycerol Monooleate.

Indications: For the relief of heartburn, sour stomach, acid indigestion and accompanying symptoms of gas.

Actions: Extra Strength Rolaids provides rapid neutralization of stomach acid while at the same time alleviating the symptoms of gas. Each tablet has an acid-neutralizing capacity of 200 ml. of 0.1N hydrochloric acid and the ability to maintain the pH of the stomach contents at 3.5 or greater for a significant period of time. Each tablet contains less than 0.4 mg of sodium and provides 40% of the adult U.S. RDA for calcium.

Warnings: Do not take more than 8 tablets in a 24-hour period or use the maximum dosage of this product for more than 2 weeks except under the advice and supervision of a physician. Keep this and all drugs out of the reach of children.

Dosage and Administration: Chew 1 or 2 tablets as symptoms occur. Repeat hourly if symptoms return or as directed by a physician.

How Supplied: Extra Strength Rolaids is available in Assorted Mint Flavors. One roll contains 10 tablets: 3-pack contains three 10-tablet rolls; one bottle contains 55 tablets; one bottle contains 110 tablets.

Shown in Product Identification Section, page 433

SOOTHERS® Throat Drops
From the makers of Halls

Active Ingredients: Each centerfilled tablet contains menthol 2 mg.

Inactive Ingredients: Colors (Including Yellow 6), Corn Syrup, Flavoring, Glycerin, High Fructose Corn Syrup, Honey and Sugar.

Indications: For temporary relief of occasional minor irritation, pain, sore mouth, and sore throat or pain associated with canker sores.

Warnings: If sore throat is severe, persists for more than 2 days, is accompanied or followed by fever, headache, rash, nausea, or vomiting, consult a doctor promptly. If sore mouth symptoms do not improve in 7 days, see your dentist or doctor promptly. Keep this and all drugs out of the reach of children.

Dosage and Administration: Adults and children 5 years of age and older: dissolve 1 drop slowly in mouth. May be repeated every 2 hours as needed or as directed by a dentist or doctor. Children under 5 years of age: consult a dentist or doctor.

How Supplied: Soothers Throat Drops are available in packages of 10 tablets each and in bags of 25 tablets. They are available in cherry and orange flavors.

Shown in Product Identification Section, page 433

Products are indexed alphabetically in the **PINK SECTION.**

Water-Jel Technologies, Inc.

243 VETERANS BLVD.
CARLSTADT, NJ 07072

WATER–JEL® Sterile Burn Dressings
One-Step Emergency Burn Care Product for all types of burns
WATER-JEL® Burn Jel™
Topical for minor burns

Key Facts: Water-Jel is a unique, patented one-step product ideal for emergency first aid burn care. The scientifically formulated gel combines with a special carrier material to: Ease pain, prevent burn progression, cool the skin and stabilize skin temperature, protect the covered wound from contamination, facilitate removal of burnt clothing or jewelry; Won't harm skin or eyes, does not require a water source to continue cooling, and is non-allergenic.
Water-Jel Burn Jel is a new topical for minor burns that works fast and provides lasting relief. It contains the active ingredient, lidocaine, thereby offering the pain relief capabilities of lidocaine, and in combination with the Water-Jel gel, also cools and soothes. It is water-based, dissipates heat and is easily removed.

Major Uses: Water-Jel Sterile Burn Dressings are used as Emergency First Aid for all types of burns. . . Fire, steam, heat, electrical, boiling water.
Water-Jel Burn Jel is a topical used for long-lasting relief of minor burns.

Safety Information: Chemical burns must be thoroughly flushed before applying Water-Jel. Consult a physician if the burn is severe, covers an area larger than your palm, or involves your face.

Description: Each Sterile Burn Dressing packet contains a gel-soaked polyester fabric.
The gel is an off-white translucent color. It has a characteristic odor. It is sterile. A freezing point of −15°C and a boiling point of +92°C. The gel is a proprietary formulation of natural gums and oils in a preserved, sterile, easily washed-off aqueous base.
Water-Jel Burn Jel is available in a 4 fl. oz. squeeze bottle or in single dose, foil packets each ⅛ oz (25 packets per dispenser box).

Indications: Water-Jel Sterile Burn Dressings provide Emergency First Aid for all burns. The Burn Dressings provide fast relief of pain due to burns. It soothes and cools the burned area and protects the covered wound from contamination. It stops burn progress and is easily removed without re-injuring the wound. It is non-allergenic.
Water-Jel Burn Jel is a topical that offers the same benefits as the Water-Jel dressings plus lidocaine for fast, lasting pain relief of minor burns.

Application: Simply open the Water-Jel Sterile Dressing package and apply the dressing to the burned area. Pour the excess gel from the package onto the dressing. Keep in place for approximately 15 to 20 minutes.
Water-Jel Burn Jel is applied directly to the wound. Simply squeeze the gel out or open the packet & pour.

Warning: In the case of chemical burns, the wound must be thoroughly flushed before applying Water-Jel. Consult a physician if the burn is severe, covers an area larger than your palm, or involves the face.

How Supplied: Water-Jel Sterile Burn Dressings are available in several sizes for use on different size burns—2″×2″; 2″×6″; 4″×4″; 4″×16″; and 8″×18″. Water-Jel is contained in heat-sealed foil packets.
Water-Jel Burn Jel is available in a 4 oz squeeze bottle and in single-dose ⅛ oz foil packets. The single-dose packets are packaged 25 to a dispenser box. Squeeze bottle and dispenser box are designed to fit first aid kits and medicine cabinets.

EDUCATIONAL MATERIAL

"Since the Dawn of Civilization . . . "
4-page, full color brochure.
Descriptive use and application of all Water-Jel® Fire Rescue, Heat Shield and Emergency Burn care products.
"At Last . . . A Burn Topical that Measures up . . . "
2-page, full-color brochure. Descriptive use and application of Water-Jel Burn Jel, a 'topical' for minor burns.
"Technical Specifications"
2-page, in-depth specifications of all Water-Jel® products.
"Presentation Video"
11-minute video on the use of Water-Jel® products.

IDENTIFICATION PROBLEM?
Consult the
Product Identification Section
where you'll find
products pictured
in full color.

Wellness International, Inc.

1501 LUNA, SUITE 102
CARROLLTON, TX 75006

FLORA-PLUS™ MULTIPLE LACTOBACILLI BACTERIUM including Acidophilus, Bulgaricus, Bifidus with "Transporters" 84 Capsules

The **FLORA-PLUS** complex uses a combination of lyophilized freeze-dried bacteria presented in 3 individual strains: 1) lactobacillus acidophilus, 2) lactobacillus bulgaricus and 3) lactobacillus bifidus, each providing no less than 500 million viable organisms per gram. To serve as a biological foundation for the lactobacillus bacterium, a high protein whey isolate is used to provide an ideal food base in which the bacteria can multiply. Whey is predigested by the lactobacilli during the processing of cheese and contains lactic acid which contributes to the acidic environment that is to be established.

Recommended Use: 1 capsule taken 3 times daily. At least a minimum of 15 minutes before each meal. REFRIGERATE AFTER OPENING.

Ingredients: 3 capsules contains:
[See table top of next page.]
Blended in a base of the following substances: Lactobacillus acidophilus, Lactobacillus bifidus, Lactobacillus bulgaricus, whey protein isolate, sodium gluconate, glycine, L-Methionine.
In defining FERMENTATIVE YIELDING REACTIONARY EFFECT, the body's internal environment sets the stage for focus. The human body is exposed to a multitude of negative or toxin-generating bacteria. These sources can interfere with absorption percentages of the health sustaining nutrients we ingest daily. The **FLORA-PLUS** formula was designed to re-introduce positive flora that our body carries but often shows a deficiency of as a consequence of poor diet, excessive toxins antibiotics, and a host of other environmental impurities. By yielding (making available), to the intestinal tract one of the body's best defense mechanisms (lactobacilli bacteria), an enhanced acidic environment is made possible to react to unwanted bacteria and related toxins effecting that response. The lactobacilli must survive the secretion of strong stomach acids on their journey through the digestive network. With **FLORA-PLUS**, a protective "TRANSPORTER" group has been used to protect the bacterium during the crucial stage of digestion, allowing for increased availability of the formula and as a result, a substantial impact in the battle of internal pollution.
KEEP IN A COOL, DRY AREA.

Manufactured Exclusively for
Wellness International Network, Inc.
Dallas, TX 75006

		%USRDA
VITAMIN C (Ascorbic Acid)	30 mg	50
VITAMIN B6 (Pyridoxal-5 Phosphate)	24 mg	1200
CALCIUM (Calcium Carbonate)	75 mg	10

NUTRA-LEAN™ NUTRITIONAL DRINK MEAL REPLACEMENT WITH 8 OZ. FORTIFIED NONFAT MILK

Nutra-Lean Nutritional Drink is scientifically designed for effective weight management which promotes the loss of body fat, while maintaining lean body mass (muscle, bone, internal organs). **Nutra-Lean Nutritional Drink** is recommended as part of a dietary plan to achieve low fat, low cholesterol, low sodium, high fiber diet.
[See table below.]

Ingredients: Protein Blend (Caseinate, Soy Protein Isolate, Whey Protein Concentrate, dl-Methionine, Chickpea Protein Flour), Fructose, Fiber Blend (Guar Gum, Oat Fiber, Cellulose Fiber, Carrageenan, Apple Fiber, Pectin), Maltodextrin, Natural Flavors, Magnesium Oxide, Dicalcium Phosphate, Lecithin, Potassium Chloride, Bee Pollen, Calcium Ascorbate, Papain, Bromelain, Vitamin E Acetate, Niacin, Vegetable Blend (Beet Root, Broccoli, Tomato, Carrot and Cauliflower Powders), Zinc Oxide, Pyridoxine Hydrochloride, Vitamin D, Folic Acid, Cobalamin.
Nutra-Lean Nutritional Drink is a delicious limited calorie drink containing unique blends of high quality protein, carbohydrate and dietary fiber, designed for weight control.

High P.E.R. Protein

Protein efficiency ration (P.E.R.) is a measure of protein quality and depends on a complete spectrum of essential amino acids with a P.E.R. of 2.5 as a standard of high quality protein. Nutra-Lean Nutritional Drink, with its unique protein blend, has a P.E.R. of 2.5.

***Essential Amino Acids**
Alanine
Arginine
Aspartic Acid
Cysteine
Glutamic Acid
Glycine
*Histidine
*Isoleucine
*Leucine
*Lysine
*Methionine
*Phenylalanine
Proline
Serine
*Threonine
*Tyrosine
*Valine

Recommended Use: Add contents of one packet of **Nutra-Lean Nutritional Drink** to 8 ounces of water, juice or nonfat milk. Add 2–3 ice cubes and mix thoroughly with a hand or power blender. For added flavor, blend in a banana and/or other favorite fruit. (Optional: sweeten to taste with a low calorie sweetener.)

Nutrition Information (Per Serving)
Serving Size .... 28.35 gm (1 oz.)
Servings Per Packet 1

		WITH 8 OZ. VITAMIN A & D FORTIFIED NONFAT MILK
Calories	100	190
Protein	9 gm	18 gm
Carbohydrate	13 gm	25 gm
Fat	less than 1 gm	1 gm
Cholesterol	0 mg	10 mg
Sodium	70 mg	200 mg
Potassium	200 mg	620 mg
Fiber	3 gm	3 gm
Percentage of U.S. Recommended Daily Allowances (% U.S. RDA)		
Protein	20	40
Vitamin A	*	10
Vitamin C	100	100
Thiamine	*	6
Riboflavin	*	25
Niacin	100	100
Calcium	25	60
Iron	*	*
Vitamin D	100	120
Vitamin E	100	100
Folic Acid	100	10
Vitamin B6	100	100
Phosphorous	15	40
Vitamin B12	100	110
Magnesium	100	110
Zinc	35	40

*Contains less than 2% of the U.S. RDA of these nutrients

Co-Nutrients:
Bee Pollen ....100 mg   Papain ....50 mg   Bromelain ....50 mg

NOTE: When mixing with one serving of **Tri-Lean,** use 12 oz. of water.

Caution: It is advisable to consult with a physician before beginning any weight loss program. Pregnant and lactating women and individuals in poor health or with known medical conditions should diet only under the supervision of a physician.

Manufactured Exclusively for
Wellness International Network, Inc.
Dallas, TX 75006

TRI-LEAN™ VITAMIN/MINERAL AMINO ACID ORANGE FLAVOR COMPLEX ADDITIVE

Tri-Lean is a delicious blend of vitamins, minerals and amino acids in an orange flavor formulation with the ideal ratios for the ultimate approach for stress related and dietary deficiencies of today's lifestyle.
Mixed with **Nutra-Lean** gives you a rich creamy serving of energy, needed nutrients in a natural orange flavored drink.
Directions: Add contents of one packet **Tri-Lean** to one serving (1 oz.) of **Nutra-Lean.**
NOTE: Tri-Lean may be mixed with 8 oz. of water and served separately. For best results, blend with 2-3 ice cubes.
This product is free of fillers, binders, corn, milk, wheat, and yeast.
[See table top of next page.]

Ingredients: Tri-lean Carbohydrate Blend (Sucrose, Maltodextrin, Fructose, and Dextrose), Tri-lean Vitamin, Mineral and Amino Acid Blend (Magnesium Oxide, L-Carnitine, Choline Bitartrate, Tricalcium Phosphate, Vitamin E Acetate, Ascorbic Acid, Potassium Chloride, Inositol, Citrus Bioflavonoids, Niacin, D-Calcium Pantothenate, Vitamin A Palmitate, Beta Carotene, Ferrous Fumarate, Zinc Oxide, L-Glutamine, Pyridoxine Hydrochloride, Riboflavin, L-Phenylalanine, Thiamine Hydrochloride, L-Methionine, Cyanocobalamin, Vitamin D, Glycine, Folic Acid, D-Biotin, Potassium Iodide, Chromium Picolinate, and Sodium Selenite), Citric Acid, Natural Orange Flavor.
Keep out of reach of children.

Manufactured Exclusively for
Wellness International Network, Inc.
Dallas, TX 75006

EDUCATIONAL MATERIAL

1. PHD Information Booklet—Available for Purchase $2.50
2. Audio Tape by Steven E. Langer, MD—Available for Purchase $5.00
3. Research Papers on Flora-Plus Product—Free

Nutrition Information Per Serving:

Serving Size	18 gm (0.6 oz.)				
Servings Per Packet	1				
Calories	60	Carbohydrate	15 gm	Sodium	0 mg
Protein	0 gm	Fat	0 gm		

PERCENTAGE OF U.S. RECOMMENDED DAILY ALLOWANCE (USRDA)

Vitamin A (Vitamin A Palmitate from Beta Carotene)	100	Vitamin E	100	*Choline	100 mg
Vitamin C	100	Vitamin B6	100	*Inositol	50 mg
Thiamine	100	Folic Acid	100	*Potassium	35 mg
Riboflavin	100	Vitamin B12	100	*Bioflavonoids	25 mg
Niacin	100	Phosphorous	5	*Chromium	70 mcg
Calcium	10	Magnesium	50	*Selenium	20 mcg
Iron	10	Zinc	25	*L-Carnitine	200 mg
Vitamin D	100	Biotin	100	*L-Glutamine	3542 mcg
		Pantothenic Acid	100	*L-Phenylalanine	1657 mcg
		Iodine	50	*L-Methonine	886 mcg
				*Glycine	500 mcg

Contains less than 2% of U.S. RDA of Protein
*No U.S. RDA Established for these nutrients

Whitehall Laboratories Inc.

Division of American Home Products Corporation
685 THIRD AVENUE
NEW YORK, NY 10017

ADVIL®
[*ad 'vĭl*]
Ibuprofen Tablets, USP
Ibuprofen Caplets
Pain Reliever/Fever Reducer

WARNING: ASPIRIN-SENSITIVE PATIENTS. Do not take this product if you have had a severe allergic reaction to aspirin, e.g.—asthma, swelling, shock or hives, because even though this product contains no aspirin or salicylates, cross-reactions may occur in patients allergic to aspirin.

Active Ingredient: Each tablet or caplet contains Ibuprofen 200 mg.

Inactive Ingredients: Acacia, Acetylated Monoglycerides, Beeswax or Carnauba Wax, Calcium Sulfate, Colloidal Silicon Dioxide, Dimethicone, Iron Oxide, Lecithin, Pharmaceutical Glaze, Povidone, Sodium Benzoate, Sodium Carboxymethylcellulose, Starch, Stearic Acid, Sucrose, Titanium Dioxide.

Indications: For the temporary relief of minor aches and pains associated with the common cold, headache, toothache, muscular aches, backache, for the minor pain of arthritis, for the pain of menstrual cramps and for reduction of fever.

Dosage and Administration: Adults: Take one tablet or caplet every 4 to 6 hours while symptoms persist. If pain or fever does not respond to one tablet or caplet, two tablets or caplets may be used but do not exceed six tablets or caplets in 24 hours unless directed by a doctor. The smallest effective dose should be used. Take with food or milk if occasional and mild heartburn, upset stomach, or stomach pain occurs with use. Consult a doctor if these symptoms are more than mild or if they persist. Children: Do not give this product to children under 12 except under the advice and supervision of a doctor.

Warnings: Do not take for pain for more than 10 days or for fever for more than 3 days unless directed by a doctor. If pain or fever persists or gets worse, if new symptoms occur, or if the painful area is red or swollen, consult a doctor. These could be signs of serious illness. If you are under a doctor's care for any serious condition, consult a doctor before taking this product. As with aspirin and acetaminophen, if you have any condition which requires you to take prescription drugs or if you have had any problems or serious side effects from taking any nonprescription pain reliever, do not take this product without first discussing it with your doctor. **IF YOU EXPERIENCE ANY SYMPTOMS WHICH ARE UNUSUAL OR SEEM UNRELATED TO THE CONDITION FOR WHICH YOU TOOK IBUPROFEN, CONSULT A DOCTOR BEFORE TAKING ANY MORE OF IT.** Although ibuprofen is indicated for the same conditions as aspirin and acetaminophen, it should not be taken with them except under a doctor's direction. Do not combine this product with any other ibuprofen-containing product. As with any drug, if you are pregnant or nursing a baby, seek the advice of a health professional before using this product. **IT IS ESPECIALLY IMPORTANT NOT TO USE IBUPROFEN DURING THE LAST 3 MONTHS OF PREGNANCY UNLESS SPECIFICALLY DIRECTED TO DO SO BY A DOCTOR BECAUSE IT MAY CAUSE PROBLEMS IN THE UNBORN CHILD OR COMPLICATIONS DURING DELIVERY.** Keep this and all drugs out of the reach of children. In case of accidental overdose, seek professional assistance or contact a poison control center immediately.

How Supplied: Coated tablets in bottles of 8, 24, 50 (non-child resistant size), 100, 165 and 250. Coated caplets in bottles of 8, 24, 50 (non-child resistant size), 100, 165, and 250. Coated tablets in thermoform packaging of 8.

Storage: Store at room temperature; avoid excessive heat (40°C, 104°F).

Shown in Product Identification Section, page 433

ADVIL® Cold and Sinus
(formerly CoADVIL®)
Ibuprofen/Pseudoephedrine Caplets*
Pain Reliever/Fever Reducer/Nasal Decongestant

***Oval-Shaped tablets**

WARNING: ASPIRIN-SENSITIVE PATIENTS. Do not take this product if you have had a severe allergic reaction to aspirin, eg, asthma, swelling, shock or hives, because even though this product contains no aspirin or salicylates, cross-reactions may occur in patients allergic to aspirin.

Indications: For temporary relief of symptoms associated with the common cold, sinusitis or flu, including nasal congestion, headache, fever, body aches, and pains.

Directions: *Adults:* Take 1 caplet every 4 to 6 hours while symptoms persist. If symptoms do not respond to 1 caplet, 2 caplets may be used, but do not exceed 6 caplets in 24 hours unless directed by a doctor. The smallest effective dose should be used. Take with food or milk if occasional and mild heartburn, upset stomach, or stomach pain occurs with use. Consult a doctor if these symptoms are more than mild or if they persist. *Children:* Do not give this product to children under 12 years of age except under the advice and supervision of a doctor.

Warnings: Do not take for colds for more than 7 days or for fever for more than 3 days unless directed by a doctor. If the cold or fever persists or gets worse, or if new symptoms occur, consult a doctor. These could be signs of serious illness. As with aspirin and acetaminophen, if you have any condition which requires you to take prescription drugs or if you have had any problems or serious side effects from taking any nonprescription pain reliever, do not take this product without first discussing it with your doctor. IF YOU EXPERIENCE ANY SYMPTOMS WHICH ARE UNUSUAL OR SEEM UNRELATED TO THE CONDITION FOR WHICH YOU TOOK THIS PRODUCT, CONSULT A DOCTOR BEFORE TAKING ANY MORE OF IT. If you are under a doctor's care for any serious condition, consult a doctor before taking this product.

Do not exceed recommended dosage because at higher doses nervousness, dizziness, or sleeplessness may occur. Do not take this product if you have high blood pressure, heart disease, diabetes, thyroid disease or difficulty in urination due to enlargement of the prostate gland, except under the advice and supervision of a doctor.

Drug Interaction Precaution: Do not take this product if you are presently taking a prescription drug for high blood pressure or depression without first consulting your doctor. Do not combine this product with other nonprescription pain relievers. Do not combine this product with any other ibuprofen-containing product. As with any drug, if you are pregnant or nursing a baby, seek the advice of a health professional before using this product.

IT IS ESPECIALLY IMPORTANT NOT TO USE THIS PRODUCT DURING THE LAST 3 MONTHS OF PREGNANCY UNLESS SPECIFICALLY DIRECTED TO DO SO BY A DOCTOR BECAUSE IT MAY CAUSE PROBLEMS IN THE UNBORN CHILD OR COMPLICATIONS DURING DELIVERY. Keep this and all drugs out of the reach of children. In case of accidental overdose, seek professional assistance or contact a poison control center immediately.

Active Ingredients: Each caplet contains Ibuprofen 200 mg and Pseudoephedrine HCl 30 mg.

Inactive Ingredients: Carnauba or Equivalent Wax, Croscarmellose Sodium, Iron Oxides, Methylparaben, Microcrystalline Cellulose, Propylparaben, Silicon Dioxide, Sodium Benzoate, Sodium Lauryl Sulfate, Starch, Stearic Acid, Sucrose, Titanium Dioxide.

How Supplied: Advil® Cold and Sinus is an oval-shaped tan-colored caplet supplied in consumer bottles of 40 and blister packs of 20. Medical samples are available in a 2's pouch dispenser.

Storage: Store at room temperature; avoid excessive heat (40°C, 104°F).

Shown in Product Identification Section, page 433

Maximum Strength ANBESOL® Gel and Liquid

[an'ba-sol"]

Oral Anesthetic/Antiseptic

Regular Strength ANBESOL® Gel and Liquid

Oral Anesthetic/Antiseptic

BABY ANBESOL®

Original and Grape Flavors

Oral Anesthetic Gel

Description: Anbesol is an oral anesthetic/antiseptic which is available in a Maximum Strength and Regular Strength gel and liquid. Baby Anbesol, available in gel, is an anesthetic only and is alcohol-free. Baby Anbesol is available in original and grape flavors.

The Maximum Strength formulations contain Benzocaine 20% and Alcohol 60%.

The Regular Strength formulations contain Benzocaine 6.3%, Phenol 0.5% and Alcohol 70%.

The Baby Anbesol Gels contain Benzocaine 7.5%.

Indications: Maximum Strength and Regular Strength Anbesol are indicated for the temporary relief of pain associated with toothache, canker sore, cold sore/fever blister, minor dental procedures, or minor injury or irritation of the mouth and gums caused by dentures or orthodontic appliances. Baby Anbesol Gels are indicated for the temporary relief of sore gums due to teething in infants and children 4 months of age and older.

Actions: Temporarily deadens sensations of nerve endings to provide relief of pain and discomfort; reduces oral bacterial flora temporarily as an aid in oral hygiene (Regular and Maximum Strengths only).

Warnings: Do not use for more than 7 days unless directed by a doctor/dentist. If sore mouth symptoms do not improve in 7 days; if irritation or pain persists or worsens; or if swelling, rash or fever develops, see your doctor/dentist promptly. Do not exceed recommended dosage. Do not use this product if you have an allergy to local anesthetics such as procaine, butacaine, benzocaine, or other "caine" anesthetics. Fever and nasal congestion are not symptoms of teething and may indicate the presence of infection. If these symptoms persist, consult your doctor. Avoid contact with eyes. Keep this and all drugs out of the reach of children. In case of accidental overdose, seek professional assistance or contact a poison control center immediately.

Maximum and Regular Strengths: EXTREMELY FLAMMABLE. KEEP AWAY FROM FIRE OR FLAME. AVOID SMOKING DURING APPLICATION AND UNTIL PRODUCT HAS DRIED.

Dosage and Administration: Maximum Strength and Regular Strength Anbesol: Gel—To open tube, cut tip on score mark with scissors. Liquid—Wipe liquid on with cotton, cotton swab, or fingertip.

Adults and children 2 years of age and older: Apply to the affected area on or within the mouth up to 4 times daily or as directed by a doctor/dentist. Children under 12 years of age should be supervised in the use of this product. Children under 2 years of age: Consult a doctor/dentist.

For gels only: For denture irritation, apply thin layer to affected area and do not reinsert dental work until irritation/pain is relieved. Rinse mouth well before reinserting. If irritation/pain persists, contact your doctor/dentist. NOT FOR USE UNDER DENTURES AND OTHER DENTAL WORK.

Baby Anbesol and Grape Baby Anbesol: To open tube, cut tip on score mark with scissors. Apply to the affected area not more than 4 times daily or as directed by a doctor/dentist. For infants under 4 months of age there is no recommended dosage or treatment except under the advice and supervision of a doctor/dentist.

Inactive Ingredients:

Maximum Strength Gel: Carbomer 934P, D&C Yellow #10, FD&C Blue #1, FD&C Red #40, Flavor, PEG-12, Saccharin.

Maximum Strength Liquid: D&C Yellow #10, FD&C Blue #1, FD&C Red #40, Flavor, PEG-8, Saccharin.

Regular Strength Gel: Camphor, Carbomer 934P, D&C Red #33, D&C Yellow #10, FD&C Blue #1, FD&C Yellow #6, Flavor, Glycerin.

Regular Strength Liquid: Camphor, Glycerin, Menthol, Potassium Iodide, Povidone Iodine.

Original Baby Gel: Carbomer 934P, D&C Red #33, Disodium EDTA, Flavor, Glycerin, PEG-8, Saccharin, Water.

Grape Baby Gel: Benzoic Acid, Carbomer 934P, D&C Red #33, Disodium EDTA, FD&C Blue #1, Flavor, Glycerin, Methylparaben, PEG-8, Propylparaben, Saccharin, Water.

How Supplied: All Gels in .25 oz (7.2 g) tubes, Maximum Strength Liquid in .31 fl oz (9 mL) bottle, Regular Liquid in two sizes—.31 fl oz (9 mL) and .74 fl oz (22 mL) bottles.

Shown in Product Identification Section, page 434

Maximum Strength ARTHRITIS PAIN FORMULA™

[är'thrīt-is' pān' for-mye-la]

Analgesic Caplets With Aspirin and Buffers

(See *1993 Physicians' Desk Reference.*)

COMPOUND W®

['käm-pound W]

Salicylic Acid Wart Remover Liquid and Gel

(See *1993 Physicians' Desk Reference.*)

Continued on next page

Whitehall—Cont.

DENOREX®
[*dĕn 'ō-reks*]
Medicated Shampoo
DENOREX®
Mountain Fresh Herbal Scent Medicated Shampoo
DENOREX®
Medicated Shampoo and Conditioner
DENOREX®
Extra Strength Medicated Shampoo
DENOREX®
Extra Strength Medicated Shampoo with Conditioners

Description: The Shampoo (Regular and Mountain Fresh Herbal) and the Shampoo and Conditioner contain Coal Tar Solution 9.0% (equivalent to 1.8% Coal Tar). The Extra Strength Shampoo and the Extra Strength Shampoo with Conditioners contain Coal Tar Solution 12.5% (equivalent to 2.5% Coal Tar).

Indications: Relieves and helps eliminate the itching, flaking, scaling and irritation associated with dandruff, seborrheic dermatitis and psoriasis.

Actions: Denorex Shampoo is an antiseborrheic and antipruritic which loosens and softens scales and crusts. Coal tar helps correct abnormalities of keratinization by decreasing epidermal proliferation and dermal infiltration.

Warnings: For external use only. Avoid contact with eyes. If contact occurs, rinse eyes thoroughly with water. If condition worsens or does not improve after regular use of this product as directed, consult a doctor. Use caution in exposing skin to sunlight after applying this product. It may increase your tendency to sunburn for up to 24 hours after application. Do not use for prolonged periods without consulting a doctor. Do not use this product with other forms of psoriasis therapy such as ultraviolet radiation or prescription drugs unless directed to do so by a doctor. If condition covers a large area of the body, consult your doctor before using this product. Keep this and all drugs out of the reach of children. In case of accidental ingestion, seek professional assistance or contact a poison control center immediately.

Directions: Shake well. Lather, rinse thoroughly; repeat. The scalp may tingle slightly during treatment. For best results use at least twice a week or as directed by a doctor.

Inactive Ingredients:
Regular Shampoo: Chloroxylenol, Lauramide DEA, Menthol, Stearic Acid, TEA-Lauryl Sulfate, Water, Alcohol 7.5% by volume.
Mountain Fresh Regular Shampoo: Chloroxylenol, Fragrance, Hydroxypropyl Methylcellulose, Lauramide DEA, Menthol, Stearic Acid, TEA-Lauryl Sulfate, Water, Alcohol 7.5% by volume.
Shampoo and Conditioner: Chloroxylenol, Citric Acid, Fragrance, Hydroxypropyl Methylcellulose, Lauramide DEA, Menthol, PEG-27 Lanolin, Polyquaternium-11, TEA-Lauryl Sulfate, Water, Alcohol 7.5% by volume.
Extra Strength Shampoo: Chloroxylenol, FD&C Red #40, Fragrance, Glycol Distearate, Hydroxypropyl Methylcellulose, Lauramide DEA, Menthol, TEA-Lauryl Sulfate, Water, Alcohol 10.4% by volume.
Extra Strength Shampoo with Conditioners: Chloroxylenol, Citric Acid, Cocodimonium Hydrolyzed Protein, FD&C Red #40, Fragrance, Glycol Distearate, Hydroxypropyl Methylcellulose, Lauramide DEA, Menthol, PEG-27 Lanolin, Polyquaternium-6, TEA-Lauryl Sulfate, Water, Alcohol 10.4% by volume.

How Supplied:
Available in 4 oz., 8 oz. and 12 oz. bottles.
Shown in Product Identification Section, page 434

DERMOPLAST®
[*der 'mō-plăst*]
Spray and Lotion
Anesthetic Pain Relief With Benzocaine

(See *1993 Physicians' Desk Reference.*)

DRISTAN ORAL PRODUCTS

[See table top of next page.]

DRISTAN® JUICE MIX-IN™
Nasal Decongestant/Analgesic/ Cough Suppressant

[See table top of next page.]

Description: Each packet contains: Acetaminophen 500 mg, Pseudoephedrine HCl 60 mg, and Dextromethorphan HBr 20 mg.

Indications: DRISTAN® JUICE MIX-IN™ contains a **cough suppressant** to temporarily relieve irritating coughs; a **decongestant** to temporarily relieve nasal congestion and sinus pressure and reduce swollen nasal passages; and an **analgesic** to temporarily relieve headache, body aches, minor sore throat pain and reduce fever.

Actions: Acetaminophen is an analgesic and antipyretic. Pseudoephedrine HCl is an oral nasal decongestant. Dextromethorphan HBr is a cough suppressant.

Warnings: Do not take this product for persistent cough such as occurs with smoking, asthma or emphysema, or if cough is accompanied by excessive secretions (mucus), unless directed by a physician. A persistent cough may be a sign of a serious condition. If cough persists for more than 1 week, recurs, or is accompanied by fever, rash or persistent headache, consult a physician. Persons with asthma, glaucoma, diabetes, heart or thyroid disease or difficulty in urination due to enlarged prostate gland should use only as directed by a physician. *Drug Interaction Precaution:* Do not take this product if you are presently taking a prescription drug for high blood pressure or depression, or a monoamine oxidase inhibitor, unless directed by a doctor. Do not exceed recommended dosage because at higher doses nervousness, dizziness, or sleeplessness may occur. If symptoms do not improve within 7 days or are accompanied by high fever, discontinue use and see a physician. If sore throat is severe, persists for more than 2 days, is accompanied by fever, headache, rash, nausea or vomiting, consult a doctor promptly. As with any drug, if you are pregnant or nursing a baby, seek the advice of a health professional before using this product. Do not give to children under 12. Keep this and all drugs out of the reach of children. In case of accidental overdose, seek professional assistance or contact a poison control center immediately. Prompt medical attention is critical for adults as well as for children even if you do not notice any signs or symptoms.
Do not mix with any juice to which you have had an allergic reaction in the past.

Directions: Adults and Children 12 years of age and over: Mix one packet in 6 oz. of your favorite juice. Stir briskly for at least 15 seconds. Drink promptly. May repeat every 4 hours, not to exceed 4 doses in 24 hours. Do not give to children under 12.

Inactive Ingredients: Hydroxypropyl Methylcellulose, Povidone, Silica, Starch, Stearic Acid, Sucrose, Tricalcium Phosphate.

How Supplied: In packages containing 1 (trial size), 5 or 10 individual use packets.
Patent Pending
Shown in Product Identification Section, page 434

DRISTAN®
[*drĭs 'tăn*]
Nasal Decongestant Spray
Menthol Nasal Spray

Description: Dristan Nasal Spray and Dristan Menthol Nasal Spray contain Phenylephrine HCl 0.5%, Pheniramine Maleate 0.2%.

Actions: Phenylephrine HCl is a sympathomimetic agent that constricts the smaller arterioles of the nasal passages producing a gentle and predictable decongesting effect.

Indications: For the temporary relief of nasal congestion due to colds, hay fever, or other upper respiratory allergies.

Warnings: Do not exceed recommended dosage because burning, stinging, sneezing or increase of nasal discharge may occur. Do not use this product for more than 3 days. If symptoms persist, consult a doctor. Do not use this

	Per Tablet/Caplet/Packet					
	Dristan Juice Mix-In Packet	**Max. Str. Dristan Cold*** Gel Caplet	**Max. Str. Dristan Cold**** Coated Caplet	**Dristan Cold*** Coated Tablet	**Dristan Allergy** Coated Caplet	**Dristan Sinus** Coated Caplet
Analgesic						
Acetaminophen	500 mg	500 mg	500 mg	325 mg	—	—
Ibuprofen	—	—	—	—	—	200 mg
Nasal Decongestant						
Pseudoephedrine HCl	60 mg	30 mg	30 mg	—	60 mg	30 mg
Phenylephrine HCl	—	—	—	5 mg	—	—
Antihistamine						
Brompheniramine Maleate	—	2 mg	—	—	4 mg	—
Chlorpheniramine Maleate	—	—	—	2 mg	—	—
Cough Suppressant						
Dextromethorphan HBr	20 mg	—	—	—	—	—

*Multi-Symptom Formula
**No Drowsiness Formula

product if you have heart disease, high blood pressure, thyroid disease, diabetes, or difficulty in urination due to enlargement of the prostate gland unless directed by a doctor. The use of this dispenser by more than one person may spread infection. Keep this and all medicines out of children's reach. In case of accidental ingestion, seek professional assistance or contact a poison control center immediately.

Dosage and Administration: With head upright, insert nozzle in nostril. Spray quickly, firmly and sniff deeply. Adults: Spray 2 or 3 times into each nostril, not more often than every 4 hours. Children under 12 years of age: As directed by a doctor.

Inactive Ingredients: Dristan Nasal Decongestant Spray: Alcohol 0.4%, Benzalkonium Chloride 1:5000 in buffered isotonic aqueous solution, Eucalyptol, Hydroxypropyl Methylcellulose, Menthol, Sodium Chloride, Sodium Phosphate, Thimerosal Preservative 0.002%, and Water.
Dristan Menthol Nasal Spray: Benzalkonium Chloride 1:5000 in buffered isotonic aqueous solution, Camphor, Eucalyptol, Hydroxypropyl Methylcellulose, Menthol, Methyl Salicylate, Polysorbate 80, Sodium Chloride, Sodium Phosphate, Thimerosal Preservative 0.002%, and Water.

How Supplied: Dristan Nasal Decongestant Spray: 15 mL and 30 mL plastic squeeze bottles.
Dristan Menthol Nasal Spray: 15 mL and 30 mL plastic squeeze bottles.

DRISTAN® ALLERGY
Nasal Decongestant/Antihistamine Caplets

[See table above.]

Description: Each Dristan Allergy Coated Caplet contains: Pseudoephedrine Hydrochloride 60 mg and Brompheniramine Maleate 4 mg.

Actions: Pseudoephedrine HCl is an oral nasal decongestant and is effective in relieving nasal/sinus congestion. Brompheniramine maleate is an antihistamine effective in the control of the runny nose, sneezing, and watery eyes associated with elevated histamine levels in disorders of the respiratory tract.

Indications: DRISTAN ALLERGY CAPLETS provide hours of effective relief of symptoms associated with allergies, hay fever or other upper respiratory problems. DRISTAN ALLERGY CAPLETS are indicated for relief of nasal congestion, sinus pressure, swollen nasal passages, sneezing, runny nose, and itchy/watery eyes. Each caplet is coated for easy swallowing.

Directions: ADULTS and CHILDREN over 12 years of age: 1 caplet every 4 to 6 hours, not to exceed 4 caplets in 24 hours.

Warnings: Avoid alcoholic beverages and driving a motor vehicle or operating heavy machinery while taking this product. May cause drowsiness or excitability especially in children. Persons with asthma, glaucoma, high blood pressure, diabetes, heart or thyroid disease, difficulty in urination due to an enlarged prostate gland, or taking an antidepressant drug, should use only as directed by a physician. Do not exceed recommended dosage because at higher doses nervousness, dizziness, or sleeplessness may occur.
If symptoms do not improve within 7 days or are accompanied by high fever, discontinue use and see a physician.
As with any drug, if you are pregnant or nursing a baby, seek the advice of a health professional before using this product. Do not give to children under 12 years of age. Keep this and all drugs out of the reach of children. In case of accidental overdose, seek professional assistance or contact a poison control center immediately. Store at room temperature.

Active Ingredients: Each caplet contains Pseudoephedrine Hydrochloride 60 mg and Brompheniramine Maleate 4 mg.

Inactive Ingredients: Ammonium Hydroxide, Calcium Stearate, D&C Yellow #10 Lake, FD&C Blue #1 Lake, Hydrogenated Vegetable Oil, Hydroxypropyl Methylcellulose, Iron Oxide, Microcrystalline Cellulose, Pharmaceutical Glaze, Polyethylene Glycol, Polysorbate 80, Potassium Hydroxide, Propylene Glycol, Silica and Titanium Dioxide.

How Supplied: Green coated caplets in blister packs of 20 and bottles of 40.
Shown in Product Identification Section, page 434

DRISTAN® COLD
[*drĭs 'tăn*]
Nasal Decongestant/ Antihistamine/Pain Reliever Coated Tablets

[See table above.]

Description: Each Dristan Cold Coated Tablet contains: Phenylephrine HCl 5 mg, Chlorpheniramine Maleate 2 mg, Acetaminophen 325 mg.

Actions: Acetaminophen, an antipyretic and analgesic, reduces elevated body temperature and relieves headache, minor sore throat pain, and body aches associated with a cold. Phenylephrine HCl, an oral nasal decongestant (sympathomimetic amine), reduces nasal/sinus congestion, sinus pressure, and swollen nasal passages. Chlorpheniramine maleate, an antihistamine, controls rhinorrhea, sneezing, and lacrimation associated with elevated histamine levels in disorders of the respiratory tract.

Continued on next page

Whitehall—Cont.

Indications: For the temporary relief of headache, nasal congestion, runny nose, sore throat, fever and minor aches and pains due to a cold and for sneezing and itchy, watery eyes due to hay fever or other upper respiratory allergies.

Warnings: May cause excitability or drowsiness, especially in children; alcohol, sedatives, and tranquilizers may increase the drowsiness effect. Avoid alcoholic beverages while taking this product. Do not take this product if you are taking sedatives or tranquilizers without first consulting your doctor. Use caution when driving a motor vehicle or operating machinery. Do not exceed recommended dosage, because at higher doses nervousness, dizziness, or sleeplessness may occur. Do not take this product if you have asthma, glaucoma, emphysema, chronic pulmonary disease, shortness of breath, difficulty in breathing, heart disease, high blood pressure, thyroid disease, diabetes, or difficulty in urination due to enlargement of the prostate gland unless directed by a doctor. DRUG INTERACTION PRECAUTION: DO NOT TAKE THIS PRODUCT IF YOU ARE PRESENTLY TAKING A PRESCRIPTION DRUG FOR HIGH BLOOD PRESSURE OR DEPRESSION, OR A MONOAMINE OXIDASE INHIBITOR, WITHOUT FIRST CONSULTING YOUR DOCTOR. Do not take this product for more than 7 days or for fever for more than 3 days. If pain or fever persists or gets worse, if new symptoms occur, or if redness or swelling is present, consult a doctor because these could be signs of a serious condition. If sore throat is severe, persists for more than 2 days, is accompanied by fever, headache, rash, nausea or vomiting, consult a doctor. As with any drug, if you are pregnant or nursing a baby, seek the advice of a health professional before using this product. Keep this and all drugs out of the reach of children. In case of accidental overdose, seek professional assistance or contact a poison control center immediately. Prompt medical attention is critical for adults as well as children even if you do not notice any signs or symptoms.

Directions: Adults: Two tablets every four hours, not to exceed 12 tablets in 24 hours. Children 6–12 years of age: One tablet every four hours, not to exceed 5 tablets in 24 hours.

Inactive Ingredients: Calcium Stearate, Croscarmellose Sodium, D&C Yellow #10 Lake, FD&C Yellow #6 Lake, Hydroxypropyl Methylcellulose, Microcrystalline Cellulose, Polyethylene Glycol, Povidone, Starch, Stearic Acid.

How Supplied: Yellow/White coated tablets in tins of 12 and blister packages of 20 and bottles of 40 and 75.

Maximum Strength
DRISTAN® COLD
[*drĭs 'tăn*]
NO DROWSINESS FORMULA
Nasal Decongestant/Pain Reliever
Coated Caplets

[See table on preceding page.]

Description: Each Maximum Strength Dristan Cold Coated Caplet contains: Pseudoephedrine HCl 30 mg and Acetaminophen 500 mg.

Actions: Acetaminophen is both an antipyretic and an analgesic. This maximum strength non-aspirin pain reliever effectively reduces elevated body temperature, headache pain and body aches associated with a cold. Pseudoephedrine HCl is an oral nasal decongestant and is effective in reducing nasal/sinus congestion, sinus pressure and swollen nasal passages.

Indications: For the temporary relief of cold symptoms such as nasal congestion, headache, sore throat, muscular aches (or minor aches and pains) and fever.

Warnings: Do not exceed recommended dosage because at higher doses nervousness, dizziness, or sleeplessness may occur. Do not take this product if you have heart disease, high blood pressure, thyroid disease, diabetes, or difficulty in urination due to enlargement of the prostate gland unless directed by a doctor. DRUG INTERACTION PRECAUTION: DO NOT TAKE THIS PRODUCT IF YOU ARE PRESENTLY TAKING A PRESCRIPTION DRUG FOR HIGH BLOOD PRESSURE OR DEPRESSION, OR A MONOAMINE OXIDASE INHIBITOR, WITHOUT FIRST CONSULTING YOUR DOCTOR. Do not take this product for pain for more than 7 days, or for fever for more than 3 days, unless directed by a doctor. If pain or fever persists or gets worse, if new symptoms occur, or if redness or swelling is present, consult a doctor because these could be signs of a serious condition. If sore throat is severe, persists for more than 2 days, is accompanied by fever, headache, rash, nausea or vomiting, consult a doctor promptly. As with any drug, if you are pregnant or nursing a baby, seek the advice of a health professional before using this product. Keep this and all drugs out of the reach of children. In case of accidental overdose, seek professional assistance or contact a poison control center immediately. Prompt medical attention is critical for adults as well as children even if you do not notice any signs or symptoms.

Directions: Adults and children over 12 years of age: 2 caplets every 6 hours, not to exceed 8 caplets in any 24 hour period. Children under 12 should use only as directed by a doctor.

Inactive Ingredients: Calcium Stearate, Croscarmellose Sodium, D&C Red #7 Lake, D&C Yellow #10 Lake, FD&C Yellow #6 Lake, Hydrogenated Vegetable Oil, Hydroxypropyl Methylcellulose, Microcrystalline Cellulose, Pharmaceutical Glaze, Polyethylene Glycol, Povidone, Starch, Stearic Acid, Titanium Dioxide.

How Supplied: Yellow coated caplets in blister packages of 20 and bottles of 40.

Shown in Product Identification Section, page 434

Maximum Strength
DRISTAN® COLD
[*drĭs 'tăn*]
MULTI-SYMPTOM FORMULA
Nasal Decongestant/Antihistamine/
Pain Reliever Gel Caplets

[See table on preceding page.]

Description: Each gel caplet contains: Acetaminophen 500 mg, Pseudoephedrine HCl 30 mg, and Brompheniramine Maleate 2 mg.

Indications: MAXIMUM STRENGTH DRISTAN® COLD GEL CAPLETS contain a decongestant to temporarily relieve nasal congestion, sinus pressure and reduce swollen nasal passages; an antihistamine to temporarily relieve sneezing, runny nose, and watery eyes; and an analgesic to temporarily relieve headache, body aches, minor sore throat pain, and reduce fever.

Actions: Acetaminophen is an analgesic and antipyretic. Pseudoephedrine HCl is an oral nasal decongestant. Brompheniramine Maleate is an antihistamine.

Warnings: **Avoid alcoholic beverages and driving a motor vehicle or operating heavy machinery while taking this product. Do not take this product if you are taking sedatives or tranquilizers, without first consulting your doctor. May cause drowsiness or excitability especially in children. Persons with asthma, glaucoma, diabetes, heart or thyroid disease, or difficulty in urination due to an enlarged prostate gland, should use only as directed by a physican.** ***Drug Interaction Precaution:*** **Do not take this product if you are presently taking a prescription drug for high blood pressure or depression unless directed by a doctor. Do not exceed recommended dosage because at higher doses nervousness, dizziness, or sleeplessness may occur. If symptoms do not improve within 7 days or are accompanied by high fever, discontinue use and see a physician. If sore throat is severe, persists for more than 2 days, is accompanied by fever, headache, rash, nausea or vomiting, consult a doctor promptly. As with any drug, if you are pregnant or nursing a baby, seek the advice of a health professional before using this product. Do not give to children under 12. Keep this and all drugs out of the reach of children. In case of accidental overdose, seek professional assistance or contact a poison control center immediately. Prompt medical attention is**

critical for adults as well as for children even if you do not notice any signs or symptoms.

Directions: Adults and children 12 years of age and over: 2 gel caplets every 6 hours, not to exceed 8 gel caplets in any 24 hour period. Do not give to children under 12 years of age.

Inactive Ingredients: Calcium Stearate, Croscarmellose Sodium, D&C Red #30 Lake, EDTA, FD&C Blue #1 Lake, FD&C Red #40 Lake, Gelatin, Glycerin, Hydrogenated Vegetable Oil, Hydroxypropyl Methylcellulose, Iron Oxide, Lecithin, Microcrystalline Cellulose, Pharmaceutical Glaze, Polyethylene Glycol, Povidone, Simethicone, Starch, Stearic Acid, Titanium Dioxide, Triacetin.

How Supplied: In packages of 4s (trial size), 16s and 36s.

Shown in Product Identification Section, page 434

DRISTAN® SALINE SPRAY
Non-Medicated Nasal Moisturizer

Description: Dristan Saline Spray is a non-medicated moisturizer for dry, irritated nasal membranes. It is safe to use with oral cold, allergy and sinus medications.

Indications: For prompt, soothing relief of dry, irritated nasal membranes due to colds, allergies, low humidity, or other nasal irritations.

Warnings: Keep this and all drugs out of the reach of children. The use of this dispenser by more than one person may spread infection.

Directions: Use as often as needed. **For Adults:** With head upright, insert nozzle in nostril and spray quickly and firmly. Spray 2 or 3 times as often as needed or as directed by a physician. **For Infants and Children:** With head back, turn bottle upside down and squeeze 2 to 3 drops in each nostril as often as needed or as directed by a physician. Wipe nozzle clean after use.

Ingredients: Water, Sodium Chloride, Benzyl Alcohol, Hydroxypropyl Methylcellulose, Sodium Phosphate, Disodium Phosphate, Benzalkonium Chloride, Disodium EDTA.

How Supplied: In ½ Fl. oz. (15 mL) plastic squeeze bottles.

Shown in Product Identification Section, page 434

DRISTAN® SINUS
Ibuprofen/Pseudoephedrine Caplets*
Pain Reliever/Nasal Decongestant

*Oval-shaped tablets

[See table on page 777.]

WARNING: ASPIRIN-SENSITIVE PATIENTS. Do not take this product if you have had a severe allergic reaction to aspirin, eg, asthma, swelling, shock or hives, because even though this product contains no aspirin or salicylates, cross-reactions may occur in patients allergic to aspirin. Use other Dristan formulas.

Indications: For temporary relief of symptoms associated with the common cold, sinusitis or flu, including nasal congestion, headache, fever, body aches, and pains.

Directions: *Adults:* Take 1 caplet every 4 to 6 hours while symptoms persist. If symptoms do not respond to 1 caplet, 2 caplets may be used, but do not exceed 6 caplets in 24 hours, unless directed by a doctor. The smallest effective dose should be used. Take with food or milk if occasional and mild heartburn, upset stomach, or stomach pain occurs with use. Consult a doctor if these symptoms are more than mild or if they persist. *Children:* Do not give this product to children under 12 years of age except under the advice and supervision of a doctor.

Warnings: Do not take for colds for more than 7 days or for fever for more than 3 days unless directed by a doctor. If the cold or fever persists or gets worse, or if new symptoms occur, consult a doctor. These could be signs of serious illness. As with aspirin and acetaminophen, if you have any condition which requires you to take prescription drugs or if you have had any problems or serious side effects from taking any nonprescription pain reliever, do not take this product without first discussing it with your doctor.
IF YOU EXPERIENCE ANY SYMPTOMS WHICH ARE UNUSUAL OR SEEM UNRELATED TO THE CONDITION FOR WHICH YOU TOOK THIS PRODUCT, CONSULT A DOCTOR BEFORE TAKING ANY MORE OF IT. If you are under a doctor's care for any serious condition, consult a doctor before taking this product.
Do not exceed recommended dosage because at higher doses nervousness, dizziness or sleeplessness may occur. Do not take this product if you have high blood pressure, heart disease, diabetes, thyroid disease or difficulty in urination due to enlargement of the prostate gland, except under the advice and supervision of a doctor.

Drug Interaction Precaution: Do not take this product if you are presently taking a prescription drug for high blood pressure or depression without first consulting your doctor. Do not combine this product with other nonprescription pain relievers. Do not combine this product with any other ibuprofen-containing product. As with any drug, if you are pregnant or nursing a baby, seek the advice of a health professional before using this product. IT IS ESPECIALLY IMPORTANT NOT TO USE THIS PRODUCT DURING THE LAST 3 MONTHS OF PREGNANCY UNLESS SPECIFICALLY DIRECTED TO DO SO BY A DOCTOR BECAUSE IT MAY CAUSE PROBLEMS IN THE UNBORN CHILD OR COMPLICATIONS DURING DELIVERY. Keep this and all drugs out of the reach of children. In case of accidental overdose, seek professional assistance or contact a poison control center immediately. Store at room temperature; avoid excessive heat (40°C, 104°F).

Active Ingredients: Each caplet contains Ibuprofen 200 mg and Pseudoephedrine HCl 30 mg.

Inactive Ingredients: Carnauba or Equivalent Wax, Croscarmellose Sodium, Iron Oxide, Methylparaben, Microcrystalline Cellulose, Propylparaben, Silicon Dioxide, Sodium Benzoate, Sodium Lauryl Sulfate, Starch, Stearic Acid, Sucrose, Titanium Dioxide.

How Supplied: Dristan Sinus is an oval-shaped white-colored caplet supplied in consumer blister packs of 20 and bottles of 40.
U.S. Patent No. 5,087,454

Shown in Product Identification Section, page 434

DRISTAN®
[*drĭs 'tăn*]
12-hr Nasal Decongestant Spray

Description: Dristan 12-hr nasal spray contains Oxymetazoline HCl 0.05%.

Actions: The sympathomimetic action of Dristan 12-hr nasal spray constricts the smaller arterioles of the nasal passages and produces a prolonged (up to 12 hours), gentle and predictable decongesting effect.

Indications: For the temporary relief of nasal congestion due to colds, hay fever or other upper respiratory allergies.

Warnings: Do not exceed recommended dosage because burning, stinging, sneezing, or increase of nasal discharge may occur. Do not use this product for more than 3 days. If symptoms persist, consult a doctor. Do not use this product if you have heart disease, high blood pressure, thyroid disease, diabetes, or difficulty in urination due to enlargement of the prostate gland unless directed by a doctor. The use of this dispenser by more than one person may spread infection. Keep this and all drugs out of the reach of children. In case of accidental ingestion, seek professional assistance or contact a poison control center immediately.

Directions: With head upright, insert nozzle in nostril. Spray quickly, firmly and sniff deeply. Adults and children 6 to under 12 years of age (with adult supervision): spray 2 or 3 times into each nostril not more than every 10–12 hours. Do not exceed two applications in any 24 hour period. Children under 6 years of age: consult a doctor.

Inactive Ingredients: Benzalkonium Chloride 1:5000 in buffered isotonic aqueous solution, Hydroxypropyl Methylcellulose, Potassium Phosphate, So-

Continued on next page

Whitehall—Cont.

dium Chloride, Sodium Phosphate, Thimerosal Preservative 0.002%, and Water.

How Supplied: Available in 15 mL and 30 mL plastic squeeze bottles.

POSTURE®
[*pos 'tūr*]
600 mg
High Potency Calcium Supplement

(See *1993 Physicians' Desk Reference.)*

POSTURE®-D
600 mg
High Potency Calcium Supplement with Vitamin D

(See *1993 Physicians' Desk Reference.)*

PREPARATION H®
[*prep-e 'rā-shen-āch*]
Hemorrhoidal Ointment and Cream
PREPARATION H®
Hemorrhoidal Suppositories

Description: Preparation H is available in ointment, cream and suppository product forms. The **Ointment** contains Live Yeast Cell Derivative, supplying 2,000 units Skin Respiratory Factor per ounce of Ointment, and Shark Liver Oil 3.0% in a specially prepared Rectal Petrolatum Base.
The **Cream** contains Live Yeast Cell Derivative, supplying 2,000 units Skin Respiratory Factor per ounce of Cream, and Shark Liver Oil 3.0% in a specially prepared Rectal Cream Base containing Petrolatum.
The **Suppositories** contain Live Yeast Cell Derivative, supplying 2,000 units Skin Respiratory Factor per ounce of Cocoa Butter Suppository Base, and Shark Liver Oil 3.0%.

Indications: Preparation H helps shrink swelling of hemorrhoidal tissues caused by inflammation and gives prompt, temporary relief in many cases from pain and itching in tissues.

Precautions: In case of bleeding, or if your condition persists, a physician should be consulted. Keep this and all drugs out of the reach of children. In case of accidental ingestion, seek professional assistance or contact a poison control center immediately.

Dosage and Administration: **Ointment/Cream:** Before applying, remove protective cover from applicator. Lubricate applicator before each application and thoroughly cleanse after use. It is recommended that Preparation H Hemorrhoidal ointment/cream be applied freely to the affected rectal area whenever symptoms occur, from three to five times per day, especially at night, in the morning, and after each bowel movement. Frequent application with Preparation H ointment/cream provides continual therapy which leads to more rapid improvement of rectal conditions.
Suppositories: Whenever symptoms occur, remove wrapper, insert one suppository rectally from three to five times per day, especially at night, in the morning, and after each bowel movement. Frequent application with Preparation H suppositories provides continual therapy which leads to more rapid improvement of rectal conditions .

Inactive Ingredients: **Ointment**—Beeswax, Glycerin, Lanolin, Lanolin Alcohol, Mineral Oil, Paraffin, Phenylmercuric Nitrate 1:10,000 (as a preservative), Thyme Oil.
Cream—BHA, Cellulose Gum, Cetyl Alcohol, Citric Acid, Disodium EDTA, Glycerin, Glyceryl Stearate, Lanolin, Methylparaben, Phenylmercuric Nitrate, 1:10,000 (as a preservative), Propyl Gallate, Propylene Glycol, Propylparaben, Simethicone, Sodium Lauryl Sulfate, Stearyl Alcohol, Water, Xanthan Gum. May also contain Glyceryl Oleate and/or Polysorbate 80.
Suppositories — Beeswax, Glycerin, Phenylmercuric Nitrate 1:10,000 (as a preservative), Polyethylene Glycol 600 Dilaurate.

How Supplied: **Ointment:** Net Wt. 1 oz. and 2 oz. **Cream:** Net wt. 0.9 oz. and 1.8 oz. **Suppositories:** 12's, 24's, 36's and 48's.
Store at controlled room temperature in cool place but not over 80° F.

Shown in Product Identification Section, page 434

PREPARATION H® Cleansing Tissues
[*prep-e 'rā-shen-āch*]

Description: Preparation H Cleansing Tissues are alcohol-free, nonburning, pre-moistened tissues that soothe, clean, and freshen.

Indications and Use: Preparation H Cleansing Tissues are formulated to moisturize and cleanse rectal or vaginal skin that is itching, burning, or irritated due to hemorrhoids, diarrhea, rashes, or rectal/vaginal surgery. FOR HYGIENE, use Preparation H cleansing tissues after each bowel movement in place of, or in conjunction with, ordinary toilet tissue. FOR MAXIMUM HEMORRHOIDAL CARE, cleanse hemorrhoidal area with Preparation H Cleansing Tissues before using Preparation H Suppositories, Ointment or Cream. TO USE AS A COMPRESS, fold Preparation H Cleansing Tissues and apply to irritated skin for 5 to 15 minutes. Preparation H Cleansing Tissues are safe and comfortable to use as often as you wish.

Directions: Gently apply Preparation H Cleansing Tissues as needed, particularly after each bowel movement, tampon change, or prior to use of Preparation H Suppositories, Ointment, or Cream.

Caution: In case of rectal bleeding or continued irritation, discontinue use and consult a physician promptly.

Ingredients: Purified Water, Propylene Glycol, Phenoxyethanol, Methylparaben, Propylparaben, Butylparaben and Citric Acid.

How Supplied: Preparation H Cleansing tissues are supplied in a portable, reusable, resealable package of 15 or a resealable package of 40 tissues.

Shown in Product Identification Section, page 434

PREPARATION H®
HYDROCORTISONE 1%
[*prep-e 'ra-shen-ach*]
Anti-Itch Cream

Description: Preparation H® Hydrocortisone 1% is an antipruritic external analgesic cream containing 1% Hydrocortisone.

Indications: For the temporary relief of external anal itch and itching associated with minor skin irritations and rashes. Other uses of this product should be only under the advice and supervision of a doctor.

Warnings: For external use only. Avoid contact with the eyes. If condition worsens, or if symptoms persist for more than 7 days or clear up and occur again within a few days, stop use of this product and do not begin use of any other hydrocortisone product unless you have consulted a doctor. Do not exceed the recommended daily dosage unless directed by a doctor. In case of bleeding, consult a doctor promptly. Do not put this product into the rectum by using fingers or any mechanical device or applicator. Do not use for the treatment of diaper rash. Consult a doctor. Keep this and all drugs out of the reach of children. In case of accidental ingestion, seek professional assistance or contact a poison control center immediately.

Directions: Adults: When practical, cleanse the affected area by patting or blotting with an appropriate cleansing tissue, such as Preparation H Cleansing Tissues. Gently dry by patting or blotting with toilet tissue or soft cloth before application of this product. Apply to affected area not more than 3 to 4 times daily.
Children under 12: consult a doctor.

Inactive Ingredients: BHA, Cellulose Gum, Cetyl Alcohol, Citric Acid, Disodium EDTA, Glycerin, Glyceryl Oleate, Glyceryl Stearate, Lanolin, Methylparaben, Petrolatum, Propyl Gallate, Propylene Glycol, Propylparaben, Simethicone, Sodium Benzoate, Sodium Lauryl Sulfate, Stearyl Alcohol, Water, Xanthan Gum.

How Supplied: Available in Net Wt. 0.9 oz. tube. Store at room temperature or in cool place not over 80°F.

Shown in Product Identification Section, page 434

PRIMATENE®
[*prīm 'a-tēn*]
Mist
(Epinephrine Inhalation Aerosol Bronchodilator)

Description: Primatene Mist contains Epinephrine 5.5 mg/mL.

Action: Epinephrine is a sympathomimetic agent which relaxes bronchial smooth muscle during an acute asthma attack.

Indications: Primatene Mist is indicated for temporary relief of shortness of breath, tightness of chest, and wheezing due to bronchial asthma. It eases breathing for asthma patients by reducing spasms of bronchial muscles.

Dosage and Administration: Inhalation dosage for adults and children 4 years of age and older: Start with one inhalation, then wait at least 1 minute. If not relieved, use once more. Do not use again for at least 3 hours. The use of this product by children should be supervised by an adult. Children under 4 years of age: Consult a physician. Each inhalation delivers 0.22 mg. of epinephrine.

Warnings: Do not use this product unless a diagnosis of asthma has been made by a physician. Do not use this product if you have heart disease, high blood pressure, thyroid disease, diabetes, or difficulty in urination due to enlargement of the prostate gland unless directed by a physician. As with any drug, if you are pregnant or nursing a baby, seek the advice of a health professional before using this product. Do not use this product if you have ever been hospitalized for asthma or if you are taking any prescription drug for asthma unless directed by a physician. Keep this and all drugs out of the reach of children. In case of accidental overdose, seek professional assistance or contact a poison control center immediately. **Drug Interaction Precaution:** Do not use this product if you are presently taking a prescription drug for high blood pressure or depression, without first consulting your physician. DO NOT CONTINUE TO USE THIS PRODUCT, BUT SEEK MEDICAL ASSISTANCE IMMEDIATELY IF SYMPTOMS ARE NOT RELIEVED WITHIN 20 MINUTES OR BECOME WORSE. DO NOT USE THIS PRODUCT MORE FREQUENTLY OR AT HIGHER DOSES THAN RECOMMENDED UNLESS DIRECTED BY A PHYSICIAN. EXCESSIVE USE MAY CAUSE NERVOUSNESS AND RAPID HEART BEAT AND POSSIBLY, ADVERSE EFFECTS ON THE HEART.

Precautions: Contents under pressure. Do not puncture or throw container into incinerator. Using or storing near open flame or heating above 120° F (49° C) may cause bursting. Store at room temperature 59° F–86° F (15° C–30° C).

Directions For Use of The Mouthpiece:
The Primatene Mist mouthpiece, which is enclosed in the Primatene Mist 15mL size (not the refill size), should be used for inhalation only with Primatene Mist.

1. Take plastic cap off mouthpiece. (For refills, use mouthpiece from previous purchase.)
2. Take plastic mouthpiece off bottle.
3. Place other end of mouthpiece on bottle.
4. Turn bottle upside down. Place thumb on bottom of mouthpiece over circular button and forefinger on top of vial. Empty the lungs as completely as possible by exhaling.
5. Place mouthpiece in mouth with lips closed around opening. Inhale deeply while squeezing mouthpiece and bottle together. Release immediately and remove unit from mouth. Complete taking the deep breath, drawing the medication into your lungs and holding breath as long as comfortable.
6. Then exhale slowly keeping lips nearly closed. This distributes the medication in the lungs.
7. Replace plastic cap on mouthpiece.
8. The Primatene Mist mouthpiece should be washed once daily with soap and hot water, and rinsed thoroughly. Then it should be dried with a clean, lint-free cloth.

Inactive Ingredients: Alcohol 34%, Ascorbic Acid, Fluorocarbons (Propellant), Water. Contains No Sulfites.

How Supplied:
½ Fl. oz. (15 mL) With Mouthpiece.
½ Fl. oz. (15 mL) Refill
¾ Fl. oz. (22.5 mL) Refill

Shown in Product Identification Section, page 434

PRIMATENE®
[*prīm 'a-tēn*]
Mist Suspension
(Epinephrine Bitartrate Inhalation Aerosol Bronchodilator)

Description: Primatene Mist Suspension contains Epinephrine Bitartrate 7.0 mg/mL.

Action: Epinephrine is a sympathomimetic agent which relaxes bronchial smooth muscle and thereby eases breathing during an acute asthma attack.

Indications: Primatene Mist Suspension is indicated for temporary relief of shortness of breath, tightness of chest, and wheezing due to bronchial asthma. Eases breathing for asthma patients by reducing spasms of bronchial muscles.

Dosage and Administration: Shake before using. Inhalation dosage for adults and children 4 years of age and older: Start with one inhalation, then wait at least 1 minute. If not relieved, use once more. Do not use again for at least 3 hours. The use of this product by children should be supervised by an adult. Children under 4 years of age: Consult a physician. Each inhalation delivers 0.3 mg. Epinephrine Bitartrate equivalent to 0.16 mg. Epinephrine Base.

Warnings: Do not use this product unless a diagnosis of asthma has been made by a physician. Do not use this product if you have heart disease, high blood pressure, thyroid disease, diabetes, or difficulty in urination due to enlargement of the prostate gland unless directed by a physician. As with any drug, if you are pregnant or nursing a baby, seek the advice of a health professional before using this product. Do not use this product if you have ever been hospitalized for asthma or if you are taking any prescription drug for asthma unless directed by a physician. Keep this and all drugs out of the reach of children. In case of accidental overdose, seek professional assistance or contact a poison control center immediately. **Drug Interaction Precaution:** Do not use this product if you are presently taking a prescription drug for high blood pressure or depression, without first consulting your physician.
DO NOT CONTINUE TO USE THIS PRODUCT, BUT SEEK MEDICAL ASSISTANCE IMMEDIATELY IF SYMPTOMS ARE NOT RELIEVED WITHIN 20 MINUTES OR BECOME WORSE. DO NOT USE THIS PRODUCT MORE FREQUENTLY OR AT HIGHER DOSES THAN RECOMMENDED UNLESS DIRECTED BY A PHYSICIAN. EXCESSIVE USE MAY CAUSE NERVOUSNESS AND RAPID HEART BEAT AND POSSIBLY, ADVERSE EFFECTS ON THE HEART.

Precautions: Contents under pressure. Do not puncture or throw container into incinerator. Using or storing near open flame or heating above 120° F (49° C) may cause bursting. Store at room temperature 59° F–86° F (15° C–30° C).

Directions For Use of The Inhaler:

1. SHAKE WELL BEFORE USING.
2. HOLD INHALER WITH NOZZLE DOWN WHILE USING. Empty the lungs as completely as possible by exhaling.
3. Purse the lips as in saying "O" and hold the nozzle up to the lips keeping the tongue flat. As you start to take a deep breath, squeeze nozzle and can together, releasing one full application. Complete taking a deep breath, drawing medication into your lungs.
4. Hold breath for as long as comfortable. Then exhale slowly, keeping the lips nearly closed. This distributes the medication in the lungs.
5. The Primatene Mist Suspension nozzle should be washed once daily. After removing the nozzle from the vial, wash it with soap and hot water, and rinse thoroughly. Then it should be dried with a clean, lint-free cloth.

Inactive Ingredients: Fluorocarbons (Propellant), Sorbitan Trioleate. Contains No Sulfites.

How Supplied: ⅓ Fl. oz. (10 mL) pocket-size aerosol inhaler.

Continued on next page

Whitehall—Cont.

PRIMATENE®
[*prīm 'a-tēn*]
Tablets

Description: Primatene Tablets contain Theophylline Anhydrous 130 mg and Ephedrine Hydrochloride 24 mg.

Actions: Primatene Tablets contain two bronchodilators, theophylline, a methylxanthine, and ephedrine, a sympathomimetic amine. The pharmacologic action of theophylline may be mediated through inhibition of phosphodiesterase with a resulting increase in intracellular cyclic AMP. The β-adrenergic ephedrine acts by a different mechanism to produce cyclic AMP. The combination of a xanthine and a sympathomimetic appears to produce more smooth muscle relaxation than when either drug is used alone.

Indications: For temporary relief of shortness of breath, tightness of chest, and wheezing due to bronchial asthma. Eases breathing for asthma patients by reducing spasms of bronchial muscles.

Warnings: Do not use this product unless a diagnosis of asthma has been made by a doctor. Do not use this product if you have heart disease, high blood pressure, thyroid disease, diabetes or difficulty in urination due to enlargement of the prostate gland unless directed by a doctor. Do not use this product if you have ever been hospitalized for asthma or if you are taking any prescription drug for asthma unless directed by a doctor. **DRUG INTERACTION PRECAUTION:** DO NOT TAKE THIS PRODUCT IF YOU ARE PRESENTLY TAKING A PRESCRIPTION DRUG FOR HIGH BLOOD PRESSURE OR DEPRESSION. IF YOU ARE PRESENTLY TAKING A MONOAMINE OXIDASE INHIBITOR, FIRST CONSULT YOUR PHYSICIAN. Do not continue to use this product but seek medical assistance immediately if symptoms are not relieved within 1 hour or become worse. Some users of this product may experience nervousness, tremor, sleeplessness, nausea, and loss of appetite. If these symptoms persist or become worse, consult your doctor. As with any drug, if you are pregnant or nursing a baby, seek the advice of a health professional before using this product. Keep this and all drugs out of the reach of children. In case of accidental overdose, seek professional assistance or contact a poison control center immediately.

Directions: Adults and children 12 years of age and over: 1 or 2 tablets initially and then one every 4 hours, as needed, not to exceed 6 tablets in 24 hours. For children under 12, consult a doctor.

Inactive Ingredients:
Croscarmellose Sodium, D&C Yellow No. 10 Lake, FD&C Yellow No. 6 Lake, Magnesium Stearate, Microcrystalline Cellulose, Silica, Starch, Stearic Acid.

How Supplied: Available in 24 and 60 tablet thermoform blister cartons.

Shown in Product Identification Section, page 434

RIOPAN®
[*rī 'opan*]
magaldrate
Antacid

Description: RIOPAN is a buffer antacid containing the unique chemical entity Magaldrate. Each teaspoonful (5 mL) of suspension contains Magaldrate 540 mg. RIOPAN is considered dietetically sodium-free [containing not more than 0.013 mEq (0.3 mg) sodium per teaspoonful].

Actions: The active ingredient in RIOPAN, Magaldrate, demonstrates a rapid and uniform buffering action. The acid-neutralizing capacity of RIOPAN is 15.0 mEq/5 mL. RIOPAN does not produce acid rebound or alkalinization.

Indications: Riopan is indicated for the relief of heartburn, sour stomach, and acid indigestion. For symptomatic relief of hyperacidity associated with the diagnosis of peptic ulcer, gastritis, peptic esophagitis, gastric hyperacidity, and hiatal hernia.

Dosage and Administration: Take two to four teaspoonfuls, between meals and at bedtime, or as directed by the physician.

Warnings: Patients should not take more than 18 teaspoonfuls in a 24-hour period or use the maximum dosage for more than two weeks, or use if they have kidney disease, except under the advice and supervision of a physician. Keep this and all drugs out of the reach of children.

Drug Interaction Precaution: Do not use in patients presently taking a prescription antibiotic drug containing any form of tetracycline.

Inactive Ingredients: Flavor, Glycerin, Potassium Citrate, Saccharin, Sorbitol, Xanthan Gum, Water.

How Supplied: In 12 fl. oz. (355 mL) plastic bottles. Store at room temperature (approximately 25°C or 77°F). Avoid freezing.

RIOPAN PLUS®
[*rī 'opan plŭs*]
magaldrate and simethicone
Antacid plus Anti-Gas

Description: RIOPAN PLUS is a buffer antacid plus anti-gas combination product containing the unique chemical entity Magaldrate. Each teaspoonful (5 mL) of suspension contains Magaldrate 540 mg and Simethicone 40 mg. RIOPAN PLUS is considered dietetically sodium-free [containing not more than 0.013 mEq (0.3 mg) sodium per teaspoonful].

Actions: The active antacid ingredient in RIOPAN PLUS, Magaldrate, provides a rapid and uniform buffering action. The acid-neutralizing capacity of RIOPAN PLUS is 15.0 mEq/5 mL. RIOPAN PLUS does not produce acid rebound or alkalinization. Simethicone reduces the surface tension of gas bubbles so that the gas is more easily eliminated.

Indications: RIOPAN PLUS is indicated for the relief of heartburn, sour stomach and acid indigestion accompanied by the symptoms of gas. For symptomatic relief of hyperacidity associated with the diagnosis of peptic ulcer, gastritis, peptic esophagitis, gastric hyperacidity, and hiatal hernia. For post-operative gas pain.

Dosage and Administration: Take two to four teaspoonfuls between meals and at bedtime, or as directed by the physician.

Warnings: Patients should not take more than 12 teaspoonfuls in a 24-hour period, or use the maximum dosage for more than two weeks, or use if they have kidney disease, except under the advice and supervision of a physician. Keep this and all drugs out of the reach of children.

Drug Interaction Precaution: Do not use in patients presently taking a prescription antibiotic drug containing any form of tetracycline.

Inactive Ingredients: Flavor, Glycerin, PEG-8 Stearate, Potassium Citrate, Saccharin, Sorbitan Stearate, Sorbitol, Xanthan Gum, Water.

How Supplied: In 12 fl. oz. (355 mL) plastic bottles. Store at room temperature (approximately 25°C or 77°F). Avoid freezing.

RIOPAN PLUS® 2
[*rī 'opan plus 2*]
magaldrate and simethicone
Double Strength
Antacid plus Anti-Gas
Mint and Cherry Flavors

Description: RIOPAN PLUS 2 is a double strength buffer antacid plus anti-gas combination product containing the unique chemical entity Magaldrate. Each teaspoonful (5 mL) of suspension contains Magaldrate 1080 mg and Simethicone 40 mg. RIOPAN PLUS 2 is considered dietetically sodium-free [containing not more than 0.013 mEq (0.3 mg) sodium per teaspoonful].

Actions: Magaldrate, the active antacid ingredient in RIOPAN PLUS 2, provides a rapid and uniform buffering action. The acid-neutralizing capacity of Double Strength RIOPAN PLUS 2 is 30 mEq/5 mL. RIOPAN PLUS 2 does not produce acid rebound or alkalinization. Simethicone reduces the surface tension of gas bubbles so that the gas is more easily eliminated.

Indications: RIOPAN PLUS 2 is indicated for the relief of heartburn, sour stomach and acid indigestion accompanied by the symptoms of gas. For symptomatic relief of hyperacidity associated with the diagnosis of peptic ulcer, gastritis, peptic esophagitis, gastric hyperacidity, and hiatal hernia. For postoperative gas pain.

Dosage and Administration: Take two to four teaspoonfuls between meals and at bedtime, or as directed by the physician.

Warnings: Patients should not take more than 12 teaspoonfuls in a 24-hour period, or use the maximum dosage for more than two weeks, or use if they have kidney disease, except under the advice and supervision of a physician. Keep this and all drugs out of the reach of children.

Drug Interaction Precaution: Do not use in patients presently taking a prescription antibiotic drug containing any form of tetracycline.

Inactive Ingredients: Flavor, Glycerin, PEG-8 Stearate, Potassium Citrate, Saccharin, Sorbitan Stearate, Sorbitol, Xanthan Gum, Water.

How Supplied: In 12 fl. oz. (355 mL) and 6 fl. oz. plastic bottles. Available in mint and cherry vanilla flavors.
Store at room temperature (approximately 25°C or 77°F). Avoid freezing.

Shown in Product Identification Section, page 434

SEMICID®
[sĕm 'ē-sĭd]
Vaginal Contraceptive Inserts

Description: Semicid is a safe and effective, nonsystemic, reversible method of birth control. Each vaginal contraceptive insert contains 100 mg of the spermicide nonoxynol-9. It contains no hormones and is odorless and nonmessy.
When used consistently and according to directions, the effectiveness of Semicid is approximately equal to other vaginal spermicides, but is less than oral contraceptives. Semicid requires no applicator and has no unpleasant taste. Unlike foams, creams and jellies, Semicid does not drip or run, and Semicid inserts are easier to use than the diaphragm. Also, Semicid does not effervesce like some inserts, so it is not as likely to cause a burning feeling.

Actions: Semicid gently dissolves within the vagina to form a protective barrier that kills sperm.

Indication: For the prevention of pregnancy.

Warnings: DO NOT INSERT SEMICID IN URINARY OPENING (urethra). If you accidentally insert Semicid into the urinary opening, you may have increased burning when urinating, difficulty in starting to urinate; you may also notice a pink color of your urine or have abdominal pain. If these symptoms occur, drink large amounts of water in order to urinate as frequently as possible (even if urinating causes discomfort), and consult your doctor or clinic immediately.
If you accidentally insert Semicid into the urinary opening and become aware of this before intercourse, do not proceed with sexual activity. If your doctor has told you that you should not become pregnant, ask your doctor if you can use this product for contraception. Any delay in your menstrual period may be an early sign of pregnancy. If this happens, consult your doctor or clinic as soon as possible. If you or your partner think you have had an allergic reaction to the spermicide (nonoxynol-9) in this product, do not use Semicid.
A small number of men and women may be sensitive to nonoxynol-9. Therefore, if you or your partner experience irritation, burning or itching in the genital area, discontinue use. If these symptoms persist, consult your doctor or clinic. If douching is desired, always wait at least 6 hours after intercourse before douching. Keep this and all drugs out of the reach of children. In case of accidental ingestion, seek professional assistance or contact a poison control center immediately.

Directions for use: Each Semicid insert is sealed in plastic. To use, just unwrap one insert. Use the forefinger and thumb to position the unwrapped insert as deeply as possible into the VAGINAL OPENING, the same opening from which the menstrual flow leaves the body (and where a tampon is placed). EXTREME CARE SHOULD BE TAKEN NOT TO INSERT SEMICID INTO THE URINARY OPENING (URETHRA), the opening from which urine passes out of the body.
It is ESSENTIAL that Semicid be inserted at least 15 minutes before intercourse so it can dissolve in the vagina. If intercourse is delayed for more than one (1) hour after insertion or if intercourse is repeated at any time, another insert must be used. It is safe to use Semicid as frequently as needed, however, "directions for use" should be carefully followed each time.
Active Ingredients: Each insert contains Nonoxynol-9, 100 mg.

Inactive Ingredients: Benzethonium Chloride, Citric Acid, D&C Red #21 Lake, D&C Red #33 Lake, Methylparaben, Polyethylene Glycol, Water.

How Supplied: Strip Packaging of 9's and 18's.
Keep Semicid at room temperature (not over 86°F or 30°C).

Shown in the Product Identification Section of the Physicians' Desk Reference (For Prescription Drugs), page 436

TODAY®
[tü-dā]
Vaginal Contraceptive Sponge

Description: Today Vaginal Contraceptive Sponge is a soft polyurethane foam sponge containing nonoxynol-9, a spermicide used by millions of women for over 25 years.
Today Sponge is Effective, Safe, and Convenient. Today Sponge provides 24-hour contraceptive protection without hormones, allowing spontaneity. Today Sponge is easy to use, nonmessy and disposable.

Active Ingredient: Each Today Sponge contains nonoxynol-9, one gram.

Inactive Ingredients: Benzoic acid, citric acid, sodium dihydrogen citrate, sodium metabisulfite, sorbic acid, water in a polyurethane foam sponge.

Indication: For the prevention of pregnancy.

Actions: Used as directed, Today Vaginal Contraceptive Sponge prevents pregnancy in three ways: 1) the spermicide nonoxynol-9 kills sperm before they can reach the egg; 2) Today Sponge traps and absorbs sperm; 3) Today Sponge blocks the cervix so that sperm cannot enter.
Today Sponge is designed for easy insertion into the vagina. It is positioned against the cervix, and while in place provides protection against pregnancy for 24 hours. The soft polyurethane foam sponge is formulated to feel like normal vaginal tissue and has a specially designed ribbon loop attached to an interior web for maximum strength.
In clinical trials of Today Sponge in over 1,800 women worldwide who completed over 12,000 cycles of use, the method-effectiveness, i.e., the level of effectiveness seen in women who followed the printed instructions exactly and who used Today Sponge every time that they had intercourse, was 89 to 91%. In women who did not use Today Sponge consistently and properly, the effectiveness was 84 to 87%.

Instructions: Remove one Today Sponge from airtight inner pack, wet thoroughly with clean tap water, and squeeze gently several times until it becomes very sudsy. The water activates the spermicide. Fold the sides of Today Sponge upward until it looks long and narrow and then insert it deeply into the vagina with the string loop dangling below. Protection begins immediately and continues for 24 hours. It is not necessary to add creams, jellies, foams, or any other additional spermicide as long as Today Sponge is in place, no matter how many acts of intercourse may occur during a 24-hour period. Always wait 6 hours after your last act of intercourse before removing Today Sponge. If you have intercourse when Today Sponge has been in place for 24 hours, it must be left in place an additional 6 hours after intercourse before removing it. It is unlikely that To-

Continued on next page

Whitehall—Cont.

day Sponge will fall out. During a bowel movement or other form of internal straining, it may be pushed down to the opening of the vagina and perhaps fall out. If you suspect this is happening, simply insert a finger into your vagina and push the sponge back. If it should fall into the toilet, moisten a new sponge and insert it immediately.
To remove Today Sponge, place a finger in the vagina and reach up and back to find the string loop. Hook a finger around the loop. Slowly and gently pull the Sponge out. Some women, especially first-time users, may have difficulty removing the Sponge. This situation may be due to tension or unusually strong muscular pressure. Simple relaxation of the vaginal muscles and bearing down should make it possible to remove the Sponge without difficulty. See User Instruction Booklet (Section 8) for details on removing Today Sponge or call the Today TalkLine 1-800-223-2329.

Warnings: Some cases of Toxic Shock Syndrome (TSS) have been reported in women using barrier contraceptives including the diaphragm, cervical cap and Today Sponge. Although the occurrence of TSS is uncommon, some studies indicate that there is an increased risk of non-menstrual TSS with the use of barrier contraceptives, including Today Sponge. Today Sponge should not be left in place for more than 30 hours after insertion. If you experience two or more of the warning signs of TSS including fever, vomiting, diarrhea, muscular pain, dizziness, and rash similar to sunburn, consult your physician or clinic immediately. If you have difficulty removing the sponge from your vagina or you remove only a portion of the sponge, contact the Today TalkLine or consult your physician or clinic immediately. Today Sponge should not be used during the menstrual period. After childbirth, miscarriage or other termination of pregnancy, it is important to consult your physician or clinic before using this product. If you have ever had Toxic Shock Syndrome do not use Today Sponge.
A small number of men and women may be sensitive to the spermicide in this product (nonoxynol-9) and should not use this product if irritation occurs and persists. If you or your partner have ever experienced an allergic reaction to the spermicide used in this product, it is best to consult a physician before using Today Vaginal Contraceptive Sponge. If either you or your partner develops burning or itching in the genital area, stop using this product and contact your physician.
A higher degree of protection against pregnancy will be afforded by using another method of contraception in addition to a spermicidal contraceptive. This is especially true during the first few months, until you become familiar with the method. In our clinical studies, approximately one-half of all accidental pregnancies occurred during the first three months of use. Where avoidance of pregnancy is essential, the choice of contraceptive should be made in consultation with a doctor or a family planning clinic. Any delay in your menstrual period may be an early sign of pregnancy. If this happens, consult your physician or clinic as soon as possible. Keep this and all drugs out of reach of children. In case of accidental ingestion of Today Sponge, call a poison control center, emergency medical facility or doctor. (For most people ingestion of small amounts of the spermicide alone should not be harmful.)
As with any drug, if you are pregnant or nursing a baby, seek professional advice before using this product.

How To Store: Store at normal room temperature.

How Supplied: Packages of 3s, 6s, and 12s.

Shown in Product Indentification Section, page 434

Wyeth-Ayerst Laboratories

Division of American Home Products Corporation
P.O. BOX 8299
PHILADELPHIA, PA 19101

Wyeth-Ayerst Tamper-Resistant/Evident Packaging

Statements alerting consumers to the specific type of Tamper-Resistant/Evident Packaging appear on the bottle labels and cartons of all Wyeth-Ayerst over-the-counter products. This includes plastic cap seals on bottles, individually wrapped tablets or suppositories, and sealed cartons. This packaging has been developed to better protect the consumer.

ALUDROX®
[al 'ū-drox]
Antacid
(alumina and magnesia)
ORAL SUSPENSION

Composition: *Suspension* —each 5 ml teaspoonful contains 307 mg aluminum hydroxide [$Al(OH)_3$] as a gel and 103 mg of magnesium hydroxide. The inactive ingredients present are artificial and natural flavors, benzoic acid, butylparaben, glycerin, hydroxypropyl methylcellulose, methylparaben, propylparaben, saccharin, simethicone, sorbitol solution, and water. Sodium content is 0.10 mEq per 5 ml suspension.

Indications: For temporary relief of heartburn, upset stomach, sour stomach, and/or acid indigestion.

Directions: *Suspension* —Two teaspoonfuls (10 ml) every 4 hours or as directed by a physician. Medication may be followed by a sip of water if desired.

Warnings: Do not take more than 12 teaspoonfuls (60 ml) of suspension in a 24-hour period or use maximum dosage for more than two weeks except under the advice and supervision of a physician. Prolonged use of aluminum-containing antacids in patients with renal failure may result in or worsen dialysis osteomalacia. Elevated tissue aluminum levels contribute to the development of dialysis encephalopathy and osteomalacia syndromes. Also, a number of cases of dialysis encephalopathy have been associated with elevated aluminum levels in the dialysate water. Small amounts of aluminum are absorbed from the gastrointestinal tract and renal excretion of aluminum is impaired in renal failure. Prolonged use of aluminum-containing antacids in such patients may contribute to increased plasma levels of aluminum. Aluminum is not well removed by dialysis because it is bound to albumin and transferrin, which do not cross dialysis membranes. As a result, aluminum is deposited in bone, and dialysis osteomalacia may develop when large amounts of aluminum are ingested orally by patients with impaired renal function. As with any drug, if you are pregnant or nursing a baby, seek the advice of a health professional before using this product.

Drug Interaction Precautions: Do not take this product if you are presently taking a prescription antibiotic drug containing any form of tetracycline.
Keep at Room Temperature, Approx. 77°F (25°C).
Suspension should be kept tightly closed and shaken well before use. Avoid freezing.
Keep this and all drugs out of the reach of children.

How Supplied: *Oral Suspension* —bottles of 12 fluidounces.

Shown in Product Identification Section, page 435

Professional Labeling: Consult *1993 Physicians' Desk Reference.*

AMPHOJEL®
[am 'fo-jel]
Antacid
(aluminum hydroxide gel)
ORAL SUSPENSION • TABLETS

Composition: *Suspension—Peppermint flavored* —Each teaspoonful (5 mL) contains 320 mg aluminum hydroxide [$Al(OH)_3$] as a gel, and not more than 0.10 mEq of sodium. The inactive ingredients present are calcium benzoate, glycerin, hydroxypropyl methylcellulose, menthol, peppermint oil, potassium butylparaben, potassium propylparaben, saccharin, simethicone, sorbitol solution, and water. *Suspension—Without flavor* —Each teaspoonful (5 mL) contains 320 mg of aluminum hydroxide [$Al(OH)_3$] as a gel. The inactive ingredients present are butylparaben, calcium benzoate, glycerin, hydroxypropyl methylcellulose, methylparaben, propylparaben, saccharin, simethicone, sorbitol solution, and water. *Tablets* are available in 0.3 and 0.6 g strengths. Each contains, respectively, the equivalent of 300 mg and 600 mg aluminum hydroxide as a dried gel. The inactive ingredients present are artificial and natural flavors, cellulose, hydrogenated vegetable oil, magnesium stearate, polacrilin potassium, saccharin, starch, and talc. The 0.3 g (5 grain) tablet is equivalent to about 1 teaspoonful of the suspension and the 0.6 g (10 grain) tablet is equivalent to about 2 teaspoonfuls. Each 0.3 g tablet contains 0.08 mEq of sodium and each 0.6 g tablet contains 0.13 mEq of sodium.

Indications: For temporary relief of heartburn, upset stomach, sour stomach, and/or acid indigestion.

Directions: *Suspension* —Two teaspoonfuls (10 ml) to be taken five or six times daily, between meals and on retiring or as directed by a physician. Medication may be followed by a sip of water if desired. *Tablets* —Two tablets of the 0.3 g strength, or one tablet of the 0.6 g strength, five or six times daily, between meals and on retiring or as directed by a physician. It is unnecessary to chew the 0.3 g tablet before swallowing with water. After chewing the 0.6 g tablet, sip about one-half glass of water.

Warnings: Do not take more than 12 teaspoonfuls (60 ml) of suspension, or more than twelve 0.3 g tablets, or more than six 0.6 g tablets in a 24-hour period or use this maximum dosage for more than two weeks except under the advice and supervision of a physician. May cause constipation. Prolonged use of aluminum-containing antacids in patients with renal failure may result in or worsen dialysis osteomalacia. Elevated tissue aluminum levels contribute to the development of dialysis encephalopathy and osteomalacia syndromes. Also, a number of cases of dialysis encephalopathy have been associated with elevated aluminum levels in the dialysate water. Small amounts of aluminum are absorbed from the gastrointestinal tract and renal excretion of aluminum is impaired in renal failure. Prolonged use of aluminum-containing antacids in such patients may contribute to increased plasma levels of aluminum. Aluminum is not well removed by dialysis because it is bound to albumin and transferrin, which do not cross dialysis membranes. As a result, aluminum is deposited in bone, and dialysis osteomalacia may develop when large amounts of aluminum are ingested orally by patients with impaired renal function. As with any drug, if you are pregnant or nursing a baby, seek the advice of a health professional before using this product.

Drug Interaction Precaution: Antacids may interact with certain prescription drugs. Do not use this product if you are presently taking a prescription antibiotic containing any form of tetracycline. If you are presently taking a prescription drug, do not take this product without checking with your physician.
Keep tightly closed and store at room temperature, Approx. 77°F (25°C).
Suspension should be shaken well before use. Avoid freezing.
Keep this and all drugs out of the reach of children.

How Supplied: *Suspension* —Peppermint flavored; without flavor—bottles of 12 fluidounces. *Tablets* —a convenient auxiliary dosage form—0.3 g (5 grain) bottles of 100; 0.6 g (10 grain), boxes of 100.

Shown in Product Identification Section, page 435

Professional Labeling: Consult *1993 Physicians' Desk Reference.*

BASALJEL®
[bā 'sel-jel]
(basic aluminum carbonate gel)
ORAL SUSPENSION • CAPSULES • TABLETS

Composition: *Suspension* —each 5 mL teaspoonful contains basic aluminum carbonate gel equivalent to 400 mg aluminum hydroxide [$Al(OH)_3$]. The inactive ingredients present are artificial and natural flavors, butylparaben, calcium benzoate, glycerin, hydroxypropyl methylcellulose, methylparaben, mineral oil, propylparaben, saccharin, simethicone, sorbitol solution, and water. *Capsule* contains dried basic aluminum carbonate gel equivalent to 608 mg of dried aluminum hydroxide gel or 500 mg aluminum hydroxide [$Al(OH)_3$]. The inactive ingredients present are D&C Yellow 10, FD&C Blue 1, FD&C Red 40, FD&C Yellow 6, gelatin, polacrilin potassium, polyethylene glycol, talc, and titanium dioxide. *Tablet* contains dried basic aluminum carbonate gel equivalent to 608 mg of dried aluminum hydroxide gel or 500 mg aluminum hydroxide. The inactive ingredients present are cellulose, hydrogenated vegetable oil, magnesium stearate, polacrilin potassium, starch, and talc.

Indications: For the symptomatic relief of hyperacidity, associated with the diagnosis of peptic ulcer, gastritis, peptic esophagitis, gastric hyperacidity, and hiatal hernia.

Warnings: Do not take more than 24 tablets/capsules/teaspoonsful of BASALJEL in a 24-hour period, or use this maximum dosage for more than two weeks except under the advice and supervision of a physician. Dosage should be carefully supervised since continued overdosage, in conjunction with restriction of dietary phosphorus and calcium, may produce a persistently lowered serum phosphate and a mildly elevated alkaline phosphatase. A usually transient hypercalciuria of mild degree may be associated with the early weeks of therapy. Prolonged use of aluminum-containing antacids in patients with renal failure may result in or worsen dialysis osteomalacia. Elevated tissue aluminum levels contribute to the development of dialysis encephalopathy and osteomalacia syndromes. Also, a number of cases of dialysis encephalopathy have been associated with elevated aluminum levels in the dialysate water. Small amounts of aluminum are absorbed from the gastrointestinal tract and renal excretion of aluminum is impaired in renal failure. Prolonged use of aluminum-containing antacids in such patients may contribute to increased plasma levels of aluminum. Aluminum is not well removed by dialysis because it is bound to albumin and transferrin, which do not cross dialysis membranes. As a result, aluminum is deposited in bone, and dialysis osteomalacia may develop when large amounts of aluminum are ingested orally by patients with impaired renal function. As with any drug, if you are pregnant or nursing a baby, seek the advice of a health professional before using this product.

Dosage and Administration: *Suspension* —two teaspoonsful (10 mL) in water or fruit juice taken as often as every two hours up to twelve times daily. Two teaspoonsful have the capacity to neutralize 23 mEq of acid. *Capsules* —two capsules as often as every two hours up to twelve times daily. Two capsules have the capacity to neutralize 24 mEq of acid. *Tablets* —two tablets as often as every two hours up to twelve times daily. Two tablets have the capacity to neutralize 25 mEq of acid. The sodium content of each dosage form is as follows: 0.13 mEq/5 mL for the suspension, 0.12 mEq per capsule, and 0.12 mEq per tablet.

Precautions: May cause constipation. Adequate fluid intake should be maintained in addition to the specific medical or surgical management indicated by the patient's condition.

Drug Interaction Precaution: Alumina-containing antacids should not be used concomitantly with any form of tetracycline therapy.

How Supplied: Suspension—bottles of 12 fluidounces.
Capsules—bottles of 100 and 500.
Tablets (scored)—bottles of 100.

Shown in Product Identification Section, page 435

Professional Labeling: Consult *1993 Physicians' Desk Reference.*

CEROSE-DM®
[se-ros 'DM]
Antihistamine/Nasal Decongestant/ Cough Suppressant

Description: Each teaspoonful (5 mL) contains 15 mg dextromethorphan hydrobromide, 4 mg chlorpheniramine maleate, and 10 mg phenylephrine hydrochloride. Alcohol 2.4%. The inactive ingredients present are artificial flavors, citric acid, edetate disodium, FD&C Yel-

Continued on next page

Wyeth-Ayerst—Cont.

low 6, glycerin, saccharin sodium, sodium benzoate, sodium citrate, sodium propionate, and water.

Indications: For the temporary relief of cough due to minor throat and bronchial irritation as may occur with the common cold or with inhaled irritants. Temporarily relieves nasal congestion, runny nose, and sneezing due to the common cold, hay fever, or other upper respiratory allergies.

Directions: Adults and children 12 years of age and over: One teaspoonful every four hours as needed. Children 6 to under 12 years of age: One-half teaspoonful every four hours as needed. Do not exceed six doses in a 24-hour period. For children under 6 years, consult a doctor.

Drug Interaction Precaution: Do not take this product if you are presently taking a prescription drug for high blood pressure or depression without first consulting your doctor.

Warnings: May cause marked drowsiness; alcohol may increase the drowsiness effect. Avoid alcoholic beverages while taking this product. Use caution when driving a motor vehicle or operating machinery. Do not take this product if you have heart disease, high blood pressure, thyroid disease, diabetes, asthma, glaucoma, emphysema, chronic pulmonary disease, shortness of breath, difficulty in breathing, or difficulty in urination due to enlargement of the prostate gland unless directed by a doctor. This product may cause excitability, especially in children. Do not exceed recommended dosage because at higher doses nervousness, dizziness, or sleeplessness may occur. Do not take this product for more than 7 days. A persistent cough may be a sign of a serious condition. If symptoms persist for more than one week, tend to recur, or are accompanied by fever, rash, or persistent headache, consult a doctor. Do not take this product for persistent or chronic cough such as occurs with smoking, or if cough is accompanied by excessive phlegm (mucus) unless directed by a doctor. As with any drug, if you are pregnant or nursing a baby, seek the advice of a health professional before using this product.

Keep this and all drugs out of the reach of children. In case of accidental overdose, seek professional assistance or contact a Poison Control Center immediately.

How Supplied: Cases of 12 bottles of 4 fl. oz.; bottles of 1 pint.

Keep tightly closed—Store below 77° F (25° C).

Shown in Product Identification Section, page 435

COLLYRIUM for FRESH EYES

[ko-lir 'e-um]

a neutral borate solution

EYE WASH

Description: Soothing Collyrium Eye Wash for Fresh Eyes is specially formulated to soothe, refresh, and cleanse irritated eyes. Collyrium Eye Wash is a neutral borate solution that contains boric acid, sodium borate, benzalkonium chloride (as a preservative), and water.

Indications: To cleanse the eye, loosen foreign material, air pollutants or chlorinated water.

Recommended Uses:

Home—For emergency flushing of foreign bodies or whenever a soothing eye rinse is necessary.

Hospitals, dispensaries and clinics—For emergency flushing of chemicals or foreign bodies from the eye.

Directions: Puncture bottle by twisting clear cap fully down onto bottle; then remove clear cap from bottle and discard. Remove the eyecup from plastic bag. Rinse blue eyecup with clear water immediately before and after each use. Avoid contamination of rim and interior surface of eyecup. Fill blue eyecup one-half full with Collyrium Eye Wash. Apply cup tightly to the affected eye to prevent the escape of the liquid and tilt head backward. Open eyelid wide and rotate eyeball to thoroughly wash eye. Rinse cup with clean water after use and recap by twisting blue threaded eyecup fully onto bottle for storage and subsequent use.

Warnings: Do not use if solution changes color or becomes cloudy, or with a wetting solution for contact lenses or other eye care products containing polyvinyl alcohol.

To avoid contamination do not touch tip of container to any surface. Replace cap after using. If you experience eye pain, changes in vision, continued redness, irritation of the eye, or if the condition worsens or persists, consult a doctor. Obtain immediate medical treatment for all open wounds in or near the eye.

The Collyrium for Fresh Eyes bottle is sealed for your protection. Prior to first use, remove cap and squeeze bottle. If bottle leaks, do not use.

Keep this and all medication out of the reach of children.

Keep bottle tightly closed at Room Temperature, Approx. 77°F (25°C).

How Supplied: Bottles of 4 fl. oz. (118 ml) with eyecup.

Shown in Product Identification Section, page 435

COLLYRIUM FRESH™

[ko-lir 'e-um]

Sterile Eye Drops

Lubricant

Redness Reliever

Description: Collyrium Fresh is a specially formulated sterile eye drop which can be used, up to 4 times daily, to relieve redness and discomfort due to minor eye irritations caused by dust, smoke, smog, swimming, or sun glare.

The active ingredients are tetrahydrozoline HCl (0.05%) and glycerin (1.0%). Other ingredients include benzalkonium chloride (0.01%) and edetate disodium (0.1%) as preservatives, boric acid, hydrochloric acid and sodium borate.

Indications: For the temporary relief of redness due to minor eye irritations or discomfort due to burning or exposure to wind or sun.

Directions: Tilt head back and squeeze 1 to 2 drops into each eye up to 4 times daily, or as directed by a physician.

Warnings: Do not use if solution changes color or becomes cloudy. Remove contact lenses before using. If you have glaucoma, do not use this product except under the advice and supervision of a physician. Overuse of this product may produce increased redness of the eye. To avoid contamination, do not touch tip of container to any surface. Replace cap after using. If you experience eye pain, changes in vision, continued redness or irritation of the eye, or if the condition worsens or persists for more than 72 hours, discontinue use and consult a physician.

Keep this and all medication out of the reach of children.

Retain carton for complete product information.

Keep bottle tightly closed at Room Temperature, Approx. 77°F (25°C).

How Supplied: Bottles of ½ fl. oz. (15 ml) with built-in eye dropper.

Shown in Product Identification Section, page 435

DONNAGEL®

[don 'nă-jel]

Liquid and Chewable Tablets

Each tablespoon (15 mL) of **Donnagel Liquid** contains: 600 mg Attapulgite, USP.

Inactive Ingredients: Alcohol 1.4%, Benzyl Alcohol, Carboxymethylcellulose Sodium, Citric Acid, FD&C Blue 1, Flavors, Magnesium Aluminum Silicate, Methylparaben, Phosphoric Acid, Propylene Glycol, Propylparaben, Saccharin Sodium, Sorbitol, Titanium Dioxide, Water, Xanthan Gum.

Each **Donnagel Chewable** Tablet contains: 600 mg Attapulgite, USP.

Inactive Ingredients: D&C Yellow 10 Aluminum Lake, FD&C Blue 1 Aluminum Lake, Flavors, Magnesium Stearate, Mannitol, Saccharin Sodium, Sorbitol, Water.

Indications: Donnagel is indicated for the symptomatic relief of diarrhea. It reduces the number of bowel movements, improves consistency of loose, watery bowel movements and relieves cramping.

	Liquid	Chewable Tablets
Adults	2 Tablespoons	2 Tablets
Children		
12 years and over	2 Tablespoons	2 Tablets
6 through 11 years	1 Tablespoon	1 Tablet
3 through 5 years	½ Tablespoon	½ Tablet
Under 3 years	Consult Physician	

Liquid should be shaken well. Tablets should be chewed thoroughly and swallowed.

Warnings: Patients are told that diarrhea may be serious. They are warned not to use this product for more than 2 days, or in the presence of fever, or in children under 3 years of age unless directed by a physician.
This product should not be taken by patients who are hypersensitive to any of the ingredients. As with any drug, women who are pregnant or nursing a baby should seek the advice of a health professional before using this product.

Dosage and Administration: Full recommended dose should be administered at the first sign of diarrhea and after each subsequent bowel movement, NOT TO EXCEED 7 DOSES IN A 24-HOUR PERIOD.
[See table above.]

How Supplied: Donnagel Liquid (green suspension) in 4 fl. oz. (NDC 0031-3017-12) and 8 fl. oz. (NDC 0031-3017-18).
Donnagel Chewable Tablets (light-green, flat-faced, beveled-edged, round tablets with darker green flecks; one side engraved AHR, obverse engraved Donnagel) in consumer blister packages of 18 (NDC 0031-3018-51).
Store at Controlled Room Temperature, between 15°C and 30°C (59°F and 86°F).
Shown in Product Identification Section, page 435

NURSOY®
[nur-soy]
Soy protein isolate formula
READY–TO–FEED
CONCENTRATED LIQUID
POWDER

Breast milk is the preferred feeding for newborns. NURSOY® milk-free formula is intended to meet the nutritional needs of infants and children who are not breast-fed and are allergic to cow's milk protein and/or intolerant to lactose. NURSOY Ready-to-Feed and Concentrated Liquid contain sucrose as their carbohydrate. NURSOY Powder contains corn syrup solids and sucrose as its carbohydrate. Professional advice should be followed.
NURSOY's fat blend closely resembles the fatty acid composition of human milk and has physiologic levels of linoleic and linolenic acid.
NURSOY contains beta-carotene, a component of human milk. The estimated renal solute load of NURSOY is relatively low.

Ingredients (in normal dilution supplying 20 calories per fluidounce): 87% water; 6.7% sucrose; 3.4% oleo, coconut, oleic (safflower) and soybean oils; 2.0% soy protein isolate; and less than 1% of each of the following: potassium citrate; monobasic sodium phosphate; calcium carbonate; dibasic calcium phosphate; magnesium chloride; calcium chloride; soy lecithin; calcium carrageenan; calcium hydroxide; L-methionine; sodium chloride; potassium bicarbonate; taurine; ferrous, zinc, and cupric sulfates; L-carnitine; potassium iodide; ascorbic acid; choline chloride; alpha-tocopheryl acetate; niacinamide; calcium pantothenate; riboflavin; vitamin A palmitate; thiamine hydrochloride; pyridoxine hydrochloride; beta-carotene; phytonadione; folic acid; biotin; cholecalciferol; cyanocobalamin.
NURSOY Powder contains corn syrup solids and sucrose. NURSOY Ready-to-Feed and Concentrated Liquids contain only sucrose. [See table next column.]

Preparation: *Ready-to-Feed* (32 fl. oz. cans of 20 calories per fluidounce formula)—shake can, open and pour into previously sterilized nursing bottle; attach nipple and feed. Cover opened can and immediately store in refrigerator. Use contents of can within 48 hours of opening.
Prolonged storage of can at excessive temperatures should be avoided.
Expiration date is on top of can.
WARNING: DO NOT USE A MICROWAVE TO PREPARE OR WARM FORMULA. SERIOUS BURNS MAY OCCUR.
Concentrated Liquid—For normal dilution supplying 20 calories per fluidounce, use equal amounts of NURSOY® liquid and cooled, previously boiled water.
Note: Prepared formula should be used within 24 hours.
Prolonged storage of can at excessive temperatures should be avoided.
Expiration date is on top of can.
WARNING: DO NOT USE A MICROWAVE TO PREPARE OR WARM FORMULA. SERIOUS BURNS MAY OCCUR.
Powder—For normal dilution supplying 20 calories per fluidounce, add 1 scoop (8.9 grams or 1 standard tablespoonful) of NURSOY POWDER, packed and leveled, to 2 fluidounces of cooled, previously boiled water. For larger amounts of formula, add ¼ standard measuring cup of powder (35.5 grams), packed and leveled, to 8 fluidounces (1 standard measuring cup) of water.

PROXIMATE ANALYSIS
at 20 calories per fluidounce
READY-TO-FEED, CONCENTRATED LIQUID, and POWDER

	(W/V)
Protein	1.8 %
Fat	3.6 %
Carbohydrate	6.9 %
Water	87.0 %
Crude fiber not more than	0.01 %
Calories/fl. oz.	20

Vitamins, Minerals: In normal dilution, each liter contains:

A	2,000	IU
D_3	400	IU
E	9.5	IU
K_1	100	mcg
C (ascorbic acid)	55	mg
B_1 (thiamine)	670	mcg
B_2 (riboflavin)	1000	mcg
B_6	420	mcg
B_{12}	2	mcg
Niacin	5000	mcg
Pantothenic acid	3000	mcg
Folic acid (folacin)	50	mcg
Choline	85	mg
Inositol	27	mg
Biotin	35	mcg
Calcium	600	mg
Phosphorus	420	mg
Sodium	200	mg
Potassium	700	mg
Chloride	375	mg
Magnesium	67	mg
Manganese	200	mcg
Iron	12.0	mg
Copper	470	mcg
Zinc	5	mg
Iodine	60	mcg

Note: Prepared formula should be used within 24 hours.
Prolonged storage of can at excessive temperatures should be avoided.
Expiration date is on bottom of can.
WARNING: DO NOT USE A MICROWAVE TO PREPARE OR WARM FORMULA. SERIOUS BURNS MAY OCCUR.

How Supplied: *Ready-to-Feed*—presterilized and premixed, 32 fluidounce (1 quart) cans, cases of 6 cans;
Concentrated Liquid—13 fluidounce cans, cases of 12 cans;
Powder—1 pound cans, cases of 6 cans.
Questions or Comments regarding NURSOY: 1-800-99-WYETH.
Shown in Product Identification Section, page 435

SMA®
Iron fortified
Infant formula
READY–TO–FEED
CONCENTRATED LIQUID
POWDER

Breast milk is the preferred feeding for newborns. Infant formula is intended to replace or supplement breast milk when

Continued on next page

Wyeth-Ayerst—Cont.

breast feeding is not possible or is insufficient, or when mothers elect not to breast feed.

Good maternal nutrition is important for the preparation and maintenance of breast feeding. Extensive or prolonged use of partial bottle feeding, before breast feeding has been well established, could make breast feeding difficult to maintain. A decision not to breast feed could be difficult to reverse.

Professional advice should be followed on all matters of infant feeding. Infant formula should always be prepared and used as directed. Unnecessary or improper use of infant formula could present a health hazard. Social and financial implications should be considered when selecting the method of infant feeding.

SMA® is close in overall nutrient composition to human milk with its physiologic fat blend, whey-dominated protein composition, and inclusion of beta-carotene and nucleotides.

SMA, utilizing a hybridized safflower (oleic) oil, became the first infant formula offering fat and calcium absorption closest to that of human milk, with physiologic levels of linoleic acid and linolenic acid. Thus, the fat blend in SMA provides a ready source of energy, helps protect infants against neonatal tetany and produces a ratio of vitamin E to polyunsaturated fatty acids (linoleic acid) more than adequate to prevent hemolytic anemia and yields a serum lipid profile close to that of the breast-fed infant.

By combining reduced minerals whey with skimmed cow's milk, SMA reduces the protein content to fall within the range of human milk, adjusts the whey-protein to casein ratio to that of human milk, and subsequently reduces the mineral content to a physiologic level.

The resultant 60:40 whey-protein to casein ratio provides protein nutrition superior to a casein-dominated formula. In addition, the essential amino acids, including cystine, are present in amounts close to those of human milk. So the protein in SMA is of high biologic value.

Five nucleotides found in higher amounts in human milk compared to infant formula have been added to SMA at the levels found in breast milk.

The physiologic mineral content makes possible a low renal solute load which helps protect the functionally immature infant kidney, increases expendable water reserves and helps protect against dehydration.

Use of lactose as the carbohydrate results in a physiologic stool flora and a low stool pH, decreasing the incidence of perianal dermatitis.

Ingredients: SMA Concentrated Liquid or Ready-to-Feed. Water; nonfat milk; reduced minerals whey; oleo, coconut, oleic (safflower or sunflower), and soybean oils; lactose; soy lecithin; taurine; cytidine-5′-monophosphate; calcium carrageenan; adenosine-5′-monophosphate; disodium uridine-5′-monophosphate; disodium inosine-5′-monophosphate; disodium guanosine-5′-monophosphate; *Minerals:* Potassium bicarbonate and chloride; calcium chloride and citrate; sodium bicarbonate and citrate; ferrous, zinc, cupric, and manganese sulfates. *Vitamins:* ascorbic acid, alpha tocopheryl acetate, niacinamide, vitamin A palmitate, calcium pantothenate, thiamine hydrochloride, riboflavin, pyridoxine hydrochloride, beta-carotene, folic acid, phytonadione, biotin, cholecalciferol, cyanocobalamin.

SMA Powder. Lactose; oleo, coconut, oleic (safflower or sunflower), and soybean oils; nonfat milk; whey protein concentrate; soy lecithin; taurine; cytidine-5′-monophosphate; adenosine-5′-monophosphate; disodium uridine-5′-monophosphate; disodium inosine-5′-monophosphate; disodium guanosine-5′-monophosphate. *Minerals:* Potassium phosphate; calcium hydroxide; magnesium chloride; calcium chloride; sodium bicarbonate; ferrous sulfate; potassium hydroxide; potassium bicarbonate; zinc, cupric, and manganese sulfates; potassium iodide. *Vitamins:* Ascorbic acid, choline chloride, inositol, alpha tocopheryl acetate, niacinamide, calcium pantothenate, vitamin A palmitate, riboflavin, thiamine hydrochloride, pyridoxine hydrochloride, beta-carotene, folic acid, phytonadione, biotin, cholecalciferol, cyanocobalamin.

[See table top right.]

Preparation: *Ready-to-Feed* (8 and 32 fl. oz. cans of 20 calories per fluidounce formula)—shake can, open and pour into previously sterilized nursing bottle; attach nipple and feed immediately. Cover opened can and immediately store in refrigerator. Use contents of can within 48 hours of opening.

Prolonged storage of can at excessive temperatures should be avoided.

Expiration date is on top of can.

WARNING: DO NOT USE A MICROWAVE TO PREPARE OR WARM FORMULA. SERIOUS BURNS MAY OCCUR.

Powder—(1 pound can)—For normal dilution supplying 20 calories per fluidounce, use 1 level measuring scoop to 2 fluidounces of cooled, previously boiled water.

Prolonged storage of can of powder at excessive temperatures should be avoided.

Expiration date is on bottom of can.

WARNING: DO NOT USE A MICROWAVE TO PREPARE OR WARM FORMULA. SERIOUS BURNS MAY OCCUR.

Concentrated Liquid—For normal dilution supplying 20 calories per fluidounce, use equal amounts of SMA® liquid and cooled, previously boiled water.

Prolonged storage of can at excessive temperatures should be avoided.

PROXIMATE ANALYSIS at 20 calories per fluidounce READY-TO-FEED, POWDER, and CONCENTRATED LIQUID:

	(W/V)
Fat	3.6 %
Carbohydrate	7.2 %
Protein	1.5 %
60% Lactalbumin (whey protein)	0.9 %
40% Casein	0.6 %
Crude Fiber	None
Total Solids	12.6 %
Calories/fl. oz.	20

Vitamins, Minerals: In normal dilution, each liter contains:

A	2000	IU
D_3	400	IU
E	9.5	IU
K_1	55	mcg
C (ascorbic acid)	55	mg
B_1 (thiamine)	670	mcg
B_2 (riboflavin)	1000	mcg
B_6 (pyridoxine hydrochloride)	420	mcg
B_{12}	1.3	mcg
Niacin	5000	mcg
Pantothenic Acid	2100	mcg
Folic Acid (folacin)	50	mcg
Choline	100	mg
Biotin	15	mcg
Calcium	420	mg
Phosphorus	280	mg
Sodium	150	mg
Potassium	560	mg
Chloride	375	mg
Magnesium	45	mg
Manganese	100	mcg
Iron	12	mg
Copper	470	mcg
Zinc	5	mg
Iodine	60	mcg

Expiration date is on top of can.

WARNING: DO NOT USE A MICROWAVE TO PREPARE OR WARM FORMULA. SERIOUS BURNS MAY OCCUR.

Note: Prepared formula should be used within 24 hours.

How Supplied: *Ready-to-Feed*—presterilized and premixed, 32 fluidounce (1 quart) cans, cases of 6 cans; 8 fluidounce cans, cases of 24 (4 carriers of 6 cans). *Powder*—1 pound cans with measuring scoop, cases of 6 cans. *Concentrated Liquid*—13 fluidounce cans, cases of 24 cans.

Also Available: SMA® lo-iron. Those who appreciate the particular advantages of SMA® infant formula close in nutrient composition to mother's milk, sometimes need or wish to recommend a formula that does not contain a high level of iron. SMA® lo-iron has all the benefits of regular SMA® but with a reduced level of iron of 1.4 mg per quart. Infants should receive supplemental dietary iron from an outside source to meet daily requirements.

Concentrated Liquid—13 fl. oz. cans, cases of 12 cans. *Powder*—1 pound cans with measuring scoop, cases of 6 cans.

Ready-to-Feed—32 fl. oz. cans, cases of 6 cans.

Preparation of the standard 20 calories per fluidounce formula of SMA® lo-iron is the same as SMA® iron fortified given above.

Questions or Comments regarding SMA: 1-800-99-WYETH.

Shown in Product Identification Section, page 435

STUART PRENATAL® Tablets Multivitamin/Multimineral Supplement

One Tablet Daily Provides

VITAMINS	**RDA***	
A	90%	4,000 IU
D	100%	400 IU
E	90%	11 mg
C	110%	100 mg
Folic Acid	200%	0.8 mg
B_1 (thiamin)	90%	1.5 mg
B_2 (riboflavin)	90%	1.7 mg
Niacin	90%	18 mg
B_6 (pyridoxine hydrochloride)	120%	2.6 mg
B_{12} (cyanocobalamin)	150%	4 mcg
MINERALS	**RDA***	
Calcium	20%	200 mg
Iron	200%	60 mg
Zinc	130%	25 mg

*Recommended Dietary Allowances (Food and Nutrition Board, NAS/NRC-1989) for pregnant and/or lactating women.

Ingredients

Active: calcium sulfate, ferrous fumarate, ascorbic acid, dl-alpha tocopheryl acetate, zinc oxide, niacinamide, vitamin A acetate, pyridoxine hydrochloride, riboflavin, thiamin mononitrate, folic acid, cholecalciferol, cyanocobalamin. Inactive: croscarmellose sodium, hydroxypropyl methylcellulose, microcrystalline cellulose, pregelatinized starch, red iron oxide, titanium dioxide.

Indications: STUART PRENATAL is a nonprescription multivitamin/multimineral supplement for use before, during, and after pregnancy. It provides essential vitamins and minerals, including 60 mg of elemental iron as well-tolerated ferrous fumarate, and 200 mg of elemental calcium (nonalkalizing and phosphorus-free), and 25 mg zinc. STUART PRENATAL also contains 0.8 mg folic acid.

Directions: Before, during and after pregnancy, one tablet daily, or as directed by a physician.

Warning: In case of accidental overdose, seek professional assistance or contact a Poison Control Center immediately. Keep out of the reach of children.

How Supplied: Bottles of 100 light pink tablets imprinted "STUART 071". A child-resistant safety cap is standard on 100 tablet bottles as a safeguard against accidental ingestion by children. NDC 0038-0071.

Shown in Product Identification Section, page 435

WYANOIDS® Relief Factor
[*wi 'a-noids*]
Hemorrhoidal Suppositories

Description: Active Ingredients: Live Yeast Cell Derivative, Supplying 2,000 units Skin Respiratory Factor Per Ounce of Cocoa Butter Suppository Base and Shark Liver Oil 3%. **Inactive Ingredients:** Beeswax, Glycerin, Phenylmercuric Nitrate 1:10,000 (as a preservative), Polyethylene Glycol 600 Dilaurate.

Indications: To help shrink swelling of hemorrhoidal tissues and provide prompt, temporary relief from pain and itching.

Usual Dosage: Use one suppository up to five times daily, especially in the morning, at night, and after bowel movements, or as directed by a physician.

Directions: Remove wrapper and insert one suppository rectally using gentle pressure. Frequent application and lubrication with Wyanoids® Relief Factor provide continual therapy which will lead to more rapid improvement of rectal conditions.

Caution: In case of bleeding or if the condition persists, the patient should consult a physician. Keep this and all medicines out of the reach of children. Do not store above 80°F.

How Supplied: Boxes of 12 and 24.

Shown in Product Identification Section, page 435

EDUCATIONAL MATERIAL

Audiovisual Programs

The ***Wyeth-Ayerst Audiovisual Catalog,*** listing audiovisual programs available through the Wyeth-Ayerst Audiovisual Library or on loan through the local Wyeth-Ayerst representative, can be obtained by writing Professional Service, Wyeth-Ayerst Laboratories, P.O. Box 8299, Philadelphia, PA 19101.

Zila Pharmaceuticals, Inc.

5227 NORTH 7th STREET
PHOENIX, AZ 85014-2817

ZILACTIN® Medicated Gel
ZILACTIN®-L Liquid
DERMAFLEX™ Topical Anesthetic Gel Coating

Description: Zilactin Medicated Gel stops pain and speeds healing of canker sores, fever blisters and cold sores. Zilactin forms a tenacious, occlusive film which holds the medication in place while controlling pain. Intra-orally, the film can last up to six hours, usually allowing pain-free eating and drinking. Extra-orally, the film can last much longer.

Zilactin-L is a non film-forming liquid that treats and relieves the pain, itching and burning of developing and existing cold sores and fever blisters. Zilactin-L is specially formulated to treat the initial signs of tingling, itching or burning that signal an oncoming cold sore or fever blister. Zilactin-L can often prevent developing cold sores or fever blisters from breaking out. If a lesion does occur, Zilactin-L will significantly reduce the size of the outbreak.

DermaFlex is a topical anesthetic gel "bandage" that provides temporary relief and protection of minor skin irritations including the pain and itching associated with scrapes, minor cuts, insect bites and minor rashes. DermaFlex forms a flexible, invisible, waterproof bandage which holds the active ingredient (pain relieving lidocaine) in place for hours while protecting the affected skin.

Clinical studies on the effectiveness of Zila's products are available on request.

Active Ingredients: Zilactin—Tannic acid (7%); **Zilactin-L**—Lidocaine (2.5%); **DermaFlex**—Lidocaine (2.5%)

Application: Zilactin: FOR USE IN THE MOUTH AND ON LIPS. Apply every four hours for the first three days and then as needed. Dry the affected area with a gauze pad, tissue or cotton swab. Apply a thin coat of Zilactin and allow 30-60 seconds for the gel to dry into a film. Outside the mouth, Zilactin forms a transparent film. Inside the mouth, the film is white.

Zilactin-L: FOR USE ON THE LIPS AND AROUND THE MOUTH. Apply every 1-2 hours for the first three days and then as needed. For maximum effectiveness use at first signs of tingling or itching. Moisten a cotton swab with several drops of Zilactin-L. Apply on lip area where symptoms are noted or directly on existing cold sore or fever blister and allow to dry for 15 seconds.

DermaFlex: FOR EXTERNAL USE. Apply as needed (not more than 3-4 times daily). Dry the affected area. Apply a coat of DermaFlex and allow 60 seconds for the gel to dry into a transparent film. Apply a second coat and allow it to dry. Additional coats are applied directly over existing film bandage.

Warning: A mild, temporary stinging sensation may be experienced when applying Zilactin, Zilactin-L or DermaFlex

Continued on next page

Zila—Cont.

to an open cut, sore or blister. DO NOT USE IN OR NEAR EYES. In the event of accidental contact with the eye, flush with water immediately and continuously for ten minutes. Seek immediate medical attention if pain or irritation persists. For temporary relief only. As with all medications, keep out of the reach of children.

How Supplied: Zila products are nonprescription and carried by most drug wholesalers, retail chains and independent pharmacies. Each product is available to physicians and dentists directly from Zila in full size and single use packages.
For further information call or write:

Zila Pharmaceuticals, Inc.
5227 N. 7th Street, Phoenix, AZ 85014-2817, (602) 266-6700

U.S. patent numbers 4,285,934; 4,381,296; 5,081,157 and 5,081,158

Shown in Product Identification Section, page 435

EDUCATIONAL MATERIAL

Samples and literature are available to medical professionals on request.

SECTION 7

Diagnostics, Devices and Medical Aids

This section is intended to present product information on Diagnostics, Devices and Medical Aids designed for home use by patients. The information concerning each product has been prepared, edited and approved by the manufacturer.

The Publisher has emphasized to manufacturers the necessity of describing products comprehensively so that all information essential for intelligent and informed use is available. In organizing and presenting the material in this edition the Publisher is providing all the information made available by manufacturers.

In presenting the following material to the medical profession, the Publisher is not necessarily advocating the use of any product.

MEDICAL ECONOMICS DATA

Lavoptik Company, Inc.

661 WESTERN AVENUE N.
ST. PAUL, MN 55103

LAVOPTIK® Eye Cups

Description: Device—Sterile disposable eye cups.

How Supplied: Individually bagged eye cups are packed 12 per box, NDC 10651-01004.

Ortho Pharmaceutical Corporation

Advanced Care Products
RARITAN, NJ 08869

ADVANCE®
Pregnancy Test

Active Ingredients: Human Chorionic Gonadotropin (HCG) antibody/colored conjugate.

Indications: An in-vitro pregnancy test for use in the home that can detect the presence of HCG in the urine as early as the first day of the missed period.

Actions: ADVANCE will accurately detect the presence or absence of HCG in urine in just five minutes. It is as accurate as pregnancy test methods used in many hospitals.

Dosage and Administration: Using the urine dropper, drop five drops of urine in the urine well of the test stick. Wait for red to appear in the End of Test window (may take about five minutes). If, after the End of Test window has turned red, two lines have formed in the center of the Result window, the patient is probably pregnant. If one line appears, no pregnancy hormone has been detected and the patient is probably not pregnant. In the unlikely event that neither sign appears, the test system has not worked properly and the patient should call the toll free number included in the package insert. The toll free number is staffed by Registered Nurses who can answer any questions the patient may have about her results, or how she performed the test. The test results may be affected by various other factors and medications such as thiazide diuretics, plurothiazine, hormones, steroids, chemotherapeutics, and thyroid drugs.

How Supplied: Each ADVANCE test contains a plastic test stick, a urine collection cup, a urine dropper, and complete instructions for use.

Storage: Store at room temperature (59°–86°F). Do not freeze.

Shown in Product Identification Section, page 417

FACT PLUS™
Pregnancy Test

Active Ingredients: Human Chorionic Gonadotropin (HCG) antibody, HCG antibody/colored conjugate.

Indications: An in-vitro pregnancy test for use in the home that can detect the presence of HCG in the urine as early as the first day of a missed period.

Actions: FACT PLUS will accurately detect the presence or absence of HCG in urine in as soon as 5 minutes using urine collected at any time of day. One step FACT PLUS is the same pregnancy test method used in many hospitals.

Dosage and Administration: Using the urine dropper, drop five drops of urine in the Urine Well of the test disk. Wait for red to appear in End of Test Window (may take about 5 minutes). If, after the End of Test Window has turned red, a plus (+) sign has formed in the center of the test disk, the patient is probably pregnant. If a minus (–) sign appears, no pregnancy hormone has been detected and the patient is probably not pregnant. In the unlikely event that neither sign appears the test system has not worked properly and the patient should call the toll free number included in the package insert. This toll free number is staffed by Registered Nurses who can answer any questions the patient may have about her results, or how she performed the test. The test results may be affected by various other factors and medications such as thiazide diuretics, plurothiazine, hormones, steroids, chemotherapeutics, and thyroid drugs.

How Supplied: Each FACT PLUS kit contains a plastic test disk, a urine collection cup, a urine dropper, and complete instructions for use.

Storage: Store at room temperature (59–86°F). Do not freeze.

Shown in Product Identification Section, page 417

Parke-Davis

Consumer Health Products Group
Division of Warner-Lambert Company
201 TABOR ROAD
MORRIS PLAINS, NJ 07950

e·p·t® STICK TEST
Early Pregnancy Test

Before You Begin the e·p·t Test:

- Please carefully read through this entire instruction insert.
- Registered nurses are available to confidentially answer your calls regarding e·p·t.
- If you have any questions, call toll-free 1-800-562-0266 or 1-800-223-0182, weekdays 9 AM to 5 PM EST.

Familiarize Yourself with the e·p·t Stick

- Remove the test stick from the foil pouch. Discard the freshness sachet and **pull the protective pink cap off the stick** (do not discard pink cap). Please note the two different sides of the stick:
- **Side One** (Square Windows) The square windows are used **TO TAKE** the test.
- **Side Two** (Test & Control Windows) The round windows are used **TO READ** the results.

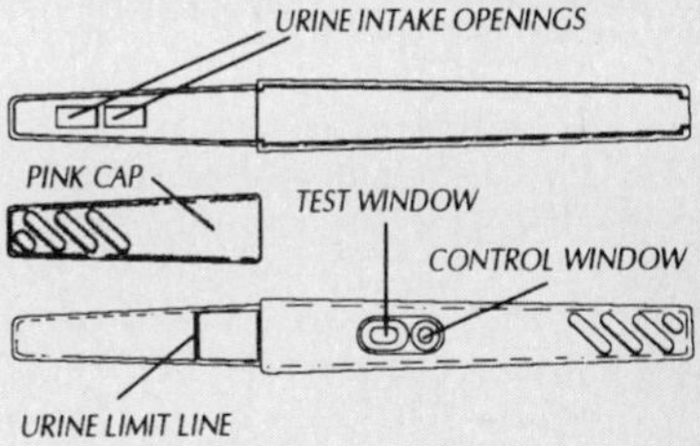

Performing the e·p·t Test

To perform the test, hold the stick with the square windows facing toward you and pointing downward (please see illustration). Important: In order to obtain accurate test results, the Test and Control Windows (round windows) must face away from you and remain dry. [See illustration on top of next page.]
Urinate on the square windows for at least 5 seconds.
If you cannot maintain a urine stream, urinate in a cup and dip the square windows exactly up to the limit line for 5 seconds.

Continued on next page

This product information was prepared in November 1992. On these and other Parke-Davis Products, detailed information may be obtained by addressing PARKE-DAVIS, Consumer Health Products Group, Division of Warner-Lambert Company, Morris Plains, NJ 07950.

Parke-Davis—Cont.

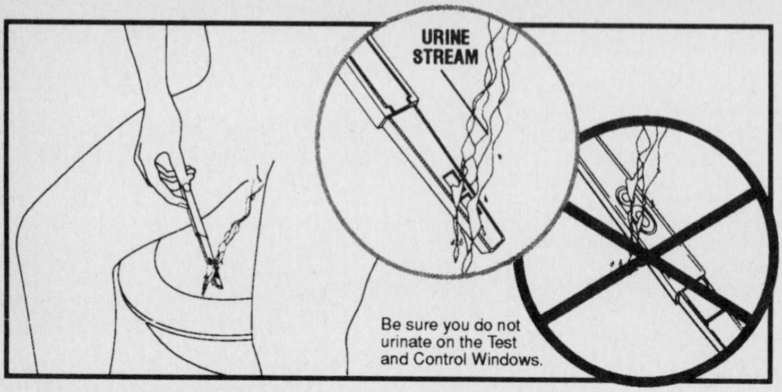

When finished, lay stick flat on counter with Test and Control Windows (round windows) facing up. Replacing pink cap is optional.

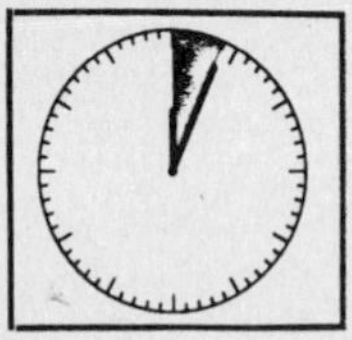

- You will notice color begining to appear in the Test and Control Windows. This is how the stick works.
- Wait at least **4 mintues** before reading the results.

Reading the Results

Both round windows will initially turn a dark pink/purple color. This color will fade after a few mintues leaving a pink/purple dot in the Control Window. This lets you know the test is working. Either a pink/purple dot or no color (white) will remain in the Test Window. This lets you know whether or not you are pregnant. To interpret results, please see illustration below.

PREGNANT

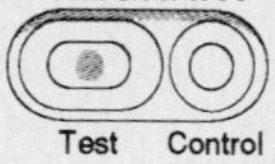

After 4 minutes, if a pink/purple dot or spot is centered in the Test Window, the test has indicated that you are **PREGNANT.** Please note, the color in the Test and Control Windows do not have to match each other.

NOT PREGNANT

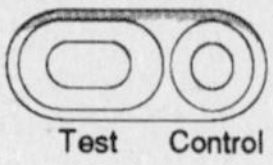

If after 4 or more minutes the color in the Test Window disappears, the test has indicated that you are **NOT PREGNANT.**

If there is no color in the Control Window, DO NOT READ the result because it may be inaccurate. Please save the stick and box and call the toll-free number 1-800-562-0266 or 1-800-223-0182, weekdays 9 AM to 5 PM EST.

Frequently asked Questions

How Does e·p·t Work?

When a woman becomes pregnant, her body produces a special hormone known as hCG (human Chorionic Gonadotropin), which appears in the urine. **e·p·t** can detect this hormone as early as the first day you miss your period. If the test indicates you are pregnant, it is detecting hCG, and you should see your doctor.

Do I Have To Test In The Morning?

No. You can use **e·p·t** any time of day. You do not have to use first morning urine.

How Soon Can I Use e·p·t?

e·p·t can detect hCG hormone levels in your urine as early as the day your period should have started. **e·p·t** can be used on the day of your missed period as well as any day thereafter.

Can I Collect The Urine In A Cup Instead?

Yes, If the cup or container is clean and dry. Immerse uncapped Test Stick into urine for at least 5 seconds, making sure that the Test Stick is immersed up to line indicated on reverse side of Urine Intake Openings. Then remove Test Stick from urine and continue with the test.

What If The Test Changes Color, But The Color Isn't The Same As The Picture In This Insert?

If the test is positive, the Test Window will retain a circle of some shade of pink/purple color after the 4-minute waiting period. The color can be ANY SHADE of pink/purple and DOES NOT HAVE TO MATCH the color pictured or the color present in the Control Window.

NOTE: e·p·t is so sensitive, it can detect pregnancy as early as the day of a missed period. However, during pregnancy, each day after a missed period results in higher levels of hCG (the pregnancy hormone) in the urine. This is why testing a few days or a week after a missed period will result in a darker test color than the first day of a missed period.

What Do I Do If The Test Result Is Positive?

If the test result is positive, you should see your doctor to discuss your pregnancy and next steps. Early prenatal care is important to ensure the health of you and your baby.

What Do I Do If The Test Result Is Negative?

If the test result is negative, no pregnancy hormone (hCG) has been detected and you are probably not pregnant. However, you may have miscalculated when you period was due. If your period does not start within a week, repeat the test. If you still get a negative result and your period has not started, you should see a doctor.

What If I Don't Wait The Full 4 Minutes Before Reading The Test Result?

If you read the test result before the full 4 minutes have passed, you may not give the test enough time to work, and the results may be inaccurate.

What If I Don't Think The Results Of The Test Are Correct?

If you follow the instructions carefully, you should not get a false result. Certain drugs and rare medical conditions may give a false result. Analgesics, antibiotics, and birth control pills should not affect the test result. If you repeat the test and continue to get an unexpected result, contact your doctor.

IF YOU HAVE FURTHER QUESTIONS ABOUT e·p·t CALL TOLL-FREE 1-800-562-0266 OR 1-800-223-0182, WEEKDAYS 9 AM to 5 PM EST.

Shown in Product Identification Section, page 418

Whitehall Laboratories Inc.

Division of American Home Products Corporation
685 THIRD AVENUE
NEW YORK, NY 10017

CLEARBLUE EASY™
Pregnancy Test Kit

Clearblue Easy is one of the easiest and fastest pregnancy tests available because all a woman has to do is hold the absorbent tip in her urine stream and in 3 minutes she can read the result. A blue line appears in the small window to show that the test is complete and the large window shows the test result. If there is a blue line in the large window, the woman is pregnant. If there is no line, she is not pregnant.

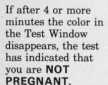

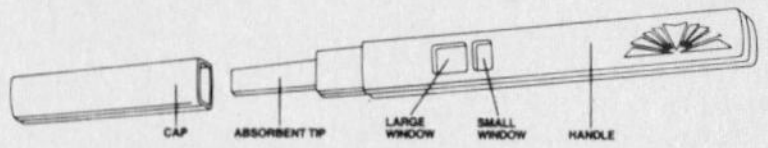

Clearblue Easy is a rapid, one-step pregnancy test for home use which detects the pregnancy hormone HCG (human chorionic gonadotropin) in the urine. This hormone is produced in increasing amounts during the first part of pregnancy. Clearblue Easy uses sensitive monoclonal antibodies to detect the presence of this hormone from the first day of a missed period.

A negative result means that no pregnancy hormone was detected and the woman is probably not pregnant. If the menstrual period does not start within a week, she may have miscalculated the day her period was due. She should repeat the test using another Clearblue Easy test. If the second test still gives a negative result and she still has not menstruated, she should see her doctor.

Clearblue Easy is specially designed for easy use at home. However, if there are

any questions about the test or results, give the Clearblue Easy TalkLine a call at 1-800-883-EASY. A specially trained staff of advisors is available to answer your questions.
Manufactured by Unipath Ltd., Bedford, U.K. Unipath, Clearblue Easy and the fan device are trademarks.
Distributed by Whitehall Laboratories, New York, NY 10017.

Shown in Product Identification Section, page 434

CLEARPLAN EASY™
One-Step Ovulation Predictor

CLEARPLAN EASY is one of the easiest home ovulation predictor tests to use because of its unique technological design. It consists of just one piece and involves only one step to get the results. To use CLEARPLAN EASY, a woman simply holds the absorbent tip in her urine stream (a woman can test any time of day) for 5 seconds, and after 5 minutes, she can read the results. A blue line will appear in the small window to show her that the test has worked correctly. The large window indicates the presence of luteinizing hormone (LH) in her urine. If there is a line in the large window which is similar to or darker than the line in the small window, she has detected her LH surge.

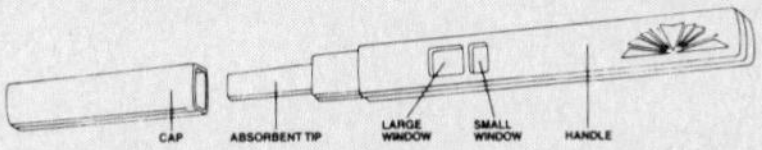

Laboratory tests confirm that CLEARPLAN EASY is over 98% accurate in detecting the LH surge as shown by radioimmunoassay (RIA).
CLEARPLAN EASY employs highly sensitive monoclonal antibody technology to accurately predict the onset of ovulation, and, consequently, the best time each month for a woman to try to become pregnant. The test monitors the amount of LH in a woman's urine. Small amounts of LH are present during most of the menstrual cycle, but the level normally rises sharply about 24 to 36 hours before ovulation (which is when an egg is released from the ovary). CLEARPLAN EASY detects this LH surge which precedes ovulation so that a woman knows 24–36 hours beforehand the time she is most able to become pregnant.
A woman will be most fertile during the 2 to 3 days after an LH surge is detected. Sperm can fertilize an egg for many hours after sexual intercourse. So, if sexual intercourse occurs during the 2–3 days after a similar or darker line appears in the large window, the chances of getting pregnant are maximized.

CLEARPLAN EASY contains 5 days of tests. If, because a woman's cycles are irregular or if for any other reason a woman does not detect her LH surge after 5 days of testing, she should continue testing with a second CLEARPLAN EASY kit. CLEARPLAN EASY offers users the support of a TalkLine (1-800-883-EASY). This service is operated by trained advisors who are available to answer any questions about using the test or reading the results.

Produced by Unipath Ltd., Bedford, U.K. Unipath, CLEARPLAN EASY and the fan device are trademarks.
Distributed by Whitehall Laboratories, New York, NY 10017.

Shown in Product Identification Section, page 434

MEDICAL ECONOMICS DATA

DRUG INFORMATION CENTERS

Centers in each state are listed alphabetically by city.

ALABAMA

Drug Information Service
University of Alabama Hospital
Birmingham
Mon-Fri 8 AM-5 PM
(205) 934-2162

Global Drug Information Center
Samford University School of Pharmacy
Birmingham
Mon-Fri 8 AM-4:30 PM
(205) 870-2891

Huntsville Hospital Drug Information Center
Huntsville
Mon-Fri 8 AM-5 PM
(205) 533-8284

ARIZONA

Arizona Poison and Drug Information Center
Arizona Health Science Center
University Medical Center
Tucson
7 days/week, 24 hours
(602) 626-6016; (800) 362-0101

ARKANSAS

Arkansas Poison and Drug Information Center
University of Arkansas for Medical Sciences
Little Rock
Mon-Fri 8 AM-9 PM
(501) 666-5532

CALIFORNIA

Alta Bates-Herrick Hospital
Drug Information Service
Berkeley
Mon-Fri 8 AM-4:30 PM
(415) 540-1503

Drug Information Analysis Center
Valley Medical Center
Fresno
Mon-Fri 8 AM-4:30 PM
(209) 453-4596

Los Angeles Regional Drug and Poison Information Center
University of Southern California
Los Angeles
Mon-Fri 7:45 AM-4:15 PM
(213) 226-7741

Drug Information Analysis Service
Veterans Administration Medical Center
San Diego
Mon-Fri 8 AM-4:30 PM
(619) 552-8585

Drug Information Center
US Naval Hospital
San Diego
Mon-Fri, 24-hour service
(619) 532-8414

Drug Information Service
University of California
San Diego
Mon-Fri 9 AM-5 PM
(619) 294-6085

Drug Information Analysis Service
University of California
San Francisco
Mon-Fri 8 AM-6 PM
(415) 476-4346

Drug Information Services
St. Johns Hospital and Health Center
Santa Monica
Mon-Fri 8 AM-5 PM
(310) 829-8243
after hours (310) 829-8250

Drug Information Center
Stanford University Hospital
Department of Pharmacy H0301
Stanford
Mon-Fri 9 AM-5 PM
(415) 723-6422

COLORADO

Rocky Mountain Drug Consultation Center
Denver
Mon-Fri 8:30 AM-3:30 PM
(303) 893-3784

Drug Information Center
University of Colorado Health Science Center
Denver
Mon-Fri 8 AM-4:30 PM
(303) 270-8489

CONNECTICUT

Drug Information Service
University of Connecticut Health Center
Farmington
Mon-Fri 8 AM-4:30 PM
(203) 679-2783

Drug Information Center
Hartford Hospital
Hartford
Mon-Fri 8:30 AM-5 PM
(203) 524-2221;
after hours (203) 524-2961

Drug Information Center
Yale-New Haven Hospital
New Haven
Mon-Fri 8:15 AM-4:45 PM
(203) 785-2248

DISTRICT OF COLUMBIA

Drug Information Center
Children's National Medical Center
Washington
Mon-Fri 8 AM-4:30 PM
(202) 745-2055; (202) 745-3171;
(202) 745-3172

Drug Information Center
Washington Hospital Center
Washington
Mon-Fri 7:30 AM-4 PM
(202) 877-6646

Drug Information Service
Howard University Hospital
Washington
Mon-Fri 8:30 AM-5 PM
(202) 865-1325

FLORIDA

Drug Information & Pharmacy Center
Shands Hospital at University of Florida
Gainesville
Mon-Fri 9 AM-5 PM
(904) 395-0408

Drug Information Service
University Medical Center
Jacksonville
Mon - Fri 8 AM-5 PM
(904) 549-4095

Drug Information Center
University of Miami/Jackson Memorial Hospital
Miami
Mon-Fri 9 AM-5 PM
(305) 585-6898

Drug Information Center
VA Medical Center
Miami
Mon-Fri 7:30 AM-4 PM
(305) 324-3237

Drug Information Service
Southeastern University of the Health Sciences
North Miami Beach
Mon-Fri 9 AM-5 PM
(305) 948-8255

GEORGIA

Emory University Hospital
Department of Pharmaceutical Services
Atlanta
Mon-Fri 8:30 AM-5 PM
(404) 727-4644

Drug Information Service
Northside Hospital
Atlanta
Mon-Fri 9 AM-4 PM
(404) 851-8676

Drug Information Center
Grady Hospital
Atlanta
Mon-Fri 8 AM-4 PM
(404) 616-7725

Drug Information Center
University of Georgia
Medical College of Georgia
Augusta
Mon-Fri 8:30 AM-5 PM
(706) 721-2887

IDAHO

Idaho Drug Information Service
Pocatello Regional Medical Center Campus
Pocatello
Mon-Fri 8 AM-4:30 PM
(208) 236-4689

ILLINOIS

Drug Information Center
Parkside Recover Center
BroMenn Life Care Center
Bloomington
Mon-Fri 24 Hours
(309) 829-0755

Drug Information Center
Northwestern Memorial Hospital
Wesley
Chicago
Mon-Fri 8:30 AM-5 PM
(312) 908-7573

Drug Information Center
University of Illinois at Chicago
Chicago
Mon-Fri 8 AM-5 PM
(312) 996-0209

Drug Information Service
Saint Joseph Hospital and Health Care Center
Chicago
7 days/week, 24 hours
(312) 975-3199

Drug Information Services
University of Chicago
Chicago
Mon-Fri 8 AM-5 PM
(312) 702-1388

Drug Information Center
Ingalls Memorial Hospital
Harvey
Mon-Fri 8 AM-4:30 PM
(708) 333-2300, ext 443

Drug Information Service
Hines Veterans Administration Hospital
Inpatient Pharmacy
Hines
Mon-Fri 8 AM-4 PM
(708) 343-3183

Drug Information Center
Lutheran General Hospital
Park Ridge
Mon-Fri 8 AM-5 PM
(708) 696-8128

Drug Information Center
Swedish-American Hospital
Rockford
7 days/week, 24 hours
(815) 968-4400, ext 4577

INDIANA

Drug Information Center
St. Vincent Hospital
Indianapolis
Mon-Fri 8 AM-4 PM
(317) 871-3200

Indiana University Medical Center
Pharmacy Department UH1410
Indianapolis
Mon-Fri 8 AM-4:30 PM
(317) 274-3581

IOWA

Drug Information Center
Mercy Hospital Medical Center
Des Moines
7 days/week, 24 hours
(515) 247-3286

Variety Club Drug and Poison
Information Center
Iowa Methodist Medical Center
Des Moines
7 days/week, 24 hours
(515) 241-6254;
(800) 362-2327 (Iowa only)

Drug Information Center
University of Iowa Hospital and Clinics
Iowa City
7 days/week, 24 hours
(319) 356-2600

KANSAS

Drug Information Center
Kansas University Medical Center
Kansas City
Mon-Fri 8 AM-4 PM
(913) 588-2328

KENTUCKY

Drug Information Center
Chandler Medical Center
College of Pharmacy
University of Kentucky
Lexington
Mon-Fri 8 AM-5 PM
(606) 233-5320

LOUISIANA

Drug Information Center- Poison Control Center
St. Francis Medical Center
Monroe
7 days/week, 24 hours
(318) 325-6454

Xavier University
Drug Information Center
Tulane Medical Center Hospital and Clinic
New Orleans
Mon-Fri 9 AM-5 PM
(504) 588-5670

MARYLAND

Drug Information Services
The Anne Arundel Medical Center
Annapolis
7 days/week, 24 hours
(410) 267-1130; (410) 267-1000

Drug Information Center
Franklin Square Hospital Center
Baltimore
Mon-Fri 8 AM-5 PM
(410) 682-7700;
after hours (410) 682-7374

Drug Information Service
Johns Hopkins Medical Center
Baltimore
Mon-Fri 8 AM-5 PM
(410) 955-6348

Drug Information Center
University of Maryland Medical System
Department of Pharmacy Services
Baltimore
Mon-Fri 8:30 AM-5 PM
(410) 328-5668

Drug Information Service
National Institutes of Health
Pharmacy Department
Bethesda
Mon-Fri 8:30 AM-5 PM
(301) 496-2407

Drug Information Services
Malcolm Grow USAF Medical Center
Camp Springs
Mon-Fri 7:30 AM-6 PM
(301) 981-4209

Drug Information Center
Memorial Hospital
Easton
7 days/week, 24 hours
(410) 822-1000, ext 5645

MASSACHUSETTS

Drug Information Service
Brigham and Women's Hospital
Boston
Mon-Fri 7 AM-5 PM
(617) 732-7166

Drug Information Service
New England Medical Center Pharmacy
Boston
Mon-Fri 8 AM-4:30 PM
(617) 956-5377

Drug Information Center
UMMC Hospital
Worcester
Mon-Fri 8:30 AM-5 PM
(508) 856-3456;
(508) 856-2775

MICHIGAN

Drug Information Service
University of Michigan Medical Center
Ann Arbor
Mon-Fri 8 AM-5 PM
(313) 936-8200;
after hours (313) 936-8251

Drug Information Center
Henry Ford Hospital
Detroit
Mon-Fri 8 AM-5 PM
(313) 876-1229

Drug Information Service
Pharmacy Department
Sinai Hospital
Detroit
Mon-Fri 8 AM-4:30 PM
(313) 493-5692

Drug Information Services
Harper Hospital
Detroit
Mon-Fri 8 AM-5 PM
(313) 745-2006;
after hours (313) 745-8638

Bronson Drug & Poison Information Center
Bronson Methodist Hospital
Kalamazoo
7 days/week, 24 hours
(616) 341-6409

Drug Information Center
Sparrow Hospital
Lansing
Mon-Fri 8 AM-4:30 PM
(517) 483-2444

Drug Information Center
St. Joseph Mercy Hospital
Pontiac
Mon-Fri 8 AM-4:30 PM
(313) 858-3055

Drug Information Services
William Beaumont Hospital
Royal Oak
Mon-Fri 8 AM-4:30 PM
(313) 551-4077

Drug Information Center
Saginaw General Hospital
Saginaw
7 days/week, 24 hours
(517) 791-4448

Drug Information Service
Providence Hospital
Southfield
Mon-Fri 8 AM-4:30 PM
(313) 424-3125

MINNESOTA

Drug Information Service
University of Minnesota Hospital and Clinic
Minneapolis
Mon-Fri 10 AM-4 PM
(612) 626-3000

Drug Information Center
St. Mary's Hospital
Rochester
Mon-Fri 8 AM-4:30 PM
(507) 255-5062;
after hours (507) 255-5732

Drug Information Center
United Hospital and Children's Hospital of St. Paul
St. Paul
Mon-Fri 9 AM-5 PM
(612) 220-8566

MISSISSIPPI

Drug Information Center
University of Mississippi Medical Center
Jackson
Mon-Fri 8 AM-5 PM; on call 24 hours
(601) 984-2060

MISSOURI

Drug Information Center
St. John's Regional Health Center
Springfield
Mon-Fri 7:30 AM-4:30 PM
(417) 885-3488

Drug Information Service
Heartland Hospital West
St. Joseph
7 days/week, 24 hours
(816) 271-7582

NEBRASKA

Drug Information Service
School of Pharmacy
Creighton University
Omaha
Mon-Fri 8:30 AM-4:30 PM
(402) 280-5101

Drug Information and Education Services
University of Nebraska Medical Center
Omaha
Mon-Fri 8 AM-4:30 PM
(402) 559-4114

NEW HAMPSHIRE

Drug Information Center
Dartmouth-Hitchcock Medical Center
Lebanon
Mon-Fri 7:30 AM-4 PM
(603) 650-5590

NEW MEXICO

New Mexico Poison & Drug Information Center
University of New Mexico
Albuquerque
7 days/week, 24 hours
(505) 843-2551;
(800) 432-6866 (NM only)

NEW YORK

Drug Information Center
Department of Pharmacy, RM BN42
Bronx Municipal Hospital Center
Bronx
Mon-Fri 9 AM-5 PM
(718) 918-4556

International Drug Information Center
Long Island University
Arnold & Marie Schwartz College of Pharmacy
Brooklyn
Mon-Fri 9 AM-5 PM
(718) 488-1000

Drug Information Center
Erie County Medical Center
Buffalo
Mon-Fri 8 AM-5 PM
(716) 898-3000

Drug Information Center
The Mary Imogene Bassett Hospital
Cooperstown
Mon-Fri 8:30 AM-5 PM
(607) 547-3686

Drug Information Center
St. John's University at Long Island
Jewish Medical Center
New Hyde Park
Mon-Fri 9 AM-3 PM
(718) 470-DRUG

Drug Information Center
Lenox Hill Hospital
New York
Mon-Fri 9 AM-5 PM
(212) 439-3190

Drug Information Center
Memorial Sloan-Kettering Cancer Center
New York
Mon-Fri 9 AM-5 PM
(212) 639-7552

Drug Information Center
Mount Sinai Medical Center
New York
Mon-Fri 9 AM-5 PM
(212) 241-6619

Drug Information Service
Bellevue Hospital Center
New York
Mon-Fri 9 AM-5 PM
(212) 561-6504

Drug Information Service
The New York Hospital
New York
Mon-Fri 9 AM-5 PM
(212) 746-0741

Drug Information Service
Department of Pharmacy
University of Rochester at Strong Memorial Hospital
Rochester
Mon-Fri 8 AM-5 PM
(716) 275-3718;
after hours (716) 275-2681

Suffolk Drug Information Center
University Hospital
SUNY-Stony Brook
Stony Brook
Mon-Fri 8 AM-4:30 PM
(516) 444-2672;
after hours (516) 444-2680

NORTH CAROLINA

Drug Information Center
University of North Carolina Hospitals
Chapel Hill
Mon-Fri 8 AM-5 PM
(919) 966-2373;
after hours (919) 966-4131, pager 3866

Triad Poison and Drug Information Center
Moses H. Cone Memorial Hospital
Greensboro
7 days/week, 24 hours
(919) 379-4105

Eastern Carolina Drug Information Center
Pitt County Memorial Hospital
Greenville
Mon-Fri 8 AM-4:30 PM
(919) 551-4257

Drug Information Service Center
North Carolina Baptist Hospital
Bowman-Gray Medical Center
Winston-Salem
Mon-Fri 8 AM-5 PM
(919) 716-2037

OHIO

Drug Information Center
Raabe College of Pharmacy
Ohio Northern University
Ada
Mon-Fri 9 AM-3 PM
(419) 772-2307

Cleveland Clinic Foundation Drug Information Center
Cleveland
Mon-Fri 8 AM-4:30 PM
(216) 444-6456

Drug Information Center
Department of Pharmacy, Doan Hall 368
Ohio State University Hospital
Columbus
Mon-Fri 8 AM-4 PM
(614) 293-8679

Drug Information Center
Riverside Methodist Hospitals
Columbus
Mon-Fri 8 AM-5 PM
(614) 566-5425

Western Ohio Poison & Drug Information Center
Children's Medical Center
Dayton
7 days/week, 24 hours
(513) 222-2227;
(800) 762-0727

Drug Information Service
The Toledo Hospital
Toledo
Mon-Fri 8 AM-4:30 PM
(419) 471-2171;
after hours (419) 471-5637

Drug Information/Poison Center
Bethesda Hospital
Zanesville
7 days/week, 24 hours
(614) 454-4221; (614) 454-4300;
(800) 686-4221

OKLAHOMA

Drug Information Center
Presbyterian Hospital
Oklahoma City
Mon-Fri 7 AM-3:30 PM
(405) 271-6226

Drug Information Service
University of Oklahoma
Health Sciences Center
Oklahoma City
Mon-Fri 8 AM-5 PM
(405) 271-8080

Drug Information Service
St. Francis Hospital
Tulsa
Mon-Fri 9 AM-5:30 PM
(918) 494-6339

OREGON

University Drug Consultation Service
The Oregon Health Sciences University
Portland
Mon-Fri 8:30 AM-5 PM
(503) 494-7530

PENNSYLVANIA

Pharmacy and Drug Information Services
Hamot Medical Center
Erie
7 days/week, 24 hours
(814) 877-6022

Drug Information Center
Temple University Hospital
Department of Pharmacy
Philadelphia
Mon-Fri 8 AM-4:30 PM
(215) 221-4644

Drug Information Center
Thomas Jefferson University Hospital
Philadelphia
Mon-Fri 8 AM-5 PM;
on call after hours (215) 955-8877

Drug Information Center
Medical College of Pennsylvania
Pharmacy Department
Philadelphia
7 days/week, 24 hours
(215) 842-6550

Center for Drug Information
St. Mercy Hospital of Pittsburgh
Pittsburgh, PA
Mon-Fri 7:30 AM-8 PM
(412) 232-7903; (412) 232-7907

Drug Information and Pharmacoepidemiology Center
University of Pittsburgh Medical Center
Pittsburgh
Mon-Fri 8 AM-6 PM; On call 24 hours*
(412) 624-3784

Drug Information Center
Allegheny General Hospital
Pittsburgh
Mon-Fri 8 AM-4:30 PM
(412) 359-3192

Drug Information Center
Crozer-Chester Medical Center
Upland
Mon-Fri 8 AM-4:30 PM
(215) 447-2843;
after hours (215) 447-2862

Drug Information Center
Williamsport Hospital and Medical Center
Williamsport
Mon-Fri 8 AM-4:30 PM;
on call 7 days/week, 24 hours
(717) 321-3289

PUERTO RICO

Centro de Informacion de Medicamentos
Colegio de Farmacia RCM
San Juan
Mon-Fri 8 AM-4 PM
(809) 758-2525, ext 1516;
(809) 763-0196

RHODE ISLAND

Drug Information Service
Department of Pharmacy
Rhode Island Hospital
Providence
Mon-Fri 8:30 AM-5 PM
(401) 444-5547

Drug Information Center
University of Rhode Island
Roger Williams Medical Center
Providence
Mon-Fri 8 AM-4 PM
(401) 456-2260

SOUTH CAROLINA

Drug Information Service
Medical University of South Carolina
Charleston
Mon-Fri 8 AM-5 PM
(803) 792-3896;
(800) 922-5250 (SC only)

Drug Information Center
Spartanburg Regional Medical Center
Spartanburg
Mon-Fri 8 AM-5 PM
(803) 560-6910;
after hours (803) 560-6779

SOUTH DAKOTA

South Dakota Drug Information Center
Brookings
7 days/week, 8 AM-4:30 PM
(800) 456-1004

Drug Information Center
McKennan Hospital
Sioux Falls
7 days/week, 24 hours
(605) 336-3894;
(800) 952-0123 (Iowa only);
(800) 843-0505 (out of state)

TENNESSEE

Drug Information Center
University of Tennessee Medical Center
Knoxville
Mon-Fri 8 AM-4:30 PM
(615) 544-9125

Drug Information Center
University of Tennessee
Memphis
Mon-Fri 8 AM-5 PM
(901) 528-5555

South East Regional Drug Information Center
VA Medical Center
Memphis
Mon-Fri 7:30 AM-4 PM
(901) 523-8990, ext 5191

TEXAS

Drug Information Center
University of Texas Medical Branch
Galveston
Mon-Fri 8 AM-5 PM
(409) 772-2734

Drug Information Center
Ben Taub General Hospital
Texas Southern University College of Pharmacy and Health Sciences
Houston
8 AM-4 PM
(713) 793-2915

Drug Information Center
Hermann Hospital
Houston
Mon-Fri 8 AM-4:30 PM
(713) 797-2073

Drug Information Center
M.D. Anderson Cancer Center
Houston
Mon-Fri 8 AM-4:30 PM
(713) 792-2858;
after hours (713) 792-2875

Drug Information Center
Methodist Hospital
Houston
Mon-Fri 8 AM-5 PM
(713) 790-4190

Drug Information Center
St. Luke's Episcopal Hospital/Texas Heart Institute
Houston
7 days/week, 24 hours
(713) 791-3098

Drug Information Center Department of Pharmacy
Wilford Hall USAF Medical Center
Lackland AFB
Mon-Fri 7:30 AM-5 PM
(512) 670-6291

Methodist Hospital Drug Information & Consultation Service
Lubbock
Mon-Fri 8 AM-5 PM
(806) 793-4012

Drug Information Center
Scott and White Memorial Hospital
Temple
Mon-Fri 8 AM-5 PM
(817) 774-4636

UTAH

Drug Information Center
Department of Pharmacy Services
University of Utah Hospital
Salt Lake City
Mon-Fri 8:30 AM-4:30 PM
(801) 581-2073

VIRGINIA

Drug Information Center
Sentara Hampton General Hospital
Hampton
Mon-Fri 7:30 AM-4 PM
(804) 727-7185

Drug Information Center
St. Mary's Hospital
Richmond
Mon-Fri 7:30 AM-4 PM
(804) 281-8058

WASHINGTON

Drug Information Center
Washington State University
College of Pharmacy
Spokane
Mon-Fri 8 AM-4:30 PM
(509) 456-4409

WEST VIRGINIA

West Virginia Drug Information Center
WVU-HSC
Morgantown
Mon-Fri 9 AM-5 PM
(304) 293-5101;
(800) 352-2501 (WV only)

WISCONSIN

Drug Information Center
University of Wisconsin Hospital and Clinics
Madison
7 days/week, 24 hours
(608) 262-1315

WYOMING

Drug Information Center
University of Wyoming
Laramie
Mon-Fri 8 AM-5 PM
(307) 766-6128